www.harcourt-international.com

Bringing you products from all Harcourt companies including Baillière Tindall, Ch Mosby and W.B. Saunders

- ▶ **Browse** for latest information on new books, journals and electronic products

- ▶ **Search** for information on over 20 000 published titles with full product information including tables of contents and sample chapters

- ▶ **Keep up to date** with our extensive publishing programme in your field by registering with eAlert or requesting postal updates

- ▶ **Secure online ordering** with prompt delivery, as well as full contact details to order by phone, fax or post

- ▶ **News** of special features and promotions

If you are based in the following countries, please visit the country-specific site to receive full details of product availability and local ordering information

USA: www.harcourthealth.com

Canada: www.harcourtcanada.com

Australia: www.harcourt.com.au

ESSENTIAL SURGERY
PROBLEMS, DIAGNOSIS AND MANAGEMENT

PUBLISHERS' NOTE ABOUT THE AUTHORS

The authorship of this book is unusual in that at the time it was first written only one of the authors was a consultant surgeon (CRGQ), while the others were junior hospital doctors. We believe this resulted in a radically new approach which has proved deservedly popular with its readers.

George Burkitt obtained qualifications in dental surgery and community medicine before studying clinical medicine as a mature student in Cambridge, England. This book was written while he was a senior house officer and represents the book he would like to have had during his training. He has a deep interest in medical education and is co-author of two other best selling student texts by the same publisher. These are *Wheater's Functional Histology*, and *Wheater's Basic Histopathology*. The former was written whilst a preclinical medical student in Nottingham, and the latter whilst a clinical student in Cambridge. On completion of the First Edition of this book, he returned to Australia working in family practice and palliative care in Newcastle NSW. During this time, he developed a deep interest in the emerging subject of men's health and wellbeing and in 1995 moved to Sydney where he now conducts a practice specialising in counselling men in crisis.

Clive Quick also trained initially as a dental surgeon but is now a consultant general and vascular surgeon at the teaching hospitals associated with the Clinical School of the University of Cambridge. He has a strong interest in computers as tools of communication. As an associate lecturer in the University, he teaches and examines clinical students in surgery. He is also heavily involved in training junior surgeons which is how he came to know his two co-authors. He has been the organiser of the Cambridge FRCS course and the Cambridge Anastomosis Workshop and was until recently a member of the Court of Examiners of the Royal College of Surgeons of England for the primary and final FRCS and the MRCS examinations.

The artist, **Philip Deakin**, first trained in physiology and later in medicine and is now a family practitioner in Sheffield, England. He had previously prepared the drawings for the afore-mentioned *Wheater's Functional Histology*. For this edition, he has redrawn all the line illustrations using computer graphics, employing his medical knowledge and artistic skill to achieve unusual accuracy and immediacy, whilst retaining an attractive economy and clarity of style.

Commissioning Editor: Laurence Hunter
Project Development Manager: Janice Urquhart
Project Management: Wendy Lee, Dilys Hartland
In-house Project Manager: Frances Affleck
Design direction: Erik Bigland

ESSENTIAL SURGERY
PROBLEMS, DIAGNOSIS AND MANAGEMENT

H. George Burkitt
BDScHons (Queensland) FRACDS MMedSci (Nottingham) MB BChir(Cambridge) FRACGP FACPsychMed

General Medical Practitioner and Medical Author, Sydney, New South Wales, Australia

Clive R. G. Quick
MB BS(London) FDS FRCS(England) MS(London) MA(Cambridge)

Consultant General and Vascular Surgeon, Hinchingbrooke Hospital, Huntingdon and Addenbrooke's Hospital, Cambridge; Associate Lecturer in Surgery, University of Cambridge; Former Examiner in Basic Sciences and Clinical Surgery for FRCS and MRCS (England)

Illustrations by

Philip J. Deakin
BSc(Hons) MBChB(Sheffield)

General Medical Practitioner, Sheffield, UK

Foreword by

Andrew T. Raftery
BSc MD MI Biol C Biol FRCS FRCS(E)

Consultant Surgeon, Northern General Hospital NHS Trust, Sheffield; Honorary Senior Clinical Lecturer in Surgery, University of Sheffield; Member of the Court of Examiners (Formerly Chairman), Royal College of Surgeons of England; Member of Panel of Examiners, Intercollegiate Specialty Board in General Surgery

THIRD EDITION

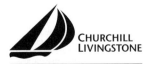
CHURCHILL LIVINGSTONE

EDINBURGH LONDON NEW YORK PHILADELPHIA ST LOUIS SYDNEY TORONTO 2002

CHURCHILL LIVINGSTONE
An imprint of Harcourt Publishers Limited

© Harcourt Publishers Limited 2002

 is a registered trademark of Harcourt Publishers Limited

The right of H. George Burkitt, Clive R. G. Quick and Philip J.
Deakin to be identified as authors of this work has been asserted by
them in accordance with the Copyright, Designs and Patents Act
1988

First published 1990
Second edition 1996
Third edition 2002

Main Edition ISBN 0 443 06375 3
International Student Edition ISBN 0 443 06408 3

British Library Cataloguing in Publication Data
A catalogue record for this book is available from the British
Library

Library of Congress Cataloging in Publication Data
A catalog record for this book is available from the Library of
Congress

Note
Medical knowledge is constantly changing. As new information
becomes available, changes in treatment, procedures, equipment
and the use of drugs become necessary. The authors and the
publishers have taken care to ensure that the information given in
this text is accurate and up to date. However, readers are strongly
advised to confirm that the information, especially with regard to
drug usage, complies with the latest legislation and standards of
practice.

The
publisher's
policy is to use
**paper manufactured
from sustainable forests**

Printed in Spain

Foreword

There have been major changes in the undergraduate course and in surgical training in the United Kingdom in the last few years. Very little basic science is now taught in the early years of the undergraduate course and therefore the candidate has less knowledge of this to carry forward and apply in the clinical years. Also, much of the undergraduate course nowadays involves problem-based learning.

Essential Surgery is written in a different way to other standard surgical texts. The pathophysiological basis of surgical disease is presented in a way that bridges the gap between basic medical science and clinical medicine. Particularly, this book describes sound principles of surgery on which to expand one's learning. The First Edition of Essential Surgery was written primarily for clinical students but with the reduction in the amount of learning in the undergraduate course, there is now sufficient in this book for the basic surgical trainee. Some of the chapters also provide good revision material for the higher surgical trainee, especially before sitting the UK Intercollegiate FRCS Examination in General Surgery.

This is an excellent book, providing a broad surgical education for both undergraduate and postgraduate. A wide variety of surgical topics is covered, together with some epidemiology and preventive medicine, which helps to integrate surgery into the health care and community setting.

When the First Edition of this book appeared in 1990 it was impressive, particularly as only one of the authors (Clive Quick) was a Consultant Surgeon at the time of writing, while the other two (George Burkitt and Dennis Gatt – the latter having retired from the Third Edition) were junior hospital doctors. I did not think that the First Edition could be improved upon but the Second Edition in 1996 was more impressive and I think that this Third Edition will excel even that.

George Burkitt, who was a mature medical student and already possessed a dental qualification, had written two successful medical books during his medical studies. I had the pleasure of teaching him as a clinical student in Cambridge and I liked to think that I taught him some of the material presented in this book. In truth, I probably learned more from him than he did from me! Clive Quick has considerable experience as an outstanding surgical teacher and examiner and has been a colleague of mine for many years on the Court of Examiners of the Royal College of Surgeons of England. Together with Phil Deakin, a family medical practitioner who has combined his medical knowledge with his considerable artistic skills to produce the excellent diagrams, they have produced an outstanding surgical text.

It is a pleasure and a privilege to have been asked to write the foreword for this Edition. I believe that readers will find it stimulating and will particularly enjoy the style of presentation. Without a doubt this book provides an excellent basis for surgical learning for undergraduate and postgraduate alike. I wish it the success that it deserves.

Andrew T. Raftery

Preface

The purpose of this book as established in the First Edition was to present the subject of surgery in a fresh, invigorating and accessible way. The continuing enthusiasm of students and teachers has highlighted the need for this updated Third Edition. In it, we have endeavoured to build on the quality of the original text without increasing its length. We have brought all of the text up to date and produced a number of new boxes and tables, a process of evolution rather than revolution for this edition. We have also radically improved the layout and the reader appeal of the book by using a larger page format and designing entirely new 'page furniture'. This means that illustrations have been made larger where necessary to better convey their message and link more harmoniously with the text. The chapter arrangement has been improved by splitting some of the larger chapters and reordering the content of several others to make them more logical. In addition, we have progressed from two tone to full colour printing for the entire book. All of the clinical and operative photographs have been regenerated in colour and the line drawings have been redrafted by the original artist Dr Phil Deakin in a more coherent style, taking advantage of a broader range of colours to improve their clarity and immediacy. Many of the radiographs have been replaced and the remaining originals have been regenerated digitally to illustrate the diagnostic points more clearly.

This book was written primarily for clinical students and is intended to cover the whole field of general surgery and urology for modern clinical courses. However, we also took the view that we should strive to present the sometimes complex ideas in ways that could be understood by anyone with a moderate understanding of human biology, and yet would not talk down to those with a more advanced level of understanding and training. We believe this is why the book has maintained a broad appeal beyond clinical medical students, ranging from nurses and others training in professions allied to medicine to higher surgical trainees. It has proved particularly useful as a textbook for trainee surgeons taking examinations such as the MRCS, which require an understanding of applied basic sciences and the essential principles of surgery rather than extensive details of operative technique. In addition this book was designed to be a continuing reference text for doctors in other specialties, including family practice. We still believe that this new edition of *Essential Surgery* will have the greatest appeal for readers who want to understand surgery rather than merely pass examinations.

There are several major differences between this book and standard surgical textbooks that have been retained for this edition. The pathophysiological basis of surgical diseases and of their management is presented to bridge the gap between basic medical sciences and clinical problems and we have adopted a problem-solving approach to diagnosis and treatment where practicable, believing that understanding how diagnoses are made and why particular treatments are used is more memorable than rote learning. With this in mind, we have tried to view the practical management of patients through the eyes of the trainee or student. Throughout the book we have used original illustrative material extensively, much of it new, to emphasise important concepts, to avoid unnecessary text, and to assist revision for exams. This includes photographs of clinical cases including operations and pathological specimens, radiographs, anatomical and operative diagrams, and tables and summaries of the text. The clinical material is largely drawn from our day-to-day practice and we have generally chosen typical rather than gross examples so the reader can see how patients most commonly present.

We have incorporated epidemiology, preventive strategies and issues affecting surgical services into the text so as to integrate surgery into the wider health care and community setting. We make no apology for including outlines of common surgical operations to enable students and trainee surgeons to explain operations to patients, to participate intelligently in the operating department, to understand and thereby prevent complications as well as to perform certain minor operations themselves. Finally, there is a major section on accident surgery as this is an important part of general surgical training and practice.

As in the last edition, major changes in the book represent the evolution and refinement in surgery over the five years since publication of the previous edition. Over this period, there have been further advances in minimal access diagnostic techniques which have simplified and expedited the diagnostic process and brought about novel therapeutic applications, most of which have increased the accuracy of diagnosis or reduced the pain and suffering previously associated with such interventions. Further consensus guidelines for managing common disorders have emerged and these have been incorporated into the text. Laparoscopic general surgery has matured over the last few years and has settled down to a range of applications with their acknowledged place in the surgical armamentarium. Meanwhile, the more experimental or fringe techniques have largely withered away.

The section on palliative care has been greatly enhanced and a new section on the ways surgeons may be involved with HIV cases has been added. In trauma surgery, further advances in the understanding of the pathophysiology of head injury have led to clearer guidelines in managing such injuries. In the chapter on prostate disorders, the section on cancer has been rewritten to include the classification and management of the various stages of the condition.

Surgeons involved in teaching are sometimes unaware of the non-surgical and social aspects of patient care, yet these are often of vital concern to doctors in training and their patients. Furthermore, only a small proportion of 'surgical conditions' such as abdominal pain, urinary tract infections and minor injuries ever reach a surgical specialist. For these reasons, we have tried to present a balanced community perspective of surgery encompassing disease prevention, primary care and the allocation of finite resources for health care.

We do not pretend that surgery can be taught entirely in a problem-orientated way, so descriptions of individual diseases have also been covered in a more conventional manner. Nevertheless, we believe that the benefits of our overall approach are self-evident. We hope our readers will continue to enjoy it and will appreciate the continuing efforts we have made to keep pace with change. Above all, it remains our ambition to stimulate the reader to a greater enjoyment and understanding of the practice of surgery.

Australia and UK 2001

H. G. B.
C. R. G. Q.

Acknowledgements

We acknowledge the contribution made to previous editions of this book, particularly the First Edition, by Mr Dennis Gatt, Consultant Surgeon in Malta, who has now retired from the authorship team. We are once again grateful for the substantial and unstinting help we have received from colleagues and friends in preparing this Third Edition. They are based at Hinchingbrooke Hospital, Huntingdon unless otherwise stated. In particular, major contributions were made by consultant radiologists Drs Tony Booth, Catherine Hubbard, Adrian Warner and Helen Taylor, who have built on their own previous revisions of the original work of Dr Graham Hurst in updating Chapter 5 as well as reviewing all other radiographs and radiological procedures in the book and providing a number of new illustrations. Dr Mike Harris, consultant histopathologist selected and prepared all of the new histology slides required by the move to full colour. In Australia, Matthew Carmody, consultant surgeon in Brisbane, reviewed more than half the book in detail, providing a fresh view on much of its content. Grant Williams and Andrew Doble, consultant urologists at Hinchingbrooke and Addenbrooke's Hospital respectively, radically revised chapters 27–33 on urology and the male genitalia, originally created by the late Andrew Higgins.

Stephen Large, consultant cardiothoracic surgeon at Papworth Hospital, revised his own material in Chapters 24 and 47, along with his colleague Stephen Tsui, who also provided several new illustrations. Professor Ted Howard, paediatric surgeon, formerly at King's College Hospital, London once again revised his sections on neonatal surgery in Chapters 44 and 45 and Dr Paul Siklos, consultant physician at West Suffolk Hospital, thoroughly revised his chapter on the medical management of surgical patients. Dr Margaret Saunders, consultant in palliative care, reviewed and revised the section on palliative care and Neville Jamieson, lecturer in Surgery and Honorary Consultant Surgeon at Addenbrooke's Hospital, completely reworked and updated chapter 4 on organ transplantation. Dr Juliet Foweraker, consultant microbiologist, revised and updated the microbiological material originally produced by Dr Mark Farrington, including disinfection and sterilisation. Dr Howard Smith, consultant anaesthetist at Peterborough District Hospital, reviewed his own material on anaesthesia and perioperative pain relief and provided a new table on resuscitation as well as valuable material on MODS and SIRS.

All who assisted with the preparation of the First and Second Editions deserve our continuing thanks, particularly those who have constructively reviewed chapters or sections in their own fields. We are also grateful to other colleagues who have advised on aspects of their expert areas. We believe their comments have helped us to keep up to date. Most of these contributors are based at Hinchingbrooke or Addenbrooke's Hospital, Cambridge, and include Dr Trevor Baglin (blood transfusion), Mr George Cormack (principles of plastic surgery), Dr Dick Dickinson (gastroenterology), Mr Richard Miller (Chs 15 and 16), Dr Michael Williams, consultant oncologist (Chs 4 and 28) and Professor John Pickard (head injuries). Another important contributor was Professor David Leaper of North Tees Hospital (Ch. 38). Mr Etienne Moore kindly allowed us to reproduce his mnemonic for severity stratification in acute pancreatitis. Some of the new clinical illustrations were provided by Mr David Adlam (oral lesions), Mr Jan Gryf-Lowczowski (colorectal polyps), Mr George Lamberty (skin disorders), Dr Nagy Antoun (CTs of head injury), Dr Suzy Forster (HIV) and Dr David Lomas (MRCP images and explanations). To all of our colleagues and contributors, we are greatly indebted.

A continuing debt of gratitude goes to all those who contributed so much to the First Edition, in particular, the late Mr Leonard Beard who prepared all the original photographs and the reproductions of radiographs and clinical slides, Dr Graham Hurst who collected and annotated all the original radiographs and the late Andrew Higgins who originated the urological chapters. Finally, we acknowledge the important work of Dr Jane Hailey, now a paediatrician in Vancouver, Canada, who as a house officer (intern), spent countless hours editing the whole text in meticulous detail, polishing the English and rendering it much more fluent and comprehensible.

Contents

Basic principles of surgical practice

1 Pathophysiological mechanisms of surgical disease: inflammation and infection

INTRODUCTION

The traditional approach to teaching surgical diagnosis is for the student to attempt to match a patient's symptoms and signs with standard sets of symptoms and signs known to characterise each disease. While most diagnoses match their classic descriptions at certain stages in their evolution, this may not be so at the particular moment the patient presents for treatment. Patients commonly present before recognisable patterns have evolved or else at a late stage, with the typical clinical picture having been missed or ignored on the way.

The diagnostic process can also be confusing if not all the symptoms and signs expected for a particular diagnosis are present or if the symptoms and signs seem inconsistent with the working diagnosis.

This book seeks to develop a more logical and reliable approach to diagnosis than simple pattern recognition by attempting to explain clinical features on the basis of the evolving pathophysiology and local anatomy. Likewise this should form the basis of understanding appropriate management strategies. This chapter provides a review of the main mechanisms of 'surgical' disease against a background of the basic medical sciences.

PRINCIPAL MECHANISMS OF SURGICAL DISEASE

These are summarised in Box 1.1

TRAUMA

Tissue trauma, literally injury, includes in its wider sense damage inflicted by any physical means, i.e. mechanical, thermal, chemical, electrical mechanisms or ionising radiation. Common usage, however, tends to imply mechanical injury, either blunt or penetrating, as caused by accidents in industry or in the home, road traffic accidents, fights, firearms and other missile injuries. Damage varies according to the nature of the causative agent, and the visible surface injuries may give little

SUMMARY
Box 1.1 Principal mechanisms of surgical disease
- Trauma
- Anatomical abnormalities—congenital or acquired
- Disorders of normal function
- Inflammation—infection, chemical and immunological mechanisms
- Ischaemia and infarction
- Metabolic and hormonal disorders
- Neoplasia—benign and malignant
- Other abnormalities of growth

indication of the extent of deep tissue damage as, for example, in head injuries or bullet wounds.

ANATOMICAL ABNORMALITIES

Anatomical abnormalities can be developmental in origin, i.e. **congenital**, or else **acquired** as a result of trauma or some other disease process.

Congenital abnormalities of surgical interest range from potentially fatal conditions such as urethral valves and various gut atresias to minor cosmetic deformities. Developmental abnormalities may become manifest at any time between fetal life and old age, although the majority are present at birth or appear in early childhood. For example, gut atresias often present with grossly excessive amniotic fluid (**polyhydramnios**) during pregnancy; urethral valves present in the neonatal period with obstructive renal failure. A patent processus vaginalis may result in an inguinal hernia at any stage from birth to early adulthood, whilst renal abnormalities such as polycystic kidney may present in middle life as an abdominal mass or with renal failure or haematuria.

Whilst many congenital abnormalities give rise to disease by direct **anatomical effects**, other abnormalities produce disease by more subtle **disruption of function**, with the underlying disorder only revealed on appropriate investigation. For example, ureteric abnormalities which allow urinary reflux from the bladder predispose to recurrent kidney infections.

Acquired anatomical abnormalities result from direct or indirect **damage** inflicted by trauma or disease, from the body's **response** to these or as an effect or side effect of **treatment**. For example, obstruction of the bladder outlet may result from benign prostatic hypertrophy, from the fibrotic response to gonococcal urethritis or from damage inflicted during urethral instrumentation.

DISORDERS OF FUNCTION

A variety of common disorders owe their origin to abnormalities of function. The gastrointestinal tract is particularly susceptible; for example, large bowel malfunction leads to constipation, irritable bowel syndrome and diverticular disease. The modern low-fibre diet is undoubtedly an important cause of these disorders, the colon having evolved on a diet high in fibre.

INFLAMMATION

Many surgical disorders result from inflammatory processes, most often stemming from infection. Surgical admissions for infection have markedly decreased since the advent of antibiotics but unfortunately, infection remains a common complication of operative surgery. Inflammation may also result from physical irritation, particularly by noxious chemical agents, e.g. gastric acid/pepsin in peptic ulcer disease or pancreatic enzymes in acute pancreatitis. Immunological mechanisms play a part in the inflammatory bowel disorders of ulcerative colitis and Crohn's disease but whether they constitute cause or effect is not yet known.

ISCHAEMIA AND INFARCTION

Obliterative atherosclerosis is a cause of enormous morbidity and mortality, particularly in later life. When the disease restricts blood flow in large distributing arteries to the point of causing chronic or severe ischaemia, it is often possible to improve flow by surgical or radiological procedures (e.g. aorto-femoral bypass grafting or angioplasty); when atherosclerosis is severe and generalised, however, reconstructive surgery may not be possible and amputation of an ischaemic limb may be the only alternative.

Arterial embolism is a cause of acute ischaemia of limbs, intestine or brain. These emboli usually originate in the heart. Surgical embolectomy can often restore flow in the femoral arteries and occasionally in the superior mesenteric artery by retrieving the occluding material. This is not possible in the brain but surgical treatment of the carotid disease may prevent further embolic episodes. Atherosclerosis of the carotid bifurcation and other extracranial arteries causes disease in two ways: firstly, by vascular narrowing or occlusion **restricting the blood supply** and, secondly, by accumulation of platelet thrombi on atherosclerotic ulcers which then **embolise** into the brain causing strokes or transient ischaemic attacks. Either type of disease may require surgical reconstruction.

When a portion of bowel becomes strangulated, the initial mechanism of tissue damage is venous obstruction and this fairly rapidly progresses to arterial ischaemia and infarction. Chronic **venous insufficiency** in the lower limb is responsible for the majority of chronic leg ulcers. The elevated hydrostatic venous pressure interferes with nutrition and gas exchange in the superficial tissues of the leg leading to tissue breakdown and retarded healing.

METABOLIC DISORDERS

The lower limb complications of diabetes, particularly neuropathy and infection, lead to the **diabetic foot** which represents an important surgical problem. In addition, diabetes predisposes to atherosclerosis and also poses special management problems in a patient undergoing surgery.

Hypersecretion of certain hormones, as in thyrotoxicosis and hyperparathyroidism, may require surgical reduction of glandular tissue. Other metabolic disorders may cause stones in the gall bladder (e.g. haemolytic diseases causing pigment stones) or in the urinary tract (e.g. hypercalciuria and hyperuricaemia causing calcium and uric acid stones respectively).

NEOPLASIA

Malignant tumours are responsible for a large part of the general surgical workload. Many surgical referrals are initiated by a fear or suspicion of cancer and many investigations and some operations are performed in the hope of refuting the diagnosis. Some malignant neoplasms can be cured by operative surgery but all too often the appearance of distant metastases or recurrent disease dashes the hope of a cure. In incurable cases, worth-while surgical palliation may improve the quality of life or even extend life expectancy.

Certain **benign tumours** such as lipomas are very common and require surgery mainly for cosmetic or mechanical reasons. Less commonly, benign tumours are removed because of obstruction of a hollow viscus or because of surface bleeding. Benign endocrine tumours may have to be removed because of excess hormone secretion, e.g. an insulinoma causing hypoglycaemia or a parathyroid adenoma causing hypercalcaemia. Finally, benign tumours may be clinically indistinguishable from malignant tumours and are removed to obtain a histological diagnosis. Neoplasia is discussed in more detail in Chapter 7.

OTHER ABNORMALITIES OF TISSUE GROWTH

In surgery, the term **cyst** is imprecisely used to describe a mass which appears to contain fluid because of its characteristic fluctuance and transilluminability. In true pathological terms, cysts are epithelium-lined cavities; most represent ducts dilated by retained secretion usually due to obstruction. In some cases there is epithelial hyperplasia, excessive secretion and structural distortion as, for example, in breast cysts. Some cysts arise from ectopic epithelial remnants or as a result of necrosis in the centre of an epithelial mass. Cysts commonly require surgical removal (or drainage) for aesthetic reasons or to exclude malignancy, e.g. epidermal cysts, epididymal cysts, breast cysts.

Other growth disturbances such as **hyperplasia** and **hypertrophy** give rise to surgical problems, in particular benign prostatic hyperplasia, fibroadenosis of the breast and thyroid goitres.

'THE SURGICAL SIEVE'

The foregoing mechanisms of surgical disease may provide a useful 'first principles' framework or *aide-mémoire* upon which to construct a differential diagnosis. This is particularly useful when the symptoms and signs do not immediately point to a diagnosis. This approach is often referred to as the 'surgical sieve'. However, it should not become a substitute for logical thought based on the clinical findings.

ACUTE INFLAMMATION

Acute inflammation is the principal mechanism by which living tissues respond to injury. The purpose of the inflammatory response is to neutralise the injurious agent, to remove damaged or necrotic tissue, and to restore the tissue to useful function. The central feature of acute inflammation is the formation of an inflammatory exudate. This has three principal components: **serum**, **leucocytes** (predominantly neutrophils) and **fibrinogen**.

Formation of the inflammatory exudate involves three vascular phenomena which are collectively responsible for the '**cardinal signs of Celsus**', i.e. redness, swelling, heat, pain and loss of function. These are as follows:

● Dilatation of local blood vessels leads to engorgement of the tissues and increased perfusion; this is responsible for the clinical signs of local redness, heat and some of the swelling
● Increased capillary permeability results in serum and plasma proteins (including immunoglobulins and fibrinogen) passing into the extracellular tissues which further increases the swelling (**oedema**). Pain is caused by swelling and by some of the substances which mediate the inflammatory process, e.g. kinins. The inflammatory exudate serves to irrigate the area, diluting toxins and organisms, which are drained away to regional lymph nodes. Fibrinogen polymerises to form fibrin in the damaged tissue which inhibits bacterial spread
● Leucocytes migrate into the area of injury and once there, the neutrophils and macrophages (both tissue-fixed and those from blood monocytes) commence phagocytosis of tissue debris. Macrophages are long-lived but neutrophils die after a burst of lysosomal activity, releasing **endogenous pyrogens** which are at least partly responsible for the fever often associated with acute inflammation

OUTCOMES OF ACUTE INFLAMMATION

The possible outcomes of the acute inflammatory process are summarised in Figure 1.1.

RESOLUTION

If tissue damage is minimal and there is no actual tissue necrosis, then the acute inflammatory response eventually settles and the tissue returns virtually to normal

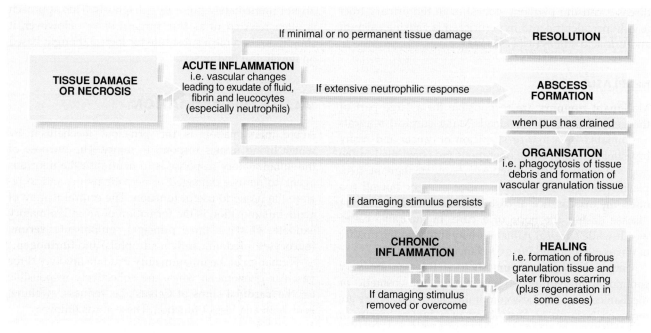

Fig. 1.1 Acute inflammation and its sequelae

with no evidence of scarring. A good example is the resolution of sunburn or transient peptic gastritis.

ABSCESS FORMATION

An abscess is a collection of pus (dead and dying neutrophils plus proteinaceous exudate) walled off by a zone of acute inflammation. Acute abscess formation occurs particularly in response to certain microorganisms which attract neutrophils and yet are resistant to phago-cytosis or lysosomal destruction. Abscess formation also occurs in response to highly localised tissue necrosis and to some organic foreign bodies (e.g. wood splinters, linen suture material), although infection may also be involved in these cases. The main **pyogenic organisms** of surgical importance are *Staphylococcus aureus*, some streptococci (particularly *Strep. pyogenes*), *Escherichia coli* and related Gram-negative bacilli ('coliforms'), and *Bacteroides* spp.

Without treatment, abscesses tend to 'point' spontaneously to the nearest epithelial surface (e.g. skin, gut, bronchus), eventually discharging their contents. Provided the injurious agent is thereby eliminated, spontaneous drainage leads to healing. If an abscess is far from a surface (e.g. deep in the breast), it progressively enlarges causing much tissue destruction. Sometimes local defence mechanisms are overwhelmed, leading to runaway local infection (**cellulitis**) and sometimes systemic sepsis.

Even with small and well-localised abscesses, showers of bacteria enter the general circulation (**bacteraemia**) but are mopped up by the phagocytic cells of the liver and spleen before they can proliferate. This process is responsible for a **swinging pyrexia** which is characteristic of an abscess. The site may not be clinically apparent if the abscess is very deep-seated (e.g. subphrenic or pelvic abscess) and the patient may be otherwise well. A typical temperature chart is shown in Figure 1.2. In the presence of an abscess, the number of neutrophils in the bloodstream rises dramatically as they are released in greater numbers from the bone marrow; thus, a marked **neutrophil leucocytosis** (i.e. white cell count greater than 15×10^9/L with more than 80% neutrophils) usually indicates a pyogenic infection. Severe infection with an excessive cytokine response spilling over into the systemic circulation causes **systemic sepsis** and rapid clinical deterioration (see Ch. 2, p. 25).

If spontaneous drainage of an abscess does not eliminate the injurious agent, the neutrophil response persists and pus continues to be formed, resulting in a **chronic abscess**. This may be manifest as a continuously discharging sinus or a surface abscess which inter-mittently forms, discharges and then heals. Alternatively a chronic abscess may be suspected only because of its systemic effects (e.g. a swinging pyrexia). From the fore-going, it follows that the essential principle of managing any abscess is to establish complete drainage, usually by incision or aspiration. Any residual necrotic or foreign material must be eliminated by curettage or excision. Indeed, before the antibiotic era, abscesses were a major cause of hospital admission and the principle of drainage was well known, with most hospitals having a separate 'septic' ward.

Antibiotics are often misused to treat abscesses. Once an abscess has fully formed, antibiotics seldom effect a

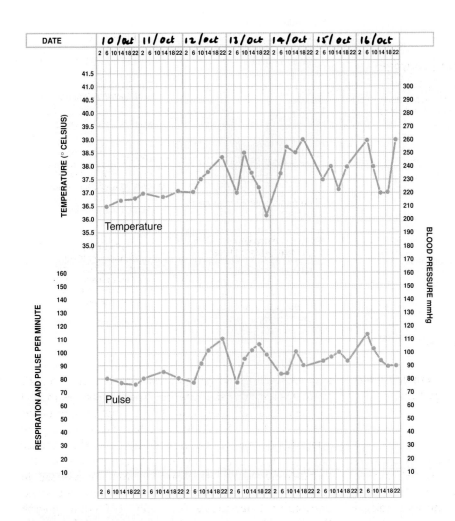

Fig. 1.2 Temperature chart showing swinging pyrexia

cure because the pus and foreign or necrotic material remain and antibiotics cannot gain ready access to the bacteria within the pus. Nevertheless, antibiotics may halt expansion or even sterilise the pus; the residual sterile abscess is sometimes known as an **antibioma**. If appropriate antibiotics are given early enough in an infection, organisms can be eliminated before the stage of abscess formation. For example, staphylococcal breast infections are common during lactation and if untreated often lead to breast abscesses; this formerly common surgical problem is now rare because of timely antibiotic treatment by family practitioners. Likewise, in surgical operations where there is known to be a particular risk of infection, prophylactic antibiotics can dramatically reduce the incidence of postoperative abscess formation and other septic complications.

ORGANISATION AND REPAIR

The most common sequel to acute inflammation is organisation, in which dead tissue is removed by phagocytosis and the defect filled by vascular connective tissue known as **granulation tissue**. This granulation tissue is gradually 'repaired' to bring about a **fibrous scar**. In some cases the original tissue may regenerate.

The simplest example of organisation and repair is healing of an uncomplicated skin incision (see Fig. 1.3). In this case, there is no necrotic tissue and the margins of the wound are brought into apposition with sutures. An acute inflammatory response develops in the immediate vicinity of the incision and by the third day, granulation tissue bridges the dermal defect. In the meantime, proliferating surface epithelium rapidly restores the epidermis. Fibroblasts invade the granulation tissue laying down collagen, so that the repair is strong enough to permit suture removal after 5–10 days. At this stage the scar is still red but the blood vessels gradually regress and it becomes a pale linear scar within a few months. This process is known as **healing by primary intention** (see Fig. 1.3).

If tissue loss prevents the wound edges from coming together, the healing process has to make good the

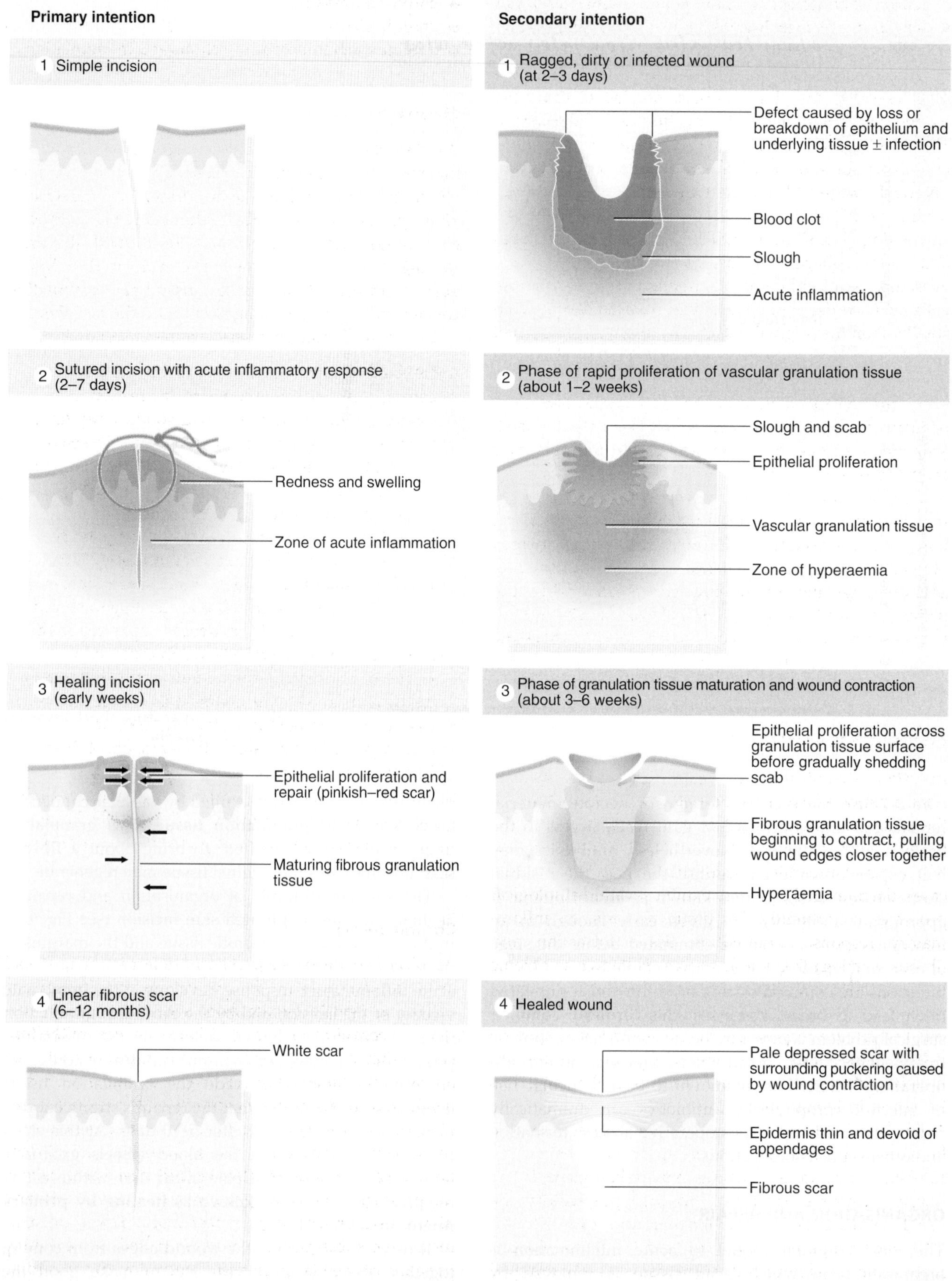

Primary intention

1 Simple incision

Secondary intention

1 Ragged, dirty or infected wound
(at 2–3 days)

Defect caused by loss or
breakdown of epithelium and
underlying tissue ± infection

Blood clot

Slough

Acute inflammation

2 Sutured incision with acute inflammatory response
(2–7 days)

Redness and swelling

Zone of acute inflammation

2 Phase of rapid proliferation of vascular granulation tissue
(about 1–2 weeks)

Slough and scab

Epithelial proliferation

Vascular granulation tissue

Zone of hyperaemia

3 Healing incision
(early weeks)

Epithelial proliferation and
repair (pinkish–red scar)

Maturing fibrous granulation
tissue

3 Phase of granulation tissue maturation and wound contraction
(about 3–6 weeks)

Epithelial proliferation across
granulation tissue surface
before gradually shedding
scab

Fibrous granulation tissue
beginning to contract, pulling
wound edges closer together

Hyperaemia

4 Linear fibrous scar
(6–12 months)

White scar

4 Healed wound

Pale depressed scar with
surrounding puckering caused
by wound contraction

Epidermis thin and devoid of
appendages

Fibrous scar

Fig. 1.3 Wound healing by primary and secondary intention

deficiency. The defect is initially filled with blood clot which later becomes invaded by vascular granulation tissue from the healthy wound base. The inflammatory exudate solidifies at the surface forming a protective scab. Fibrin in the clot contracts, helping to draw the wound edges together, reducing the size of the defect. Fibroblasts invade the granulation tissue and collagen is laid down in the extracellular spaces; contraction of myofibrils within fibroblasts shrinks the wound defect, beginning about 3 weeks after the insult. Over the succeeding weeks and months, the blood vessels regress and more collagen is formed, leaving a relatively avascular scar; gradual contraction of the mature collagen (cicatrisation) ensures that the final scar is much smaller than the original defect. The overlying epidermal defect is gradually bridged by epithelial proliferation from the wound margins. The epithelial cells slide over each other on the surface of the granulation tissue and beneath the edges of the scab which is eventually shed. This whole process is known as **healing by secondary intention** (see Fig. 1.3).

The rate and success of wound healing may be impaired by a variety of local factors including retained foreign bodies, necrotic tissue, infection, poor or damaged blood supply, continued wound contamination, unsuitable dressings and interference with the wound by the patient, as well as by systemic factors such as malnutrition, immunosuppression and uncontrolled diabetes.

CHRONIC INFLAMMATION

In certain circumstances, an injurious agent persists over a long period causing continuing tissue destruction. At the same time the body attempts to deal with both the original and the continuing tissue damage by the process of acute inflammation, organisation and repair. In these cases, the damaged area may exhibit several pathological processes concurrently, i.e. tissue necrosis, an inflammatory response, granulation tissue formation and fibrous scarring. This whole process is known as chronic inflammation and is characterised histologically by a predominance of macrophages (sometimes forming giant cells) which are responsible for phagocytosis of necrotic debris. Lymphocytes and plasma cells are also present, indicating the involvement of immunological mechanisms in chronic inflammation.

Chronic inflammation represents a tenuous balance between a persistent injurious agent and the body's reparative responses. Healing only takes place if the injurious agent is removed and then proceeds in the usual manner but often with much more scarring.

A wide range of agents can lead to chronic inflammation and the clinical patterns of disease can be grouped into three broad categories:

- chronic abscesses
- chronic ulcers
- specific granulomatous infections and inflammations

Chronic abscesses

As described earlier, a chronic abscess arises if the injurious agent causing an acute abscess is not fully eliminated. Pus continues to be formed and the abscess either persists or discharges continuously via a **sinus** or else 'points' and discharges periodically with the sinus healing over between times. The wall of the chronic abscess consists of fibrous scar tissue and granulation tissue resulting from healing attempts at the periphery.

Causes of chronic abscesses include the following:

- **Infected foreign bodies** are probably the most common cause of chronic abscess formation in modern surgical practice. Foreign bodies may have been deliberately implanted and become infected (e.g. synthetic mesh used for inguinal hernia repair, prosthetic hip joint) or have become embedded during an accident (e.g. glass fragments)
- **Dead tissue** of any sort can act as a foreign body, forming a nidus for infection. For example, diabetes may be complicated by deep infections in the foot with necrosis of tendon and bone leading to chronic abscesses and ulcers. Hairs deeply implanted in the skin of the natal cleft may be responsible for a pilonidal sinus or abscess. An infected dead tooth or root fragment may intermittently discharge via an associated 'gum boil' (see Fig. 1.4). Chronic osteomyelitis is associated with remnants of dead bone known as sequestra
- A chronic abscess can arise without a foreign body if the abscess is so deep and well circumscribed as to prevent spontaneous drainage; the best example is a subphrenic abscess

Chronic ulcers

An ulcer is defined as a persistent defect in an epithelial or mucosal surface. Except for malignant ulcers, ulceration usually results from a combination of low-grade mechanical or chemical injury to the epithelium and underlying supporting tissue together with an impaired reparative response. For example, elderly and debilitated patients are susceptible to pressure sores ('bed sores') which develop over bony prominences such as the sacrum and heels. In these cases, the patient does not regularly and automatically shift position to relieve the pressure of body weight because of immobility and diminished protective pain responses. Tissue necrosis results and subsequent healing is impaired by continuing pressure ischaemia, poor tissue perfusion (from cardiac or peripheral vascular disease) and malnutrition.

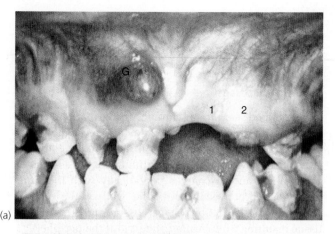

(a)

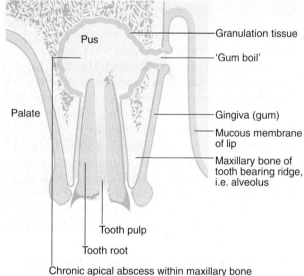

(b)

Fig. 1.4 'Gum boil' as an example of a chronic abscess
(a) Grossly neglected mouth showing widespread dental caries.
There is an inflammatory swelling on the buccal (cheek) aspect of the
alveolus **G** caused by a chronic apical dental abscess on the upper
right incisor. Note the left central incisor 1 is missing and the left
lateral incisor 2 has fractured at gum level because of caries.
(b) Sagittal section through 'gum boil' of upper incisor tooth. The
gum boil is in fact a sinus on the gum which discharges either
chronically or intermittently. Exposed to infection, the tooth pulp has
become necrotic while the apical abscess is slowly expanding due to
the continued presence of infected necrotic tissue (i.e. the tooth
pulp). The tooth root is all that remains after the crown has fractured
due to dental caries.

Another common example is the chronic leg ulcer in
chronic venous insufficiency; this fails to heal because of
local ischaemia induced by the high venous pressure,
and the problem is often exacerbated by secondary
infection.

A chronic peptic ulcer results from persistent acid-
pepsin attack upon the gastric or duodenal mucosa and
the lesion persists because the reparative response is
insufficient to tip the balance in favour of repair. The
lesion is often initiated and then exacerbated by aspirin
or other non-steroidal anti-inflammatory drugs (NSAIDs)

or alcohol. On the other hand, healing can be assisted by
neutralising the acid with antacids, by blocking acid
production with H_2 antagonists or by enhancing local
protective factors with drugs such as sucralfate.

In summary, a chronic ulcer represents a tenuous,
unresolved balance between persistent injurious factors
and an inadequate reparative response. The principle of
management is therefore to diminish or remove the
damaging factors and to promote the healing response.

The specific granulomatous infections and inflammations

Certain microorganisms such as *Mycobacterium tuberculosis*, *Mycobacterium leprae* and *Treponema pallidum*
(causing tuberculosis, leprosy and syphilis respectively)
excite a minimal acute inflammatory response and
stimulate a chronic inflammatory response almost from
the outset. The lesions are characterised by accumulation
of macrophages which form into **granulomas**, the
diseases thus being known as the **specific granulomatous
infections**.

A tuberculous **cold abscess** is a pus-like accumulation
of liquefied caseous material containing the occasional
mycobacterium. In contrast to a pyogenic abscess, the
lesion is cold to the touch since there is no associated
acute inflammatory vascular response. In developed
countries, tuberculous abscesses were once common
but are now rare. Cervical lymph node tuberculosis
('scrofula') often produced a 'collar-stud' abscess, i.e. a
superficial fluctuant abscess communicating with a deep
(and often larger) lymph node abscess via a small fascial
defect. Tuberculosis of the thoraco-lumbar spine causes
local destruction and may track down under the inguinal
ligament within the psoas sheath, presenting as a 'psoas
abscess' in the groin. A tuberculous ulcer is shown in
Figure 1.5.

Certain extremely fine particulate materials, such as
talc and beryllium, produce similar granulomatous reactions known as **foreign body granulomas**. Talc was
traditionally used as a lubricant powder in surgical
gloves and occasionally after laparotomy aroused an
intense, diffuse granulomatous peritoneal reaction causing
widespread bowel adhesions. Talc was abandoned and
replaced by starch, which in itself has been incriminated
in causing starch granulomas. For this reason, the
present trend is to use gloves without powder when
body cavities are opened.

INFECTION

GENERAL PRINCIPLES

(See also 'Principles of asepsis and infection control',
Ch. 6, pp. 66–71.)

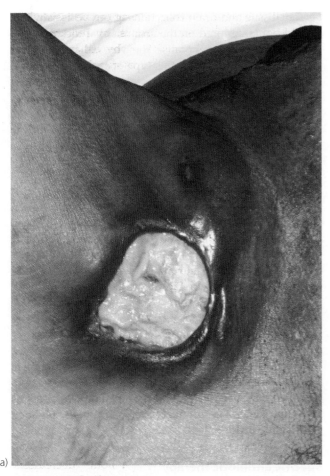

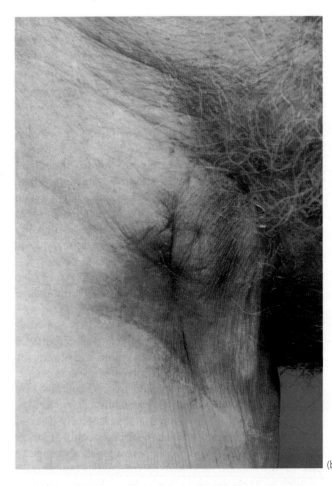

(a)

(b)

Fig. 1.5 Tuberculous ulcer
(a) This patient had lived in South Africa and had developed this painless and slowly enlarging ulcer about three months earlier. It shows the typical appearances of a 'wash leather' base and an undercut edge. Diagnosis was based on a biopsy and treatment involved draining the involved lymph nodes visible above the ulcer and a course of antituberculous chemotherapy. **(b)** Shows the healed lesion two months later.

It is important to distinguish between **infection**, which is a sustained local attack by microorganisms, and **sepsis**, which is essentially an excessive and inappropriate cytokine response to particular types of severe infection. Clinically significant infection arises when the size of an inoculum or the virulence of a microorganism is sufficient to overcome the resistance offered by protective surface phenomena, non-specific tissue defences and any specific immune responses. The virulence of an organism depends on its qualities of adherence and invasiveness and its ability to produce toxins. Tissue invasion of microorganisms may be enhanced by secretion of enzymes (e.g. hyaluronidase and streptokinase), avoidance of phagocytosis (e.g. encapsulation or spore formation), inherent resistance to lysosomal destruction or the ability to kill phagocytes. Toxins may be secreted by the organism (**exotoxins**) or released upon the death of the organism (**endotoxins**); in either case the toxin may produce local tissue damage (e.g. gas gangrene) or cause distant effects directly (e.g. tetanus) or by activating cytokine systems to cause sepsis

syndrome or disseminated intravascular coagulopathy (see Ch. 2).

Infections may be **community-acquired** (e.g. pneumococcal lobar pneumonia in a fit young adult) or **hospital-acquired**. The latter are also known as **nosocomial** infections and may follow surgery.

In **post-surgical** infections, organisms gain entry to the tissues through an **abnormal opening**, i.e. surface damage (such as a surgical or traumatic wound) or from a perforated viscus. Alternatively, physiological **protective mechanisms** may be disrupted, allowing infection to gain ascendancy. For example, neutropenia predisposes to infection, and bronchopneumonia is more liable to develop in a smoker following immobility or anaesthesia.

Furthermore, the surgical patient's **general resistance** may be impaired by malnutrition, malignancy, rheumatoid disease, corticosteroid therapy or other immunosuppressive drugs. In many cases, the infecting organisms are part of the patient's normal skin, bowel or respiratory tract flora or are normally present in the external environment. Nosocomial infection may be acquired by cross-infection from other infected patients, or from contaminated equipment or furnishings, or from 'carriers' among staff.

USE OF MICROBIOLOGICAL TESTS IN MANAGEMENT OF SURGICAL INFECTIONS

Surgical infection should be diagnosed on clinical grounds and the laboratory used to define the nature of the infection and to guide antibiotic therapy. Keen but inexperienced junior medical or nursing staff often take microbiological swabs from wounds or ulcers, which grow organisms in the laboratory, without realising that this may represent **colonisation** rather than clinically important infection. The clinical picture should always be the factor which determines a decision to begin treatment, although certain organisms such as *Strep. pyogenes* may require treatment to prevent cross-infection even if the lesion is clinically mild.

The results of specimens taken from dirty contaminated sites must be interpreted with caution. Superficial slough or discharge often contains colonising organisms of little significance. For example, in osteomyelitis caused by *Staph. aureus*, the sinus opening may be colonised by *Proteus* or *Pseudomonas* spp. The infecting organism may not be grown unless the wound is first carefully cleaned with saline and then the lesion swabbed deeply. If larger quantities of infected material are available, a syringe of pus or an excised segment of infected tissue should be sent to the laboratory for culture. Where possible, samples should be taken before antibiotics are given.

For best results, microbiological specimens should be transported quickly to the laboratory and certainly within 2 hours. If this is not possible, the specimen should be kept at 4°C. Blood culture specimens should be placed in an incubator at 35°C.

PRINCIPLES OF TREATMENT OF INFECTION

Removal of infected foci

An infected area that is poorly vascularised is effectively isolated from the body's humoral and cellular defence mechanisms as well as from circulating antibiotics. Retained infected material may over-activate cytokine mechanisms which precipitate multiple organ dysfunction syndrome. Thus, a vital first step is to remove infected necrotic tissue and drain collections of pus. This principle should not be ignored on the grounds that the patient is too ill for operation because the very ill patient may recover dramatically after this type of surgery. Common examples include draining abscesses, amputating infected necrotic limbs, removing infected foreign bodies (e.g. cannulae, prostheses, trauma debris) and draining the infected contents of hollow viscera such as bile ducts, kidneys and ureters.

Empirical antibiotic therapy

If treatment is urgent, antibiotics should be chosen according to the common pathogens likely in a given situation and with the knowledge of local antibiotic sensitivity profiles. A Gram stain performed on material from a usually sterile site can guide initial therapy until culture and sensitivity results are available. In an abdominal wound infection where hollow viscera have not been opened, *Staph. aureus* is the likely infecting organism and an anti-staphylococcal penicillin such as flucloxacillin can be commenced (see p. 13). If, however, the patient is known to carry methicillin-resistant *Staph. aureus* (MRSA)(see p. 13), vancomycin may be indicated. If bowel has been opened, Gram-negative organisms including anaerobes are likely and an antibiotic regimen is chosen to include these bacteria.

Specific antibiotic therapy

Once microbiological test results are available, therapy is modified to deal with the particular organisms grown and their antibiotic sensitivities. Specific 'narrow-spectrum' therapy is more effective and has fewer side effects than broad-spectrum 'shotgun' therapy. It also minimises the possibility of superinfection with organisms such as *Clostridium difficile* (see p. 16) and yeasts.

Nutritional support

Major sepsis results in severe catabolism (see Ch. 2) and may be associated with hypoalbuminaemia and wasting. Relatively simple measures such as nasogastric tube feeding should be considered if the patient is unable to swallow. The more complex procedure of total parenteral nutrition may be appropriate in other situations (see Ch. 50).

BACTERIA OF PARTICULAR SURGICAL IMPORTANCE

STAPHYLOCOCCI

PATHOPHYSIOLOGY

Staphylococci are **Gram-positive cocci** of which the main pathogenic species is *Staph. aureus*. This typically produces pustules, boils, breast abscesses, wound infections and osteomyelitis. Part of the virulence of *Staph. aureus* is due to its production of a variety of enzymes and toxins. *Staph. aureus* can also be part of the normal flora. About 30% of the general population are nasal carriers and 10% carry it on the perineal skin. *Staph. epidermidis*, (formerly *Staph. albus*), a **coagulase-negative** staphylococcus, is a universal skin commensal which rarely produces significant clinical infection or merits antibiotic therapy, except when it causes infections associated with exogenous materials such as prosthetic implants and intravenous cannulae.

Staphylococcal cell walls are resistant to adverse conditions such as drying, and the organism is able to persist for long periods under dry conditions such as in ward dust from where infection may spread. Some strains such as MRSA (see below) can be passed from patient to patient on staff hands if care is not taken with hand washing after every patient contact.

ANTIBIOTIC SENSITIVITIES

In the early antibiotic era, most staphylococci were sensitive to penicillin. More than 85% of strains in both family practice and hospital are now resistant. This is largely due to their ability to produce **penicillinase**. Most *Staph. aureus* strains remain sensitive to a reasonable range of commonly used antibiotics, e.g. **flucloxacillin** (a **penicillinase-resistant** penicillin), **erythromycin** and some of the **cephalosporins**; **gentamicin** is also active against *Staph. aureus*.

A relatively recent and potentially devastating problem is the emergence of strains of *Staph. aureus* resistant to flucloxacillin and all cephalosporins. Some are also resistant to gentamicin, erythromycin and chloramphenicol and sensitive only to the relatively toxic and expensive drug **vancomycin**, which has to be given intravenously. These strains are known by the term **methicillin-resistant *Staph. aureus* (MRSA)**; methicillin is the drug tested in the laboratory to predict flucloxacillin and cephalosporin resistance. Infections with this organism appear sporadically in hospitals, often where antibiotics have been used indiscriminately. The infections often originate in transplant units or intensive care units and then spread to cause serious and often fatal cross-infections. Radical measures have to be taken to prevent spread of epidemic proportions. Ward areas at greatest risk of MRSA infection are burns units, intensive care units, cardiothoracic surgical wards, neonatal units, orthopaedic wards and geriatric wards. It is often erroneously believed that MRSA is inherently more pathogenic than other *Staph. aureus* strains. In fact, the organisms excite similar inflammatory responses aimed at their elimination; the difference is that MRSA infections are more difficult to treat. MRSA may be sensitive in vitro to aminoglycoside antibiotics such as gentamicin but this is rarely of much value in clinical practice. In some cases, oral treatment with **tetracycline** or a **combination of rifampicin and fusidic acid** is appropriate; the combination prevents rapid development of antibiotic resistance to each agent alone.

A particularly worrying development is the emergence of **VISA**, which is *Staph. aureus* of intermediate sensitivity (i.e. relatively resistant) to vancomycin. Inappropriate use of vancomycin must be avoided to prevent selection of such mutants.

STREPTOCOCCI

PATHOPHYSIOLOGY

Streptococci are **Gram-positive** coccoid organisms which were first described in infected surgical wounds by Billroth in 1874.

Streptococci may be classified by their oxygen requirements into **aerobic**, **anaerobic** and **microaerophilic** (i.e. grow best in reduced oxygen concentrations) and further subdivided by their ability to produce different patterns of **haemolysis** on agar culture plates containing red blood cells.

Alpha haemolytic streptococci cause partial haemolysis with a green discoloration; important pathogens in this group include the *viridans* group of streptococci and *Strep. pneumoniae*.

Beta haemolytic streptococci produce complete haemolysis and may be grouped serologically into **Lancefield groups** A to O. The important human pathogens are group A streptococci (*Strep. pyogenes*—of major surgical importance) and group B streptococci (*Strep. agalactiae*—a common cause of serious neonatal sepsis). Streptococci in groups C and G are occasional causes of cellulitis and bacteraemia. Some streptococci and enterococci carry a group D antigen. Microaerophilic streptococci such as *Strep. milleri* carry a group F antigen.

Some streptococci are non-haemolytic and were formerly known as gamma haemolytic streptococci.

STREPTOCOCCI OF PARTICULAR SURGICAL SIGNIFICANCE

Strep. pyogenes (groups A and B beta haemolytic streptococcus)

This is the main human pathogenic streptococcus and is carried in the upper respiratory tract by about 10% of children but less often by adults. It can cause cellulitis and, less commonly nowadays, erysipelas. *Strep. pyogenes* is also a common cause of sore throat as well as post-streptococcal syndromes such as rheumatic fever which predisposes to cardiac valvular damage and subsequent infective endocarditis.

In acute **cellulitis**, a locally spreading infection involves the dermis and hypodermis, facilitated by production of hyaluronidase and streptokinase. In limb infections, organisms draining towards regional lymph nodes via lymphatics may produce perilymphatic inflammation and painful red streaks along the limb, i.e. **lymphangitis**.

13

The regional nodes react vigorously, becoming enlarged, painful and tender, a condition known as **lymphadenitis**. This may also occur in staphylococcal infections. Severe tissue damage may be caused by certain highly invasive strains of *Strep. pyogenes* leading to a **necrotising fasciitis**. If the infecting strain also produces certain exotoxins a life-threatening **streptococcal toxic shock syndrome** may develop.

Viridans streptococci

The *viridans* group of streptococci are oral commensals of low virulence but are the most common organisms causing infective endocarditis. This may occur as a complication of certain surgical procedures in the presence of pre-existing cardiac abnormalities; the subject is described in detail in Chapter 46.

Strep. pneumoniae (pneumococcus)

This organism is the most common cause of lobar pneumonia and can also cause bronchopneumonia in susceptible post-surgical patients. *Strep. pneumoniae* is a common cause of middle ear infections (otitis media); it is also involved in acute exacerbations of chronic bronchitis. Pneumococcal meningitis may occur in the young and elderly and may complicate head injury. Severe pneumococcal sepsis is particularly likely after splenectomy but may be prevented by vaccination and penicillin prophylaxis.

Strep. milleri (*anginosus* group)

Many of the *Strep. milleri* group have microaerophilic culture requirements. They are often found in abscesses in the appendix area, and the liver, lung and brain.

Anaerobic streptococci

Members of this group are bowel commensals and may form part of the mixed flora in many intraperitoneal abscesses and infection associated with necrotic tissue, e.g. diabetic foot ulcers.

ANTIBIOTIC SENSITIVITIES

Penicillin is the drug of choice for most streptococcal infections. In seriously ill patients, **benzylpenicillin** is given parenterally. For less serious infections in patients able to tolerate oral therapy, **penicillin V (phenoxymethyl penicillin)** or **ampicillin/amoxycillin** is the drug of choice. Many streptococci are also sensitive to **macrolides** (e.g. **erythromycin, clarithromycin**). Some pneumococci are now partially resistant to penicillin. Most infections, however, are still cleared with high-dose penicillin although meningitis needs alternative antibiotics such as vancomycin.

ENTEROCOCCI

PATHOPHYSIOLOGY

The enterococci are **Gram-positive cocci** closely related to streptococci. The most common species is *E. faecalis* (formerly *Strep. faecalis*). Enterococci form part of the normal bowel flora and may cause infection where bowel has been opened or infect the urinary or genital tracts.

ANTIBIOTIC SENSITIVITIES

Penicillin, **ampicillin**, **amoxycillin** or **vancomycin** is used for enterococcal infections. In serious infections such as endocarditis, a combination of penicillin and gentamicin is used to ensure bactericidal activity.

The cephalosporins are all ineffective. In hospitals where broad-spectrum (third-generation) cephalosporins are used as empirical therapy for bowel-related infections or septicaemia, enterococci are a frequent cause of nosocomial (hospital-acquired) infection. Vancomycin-resistant enterococci (VRE) are now being found. They are usually low-grade pathogens but can infect intravascular lines. Endocarditis caused by VRE is very difficult to treat.

ENTEROBACTERIACEAE

PATHOPHYSIOLOGY

The Enterobacteriaceae are a large family of **Gram-negative bacilli** (i.e. rods) which usually make up about 1% of the normal intestinal flora (see Table 1.1); these organisms are commonly referred to as 'coliforms'. The organisms can be cultured under aerobic and anaerobic conditions and, like other members of the bowel flora, grow in media containing bile salts such as McConkey or CLED agar; this helps in their identification.

Infections of surgical importance with Enterobacteriaceae are usually opportunistic in nature with the bacteria almost always arising from the patient's own bowel. Infection results from direct contamination from perforated or surgically opened bowel, perineal spread (to nearby wounds or urinary tract) or haematogenous spread.

Escherichia coli is the most common pathogen of the Enterobacteriaceae and is responsible for many surgical infections, often in synergy with other bacteria. *E. coli* is the most common cause of urinary tract infections (about 80% of all UTIs) and **Gram-negative septicaemia**. Coliform bronchopneumonia occasionally occurs in

Table 1.1 Bacteria of the family Enterobacteriaceae

Organism	Clinical Infection
Primary gut pathogens	
Salmonella, e.g. *S. typhi*, *S. enteritidis*	Typhoid fever Gastroenteritis
Shigella, e.g. *S. dysenteriae*, *S. sonnei*	Dysentery Traveller's diarrhoea
Some *Escherichia coli* strains, e.g. 0157:H7	Haemolytic uraemic syndrome
Gut colonisers that can cause infections	
Escherichia coli *Klebsiella* *Proteus* *Enterobacter* *Morganella* *Citrobacter*	Peritonitis and intraperitoneal abscesses (usually mixed infection with anaerobes) Septicaemia Urinary tract infections Ascending cholangitis (May also cause hospital-acquired infections, e.g. after instrumentation, central venous catheters, pneumonia in intensive care)
Gut colonisers that rarely cause infection	
Enterobacter *Serratia* *Morganella* *Citrobacter*	Usually hospital-acquired infections, e.g. after instrumentation, central venous catheters, in intensive care

debilitated, immunosuppressed or seriously ill patients. *Klebsiella*, *Enterobacter* and *Serratia* are being isolated more often in surgical bowel-related infections. *Proteus* is a common cause of urinary tract infections but occasionally causes other surgical infections, usually originating from the urinary tract.

ANTIBIOTIC SENSITIVITIES

Many coliforms are now resistant to ampicillin (and amoxycillin) and first-generation cephalosporins, e.g. cephalothin, but most are sensitive to **second- and third-generation cephalosporins**, e.g. **cefuroxime, cefotaxime**. Gentamicin is still a very effective and cheap agent against coliforms. Most coliforms are sensitive to ciprofloxacin. For prophylaxis in bowel and for biliary tract surgery and for treating related local and systemic infections, gentamicin or a second-generation cephalosporin (e.g. cefuroxime) is recommended, together with metronidazole for its activity against anaerobes. These accompany Enterobacteriaceae but are not in this group. Many coliforms are still sensitive to **trimethoprim** alone, which is often used to treat urinary tract infections. Resistant strains are much more frequent within hospitals than in the community. They are often found causing urinary tract infection in catheterised patients who have had repeated courses of antibiotics.

'NON-SURGICAL' ENTEROBACTERIACEAE

Other members of the Enterobacteriaceae family produce primary gut infections, although these only occasionally enter the province of the surgeon; for example, *Salmonella typhi* causes **typhoid** which may cause bowel perforations and *Shigella* causes **bacillary dysentery**. Rarely, *Salmonella* is incriminated in acute appendicitis and primary 'mycotic' aneurysms. An increasingly important, often unrecognised variety of **acute haemorrhagic colitis** is caused by *E. coli* 0157:H7; this is clinically indistinguishable from acute ulcerative colitis and should be sought bacteriologically in cases of suspected ulcerative colitis. *Yersinia* sometimes produces an acute inflammation of the ileum which may mimic the clinical picture of acute appendicitis. At laparotomy it appears similar to Crohn's disease of the terminal ileum.

PSEUDOMONAS

PATHOPHYSIOLOGY

The main pathogen in this group of **aerobic Gram-negative rods** is *Pseudomonas aeruginosa*, an uncommon cause of surgical infection. It tends to cause infections in debilitated, hospitalised patients. It is a normal commensal of the human gut in about 10% of the population. The organism is resistant to many antibiotics and therefore tends to proliferate when other flora have been suppressed by broad-spectrum antibiotic therapy. Like *Klebsiella* and *Enterobacter*, it poses a problem in institutions because of its ability to survive many chemical disinfectants and antiseptics.

Ps. aeruginosa may be responsible for fatal septicaemia (especially in terminally ill patients) and pneumonia, particularly in ventilated patients. Longstanding wounds such as compound fractures and chronic leg ulcers may become colonised by *Ps. aeruginosa*, although it is not always clinically significant. It can be recognised by the characteristic blue-green pigmentation of the discharge. The organism is also found in patients with indwelling urinary catheters. *Ps. aeruginosa* often colonises and may be a pathogen in burns infections. It can cause a fatal septicaemia when burns are extensive. Finally, it is an important complication of ophthalmic surgery and may lead to loss of the infected eye; it is also often responsible for chronic and recurrent external ear infections (otitis externa).

ANTIBIOTIC SENSITIVITIES

Treatment of pseudomonal infections often requires **combination therapy** because of its widespread antibiotic resistance and the severity of infections. Treatment usually involves an **aminoglycoside** (**gentamicin** or tobramycin) and an extended-spectrum beta lactam antibiotic such as **ceftazidime**, **piperacillin** or **imipenem**. The quinolone antibiotics **ciprofloxacin** and **norfloxacin** are active alone against *Ps. aeruginosa* and are the only effective oral antipseudomonal agents. True infection must be distinguished from colonisation where treatment is not indicated and will only encourage the development of resistance.

BACTEROIDES

PATHOPHYSIOLOGY

Bacteroides spp. and related organisms (e.g. **fusobacteria**) are **Gram-negative, non-sporing anaerobic bacilli** which make up the greatest proportion of normal gastrointestinal flora, outnumbering *E. coli* and its related coliforms by about 1000 to 1. *B. fragilis* is a small group of these, making up less than 1% of the bowel anaerobes. It is surgically important for causing pyogenic infections in combination with other gut commensals after faecal contamination of the peritoneal cavity and occasionally sepsis in debilitated patients. Because of their strictly anaerobic culture requirements, identification of these organisms as pathogens was neglected until the early 1970s. Indeed *Bacteroides* spp. were probably responsible for many so-called 'sterile' intra-abdominal abscesses in the past. The importance of *B. fragilis* as a cause of surgical infection is probably still underestimated.

ANTIBIOTIC SENSITIVITIES

Bacteroides spp. and the other Gram-negative anaerobes are highly sensitive to **metronidazole**, which can be given orally, intravenously or rectally, the last giving blood levels equivalent to those achieved by intravenous administration. Metronidazole is now given as standard prophylaxis before operation for appendicectomy and large bowel surgery, where it has dramatically reduced the incidence of postoperative peritoneal and wound infections. *Bacteroides* spp. are also often sensitive to the combination of **ampicillin/amoxycillin** and **clavulanic acid** (Augmentin).

CLOSTRIDIA

Clostridia are Gram-positive rods which are widely distributed in the soil and as intestinal commensals. The organisms form **spores** which are resistant to drying, heat and antiseptics and can survive for long periods. Clostridia are mostly **obligate anaerobes** which can only proliferate in the absence of oxygen; they are responsible for much of the putrefaction and decay of animal material in nature. The main pathological effects of

clostridial infections are caused by powerful exotoxins. The infections of surgical interest are **gas gangrene**, **tetanus** and **pseudomembranous colitis**.

GAS GANGRENE

Gas gangrene results when *Clostridium perfringens* (formerly called *C. welchii*) and other anaerobes (e.g. *Bacteroides* spp. and **anaerobic streptococci**) proliferate in necrotic tissue, secreting powerful toxins. These spread rapidly and destroy nearby tissues, generating gas at the same time which gives rise to the characteristic clinical sign of crepitus ('crackling') on palpation and the typical X-ray appearance shown in Figure 1.6. Deep traumatic wounds involving muscle, and wounds contaminated with soil, clothes or faeces are most susceptible. The condition is particularly common in battle wounds and gas gangrene was responsible for vast numbers of deaths during the First World War.

In surgical practice, the highest risk of gas gangrene is in **lower limb amputations** performed for ischaemia (infection from the patient's own bowel) and in high-velocity **gunshot wounds** (infection from the patient's own perforated bowel or by external contamination). Gas gangrene occasionally occurs in other surgical

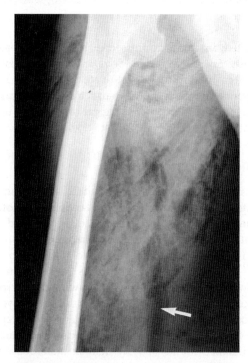

Fig. 1.6 Gas gangrene
Gas gangrene involving all the muscles of the right thigh in a 46-year-old man who sustained extensive contaminated lacerations of the medial thigh (arrowed) in a road traffic accident. Gas gangrene developed because necrotic muscle was not excised early and completely. Note the widespread streaks of radiolucent gas bubbles tracking along the muscle planes. This patient died of toxaemia despite antibiotics, surgery and hyperbaric oxygen therapy.

wounds where ischaemic tissue has become contaminated with bowel flora. The area of muscle necrosis may be small at first. Gas gangrene is recognised when the overlying skin turns black and the process spreads at an alarming rate. Within hours the underlying necrosis rages along the muscle planes. Later the skin breaks down and a thin, foul-smelling purulent exudate leaks from the wound. **Toxins** are absorbed into the general circulation and cause rapid clinical deterioration and death within 24–48 hours unless the process can be halted by timely and vigorous intervention.

C. perfringens is very sensitive to **benzylpenicillin** which should be given prophylactically by injection immediately after a traumatic injury involving muscle, or less than an hour before amputation of an ischaemic limb (metronidazole can be used for patients allergic to penicillin). Preventing clostridial infection in contaminated wounds requires meticulous surgical excision of all necrotic tissue, followed by packing of the wound rather than suturing. Further excisions are likely to be needed.

Treatment of established gas gangrene is urgent and must proceed vigorously if there is to be any hope of survival. Treatment is with penicillin and radical excision of necrotic tissue. High doses of penicillin are given intravenously to kill organisms in viable and vascularised tissue. Emergency surgery is performed to remove all necrotic tissue. This involves carving back the necrotic muscle to healthy bleeding tissue; the affected muscle is recognised by its brick-red colour and failure to contract on cutting.

Hyperbaric oxygen therapy may be used to raise the oxygen tension in the necrotic tissues, inhibiting growth of the organisms. The patient is placed in a high-pressure chamber with pure oxygen at about 3 atmospheres pressure for several hours daily. However, gas gangrene may continue to spread despite these measures, necessitating further heroic surgical interventions. Even with all this intensive treatment, the prognosis for established gas gangrene remains bleak.

TETANUS

Tetanus is caused by *Clostridium tetani* which infects dirty wounds in a similar manner to gas gangrene. The size of the entry wound may be minute, perhaps caused by a rose thorn or splinter. The organism produces an **exotoxin** which has little local effect but, even in minute quantities, has powerful remote neuromuscular effects causing widespread muscular spasm. The first signs are often **acute muscle spasms** and **neck stiffness** or **trismus** ('lockjaw'). If untreated, these progress to **opisthotonus** (arching of the back due to extensor spasm), generalised convulsions and eventually death from exhaustion and respiratory failure several days later.

Tetanus is now rare in developed countries because of widespread immunisation with **tetanus toxoid** during childhood, followed by boosters at 10-year intervals. Any patient with a penetrating injury, however trivial, should be given a booster dose if none has been given in the previous 5 years. If no booster dose has been given for 10 years, full revaccination should be carried out. The annual incidence of tetanus in developed countries is about one per million population, and is most common following trivial gardening injuries in the elderly, who are least likely to have been properly immunised. If there is doubt about satisfactory immunisation status following a major contaminated injury, **benzylpenicillin** should be given prophylactically as well as passive immunisation with **tetanus immune globulin** collected from people with known high titres. Treatment of established tetanus usually requires artificial ventilation with drug paralysis, in addition to the usual antibiotics and passive immunisation. Mortality remains high, especially in the elderly.

Globally, tetanus remains a massive problem after trauma. A particular local problem in some developing countries is neonatal tetanus resulting from the practice of applying cow dung as a dressing to the umbilical stump.

PSEUDOMEMBRANOUS COLITIS

Pseudomembranous colitis can be the most serious form of **antibiotic-associated diarrhoea** (see Ch. 21) and is caused by overgrowth of a toxigenic *Clostridium difficile*, an organism named for the difficulty of growing it in culture. Infection results in the formation of a thick fibrinous 'membrane' on the large intestinal mucosa, within which the organism proliferates. Its toxins cause a profound watery and sometimes bloody diarrhoea, leading to dehydration and loss of electrolytes.

Although pseudomembranous colitis is uncommon, it may develop after only a single dose of almost any antibiotic. Clindamycin and lincomycin were the most commonly implicated drugs but these are rarely used now; cephalosporins are now the most common cause. Diagnosis can be made by sigmoidoscopy and biopsy in the 50% of patients with left-sided colonic involvement. The best method of diagnosis is to detect the specific toxin in the stool; this can be performed by looking for a cytopathic effect on cells cultured in vitro. *Cl. difficile* can also be cultured from the stool. Although the organism is sensitive to penicillin, this fails to penetrate the pseudomembrane. **Oral metronidazole** is effective in most patients. Oral **vancomycin**, which is not absorbed from the gastrointestinal tract, can also be used but this is now discouraged because of the concern of selecting VRE (see p. 14).

The main bacteria of surgical importance are summarised in Table 1.2.

Table 1.2 Main bacteria of surgical importance and their antibiotic sensitivities

Classification	Organism	Typical infections	Antibiotic sensitivities
FACULTATIVE ANAEROBES (i.e. aerobes)	STAPHYLOCOCCI *S. aureus* (coagulase-positive)	Pustules, boils, abscesses, wound infections, osteomyelitis	Flucloxacillin Erythromycin Some cephalosporins Gentamicin Vancomycin (MRSA)
	S. epidermidis (coagulase-negative)	Skin commensal; opportunistic pathogen, especially of foreign bodies, e.g. prosthetic implants	Often resistant to multiple antibiotics. Vancomycin Flucloxacillin Erythromycin Some cephalosporins Gentamicin Rifampicin
	STREPTOCOCCI *S. pyogenes* (group A and B beta haemolytic)	Group A: cellulitis, lymphangitis, necrotising fasciitis Group B: neonatal and maternal infections, infections in diabetics	Penicillin (ampicillin/amoxicillin) Erythromycin Cephalosporins
	S. milleri	Normal gut and urogenital commensal; important cause of abscesses of appendix, liver, lung, brain	As for *S. pyogenes*
	Enterococci, e.g. *E. faecalis* and *E. faecium*	Faecal streptococci; gut commensals causing opportunistic infections, e.g. abscesses associated with bowel surgery, urinary infections, biliary infections (liver transplants), endocarditis	Innately resistant to most antibiotics with even broader acquired resistance in hospital strains. Penicillin (ampicillin/amoxycillin) +/– Gentamicin Vancomycin
	S. pneumoniae (pneumococcus)	Normal upper respiratory tract commensal; respiratory tract infections, meningitis	As for *S. pyogenes*
	Viridans streptococci	Oral and gut commensals; rare cause of infection except infective endocarditis	As for *S. pyogenes*
	OTHERS *Bacillus* spp. (rod-shaped)	Usually contaminants; multiply in biliary and wound drainage bags	
	Diphtheroids including *Corynebacterium* spp. (rod-shaped)	Skin and upper respiratory commensals; occasional opportunistic IV line infection	
GRAM-NEGATIVE Facultative anaerobes	COLIFORMS otherwise known as ENTEROBACTERIA	Urinary tract infections, Gram-negative septicaemia, bronchopneumonias in debilitated patients	Cephalosporins Gentamicin Ciprofloxacin Trimethoprim Ampicillin/amoxycillin (resistant strains frequently found)
	E. coli, *Klebsiella* spp., *Proteus*	Large bowel commensals	Usually community-acquired; tend to be antibiotic-sensitive
	Citrobacter, *Serratia*, *Enterobacter*, *Providencia* spp.	Not normal commensals in fit patients	Usually hospital-acquired; tend to be antibiotic-resistant
	Enteric: *Salmonella* and *Shigella* spp.	Gastrointestinal and systemic infections	Ciprofloxacin

Table 1.2 Continued

Classification	Organism	Typical infections	Antibiotic sensitivities
GRAM-NEGATIVE **Facultative anaerobes**	PSEUDOMONAS *Ps. aeruginosa*, *Stenotrophomonas* spp., *Acinetobacter*	Opportunistic pathogens, common in moist environments, e.g. floor mops. Rarely normal commensals. Urinary tract infections, pneumonias and septicaemias in ventilated patients, burns infections and septicaemia. Often colonise leg ulcers	Gentamicin/tobramycin Ceftazidime Piperacillin Imipenem Ciprofloxacin/norfloxacin
	Curved rod group including *Vibrio* spp. and *Campylobacter*	*V. cholerae* causes cholera; *Campylobacter* causes diarrhoea; *V. vulnificus* causes necrotising wound infections after contact with sea water	
	Fastidious group including *Haemophilus* spp.	*Haemophilus* is an upper respiratory tract commensal causing acute-on-chronic bronchitis and invasive infections in children; *Pasteurella multocida* is an oral commensal in dogs and cats and causes bite infections and septicaemia; *Neisseria* spp. include meningococcus and gonococcus	
Obligate anaerobes Non-sporing, Gram-negative			Note: virtually all are sensitive to metronidazole
	BACTEROIDES spp.	*B. fragilis* causes intraperitoneal abscesses associated with bowel surgery, genital tract infections, oral sepsis, brain abscesses	Metronidazole (Also ampicillin/amoxycillin plus clavulanic acid combination)
Non-sporing, Gram-positive	Cocci	*Peptococcus* ('anaerobic staphylococcus') and *Peptostreptococcus* ('anaerobic streptococcus'): common commensals of mucosal surfaces; components of mixed infections of mucosal surfaces	As for *S. pyogenes*
	Branching rods: *Actinomyces israelii*	Actinomycosis	Benzylpenicillin Metronidazole
Sporing, Gram-positive rods	*CLOSTRIDIA*	Faecal commensals, mostly non-pathogenic	
	Cl. perfringens	Gas gangrene, food poisoning	Benzylpenicillin Metronidazole
	Cl. tetani	Tetanus	Benzylpenicillin Metronidazole
	Cl. difficile	Antibiotic-associated diarrhoea	Metronidazole Vancomycin (orally)
MYCOBACTERIA	Slow-growing organisms with waxy cell walls	Tuberculous mycobacteria (*M. tuberculosis*, *M. bovis*) Non-tuberculous varieties: *M. avium—intracellulare* (systemic infection in AIDS), *M. marinum* (fish fancier's ulcer)	Multi-agent chemotherapy according to local sensitivities
OTHER BACTERIA	*Mycoplasma* spp., *Chlamydia* spp. and rickettsia	*Mycoplasma* and rickettsias—pneumonias; *Chlamydia*—pelvic inflammatory disease, implicated in coronary heart disease	

VIRUSES OF PARTICULAR SURGICAL IMPORTANCE

Chronic blood-borne viral infections such as **hepatitis B and C** and **human immunodeficiency virus (HIV)** are important to surgeons because of the risk of transmission to the surgeon from the patient during surgery (and vice versa), as well as cross-infection between patients. In addition, patients may need surgical intervention for complications of hepatitis or HIV infection. Preventing transmission of infection relies on **universal blood and body fluid precautions** which are described under 'Methods of infection control' in Chapter 6.

HUMAN IMMUNODEFICIENCY VIRUS (HIV)

CLASSIFICATION OF HIV INFECTIONS

The human immunodeficiency virus causes a chronic infection which usually progresses to the **acquired immune deficiency syndrome (AIDS)** over a period of 7 or more years. The illness evolves through several stages. The first is the **acute seroconversion illness** (group I—Centers for Disease Control Classification 1986). Seroconversion occurs as long as 3 months after infection is acquired, and as many as 70% of infected patients are asymptomatic at the time of seroconversion. Patients usually test negative for antibodies against HIV prior to and during the initial seroconversion illness.

Next follows the **asymptomatic period** (group II) during which the patient usually feels completely well. Later, as the disease progresses, the patient may develop generalised lymphadenopathy and wasting (**AIDS-related complex**—group III). **AIDS** (group IV) is manifest by development of unusual opportunistic infections (e.g. *Pneumocystis* pneumonia, cytomegalovirus (CMV) infections, cerebral toxoplasmosis, atypical mycobacterial infections), certain malignant diseases (Kaposi's sarcoma, generalised or cerebral lymphoma, aggressive invasive uterine cervical cancer) and neurological disease (**AIDS dementia complex**).

The use of combinations of antiretroviral drugs (high activity antiretroviral therapy) has had a dramatic effect on the natural history of the disease, with AIDS patients now surviving far longer.

SURGICAL INVOLVEMENT IN HIV CASES

Preventive measures to be adopted by medical and nursing staff and the management of needle-stick injuries are discussed in Chapter 6 under 'Methods of infection control'.

Surgeons may be involved in diagnosing bowel-related problems (e.g. oesophageal candidiasis) by oesophago-gastro-duodenoscopy (OGD). In late-stage disease, CMV infection may involve any part of the gastrointestinal tract—ranging from mouth ulcers and ulcers in the jejunum (which may perforate) to colitis. For AIDS colitis, colonoscopy and biopsy are often required for diagnosis. Treatment involves intravenous antiviral drugs.

AIDS patients may develop severe perianal herpes with secondary anal fistula or abscess formation. In a patient with known AIDS, perianal lesions should be assumed to be herpes until proven otherwise as the presentation is often atypical. Kaposi's sarcomas (see Ch. 40) may require local excision.

Surgeons may also become involved with HIV-infected patients who in late-stage disease require a long-term central venous catheter (Hickman line) with a subcutaneous infusion port. Surgeons may also be asked to place a percutaneous endoscopic gastrostomy (PEG) for feeding purposes.

Orthopaedic surgeons may be exposed to the virus when performing joint replacements in HIV-infected haemophiliacs.

VIRAL HEPATITIS

Viral hepatitis manifests clinically with anorexia, nausea and sometimes abdominal discomfort in the right upper quadrant followed by jaundice. There are many viruses that can cause hepatitis with different modes of transmission, incubation times, prognosis and complications. These include CMV, Epstein–Barr and the hepatitis viruses. Hepatitis A and E are spread by the faecal–oral route whereas hepatitis B and C can be acquired by blood and some body fluids and therefore represent a potential risk to the surgeon.

HEPATITIS A

Hepatitis A is transmitted by the faecal–oral route, has an incubation period of 2–6 weeks, rarely causes fulminating disease and never leads to chronic hepatitis or cirrhosis. Its only surgical importance is when considering the differential diagnosis of jaundice. A vaccine for preventing hepatitis A is now available.

HEPATITIS B

Hepatitis B is transmitted by blood or body fluids, including sexual intercourse, or from mother to fetus or baby (termed **vertical transmission**). Incubation is from 6 weeks to 6 months. Hepatitis B infection leads to chronic hepatitis and cirrhosis in approximately 5–10%

of cases; this cirrhosis commonly progresses to hepato-cellular carcinoma (the most common cause of hepato-cellular carcinoma world-wide). Hepatitis B is prevent-able by vaccination and this is indicated for neonates of mothers who carry the virus, all health-care workers and some high-risk groups (e.g. certain ethnic groups).

Exposure to hepatitis B virus has several possible outcomes:

● **Acute fulminant hepatitis**. This is rare but fatal
● **Acute hepatitis**. Clearing of the virus leads to lifelong immunity
● **Chronic infection**. This may lead to chronic hepatitis/cirrhosis (and possibly hepatocellular carcinoma)
● **Chronic carrier state**. This is mainly due to infection at birth or later with development of immune tolerance and no obvious active disease

Serological diagnosis of hepatitis B (see Table 1.3)

Hepatitis B surface antigen (HBsAg) can be detected in the early stages of the disease. Patients then develop antibodies to the viral core (anti-HBc); this does not confer immunity but is a marker of exposure to the virus. With clearance of the virus, patients develop surface antibodies (anti-HBs) which confer lifetime immunity. Patients who do not clear the virus remain surface antigen-positive and may become chronic carriers, i.e. remain infectious for others and prone to risk of complications themselves. In patients who are HBsAg-positive, e antigen positivity (HBeAg) is a marker of high infectivity (see 'needle-stick injury' below), but patients who are surface antigen-positive alone may still transmit the virus if there is exposure to sufficient material, e.g. by blood transfusion. Chronic carriers should be monitored for hepatocellular carcinoma by annual estimation of **serum alpha-fetoprotein** and liver ultrasound every 2 years, as partial hepatectomy can sometimes cure early cases of hepatocellular carcinoma. Hepatitis B vaccines contain the surface antigen and induce immunity by stimulating production of surface antibody; this will be the only positive serological marker in people who have been vaccinated.

HEPATITIS C

Hepatitis C is transmitted via the same routes as hepatitis B but sexual transmission is believed to be less common. The incubation period is approximately 2 months. Chronic liver disease develops in 30–50% of cases but is often of low-grade activity. Hepatitis C is also an important cause of hepatocellular carcinoma on a world-wide basis. Serological diagnosis is troublesome because of the difficulty of culturing the virus. Sero-conversion occurs late, often weeks to months after the acute illness. In most cases a positive hepatitis C anti-body test is likely to mean continuing infection.

HEPATITIS D

This is a defective virus that requires hepatitis B surface antigen for full expression and only occurs as a co-infection with hepatitis B. It can be prevented by vaccination for hepatitis B.

VIRAL INFECTION FOLLOWING SHARPS (NEEDLE-STICK) INJURY

Any sharps injury, especially from a hollow needle, may lead to transmission of viral infection if the patient carries a blood-borne virus. This is discussed in detail in Chapter 6.

To avoid such infections strategies must be adopted to reduce the risk of exposure: for example, by not re-sheathing needles. Health-care workers are given vaccination against hepatitis B. Antiretroviral drugs need to be given promptly after a significant exposure to HIV as post-exposure prophylaxis. No vaccination or treat-ment can as yet be recommended for health-care workers exposed to hepatitis C.

Table 1.3 Interpretation of hepatitis B serology

	HBsAg	anti-HBc (IgM)	anti-HBe (IgG)	anti-HBs
Acute hepatitis	+	+	– early + late	–
Immune patient following hepatitis	–	–	+	+
Chronic hepatitis (includes carrier state)	+	–	+/–	–
After effective immunisation	–	–	–	+

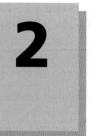

2 Systemic responses to surgery and trauma

INTRODUCTION

At the site of extensive tissue damage, local inflammatory and reparative responses take place as described in Chapter 1, but a variety of neuro-humoral systemic responses are also activated which compensate for starvation, provide additional energy and building blocks for tissue repair, and conserve sodium ions and water. There is also a massive attempt to increase glucose production by the process of **gluconeogenesis**. Adrenaline and noradrenaline are released into the systemic circulation from sympathetic nerve endings and from the adrenal medulla to play a central role in the systemic responses. In addition, there is enhanced secretion of adrenocorticotrophic hormone (ACTH), glucocorticoids (cortisol), glucagon and growth hormone, all of which contribute to the general catabolic response. At the same time increased aldosterone and antidiuretic hormone (ADH) production mediate some of the fluid and electrolyte changes. Insulin is an antagonist of most of the above hormones and is secreted in increased amounts after injury, but only from the second or third day.

FACTORS RESPONSIBLE FOR SYSTEMIC RESPONSES

Factors responsible for systemic responses to severe injury or major surgery are summarised in Box 2.1.

Fall in intravascular volume

This is one of the major factors that initiate the systemic responses. Hypovolaemia results from:

SUMMARY

Box 2.1 Factors responsible for systemic responses to severe injury or major surgery

- Fall in intravascular volume
- Reduced cardiac output and peripheral perfusion
- Pain
- Stress
- Systemic inflammatory responses and sepsis
- Inflammation
- Excess heat loss
- Secondary effects on blood
- Starvation

- Loss of fluid by haemorrhage or from the surface of burns
- Interstitial sequestration of fluid as oedema in damaged tissues and more generally as a result of the systemic hormonal responses. This process is exaggerated in systemic sepsis
- Restricted oral intake during the perioperative period or whilst in intensive care

A falling intravascular volume stimulates sympathetic activity to maintain blood pressure both by boosting cardiac output and by increasing peripheral resistance. This explains the mild tachycardia commonly seen in postoperative patients. Catecholamines also have profound metabolic effects, increasing the turnover of carbohydrates, proteins and lipids. Falling renal perfusion activates the renin–angiotensin–aldosterone system, increasing renal sodium and water reabsorption. A centrally mediated increase in ADH secretion promotes further conservation of water.

Chapter 2

Reduced cardiac output and peripheral perfusion

Circulatory efficiency may be impaired by hypovolaemia, and myocardial contractility may be depressed by anaesthetic agents and other drugs. Less commonly major events, such as sepsis, pulmonary embolism or myocardial infarction, cause cardiovascular collapse.

Pain

Pain causes increased catecholamine and ACTH secretion. Blockade of pain (e.g. by regional anaesthetic procedures) at the time of surgery greatly reduces the adverse systemic effects of pain.

Stress

Psychological stress associated with injury, severe illness or elective surgery has a similar effect to pain on sympathetic function and hypothalamic activity.

Systemic inflammatory responses and sepsis

Exotoxins and endotoxins initiate intense systemic cytokine responses with a variety of adverse metabolic effects (see p. 25). This response does not necessarily involve infection and can be initiated by a variety of adverse physiological insults.

Inflammation

Products of tissue damage and inflammation may cause systemic effects themselves or via release of cytokines and other humoral factors. The effects are similar to those involving infection.

Excess heat loss

This can occur during long operations and after extensive burns. Heat loss imposes great demands upon energy resources and may interfere with physiological processes such as blood clotting. Small babies are particularly vulnerable. Heat loss in the operating theatre is counteracted as far as possible by raising the ambient temperature, wrapping exposed parts of the body with insulating material, using warm water underblankets or warm air 'bear-huggers' and by warming fluids during intravenous infusion.

Secondary effects on blood

General metabolic responses to injury activate thrombotic mechanisms and initially depress intrinsic intravascular thrombolysis. Thus the patient is in a **prothrombotic state** and may suffer intravenous thrombosis and consequent thromboembolism.

If substantial haemorrhage occurs, clotting factors eventually become exhausted with failure of clotting. The systemic inflammatory response syndrome (SIRS—see p. 25) causes widespread intravascular thrombosis, again using up clotting factors and precipitating **disseminated intravascular coagulation** (DIC) with failure of normal clotting.

Starvation

Patients are commonly starved for 6–12 hours before operation even for uncomplicated elective surgery, and often do not start eating for 12–24 hours after operation. After major gastrointestinal surgery, food may be withheld for several days or much longer in the event of serious infective complications, anastomotic breakdown or fistula formation. Furthermore, patients with gastrointestinal tumours, malabsorption syndromes or inflammatory bowel disease may already be in a state of chronic starvation before operation.

One effect of starvation is increased susceptibility to infection. Thus, it is important to recognise and, if possible, correct starvation in surgical patients. The following are useful indicators of starvation:

- Weight loss of more than 10% of normal body weight
- Lack of nutritional intake for more than 10 days
- Low serum albumin—below 26 mg/dl is probably critical
- Low serum transferrin
- Reduced lymphocyte count
- Reduced grip strength

Effects of starvation

During starvation in the absence of illness or trauma, blood glucose is maintained by lowered insulin secretion and increased glucagon production. Other hormone levels remain normal. Initially, enhanced glycogenolysis maintains blood glucose but liver glycogen becomes exhausted within 24 hours. Gluconeogenesis in the liver and kidneys is enhanced, utilising amino acids from protein breakdown and glycerol from lipolysis as substrates. Much of the glucose thus produced is utilised by the brain; most other tissues are able to metabolise fatty acids and ketones from adipose tissue. After several weeks, the brain also adapts to using ketones. Overall energy demands fall during starvation and energy is obtained mainly at the expense of body fats. Protein is conserved until a late stage in uncomplicated starvation but this is not the case in severe trauma or surgery.

SURGICAL CATABOLISM

In most elective surgery, many of the factors mentioned above can be mitigated by accurate fluid replacement, adequate analgesia, reducing psychological stress, preventing infection and using careful operative technique to minimise tissue trauma. The result will be minimal systemic upset with rapid recovery.

On the other hand, in severe trauma and extensive operative surgery, particularly if complicated by major sepsis, the above factors will inevitably cause intense catabolism and drastic changes in fluid and electrolyte balance. Increased sympathetic activity and circulating catecholamines and insulin are the key factors in the response to major systemic insults, producing the following metabolic results:

● Enhanced hepatic glycogenolysis and gluconeogenesis
● Reduced insulin secretion and inhibition of its tissue effects block cellular utilisation of glucose
● Stimulation of glucagon secretion further enhances glycogenolysis and gluconeogenesis
● Catecholamines and glucagon stimulate lipolysis in adipose tissue releasing fatty acids; these provide the major energy source for peripheral tissues
● Breakdown of muscle protein releases amino acids, the main substrate for gluconeogenesis and the raw material for wound healing
● Increased pituitary ACTH release induces a massive rise in circulating glucocorticoids; cortisol levels can increase tenfold immediately after surgery, remaining elevated for days or weeks. Glucocorticoids also enhance gluconeogenesis and promote catabolism of muscle protein and liberation of amino acids
● Increased secretion of growth hormone and thyroid hormones, both of which inhibit the effects of insulin and promote catabolism

EFFECTS ON CARBOHYDRATE METABOLISM

The overall effect of all these hormonal actions is a rise in blood glucose levels, often resulting in **hyperglycaemia** and a **pseudodiabetic state**; blood glucose levels may reach 20 mmol/L and glucose may appear in the urine. This is in marked contrast to simple fasting, in which glucose levels are normal or slightly depressed.

EFFECTS ON BODY PROTEINS AND NITROGEN METABOLISM

In the normal healthy adult, **nitrogen balance** is maintained; protein turnover results in the daily excretion of 12–20 g of urinary nitrogen which is made good by dietary intake. In a hypercatabolic state, nitrogen losses can increase three- or fourfold. Most importantly, the metabolic environment prevents proper utilisation of food or intravenous nutrition. There is therefore an enormous and inevitable daily destruction of skeletal muscle. This state of **negative nitrogen balance** contrasts markedly with starvation, in which body protein is preserved.

EFFECTS ON LIPID STORES AND METABOLISM

The effects of major body insults upon lipid metabolism are little different from simple starvation; most of the energy requirements are met from fat stores.

Surgical catabolism only reverses as the patient recovers from the illness and therefore early parenteral nutrition (see Ch. 50) has little effect, although carbohydrates may spare some protein loss. It is worth emphasising that minimising surgical trauma and preventing perioperative complications may make the difference between recovery and death for elderly or debilitated patients.

FLUID AND ELECTROLYTE CHANGES IN MAJOR SURGERY AND TRAUMA

Major trauma, surgery and illness result in retention of sodium and water, mediated via increased secretion of aldosterone and ADH.

Aldosterone secretion

This occurs in response to a fall in renal perfusion and glomerular filtration rate that tends to accompany substantial haemodynamic disturbances. Renin is released from the juxtaglomerular apparatus of the kidney, catalysing the conversion of angiotensin I to angiotensin II in the lungs. The latter has a powerful pressor effect on the peripheral vasculature, counteracting hypotension as well as stimulating aldosterone release from the adrenal cortex. Aldosterone promotes active reabsorption of sodium ions from the distal convoluted tubules of the kidney; this is accompanied by the passive reabsorption of water. Sodium reabsorption is linked to secretion of potassium and hydrogen ions. The urine is therefore small in volume, acidic and with a low sodium concentration and raised potassium concentration. Loss of hydrogen ions causes a degree of metabolic alkalosis.

ADH secretion

This is stimulated by a rise in serum osmolality, mediated by osmoreceptors in the hypothalamus. After major trauma or surgery, however, additional factors operate. There is a reduction in circulating volume, and stress and pain promote further ADH release via other hypothalamic pathways. ADH acts on the renal collecting tubules, rendering them permeable to water which is then reabsorbed along a concentration gradient into the vasa recta of the renal medulla.

It is important to recognise the phase of **relative oliguria** and **sodium retention** that inevitably occurs after major injury or surgery as this has an important bearing on fluid management. Like surgical catabolism, described earlier, these effects are resistant to external manipulation but resolve with recovery of the patient.

SYSTEMIC INFLAMMATORY RESPONSE SYNDROME AND MULTIPLE ORGAN DYSFUNCTION

Multiple organ dysfunction syndrome or MODS (also known as multi-organ failure or MOF) came to be recognised as a distinct clinical entity in the mid-1970s when it was widely recognised that any major physiological insult could lead to failure of one or more organs remote from the initiating disease process. Later it was conceived that the underlying condition was an uncontrolled systemic inflammatory response (**systemic inflammatory response syndrome, SIRS**) initiated by a range of adverse events such as trauma, infection, inflammation, ischaemia or ischaemia–reperfusion injury. MODS is the most common reason for surgical patients to stay longer than 5 days in intensive care.

Sepsis (also known by or incorporated within the terms **septic shock, systemic sepsis, septicaemia and sepsis syndrome**) describes the early clinical features which occur when infection is the initiating factor of MODS; at this stage, the condition may be reversible. Note that the term sepsis is not synonymous with infection and should be reserved for the systemic process described here (see Box 2.2). The sequence of failure of individual organs often follows a predictable pattern with **pulmonary failure** occurring first, followed by hepatic, intestinal, renal and finally cardiac failure. Pulmonary failure is associated with acute (formerly 'adult') respiratory distress syndrome (ARDS). In hepatic failure, patients have a rising bilirubin, serum glutamic oxaloacetic transaminase (SGOT) and lactate dehydrogenase (LDH). Intestinal failure is recognised by **stress bleeding** requiring blood transfusion, renal failure by rising plasma creatinine and low urine output and, cardiac failure by low cardiac output and hypotension. Altered mental states such as confusion also occur (cerebral failure) as may DIC.

The mortality of MODS is directly related to the number of organs that fail. With one organ the mortality rate is 40%; with two, 60%; and with three organs, more than 90%.

PATHOPHYSIOLOGY OF SIRS AND MODS

SIRS involves widespread changes including endothelial injury, inflammatory cell activation, disordered haemodynamics and impaired tissue oxygen extraction. It thus

---

KEY POINTS

Box 2.2 Definitions of SIRS, MODS and sepsis

Systemic inflammatory response syndrome (SIRS)
Present if two or more of the following are found:

● Temperature > 38°C or < 36°C
● Heart rate > 90 beats/min
● Respiratory rate > 20 breaths/min or $PaCO_2$ < 4.3 kPa
● White cell count > 12 000 cells/mm^3 or < 4000 cells/mm^3 or more than 10% immature forms

Multiple organ dysfunction syndrome (MODS)

● Present if SIRS is associated with organ dysfunction, e.g. oliguria, hypoxia

Sepsis (or systemic sepsis)

● Defined as SIRS in association with bacterial infection proven by culture

Severe sepsis

● Defined as sepsis associated with signs of organ dysfunction, e.g. renal failure

Septic shock

● Defined as SIRS associated with hypotension refractory to volume replacement and requiring vasopressors

---

represents a grossly exaggerated activation of immune responses intended as host defences. The excessive unregulated release of inflammatory mediators, however, does more harm than good by causing the widespread microvascular, haemodynamic and mitochondrial changes that may eventually lead to organ failure.

Following initial tissue injury, a local inflammatory response occurs with cytokine induction. The primary response to this is endothelial activation and the expression of intercellular adhesion molecules (ICAMs). Later, neutrophils diapedese into the tissues. Complement, coagulation and other components of the inflammatory system become activated and the primary inflammatory response is amplified. All of this is normal and appropriate. However, if the injury is severe or persistent, the localised reaction may spill over into the systemic circulation producing a systemic inflammatory response, or if initiated by infection, producing the sepsis syndrome.

MEDIATORS OF SIRS AND MODS

SIRS and MODS involve complex interactions of endogenous and sometimes exogenous mediators. A range of cytokines is released from activated neutrophils as well as from endothelial and reticulo-endothelial cells. These include **tumour necrosis factor** (TNF), the **interleukins** IL1, IL2, IL6, and platelet activating factor. These mediators individually cause responses similar to those found in SIRS when injected into volunteers.

SEPSIS

The classic septic response of a hyperdynamic circulation, systemic signs of inflammation and disrupted intermediary metabolism can be induced in healthy volunteers by injecting **endotoxin** (derived from the cell walls of Gram-negative bacteria) or the cytokines TNF or interleukin 1. In Gram-negative sepsis, the lipoprotein A (lipopolysaccharide) component of the organisms has been shown to activate neutrophils and the coagulation and complement pathways. These result in endothelial activation, increasing vascular permeability and neutrophil–endothelial interaction. The final common pathway may involve migration of activated neutrophils into the interstitial space of the affected organ and the development of tissue hypoxia. In sepsis syndrome, these and other circulating factors working in synergy bring about the devastating effects of MODS.

CLINICAL CONDITIONS LEADING TO SIRS AND MODS

These include infection and endotoxaemia (50–70% of cases), retained necrotic tissue and shock. They can initiate distant organ failure by several mechanisms:

- Inducing excessive release of endogenous mediators
- Disrupting oxygen delivery to the tissues
- Impairing intestinal barrier function allowing **translocation** of intestinal bacteria and endotoxin to the portal and systemic circulations
- Damaging the reticulo-endothelial system

INFECTION

The source of infection which leads to MODS may be **acquired** (e.g. intra-abdominal abscess) or **endogenous**, i.e. from the patient's own bowel. Local infection, usually with Gram-negative bacteria, stimulates the release of a range of inflammatory mediators. A similar response is provoked by a substantial volume of necrotic tissue, e.g. gangrenous leg, and is made much worse if the tissue is infected. These **paracrine responses** are beneficial in a local sense, combating infection by increasing blood flow and vascular permeability to allow influx of phagocytes, as well as activating neutrophils to degranulate and release cytotoxic oxygen radicals. If the stimulating factor then is so great that inflammatory mediators spill over into the systemic circulation in large quantities, a cascade is initiated which may lead to sepsis and MODS. Superoxide radicals and other circulating factors then damage cells elsewhere in the body, causing widespread vasodilatation and increased vascular permeability leading to hypotension and circulatory collapse. The myocardium is depressed and cellular metabolic functions are disrupted.

Endogenous sources of infection

Bowel is a reservoir for bacteria and endotoxin which are normally safely contained. If the **intestinal barrier** is breached by splanchnic ischaemia, impoverished luminal nutrition of enterocytes or altered intestinal flora, then **bacterial translocation** can occur into the portal circulation in as little as 30 minutes. If the liver Kupffer cells are also impaired, intestinal bacteria and endotoxin are not prevented from reaching the systemic circulation. This may explain the potential for renal failure in jaundiced patients undergoing operation (hepato-renal syndrome). This endogenous source of sepsis explains the 30% of patients who suffer organ dysfunction without an obvious source of infection. Typically, patients are affected after prolonged hypotension (hypovolaemic or cardiogenic shock) or hypoxaemia (e.g. multiple trauma victims) or as a result of direct visceral ischaemia (e.g. prolonged aortic clamping and hypotension in a patient with a ruptured aortic aneurysm).

PREVENTION OF SEPSIS AND MODS

Prevention and early treatment of MODS is summarised in Box 2.3.

SURGICAL ASPECTS

When multiple organ dysfunction occurs in surgical patients, it often results from a complication such as a bowel anastomotic leak ('septic') or from severe acute pancreatitis (which may be sterile but becomes devastating if associated with pancreatic infection). Extensive tissue necrosis following trauma or death of an ischaemic limb may also precipitate the syndrome in one form or another.

Organ dysfunction often has an insidious onset. At an early stage, subclinical organ dysfunction is often suspected; at this stage active resuscitation and dealing with causative factors such as a necrotic limb are likely

SUMMARY

Box 2.3 Prevention and early treatment of multiple organ dysfunction syndrome

General prevention

- Rapid resuscitation and early definitive treatment of major injuries
- Good surgical technique
- Appropriate use of prophylactic and therapeutic antibiotics
- Early diagnosis and treatment of infective surgical complications, e.g. leaking anastomoses
- Early and thorough excision of necrotic and infected tissue

Prevention for at-risk patients and treatment of early signs

- Rapid cardiovascular resuscitation and prevention of shock (minimise splanchnic ischaemia)
- Optimisation of oxygen delivery (measure arterial PO_2 and pH and correct metabolic acidosis)
- Nutritional support via an enteral route (to nourish enterocytes)

to have beneficial effects. By 7–10 days without effective treatment, pulmonary failure (ARDS) and hepatic and renal failure appear; MODS is now present and the prognosis becomes substantially worse.

Prevention of sepsis and early management of major gut-related infection before it provokes the SIRS cascade is vital. Appropriate use of **prophylactic antibiotics** in bowel surgery or trauma is important, but intraoperative and postoperative **errors in technique** or clinical judgement are major contributing factors in more than 50% of patients with multiple organ dysfunction. Good clinical judgement, effective resuscitation, good operative technique, effective excision of necrotic tissue, minimising bacterial contamination and preventing accumulation of postoperative fluid collections (serum or blood) are all necessary factors in prevention. The purpose is to eliminate the local environment in which bacteria multiply and improve the delivery of host antibacterial defences.

Surgical complications with septic potential should be treated early, usually by definitive surgery, e.g. removal of necrotic tissue (including amputation of necrotic lower limbs), drainage of abscesses and control of peritoneal contamination by exteriorising leaking anastomoses. This helps reduce the circulating level of inflammatory mediators and limits the period of stress. In many cases it is better to perform a laparotomy on suspicion and find it normal than to 'wait and see' and risk rapid deterioration and death.

OTHER PREVENTIVE FACTORS IN AT-RISK PATIENTS

Adequate and early **fluid resuscitation** is essential in patients with hypovolaemia, whether in trauma victims, acute pancreatitis or bowel obstruction, because the loss of intravascular volume leads to deficient tissue perfusion (i.e. shock) and splanchnic ischaemia. Maintaining tissue oxygenation is also vital; at-risk patients must have arterial blood gases and pH estimated and be given supplemental oxygen or assisted ventilation as required. To help prevent intestinal bacterial translocation, enterocytes and colonocytes are best supported by **enteral feeding**, if necessary by a feeding jejunostomy or a fine-bore nasogastric tube. Glutamine, arginine and omega-3 fatty acids are believed to be particularly important components.

TREATMENT OF SEPSIS AND MODS

Septic patients need managing and careful monitoring in an intensive care unit. The longer the process continues, the more widespread and irreversible the damage; the sooner treatment is initiated, the better the chances of success. The general principles of treatment include search for and elimination of infective foci, appropriate antibiotic treatment, fluid and blood maintenance, oxygenation and enteral feeding. Treatment with new drugs designed to manipulate the endotoxin–cytokine axis has so far been unsuccessful, probably because the agents need to be given at the onset of the cascade of sepsis. Specific organ support is given as required; for example, for ARDS and renal failure. Despite all of this, the prospects for established MODS remain grim.

SHOCK

PATHOPHYSIOLOGY OF SHOCK

Shock is defined as acute circulatory failure of sufficient magnitude to compromise tissue perfusion. Cellular hypoxia and disruption of normal metabolic function, if untreated, rapidly proceed to irreversible organ damage and death. Shock may be encountered at any stage from the acute emergency through to final recovery. Treatment depends upon quick and accurate diagnosis.

There are three pathophysiological types of shock:

namely, collapse of cardiac preload (hypovolaemia), pump failure and collapse of peripheral resistance. Each may occur in a variety of circumstances.

PRELOAD COLLAPSE

Preload is defined as the rate of return of blood to the heart. Preload collapse may be due to an inadequate volume of blood to fill the venous compartment, i.e. **absolute hypovolaemia** (hypovolaemic shock) or **relative hypovolaemia** due to a rapid increase in the volume of the venous compartment relative to actual blood volume. Preload collapse is responsible for about 75% of cases of shock encountered in hospital and the majority of these are due to hypovolaemic shock.

Hypovolaemic shock

The main causes of hypovolaemic shock are:

● 'Revealed' haemorrhage, e.g. deep lacerations, large haematemesis (vomiting of blood) from a peptic ulcer, severe blood loss from a wound drain
● 'Concealed' haemorrhage, e.g. intra-abdominal bleeding from ruptured spleen or aortic aneurysm, haemorrhage from a duodenal ulcer into the small intestine, intramuscular blood loss from multiple fractures
● Extensive burns, resulting in massive loss of serum into blisters or from surface weeping
● Severe vomiting or diarrhoea, or fluid loss from small bowel fistula
● Excessive urinary loss, e.g. diabetic ketoacidosis, diuretic phase of acute tubular necrosis, powerful diuretics
● Sequestration of fluid in bowel due to obstruction
● Massive loss of fluid into interstitial tissues, as occurs in sepsis, or into the peritoneal cavity in acute pancreatitis or generalised peritonitis

PUMP FAILURE (CARDIOGENIC SHOCK)

Cardiogenic shock results from any form of 'pump failure', most commonly arising from an acute myocardial infarction or an acute ventricular arrhythmia. The condition can also be caused by cardiac valve prolapse caused by a ruptured papillary muscle. A large pulmonary embolus may also cause cardiogenic shock by obstructing blood flow through the lungs, causing secondary cardiac failure.

COLLAPSE OF PERIPHERAL RESISTANCE

Cardiac afterload or peripheral resistance is controlled predominantly by the tone of the smooth muscle of arteriolar and capillary sphincters. About 80% of capillaries are normally closed.

Septic shock

Systemic responses to severe Gram-negative infections typically cause cardiovascular collapse or **septic shock**, as described on page 29. Bacterial endotoxins activate cytokine systems and other defensive mechanisms to produce a variety of tissue effects which disrupt the normally exquisite systems of regulation of microvascular flow. This results in widespread endothelial damage, extensive peripheral vasodilatation and greatly increased capillary permeability with massive fluid leakage into the interstitial or 'third' space.

Anaphylactic shock

Anaphylactic shock is a generalised form of type I hypersensitivity reaction, occurring in response to an antigen to which the patient has previously become sensitised. The antigen binds with antibody attached to the surface of mast cells, triggering degranulation and release of histamine and other vasoactive amines. The predominant effect is extensive dilatation of the venous compartment causing marked hypovolaemia. The systemic effects are compounded by intense broncho-constriction and often laryngeal oedema which effectively halt ventilation.

In surgical practice, anaphylactic shock usually results from drug administration, particularly via the intravenous route, penicillins being the most common culprit. Anyone administering a drug should ensure the patient is not known to be sensitive. Anaphylactic reactions may also occur after intravenous injections of radiological contrast media. Insect bites (wasps, bees and hornets) and ingested nuts are also an important cause and may be seen in the accident and emergency department.

CLINICAL FEATURES OF SHOCK

The essential feature of any type of shock is a **precipitate fall in arterial blood pressure** with systolic pressure dropping by some 40 mmHg from usual levels to less than 90 mmHg. The immediate homeostatic response is **intense sympathetic activity** and catecholamine release. The heart rate increases dramatically in an attempt to increase cardiac output. Except in septic shock, there is intense cutaneous vasoconstriction in an attempt to restore intravascular volume by increasing peripheral resistance. Sudomotor activity causes profuse sweating. The hypoxic tissues revert to anaerobic respiration, producing lactic acid sufficient to cause a metabolic acidosis, and the respiratory rate rises in an attempt at compensation. The clinical picture is a cold, white, clammy patient with a rapid thready pulse and increased respiratory rate.

Septic shock presents a contrasting clinical picture in which there is a cytokine-mediated peripheral vasodilatation unresponsive to circulating catecholamines. The patient's skin is hot and flushed and cardiac output is increased to fill the dilated periphery. The pulse is typically 'bounding' in quality. Temperature, however, may be above normal or even below normal.

Without treatment, the circulation cannot support the main organ systems which fail (i.e. decompensate) one by one. Pulmonary failure leads to ARDS, and cerebral hypoxia soon causes confusion and eventually coma. Inadequate renal perfusion causes a dramatic fall in urinary output (oliguria) which, if not rapidly corrected, leads to acute tubular necrosis. If shock persists, reduced coronary flow and heart failure cause death. In septic shock, organ damage is exacerbated by endotoxins and deterioration is inexorable unless the source of infection can be rapidly eliminated and effective support measures instituted.

PRINCIPLES OF MANAGING SHOCK BY RESUSCITATION

Whatever the cause, the aim is to restore tissue perfusion and oxygenation by resuscitative measures while the diagnosis is being made and the specific treatment begun. The following steps are involved:

- Administer oxygen
- Obtain venous access and restore tissue perfusion
- Assess and monitor

RESUSCITATION

Oxygen

A mask delivering 100% oxygen should be immediately secured. The comatose patient must be intubated and positive-pressure ventilation commenced.

Venous access and tissue perfusion

An intravenous infusion should be set up immediately. Unless cardiogenic shock is likely, the circulating volume must be expanded rapidly. Plasma substitutes are preferable as they tend to draw fluid by osmosis from the extracellular tissues into the vascular compartment.

In a shocked patient, central and peripheral veins are usually collapsed and venous cannulation may prove difficult. Immediate central venous cannulation often wastes time, and the most effective method for rapid infusion is via bilateral cubital fossa cannulae. Use the shortest and largest-bore cannulae available. Unless the

doctor is experienced, a 'cut down' on the long saphenous vein at the ankle may also waste time. Fluid should be infused rapidly using an infusion pump and warmer if available, being mindful of over-rapid infusion of cold fluids. Once fluid is running, a tourniquet applied proximally causes the veins to engorge and facilitates insertion of a wider-bore cannula.

Assessment and monitoring

These involve the following procedures:

- **Basic observations** are made of temperature, pulse, blood pressure, respiratory rate and level of consciousness, monitored at frequent intervals; bounding pulse and flushed extremities will suggest the diagnosis of septic shock. Systolic blood pressure, central venous pressure and hourly urinary output are the most useful guides to success of resuscitative efforts
- **History and context** of the cardiovascular collapse, along with a knowledge of the patient's past medical history and pre-existing medical state including recent operations, will often be a valuable guide to the cause of shock
- **A general examination** is performed quickly but thoroughly to search for evidence of infection or concealed haemorrhage, particularly within the abdomen (e.g. ruptured aneurysm). A history of chest pain or the finding of an elevated jugular venous pressure suggests cardiac failure due to myocardial infarction, a cardiac murmur suggests valvular prolapse, and an expiratory wheeze is suggestive of anaphylaxis or cardiac failure
- **An ECG is performed** for evidence of myocardial infarction or pulmonary embolism. Note that the ECG changes typical of pulmonary embolism are only seen in massive embolism
- **A urinary catheter is inserted** to monitor hourly urinary output
- **A central venous line is inserted** to monitor central pressure and the response to fluid administration
- **Venous blood is taken** for measurement of haemoglobin, haematocrit, urea and electrolytes and cross-matching of blood. An arterial sample is taken for estimation of blood gas and acid–base status; blood cultures are taken if septic shock is suspected. Blood glucose should be estimated using reagent strips

SPECIFIC TREATMENTS FOR SHOCK

HYPOVOLAEMIC SHOCK

Identifying the cause of the fluid loss is top priority and immediate measures should be taken to control blood loss, e.g. pressure on a swab over a bleeding wound, a tourniquet for injured limb, laparotomy for ruptured spleen. Fluid replacement should be equivalent to the estimated fluid loss but adjusted according to the effect on central venous pressure and urine output. Where possible, fluids of similar composition to the fluids lost should be used: whole blood for haemorrhage, colloids after major burns. As a principle, however, it is not what is given but how quickly that matters. Fluids should be given in a rapid bolus, e.g. 250 ml, and the response observed. If inadequate, the bolus is repeated until shock is controlled or other measures to control blood loss are employed.

CARDIOGENIC SHOCK

The management of cardiogenic shock is best reviewed in a medical textbook; the management of pulmonary embolism (which may present as cardiogenic shock) is discussed in Chapter 47, page 643. Fluid overload is a significant hazard in cardiogenic shock and must be avoided.

SEPTIC SHOCK

Systemic sepsis leading to septic shock usually emanates from a specific focus of infection or from the patient's own intestinal organisms. The source may be obvious but, if not, a careful search must be made bearing in mind the common sites. In surgical practice, septic shock is most commonly seen either as a result of faecal peritonitis following large bowel perforation or as a result of anastomotic breakdown. In a patient who has had bowel surgery, intraperitoneal sepsis is the prime suspect but bladder or chest infection or an otherwise 'silent' infection of a central venous cannula is often the cause. In previously hypovolaemic patients, endogenous sepsis is often the cause. Debilitated patients, uncontrolled diabetics and infants are particularly vulnerable to sudden sepsis; in such cases the source of infection may not be found. Gangrene of a leg is also a potent cause.

The damaging effects of poor organ perfusion in septic shock are increased by direct and indirect endotoxic tissue damage. Treatment of septic shock is urgent and involves fluid resuscitation, oxygenation, administration of appropriate antibiotics and the tracing and elimination of the source of infection.

Blood cultures must always be taken and intravenous antibiotics administered on a 'best-guess' basis. Experience has shown that a broad-spectrum combination of gentamicin, benzylpenicillin and metronidazole is one of the most effective regimens and can be modified later if resistant organisms are isolated.

In the meantime, intravenous plasma expanders are given and the rate and volume adjusted according to blood pressure, central venous pressure and urine output. Because of 'third space', i.e. interstitial losses, volumes given may have to be large. Volume expansion helps to sustain cardiac output and tissue perfusion. Corticosteroids are known to stabilise cell membranes but evidence of their effectiveness in septic shock is lacking.

If the diagnosis of septic shock is correct, resuscitative measures should produce dramatic improvement in the patient's condition within 1–2 hours. By that time, the patient should be ready for immediate operation if an abscess or bowel perforation appears to be the cause. It cannot be emphasised too strongly that the source of infection must be urgently eliminated if the septic cascade is to be reversed.

DISSEMINATED INTRAVASCULAR COAGULATION

Another major problem in MODS and septic shock is generalised activation of the clotting cascade causing disseminated intravascular coagulation (DIC). This exhausts the supply of platelets and clotting factors V, VIII and fibrinogen (**consumption coagulopathy**) and activates the intrinsic fibrinolytic mechanisms. It becomes manifest as spontaneous bleeding or bruising and uncontrollable haemorrhage from any operation site. Diagnosis is made by finding low fibrinogen levels and high levels of D dimers (cleaved from fibrin by plasmin and evidence of fibrin lysis). Treatment includes management of the initiating cause, administration of intravenous heparin to arrest the coagulation process and infusion of necessary clotting factors, e.g. fresh-frozen plasma, cryoprecipitate.

ANAPHYLACTIC SHOCK

Anaphylactic shock, e.g. following intravenous drug administration, requires urgent treatment. Adrenaline, 1 ml of 1 in 1000 solution, is given subcutaneously, causing generalised vasoconstriction and increased cardiac output. Hydrocortisone 200–500 mg and an antihistamine such as chlorpheniramine 10 mg are given intravenously, the former stabilising the mast cells and the latter blocking histamine receptors which mediate much of the peripheral vascular response. Intravenous fluids are needed to treat the hypovolaemia.

Because of the risk of anaphylactic shock, a doctor should always administer the first dose of any intravenous agent, including radiological contrast agents and radioisotopes, and a doctor should always be available whenever parenteral drugs (including vaccinations) are being administered. The doctor is legally responsible for ensuring that resuscitation drugs and equipment are immediately available and must check this beforehand, particularly if working in an unfamiliar ward or department.

3 Principles of blood transfusion

INTRODUCTION

The ability to transfuse safely blood and, to a lesser extent, blood products revolutionised the management of major trauma. It also facilitated extraordinary advances in areas of surgery which involve heavy blood loss, such as arterial reconstruction, open heart surgery and organ transplantation.

Nevertheless, blood transfusion is not without risk— for example, from transfusion reactions, transmission of infection and potential immunosuppression in cancer patients. The problem of infection has been tragically highlighted by the development of human immuno-deficiency virus (HIV)/acquired immunodeficiency syn-drome (AIDS) in haemophiliacs and other patients after unwitting transfusion of infected blood. Indeed, several political scandals have arisen from high-level decisions not to use up-to-date methods of testing or treating donor blood for HIV.

Thus, to minimise potentially lethal effects, the decision to transfuse blood products must be based on clear indications and only after considering appropriate alternatives, such as tolerating lower haemoglobin con-centrations, using alternative infusions such as gelatin for hypovolaemia, autologous transfusion techniques or iron therapy for anaemia (see 'Reducing the need for bank blood transfusion', p. 33).

The immediate advantage of transfusing stored blood for replacing blood loss is that it remains within the vascular compartment but it should be remembered that most 'blood' for transfusion has had all useful components other than red cells removed; white cells and platelets in the transfused blood are virtually inactive and clotting factors absent. The types of transfusion currently available and the general indications for their use are as follows:

- **Stored whole blood**—less readily available now because of the demand for blood products. Most blood for transfusion is essentially red cells alone. For substantial haemorrhage, e.g. trauma, major surgery, bleeding peptic ulcer, concentrated red cells are often given together with electrolyte or gelatin solutions

- **Packed or concentrated red cells**—for substantial haemorrhage (see 'Stored whole blood' above) or for raising haemoglobin where circulating volume is adequate, especially if there is a risk of circulatory overload, e.g. chronic anaemia with cardiac failure. Most blood for transfusion is now offered in this form

- **Human albumin solution (formerly known as plasma) available as 4.5% and 20% solutions**—in terms of efficacy, mortality and cardiorespiratory function, there is little evidence that albumin solutions are any better than plasma substitutes or normal saline for resuscitating patients with burns, traumatic or septic shock, or requiring large perioperative volume replacement. Indeed, there is substantial evidence that human albumin solutions are associated with worse outcomes in some critically ill patients. Thus use of albumin solutions should probably be restricted to intensive care units for occasional use in patients critically ill with hypoproteinaemic oedema or respiratory distress syndrome. Other uses are difficult to justify in the absence of proven benefit, as albumin is expensive and is derived from human donor blood

- **Fresh-frozen plasma (FFP)**—separated from fresh blood and then frozen, FFP contains near-normal amounts of all clotting factors and other plasma proteins. It is used to replace clotting factors exhausted during major haemorrhage (due to a combination of consumption of clotting factors by attempted haemostasis and poor clotting ability of stored blood). Transfusion of FFP should be considered whenever bleeding is continuing and a clotting screen is abnormal, or in patients rapidly losing large quantities of blood. FFP is also used in patients short of clotting factors for other reasons, e.g. liver disease or for rapid reversal of coumarin-type anticoagulants. (*Note*: FFP should be blood group-compatible when possible.) Safer, cheaper products should be used for simple volume replacement

- **Platelet concentrates**—for platelet exhaustion during major haemorrhage and in thrombocytopenia

- **Cryoprecipitate, fibrinogen and other specific clotting factor concentrates**—for various specific coagulation deficiencies, e.g. haemophilia. These should only be used in consultation with a haematologist
- **Plasma substitutes**—these are solutions of macromolecules with colloid osmotic pressure and viscosity characteristics similar to plasma. Gelatin solutions (e.g. 'Haemaccel', 'Gelofusin') and etherified starch solutions (e.g. Hetastarch) have now largely replaced dextrans ('Dextran-70') and are used for initial restoration of circulating volume in haemorrhage or burns and to maintain volume, blood pressure and renal perfusion intraoperatively where blood transfusion is not indicated

LABORATORY ASPECTS OF BLOOD TRANSFUSION

BLOOD GROUPING AND COMPATIBILITY TESTING

Transfusion of incompatible blood in respect of the major blood group antigens (ABO factor) is potentially fatal. Transfusion practice has been developed to minimise this risk and involves two main steps. Firstly, the patient's ABO and Rhesus groups are established. Secondly, the patient's blood (and each unit of donor blood) is screened for antibodies. Alternatively, each unit of group-compatible donor blood intended for transfusion is cross-matched directly against the patient's serum to ensure complete compatibility. Fortunately, units of donor blood are compatible at first cross-match in about 99% of cases, and it seems likely that cross-matching will come to be regarded as unnecessary in the future; group-compatible antibody-free blood can be safely used in most cases without specific cross-matching. This would allow supply from a prepared pool of transfusion units, rather than necessitating the preparation of a patient-specific allocation, thus representing a saving in terms of both time and cost.

After the transfusion of many units of blood (e.g. massive haemorrhage from liver trauma), the patient's own antibodies are so depleted that further group-compatible blood is usually given without cross-matching. In an emergency (e.g. obstetric haemorrhage at home) where group-compatible blood is not available, then group O, Rh negative blood can be given with comparative safety, but there is a long-term risk of antibodies developing, which makes future cross-matching difficult.

STORAGE AND USEFUL LIFE OF BLOOD

Blood and blood products have exacting requirements if their quality is to be preserved. Maintaining blood quality is essentially the responsibility of the supplying laboratory; the value of blood and blood products is easily diminished if they are handled inappropriately thereafter.

Blood is stored chilled between 2 and 4°C, when it has a shelf-life of about 5 weeks. With developments in preservative solutions (e.g. CPD-A) there is little deterioration of red cell quality during storage but pH changes occur, potassium leaches out of the cells and clotting factors diminish. Blood must not normally be frozen, although expensive techniques for freezing patients' own blood in glycerol for later autotransfusion have been developed for patients with rare blood groups or unusual antibodies and, latterly, for preventing blood-borne viral infections in certain important people travelling in high-risk areas.

To ensure vitality, blood should not be removed from the laboratory or theatre refrigerator until immediately before use. If blood has been out of the refrigerator for more than 30 minutes and has not been transfused, it should be returned to the laboratory unused. Indeed, all unused blood should be returned to the laboratory as soon as it becomes apparent that it will not be required, as it may still be suitable for another patient. Empty used blood packs are often retained for 24 hours so that they can be examined and tested in the event of a transfusion reaction.

BLOOD TRANSFUSION IN CLINICAL PRACTICE

BLOOD TRANSFUSION AND ELECTIVE SURGERY

Attitudes to transfusion in elective surgery are becoming more conservative. Blood is an expensive commodity, and its use is not risk-free. In elective surgery, patients usually fall into one of three categories: transfusion not anticipated (e.g. hernia repair), transfusion possible but unlikely (e.g. cholecystectomy), and transfusion probable (e.g. major arterial reconstruction). For patients in the second category, a blood sample should be sent in advance for ABO and Rhesus grouping and antibody screening, and the serum retained in the laboratory for further compatibility testing if required later ('**group and screen**'). For patients in the third category, an appropriate number of units of blood is requested to be available for transfusion at the time of operation. In this case, the blood group and antibody screen is performed on receipt of the request and the blood is prepared a day or so before operation. If blood is then transfused and a further transfusion is required more than 2 days later, a new blood sample is needed for testing as new antibodies may have developed.

To guard against the disaster of blood being given to the wrong patient, scrupulous attention must be paid to correct and complete labelling of blood samples which are sent for grouping and cross-matching. Immediately before transfusion, the label of each unit of the supplied blood must be carefully checked against the identity and blood group of the patient.

VOLUME AND RATE OF TRANSFUSION

The volume of blood required and the rate of transfusion depend on the age of the patient, the indications for transfusion and the patient's general and cardiovascular condition.

Haemorrhage

Haemorrhage can be clinically classified according to the response to initial colloid or crystalloid resuscitation. If there is no response, such as in torrential obstetric haemorrhage from placenta previa, group O Rh negative blood is transfused as fast as necessary to maintain adequate blood pressure (i.e. systolic above 100 mmHg) and a positive central venous pressure. If there is a transient response, there may be time to check the blood group and employ group-specific blood transfusion early on. If the resuscitation response is appropriate to the blood loss, blood should be sent for group and screen; immediate transfusion is not indicated.

If rapid transfusion is required, an inflatable bag surrounding the fluid or blood pack can be used to increase the pressure. If many units are to be given, or the blood is for neonates or small children, it should be warmed by passing it through a special blood warming device.

Anaemia

Surgery can generally be performed on a patient whose haemoglobin is greater than 10 g/dl; compensated anaemia in a young person down to 8 g/dl may be tolerated with no significant increase in morbidity or mortality. Older patients are less tolerant of this level of anaemia unless the anaemia is chronic and little surgical blood loss is expected. If preoperative transfusion is needed, it should be given at least 2 days beforehand. This maximises the beneficial effects of the blood and permits fluid balance to stabilise. One unit of blood (450 ml blood + 63 ml preservative and anticoagulant solution) will raise the haemoglobin concentration by approximately 1 g/dl in an adult and is typically transfused over 3–4 hours. If a large amount of blood is required to treat anaemia, it is best to use packed cells and to transfuse slowly.

REDUCING THE NEED FOR BANK BLOOD TRANSFUSION

Deaths and serious reactions still occur from incompatible blood transfusions (particularly when blood products are administered under general anaesthesia). In addition, serious infections such as human immunodeficiency virus (HIV) can be transmitted from apparently fit infected donors with chronic latent carrier states, despite careful screening of donors and donations. The risks of side effects and complications increase in line with the number of units transfused. Risks can be reduced by rigorous scrutiny and monitoring of the indications for transfusion and by developing locally recommended blood ordering schedules for particular operations.

Autologous blood transfusion

Other methods of reducing bank blood transfusion involve 'recycling' the patient's own blood (autologous transfusion) by one of the methods described below.

Pre-donation of blood

In a pre-deposit programme, up to 4 units of blood can be collected at weekly intervals from a patient for whom major elective surgery is planned. Pre-donation can be safely achieved even in the elderly and those with cardiac disease. In the USA, such is the fear of transmitted infection that about 5% of blood now collected is for autologous transfusion. There are several drawbacks: the collection, storage and checking system is costly and complicated to administer and patients must be prepared well in advance of operation. Up to 40% of cases require additional donor blood, and about 50% of units collected are never used. There also remains the potential risk from clerical errors. Erythropoietin may be administered to increase the bone marrow response and allow a shorter donation programme but at present it is too expensive for routine use. Unfortunately, cancer surgery does not lend itself to pre-donation owing to the potential risk of transfusing malignant cells back into the circulation. Pre-donation is, however, ideal for patients due to undergo major vascular surgery.

Normovolaemic haemodilution

Normovolaemic haemodilution involves collecting blood from the patient immediately prior to surgery and replacing it with colloid. This has the advantages of autologous transfusion without the disadvantages of pre-donation or the use of cell washing and collecting equipment. Up to 2 litres of blood can be removed safely from adults without cardiac disease immediately before an operation and replaced with colloid. The procedure reduces the venous haematocrit and increases cardiac output. When about 300 ml of low-haematocrit blood have been lost at operation the normal haematocrit autologous transfusion is commenced. If blood loss is less than 2 litres, additional blood is rarely needed. The procedure is inexpensive, convenient for the patient and flexible as regards operation scheduling. The blood is fresh and contains viable platelets if kept at room temperature. It also contains significant levels of labile clotting factors. The technique has been used extensively in cardiac and vascular surgery but could be extended to other types of surgery.

Blood salvage techniques

This approach involves blood spilled at operation being collected by suction, processed and reinfused. In manual salvage, blood from suction or postoperative drainage is collected into a reservoir containing anticoagulant before being reinfused via a fine filter. This technique has been used most frequently in orthopaedic surgery.

In cases of acute massive intra-abdominal blood loss which is uncontaminated by bowel contents, e.g. multiple trauma or liver transplantation, an automated cell saver can be used. Salvaged red cells are washed, concentrated and resuspended in physiological solution, then reinfused as required at a packed cell volume of 50%. Homologous blood and blood products are often needed in addition, but the number of units of blood used is much reduced. By this method, losses of over 100 units have been recycled. Blood salvage using cell savers is generally only cost-effective where large numbers of operations requiring large volumes of blood are performed in the surgical centre.

HAZARDS AND COMPLICATIONS OF BLOOD TRANSFUSION

FEBRILE REACTIONS

Fever during blood transfusion is common and is usually due to non-red-cell immune incompatibility, e.g. proteins, white cells. If the fever is less than 38°C then the transfusion should be allowed to continue. If the fever is higher, or there are systemic symptoms (e.g. chills or rigors), then the transfusion should be stopped for 30 minutes. If the fever returns, the blood must be returned to the laboratory for testing. In most situations, febrile transfusion reactions are due to leucocyte and not red cell incompatibility.

HAEMOLYTIC REACTIONS

Massive haemolysis will occur if there is major ABO incompatibility, although this is thankfully rare. A lesser degree of haemolysis is associated with incompatibility in minor determinants. Almost all haemolytic reactions are caused by human error in transfusing incompatible blood. The clinical features of a haemolytic reaction are summarised in Box 3.1. Diagnosis is confirmed by finding

KEY POINTS

Box 3.1 Clinical features of a haemolytic transfusion reaction
- Rapidly developing pyrexia at onset of transfusion
- Dyspnoea, constrictive feeling in chest, intense headache
- Severe loin pain
- Hypotension
- Acute oliguric renal failure with haemoglobinuria (due to obstruction of tubules with haemoglobin, hypotension causing acute tubular necrosis)
- Jaundice (developing hours or days later)
- Disseminated intravascular coagulation with spontaneous bruising and haemorrhage (e.g. cerebral, gastrointestinal)

hyperbilirubinaemia and a positive Coombs test and by demonstrating an antibody on repeat screening. With massive intravascular haemolysis, haemoglobinaemia and haemoglobinuria may be found. The transfusion must be halted immediately and the patient resuscitated. Oliguria is treated by osmotic diuresis (e.g. mannitol), aided by a loop diuretic if appropriate.

ALLERGIC REACTIONS

Allergic reactions to transfusion are occasionally seen and manifest as fever, pruritus (itching), skin rashes, wheals or angio-oedema (periorbital, facial and laryngeal swelling). These tend to appear either towards the end of transfusion or else some time later. Transfusions still in progress should be discontinued and symptoms treated with antihistamines.

INFECTION

Infection may arise from three sources: the donor, contamination during the process of blood preparation and storage, or the giving set or cannula site (see Fig. 3.1, p. 36).

Infections transmitted by donor blood or blood product transfusion

Donated blood can now be screened for most significant transmissible infectious agents. Many of the tests, however, rely on detecting antibodies to viruses and therefore do not detect recently acquired disease where insufficient time has elapsed for the antibody response to develop.

Donor infections are most likely to be transmitted when a **chronic latent carrier state** can exist in the donor. Examples include:

- **Viral infections**—hepatitis B, C, and D; HIV I and II; human T-cell lymphotropic virus (HTLV) I; cytomegalovirus; Epstein–Barr virus
- **Bacterial infections**—syphilis, brucellosis
- **Protozoal infections**—malaria, Chagas' disease, and babesiosis

The most important of these infections are discussed below.

Hepatitis viruses

The 'Australia antigen' was discovered in the 1960s, together with its association with the transmissible agent for hepatitis B. This antigen was later identified as the hepatitis B virus (HBV) surface antigen (HBsAg). Donors have been screened for hepatitis B since the late 1960s by all transfusion services in the developed world and this has dramatically reduced the incidence of transfusion-related hepatitis B. Despite screening, infections occasionally occur because very low concentrations of antigen cannot be detected. Thus patients needing multiple transfusions or blood products should be vaccinated against hepatitis B. HBV is present in the plasma and is transmitted by all types of blood product except those subject to viricidal treatment.

For hepatitis B, the surface antigen HBsAg may be absent early after infection but appear later. However, transmission of hepatitis B by screened blood is uncommon.

Hepatitis C, formerly known as 'non-A, non-B hepatitis', used to be transmitted twice as often via blood transfusion as hepatitis B. The illness of hepatitis C is often mild, but up to half of all cases progress to chronic hepatitis (10% for hepatitis B) and 10% develop cirrhosis or hepatoma or both. Since 1991, all donations in the UK have been screened for hepatitis C and the incidence of post-transfusion hepatitis C has fallen from 1.3 to 0.1 per 1000 units transfused.

Human immunodeficiency virus

In 1981, the HIV epidemic and its link with blood transfusion began, with reports of opportunistic pneumonias in homosexual men and haemophiliacs. By the mid-1980s, the risk of HIV transmission via transfused blood in the USA was as high as 1 in 2500. Transmission via blood transfusion associated with surgery has been rare in the UK. Haemophiliacs were much less fortunate, being infected via clotting factor VIII preparations imported from the USA.

In the UK, all blood donors and donations have been screened for HIV antibody since 1985. About 1 in 10 000 donors is found to be HIV-positive, with new donors about four times as likely. Seropositivity implies there would be a 90% risk of HIV transmission via blood donation. Current HIV antibody detection methods are very reliable but there is a period lasting 1–3 months after infection when antibody may be undetectable. The most effective method of reducing the risk in countries where donors are unpaid is donor self-exclusion. Potential donors have the risks of infection transfer explained and are asked not to donate blood if they know they have transmissible infections or fall into high-risk categories, e.g. intravenous drug users, promiscuous homosexuals. When combined with a low prevalence of HIV in the donor pool (as in the UK), the risk of transmitting HIV via a screened blood or blood component donation is small but not negligible. The risk has been estimated at about 1 in a million units transfused.

A second virus, HIV-II, is prevalent in West Africa and has been screened for in the UK since June 1990.

Cytomegalovirus

Infection with cytomegalovirus is widespread, the virus remaining latent in leucocytes. The risk of infection is important only in immature neonates and immuno-suppressed patients who are CMV-seronegative. To minimise the risk, donated blood for these groups should be screened for CMV-specific antibody and the donation can be leucocyte-depleted in the haematology laboratory prior to transfusion.

Protozoal infection—malaria

Transfusion-transmitted malaria occurs but remains rare in developed countries. In endemic areas, however, it is common and the majority of healthy blood donors will be potentially infectious. The disease should be considered if a patient becomes ill after transfusion.

Contamination of blood or giving sets with microorganisms

Low-grade contamination of blood packs from the environment rarely has serious consequences because of the low temperatures of blood storage and the self-sterilising properties of blood. However, microorganisms may proliferate if storage conditions are inadequate or blood is left unchilled before transfusion.

Transfusion of bacterially infected blood, however, is rare but it can be catastrophic, leading to death within a very short time. Gram-negative aerobic bacilli, particularly *Pseudomonas* and *Salmonella* species, have been incriminated. The presence of exotoxins or endotoxins may also lead to life-threatening complications.

Giving sets may become contaminated unless strict aseptic technique is maintained during the setting-up or changing of any component of transfusion equipment. Finally, peripheral intravenous cannulae, and particularly central venous lines, may become infected by opportunistic skin commensals (e.g. coagulase-negative staphylococci) or contaminating pathogens (e.g. *Staphylococcus aureus*,

Escherichia coli) causing local infection (see Fig. 3.1), bacteraemia or even septicaemia. Cannula sites should be inspected daily and changed every 2 days. The same vein can then later be reused for a new infusion. In a patient with a central venous line and a pyrexia of unknown origin, the line should be removed and tested bacteriologically.

The clinical result of transfusing a bacterially contaminated donation resembles that of a haemolytic reaction, with fever, chills, hypotension, nausea and vomiting, oliguria and disseminated intravascular coagulation. Mortality is around 35%. If a patient develops adverse symptoms, investigations should include culture of the

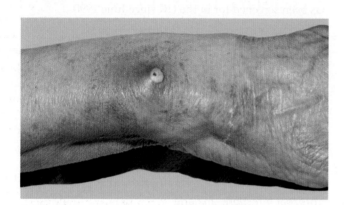

Fig. 3.1 Infected cannula site at the wrist

patient's blood and the blood product as well as re-checking compatibility.

IMMUNOSUPPRESSIVE EFFECTS OF BLOOD TRANSFUSION

Blood transfusion has been demonstrated to have a potential for immunosuppression which may influence recurrence of certain cancers, particularly colorectal, and may also have an adverse influence on postoperative infection rates. Nevertheless, the data is conflicting and as yet there is insufficient evidence of an important clinical effect.

FLUID OVERLOAD

Fluid overload is rarely a problem of blood transfusion in healthy adults but may easily develop if the cardio-vascular system is already compromised or if particularly large volumes are given or when transfusing babies and small children.

ACUTE RESPIRATORY DISTRESS SYNDROME

This may be due to anti-Fc-receptor antibodies or possibly to multiple microemboli of platelet and leucocyte aggregates. The latter is prevented by the use of a blood filter.

4 Principles of transplantation surgery

INTRODUCTION

Many patients die because of failure of a single organ system such as the kidney, liver, lungs or heart, but if the function of the failing organ could be restored, the patient would have the chance of returning to near-normal health. It is not surprising that physicians from early times have turned their attention to replacing the function of failing organs in the most direct manner, by transplanting a healthy organ from another human or an animal of another species.

The scene was set for clinical organ transplantation early in the 20th century by Alexis Carrel who was awarded the Nobel Prize for Physiology and Medicine in 1912 for his pioneering work with Charles Guthrie in vascular surgery and transplantation. Carrel, working with laboratory animals, found that **autografts** (removing and reimplanting an organ into the same animal) could be expected to function indefinitely whereas **allografts** (organs transplanted between animals of the same species) rarely functioned for more than a few days. Early attempts at transplantation in man used **xenografts** (transplantation of tissues between different species) to transfer renal tissue from pigs, goats, rabbits and apes; these were uniformly unsuccessful.

The key to organ transplantation lay in the developing field of immunology with recognition of the mechanisms involved in **graft rejection** and the elaboration and application of techniques to minimise or prevent it. The first clinically useful transplant for humans involved pig heart valves. These consist of simple avascular tissue which can be treated to render it non-immunogenic so as to avoid rejection. Porcine cardiac valve transplants have been used regularly in humans since the mid-1970s.

Progressive developments in chemical immuno-suppression to attenuate graft rejection have allowed successful grafting of many organs and tissues (see Table 4.1). Transplantation of the human cornea, kidney, liver, pancreas, heart, heart and lung, single or double lung and bone marrow is now accepted as standard, although by no means free of rejection and other complications.

Table 4.1 Numbers of transplants performed during 1990 and 1997 in Europe and the USA

Organ	Europe		USA	
	1990	1997	1990	1997
Kidney	10 383	9563	9491	8844
Heart	2134	2451	2007	2362
Liver	2139	3115	2541	4091
Pancreas	226	486	529	1063
Intestine	0	9	0	60

Promising results are now being obtained with small bowel transplants and composite grafts (known as **cluster grafts**) of several abdominal organs and sometimes the heart as well, although these are still to some extent experimental. The development of a state of **tolerance** between the graft and the host of a transplanted organ remains the goal of transplant surgeons and immunologists.

TRANSPLANT IMMUNOLOGY

MAJOR HISTOCOMPATIBILITY COMPLEX

Most tissue cells have a number of different surface **glycoproteins** which, if transplanted from one individual to another, excite a response from the recipient's immune system. These **histocompatibility antigens** are recognised by the recipient's immunocytes and the response generated involves both cell-mediated and humoral mechanisms. These responses cause destruction of the transplanted cells.

Each individual has a number of histocompatibility antigens but only one group is responsible for major graft rejection problems. These **major histocompatibility antigens** are coded for by a set of genes known as the **major histocompatibility complex (MHC)**. In humans, the MHC is located on a segment of the short arm of chromosome 6. It is present in all cells but, as it was first discovered in leucocytes, it is known as the **HLA complex** (human lymphocyte antigen system A). Within

37

the human MHC, two major groups of antigens have been described, class I and class II antigens, which have different structures and specificities. The principal class I loci are known as the A and B antigens and the principal class II loci are the DR antigens. Since each individual receives one set of genetic information from each parent there are thus six principal loci (two each for A, B and DR) and two individuals can differ at any or all of these loci. Certain HLA types are known to be associated with particular autoimmune disorders, notably ankylosing spondylitis and coeliac disease, although the reasons are unknown.

TISSUE TYPING

HLA typing of individuals is used to match the donor and recipient as closely as possible. In kidney transplantation, when donor and recipient are identical at all six loci or differ by only one A or B antigen, this has been shown to result in significantly improved graft survival; these grafts are known as **beneficial matches**. A national transplant sharing system exists in most developed countries to match donor and recipient as closely as possible. Tissue typing is usually performed serologically using specific antisera. More recently, increased accuracy using **DNA fingerprinting** has become possible but the technique is still too slow for use in clinical transplantation.

The pattern of inheritance of tissue types within families shows that each child receives one set of genetic information (**haplotype**) from each parent; siblings have a 1 in 4 chance of being **haplo-identical** and a 1 in 2 chance of having one haplotype in common. Fully HLA-matched sibling donors give the best chance of graft survival, followed by those with one haplotype in common. Other than the special case of monozygotic twins, there is still some rejection in HLA identical grafts between siblings owing to differences in minor histocompatibility antigens. ABO blood group compatibility is an obvious prerequisite for organ transplantation which must not be overlooked in the search for ever closer HLA matching.

IMMUNOSUPPRESSION

With all major organ transplants, even if there is full HLA compatibility, the recipient's immune response must be suppressed if rejection and graft loss are to be prevented. Therapy needs to be continued indefinitely, although dosage can usually be progressively reduced to **maintenance levels** following initial high-dose **induction therapy**. This is because a partly tolerant state is established as the **host-versus-graft** response diminishes. Immunosuppressive drugs are employed in various

combinations, the most common being **prednisolone**, **azathioprine** and **cyclosporin**. In many cases, **polyclonal** or **monoclonal** antilymphocyte or antithymocyte globulins are added in the initial induction period. These drugs inevitably suppress lymphocyte proliferation, antibody production and inflammation in varying degrees, and complications include impaired healing, peptic ulceration, vulnerability to infection, bone marrow suppression and occasionally development of malignancy (especially Epstein–Barr virus-related lymphoproliferative disorders). Cyclosporin represented a major advance over the earlier combination of azathioprine and steroids but has significant side effects of its own in the form of nephrotoxicity and an occasional tendency to produce hirsutism.

In the continuing search for better immunosuppressive agents, a variety of new drugs have been produced as well as new improved forms of cyclosporin. These are currently being evaluated along with several new agents including **deoxyspergualin**, **mizorbine**, **RS 61443** and the macrolides **FK506** and **rapamycin**.

GRAFT REJECTION

Graft rejection remains a major problem and can present in several ways.

Hyperacute rejection

This occurs within minutes or hours of transplantation and results from the presence of preformed antibodies, either due to previous transplantation, blood transfusions, pregnancies or ABO incompatibility. The presence of these antibodies can be detected if a cross-match is performed using serum from the potential organ recipient and cells from the donor.

Acute rejection

This cell-mediated response is common and usually occurs within 2 weeks in first-time grafts; it can usually be reversed by a temporary increase in immunosuppression, usually in the form of a short course of high-dose steroid treatment or a brief course of anti-lymphocyte globulin.

Chronic rejection

This occurs months to years after transplantation and is probably the result of antibody-mediated rejection which can occur even in the face of long-term immunosuppression. It is often associated with gradual occlusion of arteries in the graft.

PRACTICAL PROBLEMS OF TRANSPLANTATION

SOURCES OF ORGANS FOR TRANSPLANTATION

Most tissues for transplantation are derived from cadaveric donors, with the organs removed from the body as soon as possible after death has been diagnosed. Any previously fit subjects who become brain-dead following head injuries or intracranial vascular catastrophes are potential donors of intra-abdominal or intrathoracic organs. Victims have usually been resuscitated from the outset with the circulation and respiration being maintained artificially. From such **'heart-beating' donors**, multi-organ donation procedures allow all appropriate organs to be removed and maintained in optimal condition for transplantation. Non-heart-beating donors can be used for bone, skin and corneal donation and the kidneys may still be suitable for transplantation if they can be removed rapidly following cessation of the circulation.

In the case of kidney transplantation, living related family members may be donors; this gives excellent results although it has gained greater acceptance in the United States than in the United Kingdom. The risk to the donor is slight and the donor's remaining kidney hypertrophies over succeeding months, restoring renal reserve to near-normal.

'BRAIN DEATH'

In many countries, criteria have been established to form a legal definition of brain death following irreversible brain stem injury even in the presence of a continuing intact circulatory system. Once these criteria have been satisfied, and with the appropriate consent from relatives, the subject becomes eligible for 'heart-beating' organ donation. The legal criteria for brain death in the UK are summarised in Box 4.1; similar criteria are used in other countries.

The diagnosis of brain death is made on the basis of clinical criteria in the UK. Electrocardiography, cerebral blood flow and other neurophysiological tests are not required. Appropriate clinical examination must be performed by two senior doctors independent of the transplant team and must be repeated at least twice.

CONSENT

It is usual to seek the agreement of the relatives and to determine whether the potential donor expressed any objection to donation during life. The matter is simplified if the potential donor carries a donor card or has left other written instructions known to the family. The personal difficulty many doctors face in informing

KEY POINTS

Box 4.1 Legal criteria for diagnosis of brain death (UK)

1. There must be a positive diagnosis of severe structural brain damage
2. The condition causing brain damage must be irreversible
3. There must be complete loss of brain stem function—evidenced by fixed pupils, no spontaneous eye movements or response to caloric testing, absent corneal, eyelash and blink reflexes, absent laryngeal and cough reflexes, and no response to deep painful stimuli (note: some spinal reflexes may be retained despite brain death)
4. On removal of ventilatory support, there must be no spontaneous respiratory activity in the presence of a physiologically adequate increase in PCO_2
5. Any possible effects of hypothermia and drugs (e.g. muscle relaxants, respiratory depressants, alcohol) must be excluded

relatives of the death of a loved one is compounded by having to request organ donation at the same time. However, the doctor's difficulty can be eased by the knowledge that the bereaved often gain comfort from knowing that other lives will be saved by the donated organs and this gain can be set against their own loss. Awareness of the potential gains and benefits of transplantation can be increased by education and easy availability of information for the public and for the medical profession.

ORGAN PRESERVATION AND TRANSPORT

Donors are often located in hospitals many miles away from where the recipient operation is to be performed. There may also be delay in getting the recipient into hospital and ready for operation. As a result, the organ to be transplanted will usually be removed from the donor some hours before transplantation; reliable techniques for organ preservation have of necessity been developed. **Hypothermia** reduces the metabolic demands of the organ and is the mainstay of effective organ preservation. The period of **warm ischaemia** between circulatory arrest and cooling by perfusion with ice-cold preservation fluid must be kept to a minimum if irreversible damage to the organ is to be avoided. For kidneys, normal function will usually recover if warm ischaemia does not exceed 40–60 minutes but this is at the cost of a post-transplantation period of greatly impaired function due to acute tubular necrosis during which continued haemodialysis support is required. For the liver and heart, immediate function after transplantation is essential and warm ischaemia must be avoided.

Two basic methods are used for preserving organs between donation and transplantation:

- **Simple cold storage**. The organ is flushed with ice-cold preservation solution and stored at 0–4°C on ice. Using specially formulated preservation solutions with agents designed to counter hypothermic cell swelling, it is now possible to store kidneys in this way for 24–36 hours, livers for 12–18 hours and hearts for 4–6 hours
- **Continuous oxygenated hypothermic pulsatile perfusion** using special colloid-based (starch, plasma or albumin) solutions. This technique is more complex and expensive but enables kidneys to be stored for 2–3 days; the equipment is portable and can be used during transportation but the technique has not been extended to clinical preservation of other organs

SPECIFIC ORGAN TRANSPLANTS

KIDNEY TRANSPLANTS

Kidney transplantation is the longest established and most widely practised of solid organ transplants. It offers a substantial improvement in quality of life for patients with end-stage chronic renal failure who are otherwise faced with twice- or thrice-weekly haemodialysis or a regimen of continuous daily treatment using chronic ambulatory peritoneal dialysis. Donor organs can be obtained from any otherwise healthy donor up to about 70 years of age.

The kidney is transplanted into an extraperitoneal location in the iliac fossa and the renal vessels are anastomosed to the iliac artery and vein (see Fig. 4.1). The ureter is implanted into the bladder using an intramural tunnel to prevent reflux. The non-functioning kidneys are usually left in situ unless infected or causing unmanageable hypertension.

The signs of early acute rejection of the kidney are oliguria, proteinuria, and pain and tenderness of the transplanted kidney. Luckily, this relatively common form of rejection can usually be reversed easily. Overall results of renal transplantation have steadily improved owing to more effective long-term immunosuppression and better-quality organs from 'heart-beating' brain-dead donors or living related donors. The survival rate of transplanted kidneys may be as high as 90–95% at 1 year. This falls by 5–10% each year thereafter although there is evidence that the beneficial matching policy now in use may reduce the late graft attrition rate caused by chronic rejection.

HEART AND LUNG TRANSPLANTS

Cardiac transplantation has become a standard treatment for patients with ischaemic heart disease that is not amenable to coronary artery bypass grafting, as well as for patients with certain cardiomyopathies. A standard operative technique has been established employing **orthotopic** placement of the organ, i.e. replacing the diseased organ in the same anatomical location. The

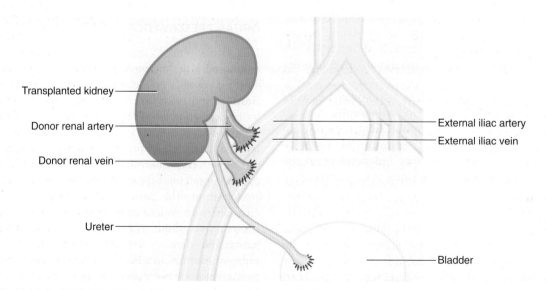

Fig. 4.1 Renal transplantation
The usual site for the transplanted kidney is in the pelvis with anastomoses between donor renal artery and vein and iliac artery and vein and between ureter and bladder

donor atria and graft vessels are sutured directly to those of the recipient. Monitoring for early rejection requires regular right-heart catheterisation and endomyocardial biopsy.

Using immunosuppressive protocols similar to those for kidney transplantation, the results of cardiac transplantation are now excellent, although the limited number of available donor organs mean that cardiac transplantation is unlikely ever to be available for all those that could benefit. Novel techniques of **genetic engineering** have raised the possibility of rearing animals such as pigs with a specially engineered genetic make-up to allow xenografts to be performed successfully. No such **transgenic** transplants have yet been performed in humans.

Combined heart and lung transplants are now also accepted as a standard treatment for patients with certain irreversible lung diseases such as cystic fibrosis, and excellent results are now obtained in specialist centres. Many cases have secondary heart disease and require a combined heart–lung transplant but in some cases the recipient's heart may be healthy and can be transplanted into another patient; this is known as the **domino heart** procedure. Single or even double lung transplants are now also performed successfully in carefully selected patients with chronic respiratory failure.

LIVER TRANSPLANTS

The indications for liver transplantation are end-stage non-malignant parenchymal liver disease, acute hepatic failure and certain inborn errors of hepatic metabolism. In children, liver-based inborn errors of metabolism and biliary atresia are the most common indications for transplantation, and the operation often needs to be performed during early infancy. Primary liver malignancies such as cholangiocarcinoma and hepatocellular carcinoma as well as liver metastatic disease are no longer accepted as indications for liver transplantation as malignancy inevitably recurs early after transplantation in the immunosuppressed patient.

The problems of rejection of the liver are less than for kidney transplantation but the operation is a more challenging undertaking. Most patients have advanced liver disease with disordered coagulation and often severe portal hypertension. A team approach has evolved, with close cooperation between surgeons and specialist liver transplant anaesthetists. The diseased liver is removed and the new liver put in its place, the vena cava, portal vein and hepatic artery being reanastomosed in turn. Careful surgical technique combined with skilled anaesthetic monitoring and intraoperative replacement of clotting factors has transformed the procedure and average blood losses are now only about 3 litres per case.

Results have improved greatly since the first liver transplant procedure in 1963 and 1-year patient survival rates of 75–85% are now standard. For paediatric cases, the problem of inadequate supply of donor organs has been solved by using reduced-size liver grafts. Either a lobe or a segment from a full-size adult organ can be transplanted thus allowing disparities in size of up to 10 to 1 between donor and recipient. In a few cases, a liver has been successfully divided so that two recipients have received grafts from a single donor organ.

The late graft attrition rate for liver transplants appears to be much lower than for kidney grafts even though matching is by blood group only without use of tissue typing. The 'Achilles heel' of liver grafting remains complications with the bile duct anastomosis. This can be performed using a direct duct-to-duct anastomosis or a roux en Y loop but despite meticulous surgical technique, the complication rate from biliary strictures or leaks remains in the 10–15% range.

PANCREAS TRANSPLANTS

Pancreas transplantation offers the tantalising hope of providing a cure for diabetes, thus avoiding its many late complications. These include myocardial ischaemia, peripheral vascular disease, peripheral neuropathy, nephropathy leading to renal failure and retinopathy leading to blindness. The pancreas presents a particular problem as the gland combines both endocrine and exocrine function. The currently favoured technique involves transplanting the whole pancreas with a small segment of duodenum. The graft is placed in the pelvis and anastomosed to the iliac vessels in the same way as a kidney graft. The attached duodenal segment is anastomosed to the urinary bladder allowing the exocrine secretions to drain into the urine. This technique has the added advantage that graft function can be readily monitored by measuring urinary amylase. Falling amylase levels provide an early indicator of rejection. Graft survival rates of 70–80% are now being obtained but long-term follow-up is needed to confirm that a technically successful graft can prevent the long-term complications of diabetes. Currently, most pancreatic transplants are combined with renal transplantation in diabetic patients with established renal failure and advanced complications of their disease.

A different approach is transplantation of pancreatic endocrine tissue alone. This is achieved by transplanting human islet cells extracted from the pancreas by collagenase digestion. The islets are then injected into the portal venous system and lodge in the liver sinusoids. The yield from extraction techniques has improved markedly, allowing a substantial percentage of the islets from a single pancreas to be recovered. However, there are only occasional reports of the technique restoring glucose tolerance to normal and no reports of long-term success.

SMALL BOWEL TRANSPLANTS

A recent advance in organ transplantation has been the development of small bowel transplantation. There is a growing number of patients who have lost all or most of their small bowel from vascular problems, volvulus, necrotising enterocolitis, atresias or Crohn's disease.

These patients have to be maintained on long-term parenteral nutrition which is expensive and inconvenient and also leaves patients at constant risk of septic complications from feeding lines as well as liver disease related to parenteral feeding. Small bowel may be transplanted alone or in combination with the liver in the case of coexisting irreversible liver disease. The technique is still in its experimental stages but results using the immunosuppressive agent FK506 are encouraging, with a substantial number of patients restored to full enteral nutrition.

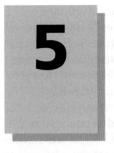

5 Imaging for surgical investigation and management

INTRODUCTION

This chapter gives an overview of investigative imaging procedures commonly used in surgery. The basis for each method of investigation is described, together with its main indications and shortcomings. As investigative equipment has developed in sophistication, an expanding field of therapeutic applications has emerged, adding to the sum of minimal access techniques. The basis of these techniques is described here and a table listing important therapeutic applications is given in Chapter 6 (Table 6.2). Examples include ultrasound and CT-guided biopsy and endoscopic placement of biliary stents.

CONVENTIONAL RADIOGRAPHY

The various tissues and constituents of the body absorb X-rays by different amounts which are related to the cube of the atomic number of their elements. This results in differential penetration of X-rays through the body and differential exposure of the silver salts in the traditional **X-ray film** or activation of the sensors in a filmless department. A radiograph is therefore a 'shadow' picture. Recent computer technology has allowed the development of 'filmless radiology' where the penetrating X-rays activate sensors in an electronic film equivalent.

On a plain radiograph, gas and fat absorb few X-rays and appear as **radiolucent** (dark) areas. Bone and other calcified tissues absorb most of the X-rays; they are thus poorly penetrated and appear as **radiopaque** (white) film images. Most urinary tract stones, some gallstones, old tuberculous lymph nodes and heavily calcified atheromatous deposits are also radiopaque. Many X-ray investigations, known as **contrast studies**, obtain their diagnostic information by imaging structures outlined with highly absorptive fluid **contrast media**.

Certain **foreign bodies** in wounds, such as metal and most glass fragments, are radiopaque, but wood and plastic fragments are radiolucent and invisible to X-rays. Gauze swabs used in operating theatres are radiolucent, but have a radiopaque strand woven into them to enable them to be located radiographically if inadvertently left inside a wound.

PERSONAL PROTECTION

Ionising radiation is potentially mutagenic and carcinogenic. Irradiation of patients and observers must therefore be kept to the minimum. This is achieved by the following:

- Giving training in radiation protection to all staff using and working near X-ray equipment

43

- Ensuring that every investigation helps with the management of the patient and that none is performed merely as 'routine'
- Improving design of X-ray equipment to minimise radiation dose whilst preserving diagnostic detail; X-ray **scatter** is reduced, and unwanted types of radiation are removed by filters
- Physical barriers to X-rays are provided in radiology suites to protect the staff. These include barium plaster in walls, lead-glass windows and lead-rubber aprons
- Workers involved in taking X-rays should keep away from the direct line of the beam and should also maintain a good distance from the X-ray source during exposure as the inverse square law determines radiation fall-off with distance
- All involved in radiography should wear X-ray-sensitive **film badges** which are regularly monitored for excess radiation

GENERAL PRINCIPLES OF RADIOGRAPHY

There are several important factors involved in producing a useful radiographic image:

- **X-ray power and exposure time** are chosen to give a diagnostically useful film exposure, with a range of image densities appropriate to the anatomical area. For example, thoracic spine views require a larger dose than lung fields

- **Different projections (views)** produce different images of the same subject. Since the X-ray tube is effectively a point source and produces a diverging beam (see Fig. 5.1), the subject is magnified. This size distortion least affects the side of the patient closest to the film, which is thus shown more clearly. The projection has important consequences for interpretation and should be recorded on the film. A frontal chest film might be labelled PA (postero-anterior) or AP (antero-posterior) with the label indicating the direction of the beam. With lateral exposures, the side nearest the film is indicated, e.g. a 'Rt' lateral chest X-ray (CXR) has the right side of the chest nearest the film
- **Patient position** during exposure (i.e. supine, prone, oblique or erect) affects the image because of the effect of gravity upon organs and other body contents such as gas or fluid. Most films are taken with a vertical X-ray beam, but a horizontal beam is sometimes necessary to demonstrate fluid levels in a cavity or in bowel (lateral decubitus), or free gas under the diaphragm

CONVENTIONAL TOMOGRAPHY

Some body structures, which would otherwise be obscured by overlying or underlying tissues on conventional X-rays, can be distinguished by the use of tomography. In tomography, the X-ray tube and film are moved in opposite directions during exposure, with the pivotal point between the two centred on the structure under investigation (see Fig. 5.2). A transverse slice at the

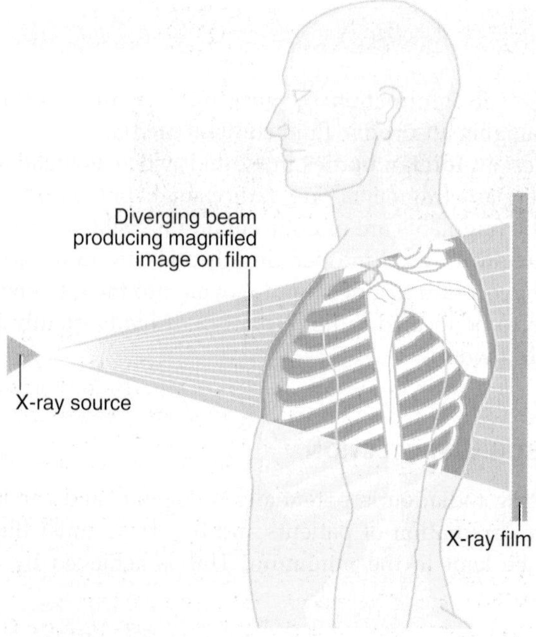

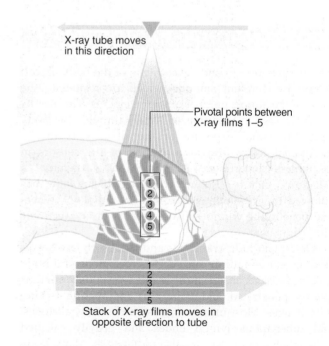

Diverging beam
producing magnified
image on film

X-ray source

X-ray film

X-ray tube moves
in this direction

Pivotal points between
X-ray films 1–5

Stack of X-ray films moves in
opposite direction to tube

Fig. 5.1 Radiological projection

Fig. 5.2 Principle of tomography

chosen depth is thus defined clearly on the film, and anything superficial or deep to it is blurred into obscurity (e.g. soft tissue, bowel gas, faeces or bones). The technique is still occasionally used—for example in intravenous urography when gas or faeces obscure the field of interest. By using a stack of films, one exposure can give a set of 'cuts' at predetermined distances from the surface. Computerised tomography is an important development of this principle and has superseded conventional tomography for most applications (see p. 56).

CONTRAST RADIOGRAPHY

When plain radiography is unsuitable for studying the area of interest, a highly X-ray-absorbing **contrast medium** can often be employed to opacify it. Contrast media work in two ways; they outline anatomical structures directly or else are concentrated physiologically in the organ they are designed to show (indirect imaging).

Direct contrast studies can be made in a variety of ways. Contrast material can be swallowed, instilled into body orifices, sinuses or fistulae, or injected into blood vessels or hollow viscera. Commonly used studies are barium enemas for examining the large bowel and arteriograms for examining the arterial system.

Indirect contrast studies are made by introducing agents into the body which are concentrated in the organs under investigation. Examples are urography (intravenous injection of contrast which is excreted in the urine) and intravenous cholangiography (injection of contrast which is concentrated in the liver and excreted in the bile).

Contrast materials

Barium sulphate is the most satisfactory agent for outlining the gastrointestinal tract. It is insoluble in water and is not absorbed. An aqueous suspension is non-irritant and very radiodense. **Gastrografin** is a water-soluble contrast medium used if contrast is likely to leak from the bowel into the peritoneal cavity—for example, for checking a recent rectal anastomosis after resection. If gastrografin is inadvertently inhaled, however, it causes

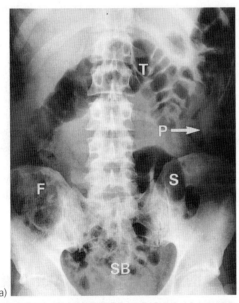

(a)

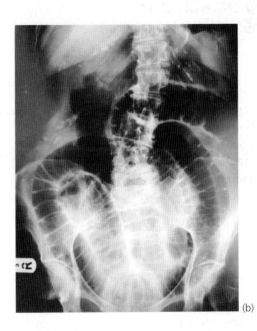

(b)

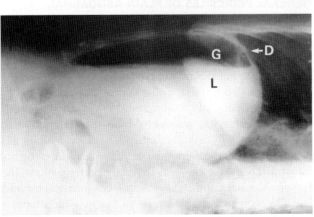

(c)

Fig. 5.3 Plain abdominal X-rays

(a) Normal supine abdominal X-ray. There is gas in most parts of the colon (transverse colon **T** and sigmoid colon **S**) and small bowel a few loops **SB** in the pelvis. Radiopaque lumps of faecal matter **F** are seen in the caecum and ascending colon. A normal pro-peritoneal fat line **P** is present on the patient's left; this would be lost if there was retroperitoneal inflammation. **(b)** Supine plain abdominal film showing gross small bowel dilatation. The clear outline of bowel in the upper left quadrant suggests perforation. The cause proved to be an obstructing carcinoma of the caecum. **(c)** Right side raised lateral decubitus X-ray (the X-ray beam was horizontal). This 78-year-old woman presented with a sudden onset of severe abdominal pain caused by a perforated duodenal ulcer. Free intraperitoneal gas **G** is seen 'floating' over the liver **L** and beneath the diaphragm **D**.

45

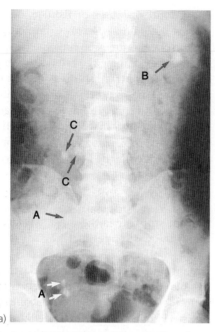 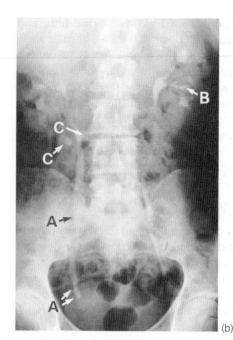

(a)   (b)

Fig. 5.4 Plain abdominal X-ray and IVU compared
(a) and **(b)** A plain abdominal film and an intravenous urogram (IVU) of the same patient showing urinary tract stones. In the plain film, several calcified opacities (arrowed) are seen. From the IVU, in which the pelvicalyceal systems and ureters contain contrast material, it can be seen that three stones **A** lie within the lower right ureter and stone **B** lies within the upper calyces of the left kidney. On the right side, two other opacities **C** are seen to lie outside the urinary tract, probably representing calcified lymph nodes in the small bowel mesentery.

pulmonary oedema and should not be used orally in patients with intestinal obstruction.

Water-soluble **iodinated benzoic acid derivatives** can be injected into vessels to opacify the circulating blood. There is also almost immediate excretion of the contrast through the kidneys into the urine. Thus, two different functions can be achieved: direct opacification of veins or arteries (venography or arteriography), and indirect demonstration of kidneys, collecting systems and bladder.

Most water-soluble contrast media have a high osmotic pressure; they are therefore irritant (particularly when used for venography) and may exacerbate pre-existing renal disease; this applies particularly at the extremes of age and in diabetic nephropathy. Since the early 1980s, new **non-ionic** agents with an osmotic pressure similar to that of plasma have been developed and are widely used. These are generally safer (although more thrombogenic) but more expensive.

Finally, care should be taken to ensure that the patient is not sensitive to the contrast medium, as this may produce an anaphylactic reaction. Resuscitation equipment and drugs should always be on hand when contrast media are injected.

DIGITAL SUBTRACTION ANGIOGRAPHY

Digital subtraction is an electronic process used in contrast vascular studies (angiography) by which the unchanging opacities of a plain radiographic image (particularly bone and gas) are subtracted from the image field produced after injection of contrast material. Modern equipment performs this process in real time. The main advantages are that lower doses of contrast media are required and, in some cases, useful images can be obtained with intravenous contrast injection. In addition, the image can be processed electronically to enhance definition, to change contrast or to concentrate on particular areas.

PLAIN ABDOMINAL RADIOGRAPHY

GENERAL PRINCIPLES OF PLAIN ABDOMINAL RADIOGRAPHY

Most abdominal films are taken with the patient supine and the X-ray beam vertical. Gut is visible when there is gas in it (see Fig. 5.3 p. 45). Normal **small bowel** is less than 3 cm in width and, in the supine position, tends to occupy the centre of the abdomen. When dilated, it can be recognised by the transverse folds (**plicae circulares**) which completely cross the lumen. The colon usually lies peripherally in the abdomen and is recognised by its **haustrations**; these are folds that only partly traverse the lumen. Normal colon is less than 6 cm in diameter and is often seen to contain lumps of faeces which have a mottled radiolucent/radiopaque appearance.

Free gas in the peritoneal cavity may be diagnostic of **bowel perforation** and is therefore an important finding. In a supine patient, free gas usually collects in the right upper quadrant. It can be confidently diagnosed when both the inside and outside of the bowel wall are outlined by radiolucent shadows, although this is uncommon. A chest or upper abdominal X-ray taken with a horizontal beam and the patient erect, usually (but not always) reveals a radiolucent gas layer under the diaphragm. This can be very small (and easily missed) but may be obvious. The best method of showing free peritoneal gas is to take an erect chest radiograph. Where the result is doubtful or if the patient is too ill to sit or stand, the patient should be placed in the **right-side raised lateral decubitus position** (i.e. lying on the left side) for 10 minutes. A horizontal beam abdominal X-ray is then taken across the table. As little as 2 mL of gas may then be demonstrable above the lateral border of the liver (see Fig. 5.3c).

The kidneys may be outlined on a plain abdominal X-ray by a radiolucent border of perinephric fat. However, overlapping bowel gas and faeces often obscure the renal outlines. Also, in a post-nephrectomy patient, the former 'renal outline' may still be visible on a plain film as bowel may fill the renal bed and be outlined by perinephric fat. Small urinary tract stones are easily obscured by overlying bowel gas or faeces; laxatives are often given prior to urography to minimise this. The liver may be visible on plain radiographs but its size cannot be accurately estimated.

When examining an abdominal X-ray, the important features to look for are:

- Calcification in areas prone to stone formation, e.g. kidney, ureters, bladder or biliary tree (see Fig. 5.4a)
- Dilated gut (stomach, small bowel or large bowel)
- Free intraperitoneal gas indicating bowel perforation. Note the importance of the patient's position when the film was taken
- Gas in abnormal places (e.g. biliary tree or urinary tract) suggesting a fistula connecting with bowel
- Non-biological objects, e.g. foreign bodies, surgical tubes or pieces of metal
- Pathological calcification, e.g. aortic aneurysm, pancreas, adrenals or uterine fibroids

The limitations of plain abdominal radiography are summarised in Box 5.1.

BOWEL CONTRAST RADIOLOGY

TECHNIQUES

Any part of the gastrointestinal tract can be demonstrated using contrast techniques. For examining the upper gastrointestinal tract, barium suspension is given orally (**barium swallow** for oesophagus and **barium**

KEY POINTS

Box 5.1 The limitations of plain abdominal radiography

- Intraperitoneal structures are not visualised unless they contain gas, displace gas-filled bowel or indent structural fat
- Non-calcified stones (90% of gallstones, 10% of urinary tract stones) are not visible
- Bowel gas and faeces easily obscure stones
- Phleboliths, calcified abdominal lymph nodes and costal cartilages readily mimic stones
- Liver and spleen size cannot be estimated accurately
- Free intraperitoneal gas is not usually visible on a supine film (a horizontal beam film is needed)

---

meal for stomach and duodenum). Progress of the contrast is observed by X-ray **fluoroscopic screening**. In screening, a technique known as **image intensification** is used to show a moving image on a television screen. The X-ray beam activates a series of sensors and the signal is converted into a video image. Screening enables the radiologist to select representative views as **spot films** to record the examination. Screening for 1 minute gives the patient a dose of X-rays equivalent to one film.

Screening is also useful to study rapid gastrointestinal motility, as in swallowing. The images are recorded on video and studied later in slow motion.

The large bowel is examined by means of contrast material given rectally (**barium enema**). It must be remembered that the lower rectum is not always well shown on this examination; a prior rectal examination and sigmoidoscopy should be performed if low lesions are not to be occasionally but disastrously missed.

For small bowel examination, a barium meal may be 'followed through' distally with serial films at intervals, but some radiologists prefer to instil contrast into the proximal jejunum through a nasal or oral tube; this is known by the confusing term **small bowel enema**.

In the early days of barium examinations, a **single contrast** technique was used. Barium was given alone and radiographs taken. However, the dense column of barium obscured much of the finer detail. Most barium studies nowadays use a **double contrast** method. Following the barium, air or carbon dioxide is used to distend the bowel, or effervescent tablets are given to distend the stomach. This separates the barium-coated bowel walls and acts as a second radiolucent contrast agent (see Fig. 5.5b). An anticholinergic agent such as hyoscine butylbromide (Buscopan) is often given at the same time to relax the bowel wall muscle and abolish spasm, thereby further improving the image. Double contrast techniques are also used for barium meal examination. With improved CT scanning, contrast CT examinations are becoming more popular for large

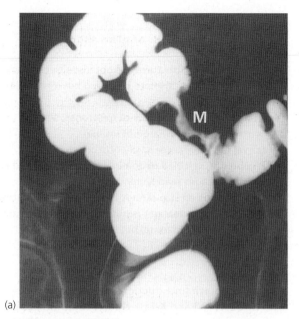
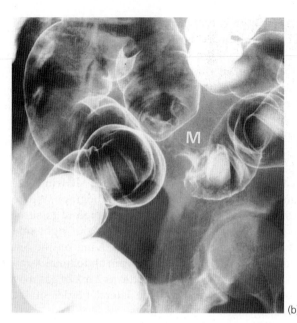

(a)   (b)

Fig. 5.5 Single and double contrast barium enemas
Typical annular carcinoma of the proximal sigmoid colon in a woman of 72. **(a)** Single contrast barium enema showing the malignant stricture **M**. Note all mucosal detail in the colon is obscured by barium. **(b)** Double contrast barium enema of the same patient also showing the stricture, but mucosal detail is outlined with a thin coating of barium. The bowel has been inflated with air.

bowel examination. Contrast is given rectally and a rapid-sequence CT scan of the abdomen performed. The procedure is quicker and less unpleasant than a conventional barium enema and is becoming the first-choice investigation for infirm patients; it may eventually supplant barium enema examination altogether. Three-dimensional images of the bowel can also be constructed to produce a virtual 'walk-through' of the colon. Whilst this technique is still in development, it holds promise for the future.

Figure 5.5 illustrates the differences between a single contrast and a double contrast barium enema in the same patient.

PREPARATION OF THE PATIENT FOR BOWEL CONTRAST STUDIES

For upper gastrointestinal contrast studies, patients should be fasted overnight except for water. For small bowel studies, laxatives are sometimes given the day before to empty the colon. This may hasten transit of contrast through the small bowel.

For a barium enema or contrast CT, prior bowel preparation is performed with laxatives (e.g. sodium picosulphate) and sometimes bowel washouts, so that artefacts are removed (faecal lumps look very similar to polyps) and small mucosal defects are not obscured. Thorough preparation of the colon is vital if important pathology is not to be missed. If a barium enema reveals inadequate preparation, further efforts should be made to clear the colon and the examination repeated. If a

right-sided colonic lesion is suspected, a barium follow-through examination may show the region satisfactorily if other methods fail.

COMPLICATIONS OF BARIUM CONTRAST STUDIES

Barium should be avoided for contrast examination if substantial peritoneal spillage is likely as, for example, when there is thought to be a perforation or anastomotic leak. In these cases, **water-soluble contrast medium** is best given initially, and if no leak is seen, barium is then substituted. This is because water-soluble materials are less radiopaque and less effective at coating the bowel wall and therefore show less surface detail than barium. For the same reasons, barium may reveal a tiny leak from the bowel which is invisible with water-soluble contrast.

Contrast studies should be used with caution in patients with bowel obstruction. Barium should not be given with suspected large bowel obstruction because if it cannot pass through, it solidifies within the bowel and can turn an incomplete obstruction into a complete one. A barium follow-through is sometimes indicated in suspected small bowel obstruction, but there is a risk that contrast material may be vomited and aspirated into the bronchial tree, causing aspiration pneumonitis (see Fig. 5.6).

Some radiologists prefer not to perform barium enema examination for several days after high rectal biopsies, believing there is a risk of perforation.

The limitations of barium contrast studies are summarised in Box 5.2.

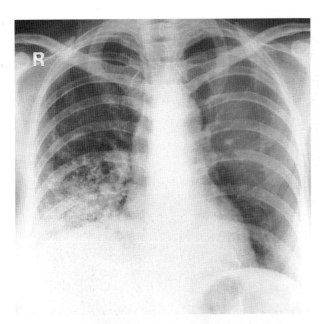

Fig. 5.6 Inhalational pneumonitis after barium meal
Right lower lobe consolidation resulting from aspiration of stomach contents including barium. The patient had undergone a laparotomy several days previously and an abdominal mass was discovered. There was still some unsuspected adynamic bowel obstruction (paralytic ileus). This barium follow-through examination was attempted too early and the patient aspirated barium into the lung after vomiting.

BILIARY CONTRAST RADIOGRAPHY

Many biliary investigative techniques described in previous editions of this book have largely been superseded because of improved equipment and experience in biliary ultrasound, increased availability of **endoscopic retrograde cholangio-pancreatography** (ERCP, see Ch. 11, p. 66) and latterly, magnetic resonance imaging techniques.

ORAL CHOLECYSTOGRAPHY

Until the mid-1980s oral cholecystography was the standard investigation for gall-bladder disease but it has now been replaced by high-resolution ultrasound scanning which is rapid, reliable and requires no contrast material. Cholecystography required the patient to be able to absorb oral contrast and images were taken 12 hours after ingestion. Cholecystography was no use in obstructive jaundice because contrast material was not excreted in sufficient concentration to register an image.

INTRAVENOUS CHOLANGIOGRAPHY

Intravenous cholangiography (IVC) used to be the standard investigation for suspected biliary stones and sometimes mild obstructive jaundice. The drawbacks are that the image is of poor resolution and the contrast

material tends to cause nausea and vomiting. The investigation is probably safer than diagnostic ERCP but still carries more risk than operative cholangiography. IVC has been largely replaced by ERCP (and less commonly percutaneous transhepatic cholangiography), both of which allow direct injection of contrast into the biliary tree. Nevertheless, intravenous cholangiography has found renewed favour with some surgeons for seeking bile duct stones prior to laparoscopic cholecystectomy. Magnetic resonance cholangiography now produces images that rival the quality of traditional techniques.

PERCUTANEOUS TRANSHEPATIC CHOLANGIOGRAPHY (PTC)

This technique for diagnosing the cause of obstructive jaundice is now rarely used where endoscopic retrograde cholangiography or magnetic resonance cholangio-pancreatography (MRCP) is available. Using a method similar to percutaneous liver biopsy, dilated intrahepatic ducts can be punctured directly with a long fine (22 G) 'Chiba' needle and injected with contrast (see Fig. 5.7c). This test can be useful if there is extrahepatic duct obstruction, when it shows the position and configuration of the obstruction.

Since a jaundiced patient is likely to have disordered blood clotting, liver bleeding is likely during the investigation, and a **clotting screen** must be performed beforehand, including prothrombin ratio and platelet count.

ENDOSCOPIC RETROGRADE CHOLANGIO-PANCREATOGRAPHY

This investigation is described in Chapter 6; its use in obstructive jaundice is described in more detail in Chapter 12. The basic technique is illustrated here in Figure 5.7.

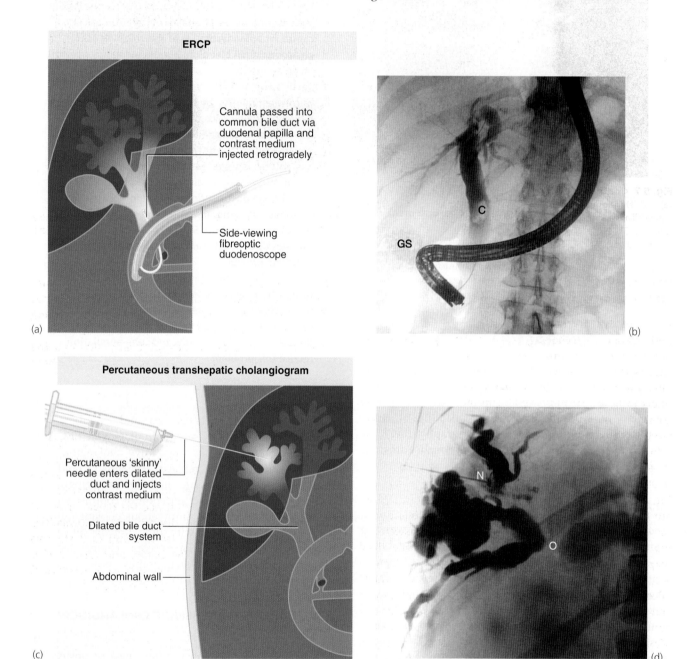

Fig. 5.7 Some techniques for demonstrating the biliary system. (a) and (b) Endoscopic retrograde cholangiography
The patient is sedated and a side-viewing gastroscope passed down into the second part of the duodenum. The ampulla of Vater is cannulated under direct vision and contrast medium injected to outline the bile ducts. A large gall stone **C** is seen within the dilated common bile duct and a collection of radiopaque gallstones **GS** is seen in the gall bladder. **(c) and (d) Percutaneous transhepatic cholangiography**. A needle **N** is passed into the liver until it encounters a dilated duct. Contrast medium is then injected to outline the ducts. This deeply jaundiced 57-year-old woman has grossly dilated intrahepatic ducts and complete obstruction of the proximal common bile duct in the porta hepatis at **O**. This was due to lymph node metastases from carcinoma of stomach. This method is employed less often nowadays because of the superior safety of other methods described here.

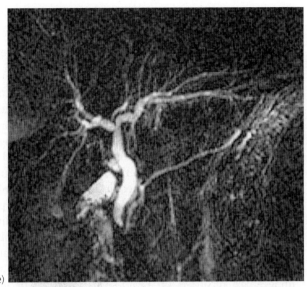
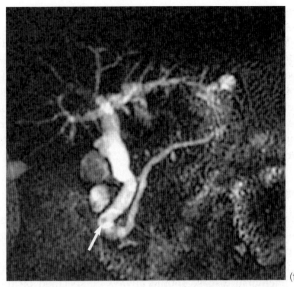

(e)   (f)

Fig. 5.7 Continued
(e) and **(f) Magnetic resonance cholangiopancreatography (MRCP)**. The technique produces images of static fluid, thus the images are of native biliary and pancreatic secretions. Each image was obtained in one second using a thick slab 'projection' method that generates images very similar to ERCP. **(e)** An example of normal biliary and pancreatic duct systems. **(f)** A small calculus in the distal common bile duct (arrowed). There is also mild dilatation of the pancreatic duct with some side branches visible.

OPERATIVE CHOLANGIOGRAPHY AND CHOLEDOCHOSCOPY

It is standard practice during open cholecystectomy to perform operative cholangiography, although the same is not yet true for laparoscopic cholecystectomy. Operative cholangiography serves several purposes; it allows the biliary anatomy to be confirmed and stones in the major ducts to be visualised, and shows whether there is free contrast flow into the duodenum. To perform an operative cholangiogram, a fine plastic cannula is introduced into a small hole cut in the side of the cystic duct and passed into the common bile duct. Water-soluble contrast material is injected in two or three stages to outline the duct system and fluoroscopic images or X-ray films are taken. If stones are demonstrated in the bile ducts, they are usually retrieved either at open cholecystectomy via a longitudinal incision in the common bile duct (**exploration of the common bile duct**) or at laparoscopic surgery using a Dormia basket via the cystic duct. (The instrument is similar to that used for ureteric stones and is illustrated in Figure 31.6, p. 416.) A further cholangiogram is often done to ensure the duct has been cleared. Many surgeons also inspect the inside of the bile ducts during the operation using a **choledochoscope**. This can be a rigid L-shaped instrument with attachments for removing stones at open surgery, or a flexible instrument around 5 mm in diameter which can be used at laparoscopic or open surgery. Choledochoscopy can markedly reduce the incidence of residual stones after exploring the bile ducts.

During laparoscopic cholecystectomy, operative cholangiography is performed routinely by some surgeons whilst others prefer preoperative intravenous cholangiography, ERCP or MRCP for selected cases. If duct stones are demonstrated by operative cholangiography during laparoscopic cholecystectomy, these may be removed by laparoscopic methods or later at ERCP, although the latter procedure risks attendant complications, e.g. biliary leakage, acute pancreatitis.

T-TUBE CHOLANGIOGRAPHY

Following exploration of bile ducts for stones, a T-tube is often left in situ to drain the duct. The transverse limb of the tube lies in the duct and the long limb drains to the exterior. About 1 week after operation, contrast can be injected along the T-tube to outline the biliary tree and confirm drainage into the duodenum. Abnormalities such as residual stones, bile leakage and duct stenosis will also be demonstrated. The mature tract formed after 2 or 3 weeks' intubation can be used to retrieve residual stones with steerable grasping instruments.

UROGRAPHY

GENERAL PRINCIPLES OF UROGRAPHY

Urography is a radiological technique for examining the kidneys and urinary collecting systems. It uses intravenous contrast medium which is concentrated and excreted by the kidneys. A plain abdominal **control film** is taken prior to contrast injection, so that any opacities can be compared with films taken after contrast. This helps to identify whether or not an opacity lies within the renal tract (see Fig. 5.4a, p. 46).

The urinary tract is examined sequentially from kidneys to bladder on films taken at intervals after injection. The renal parenchyma opacifies almost immediately. Contrast then flows successively into the renal pelvis, ureters and bladder. The kidneys can be shown in greater detail by **tomography**. This is frequently used in conjunction with ultrasound when investigating adults with haematuria.

SPECIAL PRECAUTIONS

Intravenous contrast is potentially nephrotoxic in patients with impaired renal function; patients with diabetic nephropathy are at particular risk.

Conditions which might be associated with renal parenchymal disease should always be specified on the X-ray request form to help the radiologist plan the safest investigation. The important disorders are:

● Diabetes mellitus
● Renal failure (include results of renal function tests on the request form)
● Multiple myeloma
● Heart failure

VASCULAR RADIOLOGY (ANGIOGRAPHY)

GENERAL PRINCIPLES AND HAZARDS OF ARTERIOGRAPHY AND VENOGRAPHY

The general principles of vascular radiology are described here; further detail is given in Chapter 35.

The veins or arteries of a particular anatomical region can be opacified by intravenous or intra-arterial injection of an appropriate contrast medium. This is known as **angiography**. An angiography catheter is usually inserted into a vessel some distance away from the target site and the tip manipulated into the correct position over a previously placed guide-wire. Favoured entry points to the arterial system are the femoral artery in the groin or, less commonly, the brachial artery above the elbow. Recently, the radial artery at the wrist has been employed more frequently, using smaller-diameter catheters.

If there is any suspicion of a bleeding disorder, **clotting studies** should be performed prior to vascular radiology to anticipate possible haemorrhagic complications from the vessel puncture site.

The contrast material is similar to that used for intravenous urography and therefore carries similar hazards. In addition, there is the risk of complications from the arterial or venous cannulation. These include trauma to the vessel (causing bleeding, thrombosis, wall

dissection or an arteriovenous fistula) and loss of part of the catheter into the vessel lumen.

Arteriography

In **lower limb arteriography**, the abdominal aorta and distal vessels are usually examined using a catheter placed into a femoral artery. If the aorto-iliac system is occluded and femoral pulses are impalpable, the angiography catheter can be introduced into the radial or brachial artery. Occasionally, the aorta has to be punctured directly using a long needle from the left lumbar region with the patient prone. **Translumbar aortography** gives relatively poor views of the distal lower limb vessels and carries greater risk than femoral or brachial angiography. Once the vascular catheter is in situ, water-soluble contrast is injected directly into the artery and images are recorded on rapid-sequence films or electronically. Thus stenoses or occlusions due to thrombosis, atheroma or embolism can be demonstrated. Digital subtraction angiography is now widely available for arteriography and this is discussed below.

Venography

Lower limb **venography** (**phlebography**) is used for two main purposes: to demonstrate whether there is a **deep vein thrombosis** (DVT) in a patient with a sudden onset of swelling or pain in the leg, or to investigate suspected **chronic deep venous insufficiency**. Occasionally, it is used to demonstrate reflux from deep veins into superficial varicose veins. Venography for deep venous insufficiency shows the patency of deep veins and any abnormal communications with superficial veins (incompetent perforating veins). A vein is usually cannulated in the foot to inject the contrast and a tourniquet applied around the ankle and knee to direct it into the deep veins. The diagnostic value of venography depends very much on the skill of the radiologist.

Duplex Doppler ultrasound scanning can replace both of these applications and, when available, is the first-line investigation for suspected DVT as well as chronic deep and superficial venous insufficiency. A skilled operator can demonstrate the patency or otherwise of all of the lower limb veins, the presence of thrombus and the competence of valves and perforators as well as demonstrating vein wall irregularity associated with previous DVT.

ELECTRONIC RECORDING TECHNIQUES

X-ray images can be recorded electronically in **digital** form, as opposed to the **analogue** form of conventional radiographic film. These digital images can be processed to optimise the available information; this includes subtracting background detail (thus removing bony images, for example), enhancing the contrast between tissues, magnifying areas of special interest and abstracting the best parts from a series of images. At present, this process is mainly used in angiography, where it is known as **digital subtraction angiography (DSA)** or **digital vascular imaging**.

Background subtraction in real time can produce satisfactory vascular images with much lower concentrations of contrast; indeed, when high-resolution pictures are not needed, as in screening for arterial disease or checking the patency of arterial grafts, satisfactory results can be obtained by injecting contrast **intravenously** (via a central venous line) and imaging the arteries when the contrast reaches them. However, many radiologists prefer intra-arterial injection of dilute contrast.

These electronic techniques are steadily improving and are being introduced into other areas of radiology. Already, 'filmless' X-ray departments have arrived and will doubtless become the norm, with images displayed on terminals dispersed around the hospital or even transmitted to specialists in other units or at home.

ULTRASONOGRAPHY

Medical ultrasound developed from sonar used for the detection of submarines in the Second World War. However, the technology remained an official secret until the 1960s. Since then, the principle has found many applications, from identifying shoals of fish to non-invasive imaging of body organs.

Medical ultrasound was pioneered in obstetrics where it has become an important part of prenatal assessment. As technology and electronics have improved resolution and discrimination, surgical applications have become ever wider. An important advance was **grey scale ultrasound**, which enables a whole range of tissue echogenicities to be displayed on the screen.

Interpreting ultrasound depends very much on the dynamic picture the radiologist sees during the examination, rather than what is recorded on the static films. The film record may mean little to anyone but the radiologist who performed the study!

GENERAL PRINCIPLES OF MEDICAL ULTRASOUND

Ultrasound is non-invasive, painless and almost certainly safe. An ultrasound probe containing the transducer is applied to the skin over the area of interest and the image is displayed on a screen. The probe must be 'coupled' to the skin with jelly to exclude an air interface. The probe is then moved in different directions and at different angles to best display the organ and any abnormality. 'Spot' films are taken to record the examination.

The transducer, which consists of piezo-electric crystals, both transmits and receives the ultrasound. A 1-microsecond pulse of ultrasound is emitted every millisecond, and the transducer then 'listens' for reflected ultrasound echoes over the next 999 microseconds. An image, representing a slice through the body, is gener-ated electronically, with reflections showing as bright spots on a dark screen. This is known as **B-mode** (brightness mode) and the brightness of each spot is proportional to the sound reflectivity of the tissue interfaces. The moving image is displayed on a video screen as the examination proceeds and is thus described as **real time ultrasound**.

The length and breadth of organs or lesions displayed on the screen can be accurately determined by measuring the image. Furthermore, the **volume** of some structures such as the urinary bladder or the left ventricle can be estimated. This can give useful functional information—for example, the volume of residual urine in the bladder in chronic retention, or the completeness of left ventricular emptying in cardiac failure.

Bone, stones and other calcified tissues cause an abrupt and marked change in acoustic impedance, resulting in virtually complete reflection of ultrasound. Thus the surface of hard tissue, such as a gallstone, is revealed by its echogenicity and also by the **acoustic shadow** it casts (see Fig. 13.3, p. 195). A similar, though lesser change in acoustic impedance occurs at gas/soft tissue interfaces such as that of the bowel wall and its lumen.

Minimal patient preparation is needed for ultrasound examination. For biliary ultrasound, the patient should be fasted to minimise bowel gas shadows and to reduce gall bladder contraction; for examining the pelvis, the bladder should be full of urine. This provides a fluid-filled, non-reflective 'window' for the ultrasound to reach the pelvic organs.

SPECIAL ULTRASOUND TRANSDUCERS

Special ultrasound probes have been developed for inserting into various body orifices and via endoscopic instruments and percutaneous cannulae. Rectal probes are used for examining the rectal wall and prostate gland in detail; oesophageal probes can be used to examine and monitor the heart, and vaginal probes to investigate the pelvic organs. These probes can be placed closer to the organ being examined than conventional surface probes. This allows the use of higher-frequency sound which has lower penetration but greater spectral resolution; the result is a more detailed display for laparotomy or laparoscopy. Special probes have also been developed for applying directly to the surface of tissues such as the liver to give an image with high resolution; these provide a more reliable diagnosis of liver metastases than palpation or cross-sectional imaging. Very tiny ultrasound probes on the ends of long catheters have been developed for intraluminal imaging of the vascular system. These are in an early stage of development and show future promise for visualising damaged arteries and veins.

APPLICATIONS OF ULTRASOUND IN GENERAL SURGERY

DIAGNOSTIC B-MODE (BRIGHTNESS MODE) ULTRASOUND

Ultrasound has already largely replaced cholecystography for diagnosing gall bladder disease and, for many purposes, replaces intravenous urography for examining the urinary tract.

Ultrasound is useful for:

- Distinguishing **solid** from **cystic** lesions, e.g. a thyroid cyst from a solid nodule, a renal or pancreatic cyst from a solid tumour
- Assessing palpable **abdominal masses** in the upper abdomen or pelvis
- Detecting **abnormal tissues** in a homogeneous organ, e.g. liver metastases or renal adenocarcinoma
- Detecting **damage to solid organs after trauma**, e.g. splenic or liver rupture
- Detecting **abnormal fluid collections**, e.g. pseudocyst of pancreas, ascites, pleural effusions, abscesses
- Obtaining information about the nature of lesions from the way the **echo texture** contrasts with the normal (e.g. distinguishing liver secondaries from benign lesions or normal liver)
- Detecting **movement**, such as pulsation of an aneurysm, contraction of the heart (echo shows valve morphology and movement, wall movement) and fetal movements
- Detecting **upper urinary tract dilatation** (hydronephrosis)
- **Measuring physical dimensions**, e.g. the diameter of an abdominal aortic aneurysm or a dilated bile duct, or the volume of residual urine in the bladder after micturition

- Investigating the **biliary system** for gallstones, dilated ducts, masses in the head of the pancreas, masses in the porta hepatis
- **Guiding percutaneous interventional procedures** for tissue sampling, e.g. aspiration or biopsy of liver metastases, pancreatic tumours or retroperitoneal masses, or drainage of fluid collections
- Investigating **breast lumps**, e.g. distinguishing cystic from solid lesions, suspected malignant lesions, guided cyst drainage, guided fine-needle aspiration (FNA) for cytology or core biopsy

The limitations of diagnostic ultrasound are summarised in Box 5.3.

DOPPLER-SHIFTED ULTRASOUND

Ultrasound can be used for detecting and studying blood flow by applying the Doppler principle. Simple equipment is cheap and portable, and invaluable in the vascular clinic (see Fig. 5.8). Using a special probe placed on the skin with conduction gel, a beam of ultrasound is directed at an artery or vein. Ultrasound is reflected from the red cells, the movement of which causes a frequency shift related to the velocity. The reflected ultrasound is used to generate an audible signal (for detecting blood flow) or else is electronically processed to reveal information about the nature of flow. The pitch of the audio signal is related to blood velocity and provides some qualitative assessment of whether flow is normal or abnormal. Colour flow Doppler generates false colour to provide a visual representation of the direction and velocity of blood flow (see below).

KEY POINTS

Box 5.3 The limitations of diagnostic ultrasound

- Bone almost completely reflects ultrasound and obscures any tissues beyond it. Ultrasound is therefore of little use for examining the brain and spinal cord, although it is valuable in examining for fluid collections in the chest; special transcranial Doppler probes are used for monitoring during neurosurgery and carotid artery surgery
- Bowel gas partly reflects ultrasound, which may prejudice the examination. Starving the patient and giving laxatives may help
- A thick layer of fat degrades the ultrasound image. Thus ultrasound is less accurate but is still the first choice for investigating suspected gall bladder disease in obese patients
- Ultrasound is unreliable for showing stones at the lower end of the common bile duct

veins, particularly recurrences of varicosities after surgery

DUPLEX DOPPLER ULTRASOUND SCANNING

Duplex Doppler scanning combines frequency spectral analysis of blood flow using Doppler ultrasound with real time B-mode imaging. **Colour flow Doppler** is a more advanced variant which adds false colour to show the direction of blood flow (red one way, blue the other) and the qualitative information about blood volume.

Duplex equipment is complex and expensive, while the diagnostic process is time-consuming and requires special training. However, it adds a new dimension to the investigation of blood vessels and flow and is already superseding established methods in some areas—for example, venography for deep venous insufficiency and arteriography for carotid artery disease.

Blood vessels can be imaged in longitudinal or transverse section to reveal the direction of blood flow, the velocity of flow (this rises as blood passes through a stenosis) and the presence of abnormal vessel walls or mature thrombus in the lumen. **Cardiac echo** investigation employs similar instruments and allows the study of patterns of blood flow, cardiac wall movement, cardiac output and valve movements.

Applications of duplex Doppler

- **Deep vein thrombosis**—when available, this is probably the method of first choice for detecting postoperative DVT. Thrombus more than 24 hours old can be seen and venous flow changes detected. However, the profunda vein and small calf veins are often inadequately seen
- **Chronic lower limb deep venous insufficiency**—patency and valvular competence in deep veins (e.g. femoral and popliteal) can be determined dynamically; perforator incompetence can also be detected
- **Varicose veins**—duplex ultrasound is useful for detecting and marking the short saphenous/popliteal junction before operation and for detecting communications between superficial veins and the sapheno-femoral junction in 'recurrent' long saphenous varicose veins
- **Carotid artery disease**—duplex has now become virtually the standard test for investigating extracranial vascular disease in preference to carotid angiography (which carries distinct risks). Duplex shows the morphology of diseased arteries and the velocity of flow, allowing the percentage of stenosis to be calculated. The severity of stenosis determines

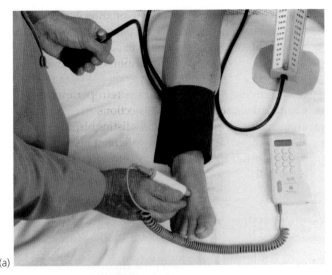
(a)

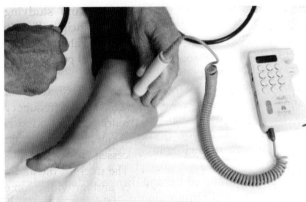
(b)

Fig. 5.8 Measuring ankle systolic pressure using a hand-held Doppler flowmeter
(a) A standard sphygmomanometer cuff is placed around the ankle just above the malleoli. Ultrasound conducting gel is applied to the tip of the probe and the probe placed lightly over the likely position of the dorsalis pedis (DP) pulse, between the first two metatarsals. The probe is moved a little at a time to obtain the strongest signal, then the cuff inflated until the pulse disappears. It is then released gradually and the systolic pressure recorded at the point of return of signal. (b) The same process is repeated at the posterior tibial pulse (PT), using the midpoint of a line between the heel and the medial malleolus to find the pulse. Note that accurate measurements require considerable experience, especially when the pressure is low. **Headphones** are recommended to reduce interference.

Main applications of Doppler-shifted ultrasound

- Measuring systolic blood pressure when it is low. This includes brachial pressure in shocked patients or in infants, and ankle systolic pressure in lower limb ischaemia. For this purpose, a sphygmomanometer cuff is placed around the arm or ankle and a portable Doppler flow detector is used as an electronic stethoscope on an artery beyond it
- Detecting the fetal heart rate
- Detecting reflux of venous blood at the sapheno-femoral or sapheno-popliteal junction in varicose

55

whether operation is required. Duplex is useful for evaluating asymptomatic bruits and following up patients after carotid endarterectomy, including the early postoperative period

- **Femoro-popliteal bypass grafts**—duplex is used for marking out the saphenous vein graft before surgery and for graft surveillance after surgery to detect remediable vein graft stenoses
- **Aorto-iliac and femoro-popliteal occlusive disease**—duplex is proving valuable for estimating the sites and severity of stenoses and occlusions. At present it

is largely a screening test but may replace arteriography in some circumstances

- **Deeper blood vessels**—these can be imaged for blood flow and obstruction, e.g. superior mesenteric and renal arteries, and renal veins for spread from renal cell carcinoma
- **Cardiac disease**—duplex is used for detecting abnormal wall movements due to ischaemia, valvular abnormalities including stenoses, congenital cardiac defects including septal defects, and intracardiac thrombus

COMPUTERISED TOMOGRAPHY (CT SCANNING)

GENERAL PRINCIPLES OF CT SCANNING

Computerised tomography involves X-raying a series of thin transverse 'slices' of the patient's head or body. A precise fan-shaped beam of X-rays is repeatedly pulsed

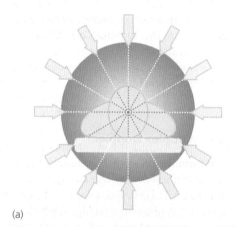

(a)

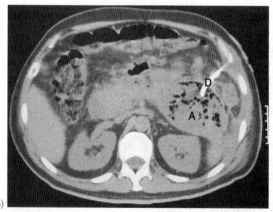

(b)

Fig. 5.9 Computerised tomography
(a) Principle of CT scanning. All images are fed into a computer and a single image produced. **(b)** CT guided drainage. This patient presented with a severe attack of acute pancreatitis and was resuscitated and gradually recovered over 2 weeks. He then developed a swinging fever, found to be due to an abscess around the tail of the pancreas. This film shows a pigtail drain **D** sited within the abscess cavity **A**.

from successive angles around the circumference of each slice and the transmitted radiation is electronically recorded on the other side (see Fig. 5.9). More modern machines spiral around the patient (spiral CT) resulting in more rapid image capture and higher resolution. Each element of the beam is attenuated according to the density of the tissue it traverses. These numerous radiation counts are analysed by a computer which builds up a picture of the tissue densities in the slice by solving many simultaneous equations. Each picture element is called a **pixel** and each volume element is known as a **voxel**. The images are displayed on a screen where they can be electronically edited and then recorded on film.

Since CT was first introduced, the pace of development has been rapid. The speed of data acquisition has dramatically improved so that spiral CT scanning produces an image of a chest or abdomen in under 1 minute. From this data, electronic multiplane or three-dimensional reconstruction can be performed to improve image quality and discrimination of abnormalities. Further information can often be gained by performing CT scanning after contrast enhancement. For example, oral or rectal contrast clearly outlines bowel, while intravenous contrast can show blood vessels, kidneys or damage to the blood–brain barrier or areas of absent blood flow such as occur in pancreatic necrosis.

At present CT and magnetic resonance imaging are competing for first place in the imaging stakes. However, it is likely that both methods will prove to have advantages in particular areas.

APPLICATIONS OF CT SCANNING

Pathological anatomy can be studied in great detail by computerised tomography and a vast array of information can be obtained to aid surgical diagnosis. Indeed, in many cases the accuracy of this information could not be rivalled by exploratory operation and yet it can be obtained non-invasively. This is particularly so in brain injury after trauma where management of serious head injuries has been transformed by head scanning. The technique enables timely and appropriate surgical intervention and avoids unnecessary exploratory operations. The best CT images are obtained in well-nourished patients because fat separates the organs.

The main indications for CT scanning are:

- Investigating areas difficult to examine by standard radiology or ultrasound. Examples include the retroperitoneal area and pancreas (deep inside the body), the lungs and mediastinum, and the brain and spinal cord (encased in bone)
- Investigating abdominal pathology when ultrasound has proved unsatisfactory or as an alternative to more invasive investigations such as barium enema examination for suspected large bowel cancer
- Pretreatment planning and follow-up in relation to radiotherapy and chemotherapy, e.g. for staging lymphomas (replaces laparotomy) and assessing intrathoracic tumours including retrosternal thyroid enlargement
- Planning surgery, e.g. establishing the extent of local invasion of oesophageal carcinoma, identifying the upper level of an aortic aneurysm, investigating the extent of lateral spread in rectal or prostatic cancer
- Assessing solid organ damage in abdominal or thoracic trauma
- Guiding needles during biopsy of masses, drainage of fluid collections or obtaining aspiration cytology specimens

MAGNETIC RESONANCE IMAGING (MRI)

GENERAL PRINCIPLES OF MAGNETIC RESONANCE IMAGING

Magnetic resonance imaging (MRI), formerly known as nuclear magnetic resonance, is a recently introduced technique, the diagnostic applications of which are rapidly expanding as the speed and resolution of the equipment improve.

MRI involves applying a powerful magnetic field to the body which causes the protons of all hydrogen nuclei to become aligned. The protons are then excited by pulses of radio waves at a frequency which causes them to resonate and emit radio signals; these are recorded electronically. Sophisticated computation then produces images which can be viewed in any plane, transverse, longitudinal or at any obliquity (see Fig. 5.10).

Lipids have a particularly high hydrogen content and are clearly seen on MRI. For this reason, the initial applications of MRI were in examining the brain and spinal cord. The technique is increasingly employed for investigating joints such as the knee, shoulder, hip and ankle, and in some cases replaces the need for arthroscopy.

An exciting new application of MRI is the study of blood flow and cardiac function, i.e. magnetic resonance angiography (MRA). Atheroma can also be demonstrated. The direction and velocity of blood flow can be

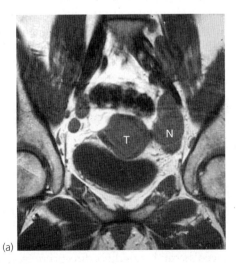

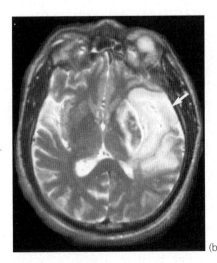

(a)   (b)

Fig. 5.10 MRI images
(a) Carcinoma of the cervix with nodal metastases in transverse section. **T** represents the cervical tumour and **N** represents involved pelvic lymph nodes. MRI is now the best method for staging carcinoma of the cervix. **(b)** T2 weighted axial MRI of the brain showing a haemorrhagic infarct in the left middle cerebral artery territory (arrowed).

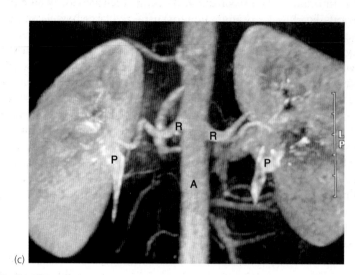

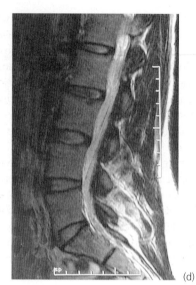

Fig. 5.10 Continued

(c) Magnetic resonance angiogram of normal kidneys showing aorta **A**, renal arteries **R**, renal substance and renal pelvis **P**. **(d)** Longitudinal MRI scan of lumbosacral spine showing normal spinal canal, spinal cord and cauda equina with no evidence of disc protrusion.

determined without the need for contrast injection, and volume flow in particular vessels can be calculated. These techniques will undoubtedly play an increasing future role in cardiac and arterial surgery.

The main technical disadvantages of MRI are claustrophobic conditions for the patient, longer scanning times and the inability to scan a patient being artificially ventilated (because of the effects of magnetism on metal fittings). These make it unsuitable for young children, the elderly or confused, patients in pain, ventilated patients and emergency patients with active bleeding. All of these disadvantages are being addressed and are likely to disappear as newer machines become available. Already scanning times have fallen, allowing good-quality imaging of chest, abdomen and pelvis. MRI is also unsuitable for imaging gas-filled organs and dense bone.

In general surgical diagnosis, MRI is useful for assessing soft tissue tumours, biliary anatomy and pelvic disease. In soft tissue tumours of the extremities, MRI is particularly important in surgical planning as it demonstrates the tumour's extent and relationship to vital structures, as well as assisting in the planning of excision margins and planes. MRI is of increasing benefit in imaging the biliary tree, producing a **magnetic resonance cholangio-pancreatogram (MRCP)**. The advantages are that sedation is not required, and, compared to ERCP there is no risk of causing pancreatitis or bleeding. As yet, the technique is not widely available. Pelvic MRI is of increasing importance in assessing complex anorectal fistulae and in certain pelvic malignancies. Of recent interest is the use of MRI spectroscopy in the assessment of breast cancer but its merits remain to be evaluated.

INTERVENTIONAL RADIOLOGY

Many of the conventional X-ray, ultrasound and CT techniques already described have been adapted to guide needles to obtain biopsy material and to place drains, thus allowing less invasive therapeutic manœuvres than were formerly required. Many of these techniques have revolutionised treatment—for example, in obliterative arterial disease—and have established the radiologist as a front-line clinician. This is a rapidly expanding field of radiology with a growing list of techniques. Some of the main surgical applications are described below.

TISSUE SAMPLING

FINE NEEDLE ASPIRATION CYTOLOGY (FNA) AND CORE BIOPSY

A fine needle (22 gauge) can be safely passed through most organs or small bowel to aspirate small fragments of tissue from a suspicious lesion. Larger-diameter needles can be used for direct core biopsy of masses. The depth and direction of the needle can now be accurately guided by ultrasound or CT to ensure a representative sample is taken. For example, pancreatic masses can be reached by transfixing bowel lying in front of the pancreas; this causes remarkably few side effects. Where practicable, many surgeons and pathologists prefer the larger specimens obtainable with **core biopsy** techniques using specially designed needles such as the **Trucut**, which is available in various configurations and dimensions.

Applications in the diagnosis of breast disease include ultrasound or mammographically guided FNA or core biopsy of asymptomatic abnormalities found on mammography, including those found on screening. Stereotactic apparatus can be employed to make this process more accurate. Mammographic guidance is also used to place a hooked wire close to an impalpable abnormality to locate it before surgical excision (**mammographic localisation**).

Guided core biopsy or FNA techniques are also important in the diagnosis of thyroid lumps, for sampling liver nodules and for taking renal biopsies in diffuse renal disease.

DRAINAGE OF ABSCESSES AND FLUID COLLECTIONS

Ultrasound and CT are often used to guide percutaneous drainage of well-defined fluid collections in the abdomen or chest, e.g. pancreatic pseudocysts or abscesses (paracolic or subphrenic). Ultrasound scanning can demonstrate the site and the dimensions of the fluid collection and can guide the least harmful route for drainage. Fluid can be drained via a needle on a once-only basis or else a self-retaining 'pigtail' drain can be put in place and drainage allowed to continue. In the first category, a subphrenic or other localised abscess can be drained; in the second category, a drain can be placed into a pseudocyst of the pancreas or locally to drain a biliary leak after surgery. In this way, many major surgical interventions can be avoided.

ENDOVASCULAR TECHNIQUES

PERCUTANEOUS TRANSLUMINAL ANGIOPLASTY (PTA)

This technique, originally known as **Gruntzig dilatation**, has rapidly become established as an alternative to surgery for overcoming many peripheral and coronary arterial stenoses. In general, short stenoses in large vessels are most suitable for this approach. The method is particularly useful for lower limb atherosclerosis (especially of the iliac and superficial femoral arteries) and for renal and coronary artery stenoses. Carotid artery disease, however, is as yet less suitable for angioplasty because of the serious consequences of embolism.

Major complications of angioplasty are rare in experienced hands but there is a small risk of precipitating

acute ischaemia. Thus, surgical salvage should always be readily available should complications develop. Unfortunately, 25–40% of angioplastied lesions undergo restenosis or occlusion within 1 year but the process can usually be repeated. For vessels which fail to remain open at the time of angioplasty, expanding wire stents can be placed within the dilated stenoses but the success rate remains to be evaluated. Angioplasty can often be performed as an extension of initial diagnostic arteriography. Overall, angioplasty causes minimal surgical and anaesthetic stress to the patient and is often performed on a day-case basis. Angioplasty is often offered when open bypass surgery would not be indicated.

Techniques of percutaneous angioplasty

Angioplasty is usually performed under local anaesthesia (see Fig. 5.11). A needle is first inserted percutaneously into an accessible artery (usually femoral, brachial or radial) and a short flexible guide-wire passed into the artery. A working sheath with a valved side-arm is passed over the guide-wire and about 15 cm into the artery. A long guide-wire is then substituted for the first and guided to and then through the stenosis under X-ray fluoroscopic control using contrast injections. An angioplasty catheter with a plastic inflatable balloon at its end is then passed over the guide-wire and manipulated into position across the stenosis. The synthetic angioplasty balloons are no wider than the catheter when non-inflated and inflate to a fixed diameter. Prior to dilatation, the arterial pressure above and below the stenosis may be measured via the catheter to determine any significant pressure gradient. The balloon is then inflated to a pressure of between 3 and 12 atmospheres to dilate the stenosis. The pressure gradient across the previously stenosed area may be measured again; if dilatation has been successful, the pressure differential across the stenosis should have been eliminated. The spreading success of angioplasty has meant that many patients can be returned to near-normal life with minimal intervention. Indeed, many more patients with claudication or coronary heart disease are now being considered for angioplasty than would formerly have been offered reconstructive arterial surgery.

LOCAL ARTERIAL THROMBOLYTIC THERAPY

An artery that is freshly occluded by thrombosis and causing ischaemia can often be recanalised by local intra-arterial infusion of thrombolytic agents. This allows high local concentrations of the thrombolytic agent with little systemic spillover and avoids most of the serious bleeding and allergic complications of systemic thrombolytic therapy. Thrombolytic agents include **streptokinase**, **urokinase** and **recombinant tissue plasminogen**

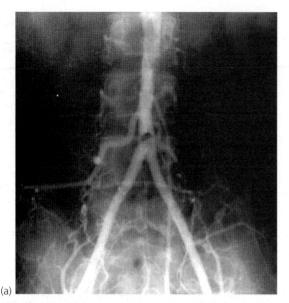
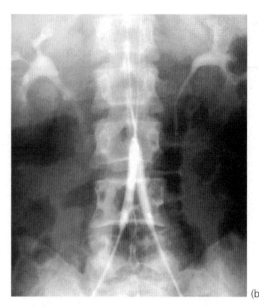

(a)　　　　　　　　　　　　　　　　　　　　　　　　　(b)

Fig. 5.11 Percutaneous transluminal angioplasty
This man of 55 presented with bilateral calf and thigh claudication. **(a)** Shows a localised severe stenosis of the distal abdominal aorta. **(b)** Shows the 'kissing balloon' technique used to dilate the stenosis. Two balloons are used to prevent asymmetrical dilatation which might compromise the opposite common iliac artery.

activator (R-tPa). The best agent has yet to be decided but tPa acts more quickly and does not cause the frequent allergic effects of streptokinase, though it is more expensive.

The main indication for thrombolysis is the acutely ischaemic limb where arteriography has demonstrated acute thrombosis superimposed upon pre-existing atherosclerotic narrowing; simple embolism is increasingly being tackled in this way too. An infusion catheter is manœuvred so as to lie within the clot and small amounts of thrombolytic agents are infused over a few hours. Arteriograms are repeated at intervals to follow progress and the clot may thus be safely dissolved. Underlying arterial stenoses may then be revealed and can often be treated by balloon angioplasty or bypass surgery. The technique can be used to lyse mature embolic material up to 2 weeks or more after embolism. Despite the foregoing, surgical embolectomy remains the best treatment for recent acute embolic ischaemia, particularly if the viability of the limb is in jeopardy.

Thrombolytic therapy can also be employed for treating pulmonary embolism although the indications and efficacy are not yet well established.

THERAPEUTIC EMBOLISATION

Highly vascular lesions, such as certain haemangiomas, which would be difficult or impossible to treat by surgery alone, can have their arterial supply reduced or obliterated by embolisation. The main supplying artery is identified by selective arteriography and a catheter

manœuvred into it, close to the lesion. A small quantity of occlusive material is injected via the catheter so as to impact in the artery where it narrows. The usual materials for embolisation are **gelatin foam, lyophilised human dura mater, minute steel coils** or **cyanoacrylate glue**. The process is repeated for all the feeding vessels.

Embolisation is sometimes used to reduce the vascularity of a lesion prior to otherwise difficult surgery (e.g. carotid body tumour) or to treat lesions not amenable to surgery (e.g. hepatic metastases or extensive arteriovenous malformations).

MINIMAL ACCESS GRAFT PLACEMENT

Increasing experience in endovascular techniques has encouraged progress towards more ambitious minimally invasive techniques—in particular, endovascular stent-grafts for abdominal aortic aneurysms, placed via femoral arteriotomies. A Dacron graft with integral metal stent is passed proximally until it lies within the neck of the aneurysm. A balloon is inflated to expand the stent into position to retain the graft. A similar mechanism is used to secure the distal limb(s). Techniques like this are still under development and clinical trials are giving promising results; however, doubts remain about long-term durability. A particular problem is **endoleakage**, i.e. continued slow bleeding into the aneurysm sac caused by failure of the graft to exclude blood from the aneurysm. The late complication rate is about 10% per year, considerably greater than that for open aneurysm grafting.

DILATATION OF GASTROINTESTINAL STRICTURES

Large balloon catheters similar to angioplasty catheters can be used to dilate benign oesophageal strictures secondary to oesophagitis. For achalasia, balloon dilatation is becoming a standard technique. Balloon dilatation is sometimes used for benign rectal strictures such as may occur at an anastomosis site, provided they are not caused by recurrent tumour. Cloth-lined expanding metal stents are now successfully employed for oesophageal, gastric outlet and colonic strictures caused by malignancy or benign conditions.

RADIOLOGICAL ACCESS TO THE UPPER URINARY TRACT

The renal pelvis can be reached percutaneously and punctured with a needle guided by ultrasound or CT scanning. The tract can be dilated to allow tubes of various sizes and types to be inserted. This access can be used to remove stones from the renal pelvis, to drain the kidney over a few days in acute distal urinary obstruction until a definitive procedure can be performed (nephrostomy drainage), and to conduct sophisticated pressure and flow measurements in suspected pelvi-ureteric junction obstruction. Gaining access to the kidney in this way is known as **percutaneous nephrostomy**.

RADIONUCLIDE SCANNING

GENERAL PRINCIPLES OF RADIONUCLIDE SCANNING

Radionuclide scanning is the diagnostic application of **nuclear medicine** techniques to identify sites of abnormal physiology, e.g. the presence of pus, abnormal phagocytic activity or areas of excessive bone turnover. Isotope scanning, however, gives poor anatomical detail. Suitable tracer agents combine a substance taken up physiologically by the target tissue and a **radioactive label**. The usual label is ^{99m}Technetium.

The tracer is either concentrated in a specific type of tissue (such as iodine in the thyroid gland) or else in tissues with similar physiological or pathological activity (such as reticulo-endothelial cells or areas of inflammation, respectively).

In the early days of nuclear medicine, tracer was detected in the body using a rectilinear scanner which tracked back and forth over the patient for 1 hour or more to build up the image. Nowadays, a gamma camera consisting of multiple detector units simultaneously collects and counts the level of radioactivity across the area of interest. This produces a complete image in one exposure (see Fig. 5.12). Several views are taken from different directions (usually anterior, posterior and oblique) and this provides more diagnostic information than a single view.

Some pathophysiological functions can be investigated by **dynamic imaging**. For this, detection of isotope continues for a period of time and the changing level of radioactivity is recorded for later computer analysis. Examples of this include estimating renal blood flow and studying renal clearance.

APPLICATIONS OF RADIONUCLIDE SCANNING

LUNG SCANNING

The most important application of lung scanning is the diagnosis of pulmonary embolism. The principle is that pulmonary emboli obliterate patchy areas of the pulmonary arterial circulation but do not interfere with lung ventilation. This is the reverse of what happens with pulmonary infection. Ideally, a **ventilation scan** and a **perfusion scan** should be performed, the two together being known as a **ventilation/perfusion scan** or **V/Q scan**. The ventilation scan is performed first. The patient inhales a gaseous radioactive tracer such as an aerosol of

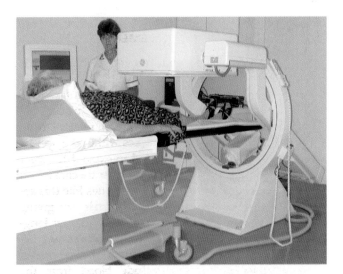

Fig. 5.12 Isotope scanning using a gamma camera
The patient has received an intravenous injection of radiolabelled tracer. The pattern of uptake is imaged by the detector array and transmitted electronically to be displayed in a monitor.

61

technetium-labelled DTPA or ^{133}Xenon, and the lungs are imaged from both front and back. Then technetium-labelled albumin microspheres are injected intravenously for the perfusion scan. These lodge in the pulmonary capillaries after traversing the chambers of the right side of the heart.

The two scans are compared for **ventilation/ perfusion mismatch**, i.e. areas that are ventilated but not perfused (embolism) and areas that are perfused but not ventilated (consolidation or collapse). An example is shown in Chapter 47 (Fig. 47.8). V/Q scanning may give a strongly positive or negative indication of pulmonary embolism, but all too often the results are equivocal. If a patient is too breathless to undergo a ventilation scan, a perfusion scan alone may be performed but accuracy is reduced.

If a right-to-left shunt is present, perfusion scanning is contraindicated because the microspheres can pass into the systemic circulation and damage critical organs. Right-to-left shunts occur in cardiac septal defects, arteriovenous malformations of the lung and sometimes within pulmonary metastases. V/Q scanning for pulmonary embolism is gradually being superseded by contrast-enhanced CT scanning.

BONE SCANNING

Phosphate-based agents (phosphates or biphosphonates) labelled with technetium are usually used for bone scanning. The tracer is taken up by areas of increased bone deposition and resorption, indicating sites of bone growth and repair (see Fig. 5.13). These include **growth plates, some primary tumours, secondary tumours, foci of bone infection, healing fracture sites, active arthritis** and **Paget's disease**. Bone scanning is highly sensitive but interpretation of the scans requires caution because of lack of specificity.

The tracer agent is injected intravenously and becomes distributed through all body fluids. The highest concentration is expected to appear at sites of osteogenesis about 6 hours later and the patient is scanned then. The tracer is also taken up in areas of **dystrophic calcification** and may sometimes reveal an unsuspected

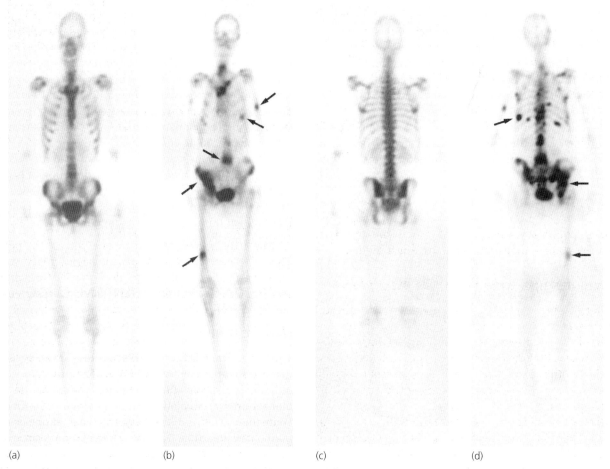

(a)   (b)   (c)   (d)

Fig. 5.13 Isotope bone scans of the whole body
(a) Anterior view of normal bone scan. **(b)** Anterior view of bone scan in a patient with multiple bony metastases (arrowed) from breast cancer.
(c) Posterior view of normal bone scan. **(d)** Posterior view of bone scan in the same patient as in **(b)**.

carcinoma of breast, an old myocardial infarction scar or a uterine fibroid.

The main indications for bone scanning are:

● Suspected bone metastases (e.g. staging breast carcinoma) or investigation of bone pain
● Biochemical abnormalities suggesting bone disease (e.g. hypercalcaemia or raised serum alkaline phosphatase)
● Suspected occult (stress) fractures of bone
● Suspected osteomyelitis
● Localising the site of unexplained skeletal pain

RENAL SCANS

Renal scanning is an important method of investigating the urinary tract. It can obtain information not available from any other source, is quick and simple to perform and allows the function of each kidney to be assessed independently. There are three main varieties of renal scan which use different isotopes. DTPA (diethylene tetramine penta-acetic acid) is excreted in the urine like urographic contrast, while DMSA (dimercaptosuccinic acid) and MAG3 remain in cortical tissue. (Aide-mémoire: DT 'Pee' A, excreted in urine; D 'Meat' SA, retained in cortical tissue.) Examples are shown in Figure 5.14.

DTPA scanning is used to follow up children with reflux nephropathy. The isotope is instilled into the bladder; the child then voids urine while being scanned and any vesico-ureteric reflux is demonstrated. DTPA is also used to diagnose ureteric obstruction and to distinguish obstructed from merely capacious non-obstructed renal tracts.

Both DMSA and DTPA can give an estimate of excretory activity when unilateral renal parenchymal disease is being investigated. The two agents can be used to estimate differential renal function when investigating renal artery stenosis or the function of a transplanted kidney. DMSA is used specifically to image the renal parenchyma to demonstrate renal scars or tumours.

SCANNING FOR GASTROINTESTINAL BLEEDING

Scanning using the patient's own isotopically labelled red cells may be employed to locate a source of continuing or intermittent gastrointestinal bleeding. This is useful where the rate of bleeding is relatively slow or in a patient with recurrent haemorrhage, particularly where the source cannot be identified by endoscopy or contrast radiology.

The patient's blood is labelled with radioactive technetium; this may be performed ex vivo or else in vivo by injecting first pyrophosphate, which binds to red cells, then technetium, which binds to pyrophosphate. The abdomen is scanned at intervals over the next 24 hours or so for 'hot spots' indicating accumulating

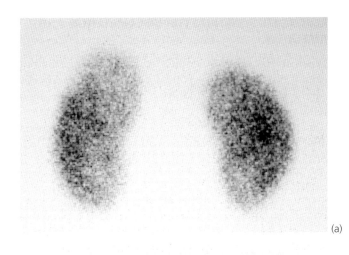

(a)

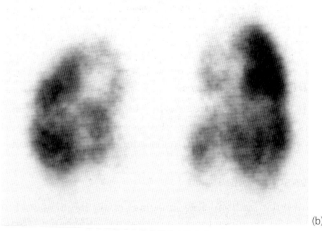

(b)

Fig. 5.14 Renal DMSA isotope scans
(a) Normal and (b) Abnormal showing patchy scarring due to episodes of pyelonephritis. In this case, there had been bilateral reflux of urine in childhood.

recent gastrointestinal haemorrhage. If the rate of bleeding is more than about 0.1 ml per minute, the scan usually reveals activity concentrated in one part of the bowel. This indicates the general area of haemorrhage rather than the precise location but does enable the surgical search to be focused—for example, on the distal stomach and duodenum, or the right side of the colon. Radionuclide scanning has the advantage of detecting an accumulation of blood over a period, whereas the alternative investigation of selective angiography is less sensitive and requires active bleeding at the moment of injection; however, the latter can reveal the site of bleeding more precisely.

In children, rectal bleeding may be due to bleeding from a Meckel's diverticulum. This is usually caused by ulceration of ectopic gastric mucosa. A radionuclide compound of technetium that is concentrated in gastric mucosa may be used to image a suspected Meckel's diverticulum.

LEUCOCYTE SCANNING FOR INFLAMMATION AND INFECTION

When an abscess or other infected focus is suspected but cannot be localised, the patient's own white blood cells can be labelled with ^{111}Indium or ^{67}Gallium citrate, then reinjected; the patient is then scanned. Typical indications for this are patients with a high swinging pyrexia after operation, or patients with sepsis of unknown origin. The process is relatively expensive because it requires a cell separator but it has a high degree of specificity and sensitivity. There is a small proportion of false negative tests, however, where a hidden abscess is not revealed by the scan.

Leucocyte scanning is also useful to determine the extent of bowel involvement in inflammatory bowel disease, both ulcerative colitis and Crohn's disease. HMPAO-labelled leucocytes migrate towards areas of inflamed bowel which are then revealed on imaging.

THYROID SCANS

Thyroid scanning is described in Chapter 43. Its use is declining in favour of fine needle aspiration and cytology except in certain disorders of thyroid function.

VASCULAR IMAGING

Vascular radionuclide imaging is in its infancy but shows promise for demonstrating differential tissue blood flow in ischaemic limbs. A radionuclide known as MUGA is beginning to provide useful information.

Radionuclide lymphangiography can also demonstrate the patency and capacity of lower limb lymphatics in chronic lymphoedema.

LIVER AND SPLEEN SCANS

Radionuclide scanning of liver and spleen is imprecise and has largely been superseded by other modalities including high-resolution CT or ultrasonography, percutaneous or laparoscopic liver biopsy and ERCP.

Reticulo-endothelial imaging ('liver scanning')

Technetium-labelled sulphur colloid is taken up by reticulo-endothelial cells in the liver (Kupffer cells) and spleen, and demonstrates the general morphology of the parenchyma. Areas of increased phagocytic activity are revealed by abnormal uptake of tracer.

Hepatobiliary imaging (HIDA scanning)

Technetium-labelled imido-diacetic acid (IDA) derivatives are concentrated by hepatocytes and excreted into bile even in the presence of jaundice. This provides a means of testing the patency of the biliary tree and cystic duct.

Hepatobiliary imaging can be used for:

- Demonstrating cystic duct obstruction in suspected acute cholecystitis
- Demonstrating bile duct obstruction in jaundiced patients to confirm the jaundice is obstructive

6 Principles of operative surgery

INTRODUCTION

This chapter outlines the essential principles of operative surgery and endoscopy and also covers a range of minor surgical techniques. These should be understood by all doctors, not just by surgeons, so as to give them an appreciation of the scope of surgery, to enable them to provide adequate explanation to patients before and after surgery and to help them participate intelligently at operations. Furthermore, most doctors are required to perform minor operations, casualty procedures or invasive investigations at one time or another and these require a knowledge of appropriate techniques.

Various suffixes derived from Greek and Latin are used in the description of certain surgical techniques; these are summarised in Box 6.1.

KEY POINTS

Box 6.1 Surgical terminology

-*oscopy* = examination of a hollow viscus, body cavity or deep structure employing an instrument specifically designed for the purpose, e.g. gastroscopy, colonoscopy, laparoscopy, arthroscopy, bronchoscopy. The general term is endoscopy

-*ectomy* = removal of an organ, e.g. gastrectomy, orchidectomy (i.e. removal of testis), colectomy

-*orrhaphy* = repair of tissues, e.g. herniorrhaphy

-*ostomy* = fashioning an artificial communication between a hollow viscus and the skin, e.g. tracheostomy, colostomy, ileostomy. The term may also apply to artificial openings between different viscera, e.g. gastro-jejunostomy, choledocho-duodenostomy (i.e. anastomosis of duodenum to common bile duct)

-*otomy* = cutting open, e.g. laparotomy, arteriotomy, fasciotomy, thoracotomy

-*plasty* = reconstruction, e.g. pyloroplasty, mammoplasty, arthroplasty

-*pexy* = relocation and securing in position, e.g. orchidopexy (for undescended testis), rectopexy (for rectal prolapse)

PRINCIPLES OF ASEPSIS AND INFECTION CONTROL

INTRODUCTION

The main bacteria and viruses involved in surgical infections have already been described in Chapter 1. The chief sources of infection are the patients themselves (particularly bowel flora), less commonly the hospital environment, food or cross-infection from other patients, and only occasionally bacteria and viruses carried by theatre personnel. Rare sources of infection are contaminated surgical instruments or equipment, dressings or parenteral drugs and fluids. The viruses causing hepatitis B and C and particularly human immunodeficiency virus (HIV) pose relatively recent and sinister risks of transmitting infection from patient to operating staff and vice versa; there is also the risk of patient-to-patient transmission. These risks of transmitting potentially serious viral diseases make it mandatory to observe **universal blood and body fluid precautions**.

The risk of postoperative bacterial infection depends on the extent of contamination of the wound or body cavity that occurs at operation or prior to it in the case of intestinal perforation. Bacteria may enter a wound by five possible routes:

- Air-borne bacteria-laden particles
- Direct inoculation from instruments and operating personnel
- From the patient's skin
- From the flora of the patient's internal viscera, especially the large bowel
- Via the bloodstream

Modern operating theatre design and aseptic procedures, if correctly observed, minimise wound contamination but infections still occur. Their results can be devastating especially in relation to artificial prostheses, skin grafts, bone and the eye. Furthermore, some patients are particularly vulnerable to infection, notably neonates, the immunosuppressed, the debilitated and the malnourished. Treatment of established infection is no substitute for prevention.

The introduction in the 1970s of perioperative prophylactic antibiotics has revolutionised the scope and outcome of certain types of operative surgery in a manner comparable to the surgical revolution of the late nineteenth century heralded by Lister's techniques of antisepsis.

METHODS OF INFECTION CONTROL

UNIVERSAL BLOOD AND BODY FLUID PRECAUTIONS

The increasing awareness of blood-borne viral infections such as hepatitis B and C and the advent of new infections such as HIV have led to the concept of **universal blood and body fluid precautions** in combating cross-infection between patients and staff. Every patient should be assumed to be a potential carrier of blood-borne infection and precautions applied whenever skin is likely to be breached and whenever instruments contaminated with blood or other body fluids are handled. Transmission of infection can occur in obvious situations such as a needle-stick injury, as well as with less obvious events such as splashes of infected material into the eye.

Disposable gloves should be worn for all procedures and physical examinations except for palpating patients' skin where there is no obvious open lesion in either patient or examiner. Staff with broken skin should apply occlusive dressings. The integrity of skin affected by minor scratches or grazes can be checked with an alcoholic skin wash, wipe or swab which causes stinging if the skin is broken. Staff often try to be particularly vigilant with known carriers of HIV or hepatitis or in other high-risk patients but relax at other times. However, research has shown that this extra care soon lapses even in known infected cases; this may explain recent publicised cases of unexpected transmission from patient to doctor, doctor to patient and patient to patient which reveal this practice to be unsound. The routine use of protective eyewear during invasive procedures to prevent conjunctival splashes is to be encouraged.

Needle-stick and other penetrating injuries

Needle-stick injuries occur when a needle already used for a patient inadvertently penetrates the skin of a health-care worker. This is a common injury which is largely avoidable. Needle-stick injuries are capable of transmitting hepatitis B but the risk for HIV is much lower. This is because the concentration of virus in HIV-positive fluids is much lower than in hepatitis and the volume of blood transmitted by needle-stick injuries is small. Needles and other disposable instruments contaminated with blood should be handled with great care and disposed of immediately after use into special plastic 'sharps' containers. These should be available wherever sharps are used so that instruments need not be passed from person to person nor carried from one place to another. It is the responsibility of the user to dispose properly of the sharp. Resheathing of used needles is the cause of some 40% of needle-stick injuries and should be avoided. Venepuncture is a high-risk procedure and should be performed with caution. The ignored needle from a cannulation left lying beside a patient might prove lethal to an unsuspecting staff member.

Hepatitis B vaccination

All staff directly involved in patient care should be vaccinated against hepatitis B. This involves three intramuscular injections—the initial injection, then 1 month and 5 months later, with booster doses at 5-yearly intervals thereafter. Hepatitis B serology should be checked 2 months after completion of vaccination. Around 5% of healthy young people fail to seroconvert and should be revaccinated. Half of these will seroconvert and the remainder are genetic non-responders.

Procedure following 'sharps' injury

If there is a definite sharps injury involving transmission of blood from an infected person, the risk of infection to the recipient is about 25% for hepatitis B, 20% for hepatitis C and 0.5% for HIV. There is also a high risk after sharps injury in a recreational environment (e.g. needles left on the beach by intravenous drug users) since hepatitis B and HIV survive well in warm, moist conditions, especially in serum and tissue debris. Thus all sharps injuries should be treated with the utmost concern. A recommended protocol is shown in Box 6.2.

THE OPERATING ENVIRONMENT

Modern **operating theatre design** plays a major role in the control of air-borne wound contamination. This is important mainly for staphylococci carried on air-borne skin scales.

The main factors influencing infection rate are:

- Concentration of organisms in the air
- Size of bacteria-laden particles
- Duration of exposure of the open wound

The first two are influenced mainly by theatre design and air supply and the last one can be minimised by avoiding unnecessarily long procedures. Operating theatre complexes are laid out so as to minimise introduction of infection from elsewhere in the hospital via air, personnel or patients. Air is drawn from the relatively clean external environment, filtered and then supplied to the operating theatres at a slightly higher pressure than outside to ensure constant outward flow. Air turnover is the most important factor; the aim is to ensure 3–15 air changes per hour which 'scrubs out' the theatre air by dilution. Standard air delivery systems aim to achieve a constant flow of clean air towards the operating table, which is then exhausted from the theatre. Despite this, convection currents allow some recirculation of air, which may have been contaminated, into the operation site.

The crucial importance of excluding infection in joint replacement surgery led to the development of sophisti-

---

KEY POINTS

Box 6.2 Protocol for managing 'sharps' injuries

1. Wash injured area immediately and encourage blood to flow from wound

2. Record all details of incident including names of persons involved

3. Test injured person (*the recipient*) serologically for HIV, hepatitis B and hepatitis C

4. Test person whose blood/body fluids contaminated the sharp (the donor) for HIV, hepatitis B and hepatitis C

5. If hepatitis B status of recipient or donor is uncertain and cannot be determined reliably within 48 hours of injury (e.g. over a weekend), administer the following to the recipient as soon as possible:
   - Hepatitis B immunoglobulin (0.06 ml/kg body weight)
   - Hepatitis B vaccine—first dose

6. The immune status of donor and recipient dictates further management as follows:
   - Recipient hepatitis B immune—no further action (or may give hepatitis B booster)
   - Recipient hepatitis B non-immune (or non-responder) and donor positive or unknown—give hepatitis B immunoglobulin and start course of hepatitis B vaccination
   - Recipient hepatitis B non-immune and donor negative—start course of hepatitis B vaccination
   - Donor HIV antibody positive or in high-risk group (e.g. homosexual, intravenous drug user, prostitute)—consult infectious diseases physician. Zidovudine therapy should be considered as soon as possible although its efficacy in preventing seroconversion is unproven and side effects are often very unpleasant (bone marrow suppression, nausea and other gastrointestinal symptoms, headache)
   - Counsel recipients on safe sex procedures to prevent possible infection of their sexual partners

7. Follow up recipients with serological testing after 3 months (hepatitis B, hepatitis C, HIV), 6 months (hepatitis B and C) and 12 months (hepatitis C); ensure completion of hepatitis B vaccination courses instituted above

---

cated **ultra-clean air delivery systems**. These have been shown to reduce postoperative infection two- to fourfold but the cost of such measures makes them difficult to justify for general surgery. Enclosure of the patient in a sterile tent in which the surgeons wear space-type suits can reduce infection rates by a further 5–7.5% but these measures are probably not warranted except in specialised joint replacement units. Despite the complexity and high cost of these special operating room arrangements, simple prophylactic antibiotics have been shown to be a more effective way of reducing infection in joint replacement surgery.

MINIMISING INFECTION FROM OPERATING THEATRE PERSONNEL

Studies of bacterial types in wound infections have shown that a modest proportion of wound infections are derived from theatre personnel. Bacteria reach the wound via the air or by direct inoculation. About 30% of healthy people carry *Staphylococcus aureus* in the nose but pathogenic organisms may also be present in the axillae and perineal area, the latter probably being the most important source. In addition, minor skin abrasions are usually infected, as are skin pustules and boils; thus personnel with these lesions must ensure that they are effectively covered with occlusive dressings or else should not enter the operating area.

Air-borne, personnel-derived infection is reduced by changing from potentially contaminated day clothes to clean theatre clothes and shoes which should not then be worn outside the theatre complex. Trouser cuffs should be elasticated or tucked into boots. Some studies suggest that females should wear trousers instead of dresses, in order to reduce 'perineal fallout'. **Face masks** are worn to deflect bacteria-containing droplets in expired air, but they become ineffective after a relatively short period, especially if they become wet. With the exception of nasal *Staph. aureus* (particularly important in infection of prostheses), bacteria derived from the head do not generally cause wound infection. The effectiveness of wearing masks and hair coverings to reduce infection is unknown.

Sterile gloves and gowns are worn by surgeons and staff directly involved in the operation to prevent direct inoculation of bacteria. Gloves are impermeable to bacteria but hands and forearms are washed before gloving and gowning with antiseptics which persist on the skin. This minimises bacterial contamination if a glove is punctured or the sleeve of the gown becomes wet. **Thorough washing** with soap and water removes extraneous contaminants but not resident flora, the numbers of which can be considerably reduced by using detergent solutions containing antiseptics such as **chlorhexidine** and **povidone-iodine**; disinfection is further improved by a final **alcohol rinse**. These are most effective if they are not rinsed off but merely dried with a sterile towel. The traditional ritual of scrubbing with a brush for 3 minutes is actually less effective than washing the hands thoroughly because it causes micro-trauma to the hands and brings more bacteria to the surface.

Despite the wearing of gloves and gown, the less the wound is handled the better. This principle particularly applies when aseptic conditions are less than ideal. On the ward, minor procedures such as bladder catheterisation or insertion of a chest drain should be performed using a **no-touch technique**.

MINIMISING INFECTION FROM THE PATIENT'S SKIN

The patient's skin, especially the perineal area, is the source of up to half of all wound infections. These can be minimised by the following measures:

- **Removing body hair**—body hair was thought to be an important source of wound contamination but this is no longer believed. Hair is removed only to allow the incision site to be seen and the wound to be closed without including hair. Shaving produces numerous small abrasions which rapidly become infected with skin commensals. If shaving is required, it should be done as close to the time of surgery as possible. Most surgeons now restrict hair removal to clipping away just enough to provide adequate skin access. An effective alternative is to use depilatory creams which avoid trauma. For small operations on the head, hair is not usually removed
- **Painting the skin with antiseptic solutions**—povidone-iodine or chlorhexidine in alcoholic or aqueous solution is applied to a wide area around the proposed operation site ('skin prep'); this is now done only when the patient is on the operating table, but in the past patients were subjected to a series of applications of antiseptics such as gentian violet for several days beforehand!
- **Draping the patient**—the standard procedure is to isolate the operating area by placing sterile drapes made of cotton or an impervious synthetic cloth over all but the immediate field of operation. However, if the drapes become soaked with blood or other body fluids, bacteria may be drawn through by capillary action. Therefore, impermeable sterile paper sheets known as **ventiles** are usually placed beforehand beneath the drapes. For high-risk surgery such as joint replacements, plastic or impermeable paper drapes with adhesive borders are often used
- **Investing the skin** at the operation site with a thin film of adherent clear plastic—the skin incision is then made through the plastic film so that little bare skin is exposed. This method has proved counter-productive because bacteria multiply beneath the film. Films impregnated with povidone-iodine may be better

REDUCING INFECTION FROM INTERNAL VISCERA

The large bowel teems with potentially pathogenic bacteria and the peritoneal cavity is inevitably contaminated in any operation at which the large bowel is opened. Therefore wherever possible, the large bowel should be mechanically cleansed prior to operation by the use of propietary bowel preparation agents such as sodium picosulphate. Pathogenic bacteria are also found in obstructed small bowel. The same applies to the stomach and small bowel of patients on H_2-receptor blocking drugs (see Ch. 14) where the normal bactericidal effect of gastric acid is lost.

STERILISATION OF INSTRUMENTS AND OTHER SUPPLIES (see Table 6.1)

In modern surgical practice, infection from instruments, swabs, equipment and intravenous fluids has been virtually eliminated by the supply of sterile packs from a central sterile supplies department (CSSD). Reusable instruments and drapes are sterilised by high-pressure steam autoclaving according to strict regulations. Most disposable items are purchased in pre-sterilised, sealed packs. Sterilisation in small autoclaves near the operating theatre should only be performed if instruments in short supply are required for successive operations. Sterilisation by any method is likely to be ineffective unless all organic material is removed from instruments by thorough cleaning first.

Problems are posed by sterilising instruments which would be damaged by heat. These include plastics, cystoscopic lenses, flexible endoscopes and electrical equipment. These can be sterilised using a variety of chemical methods such as ethylene oxide gas. Glutaraldehyde in a 2% concentration is commonly used for endoscopic instruments which need to be reused several times during an endoscopy session. They must be immersed in sterile water before use. Special precautions are required to prevent chemical injury to staff.

World-wide, many surgical instruments are prepared by boiling water 'sterilisers'. Boiling water is markedly inferior to other methods of sterilisation but is included here as it may be the only practical method in developing countries owing to cost and technical reasons. Boiling water kills most vegetative organisms within 15 minutes but spores are not killed by this method. All organic debris should, as always, be scrupulously removed, then the instruments immersed in visibly boiling water, returned to the boil and boiled continuously for at least 30 minutes to ensure hepatitis and human immunodeficiency viruses are destroyed.

SURGICAL TECHNIQUE

Surgical technique plays an important part in minimising the risk of operative infection. Non-vital tissue and collections of fluid and blood are particularly vulnerable to colonisation by infecting organisms, which may enter via the bloodstream even if direct contamination has been avoided by aseptic technique. Tissue damage should be kept to the minimum in the course of surgery by careful handling and retraction and by avoiding unnecessary diathermy coagulation. Haematoma formation is minimised by careful attention to haemostasis and placing drains into potential sites of fluid collection; **closed-drainage** or **suction-drainage** systems reduce the risk of organisms tracking back into the wound from the ward environment.

During extensive resections of bowel, ligation of its blood supply allows bacteria to permeate the wall (**translocation**) and this may contaminate the peritoneal cavity.

Gross faecal contamination is associated with a high risk of infection and great care is taken in operations where the bowel is opened. In large bowel perforation, great care is taken to physically remove faecal contamination; a planned 'second look' laparotomy after 48 hours may be advisable.

After performing anastomoses involving large bowel, a drain is often placed in the vicinity to remove collections of blood and other fluids and perhaps to minimise the danger of general peritoneal contamination should the anastomosis leak. Many surgeons now regard this as ineffective and possibly harmful.

Table 6.1 Time and temperature requirements for sterilisation by different methods

Method	Equipment to be sterilised	Temperature	Time
Steam autoclave	Unwrapped instruments and bowls Instrument sets, dressings and rubber	126°C 123°C	10 mins 3 mins
Ethylene oxide gas	Heat-sensitive materials; plastics, endoscopes, electrical equipment	55°C	2–24 hrs
Liquid glutaraldehyde	Cystoscopes and other urological equipment, plastics and heat-sensitive equipment required urgently	Room temperature	10 mins

PROPHYLACTIC ANTIBIOTICS

Despite the best aseptic techniques, some operations carry a high risk of wound infection as well as other infective complications; these can be reduced dramatically by using prophylactic antibiotics. The antibiotics chosen should be matched to the organisms likely to occur in the area of the operation and should be bactericidal rather than bacteriostatic. The relative risk of postoperative infection in different types of operation is summarised in Box 6.3.

As a general principle, prophylactic antibiotics are indicated if the anticipated risk of infection exceeds 10%, i.e. all emergency abdominal surgery, all elective colonic operations, and upper gastrointestinal operations for malignancy. Prophylactic antibiotics are also used by many surgeons for operations in the 5–10% risk category, e.g. cholecystectomy. In addition, prophylactic antibiotics are indicated in inherently low-risk cases where the consequences of infection are catastrophic, e.g. operations employing prosthetic implants or in patients with mitral stenosis or other cardiac defects at risk of subacute infective endocarditis. Prophylactic antibiotics can reduce postoperative infection rates in high-risk cases by 75%, and may almost entirely eliminate infection in lower-risk cases.

KEY POINTS

Box 6.3 Relative risk of infection in surgical wounds

Risk 2–5%

Clean operations with no preoperative infection and no opening of gastrointestinal, respiratory or urinary tracts (e.g. inguinal herniorrhaphy, breast lump excision, ligation of varicose veins)

Risk less than 10%

Clean operations with gastrointestinal, respiratory or urinary tracts opened but with minimal contamination (e.g. elective cholecystectomy, transurethral resection of prostate, excision of minimally inflamed appendix)

Risk about 20%

Operations where tissues inevitably become contaminated but without pre-existing infection, e.g. elective large bowel operations, appendicectomy where the appendix is perforated or gangrenous, fresh traumatic skin wounds (except on the face)

Risk greater than 30%

Operations in the presence of infection, e.g. abscesses within body cavities, small bowel perforation, delayed operations on traumatic wounds

Risk greater than 50%

Emergency colonic surgery (bowel unprepared) for perforation or obstruction

---

In the great majority of wound-related infections, the organisms are introduced during the operation and become established during the next 24 hours. Thus, if prophylactic antibiotics are to be effective, high blood levels must be achieved during the operation at the time contamination occurs. To achieve this, the first dose of antibiotic should be given either 1 hour before operation or preferably intravenously at induction of anaesthesia; prophylactic antibiotics should not be given any earlier as this may encourage resistant organisms to proliferate. A single preoperative dose of antibiotic is probably sufficient provided it is rapidly bactericidal and the inoculum of bacteria is small; long operations with heavy blood loss merit a second perioperative dose of antibiotics, e.g. ruptured abdominal aortic aneurysm. Many surgeons prefer to give two additional doses postoperatively but there is little evidence of additional benefit. Longer courses of prophylactic antibiotics are certainly of no advantage and may encourage resistant strains of organisms to emerge.

In general, intravenous antibiotics provide the most predictable blood levels; peak tissue levels are achieved within 1 hour of injection. For prophylaxis against anaerobes, metronidazole administered rectally gives equivalent blood and tissue levels to intravenous administration although these are not reached until 2–4 hours after administration. Oral metronidazole is usually inappropriate because of unreliable absorption and enforced perioperative starvation.

Operations involving bowel and biliary system

Patients having these operations are at risk mainly from a mixture of Gram-negative bacilli (*Enterobacteriaceae* family), faecal anaerobes (*Bacteroides fragilis*) and *Staphylococcus aureus*. Less commonly, enterococci cause surgical infection, notably *E. faecalis* (formerly *Strep. faecalis*).

The most commonly used prophylactic antibiotic regimens are:

- For biliary surgery—a cephalosporin alone (e.g. cefotaxime or cefuroxime)
- For colonic and other bowel surgery—either a combination of a cephalosporin (as for biliary surgery) and metronidazole or else a combination of gentamicin, benzylpenicillin (or ampicillin) and metronidazole. The latter combination is often preferred for bowel-related prophylaxis as it covers enterococci as well as the other organisms expected
- For appendicectomy—rectal metronidazole alone, given 2 hours before operation; this has proved as effective as any other regimen. The evidence for the beneficial effect of metronidazole in preventing infection after appendicectomy is now so strong that it may be negligent not to use it

The choice of antibiotics for prophylaxis must be kept under review because organisms change their sensitivities. An important consideration in this regard is that aminoglycosides such as gentamicin do not alter the bowel flora because their concentration in the lumen is low; this is in contrast to the cephalosporins and ampicillin. In consequence, there is a rising tide of beta-lactam-resistant bowel organisms insensitive to cephalosporins and ampicillin but sensitive to aminoglycosides. If resistant staphylococci are a problem, vancomycin may be necessary for prophylaxis.

Operations involving implantation of prostheses

Vascular grafts and joint replacements are at particular risk from *Staph. aureus* infection. Coagulase-negative staphylococci (e.g. *Staph. epidermidis*) may also be implicated and, very rarely, coliforms. Flucloxacillin is the agent of first choice for prophylaxis but gentamicin is usually added for extra protection. Cephalosporins are often used but they are less efficacious against staphylococci than flucloxacillin or gentamicin. Multiply-resistant *Staph. aureus* (MRSA) is becoming a more common cause of prosthetic infection. In areas where the risk is substantial, prophylaxis with vancomycin is appropriate.

Operations where ischaemic or necrotic muscle may remain

Lower limb amputations for arterial insufficiency and major traumatic injuries involving muscle are susceptible to gas gangrene and tetanus. **Clostridia** are highly sensitive to benzylpenicillin and metronidazole, one of which should be given in high dose as early as possible after major trauma and before major amputations for ischaemia.

PREVENTION OF CROSS-INFECTION (NOSOCOMIAL INFECTION)

Cross-infection is the term used to describe infection transmitted from other patients in the nearby hospital environment and it is rare. It should be distinguished from **colonisation** with other patients' bacteria, which is common. Cross-infection is mainly spread via food, staff, medical equipment or ward furnishings. Whenever there is patient contact which might result in transfer of infection outside of the operating theatre, the same principles of asepsis should be applied, although the achievable level of aseptic technique is lower. Doctors are probably the worst offenders as regards transfer of infection—for example, by removing dressings to inspect wounds in the open ward, by failing to wash hands between patients and by careless aseptic technique when performing ward procedures such as bladder catheterisation. Minimising patient movements between wards and hospital units also decreases cross-infection rates.

A patient with an infection which is potentially dangerous to other patients should be isolated and barrier-nursed in a single room. These infections include *Streptococcus pyogenes*, open tuberculosis and infective diarrhoeas. Infection with MRSA requires a patient to be transferred to an isolation area in the ward or, if the patient is in intensive care, transferred to an isolation room within the unit to avoid having to close to new admissions (see Ch. 1, p. 13).

ANAESTHESIA

GENERAL PRINCIPLES

Some form of anaesthesia is required for almost every surgical procedure, with the aim of preventing pain in all cases, minimising stress for the patient in most, and providing special conditions for some operations, e.g. muscular relaxation in abdominal surgery. The choice of anaesthetic techniques includes **topical (surface) anaesthesia, local anaesthetic infiltration or regional nerve block, spinal or epidural anaesthesia** and **general anaesthesia**. Methods other than general anaesthesia may be supplemented with intravenous sedation if the patient is anxious (e.g. with benzodiazepines). Intravenous sedation with these drugs produces relaxation, anxiolysis and amnesia whilst retaining protective reflexes. However, unconsciousness can be produced by these drugs and they must be carefully titrated to produce the desired effects. Intravenous sedation with benzodiazepines does not provide pain relief; if needed, this must be achieved by local anaesthesia or intravenous analgesics, for example.

CHOICE OF ANAESTHETIC TECHNIQUE

Combining local or regional anaesthesia (for pain relief) with a light general anaesthetic can minimise postoperative respiratory and cardiovascular depression compared with general anaesthesia alone, reducing postoperative morbidity. An example is the use of caudal anaesthesia in perineal operations. Local or regional anaesthesia can also be used at the end of an operation to provide postoperative pain relief; for example, intercostal nerve blocks after an abdominal operation allow more comfortable breathing and coughing, reducing the

71

likelihood of respiratory complications. Another common example is wound infiltration with local anaesthetic agents, e.g. bupivacaine. The main factors influencing choice of anaesthesia are summarised in Box 6.4

Careful selection of appropriate drug combinations for each case and close liaison between surgical and anaesthetic staff before, during and after operation greatly enhance postoperative recovery. The use of a **'high-dependency' recovery area**, where at-risk patients can be intensively nursed and monitored postoperatively, also plays an important part in early recovery from major surgery.

KEY POINTS

Box 6.4 Choice of anaesthetic technique

1. Local anaesthesia

In general, used for calm and rational patients when no autonomic discomfort is anticipated:

- Minor operations, e.g. excision of small skin lesions or dental operations
- Minor but painful procedures, e.g. insertion of chest drain, siting of peripheral venous cannulae
- Unavailability of general anaesthetic expertise, e.g. in developing countries
- Patients unfit for general anaesthesia, e.g. cardiac and respiratory cripples
- Ambulatory ('day case') surgery
- Patients unwilling to undergo general anaesthesia
- Use of combined local anaesthetic and vasoconstrictor to provide a relatively bloodless operative field (note: this must never be used in the extreme peripheries, i.e. digits, penis, nose)

2. Regional nerve block

- Minor surgery requiring wide field of anaesthesia, e.g. femoral nerve block for varicose vein surgery, pudendal block for forceps delivery
- When it is undesirable to inject local anaesthetic into the operation site, e.g. drainage of an abscess (local anaesthesia works less well in inflamed tissue)
- To avoid tissue distortion from local infiltration in delicate surgery
- Short-lived, wide-field ambulatory anaesthesia for reduction of forearm fractures or hand surgery (Bier's intravenous regional anaesthesia)

3. Epidural and spinal anaesthesia

- Lower limb surgery, e.g. amputations
- Lower abdominal, groin, pelvic and perineal surgery, e.g. caesarean sections, inguinal hernia repair, prostatectomy, bladder and urethral surgery

4. Intravenous sedation or intravenous analgesia alone

- Short-lived uncomfortable procedures where local anaesthesia is impractical, e.g. gastrointestinal endoscopy, musculoskeletal manipulation

5. Intravenous sedation combined with local anaesthesia

- Potentially unpleasant procedures despite adequate local anaesthesia, e.g. wisdom tooth extraction, toenail operations, siting of central venous lines

6. Regional analgesia with light general anaesthesia

- Caudal epidural plus general anaesthesia for operations in the perineal area, e.g. transurethral prostatectomy or resection of bladder tumours, haemorrhoidectomy, circumcision. This provides perioperative and postoperative analgesia

7. General anaesthesia

- Where all of the above are unsuitable or difficult to achieve
- Severe patient apprehension or patient preference for general anaesthesia
- Major or prolonged operations
- Abdominal or thoracic operations requiring muscle relaxation
- Where it is necessary to secure the airway by intubation
- Special indications, e.g. neurosurgery

BASIC SURGICAL TECHNIQUES

INCISION TECHNIQUE

CHOICE OF INCISION

The purpose of most skin incisions is to gain access to underlying tissues or body cavities. The first consideration when planning a surgical incision must be to achieve good access. Furthermore, the incision should be placed in a position which will allow it to be extended if necessary. Despite patients' impressions, the length of an incision (and the number of sutures required for closure) has little bearing on the rate of healing; the success of an operation should not be put at risk by inadequate access.

Secondary considerations in the choice of incision are as follows:

- **Orientation of skin tension lines (based on Langer's lines) and skin creases**—wherever possible, incisions should be made parallel to the lines of skin tension determined by the orientation of dermal collagen (e.g. a 'collar' incision for thyroid operations) as the wound is less likely to break down, there is minimal distortion, and healing with little scar tissue gives a better cosmetic result
- **Strength and healing potential of the tissues**—the nature and distribution of muscle and fascia, particularly in different parts of the abdominal wall, influences the strength of the repair. For example, a vertical lower midline incision situated in the linea alba where the abdominal wall consists of a strong layer of fascia is less prone to incisional herniation than a paramedian incision lateral to the midline
- **The anatomy of underlying structures, particularly nerves**—the incision line should run parallel to, but some distance away from, the expected course of underlying structures, reducing the risk of damage. For example, to gain access to the submandibular gland, the incision is made parallel to and 2 cm below the lower border of the mandible to avoid the mandibular branch of the facial nerve
- **Cosmetic considerations**—wherever possible, incisions should be placed in the least conspicuous position such as in a skin crease or a site that will later be concealed by clothing, e.g. a transverse suprapubic (**Pfannenstiel** or bucket-handle) incision below the 'bikini' line for operations on the bladder, uterus or ovary, a peri-areolar incision for breast biopsy

DISSECTION AND HANDLING OF DEEPER TISSUES

The skin consists of thin **epidermis** and dense, somewhat thicker **dermis**, as well as the underlying fatty **hypodermis** which may be as much as 10 cm thick in an obese individual.

Once the skin incision has been made, the scalpel is mainly reserved for incising fascia and other fibrous structures like breast tissue. Anatomical detail is exposed and displayed by a combination of blunt and sharp dissection. The purpose of dissection is to protect structures which might be damaged by bold incisions and to preserve blood supply and venous drainage. **Blunt dissection** involves teasing or stripping tissues apart using fingers, swabs or blunt instruments, following natural tissue planes. **Sharp dissection** with scissors and forceps or scalpel is used where tissues have to be cut and also to display small structures. Some surgeons prefer sharp to blunt dissection in general, believing it causes less tissue trauma. Most dissection, however, involves a combination of both.

PRINCIPLES OF HAEMOSTASIS

Bleeding is an unavoidable part of surgery. Blood loss should be minimised because bleeding obscures the operative field and hampers operative technique (the finer the surgery, the more continued bleeding interferes with visibility and quality of outcome), and because the loss has to be made up later. Excessive bleeding can be averted by judicious dissection with control of bleeding as the operation proceeds, and by minimising the area of raw tissue exposed at the operation site by accurately siting the incision and by avoiding opening unnecessary tissue planes.

CLIPPING, LIGATION AND UNDER-RUNNING

Ligation is obligatory when large vessels are divided and desirable for vessels larger than about 1 mm calibre (see Fig. 6.1). If the end of a bleeding vessel cannot be grasped by haemostat forceps, a suture can be used to encircle the vessel and its surrounding tissues, a technique often described as **under-running**. It is particularly useful for a bleeding artery in the fibrous base of a peptic ulcer.

DIATHERMY

Diathermy achieves haemostasis by local intravascular coagulation and contraction of the vessel wall caused by heating (-*thermy*) generated by particular electrical waveforms. However, enough heat is also produced to burn the tissues which may be needlessly damaged by careless use, particularly near the skin. Diathermy is ineffective for large vessels which should be ligated.

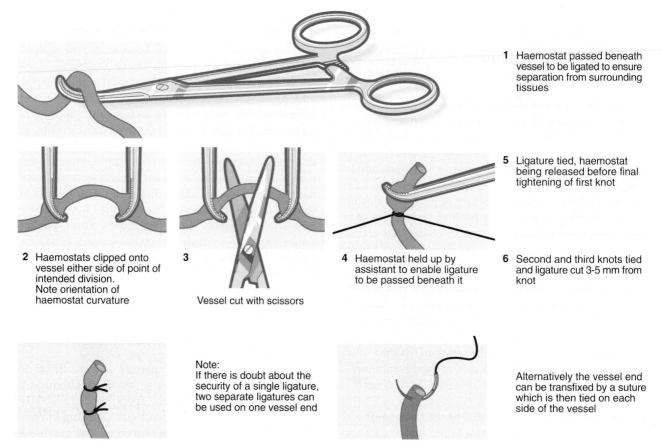

1 Haemostat passed beneath vessel to be ligated to ensure separation from surrounding tissues

5 Ligature tied, haemostat being released before final tightening of first knot

2 Haemostats clipped onto vessel either side of point of intended division.
   Note orientation of haemostat curvature

3

Vessel cut with scissors

4 Haemostat held up by assistant to enable ligature to be passed beneath it

6 Second and third knots tied and ligature cut 3-5 mm from knot

Note:
If there is doubt about the security of a single ligature, two separate ligatures can be used on one vessel end

Alternatively the vessel end can be transfixed by a suture which is then tied on each side of the vessel

Fig. 6.1 Techniques of haemostasis

There are three main variants of diathermy, illustrated in Figure 6.2, and all three modes are available on modern diathermy machines.

Monopolar diathermy is the most widely used for operative haemostasis but there is wide dispersion of the coagulating and heating effects, making it unsuitable for use near nerves and other delicate structures. Since the current passes through the patient's body, there is a risk of coagulating vessels en passant (e.g. diathermy used in circumcision may cause penile thrombosis), as well as provoking arrhythmias in patients with cardiac pacemakers. Monopolar diathermy may also result in skin burns at the indifferent electrode plate if skin contact is poor or if the plate becomes wet during operation. Current recommendations to improve contact include shaving hair from the skin where the plate is placed and using disposable self-adhesive diathermy plates.

Bipolar diathermy is used mainly for fine surgery and it requires accurate grasping of the bleeding vessel. It uses low levels of electrical power, there is almost no electrical dispersion from the tip of the forceps and much less heat is generated. The main advantages are minimal tissue damage around the point of coagulation and safety in relation to nearby nerves, blood vessels and cardiac pacemakers.

Cutting diathermy is mainly used for dividing large masses of muscle (e.g. during thoracotomy or access to the hip joint) and cutting vascular tissues (e.g. breast). The intention is a form of sharp dissection, at the same time coagulating the numerous small blood vessels as the tissue is cut; unfortunately this is not always wholly effective. A blend of cutting and coagulation is sometimes used.

TOURNIQUET AND EXSANGUINATION

This technique is used in surgery of the limbs and hands where a bloodless field is particularly desirable. For the whole limb, a pneumatic tourniquet is placed proximally around the limb. The limb is exsanguinated by elevation and spiral application of a rubber bandage (Esmark) or ring exsanguinator from the periphery; the tourniquet is then inflated. Upper limb tourniquets must not be left inflated for more than 30 minutes and lower limb tourniquets for more than about 1 hour to avoid the risk of necrosis.

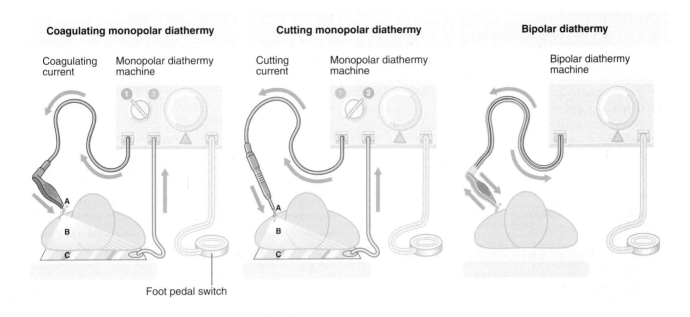

Coagulating monopolar diathermy

Coagulating current | Monopolar diathermy machine

Cutting monopolar diathermy

Cutting current | Monopolar diathermy machine

Bipolar diathermy

Bipolar diathermy machine

Foot pedal switch

Fig. 6.2 Three modes of diathermy

PRESSURE

Pressure is a useful means of controlling bleeding until platelet aggregation, reactive vasoconstriction and blood coagulation take over. It can be used for emergency control of severe arterial or venous bleeding but is equally useful for controlling diffuse small-vessel bleeding from a large raw area, e.g. liver bed after cholecystectomy. Pressure is usually applied with gauze swabs which must be kept in position for at least 10 minutes.

For intractable bleeding which is not amenable to ligature, diathermy or suture, various resorbable packing materials, e.g. oxidised cellulose, can be left in position until haemostasis occurs, allowing the wound to be closed. If bleeding simply cannot be controlled—for example, after liver injury—the bleeding cavity can be packed with gauze swabs which are left in situ and removed 48–72 hours later at a further operation. Bleeding, once controlled by this method, rarely recurs.

When a raw cavity has been created beneath the skin, external pressure dressings are sometimes a useful method of controlling potential postoperative oozing and minimising haematoma formation, e.g. after breast lump excision.

HYPOTENSIVE ANAESTHESIA

This method of anaesthesia is sometimes employed when marked diffuse bleeding is anticipated, e.g. prostatectomy, or where a bloodless field is desirable for fine dissection but where a tourniquet is impossible, e.g.

parotid surgery. The anaesthetist achieves controlled hypotension by the judicious infusion of drugs such as nitroprusside.

SUTURING AND SURGICAL REPAIR

TYPES OF SUTURE MATERIAL

Numerous types of suture are available (see Box 6.5), the most important distinction being between **absorbable** and **non-absorbable** materials. This clear-cut difference has been blurred by the advent of **slowly absorbed sutures**, e.g. polydioxanone (PDS). The groups can be subdivided into **natural** and **synthetic** materials and further subdivided into **monofilament** and **polyfilament** (braided) materials. The choice of suture material depends upon the task at hand, the handling qualities and personal preference.

Absorbable versus non-absorbable materials

The strength of absorbable sutures declines at a predictable rate for each type of material, although the suture material remains in the wound for a much longer period.

In increasing duration of useful strength, the main absorbable materials are:

● Plain catgut and chromic catgut—useful strength lasts 3 and 5 days respectively

75

KEY POINTS

Box 6.5 Suture materials and their characteristics

Typical brand names are given in brackets

Absorbable
- Plain catgut—natural monofilament
- Chromic catgut—natural monofilament
- Polyglycolic acid—synthetic braided (Dexon)
- Polyglactin—synthetic braided (Vicryl)
- Polydioxanone—synthetic monofilament (PDS, Maxon)

Non-absorbable
- Silk—natural braided
- Linen—natural braided
- Stainless steel wire—monofilament or braided
- Nylon—synthetic, usually monofilament (Ethilon)
- Polyester—synthetic braided (Ticron, and others)
- Polypropylene—synthetic monofilament (Prolene)
- Polytetrafluoroethylene (PTFE)—synthetic 'expanded' monofilament (Goretex)

- Modified polyglactin (Vicryl Rapide)—useful strength about 6 days
- Polyglycolic acid (Dexon) and polyglactin (Vicryl)— useful strength lasts about 10 days
- Polydioxanone (PDS)—retains its strength for at least 28 days

The strength of catgut declines even more quickly in the presence of infection or gastric acid, but this is not true of the synthetic absorbable sutures.

The eventual elimination of absorbable materials from the body overcomes the problem of a permanent foreign body which can harbour infection. Absorbable sutures are often used in the skin to avoid the need for removal; typical applications are minor skin operations, median sternotomies, surgery in children, circumcisions and vasectomies. Catgut sutures may give a poorer cosmetic result because of the inflammatory response they pro-voke but polyglycolic acid/polyglactin (undyed) gives good results as it is removed by hydrolysis without inflammation. The newer, modified, short-lived poly-glactin seems to have ideal properties for skin closure.

Non-absorbable sutures retain most of their strength indefinitely. They are used where the repair will take a long time to reach full strength (e.g. abdominal wall closure) or will be inherently weak (e.g. inguinal and incisional hernia repairs). Non-absorbable sutures are also widely used for skin closure; synthetic mono-filament sutures give the best cosmetic results and are most easily and painlessly removed. Subcuticular sutures, which do not penetrate the epidermis, give an excellent cosmetic result.

Natural versus synthetic materials

Catgut has been used as a suture and ligature material since before Roman times, derived from the material used for musical instrument strings. It consists mainly of collagen and is actually made from the dried small bowel submucosa of sheep or cattle. Catgut is still a widely used material, and modern manufacturing techniques have ensured a high and consistent quality. Silk and linen also have a long and distinguished history but their use is declining. Many surgeons believe that silk has the best handling and knotting properties of any material, but it provokes a strong inflammatory response exceeded only by linen. Silk is mainly used for skin sutures, where its softness means there are no sharp ends to prick the nearby skin. This is particularly important for operations involving the mouth and the perineum. Linen thread is now used rarely and mainly for ligating blood vessels. In general, natural materials are about half the price of the synthetics, a factor of importance in developing countries.

The main advantages of synthetic absorbable suture materials are that they are stronger than catgut and provoke little or no inflammatory reaction. They can be designed to meet specific requirements of absorbability, period of retention of strength, and handling properties.

Non-absorbable synthetic materials, similarly, do not provoke inflammatory reactions. Polyesters, nylon and polypropylene all retain virtually all their strength over long periods in the tissues; this is particularly important when they are used to suture arterial prostheses. All natural materials deteriorate over time and silk used for arterial prostheses has a high long-term failure rate leading to false aneurysm formation.

Monofilament versus polyfilament sutures

Monofilament materials have an extremely smooth surface and can be pulled through the tissues with minimal friction; this makes them easier to insert and remove than polyfilament braided materials. On the other hand, monofilament materials are stiff, springy and more difficult to knot. Braided materials have the best handling qualities, but their interstices provide a haven for bacteria. When used at a surface (e.g. skin or bowel wall) they tend to act as a 'wick', drawing infected material in. This problem is partly overcome by the manufacturer's application of surface coatings.

Wire sutures

Metal wire sutures have now largely been displaced by the non-absorbable synthetics. Stainless steel wire is, however, extensively used in orthopaedic surgery for bone fixation and for closure of sternotomy wounds in cardiac surgery. It is virtually inert but its main disadvantages are high rates of glove penetration and late breakage due to metal fatigue.

GAUGE OF SUTURE MATERIAL

The gauge of suture chosen for a particular task depends largely on practical experience. This takes into account the following factors:

● Strength of repair required
● Number of sutures to be placed—the greater the number, the finer can be the gauge
● Type of suture material being used—for a given gauge, the various materials have different strengths; catgut is the weakest
● Cosmetic requirements—multiple fine sutures give a better cosmetic result than fewer heavier sutures

The traditional method of describing suture gauge (US Pharmacopoeia) is confusing for the newcomer and derives from the time when sutures were much thicker than those used today. The finest suture then was designated gauge 1, with gauge 2 and upwards applying to heavier sutures. As finer and finer sutures came into use, the scale had to be taken progressively backwards from 1, i.e. gauges 0, 00 (i.e. 2/0), 000 (3/0) and so on. Nowadays, the finest suture is 10/0 which is used for extremely delicate surgery such as in the eye. A more rational metric gauge, based on suture diameter, is in use but the traditional gauge is still more widely used. A simple guide to the use of different gauges is outlined in Box 6.6.

KEY POINTS

Box 6.6 Guide to suture gauges for common procedures

Skin
● Face 5/0 or 6/0
● Hands and limbs 3/0 or 4/0
● Elsewhere 2/0 or 3/0

Abdominal wall
● Two strands of gauge 0 ('loop nylon'), gauge 1 or gauge 2

Gut anastomoses
● 2/0 or 3/0

Arterial anastomoses
● 2/0 down to 7/0 according to size of vessel

Microsurgery (e.g. eyes, microvascular, nerve repair)
● 7/0 down to as fine as 10/0

TYPES OF SUTURE NEEDLE

Vast ranges of needles have been designed to accommodate both the various different demands of general and specialist surgery and the stringent requirements of microsurgery. Characteristics of needles and broad indications for their use are summarised in Box 6.7 and illustrated in Figure 6.3.

METHODS OF SKIN SUTURING

The objective of skin suturing is to approximate the cut edges so they will heal rapidly, leaving a minimal scar. Edges to be apposed should have been cut in a clean line and perpendicular to the skin surface; ragged or angled edges should be trimmed. The cut edges should be capable of being brought together neatly and without

---

KEY POINTS

Box 6.7 Types of suture needle

1. **Method of use**
   ● Hand-held needles—routine for skin suturing; sometimes used for abdominal wall closure
   ● Instrument-held needles—necessary for deeper access and fine control

2. **Shape of needle**
   ● Straight—skin suturing
   ● Curved-half—circle used for most purposes, quarter-circle for microvascular anastomoses, three-quarter-circle for hand closure of abdominal wall

3. **Length of needle**
   ● Range from 2–60 mm—according to depth of penetration and delicacy of surgery

4. **Tissue penetration characteristics**
   ● Round-bodied with smooth pointed tip—most soft tissues, e.g. gut, fat, muscle
   ● Trocar point (semi-cutting)—moderately tough tissues, e.g. atherosclerotic arteries, fascia
   ● Cutting point—tough tissues, e.g. skin, breast tissue

5. **Means of attachment of suture to needle**
   ● Needles with an eye requiring suture material to be threaded by hand—mainly used in developing countries so that needles can be reused
   ● 'Atraumatic' needles with suture material already attached (swaged into the end)—there is no double thickness of suture material to cause extra drag and trauma as it is pulled through the tissues, and the suture material does not detach from the needle during use

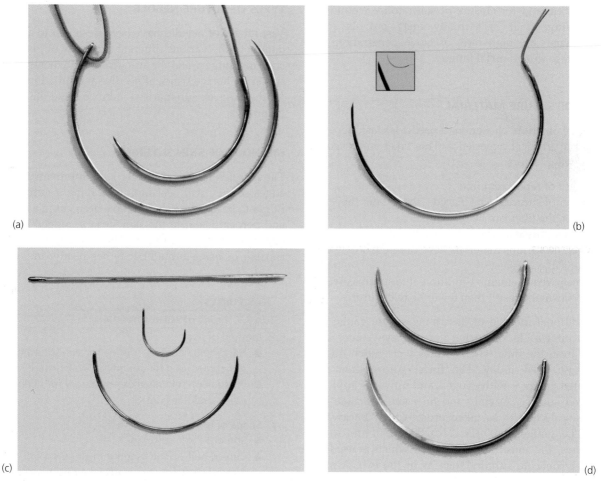

Fig. 6.3 Various types of surgical needles
(a) Two half-circle round-bodied needles, the larger with a threaded 'eye', and the smaller with the suture material swaged into it ('atraumatic' needle). Note the braided nature of the suture material. **(b)** The largest and smallest needles in common use. The larger needle is a 5/8-circle needle with a semi-cutting point, used in the hand for abdominal wall closure. Note the two strands of nylon swaged into the end. The smaller needle is used in ophthalmic surgery and has 10/0 suture material (enlarged in the inset). **(c)** Three shapes of needle. The straight needle has a cutting point and is used for skin suturing. The J-shaped needle is used mainly for femoral hernia repairs, and the large half-circle needle is for abdominal wall closure. **(d)** Two large needles showing the difference between 'round-bodied' (above) and 'cutting' ends (below).

tension; otherwise the wound may break down or the scar slowly stretch, giving an ugly result. To achieve this, it may be necessary to insert a layer of subcutaneous sutures or even mobilise the skin by undercutting in the fatty layer (see Fig. 6.4). Undue laxity should also be avoided by trimming excess skin.

There are many techniques of skin closure, the choice being governed by the nature and site of the operation and by the surgeon's personal preference. In general, facial wounds are closed with multiple fine sutures which are removed after 4 or 5 days. Abdominal and chest wound sutures are generally removed after 7 days, while sutures for wounds on the back are best left in situ for 14 days to minimise wound stretching.

Subcuticular sutures, either non-absorbable or absorbable, are often used for longer wounds in cosmetically sensitive areas, provided the risk of infection is low. Elsewhere, the choice is between interrupted and continuous suture techniques. Interrupted sutures are indicated if there is a risk of infection; if infection develops, some sutures can be removed early to facilitate drainage. If the risk of infection is high, e.g. large bowel perforation, skin wounds are better left open and closed 48–72 hours later by **delayed primary closure**. The commonly used methods of skin suturing are illustrated in Figure 6.5.

Clips and staples

Stainless steel clips (e.g. Michel clips) have been used for several decades for closing skin wounds and are popular for neck incisions after thyroidectomy. As the clips do not penetrate skin yet give good edge apposition, the cosmetic result is excellent. Staples are a relatively recent development in surgery and various instruments are used for both skin closure and bowel surgery. The skin

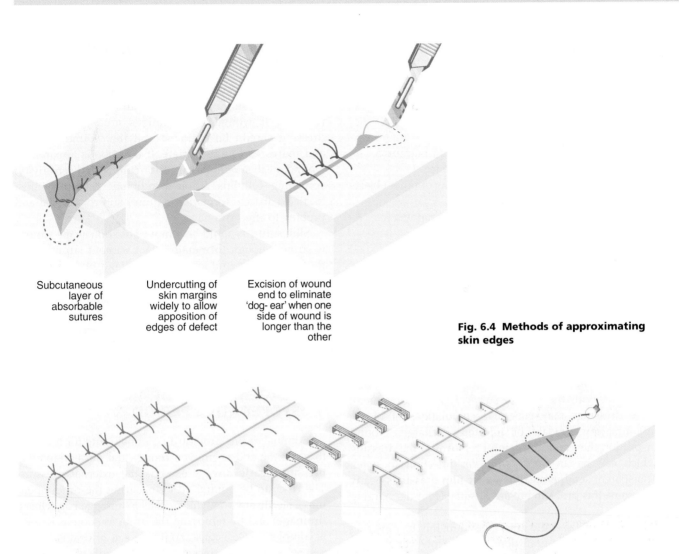

Subcutaneous layer of absorbable sutures

Undercutting of skin margins widely to allow apposition of edges of defect

Excision of wound end to eliminate 'dog- ear' when one side of wound is longer than the other

Fig. 6.4 Methods of approximating skin edges

Simple interrupted sutures

Vertical mattress sutures

Michel clips

Staples

Subcuticular

Fig. 6.5 Commonly used skin closure techniques

closure devices are similar in concept to ordinary paper staplers, with staples stored in a magazine and applied singly instead of sutures. More complex devices, which apply multiple staples simultaneously, either in a linear or circular fashion, are available for bowel anastomoses and closure of tubular viscera. Some of these devices have revolutionised surgical practice, e.g. reanastomosis of colon to rectum after Hartmann's resection or bronchial stump closure. When used for internal viscera, the staples remain in place indefinitely (see Fig. 6.6).

POSTOPERATIVE WOUND MANAGEMENT

Once a wound has been closed, the doctor has three main responsibilities: choosing the dressing, monitoring

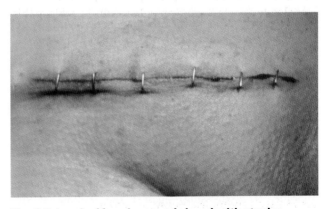

Fig. 6.6 Inguinal hernia wound closed with staples

the progress of healing and deciding when to remove the sutures.

The purposes of dressings for surgical wounds are as follows:

- To maintain the wound in a warm and moist state most conducive to healing
- To absorb or contain any superficial bleeding or inflammatory exudate
- To protect the delicate healing tissue from trauma, bacterial contamination and interference
- To prevent sutures catching on clothing or other objects
- To conceal the wound from view
- To apply pressure to the wound if haematoma formation is likely

TYPES OF WOUND DRESSING

For small surgical wounds, particularly on the face, a dressing is often unnecessary as the linear crust of inflammatory exudate performs this task admirably. In most other cases, **prepacked adhesive dressings** are used, incorporating an absorbent pad with non-stick film in contact with the wound surface. While convenient, these dressings may conceal accumulations of blood, inflammatory exudate or infected discharge. Wound inspection then requires painful removal of the dressing which can be an opportunity for infection to enter. Transparent **semipermeable plastic film dressings** neatly overcome this problem but are unsuitable for discharging wounds.

Paraffin gauze (**tulle gras**) is used mainly for covering raw areas (e.g. skin-graft donor sites). However, its non-stick paraffin content rapidly declines and blood clot and tissue proliferation soon incorporate the dressing via its open weave. As removal tends to damage the delicate new epithelium, alternative dressings such as saline-soaked gauze, **calcium alginate** (seaweed origin), **hydro-colloids** and **hydrogels** are often preferred. Newer dressings offer a more ideal wound environment with increased hydration, fewer dressing changes and greater comfort. Cost effectiveness is an issue yet to be resolved.

Gamgee is a thick cotton wool dressing material enveloped in a thin layer of gauze; this is variously used for padding sites vulnerable to trauma (e.g. amputation stumps), as pads beneath pressure bandages or as absorbent dressings for leaking wounds. **Dry dressings** are wads of dressing material (e.g. cotton gauze), usually taped or bandaged in place. Dry dressings need regular replacement and may be prevented from sticking by first placing a piece of non-adherent dressing material (e.g. Melolin, N/A dressing) against the wound. If dry dressings are used for infected wounds, exudate must not be allowed to permeate to the surface as bacteria rapidly spread from here into the environment ('strike-through').

REMOVAL OF DRESSINGS AND SUTURES

Provided the dressing remains clean and dry and the patient afebrile and generally well, there is no need to inspect clean surgical wounds until the time of suture removal. If wound complications are suspected, the dressing should be removed and the wound checked and redressed as appropriate. If infection is apparent, a wound swab should be taken for culture and sensitivity; spreading cellulitis requires antibiotic therapy, whilst localised abscess formation requires suture removal and probing to effect drainage.

Skin sutures should be removed as soon as the wound is strong enough to remain intact without support. On the back and around joints, this can take 14 days; on the abdomen, it takes about 7 days (longer in the case of steroid therapy or infection); on the face and neck healing is rapid and less influenced by functional stresses. Here, sutures can be safely removed after 3–5 days, giving a better cosmetic result.

MANAGEMENT OF DRAINS IN THE POSTOPERATIVE PERIOD

Abdominal drains provide a potential route for infection to enter the abdomen even though the intra-abdominal pressure nearly always exceeds the external pressure. The risk can be minimised by ensuring the drain opens into a sterile environment such as a drainage bag (**closed drainage**) and by removing the drain as soon as its task is completed. Decisions about removal of drains should rest with the operating surgeon who will undoubtedly have personal preferences.

The general principles of drain management are as follows:

- Suction drains help to collapse down spaces left in the tissues at operation as well as to drain blood and inflammatory exudate. These drains are mainly used after extensive excisional surgery where a large enclosed raw surface remains, e.g. after mastectomy, thyroidectomy or excision of the rectum. High-vacuum suction drains, however, should not be used near bowel for fear of suction perforation. A suction drain is usually retained only for 24 hours after operation unless substantial drainage (e.g. > 30 ml/ 24 hours) persists for longer
- Non-suction drains (e.g. large-bore silicone or rubber tubes, or corrugated drains) are mainly used for bowel and biliary anastomoses and in abscess drainage. In this case, the drain is left in place for about 5 days. Some surgeons prefer to withdraw the drain in stages so that the deep part of the drainage tract can collapse progressively, reducing the risk of leaving a deep pool of fluid

MINIMAL ACCESS SURGERY AND ENDOSCOPY

FLEXIBLE ENDOSCOPY

PRINCIPLES OF FLEXIBLE ENDOSCOPY

Strictly speaking, endoscopy applies to any method of looking into the body (see Table 6.2) through an instrument, either via an orifice such as the nose or mouth, or via an artificially created opening (e.g. laparoscopy, thoracoscopy or arthroscopy). Endoscopy using simple tubular instruments has been in use for many years and most of these methods are still in regular use, e.g. rigid sigmoidoscopy and oesophagoscopy. Developments in fibreoptics first led to a major improvement in illumination for conventional rigid endoscopes and later to the creation of flexible instruments which greatly extended the range and sophistication of endoscopic diagnostic and therapeutic techniques. The unqualified term **endoscopy** is often employed to mean gastro-intestinal endoscopy using flexible instruments with fibreoptic illumination and fibreoptic or video image transmission.

Fibreoptic illumination

Rigid endoscopes and the early flexible instruments were illuminated by tiny incandescent bulbs which were prone to failure. The amount of light they could emit was limited by the production of waste heat. These were superseded by **fibreoptic light guides** in both rigid and flexible endoscopes.

Fibreoptic light guides are used to channel light from a powerful, fan-cooled light source remote from the patient to the distal end of an endoscope. The light guides are made up of thousands of parallel glass fibres, each with total internal reflection, so that very little light is lost in transmission and no heat is transmitted. A powerful, cool light beam thus emerges from the distal end of even the longest endoscope.

Table 6.2 Summary of minimally invasive/minimal access approaches to diagnosis and treatment

Specialty area (in alphabetical order)	Diagnostic applications	Therapeutic applications
Abdomen CT or ultrasonography (note laparoscopy is covered in the adjoining text and boxes 6.8 & 6.9)	● Diagnosis of fluid collections e.g. ascites, pancreatic pseudocyst, abscess ● Percutaneous biopsy of enlarged lymph nodes, liver or pancreatic masses, other masses	● Drainage of fluid collections ● Sampling of suspected pancreatic necrosis for infection in acute pancreatitis
Anal canal	● Proctoscopy to inspect the anal canal and if necessary, biopsy lesions	● Injection or banding of haemorrhoids ● Perineal operations for rectal prolapse ● Transanal resection of tumours —'TART'
Arterial	● Arteriography (conventional or digital subtraction; magnetic resonance angiography) — demonstrating the sites and severity of arterial obstruction or aneurysms — selective or highly selective angiography for detecting the source of acute intestinal bleeding or determining the blood supply of an organ ● Ultrasound or CT diagnosis of aortic and other aneurysms ● Duplex Doppler ultrasound scanning—for carotid artery disease, peripheral arterial disease, femoro-popliteal and other graft surveillance ● Angioscopy—for direct inspection of the lumen of blood vessels	● Percutaneous transluminal angioplasty of arterial stenoses (PCTA) ● Percutaneous thrombolysis ● Embolisation for bleeding/tumours/AV malformations/preoperative treatment of vascular lesions to reduce vascularity ● Stenting of obliterative arterial disease ● Intraluminal stent grafting for aneurysms
Biliary (see also **Pancreas**)	● Distal duodenoscopy for ampullary tumours ● Diagnostic ERCP for suspected bile duct stones	● Endoscopic sphincterotomy to retrieve bile duct stones e.g. in obstructive jaundice ● Stent placement across bile duct strictures or tumours
Breast	● Fine needle aspiration cytology of solid lumps ● Stereotactic FNA or biopsy of mammographically detected lesions suspected of malignancy	● Ultrasound guided aspiration of cysts

Table 6.2 Continued

Specialty area (in alphabetical order)	Diagnostic applications	Therapeutic applications
Cardiac	• Endomyocardial biopsy for detecting rejection in heart transplants	• Angioplasty and stenting of obstructed coronary arteries • Off-pump coronary artery bypass—OPCAB (under evaluation) • Small incision or thoracoscopic approaches to standard cardiac operations using cardio-pulmonary bypass or without e,g, via partial sternotomy (under evaluation) • Percutaneous transmyocardial laser revascularisation (PMR)—cutting channels into the myocardium from lumen to attempt revascularisation—under evaluation but losing favour • Endoscopic harvesting of leg veins
Chest	• Ultrasound diagnosis of fluid collections • Thoracoscopic pleural or lung biopsy • Mediastinoscopic node biopsy	• Thoracoscopic cervico-dorsal sympathectomy for hyperhidrosis of the hands • Pleurectomy, lobectomy for benign disease
Gynaecology	• Laparoscopic diagnosis for infertility • Diagnosis of cause of acute abdomen in suspected pelvic inflammatory disease, tubal pregnancy, ovarian problems	• Laparoscopic sterilisation (tubal clipping) • Oophorectomy for palliation of breast carcinoma • Obtaining eggs for in-vitro and other forms of assisted fertilisation • Pelvic lymphadenectomy for radical cancer surgery • Operations for urinary stress incontinence
Oesophagus	• Diagnostic oesophagoscopy and biopsy—flexible instruments usually used	• Dilatation of benign oesophageal strictures • Pulsion (pushing) placement of luminal tubes and cloth covered stents for obstructing carcinoma • Palliative laser ablation of obstructing tumours—'reboring' • Injection of bleeding ulcers • Balloon compression and endoscopic sclerotherapy injection of varices • Balloon dilatation of narrow cardia in achalasia • Thoracoscopic myotomy for achalasia (Heller's operation) • Laparoscopic anti-reflux surgery
Orthopaedics	Diagnostic arthroscopy—hip, knee, ankle, shoulder, elbow and wrist	• Therapeutic arthroscopy: • Knee—removal of loose bodies; articular cartilage & menisceal surgery; cruciate reconstruction; irrigation for infection. • Shoulder—impingement decompression; shoulder stabilisation; rotator cuff repair. • Hip, elbow and ankle—removal of loose bodies; articular cartilage surgery • Wrist—percutaneous screw for scaphoid fracture
Pancreas	• Endoscopic pancreatography for suspected duct abnormalities • Endoscopic collection of exocrine secretions for cytology	• Early sphincterotomy and trawling of biliary and pancreatic ducts to relieve stone induced pancreatitis
Rectum and Colon	• Diagnostic flexible sigmoidoscopy or colonoscopy (including biopsy) for bleeding, suspected tumour, inflammatory bowel disease • Endoluminal ultrasound imaging for staging rectal cancer and determining sphincter damage • Magnetic resonance imaging for detailing the anatomy of complex fistulae	• Snare excision of polyps and adenomas • Diathermy to bleeding angiodysplasias • Diathermy loop resection of inoperable rectal tumours for palliation, or benign rectal strictures

Table 6.2 Continued

Specialty area (in alphabetical order)	Diagnostic applications	Therapeutic applications
Stomach and Duodenum	● Diagnostic inspection for ulcers and cancer ● Biopsy of ulcers and tumours ● Biopsy to diagnose *Helicobacter* infection as a cause of ulceration	● Injection treatment of acutely bleeding ulcers ● Endoscopic retrieval of foreign bodies ● Combined percutaneous and endoscopic placement of feeding gastrostomy tubes ('PEG')
Urology *Endoscopic*—usually rigid but latterly flexible	● Haematuria (staging, treatment and follow-up of bladder tumours) ● Poor urinary stream (assessment of bladder neck and prostatic obstruction) ● Ureteric obstruction (ureteroscopy or retrograde ureterography)	● Fulguration or resection of bladder tumours ● Resection of bladder neck or prostate ● Stenting of ureter to relieve stone obstruction, strictures or external compression ● Balloon dilatation of stenosed pelvi-ureteric junction via transurethral route
Percutaneous		● Direct endoscopic stone destruction and removal; indirect stone destruction using lithotripsy ● Placement of suprapubic catheters
Venous system	● Duplex Doppler ultrasound scanning—for diagnosing deep and superficial venous insufficiency	● Subfascial endoscopic perforator surgery (SEPS) for treating venous ulceration

Image transmission

The second development that was crucial in the design of flexible endoscopes was the manufacture of **coherent viewing bundles**. In these bundles, the orientation of fibres at the distal end exactly matched that at the proximal viewing end. Each fibre thus transmitted a tiny part of the distal scene to the viewing end. Here it could be inspected or photographed with a still or video camera. The view is not altered by angulation of the flexible conduit between the ends. The distal end of most flexible endoscopes allowed a viewing angle of over 100°, and the lenses gave a remarkable depth of focus. The image was so clear that accurate diagnosis could often be made on inspection alone. A later development is the CCD **(charge-coupled device) video camera**, a light- and colour-sensitive microchip placed at the distal end of a flexible endoscope. The image is transmitted via an electrical cable and is viewed on a large colour television monitor and not through an eyepiece. This system has now largely replaced the older direct viewing system.

Structure of flexible endoscopes

Most flexible endoscopes include a mechanism to steer the distal end in four directions (except for specialised ultra-slender scopes for intravascular use, for example); a distal imaging chip for video endoscopy; one or two fibreoptic light guides; a suction channel; and a channel for inflating the hollow viscus under inspection with air, doubling as a lens washing channel (see Fig. 6.7). The suction channel is also used to pass slender flexible operating tools such as tiny forceps for taking biopsies, grasping forceps for retrieving foreign bodies, laser guides for therapy (haemostasis or tumour destruction), snares for excision polyps, diathermy wires, scissors for cutting sutures and needles for injecting haemostatic agents.

APPLICATIONS OF FLEXIBLE ENDOSCOPY

Flexible endoscopes were first used to inspect the stomach in the late 1960s and the range of available instruments has progressively expanded since. There are now instruments available to inspect and cannulate the duodenal papilla, to examine all or part of the large bowel, to inspect the interior of the bile ducts at operation and to examine the bladder interior using only local anaesthesia, as well as many others.

Choledochoscopes are rigid or flexible instruments used to inspect the interior of the bile ducts at open or laparoscopic operation to ensure any stones are cleared. Their use has improved the rate of stone clearance during exploration of the common bile duct.

Narrow fibreoptic **bronchoscopes** can be passed under simple topical anaesthesia. They are used to inspect bronchi for disease and can be used to aspirate mucus plugs responsible for postoperative lobar collapse.

Angioscopy was developed for inspecting and guiding procedures within arteries. It employs slender flexible endoscopes 2–4 mm in diameter with a constant flow of saline to exclude blood. Unfortunately, they have proved to have little clinical application.

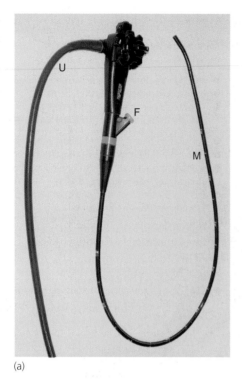

(a)

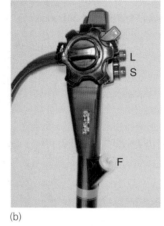

(b)

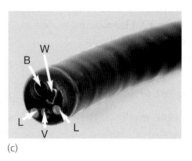

(c)

Fig. 6.7 Flexible fibreoptic gastroscope
(a) This end-viewing gastroscope is composed of a flexible main shaft **M** which is 1 m long and marked at 10-cm intervals; the distal 10 cm can be flexed in four directions to steer the instrument and obtain the best view. There is also an 'umbilical cord' **U** which is plugged into the control box and carries air to inflate the viscus, water to wash the viewing lens and suction to aspirate fluid from the lumen. There is a flush tube **F**, through which fluid can be injected to wash the stomach wall. The steering controls are better seen in photograph (b). **(b)** The steering controls consist of two concentric wheels labelled respectively **D** and **U** (down and up) and **L** and **R** (left and right). The channel **F** is also used to pass instruments, buttons to control suction **S** and air inflation and lens washing **L**. **(c)** shows the tip of the instrument in detail. The two light guides are marked **L**, **V** is the lens for the imaging chip, **W** is the exit for the inflation air and lens washing water and **B** is the channel for passing instruments and for suction. Note that the video image is transmitted up the 'scope and along the umbilical cord to the processor unit, from where it is displayed on a video monitor.

Further applications of flexible endoscopy will undoubtedly appear as endoscopes become smaller and more sophisticated.

DIAGNOSTIC UPPER GASTROINTESTINAL ENDOSCOPY

Oesophago-gastro-duodenoscopy, also known as **OGD** or **gastroscopy**, involves inspection of the upper gastrointestinal mucosa using a steerable, flexible fibreoptic endoscope. It is usually carried out under intravenous sedation on a day-case basis. Among other applications, gastroscopy enables the whole area prone to peptic ulcer disease and cancer to be directly and comprehensively examined.

Flexible endoscopy has the following advantages over gastrointestinal contrast radiology:

● Structural abnormalities such as chronic ulcers can be directly inspected whereas radiology provides only a two-dimensional image which gives little information about surface characteristics

● Benign ulcers and early malignancies are indistinguishable on radiology whereas suspicious lesions such as ulcers can be inspected and biopsied at endoscopy
● Shallow mucosal abnormalities like superficial ulceration or vascular malformations can be inspected at endoscopy
● Bile reflux through the pylorus may be visible at endoscopy
● Fibrosis and anatomical distortions from previous disease or surgery interfere much less with recognition of what is abnormal on endoscopy than on radiology
● Endoscopy can often identify the exact site of the lesion causing acute upper GI haemorrhage and give an indication of the rate of haemorrhage and the likelihood of rebleeding. Tracing the source is often impossible radiologically
● During endoscopy, therapy may be applied during the same procedure, e.g. injection of source of acute bleeding, retrieving swallowed foreign body, placement of feeding gastrostomy tube

THERAPEUTIC UPPER GASTROINTESTINAL ENDOSCOPY

Treatment of upper GI haemorrhage

First-line therapy for upper GI haemorrhage due to bleeding ulcers typically involves the injection of the ulcer using adrenaline solution alone or in combination with sclerosants. Other treatments such as laser or direct heat coagulation have proved less effective, but are still used. With such techniques, the need for urgent surgery has been substantially reduced. Patients who have acute haemorrhage from benign lesions arrested by these methods can often be managed in the long term without resort to surgery. The subject is discussed in more detail in Chapter 12. Haemorrhage due to oesophageal varices is now treated preferentially by endoscopic rubber-band ligation or injection sclerotherapy.

Treatment of oesophageal strictures

Endoscopic methods are often used for dilating benign oesophageal strictures. The endoscope is passed until the stricture is visible and then a flexible wire is passed through it into the stomach. The endoscope is removed, leaving the wire in situ. Plastic (**Celestin**) or metal (**Eder–Puestow**) dilators of increasing size are then passed over the wire which guides them safely through the stricture until sufficient dilatation has been achieved. The technique is relatively safe, can easily be repeated and avoids the need for a general anaesthetic, which is necessary when a rigid oesophagoscope is used. There is a small risk of oesophageal perforation but this is uncommon (see Fig. 6.8).

Dysphagia caused by an inoperable malignant stricture can be improved by creating a pathway through the tumour with endoscopically guided laser fulguration. Unfortunately the tumour inevitably recurs and multiple treatments are likely to be necessary. However, swallowing can be maintained and the patient's quality of life thereby improved without major surgery. In other cases, a stent can be placed endoscopically to keep the oesophagus open. This involves first dilating the stricture as for a benign stricture and then pushing a collapsed metal expanding stent covered with cloth down the oesophagus until it lies across the stricture. The cover is removed from the stent as it is deployed and it expands outwards. It also avoids a risky operation and may provide worthwhile palliation for an obstructing tumour.

DIAGNOSTIC AND THERAPEUTIC DUODENOSCOPY

A side-viewing duodenoscope can be used to inspect the duodenal papilla and guide insertion of a cannula or a variety of therapeutic tools. Cannulation allows injection of contrast material into the common bile duct and

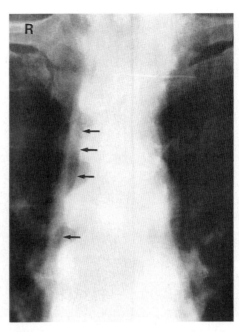

Fig. 6.8 Pneumomediastinum following perforation of an oesopheageal tumour during endoscopy
This 56-year-old man who was being investigated for difficulty in swallowing complained of chest pain after the examination. Crepitus was found in the neck due to surgical emphysema resulting from oesophageal air leaking out of the perforation and tracking up the mediastinum in to the neck.

separately into the pancreatic duct. The technique is known as ERCP (**endoscopic retrograde cholangio-pancreatography** (see Fig. 6.9 and Ch. 11)) and is now an important part of gastroenterological investigation. It is used to image the biliary duct system in preference to percutaneous transhepatic cholangiography.

ERCP can be thought of as diagnostic and therapeutic. Indications for diagnostic ERCP may be decreasing, as newer and safer techniques such as MRCP (**magnetic resonance cholangio-pancreatography**) become available. A therapeutic ERCP allows management of many disorders of the bile ducts, allowing minimal-access techniques and short hospital stays for problems that would previously have required difficult, time-consuming and dangerous operations. For example, bile duct stones can often be removed endoscopically by slitting the sphincter at the lower end (**sphincterotomy**) and retrieving them with a balloon catheter or a Dormia basket. Other therapeutic measures include insertion of stents for palliation of malignant biliary obstruction (cancer of pancreatic head, bile duct or duodenum) and for managing a postoperative bile leak.

LARGE BOWEL ENDOSCOPY (COLONOSCOPY)

Flexible endoscopes of different lengths are available for large bowel examination (see Fig. 6.10). The shortest, the

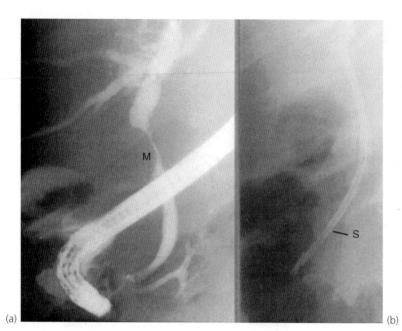

(a)

(b)

Fig. 6.9 Stenting of biliary structure
(a) ERCP showing malignant stricture of common bile duct **M** due to cholangiocarcinoma. **(b)** Stent **S** placed endoscopically across stricture for palliation.

fibreoptic sigmoidoscope, is about 60 cm long. It is simple to use and allows examination of the rectum, sigmoid and descending colon with minimal bowel preparation. Longer colonoscopes enable inspection of the entire large bowel including the caecum. Colonoscopy affords visualisation of pathological lesions, and offers an opportunity to biopsy the suspicious lesions or resect lesions such as polyps. Its use in the follow up of patients with colorectal cancer allows the search for new tumours or polyps (metachronous lesions) as well as assessing the original site of the surgery. It use in the screening of asymptomatic patients for colorectal carcinoma is controversial, mainly because of lack of patient compliance. Colonoscopy is indicated in the surveillance of patients with long-standing ulcerative colitis. It is here that the development of dysplasia is sought by taking multiple biopsies. Acutely bleeding angiodysplastic lesions can be treated with diathermy.

UROLOGICAL ENDOSCOPY

Endoscopic urology is becoming a progressively larger part of urological surgery. Most is still performed with rigid instruments but flexible instruments are being increasingly used for diagnostic cystoscopy and ureteroscopy.

Cystourethroscopy (cystoscopy) using a rigid instrument is the main diagnostic and therapeutic tool for disease of the urethra, prostate and bladder. Transurethral resection of the prostate has virtually eliminated the need for open retropubic prostatectomy and most early bladder tumours can be treated endoscopically. A similar but longer instrument, the **ureteroscope**, can now be used

for retrieving stones from the lower half of the ureter.

Endoscopic methods of percutaneous stone removal from the renal pelvis have become increasingly available (**percutaneous nephrolithotomy**). This involves creating a channel from the skin into the renal pelvis and dilating it until an endoscope can be passed. When the stone is seen, various instruments can be used to fragment it and effect removal.

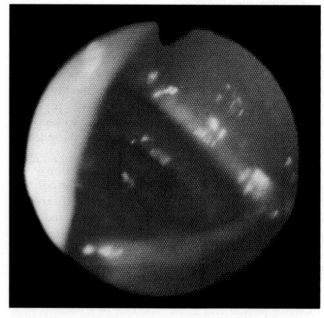

Fig. 6.10 Colonoscopic view of normal transverse colon
The transverse colon is typically triangular in cross-section when seen colonoscopically; the taenia coli form the apices.

LAPAROSCOPIC SURGERY

MINIMAL ACCESS SURGERY

After many years of sporadic attempts to reduce the trauma caused to patients by open surgery, the last few years have seen an explosion in interest and rapid development of techniques to achieve accurate diagnosis and provide treatment with the least possible tissue injury. Laparoscopic surgery was the first to catch the public's imagination but other techniques such as lithotripsy, percutaneous stone removal and angioplasty advanced in parallel. Initially called **minimally invasive surgery**, the principle of minimal access surgery is that if less tissue is damaged by avoiding or minimising surgical incisions, then less pain is likely to be experienced afterwards and the physiological responses to injury which retard recovery will be reduced. The result was intended to cause less patient suffering and allow a more rapid return to normal life. Gynaecologists led the way with laparoscopic diagnosis and procedures, particularly tubal ligation, but little development in instrumentation occurred until laparoscopic cholecystectomy emerged as a viable and extremely popular option. The pioneers stimulated the interest of general surgeons, and enthusiasm for these novel techniques (untested by the usual scientific criteria) was shared by uncritical popular media and the public. As interest and demand grew, commercial companies invested heavily to develop and improve laparoscopic equipment. 'Chip' CCD cameras appeared which allowed superior full-colour images, and practical courses proliferated rapidly to teach the techniques to surgeons.

Progress and diversity in minimal access surgery and radiology is unstoppable because of demand from interested clinicians and patients, as well as from health economists who believe some of these techniques save money by reducing hospital stay. On the negative side, the high cost of equipment, particularly if disposable instruments are used, the additional time taken for some procedures, as well as reports of high rates of serious complications, demand that proper controlled studies are performed and the techniques evaluated without emotional pressure. The phase of extreme enthusiasm has now passed and each technique is being critically evaluated against previous standards of open surgery. The expected result is that some techniques will become standard practice, some will disappear altogether and others will find favour for particular groups of patients.

An example of rapid progress in minimal access surgery is provided by cholecystectomy. Early laparoscopic cholecystectomy was hampered by poor equipment, poor imaging and lack of experience. Now that equipment is first class, experience has disseminated and audit is in place, the indications, contraindications and risks have largely become clear.

LAPAROSCOPY

Laparoscopy or peritoneoscopy has been in wide use clinically by gynaecologists since the early 1970s for diagnosing pelvic disorders and for sterilisation by tubal ligation. In the early days, laparoscopy had limited application in general surgery and was largely confined to visually guided liver biopsies. The first therapeutic gastrointestinal procedure was probably an appendicectomy performed by Semm in 1983; in 1987, Mouret first removed a diseased gall bladder laparoscopically in France. Since then, the techniques have been adopted on a broad scale by general and thoracic surgeons as a method of performing abdominal and thoracic operations via a series of small abdominal punctures rather than through large incisions.

Laparoscopy in general surgery has both diagnostic and therapeutic applications. The **diagnostic applications** are well recognised and are used increasingly as surgeons gain experience. As regards **therapeutic applications**, the advantages and potential complications of laparoscopic-guided biliary tract surgery and thoracoscopic thoracodorsal sympathectomy are now well understood. However, some of the results of 'this great uncontrolled experiment' have been catastrophic in inexperienced hands, prompting more intense scrutiny of other novel applications such as appendicectomy, inguinal hernia repair, laparoscopic-assisted colectomy and many others. These are at various stages of investigation, controversy and acceptance.

Thoracoscopy is a variation on laparoscopy and uses similar instruments for diagnostic and therapeutic applications in the thorax (see details in Ch. 24).

TECHNIQUE OF LAPAROSCOPY

Laparoscopy is usually performed under general anaesthesia. A pneumoperitoneum is first created to allow visualisation of the peritoneal cavity by introducing carbon dioxide under controlled pressure. This is done most safely by direct visualisation of the peritoneal space and placement of a Hasson-type cannula. The use of an insufflation needle (Verress needle) is still popular, especially among gynaecologists, but it requires gas to be insufflated without confirmation of the correct anatomical location. The needle is replaced with a 10 mm working laparoscope with a video camera attached to display the image on video monitors before placing further cannulas.

Most laparoscopic procedures need additional abdominal punctures for instruments such as diathermy hooks, graspers, needle holders, clip appliers and linear staplers. These secondary trocars are inserted under direct laparoscopic vision to prevent visceral injury.

The operation is performed by the operator and one or more assistants, observing progress on video monitors. Dissection is performed using laparoscopic scissors and diathermy hooks rather than lasers which are expensive and hazardous. Grasping forceps, probes or retractable 'fans' are used for retraction whilst blood vessels can be diathermised if small or clipped using clip applicators if larger. Repairs and other operative procedures are completed using laparoscopic sutures or staples and resections performed using linear or circular staplers. In laparoscopic-assisted surgery—for example, for colectomy—the major dissection is performed laparoscopically, then a small abdominal incision made to deliver the specimen.

After operation, patients experience abdominal discomfort at trocar insertion sites and shoulder discomfort from retained gas in the peritoneal cavity. Few restrictions are placed on the patient after discharge, who can return to work as soon as comfortable, often after a few days. Hopes for extremely rapid return to work, however, have not been borne out by controlled studies comparing laparoscopic cholecystectomy or hernia repair against conventional open techniques. Overall pain experienced is less but the cost/benefit ratio remains to be ascertained.

DIAGNOSTIC LAPAROSCOPY

Diagnostic laparoscopy has long been used by individual surgeons for assessing chronic liver disease and ascites of unknown origin. Recent advances in instrumentation and imaging now allow surgeons to perform abdominal exploration almost as thoroughly as through a long laparotomy incision. Key applications are in staging gastric and pancreatic cancer to assess operability by inspection, obtaining peritoneal washings and performing biopsies. By this method, patients with incurable disease are spared the trauma of exploratory open surgery (Box 6.8).

THERAPEUTIC LAPAROSCOPY

As mentioned earlier, therapeutic laparoscopy was slower in becoming accepted in general surgery than in gynaecology. Strong public interest and rapidly developing experience in laparoscopic biliary tract surgery have enhanced its use but some techniques have yet to be properly evaluated.

Thorough training and supervised experience are vital for would-be laparoscopic surgeons. The lack of 'feel' inherent in laparoscopic surgery and the two-dimensional view remove much of the feedback of open surgery and novel techniques have to be learned. Patients undergoing laparoscopic surgery sometimes have to be 'converted' to open surgery if progress is slow, if

KEY POINTS

Box 6.8 Potential indications for diagnostic laparoscopy
- Evaluation of acute or chronic liver disease
- Diagnosis of ascites of unknown cause
- Evaluation of acute or chronic abdominal pain, e.g. suspected appendicitis, gynaecological pain
- Diagnosis and staging of intra-abdominal malignancies (including evaluating the effects of chemotherapy or radiotherapy on intra-abdominal malignancies)
- As a 'second-look' procedure in patients operated on for mesenteric ischaemia
- Assessing blunt or penetrating abdominal trauma in stable patients with positive peritoneal lavage
- Exclusion of acute acalculous cholecystitis after major trauma or surgery in ICU patients

visibility is impaired or if complicating factors such as adhesions make it too difficult to evaluate the anatomy. This means that any surgeon undertaking laparoscopic procedures must have the experience to perform the procedure 'open'. As more surgery is performed laparoscopically, available experience becomes scarce and this represents a potential problem for the future.

CRITICISMS

Criticisms of laparoscopic surgery include the following:

- Procedures tend to take longer than open surgery (the difference becomes smaller as the team's experience increases)
- The capital cost of laparoscopic equipment and the revenue costs of disposable equipment are high; these can to a certain extent be justified by reduced time spent by the patient in hospital and by the use of non-disposable equipment
- Cleaning and sterilising of the delicate equipment requires dedicated and organised theatre staff and strict quality control
- Complication rates may be higher than for open surgery and some complications such as bile duct injury may be catastrophic

COMPLICATIONS

The potential for complications is greater in laparoscopic surgery than for the equivalent procedure performed 'open'. Problems include the following:

- Raised intra-abdominal pressure and head-down positioning lead to the need to ventilate patients at higher inflation pressures. This reduces venous return and cardiac output. Intra-abdominal pressures should be kept to a minimum, e.g. 15 cm H_2O

- The inducing of a pneumoperitoneum (needle injury to bowel or blood vessels, compression of venous return predisposing to deep venous thrombosis, subcutaneous emphysema, shoulder tip pain)
- Inadvertent injury can occur to many structures and may be unrecognised because the procedure is concealed. This includes injury to the abdominal wall (including the diaphragm) during needle or trocar insertion; trocar injury to intra-abdominal organs and blood vessels; or direct organ damage by dissection, diathermy or laser. Colonic resections have caused damage to nerves controlling urinary continence
- Uncontrollable haemorrhage may necessitate conversion to open operation
- Complications related to the duration of anaesthesia which may be twice as long as equivalent open surgery. Long anaesthetics have a longer recovery time and the diaphragm is 'splinted' by abdominal inflation and can precipitate cardiorespiratory complications in compromised patients. There may be an increased rate of deep vein thrombosis
- Later, bowel may strangulate through peritoneal punctures and incisional hernias can occur through puncture wounds

SPECIFIC APPLICATIONS OF THERAPEUTIC LAPAROSCOPY

Laparoscopic cholecystectomy is widely practised and is already a standard operation. Laparoscopic appendicectomy is also accepted but is performed less commonly. Laparoscopic inguinal hernia repair is widely performed, and controlled trials show that in expert hands it can have better results than some open hernia repair techniques. Other procedures described below and listed in Box 6.9 have yet to become incorporated into the standard repertoire of the general surgeon.

Laparoscopic fundoplication

Laparoscopic fundoplication allows a rapid return to normal levels of activity for patients. The technique involves in part, the dissection of the gastro-oesophageal junction at the hiatus, and the wrapping of the gastric fundus around the lower oesophagus. This 'wrap' is then sutured in place over a bougie to size the new valve. Clinical trials show it to offer a durable result which is comparable to open fundoplication. However, the availability of the technique should not replace the need to apply normal standards for electing for surgery rather than conservative management.

KEY POINTS

Box 6.9 Current and experimental therapeutic applications of laparoscopy
- Cholecystectomy (described in Ch. 13)
- Appendicectomy
- Colonic resection—benign and malignant disease
- Division of symptomatic adhesions
- Inguinal and femoral hernia repairs
- Small bowel surgery—including resection and enteral access procedures
- Peptic ulcer disease (vagotomy and plugging of duodenal perforations)
- Symptomatic oesophageal reflux (Angelchik prosthesis; round ligament sling; Nissen fundoplication)
- Nephrectomy
- Splenectomy

Laparoscopic appendicectomy

Appendicectomy for acute appendicitis is one of the most frequently performed operations by general surgeons. Laparoscopic appendicectomy offers improved diagnosis with the ability to examine the entire abdomen if the appendix is normal, a lower rate of wound complications, reduced postoperative pain and hospital stay, and perhaps more rapid return to normal activities. Laparoscopic appendicectomy may offer a lower rate of pelvic adhesions because of reduced trauma; this is an advantage in young females. Conversion to open surgery is around 2.5% in experienced hands. The main problem is that an experienced laparoscopic surgeon needs to be available to perform the operation.

Laparoscopic management of duodenal ulcer perforations

Duodenal ulcers usually perforate anteriorly and can easily be seen with the laparoscope. Under laparoscopic vision, the ulcer is closed laparoscopically using a long-term monofilament absorbable suture such as PDS. To further shore up the repair, a piece of greater omentum may be secured to the duodenum with laparoscopically placed sutures. The peritoneal cavity is irrigated using a pressure irrigator and the fluid sucked out. The initial enthusiasm for this technique has faded in recent years.

Laparoscopic placement of enterocutaneous jejunostomy tube

For long-term enteral feeding where a gastrostomy is unsuitable, a fine-bore feeding tube can be placed into the jejunum using laparoscopic techniques. This avoids the need for laparotomy.

Laparoscopic inguinal hernia repair

The standard open techniques for inguinal hernia repair are based on Bassini's extraperitoneal groin approach described in 1884. Open transabdominal repairs were performed in the 1930s but carried the increased morbidity associated with abdominal operations. Renewed interest has arisen in laparoscopic transperitoneal and, latterly, extraperitoneal approaches which may involve even less dissection than the open groin approach; they

are believed to reduce the likelihood of damage to testicular vessels, bladder and ilio-inguinal nerve (particularly for recurrent hernias). The promise of less postoperative pain and faster recovery than the open groin approach has not been fulfilled for unilateral primary hernia repairs. Furthermore, disturbing complications such as femoral artery damage have been reported. In addition, laparoscopic repairs take longer than open techniques in most hands. Although inguinal hernia repairs are increasingly performed laparoscopically, evidence about long-term recurrence rates does not yet exist. It seems likely that laparoscopic repair will be of particular value for recurrent hernias and bilateral hernias.

SOFT TISSUE SURGERY

METHODS OF OBTAINING TISSUE FOR DIAGNOSIS

Biopsy

If major surgery or other therapy is being contemplated for a suspected malignant lesion, an accurate **tissue diagnosis** should be made wherever possible.

Skin lesions can be biopsied by incision under local anaesthesia. Rectal lesions can be biopsied using forceps through a rigid sigmoidoscope, while gastric and colonic lesions can be biopsied via a flexible endoscope. Breast lumps or suspicious mammographic lesions can be sampled using percutaneous core needle biopsy or by fine needle aspiration cytology (see below).

Enlarged lymph nodes can often be diagnosed by removing one or more completely for histological examination (**excision biopsy**), although many units can now obtain satisfactory results by needle biopsy. Lymphadenectomy often requires general anaesthesia, particularly for lumps in the neck.

Biopsy guided by ultrasound or CT scanning
Abdominal masses such as liver metastases or pancreatic lesions can be biopsied percutaneously with the aid of ultrasound or CT scanning. The suspicious lesion is first located as an image and then a biopsy needle is guided into it with the help of further imaging. Guided biopsy techniques have greatly assisted surgical diagnosis and have saved many patients from unnecessary exploratory

laparotomy in the case of benign lesions and inoperable tumours. The technique can be used to sample abdominal masses or suspicious para-aortic lymph nodes in staging lymphomas or following treatment for testicular germ cell tumours.

Cytology

Special staining techniques for malignant cells can be applied to material obtained by fine needle aspiration. Cytological diagnosis requires special laboratory skills but often permits accurate diagnosis (e.g. of malignancy), which renders more invasive investigations unnecessary. A negative cytological result, however, must be interpreted with great caution because it may be due to sampling error.

Cytological diagnosis can be useful for the following:

- Examining cells aspirated from solid masses. This is particularly useful for thyroid nodules (see Ch. 43), breast lumps and mammographically detected lesions and pancreatic masses
- Examining ascitic fluid obtained from the abdomen by **paracentesis**, or pleural effusions aspirated from the chest. Fluid may also be sent for microbiological analysis
- Examining cellular material scraped from surfaces, e.g. uterine cervical smears, or fluid obtained from within hollow viscera, e.g. urine, pancreatic secretions, sputum

'MINOR' OPERATIVE PROCEDURES

Many skin lesions are amenable to simple excision or biopsy, often under local anaesthesia. These may be performed in family medical practice or in dermatological or surgical outpatient departments. A strict aseptic technique must be employed.

LOCAL ANAESTHESIA

The usual method is by infiltration of local anaesthetic (e.g. lignocaine 0.5% or 1%) into the skin surrounding the lesion. Between 1 and 10 ml of solution is usually required, but care must be taken to remain within recommended maximum safe dosages (see Table 6.3). A vasoconstrictor (e.g. adrenaline 1 in 200 000) may be incorporated to reduce vascularity in the operative field, but this must **never** be used on the extreme peripheries, i.e. fingers, toes, penis or nose, because of the high risk of ischaemic necrosis. The injecting needle should be as fine as possible and inserted into the skin as few times as possible to avoid causing unnecessary pain. Before each injection, aspiration should be attempted to ensure that the solution is not injected directly into a blood vessel as intravascular injection may cause systemic toxicity. Methods of infiltration of local anaesthetic are illustrated in Figure 6.11.

BIOPSY TECHNIQUES

EXCISION BIOPSY

The technique of excision biopsy illustrated in Figure 6.12 is appropriate for most small lesions not considered to be malignant. The lesion is removed with a fusiform piece of normal skin, with the long axis orientated along skin creases and tension lines. The specimen should include a millimetre or two of normal skin on either side of the lesion and should include the full depth of the dermis down to the subcutaneous fat.

Table 6.3 Maximum safe doses of local anaesthetic agents for infiltration in fit patients

Lignocaine	Bupivacaine (Marcain)
2% lignocaine is probably no more effective than 1% or even 0.5%	0.5% bupivacaine is probably no more effective than 0.25%
10 ml of 1% lignocaine contains 100 mg	10 ml of 0.5% bupivacaine contains 50 mg
The maximum safe dose of **plain lignocaine** is 4 mg/kg body weight	The maximum safe dose of **plain bupivacaine** is 2 mg/kg body weight
For a fit 60 kg adult, the maximum safe dose of 1% *plain* lignocaine is 16–24 ml	For a fit 60 kg adult, the maximum safe dose of 0.5% bupivacaine is 24 ml
With adrenaline, this dose can be increased to 7 mg/kg body weight	Addition of adrenaline does **not** increase the safe dose of bupivacaine and there is little point in using it for infiltration
For a fit 60 kg adult, the maximum safe dose of 1% lignocaine *with adrenaline* is 30–40 ml	No increase

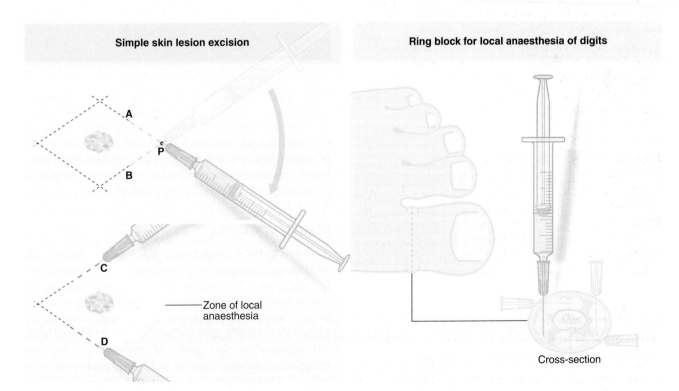

Simple skin lesion excision

A

P

B

C

D

———Zone of local anaesthesia

Ring block for local anaesthesia of digits

Cross-section

Fig. 6.11 Local anaesthetic infiltration techniques

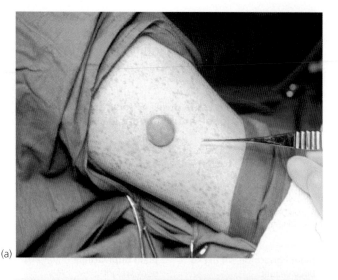

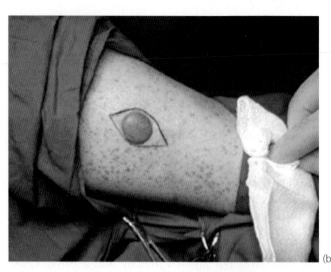

(a)

(b)

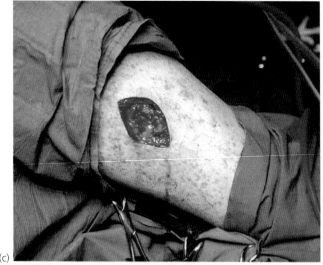

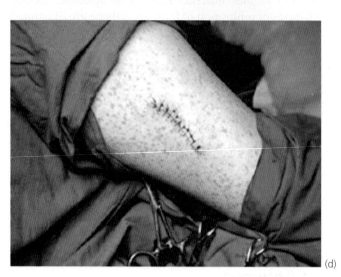

(c)

(d)

Fig. 6.12 Excision biopsy technique

INCISION BIOPSY

Incision biopsy is a technique of obtaining a tissue sample from a lesion too large or anatomically unsuitable for excision biopsy, e.g. a skin rash or a suspected malignant tumour. Major surgical procedures or radiotherapy should not be performed without histological confirmation of the diagnosis. The objective is to obtain a representative sample of the full depth of the lesion, including an area of the margin and adjoining normal tissue (see Fig. 6.13).

Destruction of lesions by diathermy, electrocautery, cryocautery or curettage

These techniques are used for small lesions where there is no clinical suspicion of malignancy or for small basal cell carcinomas and a histological diagnosis is not required; the lesion is destroyed in the process of removal. Local infiltration of anaesthetic is necessary except for cryocautery which is relatively painless.

REMOVAL OF CYSTS

A cyst is a fluid-filled lesion, lined by epithelium and usually encapsulated by a condensation of surrounding fibrous tissue. The aim of treatment is to remove the whole epithelial lining because any remnant will lead to recurrence. The technique of removal is outlined in Figure 6.14. Ideally, the cyst is dissected out intact without puncturing the cavity. If this occurs, the cyst collapses, making it difficult to identify and remove the epithelial lining. Inflamed cysts are best simply drained and excised later when the inflammation has settled.

MARSUPIALISATION

This technique is usually employed for the treatment of cysts or other fluid-filled lesions which are too large, inaccessible or technically difficult to remove. It is rarely appropriate for skin lesions but is often used for large salivary retention cysts in the floor of the mouth, cysts in the jaw and pancreatic pseudocysts. The technique is illustrated in Figure 6.15. The surgeon removes a disc from the wall of the cavity and sutures the lining to the overlying epithelium around the cut edge. This leaves a pouch, which slowly fills from below once the pressure of the cyst contents has been removed.

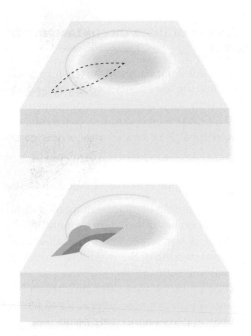

Fig. 6.13 Incision skin biopsy technique

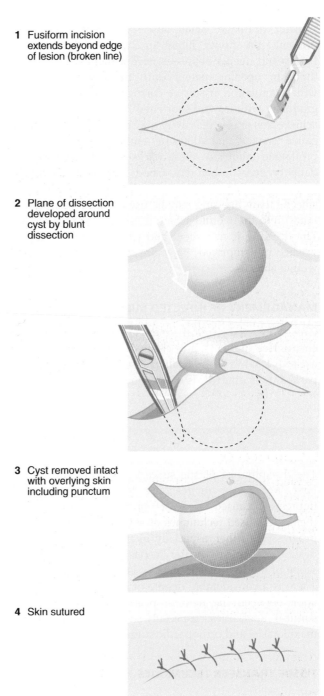

1 Fusiform incision extends beyond edge of lesion (broken line)

2 Plane of dissection developed around cyst by blunt dissection

3 Cyst removed intact with overlying skin including punctum

4 Skin sutured

Fig. 6.14 Technique of excision of an epidermal cyst

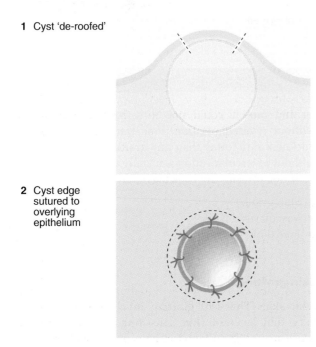

1 Cyst 'de-roofed'

2 Cyst edge sutured to overlying epithelium

Fig. 6.15 Marsupialisation of a cyst

SURGERY INVOLVING INFECTED TISSUES

MANAGEMENT OF ABSCESSES

The first principle of managing an abscess is to establish drainage of the pus. When an abscess is 'pointing' to the surface, this involves a skin incision at the site of maximum fluctuance followed by blunt probing with sinus forceps or a finger (usually under general anaesthesia) to ensure that all loculi are drained; necrotic material is removed at the same time.

After drainage, small abscesses need only a dry dressing, the cavity filling in rapidly from beneath. Larger and deeper abscesses need a method of keeping the skin opening patent until the cavity has filled with granulation tissue. A corrugated drain, which is gradually withdrawn ('shortened') over a few days, will achieve this or else the cavity may be packed with ribbon gauze soaked in saline or antiseptic solution, e.g. proflavine emulsion; these packs are usually changed daily or every other day. Good analgesia is required in the early stages. When the cavity is granulating, a silicone foam dressing may be used. This is poured as a liquid into the wound where it rapidly foams and sets. The dressing is absorbent and can easily be removed, washed and replaced. New dressings are made as the wound shrinks.

MANAGEMENT OF INFECTED SURGICAL WOUNDS

Grossly infected surgical wounds must be opened up to ensure free drainage, and cleaned. All necrotic tissue is excised leaving only healthy tissue, and the wound packed daily afterwards with saline-soaked or antiseptic-soaked gauze. The wound is usually allowed to heal by secondary intention (see Ch. 1, p. 8), although a large wound can be sutured later when infection is no longer a problem (**delayed primary closure**). In the case of deep, slowly healing wounds, a **silicone foam dressing** can be employed.

MANAGEMENT OF DIRTY OR CONTAMINATED WOUNDS

Major soft tissue injuries result in crushing and tearing of tissues, leaving devascularised areas and deep impregnation with soil, road grit or fragments of clothing. If such a wound is merely sutured, pyogenic infection is certain, and there is a serious risk of gas gangrene or tetanus.

The principles of managing these wounds were first established during the First World War, as follows:

- Thorough cleansing of all foreign material from the wound (sometimes called '**debridement**')
- Excision of all non-viable tissue ('necrosectomy')
- Loose open packing of the wound with dry cotton gauze without suturing
- Inspection of the wound under anaesthesia 2–4 days later, drainage of any new abscesses and removal of any newly apparent non-viable tissue
- Suturing of the wound when it looks clean, but avoiding tension; this is known as **delayed primary closure**. Alternatively, split skin grafting may be employed

PRINCIPLES OF PLASTIC SURGERY

The discipline of plastic surgery was born during the First World War in response to the appalling disfigurement caused by blast injuries and burns. Since then, specialised techniques of skin reconstruction have progressed further, especially in the fields of axial flap design and microvascular reconstructive surgery. The scope of modern plastic surgery is outlined in Box 6.10. There is a considerable degree of overlap and collaboration between the field of plastic surgery and other surgical specialties, especially ear, nose and throat, maxillofacial and orthopaedic surgery.

TISSUE TRANSFER TECHNIQUES

Obtaining satisfactory skin cover is one of the major problems in plastic surgery and other tissues such as fat and muscle could not be satisfactorily transferred without revascularisation. Free transplantation of full-thickness skin (other than tiny grafts) or any other tissue without revascularisation is usually unsuccessful.

Tissue transfer can be achieved in three main ways:

- Skin grafts
- Vascularised flaps
- Free flaps

Skin grafting

Split skin (Thiersch) grafting involves transplanting a very thin layer of skin consisting of little more than epidermis with no blood supply of its own. It depends on nutrition from the recipient bed for survival. Split

KEY POINTS

Box 6.10 The scope of plastic surgery

Congenital problems

● Correction of congenital defects, e.g. cleft lip and palate, syndactyly and polydactyly, prominent ears, hypospadias, vascular malformations, craniofacial deformities, congenital skin conditions, e.g. 'port wine stains'

Trauma

● Reconstruction after mutilating surgery or trauma, e.g. skin cover for compound lower limb fractures, vascularised bone transfer
● Management of facial soft tissue trauma
● Management of burns—grafting, management of scars and deformities
● Hand trauma—tendon repairs, microsurgical nerve and artery repairs, replantation surgery, e.g. digits and limbs (p. 124)

Elective hand surgery

● Dupuytren's contracture, nerve decompressions, rheumatoid disease

Cancer

● Cutaneous malignancies—excision and reconstruction with grafts or local flaps
● Major cancer surgery of the head and neck—excision and reconstruction with free tissue transfer
● Breast reconstruction after mastectomy

Aesthetic (cosmetic) surgery

● Scar removal, breast reduction and augmentation, 'face-lifts', eyelid skin reduction, nasal adjustment including after trauma
● Surgery for obesity, e.g. abdominal skin reduction, liposuction, apronectomy (for pendulous abdomen)

Miscellaneous, including reconstruction of large defects

● Reconstruction for facial palsy, decubitus (pressure) sores, soft tissue sarcoma excision, leg ulcers, reconstruction of skin after radiotherapy, destructive infections, e.g. necrotising fasciitis, compartment syndromes

skin grafts are commonly employed for burns and after wide excision of skin lesions, provided there is a recipient base of healthy tissue. The donor site heals rapidly since small islands of epithelium are left behind (see Fig. 6.16). The donor site is potentially more painful than the recipient but pain is well controlled if the donor site is dressed immediately with calcium alginate or plastic film dressings. These may be left in position for several days until the wound has epithelialised. Creating a 'mesh' of the graft helps it to take in certain circum-

stances as it allows free drainage through the perforations. Small full thickness (Wolfe) grafts may survive in certain circumstances. Examples include skin from behind the ear transferred to a severed finger tip and pinch grafts for leg ulcers.

Vascularised flaps

A flap has a blood supply of its own; a flap is not a graft. The blood supply reaches the flap via its base and is known as the vascular pedicle. Flaps can be advanced, rotated or transposed into the defect to be filled and this may provide sufficient mobility to close a moderate-sized defect. If a new defect is produced as a result of flap rotation, this clean area can usually be covered with a small split skin graft. Most flaps now used are **axial flaps** which employ established anatomical sites to ensure a blood supply running along the long axis of the flap. The early **random flaps**, devised by Gillies, were limited in scope because there was no dominant blood supply and this prevented construction of a flap which was longer than its width. Another early technique was the use of **pedicle flaps** in which a flap of skin was raised and formed into a tube while remaining attached to its site of origin at both ends. Later, one end of the tube was divided and transposed to the recipient site; later still the other end of the tube was divided and the flap opened out, shaped and sutured at the recipient site to reconstruct the defect. This, however, was a prolonged procedure necessitating long periods in hospital and uncomfortable immobilisation of the parts involved.

Axial flaps are selected according to the site of the defect and the tissues needed. A series of flaps are now described, based on detailed anatomical studies of blood supply. Flaps may be **cutaneous**, e.g. forehead flap, **fascio-cutaneous**, e.g. the 'Chinese' radial forearm flap, **myocutaneous**, e.g. latissimus dorsi, pectoralis major, **TRAM** (transverse rectus abdominis myocutaneous)—often used for breast reconstruction, and **osseous**, e.g. fibula, radius, iliac crest and rib.

Free flaps

In free tissue transfer, a carefully planned piece of tissue is first dissected out, complete with at least one main artery and vein; axial flap sites are often suitable. The whole flap is then relocated to the recipient site where the vessels are connected to a suitable local artery and vein by microvascular anastomoses. The donor site can often be closed primarily or else covered with a split skin graft. Examples are the **radial forearm flap** which supplies bone, muscle and skin, and the big toe which can be used to replace a lost thumb.

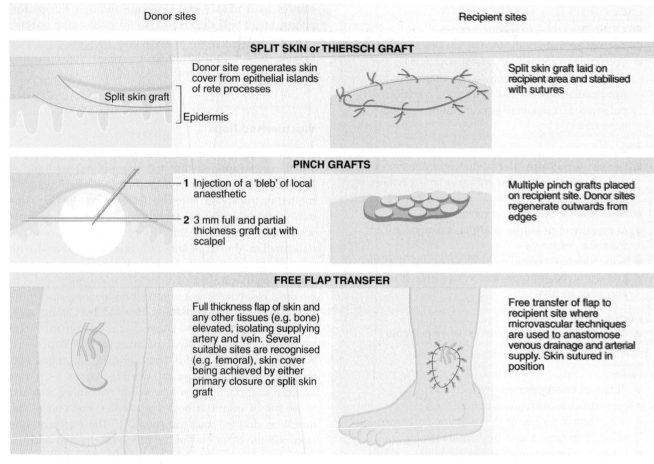

Fig. 6.16 Methods of skin grafting

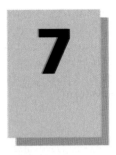

7 Principles of cancer management

INTRODUCTION

In developed countries, people are living longer. This is mainly due to public health measures which have improved infant mortality and reduced the burden of infectious diseases. Mortality from cardiovascular disease continues to dominate in late middle life but beyond that malignant disease becomes an almost equal killer. Huge strides have been made in recent years in understanding the molecular basis of cancer. Translating this into improved prevention, detection and treatment remains elusive but important developments in the foreseeable future are promised.

Malignant disease afflicts about one-third of all people in their lifetime and about one in four will die of it. Patients with malignant disease form a major part of the surgical workload and are responsible for as much as 40% of general surgical bed occupancy. Cancer patients impose disproportionate demands on services, since operations are often extensive and the patients are generally older, slower to recover and more prone to complications. At the same time, the total number of patients with malignant disease is rising because of increasing life expectancy and an increased incidence of some cancers. In the younger age groups, surgical workload from cancer is also expanding because of earlier detection, increased technical sophistication and increasing patient expectation. The incidence of common malignancies in Western countries is shown in Table 7.1.

Table 7.1 Incidence of common malignancies in men and women as a proportion of all malignancies*

Males	%	Females	%
Lung	20	Breast	29
Prostate	20	Colorectal	15
Colorectal	15	Lung	11
Urinary	10	Uterus and ovary	13
Head and neck	6	Head and neck	6
Stomach and pancreas	6	Urinary	4
Leukaemias and lymphomas	7	Leukaemias and lymphomas	7
All others	16	All others	15

*UK and USA 1990. Statistics from Australia are similar except there is a higher incidence of melanoma amounting to 7% of malignant tumours

Screening for malignant disease, notably cervical, breast and colorectal cancer, has had a significant but limited impact on mortality, partly because of lack of patient compliance (particularly in cervical and colorectal cancer) but also because of a relative inability to detect biologically early disease (in breast cancer).

Effective treatment depends on the nature of the primary cancer (i.e. tissue type, metastatic potential) and the extent of spread, as well as other physiological factors such as the patient's hormone status. Management of particular cancers is becoming more protocol-driven as the results of carefully conducted randomised trials have identified the most effective treatment regimes which increasingly involve a combination of surgical with other treatment modalities, particularly radiotherapy, chemotherapy, hormone manipulation and palliative symptom control.

Whilst the management of cancer is rapidly developing, dramatic press claims of breakthrough cures are often premature and raise false hopes. It is unlikely that a universal preventative or cure for cancer will appear. Instead, advances will be incremental and type-specific rather than encompassing the whole spectrum.

NEOPLASIA

The main characteristic of neoplasms is uncontrolled growth that persists after removal of the initiating stimulus. Most neoplasms can readily be categorised as **benign** or **malignant** according to histological pattern and in most cases it is possible to predict the likelihood of invasion or metastasis associated with malignancy. Sometimes it is difficult—for example, distinguishing between leiomyoma and leiomyosarcoma may only be possible by following the long-term behaviour of the individual tumour. Neoplasms may also be difficult to distinguish clinically from other **tumour-like disorders** such as hyperplasia (e.g. parathyroid adenoma from parathyroid hyperplasia) and hamartomata (e.g. liver secondaries from haemangiomas of the liver).

BENIGN NEOPLASMS

Benign tumours are typically well demarcated and often encapsulated, with a histological appearance reminiscent of the tissue of origin; they usually grow slowly. Benign tumours present to the surgeon in a variety of ways as summarised in Box 7.1.

MALIGNANT NEOPLASMS

Malignant tumours are typically non-encapsulated with a poorly defined, irregular outline due to local tissue invasion. Histologically, both cells and their nuclei often vary widely in shape and size, and the extent of this **pleomorphism** tends to correlate with the degree of malignancy and the future clinical behaviour of the tumour. Malignant tumours usually grow progressively and may grow rapidly. In **anaplastic tumours**, there is such loss of differentiation that little resemblance to the parent tissue remains. The supporting tissue stroma of some malignant tumours may undergo fibrous hyperplasia, which accounts for some of the characteristic clinical features of cancer; these include hardness to palpation (induration), intestinal obstruction by annular carcinomas of the large bowel and retraction of skin overlying breast cancer. On the other hand, in highly aggressive tumours, the supporting tissue stroma may be inadequate for

> **KEY POINTS**
>
> **Box 7.1 Principal modes of presentation of benign tumours**
>
> - Lesion suspected by the patient to be malignant, e.g. breast lump
> - Overt bleeding or occult blood loss causing anaemia, e.g. bowel polyps
> - Local obstructive effects, e.g. leiomyoma of small intestine
> - Pressure causing pain or dysfunction, e.g. neurofibroma
> - Unacceptable cosmetic appearance, e.g. subcutaneous lipomas
> - Production of excessive amounts of hormone by endocrine neoplasms, e.g. parathyroid adenoma, insulinoma, phaeochromocytoma

nutritional support, leading to necrosis and patchy haemorrhage within the tumour. This often presents as a sudden onset of pain and a mass.

Malignant tumours present in a variety of ways as summarised in Box 7.2.

CARCINOGENESIS

Multiple primary lesions and recurrences

Most cancers are probably caused by a combination of environmental factors and factors intrinsic to the patient. It has been estimated mathematically that about two-thirds of cancers can be attributed in some way to external factors such as ionising radiation, virus infections and carcinogens in air, food and water. Many such factors are yet to be discovered but cigarette smoking is now well recognised to be the most common carcinogen for lung, bladder and head and neck cancers. When cancer develops, it is likely that the whole of the affected organ or tissue has been altered in the same way by the carcinogen. Consequently, new primary tumours, as distinct from local recurrences, may develop later; clear distinction between these is often impossible. Certain tissues, particularly those of the bladder, breast, skin, head and neck and large

KEY POINTS

Box 7.2 Principal modes of presentation of malignant tumours

The primary lesion:

- Palpable or visible mass, e.g. breast or thyroid cancer
- Obstruction or other disruption of function of a hollow viscus, e.g. bowel obstruction by colorectal carcinoma, stridor in bronchial carcinoma
- Overt bleeding, e.g. bladder or left-sided large bowel cancer
- Occult blood loss causing anaemia, e.g. carcinoma of stomach or caecum
- Obstructive jaundice, e.g. carcinoma of head of pancreas or extrahepatic bile ducts
- Skin lesion, often ulcerated, e.g. basal and squamous cell carcinomas, malignant melanoma, breast cancer
- Nerve invasion, e.g. facial nerve palsy from parotid carcinoma, recurrent laryngeal palsy from anaplastic carcinoma of thyroid

Pain is not a common presenting feature of primary malignancy except in the pancreas, lung and nasopharynx; pain is more often associated with metastatic disease

Metastatic deposits

- Enlarged lymph nodes (nodes tend to be hard, matted and non-tender)
- Hepatomegaly, e.g. stomach, large bowel and pancreatic carcinomas
- Obstructive jaundice (usually due to lymph node mass in the porta hepatis compressing the bile ducts, but sometimes extensive liver deposits), e.g. stomach, large bowel and pancreatic carcinomas
- Abnormal masses distant from the primary lesion, e.g. abdomen, pelvis and skin
- Bone invasion causing bone pain or pathological fractures, e.g. prostatic and breast cancers
- Malignant effusions, e.g. pleural effusion in breast cancer, ascites with peritoneal deposits from intra-abdominal malignancies
- Pulmonary metastases—usually asymptomatic and found on chest X-ray
- Brain metastases—behavioural or personality changes, headache, fits, paresis, ataxias etc.
- Nerve invasion—backache and abdominal pain in abdominal lymph node metastases

Generalised systemic manifestations (uncommon except for cachexia)

- Malignant cachexia (severe weight loss and wasting)—probably caused by the production of catabolic agents by the tumour
- Fever—characteristic of lymphomas and renal adenocarcinoma; also occurs when there is extensive tumour necrosis
- Migrating thrombophlebitis and chronic disseminated intravascular coagulation (DIC)
- Peripheral neuropathies, myopathies and rare autoimmune neuromuscular phenomena, e.g. myasthenic syndrome
- Other rare autoimmune phenomena, e.g. haemolysis
- Ectopic hormone production, e.g. antidiuretic hormone (ADH), adrenocorticotrophic hormone (ACTH), parathyroid hormone (PTH) and gonadotrophins (all rare in malignancies seen in general surgery)
- Production of fetal and embryonic proteins, e.g. carcino-embryonic antigen (CEA) produced by testicular tumours and colorectal and pancreatic carcinomas; alpha-fetoprotein (AFP) produced by testicular teratomas and hepatocellular carcinomas; prostate-specific antigen (PSA) in prostatic carcinoma—may be useful as tissue markers for diagnosis, monitoring treatment and long-term follow-up

bowel, are at particular risk of new primary carcinomas. The clinical significance is that prolonged surveillance is required after an initial tumour has been treated in these areas.

Growth and spread of malignant tumours

Malignant tumours spread by local **infiltration** and by **distant metastasis** via lymphatics and the bloodstream and across coelomic cavities. Carcinogenesis, however, is not a single pathological event. Rather, the onset of

uncontrolled proliferation and the capacity for distant spread evolve in a series of mutations over successive cell divisions. Many malignancies probably arise from a single cell line (i.e. are monoclonal) and the initial event is the acquisition of the capacity to grow progressively in the native tissue. About 30 cell division cycles are probably needed to produce a clinically detectable lesion of 1 cm diameter containing 1000 million cells. The cellular properties that allow a tumour to invade surrounding tissues and lymphatic or blood capillaries and then 'take root' in regional lymph nodes or other distant tissues are probably also products of multiple mutations which have given selective survival advantages. As time passes, the constituent cells of the tumour often become increasingly heterogeneous, genetically and behaviourally.

These pathophysiological considerations have several important clinical ramifications. Firstly, the earlier the primary tumour is detected and removed (i.e. the fewer cell division cycles), the greater the chance of complete cure. Unfortunately, mutations allowing metastasis may appear very early, i.e. by about 20 cell division cycles, when the primary lesion is too small to be detected (about 1 mm diameter).

There are two conflicting theories about the significance of regional lymph node involvement in carcinoma. Both views recognise that lymph node involvement implies a worse prognosis. **Halsted** believed that lymph nodes have an important function in halting spread, at least for a time, and that radical surgery offers the potential for a cure. In more than 50% of large bowel cancers, Halsted's view is probably correct and radical surgery remains the treatment of choice, offering a potential cure even in the presence of involved lymph nodes. In many other cancers, blood-borne (haematogenous) spread, often occult, probably occurs at an early stage, rendering the disease incurable by surgery. Unfortunately, identifying which patients have metastatic disease remains elusive.

An alternative view, expressed by **Fisher**, is that lymph node metastases indicate failure of the host defences and are therefore a manifestation of systemic metastasis. In the case of breast cancer, this has led to the increased use of systemic treatment with cytotoxic and hormonal therapy with the intention of eliminating or suppressing the growth of micrometastases. This has improved survival rates. Nevertheless, radical local surgery remains important in controlling loco-regional disease in the breast, chest wall and axilla.

The probability of surgical cure when lymph node metastases are already present depends on when the cancer develops the capacity for haematogenous spread. This is often about the same time as the capacity for lymph node metastasis develops. In these cases, surgical removal of metastases is ineffective because haematogenous metastases are usually already multifocal. Occasionally blood-borne metastasis appears to be a solitary, isolated event, and a cure can sometimes be achieved—for example, by partial hepatectomy in colorectal cancer or pulmonary lobectomy for renal cell carcinoma, as well as in some paediatric malignancies. The liver, lungs, bone and brain are common target organs for haematogenous spread. Multiple metastases often respond temporarily to palliative chemotherapy, radiotherapy or hormone manipulation (e.g. carcinomas of breast, uterus, kidney and prostate) but complete cure is very rarely achieved.

This model of the development of metastatic potential means that future advances in cancer management need to focus on three factors: primary prevention, very early diagnosis and research to find effective medical (i.e. non-surgical) approaches to treatment of metastases, e.g. radiotherapy, chemotherapy and hormonal manipulation.

Sarcomas, malignancies derived from cells of mesodermal origin, are relatively uncommon and usually metastasise early via the bloodstream.

BASIC PRINCIPLES OF CANCER MANAGEMENT

Two broad considerations determine the approach to treatment for any cancer patient. The first is whether an attempt should be made to achieve a **cure** or whether **palliation** is more appropriate; the choice depends on the nature of the tumour, the extent of local spread and whether distant metastases are believed to be present. The second consideration is the **prognosis**. This takes further factors into account, including the likely natural history of the type of cancer and the patient's age and general state of health. Systems of **staging** have been devised for each tumour type, many based on the **TNM system** which scores characteristics of the **T**umour, the extent of regional lymph **N**ode involvement and the presence of **M**etastases. Staging is used in planning treatment, as a guide to prognosis and as a standardised descriptive tool for comparing efficacy of treatment in different patients and in different centres.

Cancer can recur at a later stage and the success of treatment is often described in terms of patient survival after a given number of years rather than 'cure'. **Five-year survival** is often used as the yardstick of success in cancer therapy and in many cases can be taken to imply cure. Nevertheless, some tumours, particularly breast cancer, may recur in a disseminated form as long as 30 years after apparently successful eradication. Conversely, colorectal cancer and testicular teratoma and seminoma rarely recur after the patient has survived 5 years.

TREATMENT OPTIONS

The main treatment options for malignant disease are **surgical excision, radiotherapy, cytotoxic chemotherapy** and **hormonal manipulation**, with two or more modalities of treatment often used in combination. The treatment offered to an individual patient will depend on tumour type, tumour extent and the patient's overall condition. A radical or aggressive approach to treatment, using a combination of therapies (e.g. surgery and postoperative radiotherapy or chemotherapy) may well be recommended where the aim is to cure, provided the scientific evidence supports this approach. In other patients where cure is not possible, or where disease has relapsed after radical treatment, the aim is to alleviate the symptoms of disease, i.e. to palliate.

Palliative care focuses on the quality of life rather than the quantity, and individual assessment is required as any available modality of treatment may be appropriate for relieving symptoms. Care and relief of symptoms must continue to be given as much importance in the terminal phase of the illness as during active treatment.

Most cancer treatments involve unpleasant **side effects** which may easily be overlooked by both doctor and patient in their enthusiasm for treatment. Thus it is essential that the benefits and disadvantages are carefully considered in every case, and where possible and where different options are feasible, the patient should be involved in reaching decisions. There are few circumstances where a diagnosis of cancer should be concealed from a patient; suspicion and fear of the unknown often cause more distress than a frank explanation of the diagnosis and its ramifications. Time should be allowed for the patient to formulate further questions and a follow-up consultation arranged in a few days. It often helps the patient to have a friend or relative present, but relatives should rarely be told more than the patient. Patients are also helped by well-constructed printed information, self-help groups and by specially trained cancer nurses who can spend longer with the patient and act as an intermediary if necessary.

EARLY DETECTION OF CANCER

As a general principle, the earlier in its natural history that malignancy is diagnosed and treated, the better the prognosis. The ideal is to detect cancer before invasion or metastasis has occurred, i.e. during the pre-invasive stage. Where this applies, health education can play an important part in alerting the public to early symptoms and warning signs. In the case of skin and testicular tumours, this should include regular self-examination. Although self-examination is promoted for breast cancer, there is little evidence that it is a useful screening test.

GENERAL PRINCIPLES OF SCREENING

Medical screening involves examination or investigation of an asymptomatic population with the objective of making diagnoses at an earlier stage than would otherwise be the case. For screening to have any benefit, it is a prerequisite that earlier diagnosis significantly improves

morbidity and mortality from the disease when evaluated on a population basis. In general, screening is carried out on a selected group of the population at increased risk. In the case of breast cancer, only older females are screened.

The high cost of screening large numbers of healthy individuals must be justified by the **yield** and, of course, the **effectiveness of treatment**. Within this debate, imponderables such as the economic value of a human life saved or of a period of enhanced survival need to be considered. For example, screening for pulmonary tuberculosis by mass miniature X-ray was highly successful in the 1950s and 1960s but was abandoned in the 1970s when the number of new cases discovered on screening fell to such a low level that the cost could no longer be justified. Conversely, screening for cancer of the uterine cervix was widely introduced in the late 1970s and has proved successful, despite the reluctance of many women at greatest risk to be screened.

The efficacy of any medical screening programme depends mainly on the following factors:

- The reliability of the screening procedure; this is defined by two factors, namely **sensitivity** and **specificity**. Sensitivity describes the ability of the screening procedure to identify affected individuals in the screened population, i.e. the proportion of affected individuals for whom the test result is positive. Specificity describes the degree to which a positive test result correlates with the presence of the disease; in other words, the more false positive results, the lower the specificity
- The **prevalence** (the proportion of cases already in a population) and the **incidence** (the proportion of new cases) of the disease in the population at risk
- The risks associated with untreated disease (does it need treating?)
- The potential benefits of medical or surgical intervention prompted by earlier diagnosis (is 'cure' more likely, is survival longer, is earlier treatment easier?)
- The cost and ease of screening and the inconvenience and acceptability to the population at risk
- The availability and cost of treatment

Screening for breast cancer

Screening for breast cancer by radiography (**mammography**) was introduced nationally in the UK in the late 1980s following the Forrest report of 1986. Most developed countries have employed a similar strategy. This followed results from the HIP study of New York and the Swedish two-county study which demonstrated a 30% reduction in mortality from breast cancer in screened women. In the UK, national screening policy is to invite women aged 50–65 to be screened every 3 years with single-film mammography. Results so far appear to demonstrate a 20% survival advantage for screened women, although results from Scandinavia (1999) put this figure much lower.

Mammographic screening detects breast cancers of smaller size and at an earlier stage than when symptomatic. Around 30% of cancers identified by screening are carcinoma in situ or small invasive cancers less than 0.5 cm in diameter; only about 20% have axillary nodal spread compared with 40% for symptomatic breast cancer. However, the evidence that screening for breast cancer saves significant numbers of lives is controversial. Earlier detection by screening may not in fact be significantly earlier in biological terms, i.e. detecting cancers before they metastasise, and large-scale screening remains to be convincingly translated into better outcomes.

The experience gained from breast screening and managing patients so detected has brought about rapid improvements in mammographic equipment, technique and interpretation as well as perhaps a more sensitive approach to breast disease. In addition, it has generated much scientific study of the management of early breast cancer. All of this will undoubtedly bring about benefits for all women with breast cancer and for people with other types of cancer. New breast cancer screening programmes are certain to be implemented in developed countries and these will be monitored by computer call and recall systems to overcome some of the obvious inadequacies of earlier screening programmes.

SURGERY FOR CANCER

GENERAL PRINCIPLES OF CANCER SURGERY

The ideal result of cancer surgery is the complete eradication of malignant disease without radically interfering with function. Nearly a third of cancer patients can be cured in this way; these are mainly patients with only primary disease. Whether to embark on major elective surgery depends on careful assessment of the nature of the disease and ideally of its stage. Modern techniques of cross-sectional imaging, laparoscopy and intraoperative ultrasound greatly assist in this endeavour and may save patients from fruitless radical surgery. More critical review of the results of different operations in particular malignancies has also helped to guide the indications for surgery. For example, adenocarcinoma of the pancreas is rarely treated by pancreatectomy nowadays because of the high complication rate coupled with dismal 'cure' rates.

Where metastases appear confined to local lymph nodes, these nodes are usually excised along with the primary tumour or at a second operation. Even in the presence of incurable metastases, surgical excision of the primary lesion is often required to relieve the local effects of the tumour, e.g. bleeding, pain or bowel obstruction. Palliative surgery may also be required for locally advanced or metastatic disease to deal with specific distressing symptoms (e.g. severe haemorrhage from a bladder tumour) or some emergency problem (e.g. acute bowel obstruction).

Sometimes surgery is used to **debulk** a tumour; this is combined with chemotherapy in an attempt either to improve the efficacy of chemotherapy (as in ovarian carcinoma) or to avoid leaving unstable tissue in abdominal lymph nodes (as in testicular teratoma).

RADIOTHERAPY

GENERAL PRINCIPLES OF RADIOTHERAPY

The value of ionising radiation in treating malignant tumours was recognised soon after the discovery of X-rays in 1895 and radiotherapy is now employed at some stage in managing about half of all patients with malignant disease. **Orthovoltage** X-rays (up to 250 kV) were the basis of conventional radiotherapy until the development of **megavoltage** irradiation in the late 1950s. Cobalt-60 machines provided more penetrating radiation initially, but these have been succeeded by **linear accelerators** which provide photon beams with an energy of 5–20 MeV. The radiation dose peaks below the skin, thus avoiding the former severe skin reactions. Absorption of radiation by the target tissue causes highly reactive free radicals to appear which damage DNA and cause cell death at subsequent mitosis. With their high rate of proliferation, cancer cells are particularly sensitive, but normal tissues with a high rate of cell turnover (e.g. gut mucosa and bone marrow) are also vulnerable. The total dose administered depends on the aims of treatment, the site and volume of the tumour and its relationship to important normal tissues. Treatment is given in a variable number of sessions or **fractions** over a period of weeks to allow normal tissues to recover between treatments.

The larger the volume of tumour, the greater the dosage of irradiation required for its destruction. Since the dose is limited by the tolerance of normal tissues, radiotherapy is more effective for small lesions. Radiation dose is measured in **gray** (Gy). A common daily dose is around 2 Gy and is sufficient to destroy about 50% of viable cells in the average tumour; each subsequent dose destroys 50% of the remainder causing a logarithmic decline in viable cell numbers as treatment proceeds. Planning radiotherapy for lesions deep within the body has improved markedly as a result of better planning using computed tomography (CT scanning) and magnetic resonance imaging (MRI)—for example, for bladder tumours or head and neck cancers.

Radiation can be directed to a tumour in three ways:

- **External beam irradiation**—this is the method most commonly employed for both skin and deeply located tumours
- **Local application of radioisotopes (brachytherapy)**—this involves placing the radiation source upon or within the tissue to be irradiated. Plaque sources of radiation can be employed for skin malignancies, and radioactive iridium wires or caesium needles can be implanted in the oral cavity, perineum, skin and sometimes breast, giving high-dose local irradiation. Implantation is usually performed under general anaesthesia. For cancer of the uterus and cervix, the radioactive source is placed in a sealed container within the uterine or vaginal cavity; it can be inserted without risk to staff via a flexible tube from the radiation safe under computer control
- **Systemic radioisotope therapy**—radioactive iodine given by mouth is a well-established treatment for non-neoplastic thyrotoxicosis and can also be used for treating metastases from well-differentiated thyroid tumours provided the thyroid has been removed. Attempts are still being made to direct radioisotopes precisely to cancer cells by attaching them to tumour-specific monoclonal antibodies, thus realising the dream of a 'magic bullet'; alas, this technique remains in the experimental stage

MAJOR APPLICATIONS OF RADIOTHERAPY

Radiotherapy has three major applications in cancer treatment: as a primary cure, as adjuvant treatment or as palliation. The objective must be clearly defined before treatment is begun.

PRIMARY CURATIVE RADIOTHERAPY

This application, also known as **radical radiotherapy**, is widely used for basal cell and squamous cell carcinomas of the skin. It is also used for certain tumours which are technically difficult to remove or where surgery would be particularly mutilating, as in the head, neck and larynx. Radiotherapy can be directed at the primary lesion and regional lymph nodes if appropriate and rates of cure are comparable to those achieved by surgical excision. For example, in head and neck cancers without distant metastases, cure rates of 50–90% can be achieved with radiotherapy alone; similar results can be obtained in carcinoma of the cervix. Radiotherapy is employed in the treatment of most common solid tumours and in early cases of Hodgkin's and non-Hodgkin lymphomas. The efficacy and application of radiotherapy for various tumour types is summarised in Table 7.2.

Radiotherapy can also achieve cure in up to 50% of bladder cancers, with cystectomy reserved for salvage of recurrences.

ADJUVANT RADIOTHERAPY

The principle underlying **adjuvant therapy**, whether radiological, chemical or hormonal, is that clinically undetectable micrometastases are often present in tissue surrounding a primary lesion, in regional nodes and in remote locations. These are believed to be responsible for local, regional and systemic recurrence after a primary lesion has apparently been completely removed.

Adjuvant radiotherapy can be applied to local tissue and regional nodes after (or occasionally before) surgery to try to eliminate micrometastases. The technique is most widely employed for cancer of the breast after removing the primary lesion locally or by mastectomy. Nowadays, there is a trend towards avoiding irradiation of the axilla if the lymph nodes are histologically free of cancer. If axillary nodes are involved, radiotherapy can be used as an alternative to radical lymph node clearance; survival rates are comparable to those achieved after more extensive surgery. However, the trend of opinion favours radical lymph node clearance for the improved diagnostic accuracy it provides and the prognostic value of knowing the number of nodes involved. The preference for surgery or radiotherapy remains one of local choice. Radiotherapy is also highly effective adjuvant therapy in seminoma of the testis.

Neoadjuvant radiotherapy

In certain cancers, treatment a short time before surgery with either radiotherapy or chemotherapy or both can

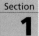

Table 7.2 Applications of radiotherapy for treating malignant disease

Tumour type	Radiosensitivity	Indications
Head and neck	Moderate	Highly effective for localised lesions especially larynx
Lung		
Small cell	High	Enhances efficacy of chemotherapy but overall cure rate less than 10%
Non-small cell	Low to moderate	Worth a trial in patients with inoperable disease for palliation
Breast	Moderate	Usually as adjuvant to surgery or to treat axillary nodal involvement or advanced local breast cancer
Thyroid		
Well differentiated	High	High cure rate in combination with surgery (systemic radioiodine therapy)
Poorly differentiated	Low	Rarely useful
Renal cell carcinoma	Low	Rarely appropriate
Transitional cell carcinoma of bladder	Moderate	Good cure rate for localised lesions
Testis	Moderate to high	Good (especially seminoma) but chemotherapy generally better (for teratoma)
Ovary	Very low	Rarely applicable
Uterus		
Cervix	Moderate	High cure rate for localised tumours; also as adjuvant therapy
Body	Moderate	Adjuvant or palliative therapy
Gastrointestinal tract	Low to moderate	Increasingly used for adjuvant therapy in advanced rectal cancers. Definitive treatment for anal carcinomas
Lymphoma		
Hodgkin's	High	Excellent cure rate for stage I & II disease
Non-Hodgkin's	High	High cure rate when used with chemotherapy
Multiple myeloma	High	Mainly used for palliation
Skin		
Basal or squamous cell carcinoma	High	Highly curable
Melanoma	Low	Used to palliate metastases
Adult central nervous system	Low to moderate	Adjuvant therapy in well-differentiated gliomas. Palliation of cerebral metastases
Paediatric malignancies	Variable	Often curative for brain tumours and effective for Wilms' tumour but limited by long-term effects on growth and development

bring benefits. This may enhance the cure rate for surgery or it may be used to 'down-stage' a cancer to make surgery possible, e.g. locally advanced rectal cancer.

PALLIATIVE RADIOTHERAPY

Palliative radiotherapy is employed for local control of primary or metastatic lesions with the intention of treating serious symptoms with the minimum of side effects or preventing impending complications, e.g. spinal cord compression. Much lower total doses are used for palliation than for attempts at cure; short courses or **single high-dose fractions** are usually adequate and are comfortable and convenient for the patient. Clearly, palliative radiotherapy can only be justified if therapeutic benefits are likely to ensue.

Radiotherapy is particularly effective in controlling metastatic deposits in bone and brain. The pain of bone metastases can often be completely relieved by radiotherapy, as can some of the neurological manifestations of brain secondaries.

Radiotherapy is also valuable in providing symptomatic relief in advanced disease. In ulcerating breast cancer, radiotherapy can shrink the primary lesion, controlling exudation and bleeding and permitting healing of overlying skin. Similarly, the distressing symptoms of cough, haemoptysis and pleuritic pain from advanced lung cancer can be eased by palliative radiotherapy. Symptoms associated with local tumour recurrence can often be controlled, e.g. haematuria from advanced bladder cancer or pain from rectal carcinoma. In abdominal malignancy, the main factor limiting the use of radiotherapy is incidental radiation injury to normal bowel. This can cause stricture formation, obstruction and continual bleeding, often years later. Indications for palliative radiotherapy are summarised in Box 7.3.

COMPLICATIONS OF RADIOTHERAPY

Despite the precise use of high-energy radiotherapy, side effects and complications still occur; the main early effects are outlined in Table 7.3.

LONG-TERM SIDE EFFECTS OF RADIOTHERAPY

Modern radiotherapy using high-energy sources and meticulous treatment, planning and delivery causes fewer side effects than the often empirical orthovoltage treatment used in its early days. Side effects such as osteoradionecrosis are rare these days (see Fig. 7.1) but **endarteritis obliterans** may be a long-term complication affecting any tissue subjected to radiotherapy. The effect is progressive impairment of blood supply, loss of specialised tissues and replacement with fibrosis. In the chest, radiotherapy can cause pulmonary fibrosis and, in women treated for left-sided breast cancer, there is an increased long-term risk of cardiac events; treatment techniques have been modified as a result. In the gastrointestinal tract, the effects of radiation on bowel (**radiation enteritis**) can be particularly serious with continued bleeding (in large bowel) and stricture formation (in small bowel). The same pathophysiological reaction probably accounts for delayed or incomplete healing after surgery with breakdown of intestinal anastomoses or formation of internal fistulae. **Radiation colitis** most commonly results from treatment of uterine cervical cancer.

KEY POINTS

Box 7.3 Indications for palliative radiotherapy

Pain control
- Bone pain (especially breast, prostate and lung metastases)
- Nerve root and soft tissue infiltration (e.g. head and neck, brachial plexus)

Dyspnoea
- Shrinkage of tumour obstructing or compressing a large airway

Ulcerating and fungating lesions
- Breast, skin, head and neck tumours

Haemorrhage
- Haemoptysis
- Haematuria
- Rectal and cervical bleeding

Emergency complications
- Spinal cord compression
- Superior vena caval obstruction
- Raised intracranial pressure
- Obstruction of tubular viscera (e.g. oesophagus, upper gastrointestinal tract, ureters)

Space-occupying lesions caused by symptomatic brain metastases
- Brain metastasis causing hemiparesis

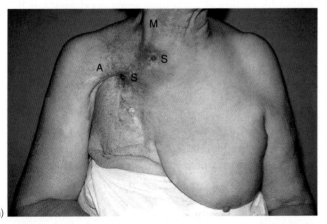
(a)

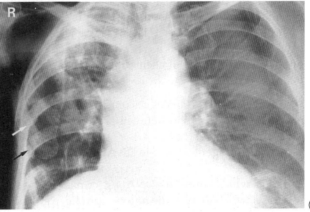
(b)

Fig. 7.1 Osteoradionecrosis after early orthovoltage radiotherapy for breast cancer
This 75-year-old woman had a radical mastectomy and orthovoltage irradiation for carcinoma of the right breast in 1949, 40 years before this photograph. She presented with two discharging skin sinuses below the clavicle. **(a)** Gross deformity of chest wall caused by excision of pectoral muscles at radical mastectomy (axilla **A**, sternomastoids **M**). Note sinus openings **S** leading down to sequestra, and widespread telangiectasia, a late result of radiotherapy. **(b)** Chest X-ray showing osteoradionecrosis of the ribs and scapula on the right side. There is typical patchy osteoporosis and osteosclerosis. Several healing pathological fractures are also evident (arrowed). Irradiation has induced lung fibrosis and pulmonary contraction resulting in a shift of the mediastinum towards the right.

Table 7.3 Early reactions and complications of radiotherapy

Reaction/complication	Management
Systemic side effects	
Malaise and fatigue—very common	These settle spontaneously with rest
Nausea, vomiting and anorexia	Anti-emetics
Effects occurring in irradiated tissues	
Skin (especially axilla, groin and perineum)	
Redness, itching and mild pain	Mild or moderate-strength topical steroids
Skin breakdown (in treatment of skin cancers, this heals after 3–4 weeks)	Moisture-retaining non-adherent dressings Silver-sulphasalazine cream
Abdomen and pelvis	
Nausea, vomiting, diarrhoea	Anti-emetics, antidiarrhoeals
Frequency, dysuria, haematuria (radiation cystitis)	Urinary alkalinising agents; exclude infection
Head and neck	
Dry mouth (xerostomia) due to salivary gland injury	Frequent oral fluids, moist oral swabs, careful attention to oral hygiene
Painful mouth, dysphagia and altered taste. This is due to inflammation and atrophy of oral mucosa (mucositis) and may also involve nasal mucosa	Topical steroids for ulcers, topical anaesthetic gels, antifungal agents for candidiasis, artificial saliva
Chest	
Painful dysphagia (radiation oesophagitis)	Local anaesthetic gel Compound antacid/alginate preparations, e.g. Gaviscon
Head	
Hair loss (alopecia)	Provision of wigs ('wig library')
Bone marrow	
Myelosuppression	Discontinue therapy, prophylactic antibiotics, platelet transfusion

CHEMOTHERAPY

GENERAL PRINCIPLES OF CHEMOTHERAPY

Success with chemotherapeutic agents in curing many haematological and childhood malignancies has encouraged the use of similar drugs to treat solid tumours previously treated only by surgery or radiotherapy.

Drugs destroy tumour cells in a variety of different ways, capitalising on their increased mitotic and metabolic rates. The main types of chemotherapeutic agent are as follows:

- **Antimetabolites**—analogues of normal cellular nutrients, e.g. methotrexate acts as a substitute for folinic acid
- **Alkylating agents**—bind to DNA, e.g. nitrogen mustards
- **Drugs which cross-link DNA**, e.g. cisplatin
- **Drugs which disrupt the mitotic spindle**, e.g. vinca alkaloids

These same cytotoxic mechanisms also affect normal tissues, though usually to a lesser extent, and are responsible for many of the side effects of chemotherapy. For many cancers, the best results are obtained by combinations of cytotoxic drugs. Particular combinations are chosen so the toxic effects of each drug impact on a different organ system; this means that each drug can be given in full tumour-toxic dose without excessive damage to normal tissues. The most effective drug combinations and doses for each tumour type have been established mainly by empirical trials (and some good luck!). It has been difficult to find regimens that give better results than combinations developed in the 1970s and 1980s, e.g. CMF for breast cancer, CHOP for lymphoma and BEP for testicular cancer. Drugs are usually given intravenously, in a series of four to six short courses separated by 3–4 weeks to allow recovery of normal tissues.

Experience has revealed a wide spectrum of sensitivities of different malignant tumours to cytotoxic therapy. These range from total destruction to no therapeutic effect. The sensitivities of different tumour types are summarised in Box 7.4.

MAJOR APPLICATIONS OF CHEMOTHERAPY

PRIMARY CURATIVE TREATMENT

This is mainly indicated for highly sensitive **germ cell tumours**, high-grade **lymphomas** and **solid tumours of**

KEY POINTS

Box 7.4 Tumour sensitivity to cytotoxic chemotherapy

Highly sensitive tumours—reasonable prospect of cure
- Hodgkin's disease
- High-grade lymphomas
- Testicular tumours
- Choriocarcinoma
- Childhood leukaemias
- Wilms' tumour (nephroblastoma)
- Ewing's sarcoma
- Osteogenic sarcoma (lung metastases)

Moderately sensitive tumours—palliation is the main objective
- Breast cancer
- Ovarian malignancies
- Small-cell (oat-cell) carcinoma of lung
- Multiple myeloma
- Acute and chronic leukaemias in adults
- Low-grade lymphomas
- Colorectal cancer

Relatively insensitive tumours—cytotoxic therapy only indicated in special circumstances or with techniques of regional infusion
- Carcinoma of lung other than small-cell type
- Squamous carcinomas of the head and neck
- Carcinoma of uterus and cervix
- Melanoma
- Hepatocellular carcinoma
- Osteogenic sarcoma (primary lesions)
- Renal adenocarcinoma
- Bladder carcinoma

childhood. Chemotherapy may be used alone after obtaining a histological diagnosis (e.g. Hodgkin's disease), or it may follow removal of the primary tumour (e.g. teratoma, Wilms' tumour), or it may be used first and then any residual tumour resected to achieve complete remission (e.g. abdominal para-aortic nodes in testicular teratoma).

ADJUVANT CHEMOTHERAPY

This involves systemic chemotherapy in addition to local treatment of the primary lesion in an attempt to destroy already disseminated but undetectable micrometastases. Adjuvant chemotherapy is often used for breast cancer where axillary lymph nodes are involved, particularly in women less than 50 years old. These patients are at high risk of developing widespread metastases later and adjuvant therapy is given in the hope of reducing the

risk. In node-positive patients, both 5- and 10-year survival rates have been improved by between 6 and 11%. Similar results can be obtained in breast cancer by ovarian ablation. In recent years, treatment has become more acceptable to patients; adjuvant chemotherapy has become more widely employed as outcomes have improved with fewer toxic side effects and better drugs to control nausea. Adjuvant chemotherapy, mainly using 5-fluorouracil (5FU) with folinic acid, appears to have a role in extending recurrence-free survival and possibly life expectancy in cancer of the colon and rectum but the results of a large UK trial (QUASAR) are awaited. Current information on this and other trials can be obtained from the UK Coordinating Committee on Cancer Research (web site: http://ukcccr.icnet.uk). For cancer of the anal canal, chemotherapy plus radiotherapy (**chemo-radiotherapy**) adds to the benefits of radiotherapy alone, often replacing the need for radical surgery.

GENERAL PALLIATIVE TREATMENT

General palliation is the rationale for using chemotherapy for disseminated malignancy in highly sensitive and moderately sensitive tumours. Cure is rarely achieved but quality of life may be greatly improved and, in some cases, life may be prolonged.

PALLIATION OF DISTRESSING LOCAL SYMPTOMS

Cytotoxic therapy may sometimes be indicated for relatively insensitive tumours if local tumour effects are so distressing that even a small reduction in tumour mass might relieve them, e.g. breast cancer causing lymphatic obstruction. The objective is not to prolong life but to improve its quality.

DIRECT ADMINISTRATION OF CYTOTOXIC AGENTS TO THE TUMOUR

In isolated primary or secondary tumours in the liver or kidneys, it is sometimes possible to cannulate the arterial supply of the lesion and administer the cytotoxic agent directly. This may successfully shrink the tumour. For superficial bladder tumours with widespread carcinoma in situ, the poor prognosis can be improved by instillation of chemotherapeutic drugs into the bladder. In early disease, this treatment may be curative.

SIDE EFFECTS OF CHEMOTHERAPY

Chemotherapy is toxic to tumour cells but also to normal body cells, especially those with rapid rates of turnover, e.g. bone marrow and gastrointestinal epithelium. Toxic effects are summarised in Box 7.5. Side effects are common but are rarely so severe that treatment is abandoned.

Chemotherapy offers substantial benefit and a chance of cure in some well-defined malignancies, as shown in Box 7.4. However, clinicians treating cancer need to have clear management objectives, i.e. cure or palliation, based on published clinical trials. Given the potential for side effects and the cost, there is no place for speculative chemotherapy where there is a lack of scientific evidence of benefit.

KEY POINTS

Box 7.5 Toxic effects of chemotherapy

Bone marrow suppression
- Causes anaemia, thrombocytopenia and leucopenia (potentially fatal)

Immunosuppression
- Causes diminished resistance to opportunistic infections

Nausea and vomiting
- Tend to occur within an hour or two of chemotherapy
- Modern anti-emetics can usually control these symptoms but delayed nausea over the ensuing days remains a problem

Disruption of gastrointestinal epithelial turnover
- Causes diarrhoea and oral ulceration

Toxicity to hair follicles
- Particularly etoposide, cyclophosphamide and doxorubicin
- Causes hair loss (recovers 6 months after treatment)

Gonadal injury
- Loss of libido, sterility and possible mutagenesis

Long-term risk of inducing other malignancies
- 20–30 times the normal risk (but still low)

Rapid tumour destruction on a massive scale
- Leads to release of purines and pyrimidines (only a problem in leukaemias and lymphomas) which cause hyperuricaemia, presenting as obstructive uropathy and renal failure
- Can be prevented by giving prophylactic allopurinol

HORMONAL MANIPULATION

GENERAL PRINCIPLES OF HORMONAL MANIPULATION

The growth of certain tumours, notably carcinoma of the prostate and some breast cancers, is partially dependent on sex hormones. Removal of the gonads or use of drugs which block or antagonise the appropriate hormone can have a valuable inhibitory effect on tumour growth.

MAJOR APPLICATIONS OF HORMONAL MANIPULATION

PROSTATIC CANCER

Surgical removal of the testes (**orchidectomy**) is one of the preferred treatments for metastatic carcinoma of the prostate and is the most cost-effective solution. **Stilboestrol** is a synthetic oestrogen and remains a standard alternative to orchidectomy. It partly works by suppressing **luteinising hormone releasing hormone** (LHRH) at hypothalamic level but may be cytotoxic to prostatic cancer cells in its own right. However, it is associated with a high risk of arterial and venous thrombosis and has fallen out of favour. LHRH analogues (gonadorelins) are as effective as orchidectomy for treating disseminated prostatic cancer. These drugs are given at intervals of several weeks; initially they cause release of luteinising hormone from the anterior pituitary, followed by inhibition. **Anti-androgen drugs** alone (e.g. cyproterone, flutamide) have proved less effective and more toxic than gonadorelins but are usually administered initially to block the testosterone 'flare'.

BREAST CANCER

Oral **tamoxifen**, an anti-oestrogen, has been shown to prolong survival after standard local treatment of breast cancer. Its effect is beneficial at all ages but greatest in postmenopausal patients, and its use for 2–5 years post-diagnosis has consistently given significant survival benefits. Tamoxifen can also give useful palliation in recurrent and metastatic breast cancer and is usually worth a trial of treatment as the drug has few side effects. Advances in hormonal treatments now allow the use of second- and even third-line hormones after relapse on tamoxifen. Duration of response to the second- and third-line treatments is often of shorter duration than the initial treatment. However, useful symptom relief may well be obtained with minimal side effects; for example,

progestogens (megestrol, Provera) can induce a useful, though temporary, response.

In metastatic breast cancer, particularly with bony metastases, **oophorectomy** brings relief from pain in about 50% of cases. This may be achieved chemically with LHRH (gonadorelin) antagonists, producing a reversible menopausal state, surgically (usually laparoscopically) or by radiotherapy. In former days, **surgical adrenalectomy** was sometimes performed following relapse after oophorectomy, with the aim of eliminating all sex hormone production. Nowadays, **aromatase-inhibiting drugs** are sometimes given to perform a 'medical adrenalectomy' after failure of tamoxifen. These are more effective and cause fewer side effects than previously used drugs such as aminoglutethimide.

PALLIATIVE CARE

GENERAL PRINCIPLES OF PALLIATIVE CARE

The principles of palliative care are outlined in Box 7.6.

Improvements in detection, diagnosis and treatment have led to increased cure rates for some cancer patients and improved survival rates for many. However, many patients with malignant tumours eventually die from progression of the primary tumour or widespread metastases. The management of incurable disease should be given as much attention as attempts at cure. In an effort to 'do all that is possible', the mistake can be made of concentrating on the primary disease while failing to treat the patient as a whole. Most patients with disseminated malignancy gradually deteriorate until they reach the terminal phase, when it becomes obvious that death will occur within the foreseeable future. A doctor's duty includes 'doing no harm' as well as trying to do some good and there should be no ethical dilemma in withdrawing treatment likely to give no benefit.

Increasingly, patients are living longer, with an increased tumour load. Patients often experience complex symptoms with possible multiple aetiologies, resulting in multiple drug use. Diagnostic tests should be used judiciously to identify those causes which are remediable, but tests which will not alter patient management should be avoided. Proposed treatments should be negotiated with the patients and families, and time must be made available for clear and honest explanation. Palliative care focuses on **quality of life**, and addresses both physical and psychological needs of the patient and the family. Many clinicians, including family practitioners, are both keen to look after their patients at the end of their lives and capable of doing so, ensuring a comfortable and dignified demise. However, specialist palliative care

KEY POINTS

Box 7.6 Principles of palliative care

1. Assess prognosis and the most likely sequence of terminal events
2. Discuss prognosis and life expectancy with the patient and close relatives (but avoid precise predictions of survival time or terminal events). Ensure the patient understands the commitment to maintaining quality of life and the relief of pain and distress
3. Explore the patient's concerns by asking open questions, e.g. what is your greatest worry or fear?
4. Arrange regular consultations by the patient's family practitioner, who should ideally be personally available to be called at any time
5. Ensure immediate availability of hospital or hospice medical care or advice in the event of sudden deterioration or onset of new symptoms, i.e. 'open door' policy
6. Identify future nursing requirements and make contingency plans, e.g. home aids (commodes, incontinence devices etc.), community nursing care, hospital relief
7. Anticipate the development of symptoms and initiate treatment before problems get out of hand. This often prevents premature or unnecessary admission to hospital or hospice
8. Pay particular attention to prevention and early treatment of pain, diarrhoea and constipation, nausea and vomiting by using appropriate drugs
9. Continually review drug therapy, titrating doses against new and changing symptoms to minimise side effects

physicians and nurses can now offer more comprehensive management, both in patients' homes and in palliative care homes, for patients with difficult management problems.

COMMON SYMPTOMS OTHER THAN PAIN REQUIRING PALLIATION

Palliative pain relief is covered in the next section. Other common symptoms requiring palliation are detailed in Table 7.4.

Effective management of the symptoms of advancing cancer requires frequent reassessment of the patient's condition, and frequent discussion with the patient to assess priorities and the acceptability of treatment offered. At all times the focus on quality of life must be retained. Patients and families are reliant on the doctor to guide them as to whether the benefit of treatment outweighs its

disadvantages. Doctors must not hesitate to discuss complex situations with other colleagues and specialists to ascertain the best course of action for their patient.

A multidisciplinary team approach to cancer patient management is known to be more successful in achieving symptom relief. Approaches other than drugs—for example, acupuncture or relaxation techniques—may help in relieving symptoms and diminish the requirement for medication. It may sometimes be necessary to administer drugs by a variety of routes and formulations (e.g. subcutaneous, transdermal) or to use unusually large doses. Long-term sequelae are often not an issue and it may be reasonable to stop drugs usually used as long-term prophylactic treatments to reduce overall medication load.

In addition to physical symptoms, psychological aspects of dying must be addressed. Patients are often reluctant to voice their concerns. Giving the patient real opportunities to talk to sympathetic carers about difficult and

Table 7.4 Common symptoms other than pain requiring palliation

Symptom	Causes	Management
Fatigue/asthenia (lack of energy)	Circulating factors released by tumour, chemotherapy, radiotherapy Pain, poor sleep, depression, anxiety	Open discussion with patient and family Encouraging gentle, regular exercise within limitations and a daily routine Address and treat remediable causes
Loss of appetite (anorexia) and weight loss	Circulating factors released by tumour, chemotherapy, radiotherapy, chronic pain and nausea, fear, depression, anxiety, 'squashed stomach' syndrome, sore mouth, dysphagia	Explanation to patient and family of known causes Meticulous attention to oral hygiene Correct remediable factors
Dysphagia and painful swallowing (odynophagia)	Tumours of pharynx, oesophagus and stomach Compression of oesophagus by extrinsic tumour (e.g. mediastinal lymph nodes) Oesophageal candidiasis Bulbar and pseudobulbar palsy	Options include insertion of stents, laser ablation, cryotherapy, brachytherapy (local radiotherapy) Radiotherapy, high-dose steroids Suspect in immunosuppressed, patients on steroids; diagnosis may require gastroscopy; may require prolonged treatment with oral antifungal agent Multidisciplinary assessment; possible fine-bore tube feeds or feeding gastrostomy
Nausea and vomiting	Drugs: opioids, NSAIDS and others Metabolic causes, e.g. hypercalcaemia, uraemia, liver failure Radiotherapy/chemotherapy Intracranial lesions Gastric outlet obstruction, intestinal obstruction Constipation	Explanation to allay anxiety; review prescriptions Anti-emetic medication e.g. metoclopramide, haloperidol, parenterally administered until vomiting controlled; continue orally whilst cause remains Anti-emetic drugs: short courses of 5HT3 antagonist and/or high-dose steroids High-dose steroids reducing to minimal maintenance dose Avoid nasogastric tube wherever possible Minimise vomiting and reduce gastric/intestinal secretions with hyoscine butylbromide May benefit from short-course high-dose steroids (for extrinsic compressive lesions) or octreotide Occasionally, percutaneous endoscopic gastrostomy (PEG) may be required to vent stomach Prophylactic laxatives for all patients prescribed opioids; generally avoid bulk laxatives in preference to softening and prokinetic agent

Table 7.4 Continued

Symptom	Causes	Management
Breathlessness (dyspnoea), cough, choking	Pleural effusion, cardiac failure, infection, anaemia	Investigate and treat all reversible causes with regard to patient's overall condition (avoid nasogastric aspiration, i.v. infusion and antibiotics in terminally ill)
	Laryngeal tumour, pulmonary tumour or major airway obstruction	May require stenting or local treatment e.g. radiotherapy/laser/cryotherapy
	Lymphangitis carcinomtosa, multiple pulmonary metastases or infiltration	Trial of high-dose dexamethasone 16 mg daily; if beneficial reduce to maintenance dose, e.g. 2–4 mg daily
	Bulbar or pseudobulbar palsy (choking)	Investigate, modify oral intake; if necessary avoid oral route
	Multifactorial: disease and debilitation	Explanation to patient and family; continue bronchodilator therapy; add intermittent oral morphine or continuous subcutaneous diamorphine terminally; oxygen if beneficial
	Anxiety—all breathless patients are anxious	Clear explanation, appropriate reassurance; anxiolytic drugs if appropriate
Constipation (be alert to possibilities of (a) constipation presenting as spurious diarrhoea due to leakage of watery faeces passed as solid faecal mass; (b) constipation as the presenting feature of low bowel obstruction)	Immobility, weakness and general debility Poor nutrition and low dietary fibre intake Opioids and other drug effects (e.g. tricyclic antidepressants) Dehydration, biochemical disturbances (hypercalcaemia, hypokalaemia)	Discuss nutritional options, encourage increased fluid intake, prescribe anti-emetic where nausea contributes to poor intake Laxatives: ● Bulking agents—should be reserved for moderately active patients with good fluid intake who are not on opioid medication ● Osmotic laxatives—lactulose (may cause flatulence and abdominal cramp); magnesium salts (sometimes unpalatable) ● Stimulants—senna, bisacodyl, danthron, docusate ● Lubricants—liquid paraffin often necessary to combine softening and stimulant agents Self-administered suppositories (glycerol and/or bisacodyl) are often acceptable to patients Enemas and manual evacuation of faeces are distressing but occasionally necessary
Confusion	Unfamiliar stimuli Cerebral metastases Infection Drugs, e.g. opioids, anticonvulsants, tricyclics Metabolic causes, e.g. uraemia, hypercalcaemia, hyponatraemia Anxiety Cerebral hypoxia	Explanation and calming reassurance to patient and family Investigation and treatment of any reversible causes Medication if necessary: distressed patient may respond to oral or parenteral benzodiazepines, e.g. diazepam 5 mg b.d., or midazolam by continuous infusion; paranoid or hallucinating patients may require haloperidol orally or subcutaneously, up to 20 mg/24 hours
Terminal restlessness (also known as terminal agitation/agitated delirium/terminal anguish/terminal distress)	As patient's level of consciousness diminishes, abnormal movements, twitching myoclonus and incomprehensible speech/noise may prove distressing for the family. Causes may include underlying psychological problems which remain unresolved, plus disease, metabolic disturbance and drug accumulation. N.B. Coordinated movements may have remediable underlying cause, e.g. pain, bladder distension, pruritis etc.	Explanation to family Identify cause of any purposeful movement and resolve, e.g. catheterise Sedation; often requires subcutaneous infusion with, e.g., midazolam (benzodiazepine) 30–90 mg/24 hours
'Death rattle' (i.e. distressing sounds of impaired breathing in terminal stage of disease)	Accumulation of bronchial secretions and loss of control of muscles of larynx and phyrynx	Explanation to family Positioning of patient often reduces sound and respiratory effort Early and continued use of antisecretory agent, e.g. hyoscine hydrobromide subcutaneously in divided doses or continuous infusion up to 3.6 mg/24 hours

distressing topics such as the fear of dying or the process of dying, or aspects of life perceived not to have been resolved when healthy, can relieve much suffering and allay needless anxiety.

Ideally, patients will spend most of their time at home, away from hospital, supported by the primary health-care team. Increasingly, patients are remaining at home to die. Arrangements must be in place, such that the patient and family are clear about who they can contact, day or night, about problems if they arise. Many general practitioners make arrangements to review their patients at home at frequent intervals. It is important that hospital professionals liaise frequently with community carers and specialists about the patient's condition, and vice versa. There must be immediate availability of specialist services and support whether for admission or advice, whenever required. If palliative care is handled well, it can bring rich rewards to both patient and doctor.

CANCER PAIN

Pain is a common feature of advanced malignant disease but is by no means universal or severe. The severity of pain usually increases as disease progresses and is often caused by multiple factors. Pain and fear of pain or both often dominate the thoughts of the patient and family and its effects are compounded by other distressing symptoms such as nausea, anxiety, depression and other psychological and spiritual factors. Pain is what the patient perceives it to be and management must involve a holistic and not merely disease-oriented approach.

ASSESSMENT OF PAIN

The successful treatment of pain requires accurate diagnosis of its cause or causes, each of which may require different management. Pain of organic origin may be caused by four mechanisms, the first three being **nociceptive** in origin (i.e. involving stimulation of sensory nerve endings):

- **Superficial somatic pain**—this pain is derived from tumour involvement of skin, subcutaneous tissues, or mucosa of mouth, anus, urethra, bladder etc. Examples include malignant ulceration, stomatitis and cystitis. The pain is often stinging or burning in character and highly localised. Examination usually reveals an inflammatory component to the local pathological process
- **Deep somatic pain**—musculoskeletal elements (periosteum, joints, muscles, tendons, ligaments), superficial lymph nodes, mesothelial membranes (pleura and peritoneum) and the liver capsule make up this category; common examples are bony metastases and liver capsule distension. Pain is dull and aching in character, well defined and aggravated by movement
- **Visceral pain**—this pain originates from solid or hollow abdominal organs (e.g. intestinal, biliary or ureteric obstruction), deep masses of tumour or lymph nodes (e.g. retroperitoneal tumour, para-aortic or mediastinal lymph nodes) or large muscle groups.

The pain is dull, deep, poorly defined and poorly localised, and is often accompanied by autonomic effects such as nausea, vomiting, sweating and cardiovascular changes
- **Neurogenic pain**—this pain does not derive from direct involvement of nerve endings but rather from tumour invasion or compression of nerves. Common causes are tumour involvement of the brachial plexus, chest wall (intercostal nerves), lumbosacral plexus, spinal cord compression and perineural tumour spread. Post-herpetic neuralgia, post-thoracotomy pain and phantom limb pain represent neurogenic pain in its most clear-cut form, and similar pain may be found in patients with malignant disease. Dysaesthesia (abnormal sensation, pins and needles, tingling, burning, painful numbness) is characteristic of neurogenic-type pain. It may be provoked by stimuli which would not usually provoke pain and this is known as **allodynia**. Pain is often **paroxysmal** (shooting, lancinating) and occurs in a recognisable peripheral nerve or dermatomal distribution in which there are often autonomic signs (e.g. sweating, coldness, pallor, cyanosis)

GENERAL PRINCIPLES OF CANCER PAIN MANAGEMENT

- **Elimination of pain** and restoration of patient activity should be the aim, whenever possible
- **Regular medication** is essential and should be based on a knowledge of duration of action of drugs and consideration of physiological factors affecting drug absorption and elimination (e.g. intestinal stasis, renal and hepatic failure)
- **Titration of the analgesic** against the severity of pain using the three-step analgesic ladder developed by the World Health Organisation (see Fig. 7.2)
- **Supplementing analgesics with other drugs** and therapies (adjuvants) appropriate to the mechanisms causing the pain (see Table 7.5)

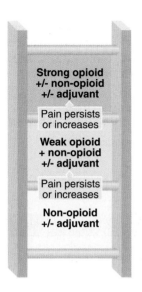

Strong opioid analgesics
Paracetamol
Aspirin
Non-steroidals

Weak opioid analgesics
Codeine
Codeine paracetamol mixtures
Others, e.g. dextropropoxyphene

Non-opioid analgesics
Morphine and related compounds,
e.g. fentanyl, methadone

Fig. 7.2 Three-step analgesic ladder for cancer pain control (WHO 1986)
Remember:
(i) by the mouth—oral medication if possible
(ii) by the clock—regularly *not* 'as required' (p.r.n.)
(iii) by the ladder—increasing potency of analgesia for increasing severity of pain.

OPIOID ANALGESIA

Morphine is the strong opioid of choice for treating cancer pain. A majority of patients will be able to take oral morphine for their pain relief, increasing the dose when required throughout their illness. Addiction is not a problem amongst cancer patients, where morphine dose has been titrated against the pain. Patients who have been on morphine whose pain has improved—for example, after radiotherapy—are able to reduce and sometimes stop morphine without difficulty. (Obviously abrupt cessation is to be avoided as physical withdrawal symptoms will occur.)

Tolerance is uncommon, even among patients who take morphine for many months. Where the patient who has been on a stable dose of morphine requires an increased dose, this usually reflects an increase in pain due to progression of disease.

Titrating the dose of morphine against the pain and increasing the dose gradually also avoid respiratory depression. Respiratory depression is only likely to be clinically significant where the dose prescribed is excessive (exceeding analgesic requirements), or where the patient's condition has deteriorated such that morphine accumulates due to reduced elimination.

When commencing morphine it is important to discuss its use with the patient and family to allay fears and misconceptions. Some patients and families equate the need for morphine with imminent death, while others fear addiction or side effects; these anxieties will usually be overcome by careful explanation. The use of parenteral morphine is generally confined to seriously ill patients unable to tolerate oral administration or the occasional patient who is intolerant of oral morphine. The **subcutaneous route** is preferred and is suitable for both single 'breakthrough' doses and for continuous subcutaneous infusions via an indwelling 'butterfly' needle. Infusions are usually controlled and delivered via a small battery-operated syringe driver holding sufficient solution for 24 hours. Morphine sulphate causes less inflammation at the infusion site than morphine tartrate, as does diamorphine (heroin) which is widely used in countries such as the UK where it is legally available. For morphine, the dose for subcutaneous use is between one-third and one-half of the equivalent oral dose. Subcutaneous bolus doses for breakthrough pain are much less painful than intramuscular injections. Morphine should not be given intravenously as this appears to induce rapid tolerance and cause escalating dose requirements and greater side effects. For patients with intractable pain in the lower body or lower limbs, morphine is sometimes administered via an epidural catheter with a subcutaneous tunnel and port (e.g. Portacath).

Remember when commencing morphine:

● Constipation will always occur in patients with a normal bowel; always prescribe a laxative and explain the need for its regular use
● Nausea may occur at the beginning of treatment and whenever the dose is increased. Nausea usually resolves over 48–72 hours but an anti-emetic—for example, metoclopramide 10 mg q.d.s.—should be prescribed on an 'as required' basis
● Drowsiness may also occur initially. This should resolve over 48–72 hours but if it persists the morphine dose should be reduced or where necessary an alternative opioid used
● Confusion may occur, especially in the elderly, where the starting dose is too high or the dose is increased too rapidly

113

Table 7.5 Adjuvant analgesics and other treatments for management of cancer pain

Treatment method	Indications
Non-steroidal anti-inflammatory agents—via oral/rectal/transdermal routes	Reduce inflammatory component in superficial and deep somatic pain. Excellent for bony and other musculo-skeletal pains
Low-dose tricyclic antidepressants (usually as single evening dose)	Used in treatment of neurogenic pain. Promotes sleep and may improve sense of well-being
Anticonvulsants (e.g. carbamazepine, sodium valproate)	Valuable for neurogenic pain especially if lancinating in quality. May be combined with other adjuvant analgesics
Antispasmodics (e.g. hyoscine butylbromide)	Reduces visceral contractions in colicky visceral pain (intestinal, biliary, ureteric) and overt bowel obstruction
Muscle relaxants (e.g. diazepam)	Relieve muscle spasms, e.g. lumbosacral, cervical, psoas
Anxiolytics/antidepressants	Where anxiety or depression are found to be contributing to the cancer pain and preventing its resolution
Antibiotics (e.g. metronidazole tablets or gel)	Help treat infected superficial lesions, e.g. ulcerated skin, breast or head and neck tumours (usually involve Gram-negative organisms)
Corticosteroids (e.g. dexamethasone 4–8 daily, prednisolone 30–60 mg daily)	Shrink inflammatory zone associated with tumour to relieve pressure effects, e.g. cerebral tumours, spinal cord and peripheral nerve compression, liver capsule stretching, tumour swelling causing obstruction to bowel, biliary or urinary tracts
Topical anti-inflammatory agents (e.g. steroid creams)	For oral and nasal mucositis, ulcerated skin lesions, radiation proctitis
Local palliative radiotherapy	For bone metastases, compressive lesions of brain and spinal cord, large airway and superior vena caval obstruction, fungating or bleeding superficial lesions
Bisphosphonates (e.g. pamidronate, clodronate)	Predominantly used for the relief of bone pain in metastatic breast cancer, and multiple myeloma. Can be given parenterally as bolus or continuously as oral therapy
Radioactive isotope therapy	Used for the relief of bone pain due to metastatic disease
Palliative chemotherapy	Sometimes relives pain by shrinkage of chemosensitive tumours
Nerve blocks (often under radiological guidance)	Very helpful in treating pain in specific areas, e.g. intercostal blocks for chest wall pain; coeliac plexus blocks for pancreatic and other 'foregut' pain. Often reduce the overall requirement for systemic analgesia
Physiotherapy and associated physical modalities (e.g. massage, TENS, hot or cold packs)	Muscle spasm, inflammatory component of nociceptive pain mechanisms. Massage for muscle spasms and lymphoedema. TENS may help neurogenic pain
Skeletal immobilisation	Elective internal fixation of long bones for incipient or actual pathological fracture of long bones

● Myoclonic jerks may be seen when using higher doses of morphine or when the patient's condition deteriorates, causing accumulation of metabolites. A reduction in dose of morphine or an alternative strong opioid may be required

● Itch, bronchospasm and hallucination occur in a few patients and require explanation and a change to an alternative opioid

ESTABLISHING TREATMENT

Once the use of morphine has been discussed and agreed with the patient, the preferred method for establishing dosage is by **titration**. The usual starting dose will be 5–10 mg of immediate-release morphine 4-hourly; this can be reduced to 2.5–5 mg for elderly patients. Occasionally, for those with renal or liver impairment or in the very elderly, the duration of analgesic effect will be prolonged and a 6–8-hourly interval may be required. It may be appropriate to 'double-dose' at night to avoid the patient waking in the early hours. The regular 4-hourly dose must always be accompanied by the same dose on an 'as required' basis for pain which 'breaks through' before the next dose is due. It is usual to allow 24 hours before considering dose increases. Increments should be 50% at the lower-dosage range of morphine—for example, 20 mg should be increased to 30 mg—but 33% in the higher-dose range—for example, 120 mg should be increased to

160 mg. Once the total 24-hour dose required has been determined, i.e. the regular 4-hourly doses plus breakthrough doses which completely control pain, an alternative formulation may be substituted. To determine doses of b.d. formulation the total 24-hour dose is divided by two; for formulations which last 24 hours, the total dose is given once daily. 'As required', immediate-release morphine must still be available for breakthrough pain.

Many patients have their pain successfully and readily treated throughout their disease by regular morphine at doses which occasionally need to be increased by their family practitioner. As the disease progresses, the tumour may advance to involve adjacent or distant structures causing an increase or change in character of the pain. Some pain may be only **partially opioid-responsive**; that is to say, adjuvant analgesia will be required to achieve pain control (see Table 7.5). Whenever pain is difficult to control it is helpful to revert to 4-hourly titration of morphine. It is important for the doctor to ascertain whether there is any benefit from incrementally increasing the doses of morphine. Where an increased dose does not reduce pain or causes additional side effects, it is likely that the pain is only partially opioid-responsive and other means of treating it must be sought. Continuing to escalate opioid doses without improving analgesia will lead to unnecessary side effects and possibly toxicity and confusion.

INCIDENT PAIN

A particularly difficult area of pain treatment is that of **incident pain**. As the name suggests, this is pain which occurs during a particular activity such as that arising from movement or due to changing a dressing. This pain is of limited duration and is not best treated by increasing the regular systemic medication, as this may lead to side effects at times other than the precipitating incident. Incident pain is best treated using an analgesic with a quick, predictable onset of action and a short duration of action (for example, dextromoramide sublingual or PR). Using additional analgesia in this way often allows the 'incident' to take place comfortably but also permits the patient to remain on the already established 24-hour opioid dose.

Successful treatment of cancer pain throughout the patient's life depends on regular reassessment, detailed examination and documentation (using a pain chart wherever appropriate), and carefully listening to the patient and carers to understand the full situation. Where the doctor works with a multidisciplinary team using all his or her skills, effective, acceptable pain relief will be achieved. The reward will be that the patient can then concentrate on what truly constitutes quality of life.

A variety of other opioids are used less commonly in palliative care and usually for specific indications. These are summarised in Table 7.6, p. 116.

SIDE EFFECTS OF MORPHINE AND OTHER OPIOID DRUGS

- **Nausea and vomiting**—commonly occur with initial administration or rapid increase in dose; therefore use a prophylactic anti-emetic with morphine initially (it may be discontinued later)
- **Constipation**—almost inevitable due to depression of gut peristalsis; use prophylactic faecal bulking agents (e.g. dietary fibre supplements, methyl cellulose preparations), osmotic agents (e.g. sorbitol, lactulose), stool softeners (e.g. dioctyl sodium) and peristaltic stimulants (e.g. senna, bisacodyl)
- **Confusion, hallucinations**—mainly a problem for high opioid doses, rapidly increasing doses and in the elderly (especially if vulnerable to toxic confusional states because of other pathological processes); reduce the dose if possible and/or treat with tranquillisers, e.g. haloperidol
- **Myoclonic spasms**, e.g. jerking—often incorrectly attributed to morphine and may be due to concomitant use of phenothiazines or similar drugs (e.g. prochlorperazine, haloperidol); they may occur due to accumulation of toxic metabolites especially in patients with renal failure

Table 7.6 Opioid drugs used in palliative care

Analgesic	Equianalgesic dose of oral morphine	Duration of action	Indications
Codeine 60 mg	5 mg	6 hours	Codeine or dihydrocodeine alone or in combination with paracetamol are used to treat mild to moderate pain. May cause nausea or constipation
Tramadol 50 mg	10 mg	6 hours	Used in moderate pain. Can be helpful where codeine preparations ineffective or not tolerated
Dextromoramide (Palfium) 5 mg	10 mg	1–2 hours	Useful sublingually or PR for rapid-onset, short-action analgesia during procedures, e.g. turning, washing, changing dressings
Diamorphine injection 10 mg	20–30 mg	4 hours	Where local regulations permit preferred to morphine, which requires the parenteral route owing to high solubility. Side effects identical to morphine
Fentanyl 25 µg/hr transdermal 'patch'	120 mg over 24 hours	72 hours	Important to establish opioid requirements by titration with morphine first. Fentanyl can be advantageous in patients intolerant of side effects of morphine, or where oral route is chronically unavailable
Methadone 5 mg syrup	10–15 mg	8–12 hours	Used in specialist units; initial titration often complex owing to prolonged and variable half-life. Used in low dose, e.g. 2–5 mg nocte or b.d. for cough suppression
Oxycodone suppository 30 mg; also available as tablets	30 mg	6–8 hours	May be useful in short term for some patients where oral route not available, e.g. postoperatively. Oral formulation sometimes used in patients intolerant of morphine
Phenazocine 5 mg	25 mg	6–8 hours	Can be used sublingually; sometimes better tolerated in elderly patients than morphine. Limited to patients where morphine dose already established, no low dose preparation is available

N.B. There is no role for buprenorphine, meptazinol or pethidine in the long-term treatment of cancer pain as they all have limitations, e.g. analgesic ceiling, short duration of action, or cumulation of toxic metabolites, which render them unsuitable for regular long-term use

Principles of accident surgery

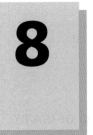

8 Accident surgery: general principles and soft tissue injuries

INTRODUCTION

Trauma patients constitute up to 20% of general surgical admissions in an average district general hospital, the percentage varying with local policies as to which department is responsible for head injuries. In most centres, head injuries are the responsibility of either general surgeons or orthopaedic surgeons; in regional neurosurgical centres, all head injuries are usually admitted directly to neurosurgery.

This chapter discusses the principles of management of serious and multiple injuries, the management of soft tissue injuries and burns.

PRELIMINARY HOSPITAL MANAGEMENT OF MULTIPLE AND SERIOUS INJURIES

There are two peaks of death after surviving trauma, the first occurring within the 'golden hour' after the accident and the second over the next few hours. Survival immediately after the accident depends on the severity of injury, the competence of immediate care and the speed of transfer to an accident unit. Deaths in the second category are usually caused by treatable conditions in which death is largely avoidable. By the time the seriously injured patient has arrived at the resuscitation room, the first peak has passed and the main danger of death is from hypovolaemia (intrathoracic or intraperitoneal haemorrhage and blood loss from multiple fractures) or from an expanding intracranial haematoma.

Most injured patients arrive at hospital with relatively trivial injuries and only a small minority require the extensive initial care described here. For the potentially seriously injured, the immediate priority after arriving at hospital is rapid initial assessment combined with resuscitation, followed by a secondary survey and prioritisation and treatment of individual injuries. Training in this process has standardised through **Advanced Trauma Life Support** (ATLS) courses, initiated by the American College of Surgeons and now run in many countries. These courses employ well-trained volunteers as 'patients' and partici-pants are given training and assessment in real-life simulations using the 'ABC system' shown in Box 8.1.

INITIAL CARE IN THE ACCIDENT DEPARTMENT

ORGANISATION OF THE ACCIDENT DEPARTMENT

The accident department is usually given prior warning by the ambulance service when seriously injured patients are on the way to hospital. This alerts the surgical and anaesthetic teams to be standing by when the patient arrives. The resuscitation room and its essential equipment are made ready for immediate use, e.g. infusion sets run through, drugs laid out. Success in managing life-threatening injuries depends on good organisation. One doctor must take overall medical responsibility and coordinate the activities of any other specialties involved. This is of paramount importance in patients with multiple injuries.

MAJOR DISASTERS

For major disasters such as train or air crashes where many casualties can be expected, each hospital designated to receive casualties should have a detailed and rehearsed **major accident plan**, defining exactly who is responsible for each of the main functions (e.g. medical coordinator, field triage officer—see below) and their precise duties, together with details of the actions required of all other team members. Parts of the plan can be summarised on action cards, distributed to designated staff when a major accident is declared.

An important task in managing major disasters is to sort patients into management priority groups on arrival, a process known as **triage**.

The usual triage categories are:

● Critical—require immediate surgery
● Serious—require surgery but can wait

● Minor injury
● Expectant—severely injured and unlikely to survive even if treated aggressively (only used in a mass casualty scene)
● Dead

PROTOCOL FOR INITIAL ASSESSMENT OF INJURY

Many patients brought to the resuscitation room have already received 'on-site' first aid from an accident team. Nevertheless, all patients need an initial rapid **primary survey** and appropriate **resuscitation**. This includes simultaneous assessment, identification and management of immediately life-threatening problems. Most deaths result

---

KEY POINTS

Box 8.1 Management priorities for the patient with multiple injuries*

1. Resuscitation and support of cardiovascular and respiratory function

A. Is the **AIRWAY** obstructed?

● Remove any oropharyngeal obstructions, e.g. teeth, dentures or blood
● Intubate trachea or perform cricothyroidotomy if necessary, especially if the patient is unconscious or has multiple jaw fractures

B. Is the patient **BREATHING** spontaneously and adequately ventilated?

● Ventilate artificially if necessary, e.g. for flail chest or serious head injuries
● Seal any open chest wounds allowing air into the pleural cavity in order to limit mediastinal 'flap' movement with each breath
● Relieve tension pneumothorax, drain haemothorax
  by chest drainage

C. What is the state of the **CIRCULATION** as assessed by pulse rate and blood pressure, and is there any obvious external haemorrhage?

● Ensure adequate circulating volume by controlling haemorrhage and replacing lost fluids by intravenous infusion
● Relieve cardiac tamponade by long needle aspiration
● Apply external cardiac massage in the case of cardiac arrest
● Catheterise the bladder to monitor urine production and to provide a guide to renal perfusion

D. Is there any **DISABILITY** of the central nervous system? Glasgow Coma Scale and brief neurological examination assess the level of consciousness and other neurological deficits

E. **EXPOSURE** of the whole patient, including removal of all clothing, to allow a rapid 'top to toe' assessment for external injury

2. Treat life-threatening injuries revealed during the primary survey

● Relieve rising intracranial pressure, e.g. surgical decompression of extradural haemorrhage
● perform thoracotomy for major heart and great vessel injuries
● perform laparotomy for gastrointestinal perforation or splenic rupture
● Investigate and repair major peripheral vascular injuries, e.g. penetrating groin injury

3. Treat major fractures and dislocations including spinal injuries

4. Treat less serious injuries after secondary survey

● Perform wound toilet of soft tissue injuries, suturing or packing as appropriate
● Reduce other fractures and dislocations
● Repair tendon and peripheral nerve injuries

---

*Based on the Advanced Trauma Life Support system of the American College of Surgeons

from head injuries or from multiple injuries involving chest, abdomen and limbs. Management priorities for the multiply injured patient are summarised in Box 8.1. Primary survey and resuscitation is followed by a **secondary survey** designed to assess the potential for developing other life-threatening problems or complications. In the critically injured patient, the urgency of initial treatment may delay progress to the secondary survey.

PREVENTION OF SECONDARY INJURIES

Primary injuries are those which result directly from the trauma. Secondary injuries occur as an indirect result of the trauma, e.g. brain damage from hypoxia, spinal cord injury due to poor handling of an unstable spinal injury. These are largely preventable with good immediate care, careful handling, rapid resuscitation and elective ventilation if needed. Early stabilisation of long bone fractures

minimises the risk of later multiple organ failure and provides stable conditions in which a formal assessment of any less urgent head, chest or abdominal injuries can be made.

Cervical spine injury

Any unconscious patient may have sustained an unstable vertebral injury, and secondary spinal cord injury may occur unless the patient is nursed and moved with extreme care. Unconscious trauma patients should always have X-rays of the cervical spine (see Fig. 8.1). Conscious patients with suspected cervical spine injuries should be moved with extreme caution. Passive neck movements must not be attempted but the patient should be allowed to perform active movements unaided; spasm or pain will restrict movement if there is a significant injury. Patients should be 'log-rolled' by several people together in order to move them.

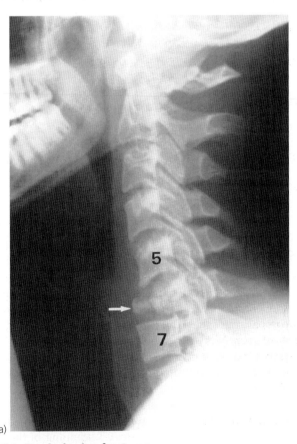
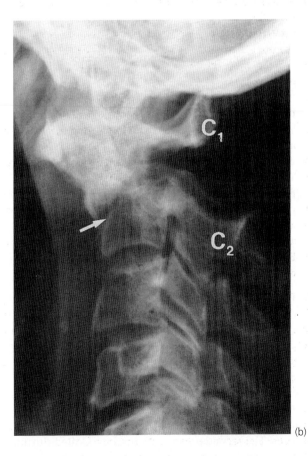

(a) (b)

Fig. 8.1 Cervical spine fractures

(a) Lateral cervical spine X-ray of a 17-year-old boy admitted semi-conscious after coming off his motor-cycle and landing head-first in a ditch. On examination he was not moving his lower limbs or hands although there was some movement at the shoulders. The X-ray shows a burst fracture of the body of C6 (arrowed) with fragments in the spinal canal; there is also some posterior subluxation of C5. **(b)** Left lateral cervical spine X-ray from another unconscious young patient showing a fracture (arrowed) of the body of C2 and severe anterior subluxation of C1.

INITIAL ASSESSMENT OF THE SERIOUSLY INJURED PATIENT

Despite the urgency of the situation, primary assessment of the trauma patient must be performed in a systematic manner, i.e. history, examination and special tests.

HISTORY

A rapid history is obtained from the patient if possible and from ambulance personnel and other witnesses. The history should include the following details:

- Time of the accident
- Nature and speed of impact
- Fate of other travellers in the same vehicle
- Conscious level of patient when discovered and later changes in conscious level
- An estimate of blood loss at scene of accident
- Details of drugs, fluids and other treatments administered at scene of accident
- Previous state of health including past medical history, drug history and drug allergies
- Details of prior food, alcohol or drug intake

EXAMINATION

A rapid preliminary examination or **primary survey** is performed as soon as the patient arrives.

The main observations are:

- Airway, breathing, circulation, neurological disability (including the ability to move all limbs) and full exposure (see Box 8.1)
- State of consciousness (Glasgow Coma Score, see p. 137)
- Signs of distress—difficulty in breathing, obvious pain
- Appearance of the skin for evidence of pallor and cyanosis
- Vital signs—pulse rate, blood pressure, respiratory pattern
- The presence of gross injuries

From this, immediate management priorities can be identified and resuscitation implemented. Once this has been done, a detailed 'head to toe' secondary survey is then performed for signs of serious head, spine, chest, abdominal, pelvic and limb injuries. The particular observations are summarised in Box 8.2; details for individual systems are described later. The examination findings and the time of examination must be carefully recorded in the patient's notes, not least for medicolegal purposes. The secondary survey must be repeated during hospitalisation as some major and many lesser injuries are missed because of the urgency of the serious injuries. Up to 20% of multiple injury patients have injuries missed in the early stages.

KEY POINTS

Box 8.2 Special points to note in systematic examination of the seriously injured patient

Head and neck
- Lacerations
- Depressed vault fractures
- Facial and jaw fractures
- Pupil size and responsiveness
- Range of active neck movements

Chest (front and back)
- Penetrating injuries
- Bruising and skin imprinting
- Pattern and rate of respiration
- Symmetry of chest movement
- Gross mediastinal shift
- Pattern of air entry throughout lung fields
- Crepitus (subcutaneous air)

Abdomen
- External injuries as for chest
- Distension by gas or fluid
- Abdominal girth
- Tenderness
- Presence of palpable or percussible bladder
- Pelvic fractures
- Bleeding from urethral meatus

Limbs
- Neurovascular status of each limb
- Lacerations
- Deformities
- Soft tissue swelling
- Fractures and dislocations

X-RAYS AND OTHER INVESTIGATIONS

In most seriously injured patients, the chest and cervical spine are X-rayed in the resuscitation room using portable equipment. The diagnostic quality of chest films must be good enough to exclude major chest wall, mediastinal and lung injuries and also to provide a baseline for comparison if the patient subsequently deteriorates. Cervical spine X-rays often fail to include C1, C7 and T1 and poor films must be interpreted with caution; if necessary they should be repeated or a CT scan of the area should be ordered.

Portable skull X-rays should only be performed if this is likely to affect immediate management as diagnostic quality tends to be inadequate. CT scanning of the skull may be required urgently in head-injured patients. All other X-rays are performed later in the radiology department once the patient has been stabilised.

Initial blood tests should include haemoglobin and

blood grouping and antibody screen and an appropriate number of units of bank blood should be ordered. In a desperate emergency, universal donor blood (group O, Rh negative) can be transfused without grouping or cross-matching, although plasma substitutes will usually suffice until compatible blood becomes available. Plasma electrolytes and glucose are usually measured, and arterial blood gases are estimated if there is any suspicion of respiratory failure.

Further investigations are guided by the nature of the individual injuries, as detailed below and in the following chapters.

MANAGEMENT OF SOFT TISSUE INJURIES

The detailed management of a particular injury depends on its site, the tissues involved, the extent of contamination and the possibility of retained foreign bodies. In every case, the danger of tetanus must be considered and tetanus toxoid administered if immunisation is inadequate. Deep, soil-contaminated wounds (however small) in an unimmunised patient warrant prophylactic penicillin.

The majority of wounds can be cleaned and sutured immediately, particularly on the face, but contused or contaminated wounds require cleansing and excision of dead tissue (debridement) followed by delayed primary suture a few days later. Less commonly, they are allowed to heal by secondary intention (see Ch. 6).

FOREIGN BODIES

The history of the injury gives a clue as to the likelihood of a foreign body being present. The main foreign bodies are road dirt and gravel, wood splinters, glass and metal fragments. Radiology will show metal and usually glass (see Fig. 8.2). The radiopacity of glass, however, depends on its lead content and a negative X-ray does not exclude its presence. It is important to remember that an unrecognised foreign body may result in litigation!

As a general principle, foreign bodies should be removed, especially if they are organic or likely to be contaminated. Glass and metal fragments are often small, multiple and deeply embedded and may be difficult or impossible to locate at operation despite X-ray diagnosis. In this case, it is not appropriate to embark on extensive exploratory surgery but to leave the fragments in situ where they rarely cause much problem. The patient must be informed about what has been left and warned that superficial fragments usually work their way to the surface and are shed spontaneously. The patient must be instructed to return if problems occur later. All of this information should be recorded in the notes in case of future legal action.

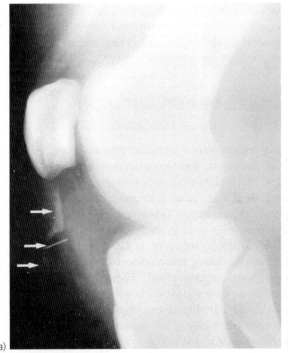

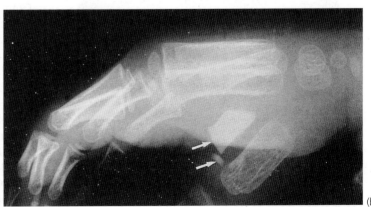

(a)   (b)

Fig. 8.2 Glass in soft tissue wounds
(a) A 19-year-old woman with lacerations near the knee after falling on to broken glass. Note several fragments of glass (arrowed) in the infrapatellar soft tissues. **(b)** Fragments of glass (arrowed) in the palm of a 12-year-old boy after he fell through a glass door. In both these cases, the fragments were missed by casualty officers because X-rays were not requested despite a history of glass injury.

FACIAL LACERATIONS

Facial lacerations heal well. Provided they are cleaned meticulously, they can be sutured primarily and expected to heal. Infection is rarely a problem because of the excellent blood supply. Even ragged skin edges do not become devitalised and trimming is rarely necessary. The main consideration is the likely cosmetic outcome and great care should be taken with suturing technique, employing general anaesthesia if necessary. Complex lacerations or skin loss, especially on children and young men or women, should be sutured by a plastic surgeon.

SCALP LACERATIONS

Apart from associated brain injury or skull fracture, the main considerations in dealing with scalp lacerations are haemostasis and whether the aponeurotic layer has been breached. Assessment and proper exploration are difficult without shaving the wound edges; large lacerations should be explored under general anaesthesia. If the aponeurosis (galea) has been breached, this layer must be sutured separately to prevent accumulation of a subaponeurotic haematoma which is vulnerable to infection. The major scalp vessels lie in the superficial

fascia between the dermis and the aponeurosis. Dense collagenous bands traverse the superficial fascia and may inhibit vascular contraction and the expected spontaneous arrest of bleeding. These vessels should be individually ligated or sutured. The extent of blood loss from scalp lacerations is easy to underestimate and may be sufficient to cause hypovolaemic shock.

LACERATIONS TO THE LIMBS AND HANDS

The main considerations with this type of injury are as follows:

- **Possible nerve, tendon or vascular injury**—assessment includes testing sensation, movement, peripheral pulses and tissue perfusion (i.e. pulses, warmth, colour, capillary refilling after blanching)
- **Tissue viability**—this is particularly important in the case of crush injuries and flap lacerations, especially of the pretibial area
- **Risk of infection**—the fingers and hands are vulnerable to infection of the pulp spaces and deep palmar spaces. These wounds need meticulous exploration, cleansing and antibiotic prophylaxis against staphylococci and streptococci (e.g. flucloxacillin plus amoxycillin). Potential for **gas gangrene** must be considered in the case of large contaminated and contused wounds involving muscle. Dead tissue should be thoroughly excised, benzylpenicillin given prophylactically, and delayed primary closure planned. Injuries from bites (especially by dogs or humans) and bones (usually in meat workers) almost invariably become infected unless antibiotic prophylaxis is given.

PRINCIPLES OF REPLANTATION SURGERY

Complete amputation of digits is common, especially in industrial accidents, but sometimes whole limbs are severed. With clean-cut injuries, it is possible to reattach the amputated part using microsurgical techniques to join the vessels and nerves. This cannot be done after crush or avulsion injuries or in grossly contaminated wounds. Even in ideal cases, recovery is slow and usually incomplete, necessitating many months away from work and much rehabilitation effort. Therefore, replantation should never be undertaken without carefully evaluating the likely benefits. In digital amputation, the greatest disability results from loss of the thumb. There is no place for replantation of a single finger, even the index finger, because the remaining fingers rapidly adapt to the loss.

Replantation should only be considered if there has been no major crushing or degloving injury. Indications for replantation include:

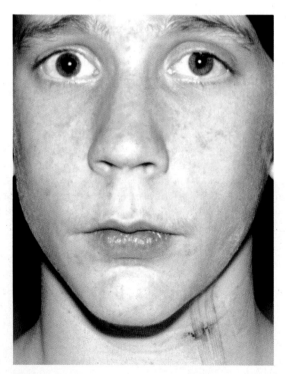

Fig. 8.3 Horner's syndrome caused by stab wound in the neck. This 19-year-old was stabbed in the neck: the knife missed the great vessels but succeeded in damaging the cervical sympathetic chain, causing miosis (contraction) of the pupil as a result of unopposed parasympathetic activity.

- Loss of whole upper limb or hand
- Loss of thumb alone
- Loss of all digits (replant thumb and one or two fingers)
- Loss of all fingers (replant one or possibly two fingers)

At the scene of the injury, the severed digit should be washed and placed in a plastic bag which is then placed inside a second plastic bag containing ice or frozen peas. In this way it can be successfully preserved for up to 12 hours.

BURNS

Burns and scalds are common injuries, resulting in 12 000 hospital admissions annually in England and Wales. Many times this number are treated on an out-patient basis. Two-thirds of burns occur in the home, the rest largely occurring in industrial accidents. The vast majority are preventable. Young children and the elderly are at greatest risk from burns and also suffer disproportionate mortality from them. Among the most common burns are those involving toddlers who pull containers of hot fluid over themselves from cookers and tables. These result in scalds to the outstretched arm, face, neck and front of the chest (see Fig. 8.4).

PATHOPHYSIOLOGY OF BURNS

THERMAL BURNS

For thermal burns of the skin, the depth of tissue destruction is an important determinant of outcome. Skin burns are divided into **partial** or **full thickness**. Partial thickness burns are those in which epidermal elements are spared, allowing spontaneous healing without skin grafting. In deep partial thickness burns, the only epithelial remnants may be hair follicles and sweat glands which extend into the hypodermis; thus with deep partial thickness burns, regeneration is slower. Full thickness burns are those in which all the epidermis has been destroyed. Skin grafting is usually necessary because epithelialisation from the margins is slow and prone to complications, in particular infection, fibrotic scarring and contractures.

The extent of damage caused by a thermal burn is related not only to the temperature of the burning agent but also to the duration of contact. Water at a temperature of only 45°C, if applied for long enough, will cause full thickness burns (scalds). This is often the mechanism of tragic burns in childhood. Thus first aid includes removing clothing soaked in hot fluid and drenching the burned area in cold water for many minutes.

Loss of the epidermis in extensive burns removes the normal barrier to evaporation of body water, and evaporation is increased because of inflammatory exudation of protein-rich fluid. Large volumes of fluid can be lost, the amount depending on the area rather

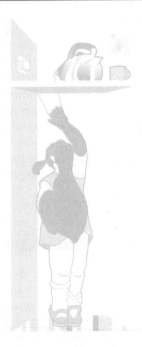

Fig. 8.4 Typical pattern of burns in a young child
The child pulls a teapot or cup of hot liquid from a table or when being held by a seated adult. The area shaded pink is typically burned.

than the depth of the burn. In large burns, vasoactive amines from the inflammatory response are released into the general circulation, causing a generalised increase in capillary permeability, increasing the volume of plasma leaving the circulation. Burns involving 15% or more of the body surface in adults and 10% in children result in hypovolaemia sufficient to cause shock.

Extensive epidermal loss and the presence of necrotic tissue place the patient at particular risk of infection and organ failure. The main organisms are *Streptococcus pyogenes* during the first week and *Pseudomonas aeruginosa* thereafter. *Pseudomonas* septicaemia is responsible for considerable mortality, even in this antibiotic era.

ELECTRICAL BURNS

Electrical burns are caused by the conversion of electrical energy into heat, and the severity of burning is proportional to the electrical resistance of the tissue through

125

which the current is transmitted. Bone offers the highest resistance. If current passes through a limb, the bones become heated and nearby structures such as muscle and blood vessels suffer greatly. Consequently, the extent of damage is often much greater than is immediately apparent. Deep tissue necrosis may not become clinically apparent until some days after an electrical burn.

INHALATIONAL INJURIES

Respiratory and systemic damage from inhalation of hot air, smoke and toxic gases (e.g. carbon monoxide or cyanides from burning upholstery) is a major cause of death and complications even when skin burns are slight. The heat of inhaled gases is often sufficient to cause inflammatory oedema of the oral, nasal and laryngeal mucosa or even serious burns. Blackening by smoke around the nasal or oral cavities warns of inhalation injury. In addition, noxious gases injure the lung parenchyma, resulting in pulmonary oedema, atelectasis and secondary pneumonias.

ASSESSMENT OF THE BURNED PATIENT

The history should include information about the source of the burn, the temperature and the duration of contact and whether there was any inhalation of noxious gases. The percentage of skin area burned must be estimated accurately for purposes of fluid replacement. The usual method is the 'rule of nines' and is illustrated in Figure 8.5. Another method is to compare the burned area with the patient's palm, which is equivalent to about 1% of total body area. The depth of burn is often difficult to assess at the time of presentation. Signs of partial thickness burns are skin redness with blanching to finger pressure and normal pinprick sensation; charred skin or thrombosed skin vessels invariably indicate a full thickness burn.

PRINCIPLES OF MANAGEMENT

One of the first management decisions is whether the burned patient requires hospital admission. Suggested criteria are summarised in Box 8.3. Patients with extensive burns, i.e. involving more than 30% of body surface, should generally be transferred to a specialist burns unit as soon as initial treatment has been carried out.

OUTPATIENT MANAGEMENT OF MINOR BURNS

The main objective is to prevent dehydration and infection of the burn site. Any blisters are punctured and a

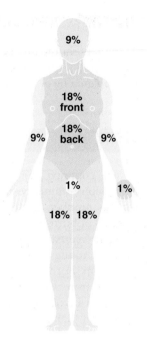

Fig. 8.5 Rule of nines
Wallace's rule for estimating the percentage of the skin surface area burned. A useful alternative estimate is that the area of the patient's own palm is approximately 1% of the total skin area.

KEY POINTS
Box 8.3 Criteria for hospital admission after burns
● Adults with burns involving 15% or more of total skin area, and children with 10% or more
● Full thickness burns
● Circumferential burns on the limbs
● Suspicion of inhalation of hot gases or smoke
● Burns to face, hands, feet or perineum (difficult to manage at home)
● Electrical burns

non-stick dressing applied. Tulle gras (paraffin gauze) impregnated with chlorhexidine or povidone-iodine may be used or alternatively silver sulphadiazine cream (Flamazine). Either dressing is then covered by a thick absorbent layer of gauze and wool or gamgee. Burns on the fingers and hands are best treated with a liberal coating of silver sulphadiazine cream and enclosing the hand in a plastic bag. The patient should be reviewed at least every second day and skin slough excised as it separates. Partial thickness burns re-epithelialise within 14–21 days. If this does not occur, the burns are full thickness and require skin grafting.

Application of the dressing gives considerable relief from pain but even minor burns are extremely painful and require suitable analgesia.

MANAGEMENT OF EXTENSIVE BURNS

The main aspects of early management of serious burn victims are fluid replacement, assessment and treatment of inhalational respiratory problems and local management of the burns.

Fluid management

As described previously, adults with 15% and children with 10% body involvement lose sufficient fluid to be at risk of hypovolaemic shock. Most fluid is lost in the first 12 hours but substantial fluid losses continue for at least another 36 hours. Since much of the fluid lost is essentially plasma, the mainstay of fluid replacement is plasma substitute (gelatin solutions) although 4.5% human albumin is still sometimes used. The remainder consists of isotonic electrolyte solutions, e.g. Hartmann's solution.

Fluid requirements should be calculated by reference to a well-tried formula, such as that of Muir and Barcley shown in Figure 8.6. With this formula, the anticipated fluid loss in each of the three 4-hour periods immediately following the burn is half the product of the percentage area of the burn and the body weight in kilograms. By way of example, for a 20% burn in a 70 kg patient, 700 ml fluid replacement is a reasonable estimate for each of the first three 4-hour periods. After the first 12 hours, the same volume is again administered in each of the next two 6-hour periods and then again over the following 12-hour period. Fluid balance must also be monitored according to pulse, blood pressure and urine output. For the last, catheterisation is usually necessary in an extensively burned patient.

Management of inhalational injuries

If there is a history of possible smoke or gas inhalation, the patient must be carefully examined for evidence of soot or skin burning around the mouth, nostrils and throat. These usually indicate serious inhalation injury. Investigations include chest X-ray, blood gas and carbon monoxide estimations and flexible bronchoscopy.

Treatment involves administration of humidified air by mask and antibiotics to prevent chest infection. If hypoxia and pulmonary oedema develop, endotracheal intubation and artificial ventilation are likely to be required.

Local management of the burn

The principles of local management of extensive partial thickness burns are the same as for minor burns. Full thickness burns will require skin grafting at some stage. Fingers, eyelids, limb flexures and genitalia nearly always require primary grafting soon after injury. In specialist centres, smaller burns are excised and grafted at the outset before infection can develop. Otherwise grafting is usually delayed for 2 weeks or so but the wounds must be free of infection. Sometimes grafting has to be performed in several stages.

Full thickness circumferential burns of the limbs and thorax begin to contract early and may restrict blood flow and respiratory movements. If these signs develop, a procedure known as **escharotomy** is performed, involving incision of the eschar longitudinally down to bleeding tissue.

Long-term problems

Even after grafting, full thickness burns across joint flexures, including the neck, may undergo severe fibrotic contraction so that movement becomes seriously limited. This difficult problem may require multiple plastic operations.

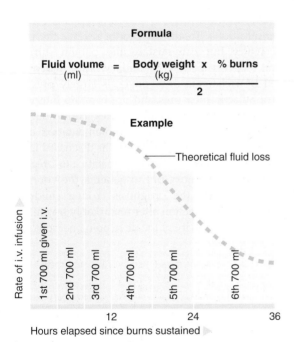

Fig. 8.6 Serious burns—a method for estimating fluid requirements over the first 36 hours (after Muir and Barcley)
The lower panel shows an example of a fluid replacement regimen for a 70 kg man with 20% burns.
Unit fluid volume = $\frac{70 \times 20}{2}$ = 700 ml.

9 Head and maxillofacial injuries

HEAD INJURIES

INTRODUCTION

Head injuries are a devastating problem with an enormous social and economic cost. They cause approximately 3500 deaths each year in the UK, about 0.6% of all deaths. Figure 9.1 demonstrates that serious injuries represent only a small proportion of head injuries; the main problem lies in the huge volume of head injuries, the medical and nursing care they require, and the chronic disability the injuries cause.

The vast number of head injury patients is a major problem in providing satisfactory trauma services. Less than half require hospital admission and of these, only a small proportion need specialist neurosurgical investigation and care. Those with serious and moderate injuries can readily be identified and monitored closely in hospital, but a small proportion of minor head injuries will deteriorate seriously later. The difficulty is to recognise those at risk without investigating and admitting every single case to hospital.

PATHOPHYSIOLOGY OF TRAUMATIC BRAIN INJURY

Traumatic brain injuries can be divided into **primary brain injuries**, the immediate result of the trauma, and **secondary brain injuries** which develop later as a result of complications. Treatment cannot reverse the primary brain injury but can sustain the patient during the natural recovery period. Secondary brain injury, mostly caused by ischaemia or hypoxia, is largely preventable by prophylactic measures and appropriate intervention. The death rate from head injuries could be greatly reduced by more widespread implementation of well-recognised management protocols, as discussed later.

The brain has minimal capacity to regenerate functionally after injury but in general, the younger the patient, the better the prognosis. Young children can often recover full function after remarkably severe injuries because of the plasticity of the developing nervous system.

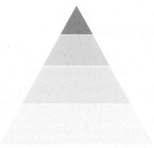

Serious head injuries requiring intensive care and often neurosurgical procedures

Head injuries admitted to hospital and discharged within 48 hours

Minor head injuries attending accident and emergency and discharged ± skull X-rays

Minor head injuries not seen in hospital

Fig. 9.1 Workload caused by head injuries

With increasing age, the consequences of the primary injury are likely to be more severe; the brain shrinks in relation to the cranial vault, allowing greater mobility under impact and a greater chance of tearing intracranial veins leading to subdural haemorrhage.

PRIMARY BRAIN INJURY

CONCUSSION

Concussion is a brain injury associated with brief loss of consciousness, usually for only a few minutes; it causes minor cognitive disturbances such as temporary confusion or amnesia. By definition there are no persistent abnormal neurological signs.

DIFFUSE AXONAL INJURY

Axonal injury occurs in mild, moderate and severe head injuries, the number of axons damaged increasing with the severity of the injury. Causative factors are similar to those that produce intracranial haematomas (described on p. 131) but the trauma is usually initiated by contact with a broader object with less force and often with lateral movement. This condition does not cause raised intracranial pressure and treatment is supportive. Sequelae include organic and psychological dysfunction including loss of concentration, memory disturbances and personality changes such as depression or disinhibition. Higher cortical functions are affected most and take longest to recover. Many of these clinical features were formerly attributed to brain-stem injury.

FOCAL BRAIN INJURIES

Focal injuries involve gross damage to localised areas of the brain and are readily visible on CT scanning. The main lesions are **cerebral contusion** or sometimes **laceration**, **haemorrhage** and **haematoma**, all of which may act as space-occupying lesions and result in secondary brain injury. The site and extent of the primary injury depends on the nature of the damaging force (see Fig. 9.2). Contusions may be small or large and occur beneath the area of impact (coup) or at the tips of the frontal or temporal lobes remote from the injury (contre-coup) as a result of the force vectors caused by deformation of the skull at the time of impact. Large contusions are associated with prolonged coma, small ones with lethargy and subtle focal deficits.

Brain injury is much more likely to have occurred if there is a skull fracture but skull fracture itself does not necessarily indicate brain injury. With overt brain injury, there is usually a period of coma followed by a period of cognitive disturbance related to the extent of diffuse axonal injury or focal injury.

SECONDARY BRAIN INJURY

Secondary brain injury may be caused by cerebral hypoxia, intracranial bleeding or infection. These are discussed in detail below.

CEREBRAL HYPOXIA

Oxygen deprivation to the brain after head injury is the most important and most easily preventable cause of secondary brain injury. It stems from ischaemia (lack of blood) or hypoxia (lack of oxygen in the blood). Damage is caused by **cellular hypoxia** or **raised intracranial pressure** due to cerebral oedema, or both. The most common cause is inadequate pulmonary oxygenation due to airway obstruction, alcohol or drug overdose, chest injury, inhalational pneumonitis, acute respiratory distress syndrome or central respiratory depression. Hypotension due to hypovolaemia may also contribute to cerebral hypoxia by reducing cerebral perfusion. Resuscitation is designed to treat both of these problems.

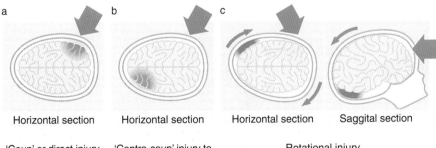

a — Horizontal section
'Coup' or direct injury. Mechanism similar to deceleration injury

b — Horizontal section
'Contra-coup' injury to side opposite blow because of rebound

c — Horizontal section — Saggital section
Rotational injury. Inertia of brain suspended within cranium leads to tearing of surface vessels and subdural haemorrhage

Fig. 9.2 Mechanisms of brain injury
(a) The mechanism of 'coup' or direct injury is similar to a deceleration injury (horizontal section). **(b)** A 'contre-coup' injury affects the side opposite to the blow because of rebound (horizontal section). **(c)** In rotational injury the inertia of the brain suspended within the cranium leads to the tearing of surface vessels and subdural haemorrhage (horizontal and sagittal sections).

INTRACRANIAL BLEEDING

Post-traumatic intracranial bleeding is traditionally classified into extradural (epidural), subdural or intra-cerebral (see Fig. 9.3) but is has recently become established that subarachnoid haemorrhage is also a common occurrence after moderate or severe head injury and carries a poor prognosis. Local brain compression causes focal neurological effects as well as a general rise in intracranial pressure. The latter may cause **temporal lobe herniation** under the tentorium cerebelli or '**coning**' of the brain stem through the foramen magnum, or both.

An acute rise in intracranial pressure manifests as:

● Deteriorating level of consciousness
● An enlarging, unresponsive pupil
● Central respiratory depression
● Falling pulse rate (late sign)
● Rising blood pressure (late sign)

Extradural haemorrhage

About 10% of severe head injuries result in extradural haemorrhage and this is most common in children, adolescents and young adults. It is most likely when there is a skull fracture in the temporal region but can occur without a fracture. It is usually caused by rupture of an artery, the middle meningeal; consequently the haematoma develops rapidly and needs urgent surgical intervention. Death will quickly follow unless the haematoma is evacuated post-haste. Emergency CT scanning is indicated, both to confirm the diagnosis and to show the position of the haematoma. With increased awareness of the problem and the more widespread availability of CT scanning, emergency burr hole drain-age of an extradural haemorrhage by a general surgeon is rarely required. Transfer to a neurosurgeon for con-sideration of craniotomy is usually the most appropriate course of action.

Pathologically, there is rapid accumulation of (arterial) blood between the skull vault and the tough dura mater with the extent of lateral spread limited by dural attach-ments. The mass bulges into the underlying brain sub-stance causing local compression and a rise in intracranial pressure.

The classic clinical picture in extradural haemorrhage is as follows:

● Loss of consciousness
● Frequently a **lucid interval** with severe headache and drowsiness
● Secondary decline in consciousness following any lucid interval
● Rapid development of a fixed, dilated pupil on the side of the injury and a hemiparesis on the opposite side

In some cases, unconsciousness is continuous from the outset. Extradural haematomas nearly always present within 24 hours of trauma.

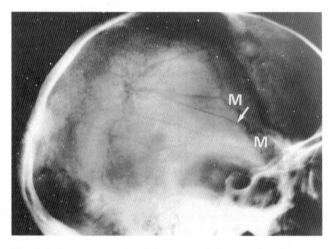

Fig. 9.4 Temporo-parietal fracture with extradural haematoma
This 20-year-old man was admitted fully conscious after being knocked off a bicycle but deteriorated rapidly 2 hours later. **(a)** Lateral skull X-ray showing a linear fracture of the right temporo-parietal bones (arrowed) crossing the course of the anterior branch of the middle meningeal artery **M** on the temporal bone.

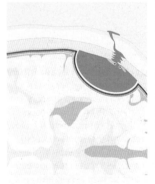

Extradural haemorrhage

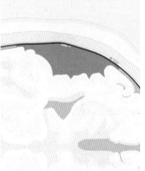

Subdural haemorrhage

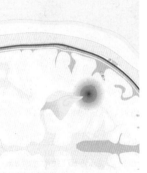

Intraventricular and intracerebral haemorrhage

Fig. 9.3 Types of post-traumatic intracranial bleeding

Subdural haematoma

Subdural haematomas are more common than extradurals and occur in about 30% of severe head injuries. Subdural haematoma usually results from the tearing of veins passing between the cerebral cortex and dura, or from laceration of the brain or cortical arteries. Blood accumulates relatively slowly in the large potential space between dura mater and arachnoid mater. The haematoma tends to spread laterally over a wide area. In contrast to extradural haemorrhage, there is usually underlying primary brain injury and the mortality is up to 50%. Subdural haematomas commonly occur in more than one site, either on the same side or on both sides (see Fig. 9.6).

In an acute subdural haemorrhage, there is usually clinical evidence of significant brain injury at the outset, with later deterioration. A lucid interval is rare. Acute subdural haemorrhage is more common in older adults because of increased brain mobility within the skull. Surgical evacuation of the clot may halt deterioration but recovery is often incomplete; most elderly patients die from this condition despite expeditious treatment. With increasing use of warfarin anticoagulation, acute subdural haematoma is seen more commonly after trivial injury.

Chronic subdural haematoma

Subdural haematomas may develop gradually in the elderly following trivial, often unrecalled, head injury. This may become manifest weeks or months later as non-specific neurological deterioration, chronic headache or coma. Most patients do not present with a history of head injury and the diagnosis is made on investigation of neurological symptoms.

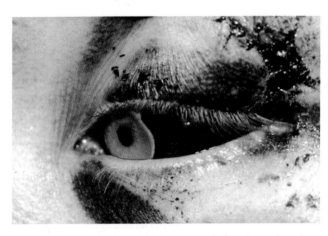

Fig. 9.6 Subconjunctival haematoma following a head injury
This 14-year-old boy fell off his bicycle and momentarily lost consciousness. This photograph shows a subconjunctival haematoma with no posterior limit indicating a fracture of the orbital wall, in this case the petrous temporal bone of the base of the skull.

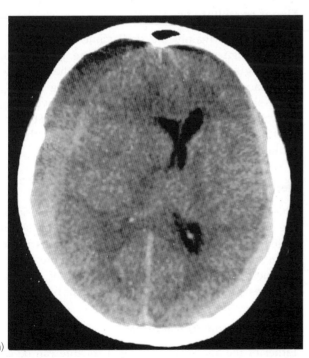
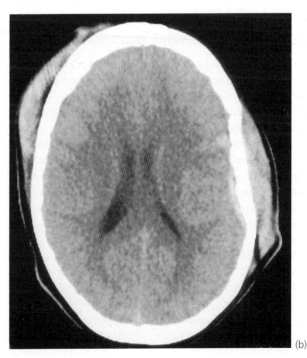

(a)　(b)

Fig. 9.5 (a) CT scan of an elderly man 48 hours after a head injury in a road traffic accident. The CT scan was performed because of a deteriorating conscious level. There is a large subdural haematoma on the right side and a smaller one on the left. The midline is shifted to the left by the mass effect of the larger haematoma and there is compression of the lateral ventricles. the patient required neurosurgical drainage. **(b)** CT scan of skull after head injury in a cyclist knocked off his bike by a car. Note the signs of external injury in the left temporal region and the right fronto parietal region. There is a depressed segment of skull bone in the left temporal region and signs of intracerebral contusion beneath both areas of injury.

Intracerebral haemorrhage

Haemorrhage into the brain parenchyma is caused by primary brain injury. Small deep lesions are often associated with diffuse axonal injury and should be monitored for expansion using serial CT scans. A larger lesion or continuing haemorrhage produces an expanding mass lesion which should be evacuated early to prevent secondary brain damage.

INFECTION

Meningeal infection may cause secondary brain injury, with organisms entering via compound skull fractures. Fractures underlying scalp lacerations are easily diagnosed as compound but others may be deceptive; for example, fractures of the skull base may communicate with the sphenoid or ethmoid sinuses, the nasal cavity or the external auditory canal. Similarly, fractures of the frontal bone often involve the frontal sinuses. Fractures of this type are thus always assumed to be compound.

Early debridement of compound depressed fractures is essential to minimise the risk of infection. There is no evidence to support the use of prophylactic antibiotics, which should be reserved for use when clinical infection is manifest; this usually becomes evident several days after injury.

SKULL FRACTURES

THE IMPORTANCE OF SKULL FRACTURES

A skull fracture indicates a severe impact. Consequently, patients with fractures are much more likely to sustain primary brain damage than those without (see Table 9.2, p. 136). In addition, patients with skull fractures are 30 times more likely to suffer secondary brain damage by the mechanisms described earlier. All patients with skull fractures therefore merit hospital admission for close observation (even if fully conscious) as well as CT scanning. Depressed fractures are often associated with some primary injury to the underlying brain but, paradoxically, the process of fracture may absorb some of the energy of impact and protect the brain.

Most skull fractures can be diagnosed only on skull X-rays or CT scanning, although basal fractures can be difficult to demonstrate. Routinely ordering plain X-rays for every patient with a head injury, however trivial, is expensive, time-consuming and inappropriate. Clinical criteria have been identified to identify those at significant risk of a skull fracture so that radiological resources can be employed cost-effectively, the criteria shown in Box 9.1 are widely employed in the UK. CT scanning is more accurate than plain films, and can rule out not only fracture, but also significant injury to the underlying brain.

KEY POINTS

Box 9.1 Indications for skull X-ray after recent head injury*

Orientated patient

- History of loss of consciousness or amnesia
- Suspected penetrating injury
- Cerebrospinal fluid or blood loss from nose or ear
- Scalp laceration (down to bone or more than 5 cm long), bruising or swelling
- Any injuries resulting from interpersonal violene
- Persisting headache and/or vomiting
- In a child, fall from a significant height (which depends in part on the age of the child) and/or on to a hard surface; tense fontanelle; suspected non-accidental injury

Patient with impaired consciousness or neurological signs

- All patients unless urgent CT is performed or transfer to neurosurgery is arranged

Note: skull X-ray is not necessary if CT is to be performed

*Based on guidelines of the working party on head injuries, Society of British Neurological Surgeons, 1998

TYPES OF SKULL FRACTURE

Linear or stellate fractures

These involve mainly the skull vault, often with little external sign of injury, although there may be some overlying scalp bruising or swelling. If there is a deep scalp laceration or a history of penetrating injury, the scalp should be deeply probed with a gloved finger, which may reveal a small bony defect or step. Linear fractures rarely exhibit displacement unless there are multiple fracture lines.

Depressed fractures

These fractures are usually caused by blunt injuries and the overlying scalp is usually lacerated or severely bruised; such fractures rarely produce serious primary brain injury unless they are depressed more than the thickness of the skull vault. Elevation of depressed fractures is usually performed for cosmetic reasons.

Compound (open) fractures

Either of the above types of skull fracture can be compound. If the dura is torn, there is a direct communication with the brain and a high risk of infection. Early debridement and dural closure are indicated. Compound fractures of the base of the skull are diagnosed clinically and with CT scanning.

Fractures of the base of the skull

These usually involve the anterior or middle cranial fossae. The characteristic clinical features are summarised in Box 9.2.

X-RAYS USED FOR DIAGNOSIS OF SKULL FRACTURES

A standard set of three X-ray films is normally taken to diagnose a skull fracture: lateral skull, AP skull and Towne's view (see Figs 9.7 and 9.8). The X-rays should be examined for the presence of fractures and also for pineal shift and fluid levels in the sphenoid and frontal sinuses. Fluid levels indicate a basal skull fracture. For suspected facial and orbital fractures, a 30° **occipito-mental** view is the standard investigation.

MANAGEMENT OF HEAD INJURIES

ASSESSING ACTUAL OR POTENTIAL BRAIN DAMAGE

History

The history is of great value in deciding whether minor head injuries need skull X-rays or admission to hospital for observation (Fig. 9.9). The most important factors which indicate brain injury and a risk of future complications are a history of unconsciousness, and amnesia

KEY POINTS

Box 9.2 Clinical signs of a fracture of the skull base

Anterior fossa fractures
● Periorbital haematoma (see Fig. 9.6)—usually bilateral and limited by the margins of the orbicularis oculi
● Subconjunctival haemorrhage (see Fig. 9.6)—the blood tracks from behind forward and therefore no posterior limit can be seen (unlike the localised subconjunctival haematoma which results from direct trauma)
● Cerebrospinal fluid rhinorrhoea—clear fluid running from the nose

Middle fossa fractures, i.e. involving petrous temporal bone
● Cerebrospinal fluid otorrhoea—clear fluid running from the ear
● Bruising over the mastoid area behind the ear (Battle's sign)

for events around the time of the accident. Amnesia for events after the accident (**post-grade amnesia**) may be more significant than for events before it (**retrograde amnesia**). The duration of unconsciousness and amnesia

(a) AP, Towne's and lateral views of the skull

A-P view

Towne's view

Lateral view

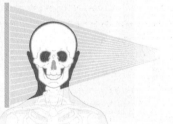

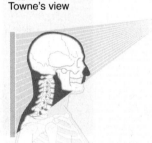

(b) 30° occipito-mental view of the facial bones

X-ray tube angled perpendicular to film

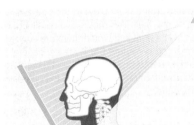

Fig. 9.7 The standard set of skull X-rays
(a) The standard set of skull X-rays includes three views: anterior-posterior (AP), Towne's view and lateral. For potential facial fractures, a 30° occipito-mental view may be added **(b)**. The AP view is the standard frontal view of the skull. A calcified pineal may show a midline shift. The Towne's view shows the occipital bone, the zygomatic arch and the mandibular condyles if the mouth is open. The occipito-mental view of the facial bones shows the middle third of the face, fluid levels in the maxillary sinuses as well as the orbits and fractures of the orbital floor.

133

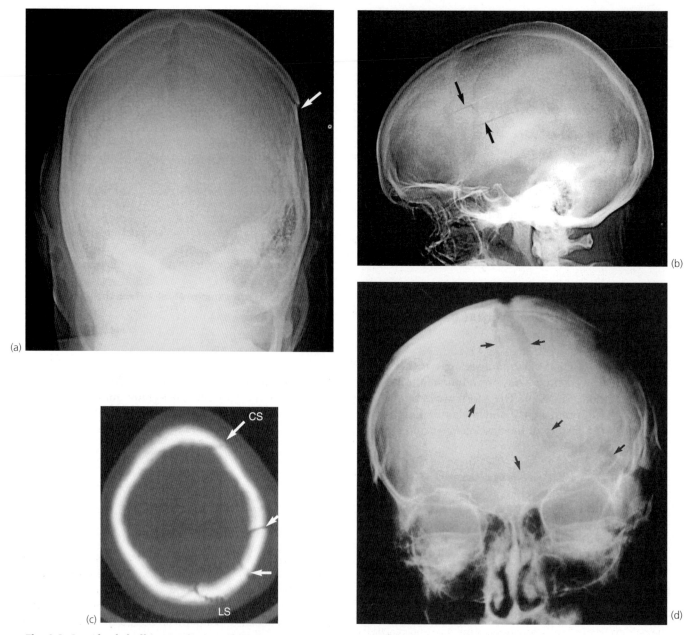

Fig. 9.8 Standard skull X-ray views and CT scan showing skull fractures
(a) Towne's view from a fully conscious 19-year-old woman after a blunt blow to the side of the head. This shows a depressed fracture in the left parietal bone (arrowed). **(b)** Lateral view of the same patient's skull. This shows two parallel fracture lines (arrowed). The segment of bone between them is depressed by more than the thickness of the skull and would therefore need elevating. **(c)** CT scan of the upper part of the skull vault in a different patient after an RTA showing a normal coronal suture **CS**. There are parietal fractures (arrowed) and **diastasis** (partial separation) of the lambdoid suture **LS**. **(d)** AP view from an unconscious 24-year-old woman after a high speed impact road traffic accident (RTA). There were deep scalp lacerations; the X-ray shows extensive fractures (arrowed) in the parietal, occipital and squamous temporal bones. Because of the lacerations, these fractures were considered compound.

are proportional to the severity of brain injury. Witnesses should be questioned as to whether or not the patient was 'knocked out'. In practice, however, the evidence is often equivocal. If the patient was travelling in a car, the extent of injuries to others in the car may give an indication of the energy transfer in the accident. Careful questioning of the patient about events leading up to the accident will usually reveal the duration of retrograde amnesia; post-grade amnesia is more difficult to assess because cerebral function tends to recover gradually.

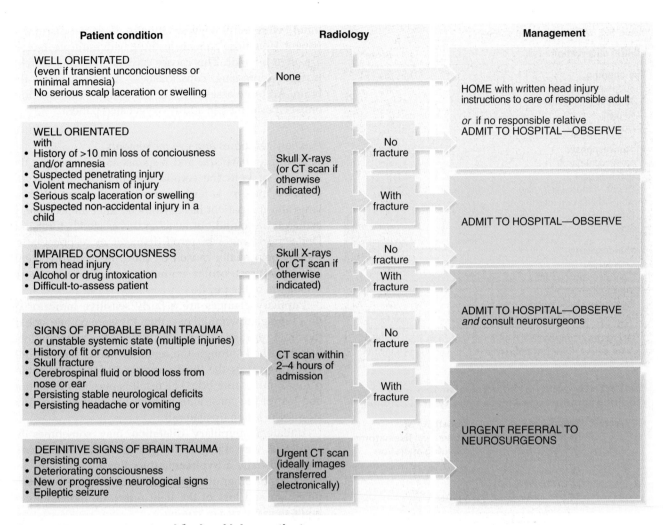

Patient condition	Radiology		Management

Fig. 9.9 Management protocol for head injury patients

Examination

In addition to a general examination, a systematic neurological examination must be performed in every case of head injury, however trivial. Particular attention should be paid to level of consciousness, pupil size and reactivity, eye movements and motor power in the limbs.

Level of consciousness

The level of consciousness is the most important single observation in head injury patients. However, unstructured clinical judgement is prone to error and lacks reproducibility. The **Glasgow coma scale** (GCS – see Table 9.1) overcomes these problems and is used world wide for assessing severity and for monitoring progress. Level of consciousness can be categorised simply and reproducibly by this method. Initial assessment should take place after resuscitation and before intubation if possible, and should take into account any sedative drugs or alcohol taken and any direct orbital injuries. If eye and verbal responses cannot be used, the motor response is the most important observation—a patient unable to follow commands has a serious head injury. In patients with impaired consciousness, pressure over the supraorbital nerve at the orbit is usually employed to elicit pain. To be scored as localising the pain, the patient's hand should rise above the clavicle. A flexion response to pain is manifest by the hand moving but not rising above the clavicle. The Glasgow coma scale can roughly sort patients into *severe* (a score of 3–8), *moderate* (9–13) and *mild* (14–15) head injuries, which helps determine appropriate investigation and treatment. The probability of intracerebral haemorrhage likely to need surgery in these groups is shown in Table 9.2. Table 9.3 shows the influence on this risk of post-traumatic amnesia and the presence of a skull fracture.

After most minor head injuries, the patient is fully conscious by the time of assessment. If there is any depression of conscious level, the patient must be admitted to hospital for observation. The extent to which brain injury is responsible for depression of consciousness is difficult to assess if the patient is intoxicated with

135

Table 9.1 Glasgow coma scale

Clinical observation	Score*
Eye opening	
Spontaneous	4
To verbal command	3
To pain	2
None	1
Motor response	
Obeys commands	6
Localises pain	5
Flexion withdrawal to pain	4
Abnormal flexion (decorticate)	3
Extension to pain (decerebrate)	2
None	1
Verbal response	
Orientated	5
Confused conversation	4
Inappropriate words	3
Incomprehensible words	2
None	1

*The Glasgow coma score is the sum of the scores from the three sections below. The worst total score is 3, the best is 15

Table 9.2 Probability of intracranial haematoma requiring surgery according to severity of head injury

GCS score	Severity of head injury	Probability of intracranial haematoma requiring operation
3–8	Severe head injury	1 in 7
9–13	Moderate head injury	1 in 51
14–15	Mild head injury	1 in 3615

alcohol or other drugs and such patients must be admitted to hospital even if the history of head injury is doubtful.

Aggressive behaviour in patients smelling of alcohol must **not** be assumed to result from intoxication (i.e. removal of social inhibition) because this behaviour also commonly arises from brain injury or hypoxia. A thorough examination must be performed with this in

mind before employing sedation to quieten a disruptive patient. Comatose patients or those with multiple injuries are often hypoxic. This causes cerebral swelling, thereby further depressing consciousness and damaging the brain. Accurate assessment of brain injury can therefore only be performed in a fully oxygenated patient.

Pupillary responses and eye movements
Normal pupillary size and response to light require the integrity of both the second and third cranial nerves. Pupil asymmetry is fairly common in the population at large and if a patient has asymmetry after an accident, it is important to find out whether this existed beforehand. Unilateral changes in pupil diameter or response after trauma are usually caused by third nerve involvement, although direct ocular trauma can cause a mydriasis (dilatation of the pupil).

Pupillary changes are a fairly sensitive indicator of developing intracranial bleeding. Pressure on one side of the brain results in the medial edge of the temporal lobe being pushed through the tentorial hiatus (herniation). This compresses the third nerve in its long intracranial course on the same side. The result is pupillary dilatation and loss of the constrictor response to light on the same side as the lesion (ipsilateral).

Unilateral pupillary dilatation may sometimes be associated with injury to the eye itself, but in this case, there is usually a **hyphaema** (bleeding into the anterior chamber) or other obvious eye injury. Bilateral pupillary dilatation and loss of the light reflex are indications of brain-stem injury, i.e. 'coning'.

If possible, the full range of eye movements and the visual fields should be checked.

Limb movements and responses
In a fully conscious patient, tone, power and coordination can be readily assessed in the standard manner. If a subtle abnormality is suspected, the patient should be asked to close his or her eyes and hold the arms outstretched, palms upwards, for 1 minute. Pronation or

Table 9.3 Influence of skull fractures and post-traumatic amnesia (PTA) on probability of intracranial haemorrhage requiring operation according to GCS group

GCS	Other features	Probability of operation being needed for intracranial haemorrhage	Multiplier effect of other clinical features on probability
14–15 (overall risk 1 in 3615)	None	1 in 31 300	
	PTA	1 in 6700	5x
	Skull fracture	1 in 81	400x
	Skull fracture and PTA	1 in 29	1000x
9–13 (overall risk 1 in 51)	No fracture	1 in 180	
	Skull fracture	1 in 5	36x
3–8 (overall risk 1 in 7)	No fracture	1 in 27	
	Skull fracture	1 in 4	7x

downward drift on one side is indicative of brain injury. For the semi-conscious or unconscious patient, the pattern of limb response to painful stimuli (the standard is pressure over the supraorbital nerve) provides a useful indication of the conscious level, as indicated in the Glasgow coma scale (see Table 9.1).

MANAGEMENT OF MINOR HEAD INJURIES

A management scheme for head injury patients is shown in Figure 9.9. For most patients presenting with head injury, only two immediate decisions have to be made: whether to perform skull X-rays or CT and whether to admit to hospital for observation. Suggested criteria for skull X-rays are shown in Box 9.1 (p. 132) and for hospital admission in Box 9.3.

The purpose of admission after minor head injury is to monitor the patient's condition for about 24 hours, during which period the majority of complications, particularly intracranial bleeding, will become apparent. Those who do not need admission should spend the first night with a responsible adult who can return the patient to hospital in the unlikely event of deterioration. A printed sheet with details of warning symptoms and signs should always be given to the accompanying adult. If a responsible adult is unavailable, hospital admission is advisable.

Box 9.4 gives the suggested criteria for arranging CT scans after head injury. As CT scanners have become more readily available, these criteria now include patients with uncomplicated skull fractures. Early CT scanning allows prompt recognition of significant intracranial injury and more efficient use of scarce high-dependency beds and neurosurgical services by indicating when specialist referral is unnecessary.

Head injury observations

The important observations for head injury patients admitted to hospital are shown in Table 9.4. These are sufficiently sensitive to provide early warning of developing complications. Observations are performed

---

KEY POINTS

Box 9.4 Criteria for CT scan and consultation with a neurosurgical unit after head injury*

Indications for CT scan in a general hospital
- Skull fracture
- Fit or convulsion
- Confusional state
- Neurological signs persisting after initial assessment and resuscitation
- Unstable systemic state precluding transfer to neurosurgery
- Diagnosis uncertain
- Tense fontanelle or suture diastasis in a child

Note: CT should be performed urgently, i.e. within 2–4 hours of admission.

Indications for prompt neurosurgical referral
- Coma persisting after resuscitation
- Deteriorating consciousness or progressive neurological signs
- Fracture of skull accompanied by
  — confusion or worsening impairment of consciousness
  — epileptic seizure
  — neurological symptoms or signs
- Open injury with any of the following
  — depressed compound fracture of skull vault
  — fracture of base of skull
  — penetrating injury
- Abnormal CT scan
- CT scan normal, but clinical progress unsatisfactory

Note: neurosurgical opinion should be sought based on clinical information; ideally, the CT images should be transferred electronically to the neurosurgical unit

*Based on the guidelines of the working party on head injuries, Society of British Neurological Surgeons, 1998

KEY POINTS

Box 9.3 Criteria for admission to a general hospital after head injury*

Orientated patient
- Skull fracture or suture diastasis (separation)
- Persisting neurological symptoms or signs
- Difficulty in assessment, e.g. suspected drugs, alcohol, non-accidental injury, epilepsy, attempted suicide
- Lack of a responsible adult to supervise the patient
- Other medical condition, e.g. coagulation disorder

All patients with impaired consciousness

Notes: 1. Transient unconsciousness or amnesia with full recovery is not necessarily an indication for admission of an adult, but may be so in a child
2. Patients with head injuries may have other serious internal injuries which are easily overlooked

*Based on the report of the working party on head injuries, Society of British Neurological Surgeons, 1998

Table 9.4 Essential observations for head injury patients

Observation	Sign of neurological deterioration
Conscious level (Glasgow coma scale)	Falling score
Pupil size and light response	Dilatation, loss of light reaction or developing asymmetry
Respiratory pattern and rate	Irregularity, slowing or reduced depth of breathing
Developing neurological signs	Focal signs point to localised intracranial damage
Pulse rate	Falling pulse rate (late sign)
Blood pressure	Rising blood pressure (late sign)

by nursing staff, the frequency depending on the state of the patient. If there is a skull fracture or any suggestion of reduced consciousness, confusion, disorientation, alcohol or drug effects, observations should be made at 30-minute intervals, at least for the first night, otherwise hourly. Observations are recorded or plotted on a special **head injury chart** so that deterioration will be immediately obvious and can be reported to medical staff at once.

Patients with minor uncomplicated head injuries who are fully alert can be safely allowed to go home after 24 hours even if there is a simple skull fracture. Patients should be advised to rest at home for about 1 week as some cognitive functions such as power of concentration may not completely recover for some days ('**post-concussion syndrome**').

MANAGEMENT OF MORE SEVERE HEAD INJURIES

Initial management

Any patient who is unconscious, has focal neurological signs or whose conscious level is moderately depressed (Glasgow coma score 14 or less) must be considered to have a moderate or serious head injury. Nowadays, these patients should have a CT scan even without evidence of skull fracture. The patient should be resuscitated and decisions made about the management of other injuries and the timing of CT scanning if other injuries need immediate treatment. If the receiving hospital does not have CT scanning facilities, the patient may need to be transferred to a regional centre after resuscitation. If

the patient is deteriorating rapidly and an extradural haemorrhage is suspected, burr holes in the temporal region must be made immediately if the patient's life is to be saved. However, with early use of CT scanning, emergency burr holes made by a general surgeon are now rarely indicated.

Continuing care

The management of intracerebral haemorrhage and other major head injury complications is highly specialised. Many of these patients have other serious injuries and may need to be nursed and monitored in an intensive care or high-dependency unit with the assistance of anaesthetic staff.

The continuing care of the patient with stable serious brain injury involves some or all of the following procedures:

- **Intensive monitoring** of vital signs and neurological status
- **Endotracheal intubation and artificial ventilation** if hypoxaemic
- **Nasogastric aspiration** for all unconscious patients to prevent inhalation of stomach contents
- **Monitoring of fluid and electrolyte balance** (hyponatraemia and hypoproteinaemia exacerbate cerebral oedema)
- **Monitoring of intracranial pressure** using a surgically implanted extradural catheter
- **Measures for the temporary control of raised intracranial pressure**, e.g. intravenous mannitol (for its osmotic effect in reducing cerebral oedema) or controlled hyperventilation (reducing pCO_2 causes cerebral vasoconstriction, reduced cerebral oedema and hence reduced intracranial pressure). Maintaining the cerebral perfusion pressure is important and may require intravenous infusion of fluids and perhaps inotropic cardiac support

Long-term recovery of intellectual function after serious brain injury is slow and cannot be hastened, although physiotherapy and occupational therapy can aid physical recovery. Patients may easily languish in the community and should therefore be encouraged to join self-help groups (such as Headway in the UK and other countries).

MAXILLOFACIAL INJURIES

GENERAL PRINCIPLES

Fractures of the facial skeleton are common, particularly after sporting injuries, road accidents and fights. The

main fractures involve the mandible, the middle third of the face, the nasal bones, the orbit and the zygoma. Facial fractures rarely pose urgent management problems except for major middle third fractures (in which the upper jaw becomes detached from the base of the skull) and multiple mandibular fractures; both may result in upper airway obstruction, and these patients may require endotracheal intubation or cricothyroidotomy to safeguard the airway. Facial fractures are generally managed by maxillofacial surgeons who may not be available in smaller hospitals. In most cases, delaying treatment for a few days does not adversely affect the outcome.

EXAMINATION FOR FACIAL FRACTURES

If there is any facial injury, the contour of the facial bones should be carefully palpated before oedema develops and obscures underlying bony deformities. The extraocular muscle attachments may be disrupted by orbital wall fractures so the full range of eye movements must be formally examined and the patient questioned about diplopia in all positions. The patient should be asked if 'the teeth bite together normally', and the mouth should be examined both for missing or displaced teeth and for the state of the dental occlusion. Abnormalities of occlusion are a common and sensitive sign of a jaw fracture which might otherwise be missed. The full range of mandibular movements should also be checked to exclude fractures or dislocations involving the mandibular condyles.

RADIOLOGY

If facial fractures are suspected, X-rays should be taken of the facial bones with the particular views chosen according to the bones under suspicion. Interpretation of facial radiographs can be difficult for the non-specialist but most fractures can be identified if the main bony contours are carefully traced and compared with the opposite side. Opacities or fluid levels in the maxillary sinuses usually represent haematoma. This commonly follows fractures of the bones surrounding the maxillary sinuses, e.g. zygoma or orbital floor.

MANDIBULAR FRACTURES

The common sites of mandibular fractures are shown in Figure 9.10. Because of the effects of oblique trauma, a fracture on one side is often accompanied by a fracture on the other side in a different position, e.g. body of mandible on one side and condylar neck on the other. Fracture lines tend to occur through points of weakness, e.g. mental foramina, unerupted third molar teeth or condylar necks. Most undisplaced mandibular fractures need no active intervention but displaced fractures require fixation. This can be achieved by wiring the lower teeth to the upper teeth or by direct wiring of the bones (see Fig. 9.11). Any fracture passing through a tooth socket defines the fracture as 'compound' and prophylactic antibiotics should be used.

FRACTURES OF THE MIDDLE THIRD OF THE FACE

Fractures of the middle third of the facial skeleton range from detachment of the palate and dental arch to complete separation of the middle third complex from the base of the skull. Diagnosis is based on clinical assessment. A simple test is to grasp the upper teeth or jaw between

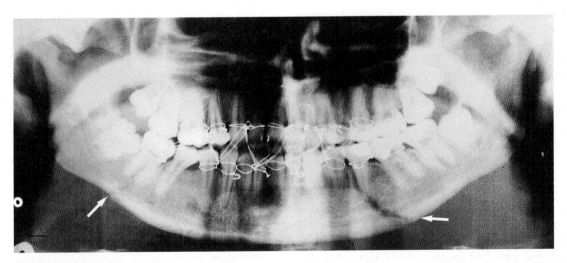

Fig. 9.10 Mandibular fractures
Oral pantomograph (OPG) showing mandible fractured in two places. Oblique fracture lines (arrowed) can be seen running down from between the left first and second premolars and between the roots of the first right molar. The fractures have been immobilised by interdental wiring, visible on the teeth in both jaws.

Oblique blow, e.g. punch

Frontal blow

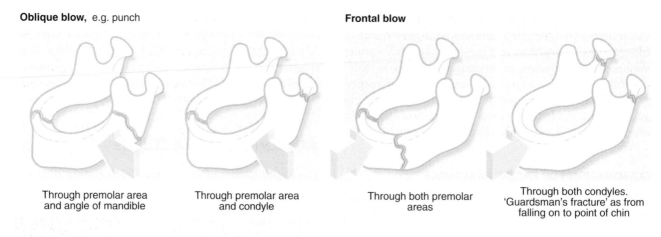

Through premolar area and angle of mandible

Through premolar area and condyle

Through both premolar areas

Through both condyles. 'Guardsman's fracture' as from falling on to point of chin

Fig. 9.11 Common sites of mandibular fractures

the fingers and attempt to move them independently of the skull. Treatment may involve disimpaction and usually requires sophisticated external fixation to the skull afterwards.

FRACTURES OF THE NASAL BONES

Trauma to the nose is extremely common and often results in nasal bone fracture. Less often, fracture dislocation of the septum occurs which may interfere with the nasal airway. Diagnosis is made on clinical grounds and the main features are flattening or lateral displacement of the nasal bridge. Bleeding from the nose often indicates a nasal fracture. The fracture is usually reduced several days later by an ENT or maxillofacial surgeon.

FRACTURES OF THE ORBIT AND ZYGOMA

DEPRESSED FRACTURES OF THE ZYGOMA

A depressed fracture of the zygoma (see Fig. 9.12) is the most common fracture in relation to the orbit and results from a blow to the cheek. The fracture line usually passes through the infraorbital foramen and causes a palpable step in the inferior orbital margin. The infraorbital nerve becomes compressed with any substantial degree of depression causing paraesthesia or numbness in its area of sensory innervation, i.e. the upper lip, upper teeth and buccal mucosa. Diagnosis may be suspected by flattening of the cheek contour; this is best seen from above and behind the patient. Overlying oedema may obscure a depressed fracture, and these patients warrant radiological examination. An associated fracture of the lateral orbital wall may produce enough bleeding for it to track forward under the conjunctiva. This type of sub-

conjunctival haemorrhage has no visible posterior limit and is the characteristic sign of an orbital wall fracture.

Treatment is indicated if there is inferior orbital nerve compression or a cosmetically unacceptable deformity. Reduction is usually accomplished via a temporal approach, sliding an elevator under the root of the zygoma, deep to the temporalis fascia.

BLOW-OUT FRACTURES OF THE ORBIT

A direct frontal blow to the orbit from an object about the size of a squash ball (3–4 cm) may act like a plunger, causing a **'blow-out' fracture** of the orbital wall without damaging the orbital margin. The blow-out most commonly involves the floor of the orbit where the bony walls are thinnest. This causes herniation of peribulbar fat into the maxillary antrum and disrupts the function of the extraocular muscles, causing diplopia and restricted upward gaze (see Figs. 9.13 and 9.14). Hence it is important to test eye movements in any patient with a facial injury. Diagnosis is suggested by finding an antral opacity (haematoma) on occipito-mental X-ray, but CT scanning of the orbit is required if the bony defect needs to be demonstrated. Treatment involves exploring the orbital floor and may require a bone graft or silicone implant.

INJURIES TO THE TEETH

Fractures and avulsions of the anterior teeth are common and may require immediate treatment in the accident and emergency department. Correct first-aid treatment may preserve teeth which would otherwise be lost.

Fractures involving the loss of more than one-third of the crown should be seen urgently by a dental surgeon as the dental pulp may be exposed or endangered. Partially avulsed teeth need to be pushed back into

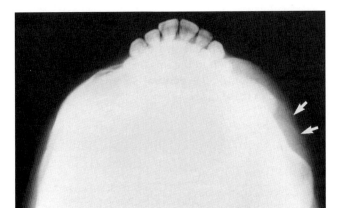

(a)

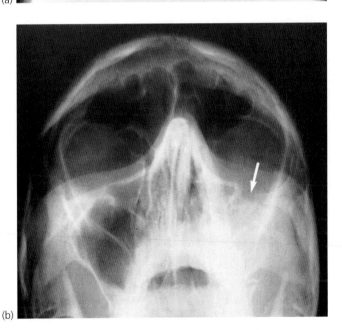

(b)

Fig. 9.12 Depressed zygomatic fractures
(a) Submento-vertical projection of a 43-year-old man who had been punched on the left cheek showing a depressed fracture of the zygomatic arch (arrowed). **(b)** 30° occipito-mental radiograph after a similar injury in a different patient. This patient had a depressed 'tripod' fracture of the zygoma manifest by discontinuity of the lower orbital margin (arrowed). Note that since the roof of the maxilla is involved, the maxillary sinus (the antrum) has typically filled with blood and is rendered radiopaque. **(c)** 3-D reconstruction of CT scans showing a severely depressed fracture of right lower orbital rim involving maxilla and zygomatic body (arrowed). The left lower orbital rim is also fractured and displaced.

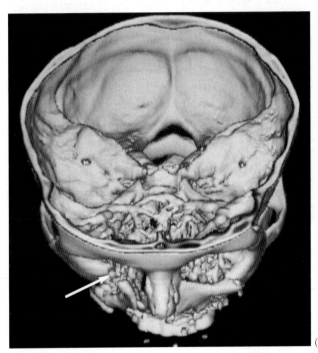

(c)

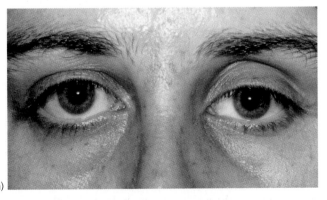

(a)

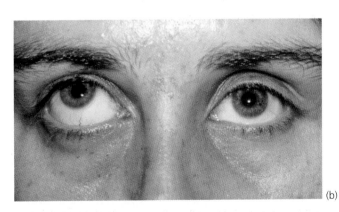

(b)

Fig. 9.13 Blow-out fracture of orbital floor
(a) This young man was punched in the left eye, causing a blow-out fracture of the orbital floor. **(b)** Note failure of upward gaze on the left due to trapping of the extraocular muscles in the fractured orbital floor.

position. This can usually be done with the fingers after local anaesthetic infiltration. Urgent dental referral for tooth splintage and root canal treatment is then required.

If a tooth is completely avulsed, it can often be successfully reimplanted by a dentist if the tooth has been carefully cleaned and wrapped in a sterile, saline-soaked swab. Discovering missing or broken teeth in an unconscious patient should alert the examining doctor to the possibility of inhalation of tooth material into the bronchi or impaction in the lips or pharynx. Chest X-ray and examination of the perioral soft tissues should be performed in these cases.

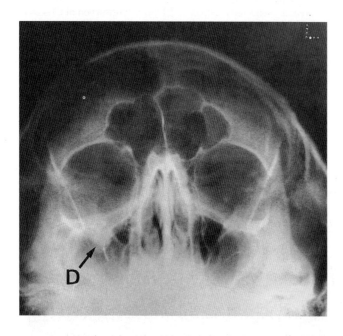

Fig. 9.14 X-ray appearance of blow-out fracture of orbital floor
This 30-year-old man was hit on the right eye by a squash ball, causing a blow-out fracture of the orbital floor by hydraulic pressure. Orbital fat and extraocular muscles have been forced into the maxillary antrum and held there by the fractured bone edges. This causes the characteristic 'hanging drop' sign **D**. Upward gaze is restricted, resulting in vertical diplopia.

10 Abdominal and chest injuries

INTRODUCTION

Abdominal and thoracic injuries co-exist fairly often and it is logical to think in terms of **torso trauma**, as both **penetrating** and **closed** (blunt) injuries can affect both cavities. Major injuries to the torso are a common cause of death at the scene of the trauma—for example, from rupture of the thoracic aorta, cardiac injury or massive liver injury. However, rapid treatment may save lives in these potentially fatal injuries.

ABDOMINAL INJURIES

Abdominal injuries are uncommon compared with head and chest injuries and mortality is low if they are managed promptly and appropriately. When death occurs, the principal causes are unrecognised injury or uncontrollable bleeding from bursting injuries of the liver or spleen or from major arteries after penetrating injury, particularly gunshot wounds. In blunt injuries, making the diagnosis can be difficult because overt signs of bleeding or perforation of a hollow viscus may not develop until several hours after the injury.

Suspected intra-abdominal injury can be confirmed by **diagnostic peritoneal lavage** (DPL). This involves instillation of 0.5–1 L normal saline into the abdominal cavity via a peritoneal dialysis catheter which is then allowed to run out. Staining with blood indicates intra-abdominal injury although a negative result does not exclude serious injury.

It is important to remember that areas of the abdomen other than the main peritoneal cavity may be injured; pelvic viscera lie within a bony cage but extend low enough to be injured by wounds in the buttock or preineum. Similarly, the retroperitoneal viscera appear to be protected, but are vulnerable to flank or back wounds, or to deep anterior stab wounds and any gunshot wounds. This area is not easily palpated; peritoneal lavage is likely to be negative and may give false reassurance.

Overall, 20% of patients with closed abdominal trauma require operation, penetrating abdominal injuries even more so; for example, 30% with stab wounds require operation and close to 100% with gunshot wounds.

PENETRATING ABDOMINAL WOUNDS

STAB WOUNDS AND OTHER SHARP ABDOMINAL WOUNDS

Stab wounds may or may not penetrate the peritoneum and often cause little damage unless the blade penetrates the retroperitoneal area and injures the great vessels or pancreas. At one time, it was thought that all abdominal stab wounds required surgical exploration but current policy is towards more conservative management in most cases. A large series from Baragwanath Hospital, Soweto, South Africa, demonstrated that 70% or more patients could safely be observed in hospital for 24 hours and explored only if there were signs of deterioration. This is because many bowel perforations seal spontaneously without causing peritonitis, and bleeding from some internal wounds also stops by normal haemostasis. The haemodynamically unstable patient and those with extensive or potentially contaminated penetrating wounds must be explored without delay.

For most patients, the first step is to determine whether the peritoneum has been breached by exploring the wound under local anaesthesia. If it has, then peritoneal lavage should be employed. If the peritoneum has not been breached or lavage is negative (as in most cases), conservative management is appropriate. However, about one-third of those who later prove to have significant intra-abdominal injury are free of signs initially, thus emphasising the need for clinical reassessment at frequent intervals.

143

BULLET AND OTHER MISSILE INJURIES

The severity of injury depends on the path and the mass of the missile and to a large extent on its velocity. Low-velocity missile wounds (e.g. hand-gun bullets) cause damage confined to the wound track, whereas high-velocity (i.e. rifle) bullet wounds injure widely and deeply. This is because the very much higher kinetic energy is dissipated in the tissues. In addition, **cavitation** is caused within the body and debris is sucked into the wounds causing contamination with clothing and soil. If the bullet hits bone, secondary missiles are created causing further injury. The size of the entry wound is no guide to the extent of injury because of the elastic recoil of the skin. Because of the unpredictable extent of the injuries, all gunshot wounds must be explored to check for visceral organ, intestinal and vascular damage. Buttock wounds should be treated in the same way as abdominal wounds.

CLOSED ABDOMINAL INJURIES

Closed abdominal injuries usually result from road traffic accidents, falls, contact injuries and accidents involving horses. Following blunt injury, about 20% of patients will require laparotomy. The **spleen** is the most vulnerable organ, especially in left-sided injuries to the lower chest or upper abdomen (see Fig. 10.1). **Liver injury** requires greater impact, usually from the front or right side. **Pancreatic injuries** are uncommon and usually result from a massive central abdominal impact, transsecting the pancreas across the vertebral bodies. The **kidneys** are vulnerable to punches or kicks in the loins.

Bowel tends to be damaged by rapid deceleration or crushing injuries, tearing in areas where freely mobile bowel is attached to the retroperitoneum, e.g. each end of the transverse colon, the duodeno-jejunal flexure, the ileocaecal area. A full **bladder**, common after a bout of heavy drinking, may rupture into the peritoneal cavity after abdominal impact. The **bladder** and **urethra** are also liable to be torn in association with displaced pelvic fractures. The clinical features and investigation of closed abdominal injuries are shown in Box 10.1.

PRINCIPLES OF MANAGEMENT OF CLOSED (BLUNT) ABDOMINAL INJURIES

Urgent laparotomy

All patients with abdominal trauma should be admitted to hospital and closely observed. Following blunt abdominal trauma, **immediate laparotomy** is indicated after initial resuscitation for cases with hypotension and evidence of abdominal injury, continuing intra-abdominal haemorrhage, overt peritonitis and those with abdominal gun-

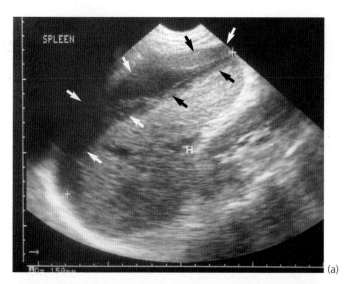

(a)

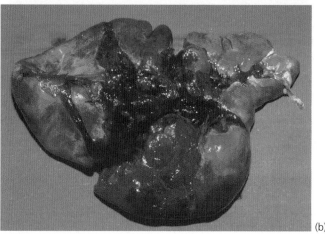

(b)

Fig. 10.1 Ruptured spleen

(a) This 67-year-old woman sustained fractures of the left lower ribs in a fall. She was discharged from hospital the following day but presented again 6 weeks later with abdominal swelling, tenderness and anaemia. This ultrasound scan shows a large subcapsular splenic haematoma (arrowed), which had presumably developed slowly over the intervening period. The scan also shows intrasplenic haemorrhage **H**. She rapidly recovered after splenectomy. **(b)** This operative specimen comes from a 15-year-old girl who fell off her pony, which then trod on the left side of her chest. She was admitted to hospital with bruising over the lower ribs and tachycardia. At laparotomy, her spleen was found to be split completely in half, necessitating removal.

shot wounds. Less urgent laparotomy may be required after investigation or observation. Indications include positive DPL, signs of gastrointestinal perforation (e.g. free gas on abdominal X-ray, developing signs of peritonitis) and specific visceral injuries not amenable to conservative treatment, e.g. splenic rupture.

Diagnostic procedures

Diagnostic procedures are needed if early laparotomy is not indicated but the accident is judged to have been one

KEY POINTS

Box 10.1 Clinical features of closed abdominal injury that suggest visceral injury

1. History
- Substantial trauma to the abdomen or lower chest
- Seat belt not worn in road traffic accident
- Abdominal pain after trauma
- Haematuria particularly following trauma to the back or loin

2. Physical signs
- Skin bruising immediately after injury—suggests impact of sufficient force to cause internal damage
- Imprinting of cloth pattern on skin (**cloth printing**)—caused by compression of skin against vertebral bodies; implies a high energy transfer impact
- Unexplained hypotension—suggests concealed haemorrhage into the abdominal cavity or elsewhere
- Abdominal distension, i.e. increasing abdominal girth—from accumulating blood, urine or gas in the peritoneal cavity
- Increasing abdominal tenderness, guarding and rigidity (difficult to assess in the presence of abdominal wall bruising)—may indicate intestinal perforation or intra-abdominal bleeding
- Lateral lower rib fractures—may be associated with injury to spleen, liver or kidney
- Pelvic fractures, especially 'butterfly' fractures of all four pubic rami—often associated with bladder or urethral injury (especially in males) and pelvic vein injury
- Inability to pass urine and the findings of blood at the urethral meatus and/or perineal bruising—imply rupture of the urethra, usually at the pelvic diaphragm, i.e. post-membranous urethra (urethral catheterisation must not be performed); rectal examination may reveal a 'high-riding' prostate
- Damage to the anus or rectum may be palpable on rectal examination, the presence of blood suggesting ano-rectal injury. If anal sphincter tone is low, this suggests neurological damage from a spinal injury

3. Investigation
- Plasma amylase level should be checked and, if raised, pancreatic injury investigated by CT scanning
- Chest and plain abdominal X-rays (supine and erect or lateral decubitus views) may show free intraperitoneal or retroperitoneal gas, rib or pelvic fractures associated with specific visceral injuries and radiopaque missiles such as bullets, shotgun pellets and glass
- Peritoneal lavage—blood-staining indicates intra-abdominal injury but a negative result does not exclude serious injury
- Ultrasound and CT scanning—particularly useful in investigating solid organs, i.e. spleen (see Fig. 10.1), liver, kidneys, pancreas. Intravenous contrast CT useful for large vessel injuries
- Intravenous urography/cystography—investigation of haematuria
- Urethrography—investigation of suspected urethral rupture
- Laparoscopy—increasingly important in investigation of closed abdominal trauma in stable patients. Can be performed under local anaesthesia

of high-energy transfer and the abdominal signs are equivocal. Investigation is also necessary where there is suspicion of an intra-abdominal injury in the following groups of patients:

- Those with impaired consciousness
- Those with thoracic, pelvic or abdominal wall injuries
- Those who are to be transferred to other units, e.g. by helicopter
- Where prolonged investigation or treatment of non-abdominal injury is needed

Diagnostic peritoneal lavage (DPL)

Diagnostic peritoneal lavage is often the first investigation. Its greatest use is in unstable polytrauma victims to confirm intra-abdominal haemorrhage; this helps determine management priorities. The test has a high sensitivity (99%) and a low false positive rate; it is best performed by mini-laparotomy under local anaesthesia using a small subumbilical incision similar to Hasson's open technique of access for laparoscopy. Patients with a positive result are explored by laparotomy or perhaps laparoscopically.

CT scanning

If DPL is equivocal, CT scanning should be performed to investigate the retroperitoneum for solid organ injury as well as for free fluid. The examination can often identify the source of haemorrhage in solid organ injuries and may allow conservative management of certain liver injuries. CT is also valuable for defining the extent and configuration of complex pelvic fractures. The investigation should also be performed in stable patients with abnormal abdominal signs or where signs appear later.

Ultrasound

Ultrasound can demonstrate free intraperitoneal fluid and the location and extent of solid organ haematomas. In pregnant patients it avoids the use of ionising radiation. However, even in expert hands ultrasound misses substantial injuries in about 10% of cases.

Clinical observation

If surgical intervention is not judged necessary, nursing observations such as pulse and blood pressure are made at regular intervals and the patient re-examined frequently by a doctor for developing signs of peritonitis or intra-abdominal bleeding. Measurements of abdominal girth are unreliable and may give a false sense of security while the patient exsanguinates; the test is to be condemned. Significant injuries will almost always become manifest within 24 hours.

INJURIES TO SOLID ORGANS

Splenic rupture is treated by urgent laparotomy and splenic repair or splenectomy. In contrast, isolated **liver injury** may be treated by surgical repair or local resection if the injury is small but is often best treated conservatively, particularly when there is major injury. This is because surgery may be incapable of controlling bleeding from hepatic vessels deep within its substance, particularly the hepatic veins that enter the inferior vena cava directly. For conservative management, large-volume blood transfusions are given until abdominal tamponade stops the bleeding. If a major liver injury is encountered at surgical exploration of the abdomen and haemorrhage cannot be arrested, it should be packed with gauze and the abdomen closed. The packs can usually be removed safely about 48 hours later.

Pancreatic transection is treated by surgically removing the distal half and oversewing the stump. A crushing pancreatic injury may have to be treated with drainage alone.

Renal injuries are usually managed conservatively unless nephrectomy is required for uncontrollable bleeding.

BOWEL INJURIES

Injuries to the small bowel are dealt with by simple suture or by resection and reanastomosis if the mesenteric vascular supply is impaired. Conventional treatment for large bowel injuries on the right side is resection and anastomosis to small bowel. Localised injuries to the rest of the colon without substantial intra-abdominal faecal contamination can usually be resected and joined end-to-end. After knife or gunshot wounds, simple repair gives good results provided there is minimal peritoneal contamination. Extensive injuries with contamination require **exteriorisation** of the damaged ends, the proximal end as a colostomy and the distal end as a mucous fistula (see Ch. 20, p. 274).

High-velocity penetrating injuries wreak havoc upon the gut, causing extensive devascularisation and multiple perforations; all necrotic or ischaemic tissue must be excised. The immediate dangers are peritonitis and sepsis syndrome from gross contamination. Exteriorisation of viable bowel ends is mandatory for this type of injury.

LOWER URINARY TRACT INJURIES

Intraperitoneal rupture of the bladder is treated by laparotomy and suturing of the bladder with a urethral catheter left in situ for about 1 week until the defect is healed. Extraperitoneal bladder rupture is treated conservatively with prolonged urethral or suprapubic catheterisation. Urethral tears require specialist urological management. If the urethral wall is partly intact (as shown on urethrography), it can be treated by catheterisation (usually suprapubic). Complete urethral avulsion injuries are usually treated by suprapubic catheterisation, with formal repair after local inflammation has settled. Formerly, attempts used to be made to 'rail-road' a catheter through the disrupted urethra at operation, by passing instruments down the urethra from the bladder and up the urethra from below. This treatment is no longer in vogue.

CHEST INJURIES

GENERAL PRINCIPLES

Chest injuries are a common cause of death in patients with multiple injuries, although the death rate has fallen dramatically in countries where the wearing of seat belts is compulsory. Seat belts, however, often cause typical **sash pattern bruising** obliquely across the chest and minor rib and sternal fractures (Fig. 10.2).

Serious chest injuries, particularly tearing injuries of the mediastinal contents, e.g. aorta, bronchi and oesophagus, may be present even without evidence of external injury. Diagnosis of serious chest injuries goes hand in hand with urgent resuscitative measures. Clinical signs may provide clues to the nature of the injury but the various diagnostic possibilities must all be considered or they may be missed. Good-quality chest X-rays are mandatory and will usually clinch the diagnosis (see Fig. 10.3).

The types of chest injury, their clinical features and their treatment are summarised in Table 10.1. The main mechanisms of chest injury are penetrating trauma, blunt impact and crush injuries, deceleration injuries and rupture of the diaphragm by abdominal compression. Fewer than 10% of chest injuries require thoracic surgery but early recognition may be life-saving.

TECHNIQUE OF INSERTING A CHEST DRAIN

Following trauma chest drains are usually placed in the fourth or fifth intercostal space in the mid-axillary line. The technique is shown in Figures 24.4 and 24.5, p. 331.

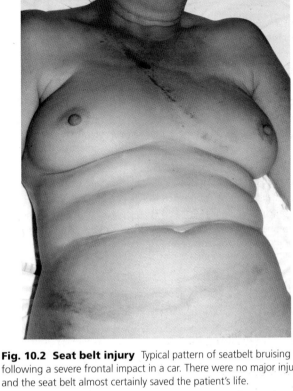

Fig. 10.2 Seat belt injury Typical pattern of seatbelt bruising following a severe frontal impact in a car. There were no major injuries and the seat belt almost certainly saved the patient's life.

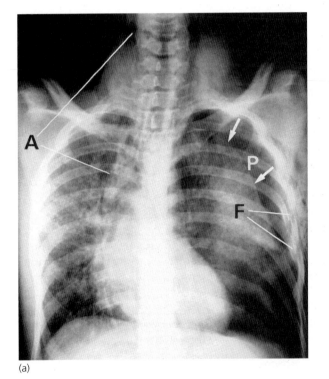

(a)

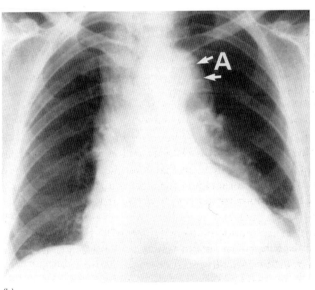

(b)

Fig. 10.3 Serious chest injuries
(a) A 20-year-old driver of a car involved in a head-on road traffic accident. He was not wearing a seat belt and his chest hit the steering wheel with great force. The chest X-ray shows multiple rib fractures **F** on the left side, associated with a flail segment which moved paradoxically on breathing. A left pneumothorax **P** is also shown, with the lung border clearly visible (arrowed). Mediastinal shift towards the right strongly suggests a tension pneumothorax; the lung would not be expected to collapse completely because of extensive contusion. Lung contusion on both sides is manifest by the patchy shadowing. There is also a pneumomediastinum with air **A** tracking from ruptured alveoli alongside the airways to the mediastinum and thence into the soft tissues of the neck causing surgical emphysema. **(b)** This chest X-ray was taken following a crushing central chest injury. The patient appeared relatively unaffected, but the X-ray shows that the aortic knuckle has a double shadow **A** and is wider than normal. CT scanning confirmed a ruptured aortic arch, the blood being contained only by a thin layer of adventitia.

Table 10.1 Types of chest injury and their management

Natural of the injury	Clinical features	Treatment
Rib fractures	Localised pain on respiration or coughing; tenderness over fractures; usually visible on chest X-ray	Analgesia, intercostal blocks, physiotherapy, prophylactic antibiotics in chronic bronchitics
Flail chest, i.e. multiple rib fractures producing a mobile segment	Respiratory embarrassment; 'paradoxical' indrawing of the flail segment on inspiration	Intercostal block analgesia; endotracheal intubation and ventilation if hypoxic
Pneumothorax, i.e. air in pleural cavity causing lung collapse	Unilateral signs: loss of chest movement and breath sounds, percussion note resonant; sometimes chest wall emphysema; confirmed by chest X-ray	Intercostal drain with underwater seal
Sucking chest wound, i.e. open pneumothorax with mediastinum 'flapping' from side to side with each respiration	Gross respiratory embarrassment, audible sucking of air through chest wound	Sealing of chest wound with impermeable dressing; intercostal drainage
Tension pneumothorax, i.e. expanding pneumothorax causing progressive mediastinal shift to the opposite side and tracheal deviation	Signs of pneumothorax with disproportionate and increasing respiratory distress and hypoxaemia	Urgent chest drainage
Lung contusion	Deteriorating respiratory function; opacification of affected lung field on chest X-ray	Oxygenation, physiotherapy, mechanical ventilation in severe cases
Rupture of bronchus (uncommon)	Respiratory distress, surgical emphysema in the neck; suggested by air in mediastinum on chest X-ray (see Fig. 10.3); confirmed by bronchoscopy	Operation by thoracic surgeon
Rupture of oesophagus (very rare)	May have surgical emphysema in the neck and pneumomediastinum on chest X-ray but diagnosis often missed until mediastinitis or empyema develops	Surgical repair if recognised early; surgical drainage and diversion for a late presentation
Haemothorax, i.e. blood in the pleural cavity usually from a chest wall injury; usual cause is a ruptured intercostal or internal mammary artery	Dull percussion note, breath sounds absent, tachycardia and hypotension due to blood loss	Urgent intercostal drain, even before X-ray (in sixth intercostal space in mid-axillary line), blood transfusion, thoracotomy if excessive bleeding
Cardiac tamponade, i.e. bleeding into pericardial cavity (usually penetrating trauma)	Hypotension, inaudible heart sounds, distended neck veins with systolic waves; enlarged, rounded heart shadow on chest X-ray; confirmed with ultrasound	Long needle aspiration via epigastric approach; operation if tamponade recurs
Cardiac contusion	May have arrhythmia or ECG changes similar to myocardial infarction	Conservative management
Rupture of aorta (usually results from deceleration injury)—fatal unless false aneurysm develops in mediastinum	Back pain, hypotension; systolic murmur or signs of tamponade in some cases; characteristic widening of mediastinum on chest X-ray; diagnosis confirmed by arteriography	Urgent thoracotomy and Dacron graft
Rupture of diaphragm, linear split usually in left diaphragm with herniation of gut into chest (penetrating or abdominal crush injury)	Respiratory distress, bowel sounds heard in the chest; diagnosis by chest X-ray and confirmed by barium meal; however, many cases are missed and only discovered much later; diagnosis may be made by laparoscopy or at laparotomy	Repair of diaphragm, usually via an abdominal approach

Symptoms, diagnosis and management

11 Non-acute abdominal pain and other abdominal symptoms

INTRODUCTION

The diagnosis and management of abdominal complaints is an important part of the workload of a general surgical outpatient clinic. The proportion of abdominal problems varies from one clinic to another depending on the availability of a medical gastroenterology service and specialist gastroenterological surgical services. Most patients with abdominal complaints are investigated and treated as outpatients and only a proportion eventually need hospital admission or operation.

The diagnoses made in patients seen in a surgical clinic are quite different from those in emergency surgical admissions to hospital. Nevertheless, the surgeon in the clinic must remain alert to unfamiliar presentations of common conditions which usually present acutely, e.g. an appendix mass.

The principal presenting symptoms of non-acute abdominal disorders are abdominal pain, difficulty in swallowing (dysphagia), loss of appetite (anorexia), weight loss, nausea and intermittent vomiting, changes

in bowel habit and anal or perianal symptoms, including rectal bleeding. In addition, patients are often referred to a surgeon after discovery of an **abdominal mass**, **obstructive jaundice** or an **iron deficiency anaemia** caused by chronic blood loss. The history can provide 70% or more of the clues to the diagnosis and so must be taken accurately and with great care.

The main presenting features of non-acute abdominal disorders are summarised in Box 11.1.

SUMMARY

Box 11.1 Main presenting features of non-acute abdominal disorders

- Abdominal pain
- Difficulty in swallowing (dysphagia)
- Weight loss, anorexia and associated symptoms
- Change in bowel habit, including rectal bleeding
- Anal and perianal symptoms
- Iron deficiency anaemia
- Obstructive jaundice
- Abdominal mass or distension

PAIN

CHARACTER, TIMING AND SITE OF THE PAIN

Pain is described by patients in many different ways, although each pathological entity tends to have its own pain characteristics. The pattern will only come to light if a thorough history is compiled. Pain is, however, a highly subjective phenomenon and the history will be coloured by the patient's own perception of the pain and its possible significance. Patients often use vague terms such as 'indigestion' and 'dyspepsia' to describe upper abdominal pain or discomfort associated with food. These terms should have little place in medical terminology, and what the patient actually means should be clarified by further questioning.

The time-related features of the pain are highly significant in working towards a differential diagnosis and may only be elicited by diligent enquiry. It is important to establish when a pain first began, how frequently it occurs (minutes, hours, days, weeks or even constantly), and whether the frequency and severity vary. The key points to be covered in taking a history of abdominal pain are summarised in Box 11.2.

KEY POINTS

Box 11.2 Assessing abdominal pain from the history

Location of pain

- Where did the pain start and where is it now, e.g. central, epigastric, right or left subcostal (hypochondrial), in right or left iliac fossa, suprapubic, 'lower abdominal', or loin pain?
- Is pain well or poorly localised (i.e. is parietal peritoneum with its somatic innervation involved)?
- Is there any radiation of the pain?

Severity and character of pain

- e.g. Discomfort, moderate or severe pain?
- What descriptive words are used by the patient: 'sharp', 'blunt', 'burning', 'crushing', 'deep', 'gnawing', 'boring', 'bloating', 'knife-like', 'stabbing'?
- How much does the pain interfere with normal living?
- Is the pain physiological (e.g. pre-defaecation colic or dysmenorrhoea) or pathological?
- Are there any changes in the character of the pain during the attack?

Variation of pain severity with time

- e.g. Constant, intermittent or episodic, 'colicky' (i.e. coming in severe cramp-like waves), background pain with exacerbations?

Overall duration of pain

- i.e. When did the pain really begin?

Periodicity

- e.g. Weekly, monthly, hourly?
- Daytime or night-time?
- Any periods free from pain?
- Any previous similar episodes or attacks?

Exacerbating and relieving factors

- e.g. Improved or made worse by food, posture or drugs?

Associated symptoms

- e.g. Vomiting, change in bowel habit

Table 11.1 Anatomical significance of the site of abdominal pain

Site of pain	Clinical significance
Right upper quadrant	Biliary tract, liver
Epigastrium	Usually foregut structures, i.e. stomach, duodenum, lower oesophagus, biliary tract, pancreas (Note: cardiac pain can also present in the epigastrium)
Left upper quadrant	Rarely directly related to anatomical structures, occasionally spleen or stomach
Central	Midgut structures, i.e. small and large bowel or pancreas (deep pain radiating to the back)
Right iliac fossa	Caecum and appendix (when parietal peritoneum is involved), ovary, right kidney and ureter, mesenteric adenitis
Suprapubic area	Bladder, uterus and adnexae
Left iliac fossa	Sigmoid colon, left kidney and ureter, ovary
Loins	Kidneys and ureters

DISEASES CAUSING NON-ACUTE ABDOMINAL PAIN

The following conditions cause non-acute abdominal pain. Each has certain characteristic features:

- **Gallstones and gall bladder dysfunction**. Biliary colic presents with irregularly recurrent bouts of severe pain, lasting 1–12 hours. Some episodes are more severe and prolonged than others and often a particularly severe bout brings the patient into hospital. The pain is usually located in the upper abdomen—often on the right side, less often in the epigastrium—and may radiate to the back on the right. It is often precipitated by rich or fatty foods and may be associated with vomiting late in the attack

- **Peptic ulcer disease**. This is typically associated with intermittent 'boring' epigastric pain which recurs several times a year and lasts for days or weeks at a time; it is not as severe as biliary colic unless there is perforation, which usually presents acutely. Retrosternal 'burning' occurs in peptic oesophagitis and tends to occur after large meals and on lying down. The association of pain with food varies according to the site of the disease; duodenal ulcer pain tends to be relieved by bland food and recurs 3–4 hours afterwards, typically in the early hours of the morning, whereas the pain of gastric ulcer and oesophagitis tends to be aggravated by food, especially if acidic or spicy. Peptic pain is generally relieved by

The **site of origin** of the pain, particularly the site at which it first manifested, suggests the anatomical structures most likely to be involved. These are shown in Table 11.1. The **distribution** and **radiation** of the pain provide further clues. Pain that extends through to the back suggests involvement of retroperitoneal structures, e.g. pancreas (carcinoma or chronic pancreatitis) or abdominal aorta (aneurysm). Gall bladder pain tends to radiate from the right hypochondrium around to the back on the right side. Renal pain tends to radiate from the loin down towards the groin and occasionally to the genitalia.

antacids and virtually always by H₂-blocking drugs (e.g. ranitidine) or proton pump inhibitors (e.g. omeprazole)

- **Chronic pancreatitis and carcinoma of pancreas**. These are typically associated with severe 'gnawing', persistent, poorly localised central pain which usually radiates through to the back and is often associated with anorexia and weight loss. The pain may be relieved by leaning forwards ('pancreatic position'). Early carcinoma of the pancreas, however, is often painless
- **Irritable bowel syndrome, constipation, diverticular disease and Crohn's disease**. These conditions may all produce a chronic symptom complex mimicking a partial obstruction of the bowel manifest by episodes of colicky pain. This is poorly localised, often 'bloating' pain, particularly post-prandially (after meals). It is of variable intensity and is often associated with transient disturbances of bowel function, particularly alternating diarrhoea and constipation. Passage of flatus or stool often temporarily relieves the symptoms
- **Chronic renal outflow obstruction (hydronephrosis) caused by stone, tumour or fibrosis**. There is 'dull', poorly defined, fairly constant loin pain which may be accompanied by typical urinary tract symptoms, e.g. haematuria and dysuria. It is often aggravated acutely by a high fluid intake
- **Gynaecological conditions**, particularly chronic pelvic inflammatory disease and ovarian tumours. These may reach the surgeon because of poorly defined lower abdominal pain. A gynaecological history should be taken in female patients; pelvic examination may reveal the cause
- **Non-surgical (i.e. 'medical') disorders causing abdominal pain**. These include liver congestion in heart failure (common), splenic infarcts or diabetes (both uncommon but important), acute intermittent porphyria, sickle-cell anaemia or tertiary syphilis (very rare). Patients sometimes present with abdominal pain for which no organic cause can be found despite extensive investigation. In these, irritable bowel syndrome or sensitivity to certain foods, e.g. gluten, need to be considered. Only as a last resort should the pain be attributed to psychological disturbance and only then if diagnostic psychological features are present. Unnecessary operations may be performed on these patients (**Munchausen syndrome**)

Note that non-acute abdominal pain in children is uncommon; the main organic causes are constipation, irritable bowel syndrome and sometimes hydronephrosis. The so-called 'periodic syndrome' is characterised by recurrent episodes of poorly defined and inconsistent

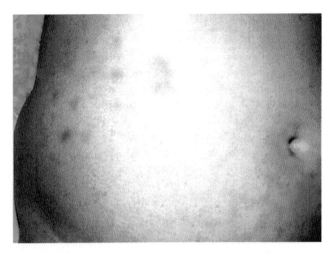

Fig. 11.1 Erythema ab igne
This woman of 45 had experienced chronic pain in the right loin area and had obtained some relief from regularly applying a hot water bottle to the area. This has resulted in typical skin damage.

abdominal pain, sufficiently severe for the child to avoid school. There are no other consistent features; psychological and environmental factors are the usual underlying causes (see Ch. 44).

APPROACH TO INVESTIGATION OF NON-ACUTE ABDOMINAL PAIN

A differential diagnosis must first be made on clinical grounds. The choice (and order) of the numerous possible investigations should be efficient and economical, after considering how each one will support or help eliminate the most probable (and common) diagnoses and influence the management. Rarer diagnoses usually need further investigation.

The following example shows the diagnostic pathway in a patient presenting with chronic epigastric pain:

1. Once the main complaint has been stated, a preliminary differential diagnosis forms in the clinician's mind even before a detailed history is completed. Acid-peptic disorders of oesophagus, stomach or duodenum (ulcers or 'non-ulcer dyspepsia') or alternatively, gall bladder disease are statistically the most likely. Irritable bowel syndrome and angina pectoris are less likely
2. A detailed history and direct questioning strengthen the possibility of certain diagnoses and diminish the likelihood of others; rarer conditions such as chronic pancreatitis might now enter the differential diagnosis
3. Physical examination may add further weight to one diagnosis over another. The clinician will particularly be seeking signs of anaemia, jaundice, tenderness or a mass (see Box 11.3)

153

KEY POINTS

Box 11.3 21 points to remember in examining a patient with abdominal symptoms

General examination

1. Well-looking or ill (thin, emaciated, weak)?
2. Alert and responding normally or obtunded and slumped?
3. Dehydrated (poor skin tone, sunken cheeks)?
4. Abnormal colour (pale, jaundiced, grey)
5. Signs of surgical wounds/dressings
6. 'Medical accessories'—i.v. infusion, urinary catheter, parenteral nutrition, monitoring apparatus, oxygen
7. End-of-bed charts—fever, tachycardia, fluid balance, trauma chart, pain chart, drug chart (e.g. strength and frequency of analgesia)

Abdominal inspection

1. Position the patient correctly (comfortable, near-flat, arms by sides) and expose the whole abdominal field ('nipples to knees' but not all at once)
2. Distended or scaphoid (sunken) abdominal shape
3. Wounds and scars
4. Bruising—umbilical or flank in acute pancreatitis; cloth printing (trauma cases)
5. Herniation (including usual sites or incisional hernias)
6. Redness or other signs of infection, erythema ab igne (see Fig. 11.1)
7. Jaundice and scratch marks resulting from pruritus (itching)

Abdominal palpation

Do not hurt the patient; watch the face for signs of discomfort

1. Gentle overall palpation for obvious abnormalities
2. Detailed examination of abnormal masses found—relationship to abdominal wall, size, shape, position, mobility, texture, hardness, fixation posteriorly or anteriorly, tenderness. Likely site or organ of origin?
3. Specific organ palpation—press in first, *then* ask the patient to breathe in deeply; gradually relax your pressure and seek the descending lower edge of the organ; repeat at 3 cm intervals moving upwards:
   - *Liver*—start as low as it might have reached, e.g. right iliac fossa, and work upwards. Percuss for upper border to gauge liver size. If large, palpate surface for irregularities, e.g. metastases
   - *Spleen*—tilt patient slightly towards right side, place left hand behind lower left ribs and gently lift. Start as low as enlargement might have reached, e.g. right iliac fossa, and palpate as for liver. Seek notch in lower edge. Percuss for resonant band of overlying colon
   - *Kidneys*—as for liver plus bimanual palpation. Place left hand in loin and attempt to push enlarged organ on to examining hand anteriorly
4. Examination for ascites (see Fig. 11.12)
5. Hernial orifices—inguinal and femoral for cough impulse; reducibility (see Ch. 25, p. 339)
6. Rectal and/or vaginal examination if appropriate
7. Percussion and auscultation if appropriate

4. A narrower and weighted set of diagnostic probabilities will by now have evolved and will form the basis for planning special investigations
5. If the most likely diagnosis is acid-peptic disorder, gastroscopy (oesophagogastroduodenoscopy, or OGD) will be considered, although if the symptoms are mild, a diagnostic trial of antacid therapy might be more appropriate. A full blood count is performed if anaemia is suspected and specimens of faeces tested for occult blood. If biliary tract disease seems most likely, ultrasound of the biliary tree, liver and pancreas is performed. The kidneys and aorta are usually examined by ultrasound at the same time

6. By this stage, investigation will usually have confirmed or eliminated the most likely diagnoses. If no diagnosis has been confirmed, alternative diagnoses are considered, usually at a subsequent visit, by further history-taking and examination. Symptoms and physical signs may have persisted unchanged, they may have changed or they may even have resolved completely during the period of investigation. Changed symptoms may suggest new diagnostic possibilities and new lines of investigation. If the symptoms have decreased, a less serious disorder such as irritable bowel syndrome might become the working diagnosis and a trial of treatment

initiated. Further investigation will depend on the patient's response to treatment or to reassurance. Often cross-sectional imaging (computed tomography or magnetic resonance imaging) is indicated, particularly in older patients, where organic disease is likely but symptoms and signs are not diagnostic

DYSPHAGIA

CLINICAL PRESENTATION

Dysphagia is the term used to describe difficulty in swallowing. The most common symptom is inability to swallow solid food, which the patient will describe as 'becoming stuck' or 'held up' before it either passes on into the stomach or is regurgitated. The patient usually reports that particular types of food are more difficult than others; fibrous foods, such as chunks of meat, usually cause the most trouble. The patient can usually indicate a precise level for the perceived obstruction. The true level of obstruction is usually some distance below that point.

Dysphagia is almost always caused by disease in or adjacent to the oesophagus but occasionally the lesion is in the pharynx or stomach. Oesophageal narrowing usually causes symptoms only when the lumen is unable to expand beyond a diameter of about 10 mm—the narrower the lumen, the more severe the symptoms. In many of the pathological conditions causing dysphagia, the lumen becomes progressively constricted and indistensible. Initially only fibrous solids cause difficulty but later the problem extends to all solids and later, even to fluids. Because narrowing is a gradual and insidious process, patients often compensate to a surprising degree (e.g. by liquidising all food) and may only present when they have difficulty in swallowing fluids or even their own saliva. By this time there is usually marked weight loss.

The common causes of dysphagia are outlined in Box 11.4. **Pain** on swallowing (usually provoked by both food and drink, particularly if hot) is a distinctive symptom which is highly suspicious of carcinoma.

Achalasia is a major exception to the usual pattern of dysphagia in that swallowing of fluids tends to cause more difficulty than swallowing solids. In achalasia, there is idiopathic destruction of the parasympathetic ganglia in Auerbach's (submucosal) plexus of the entire oesophagus, which results in functional narrowing of the lower oesophagus and peristaltic failure throughout its length. Thus the oesophagus becomes markedly distended and dilated, with solids settling towards the lower end and fluids spilling over into the airways causing **spluttering dysphagia**. This overspill and consequent symptoms tend to occur when the patient is lying flat at night. Achalasia often presents with chronic chest

infection rather than dysphagia and the diagnosis is often reached late. Similar symptoms of overspill into the airways can be provoked by bulbar palsy, most commonly provoked by a stroke.

Bolus obstruction is an acute form of dysphagia, where a lump of food sticks at a narrowed part, completely obstructing the oesophagus.

APPROACH TO INVESTIGATION OF DYSPHAGIA

Dysphagia, particularly of recent onset, must be regarded seriously and fully investigated. A plain chest X-ray should be taken to exclude bronchial carcinoma; occasionally an oesophageal fluid level behind the heart is seen, resulting from an oesophageal stricture due to hiatus hernia or achalasia. In high dysphagia, a barium swallow and meal is usually the next investigation (OGD risks perforating a pharyngeal pouch). In lower dysphagia, flexible endoscopy (OGD) is usually performed. Both OGD and contrast radiography are often required. If a lesion has been demonstrated radiologically, endoscopy allows direct inspection and biopsy to confirm (or change) the diagnosis. In disorders of function, swallowing of

---

KEY POINTS

Box 11.4 Causes of dysphagia

Obstruction arising in the oesophageal wall

- Peptic oesophagitis (often associated with hiatus hernia)—common (sometimes causes fibrous stricture)
- Carcinoma of oesophagus or cardia (uppermost part) of the stomach—common
- Candida oesophagitis particularly after major surgery—uncommon
- Pharyngeal pouch—extremely rare
- Oesophageal web (Plummer–Vinson/Paterson–Kelly syndrome)—extremely rare
- 'Oesophageal apoplexy' due to haematoma in the wall—extremely rare
- Leiomyoma of the oesophageal muscle—extremely rare

Disorders of neuromuscular function

- Achalasia—uncommon
- Bulbar or pseudobulbar palsy—rare
- Myasthenia gravis—rare

External compression of the oesophagus

- Subcarinal lymph node secondaries from carcinoma of the bronchus—fairly common
- Left atrial dilatation in mitral stenosis—rare
- Dysphagia lusoria (compression from abnormally placed great arteries)—very rare

barium-soaked bread or a video record of a barium swallow may be helpful in reaching a diagnosis. Oesophageal physiology measurements using manometry and pH are important in reaching a diagnosis of achalasia, especially in its early stages.

WEIGHT LOSS, ANOREXIA AND ASSOCIATED SYMPTOMS

Marked weight loss (**cachexia**) and loss of appetite (**anorexia**) are frequently manifestations of serious, insidious, often malignant abdominal disorders. They may be associated with a variety of other symptoms such as malaise, bloating, nausea, sporadic vomiting and regurgitation. These symptoms may have been unnoticed or dismissed as trivial by the patient and are only elicited by direct questioning.

The diseases which cause these symptoms may be grouped into four broad categories:

- **Intra-abdominal malignancies**, e.g. carcinoma of the stomach or pancreas, metastatic disease in the liver or widespread in the peritoneal cavity (arising particularly from stomach, large bowel, ovary, breast or bronchus), bowel lymphomas
- **'Medical' conditions**, e.g. alcoholism and cirrhosis, viral diseases (e.g. hepatitis or infectious mononucleosis), uncontrolled diabetes or thyrotoxicosis, malabsorption, renal failure, cardiac cachexia
- **Psychological disorders**, e.g. anxiety, depression, anorexia nervosa, bulimia
- **Chronic visceral ischaemia**, a very uncommon condition resulting from atherosclerotic narrowing of at least two of the three main visceral arteries: the coeliac axis, and the superior mesenteric and the inferior mesenteric arteries

APPROACH TO INVESTIGATION OF WEIGHT LOSS, ANOREXIA AND ASSOCIATED SYMPTOMS

In many patients, there may be other clinical clues to the main diagnosis or which suggest a line of investigation, e.g. pain, signs of anaemia or jaundice, or a palpable abdominal or rectal mass. More difficult are those cases where the symptoms occur alone. In this situation, basic screening investigations (full blood count and erythrocyte sedimentation rate, urea and electrolytes, liver function tests and urinalysis) begin to differentiate 'medical' conditions from 'surgical' ones. If these screening tests fail to produce a lead, abdominal imaging using ultrasound or CT scanning may be indicated to exclude liver metastases or an occult intra-abdominal malignancy.

If investigations still reveal no cause, a psychological cause should be seriously considered. Before such a diagnosis can be accepted, there must be positive evidence of psychiatric disturbance. In practice, by this stage, previously concealed psychiatric features often become apparent; except for anorexia nervosa or bulimia, these are rare.

CHANGE IN BOWEL HABIT, RECTAL BLEEDING AND RELATED SYMPTOMS

Normal bowel habit varies widely between different individuals in both frequency of defaecation and consistency of stool. For an individual, transient changes in bowel habit are usually insignificant but persistent change often leads to the patient seeking medical advice. Departure from the norm may have several different aspects, occurring in various combinations. The differential diagnosis of a change in bowel habit is summarised in Box 11.5.

FREQUENCY OF DEFAECATION AND STOOL CONSISTENCY

Chronic constipation or diarrhoea marks the extremes of change, although some patients develop an erratic pattern of bowel action. All may signify serious disease and deserve investigation. The index of suspicion is further raised if there is rectal bleeding or tenesmus (for definition, see p. 160). Waking from sleep to evacuate the bowels should be treated seriously, especially if it occurs frequently.

SUMMARY

Box 11.5 Differential diagnosis of change in bowel habit

- Carcinoma of colon, rectum or anus
- Diverticular disease
- Irritable bowel syndrome
- Crohn's disease of small or large bowel
- Ulcerative colitis
- Drug effects, e.g. codeine phosphate, iron, laxative abuse
- Reduction in fibre content of diet
- Parasitic infestations, e.g. giardiasis
- Following acute bacterial or parasitic colitis
- Changes in resident bacterial flora, e.g. antibiotic-associated diarrhoea
- Malabsorption syndromes
- Thyrotoxicosis

Note: in many cases, no cause is found, particularly with isolated early morning diarrhoea

Stool consistency varies according to diet but the stool is usually 'formed'. Persistently unformed stools, i.e. 'looseness', is only abnormal if it represents a change from the patient's usual habit.

Constipation

Constipation arises for four main reasons:

- Incomplete bowel obstruction, e.g. faecal impaction, an obstructing carcinoma or stricture in the bowel wall, or occasionally an extrinsic lesion such as ovarian cancer
- Loss of peristalsis, e.g. acutely due to drugs such as narcotics, antidepressants or iron, chronic diverticular disease, chronic laxative abuse
- Inadequate fibre intake or poor fluid intake, which decrease faecal volume and prolong intestinal transit time
- In bed-bound patients, multiple factors including immobility, diet, inadequate fluid intake, drug effects

Diarrhoea

Chronic diarrhoea is most often caused by irritation or inflammation of the small or large bowel. The inflammatory bowel diseases (ulcerative colitis and Crohn's disease) are important diagnoses. Chronic parasitic infestations of the large bowel with amoebae or of the small bowel with *Giardia lamblia* are easily overlooked. In areas where these diseases are not endemic, patients may give a history of foreign travel. Chronic diarrhoea may follow an acute attack of *Salmonella* or other coliform infection. Less commonly, a blind loop of small bowel remaining after bypass surgery becomes colonised with gut flora, causing changes in intraluminal metabolism (**blind loop syndrome**). The most common diagnosis in diarrhoea after intestinal infection is irritable bowel syndrome.

Bile salts irritate the bowel. Therefore if the enterohepatic circulation is disrupted, e.g. after distal small bowel resection, defective reabsorption of bile salts may cause diarrhoea. A less common cause of diarrhoea is the increased volume of bowel contents in various malabsorption syndromes. Finally, when no physical cause can be found, concealed laxative abuse or an anxiety state should be considered. Early morning diarrhoea on its own rarely indicates serious disease.

Erratic bowel habit

Some patients develop an erratic bowel habit with bouts of constipation interspersed with episodes of frequency and looseness of stool. The most common cause is **irritable bowel syndrome**, which can be attributed to a heightened pain response in conjunction with a possible over-production or change in production of normal enteric gas. In particular the symptoms include a marked gastrocolic reflex, i.e. a call to stool immediately after eating. In **diverticular disease**, constipation and 'rabbit-pellet' faeces are the dominant characteristics but there may be episodic diarrhoea, often during periods of inflammation. This may be caused by intermittent release of proximal liquefied stool past the partially obstructed solid faeces (**spurious diarrhoea**). Incomplete bowel obstruction of this type may also occur in carcinoma of the left colon, Crohn's disease or faecal impaction.

Patients treated with broad-spectrum antibiotics, particularly the cephalosporins, may develop **antibiotic-associated diarrhoea** (usually caused by *Clostridium difficile*); the symptoms are due to changes in colonic bacterial flora (see Ch. 49, p. 658).

CHANGES IN THE NATURE OF THE STOOL

Stools are normally brown owing to the presence of urobilin, a breakdown product of bile. In biliary obstruction, bilirubin does not reach the gut and the stools become pale. Stools in obvious jaundice are often described as 'putty-coloured'.

Stools may also be pale when they contain excess fat as in various malabsorption syndromes. In coeliac disease (gluten enteropathy) the stool is often loose and offensive. In fat malabsorption, the stools tend to float because of the excessive fat content and the patient has difficulty flushing them away. This is known as **steatorrhoea**.

Undigested food in the stool indicates failure of digestion and absorption. This can be normal when the diet is extremely high in fibre. It may, however, indicate malabsorption or a 'short-circuit' in the bowel due to previous bowel resection or a fistula between bowel loops.

PRESENCE OF FRANK BLOOD, ALTERED BLOOD OR MUCUS IN THE STOOL

Note: acute gastrointestinal haemorrhage is covered in Chapter 12.

Frank rectal bleeding

When a patient has seen blood in the stool, a careful history should be taken regarding the colour, i.e. fresh or altered blood, and also the relationship of the blood to the stool. Blood alone may be passed, or it may appear before or after the stool. There may be blood mixed with the stool or coating it. The only evidence may be blood-staining of the stool after defaecation.

Bright red blood usually indicates a lesion in the rectum or anus. When blood is clearly separate from the stool it suggests an anal lesion, most commonly haemorrhoids but occasionally proctitis or a carcinoma. If the blood is on the surface of the stool it suggests a lesion such as a polyp (see Fig. 11.2) or carcinoma further proximally, either in the rectum or descending colon. These observations have little diagnostic reliability. As a general rule, rectal bleeding should be assumed to be caused by tumour until proven otherwise!

When blood is mixed with the stool, it usually indicates even more proximal disease. This is usually in the left side of the colon or occasionally in the transverse colon. Carcinoma or inflammatory ulceration is often the cause. In such cases the blood, being 'older', is darker.

When the blood originates further proximally in the gastrointestinal tract, e.g. peptic ulcer, it is so altered by 'digestion' that it may not be recognised as blood by the patient. The stool is typically shiny black or plum-coloured. In rapid bleeding from stomach or duodenum, the stools become fluid and are described as 'tarry'. This is known as **melaena** and has a characteristic odour. Patients on iron therapy have greenish-black, formed stools which should not be mistaken for altered blood. In this case, faecal occult blood testing should be negative.

Occult faecal blood loss

A persistent trickle of blood from the gastrointestinal tract may not alter the appearance of the stool. This 'occult' blood may be detectable only in the laboratory. Despite the small daily quantities involved, this hidden blood loss can cause serious iron deficiency anaemia. This test can be done either at the bedside or in the laboratory.

Rectal passage of mucus or pus

Mucus ('slime') or pus may be passed alone or with the stool. Patients rarely volunteer this information but will report it when asked. The most common cause is irritable bowel syndrome. **Villous adenomas** typically secrete copious mucus, but this may also occur with frank carcinoma of the rectum. Mucus and pus may be noted in the inflammatory bowel disorders and occasionally in diverticular disease. An anal leak of mucus may be a feature of haemorrhoids and causes itching (**pruritus ani**). A patient sometimes reports passing a mass of purulent material. This usually represents spontaneous discharge of a perianal or pararectal abscess, and will often have been preceded by anal or perineal pain.

TENESMUS

Tenesmus is an unpleasant sensation of incomplete evacuation of the rectum. The sensation causes the patient to attempt defaecation (often with straining) at

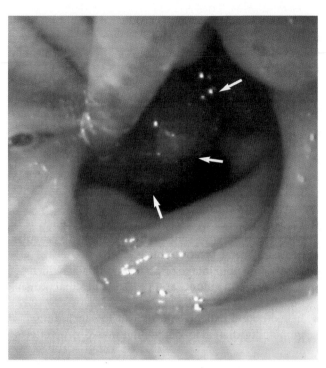

Fig. 11.2 Colonoscopic appearance of a polyp in the sigmoid colon
This 2 cm polyp (arrowed) was found to be the cause of rectal bleeding. It was easily removed with a colonoscopic snare soon after this photograph was taken.

frequent intervals. The most common cause is probably irritable bowel syndrome. Another common cause is an abnormal mass in the rectum or anal canal. This may be a carcinoma, polyp or thrombosed haemorrhoid. Occasionally a prostatic carcinoma invades around the lower rectum producing tenesmus. In some cases, despite extensive investigation, no organic cause is found for tenesmus.

APPROACH TO INVESTIGATION OF CHANGE IN BOWEL HABIT

The first step in investigation after rectal palpation is sigmoidoscopy (rectoscopy). Rigid sigmoidoscopy permits direct visual examination and biopsy of the mucosa up to the rectosigmoid junction; the term sigmoidoscopy is misleading in this case as it does not include the sigmoid colon proper. Flexible sigmoidoscopy, on the other hand, allows examination to the splenic flexure. The majority of large bowel lesions responsible for altered bowel habit occur in this region. In the case of chronic diarrhoea, stool specimens should be examined for ova and parasites and cultured for *Shigella* and *Salmonella* species. Biopsies of the rectal wall should always be taken both for histology (e.g. for Crohn's disease) and for microbiological examination.

Further investigation is based on the differential diagnosis assembled during clinical examination. Barium enema X-ray, contrast CT scanning or colonoscopy is indicated in the majority of cases. Note that in some centres, low rectal lesions cannot be reliably demonstrated on barium enema and preliminary sigmoidoscopy is mandatory. If Crohn's disease is suspected, barium studies of the small bowel may also be required.

Flexible fibreoptic endoscopes of different lengths are used to examine the colon above the rectosigmoid junction. The shortest, the flexible sigmoidoscope, may be employed with no preparation or following a simple enema and can thus be used in the outpatient clinic. An excellent view can be obtained as far as the splenic flexure, allowing examination of the area in which over 50% of large bowel cancers occur. The longer instruments, colonoscopes, require prior bowel clearance with purgatives. In some centres, they tend to be reserved for detailed inspection and biopsy of lesions already demonstrated or suspected on barium enema. Since colonoscopy is a time-consuming and rather uncomfortable procedure, patients usually require intravenous sedation and analgesia, and occasionally general anaesthesia. Therefore colonoscopy is usually performed in hospital or dedicated units as short-stay day cases.

ANAL AND PERIANAL SYMPTOMS

Anal symptoms generate a large number of surgical outpatient referrals. Symptoms include bleeding and discharge, pain and itching, local swelling and a sensation of 'something coming down'. They often cause distress out of proportion to their pathological importance. The most common diagnoses are haemorrhoids, anal fissures and local abscesses, although the occasional infiltrating anal carcinoma or low rectal carcinoma or polyp must not be overlooked.

ANAL BLEEDING

This is an extremely common symptom. It is well tolerated by patients who usually believe that 'piles' (haemorrhoids) are responsible. Patients often present when the bleeding becomes excessive or when new and different symptoms develop. The characteristic feature of anal bleeding is fresh blood separate from the stool which may only be seen 'on the paper'. Fresh bleeding, however, may arise from malignancy in the rectum, sigmoid colon or anal canal and must be treated seriously. In addition to digital examination and proctoscopy, all patients require at least sigmoidoscopy; patients over 40 require colonoscopy, barium enema or contrast CT examination to exclude large bowel cancer, whether or not a benign anal cause, such as haemorrhoids, has already been found.

ANAL PAIN AND DISCOMFORT

The principal causes of chronic anal pain and discomfort are haemorrhoids and anal fissure. Haemorrhoids usually cause periodic anal discomfort and other anal symptoms rather than severe pain. Anal carcinoma is usually painless but may present with haemorrhoid-like pain. The difference is obvious on rectal examination.

Severe perianal pain which follows each episode of defaecation usually indicates a fissure in ano. This is a longitudinal tear typically in the posterior anal mucosa ending externally in a characteristic '**sentinel pile**', a small skin tag visible at the posterior anal margin. An anal fissure is often initiated by a bout of unaccustomed constipation. A perianal abscess may be responsible for anal pain even before the abscess is clinically detectable; the rare **intersphincteric abscess** may cause chronic pain and elude detection for weeks.

An acute onset of anal pain may be caused by a **perianal haematoma**, clearly visible at the anal margin, by strangulated or thrombosed haemorrhoids or by a perianal abscess.

Proctalgia fugax describes recurrent shooting pains in the anal area. Investigations should be performed to find local causes but in many cases no cause is found.

PERIANAL ITCHING AND IRRITATION

The most common cause of these symptoms is inadequate hygiene which results in local skin irritation. This is often exacerbated by scratching or application of various topical medications. The discharge associated with haemorrhoids, fistulae or tumours tends to keep the perianal skin moist, predisposing to low-grade fungal and bacterial infections. The longer these symptoms persist, the more difficult they are to eradicate and in fastidious patients a 'fixation' can develop. In children, threadworm infestation is a common cause of perianal itching; the itching is usually worse at night.

'SOMETHING COMING DOWN'

Haemorrhoids, skin tags ('memorials to past haemorrhoids') and occasionally mucosal or rectal prolapse cause this symptom. It is exacerbated by defaecation. Many patients tolerate the condition for some time before seeking medical advice and may have to push the lumps back manually after defaecation, presenting only when this becomes impossible. A pedunculated low rectal polyp may occasionally come through the anus and be confused with prolapsed haemorrhoids. Perianal warts are occasionally mistaken for lumps arising from within the anal canal.

PERIANAL DISCHARGE

A perianal discharge results from leakage of pus, inflammatory exudate or mucus from the anus or anal area. Pus may arise from a pilonidal sinus in the natal cleft or from an anal fistula. Inflammatory exudate or excess mucus may be produced by haemorrhoids, anorectal mucosal inflammation (proctitis), a villous adenoma or an ulcerating carcinoma.

APPROACH TO INVESTIGATION OF ANAL AND PERIANAL SYMPTOMS

Proctoscopy is mandatory and should be conducted after inspection and digital rectal examination. Further examination follows the principles described earlier, but usually includes at least a rigid sigmoidoscopy. If pain makes these examinations impossible, a young patient can usually be assumed to have a fissure. In an older person, carcinoma of the anus must be excluded by examination under anaesthesia. Haemorrhoids appear as bulging bluish masses beneath the anal mucosa. They all arise above the squamocolumnar junction or dentate line ('internal piles') but may later extend beneath the perianal skin ('external piles') or prolapse through the anus ('intero-external piles').

A typical **anal fistula** appears as an inflammatory 'nipple' near the anal margin (see Fig. 11.3); it often

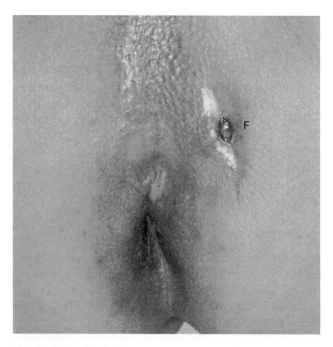

Fig. 11.3 Anal fistula
This man of 39 had presented with a perianal abscess 3 months previously that had been drained. He complained of persistent discharge which was found to be emanating from a fistulous opening **F** within the drainage scar. This proved to be a low fistula on further examination under anaesthesia.

exudes a discharge. A **pilonidal sinus** arises in the natal cleft and usually presents as a swelling with one or more associated sinuses, often with hairs protruding. In **proctitis**, the rectal mucosa is granular and reddened when seen on proctoscopy, and often bleeds to the touch (friability). An anal or low rectal carcinoma is a discrete ulcerated lesion with an indurated (firm, woody) base and a thickened margin. Diagnosis is confirmed by histological examination of a biopsy taken with special forceps. Typically, the pain of an anal fissure precludes a full examination.

The lymphatic drainage of the anal canal below the dentate line is to the inguinal lymph nodes and these should always be examined when a suspicious anal lesion is found.

IRON DEFICIENCY ANAEMIA

A common reason for surgical referral is persistent or severe anaemia believed to be caused by chronic blood loss. The patient may have presented initially with symptoms of chronic anaemia, namely lethargy, generalised weakness, breathlessness or even angina. Just as often, the anaemia has been recognised during general physical examination or on a blood count.

Chronic anaemia has many causes. Iron deficiency is the commonest and is the only one with a cause likely to need surgical treatment. In blood films, iron deficiency anaemia is characterised by hypochromic, microcytic red blood cells. Serum iron level is low and transferrin elevated. Iron deficiency anaemia can be caused by chronic low-grade blood loss (which is often occult), inadequate dietary iron intake or absorption, or a combination of both. In some patients, the pattern of iron deficiency may be complicated by a coexisting anaemia from another cause, particularly the 'anaemia of chronic illness'. For example, an elderly patient with rheumatoid arthritis may have a chronic normochromic, normocytic anaemia due to chronic disease, as well as an iron deficiency anaemia caused by gastric bleeding provoked by non-steroidal anti-inflammatory drugs.

APPROACH TO INVESTIGATION OF ANAEMIA

Investigation of a patient with suspected iron deficiency anaemia has five main components:

● History—seeking sources of blood loss from the various tracts (see Box 11.6) and excluding inadequate dietary iron intake. Previous gastrectomy may cause vitamin B_{12} deficiency and also diminished acid output, which may prevent adequate iron absorption
● Physical examination—seeking an abdominal mass, an enlarged Virchow's node in the left supraclavicular

Box 11.6 Conditions causing chronic occult blood loss

Lesions in the gastrointestinal tract

- Ulcerating tumours or polyps of the following (in order of frequency): caecum, stomach, the rest of the large bowel, and (rarely) connective tissue tumours of small bowel, e.g. leiomyosarcoma
- Chronic peptic ulceration, i.e. hiatus hernia with reflux oesophagitis, gastric and duodenal ulcers or stomal ulceration following gastric surgery. All may be induced or aggravated by ingestion of aspirin and other non-steroidal anti-inflammatory drugs. These drugs can also cause chronic gastric haemorrhage from superficial erosions
- Other 'ulcerating' lesions of the bowel, e.g. haemorrhoids, angiodysplasias of colon or small bowel
- Chronic parasitic infestations, e.g. hookworm (extremely common in some developing countries)

Lesions in the female genital tract

- Heavy menstrual loss (menorrhagia is an extremely common but easily overlooked cause)
- Carcinoma of uterus or cervix (usually presents as abnormal vaginal bleeding rather than anaemia)

Lesions in the urinary tract (rarely sufficient to cause anaemia)

- Transitional cell carcinoma of bladder, pelvicalyceal systems or ureters
- Renal cell carcinoma (may cause haematuria but rarely anaemia)
- Chronic parasitic infestations, e.g. schistosomiasis (common in some developing countries)

area (indicative of intra-abdominal malignancy), a rectal lesion or signs of a 'medical' cause
- Confirmation of iron deficiency anaemia and exclusion of common 'medical' causes of anaemia such as rheumatoid arthritis or chronic leukaemias—examine blood film, measure ESR, serum iron and transferrin, B$_{12}$ and folate. When there is a 'mixed' anaemia, measuring iron stores in a bone marrow biopsy is the definitive method of diagnosing iron deficiency. Small bowel biopsies may demonstrate coeliac disease in a proportion of patients with simple anaemia without bowel symptoms
- Testing of specimens of stool for occult blood (at least three specimens should be tested)
- Pursuing clues that suggest the origin of bleeding by using special investigations such as endoscopy and contrast radiology. When occult blood is found in the

faeces and there are no digestive symptoms, colonoscopy is usually performed first, looking for tumours, polyps, inflammatory bowel disease or angiodysplasias. If negative, this is followed by gastroscopy. Both may be performed in the one session. If both are negative, it may be appropriate to proceed to small bowel contrast radiography

Occasionally, gastrointestinal bleeding continues, even though all investigations appear normal. The next step is often to repeat the appropriate investigations. If bleeding is rapid and serious enough to merit operation and no obvious lesion is found, the whole small bowel may be examined by operative endoscopy (enteroscopy). The small bowel is opened and a colonoscope threaded along its full length, transilluminating the bowel in the process. Small bowel angiodysplasias can only be reliably located by this method.

OBSTRUCTIVE JAUNDICE

Patients with jaundice usually reach the surgeon when a provisional diagnosis of obstructive jaundice has already been made. There is often evidence that the obstruction involves the bile ducts (i.e. posthepatic obstruction).

THE NORMAL ENTEROHEPATIC CIRCULATION

The **haem** component of spent red cells is normally broken down to bilirubin (mainly in the spleen and bone marrow), bound to albumin and transported to the liver. This relatively stable protein-pigment complex is insoluble in water and is not excreted in the urine. In the liver, the complex is split and the bilirubin conjugated with glucuronic acid which makes it water-soluble, before it is excreted into the bile canaliculi. The normal concentration of both conjugated and unconjugated bilirubin in the blood is very low. Bacterial action in the bowel converts conjugated bilirubin into colourless **urobilinogen** and pigmented **urobilin** which imparts the brown colour to normal faeces. Some urobilinogen is reabsorbed, passing to the liver in the portal blood, and is then re-excreted in the bile. The entire process is called an **enterohepatic circulation** (see Fig. 11.4). A small amount of urobilinogen escapes into the systemic circulation and is excreted in the urine.

Bile acids (**salts**) are synthesised in the liver from cholesterol-based precursors. These are excreted in bile to the duodenum and facilitate lipid digestion and absorption in the small intestine. About 95% of the bile acids are reabsorbed in the distal ileum and return to the liver via the portal vein, only to be re-excreted in the bile. Thus both bilirubin and bile acids are involved in enterohepatic circulations.

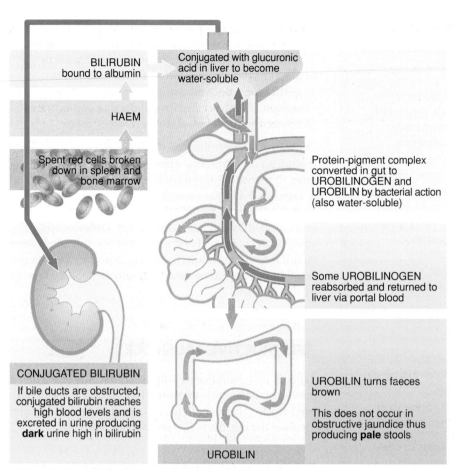

BILIRUBIN
bound to albumin

Conjugated with glucuronic
acid in liver to become
water-soluble

HAEM

Spent red cells broken
down in spleen and
bone marrow

Protein-pigment complex
converted in gut to
UROBILINOGEN and
UROBILIN by bacterial action
(also water-soluble)

Some UROBILINOGEN
reabsorbed and returned to
liver via portal blood

CONJUGATED BILIRUBIN

If bile ducts are obstructed,
conjugated bilirubin reaches
high blood levels and is
excreted in urine producing
dark urine high in bilirubin

UROBILIN turns faeces
brown

This does not occur in
obstructive jaundice thus
producing **pale** stools

UROBILIN

**Fig. 11.4 Normal dynamics of
bilirubin excretion and the effects
of obstructive jaundice**
Note that urobilinogen will appear in
substantial quantities in the urine if large
amounts are produced because of
haemolytic anaemia, or if there is liver cell
damage.

PATHOPHYSIOLOGY OF OBSTRUCTIVE JAUNDICE

If biliary outflow becomes obstructed, conjugated bilirubin is dammed back in the liver where it enters the bloodstream and causes a gradual rise in plasma bilirubin. Once the plasma bilirubin level exceeds about 30 μmol/L, jaundice should be clinically detectable. Above 60 μmol/L, jaundice is obvious. Conjugated bilirubin, being water-soluble, is excreted in the urine, turning it dark. The presence of bilirubin in the urine, together with an indication of its concentration, is easily established by ward dipstick testing. Significant quantities usually mean biliary obstruction.

In obstructive jaundice there is diminished or absent excretion of bile into the bowel, causing changes in the faeces. There is less urobilin to darken the stool and fewer bile acids, resulting in defective fat absorption. The two combine to give the stool a characteristic 'putty' colour.

A particular consequence of poor dietary fat absorption is malabsorption of vitamin K. This leads to decreased hepatic synthesis of clotting factors, notably prothrombin. Impairment of blood clotting is not so great as to cause spontaneous haemorrhage or bruising but there is a significant risk of haemorrhage during surgery or after liver biopsy. Thus the coagulation profile must be checked before any invasive procedure. The coagulopathy is corrected with parenteral vitamin K or, in the case of an urgent procedure, fresh, frozen plasma. Biliary obstruction also dams back bile acids, which raises their blood concentration leading to deposition in the skin; this in turn sometimes causes intense itching.

Blood tests in obstructive jaundice

Obstructive jaundice is manifest biochemically by an elevated level of plasma bilirubin, predominantly in the conjugated form. There is marked elevation of plasma alkaline phosphatase (liver isoenzyme) which is derived from bile canaliculi, but the transaminases, derived from hepatocytes, are usually only mildly elevated. When biliary obstruction is intrahepatic (e.g. cholangiocarcinoma obstructing only one duct) there may be a mixed biochemical picture with evidence of hepatocyte damage as well as duct obstruction. Liver function tests are, however, an unreliable guide and ultrasonography of the liver is mandatory.

HISTORY AND EXAMINATION OF PATIENTS WITH OBSTRUCTIVE JAUNDICE

History-taking should include enquiry about episodes of pain typical of gallstone disease, previous episodes of obstructive jaundice which resolved spontaneously, or previous biliary tract surgery. Attacks of acute pancreatitis also suggest gallstone disease. A history of anorexia, weight loss and non-specific upper gastrointestinal disturbances is common in carcinoma of the pancreas, a disease more common in the elderly. Inflammatory bowel disease predisposes to **sclerosing cholangitis** although this is relatively rare.

There are several notable points in the examination of the jaundiced patient. Early jaundice is a subtle physical sign and will be missed unless the patient is examined in a good light, preferably daylight. Jaundice is first detectable in the conjunctivae and soon afterwards in the skin of the abdominal wall. In some cases of obstructive jaundice, the patient develops generalised itching (pruritus) and scratch marks may be apparent. The general stigmata of liver disease, such as spider naevi and liver 'flap', are only found when jaundice is caused by primary liver disease rather than extrinsic obstruction.

The abdomen should be examined, particularly for ascites, an enlarged liver or spleen, abnormal masses or a palpable gall bladder. An enlarged liver may be caused by primary or secondary malignancy. Splenomegaly with hepatomegaly is an important sign of chronic parenchymal liver disease (usually cirrhosis) and indicates portal hypertension. Ascites in a patient with obstructive jaundice is almost always due to disseminated intra-abdominal malignancy.

Courvoisier's 'law' (see Fig. 11.5) was formulated in 1890 and states that obstructive jaundice in the presence of a palpable gall bladder is not due to stone (and is therefore likely to be caused by tumour). The argument is that gallstones cause chronic inflammation leading to fibrosis of the gall bladder which prevents its distension. An alternative explanation is that intermittent stone obstruction leads to thickening of the gall bladder wall which prevents distension. In malignancy, progressive obstruction occurs over a short period and the gall bladder distends easily.

Particular attention is paid to the colour of the stool found on rectal examination, as a pale stool is characteristic of obstructive jaundice. The urine should also be inspected. In obstructive jaundice, it is usually dark yellow or orange from the presence of conjugated bilirubin, and froths when shaken due to the detergent effect of bile acids.

Conditions causing obstructive jaundice are listed in Box 11.7.

APPROACH TO INVESTIGATION OF JAUNDICE

Jaundice is usually investigated step by step as follows:

- Exclude infective hepatitis by screening for hepatitis B and C (see Table 1.3, p. 21). Other antigen and antibody tests may be carried out if suspicion of infective hepatitis is high. A history of transfusion, intravenous drug abuse or travel may increase the likelihood of an infection
- Confirm that the jaundice is obstructive if possible by means of liver function tests (see Fig. 11.6) (although there are not completely reliable). Mild jaundice is commonly found in patients with Gilbert's syndrome, due to a mild congenital abnormality of haemoglobin metabolism with no serious significance. Obstructive jaundice is characterised by a predominance of conjugated bilirubin and a high alkaline phosphatase level (liver isoenzyme); transaminase levels are only moderately elevated
- Hepatobiliary ultrasonography is the simplest means of demonstrating dilated intrahepatic ducts (see Fig. 11.7), liver secondaries, a dilated extrahepatic biliary system or gall bladder abnormalities including stones. Ultrasound may reveal the cause of

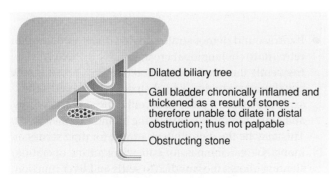

— Dilated biliary tree

— Gall bladder chronically inflamed and thickened as a result of stones - therefore unable to dilate in distal obstruction; thus not palpable

— Obstructing stone

Obstructive jaundice due to stone

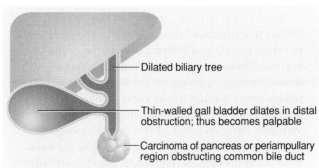

— Dilated biliary tree

— Thin-walled gall bladder dilates in distal obstruction; thus becomes palpable

— Carcinoma of pancreas or periampullary region obstructing common bile duct

Obstructive jaundice due to carcinoma

Fig. 11.5 Courvoisier's law

KEY POINTS

Box 11.7 Conditions causing obstructive jaundice

Stones in the common bile duct

- Very common
- Suggested by a history of pain typical of biliary colic. Jaundice may be progressive (if a stone is firmly impacted), fluctuant without ever disappearing altogether (if a stone alternately impacts and disimpacts), or intermittent (if multiple small stones successively impact then pass through the lower end of the common bile duct)

Carcinoma of the head of the pancreas

- Common
- Typically causes painless jaundice which is persistent or progressive. The gall bladder may be palpable (Courvoisier's law, see Fig. 11.5)

Acute or chronic pancreatitis

- Uncommon
- Common bile duct is obstructed

Mirizzi's syndrome

- Rare
- Chronic cholecystitis extending to involve the common bile duct

Periampullary tumours

- i.e. of ampulla, bile duct or duodenum (uncommon)
- Clinical features similar to carcinoma of head of pancreas

Benign strictures of the common bile duct

- May be due to surgical damage (fairly common) or previous stone (uncommon)
- Clinical features similar to carcinoma of head of pancreas

Other malignant tumours

- May cause bile duct obstruction above the ampulla, e.g. secondaries in the porta hepatis (fairly common), cholangiocarcinoma (uncommon), carcinoma of the gall bladder (rare)

Intrahepatic bile duct obstruction

- e.g. Cholangiocarcinoma, sclerosing cholangitis (rare)

Intrahepatic cholestasis

- Diagnosed when jaundice is obstructive but the duct system is normal
- Viral hepatitis is a common cause
- Systemic sepsis often causes low-grade jaundice (liver dysfunction)
- Idiosyncrasy to certain drugs (including chlorpromazine, oral contraceptives and chlorpropamide) interferes with bile excretion from hepatocytes, presumably by affecting membrane transport
- Hepatic lymphoma is another classic but rare cause of intrahepatic cholestasis

obstructive jaundice to be a tumour in the head of the pancreas or enlarged lymph nodes in the porta hepatis. Ultrasound, however, is unreliable for demonstrating pathology in the lower portion of the biliary tree; although it may show gallstones, it is unreliable for excluding them. In particular it may not visualise common bile duct stones or lesions in the head of the pancreas. CT scanning may be the next stage if the findings are equivocal. This is particularly useful for demonstrating primary or secondary tumours but may miss a small carcinoma at the lower end of the common bile duct

- If ultrasound demonstrates dilated ducts, endoscopic retrograde cholangiopancreatography (ERCP) is frequently the next investigation (see Fig. 11.8). It is now usual practice to drain an obstructed bile duct at the same procedure if practicable, either by sphincterotomy and stone removal or by placing an intraluminal **stent**. This may be the definitive treatment for duct stones or inoperable carcinomas; for patients requiring operation, stenting allows the jaundice to settle and liver function to improve. The role of non-therapeutic ERCP is gradually being supplanted by magnetic resonance cholangiopancreatography (MRCP).

Non-acute abdominal pain and other abdominal symptoms

SPECIMEN *Venous blood*		DATE TAKEN		Status Please Tick Box	Surname		Unit No.	
EXAMINATION REQ'D *LFTs*		LAB No		NHS	First Names		Date of Birth *9ᵗʰ Mar '13*	
CLINICAL DETAILS RELATING TO REQUEST *Obstructive Jaundice*				PRIVATE		M/F		
				OSV	Cons/GP		Ward/Dept/Research Code	
SIGNED				CAT 2				
					USE BALLPOINT PEN – PRINT FIRMLY			
Tot. Protein	**64** g/L	Na	mmol/L	Ca		mmol/L	Arterial [H⁺]	nmol/L
Albumin	**24** g/L	K	mmol/L	Phos		mmol/L	PCO₂	kPa
	40 g/L	HCO₃	mmol/L	Uric Acid		mmol/L	Std. HCO₃	mmol/L
Bili Tot	**206** μmol/L	Urea	mmol/L	Magnesium		mmol/L	Base Excess	mmol/L
Conj	**166** μmol/L	Creatinine	mmol/L	Iron		μmol/L	O₂ Sat.	%
Alk. Phos.	**1835** U/L	Glucose	mmol/L	IBC		μmol/L	PO₂	kPa
ALT	**188** U/L							
γGT	U/L							
CK	U/L							
HBD	U/L							
Cholesterol	mmol/L							
Triglyceride	mmol/L							
T₄	mmol/L							
FT₄	mmol/L							
FSH	mU/L	Signed	Reported		Received		**CHEM**	

Fig. 11.6 Typical liver function test result in obstructive jaundice

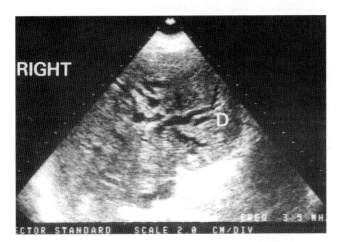

Fig. 11.7 Ultrasonogram showing dilated intrahepatic ducts
An ultrasound scan in an 80-year-old man with obstructive jaundice. This transverse section through the liver shows the characteristic 'double-barrel shotgun sign' **D**, with two parallel tubular structures representing major branches of the bile duct and portal vein. Normally, the portal vein is four times wider than the corresponding bile duct. Here they are the same diameter.

Alternatively, percutaneous Chiba needle ('skinny needle') transhepatic cholangiography can be performed. Both tests show the site and often the nature of an obstruction although the latter test is more invasive. If bile ducts are not dilated, liver biopsy or biopsy of demonstrated secondaries may be performed (with ultrasound or CT guidance). Because clotting is frequently abnormal, clotting studies must be performed before any invasive procedure. Abnormalities are corrected by giving daily vitamin K injections and if a clotting defect remains, infusing

fresh-frozen plasma before and during any invasive procedure. Laparoscopy may be used to visualise the liver directly and to obtain biopsy specimens from suspicious areas.

Occasionally, a firm diagnosis cannot be made before operation; abdominal exploration and frozen section histology may provide the answer. Laparotomy provides an opportunity for treatment at the same time.

PRINCIPLES OF MANAGEMENT OF OBSTRUCTIVE JAUNDICE

The primary aim of treatment is to relieve the obstruction of the biliary tract. Obstructed bile is often infected and a fulminant **acute cholangitis** can develop at any time. Back pressure interferes with other liver functions such as synthesis of albumin and clotting factors. Eventually structural liver damage ensues.

Three categories of obstruction may be defined according to surgical treatment options:

- Potentially curable obstructions
- Obstruction due to incurable tumour
- Terminal disease

Potentially curable obstructions

These include bile duct stones and strictures as well as small tumours of the lower bile ducts, duodenum or ampullary region (periampullary tumours) (see Fig. 11.9). If an operation is needed, it is better to relieve the jaundice beforehand and allow liver function to recover by stone removal or endoscopic placement of a tube

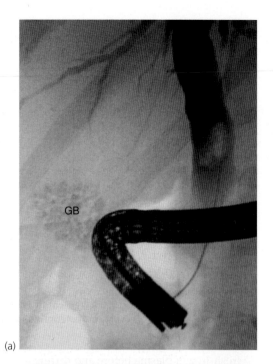

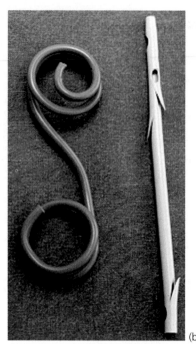

(a)

(b)

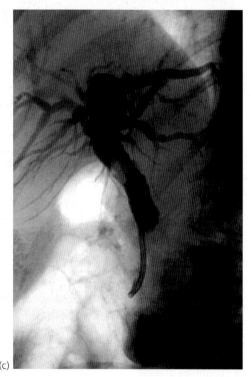

(c)

Fig. 11.8 Endoscopic stenting
(a) Diagnostic endoscopic retrograde cholangiogram (ERC) showing an enlarged common bile duct containing a single large stone. A collection of radiopaque gallstones is seen in the gall bladder **(GB)**. **(b)** Two types of biliary stent: the pigtail type on the left and the notched variety on the right, as used in this patient. **(c)** Despite endoscopic sphincterotomy, the bile duct stone could not be retrieved so a tubular self-retaining stent has been placed to relieve the obstructive jaundice. The stone was successfully removed endoscopically on a later occation.

within the bile duct. These tubes are known as **stents**, named after the inventor of earlier devices of this kind. Current large-bore duodenal endoscopes allow per-oral placement of stents up to 4 mm in diameter.

The number, size and position of **bile duct stones** may have been identified before operation by ERCP (or by percutaneous transhepatic cholangiography). Stones may be removed at ERCP by dividing the ampullary

sphincter using a 'bow-string' diathermy wire via the duodenal endoscope. Sometimes if the stone is very large or impacted the obstructed bile may be drained by placing a stent without stone removal.

Where it is available, sphincterotomy or stent placement is the initial treatment of choice for virtually all patients with common bile duct stones causing obstructive jaundice but particularly so for the following groups:

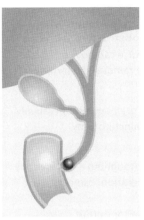
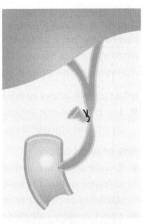

Stone in common bile duct

Benign stricture, e.g.
following trauma at
cholecystectomy

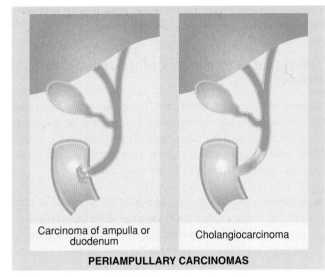

Carcinoma of ampulla or
duodenum

Cholangiocarcinoma

PERIAMPULLARY CARCINOMAS

Fig. 11.9 Some potentially curable causes of obstructive jaundice

- Acute cholangitis where it may represent an emergency
- Patients who have previously had a cholecystectomy
- If laparoscopic cholecystectomy is planned
- Debilitated elderly patients where laparotomy would be specially hazardous

If open cholecystectomy is the chosen treatment, bile duct stones can be identified by X-ray cholangiography performed during the operation (**peroperative cholangiography**) and removed surgically. This can also be achieved during laparoscopic cholecystectomy, but is less widely practised. Operative **choledochoscopy** is one technique where a flexible or rigid 'scope allows a visual check for completeness of stone removal.

Many surgeons undertaking laparoscopic cholecystectomy routinely perform operative cholangiography but only a small proportion undertake laparoscopic exploration of the common bile duct as this is a difficult and time-consuming procedure.

Bile duct strictures can be treated by long-term stenting. Strictures are usually due to post-surgical fibrotic scarring but occasionally result from inflammatory scarring due to cholecystitis with jaundice (**Mirizzi's syndrome**). The 'gold standard' for more severe strictures or for iatrogenic division or ligation of the common bile duct is surgical reconstruction of the bile ducts.

Small **tumours in the periampullary region** may be amenable to complete excision, thereby relieving biliary obstruction. A complete cure is often achieved. **Adenocarcinoma of the head of the pancreas** is a common cause of obstructive jaundice but the long-term prognosis is poor even after a successful radical pancreaticoduodenectomy (which itself has a high mortality rate). This may get better as specialist surgical centres improve preoperative staging and achieve better surgical out-

comes. At present, the trend is towards palliative treatment with stenting, together with gastro-jejunostomy if the duodenum becomes obstructed by invading tumour.

Obstruction due to incurable tumour

This commonly occurs in carcinoma of the head of the pancreas, less often with lymph node metastases in the porta hepatis and rarely from carcinoma of the gall bladder. Stenting is the palliative treatment of choice but if this proves impossible, various operations can bypass the obstruction by joining small bowel to the gall bladder or bile duct proximal to the obstruction or to dilated ducts within the liver. For carcinoma of the head of the pancreas **triple bypass** (see Ch. 17) is the classic palliative operation but stenting to provide internal biliary drainage has markedly reduced the need for this operation.

All these techniques merely overcome the problem of obstructive jaundice and have no influence on the course of the disease. Eventually and often within a few months, the patient succumbs to other manifestations of the cancer. Percutaneous **coeliac ganglion blockade** provides effective palliation for intractable pain.

Terminal disease

By the time obstructive jaundice has developed, some patients have reached a terminal stage of their cancer. In these cases, stenting may still be indicated but surgical interference may be difficult to justify; the aim should be to relieve distress and allow a dignified death. Some patients experience severe itching which may be lessened by drugs such as antihistamines or chlorpromazine. Oral

167

Section 3

cholestyramine is not indicated because it only removes bile salts which are able to reach the bowel.

SPECIAL RISKS OF SURGERY IN THE JAUNDICED PATIENT (see Box 11.8)

Despite the fact that most obstructive jaundice can now be relieved preoperatively by stone removal or stenting, surgery must still be performed in a jaundiced patient. This poses a greater risk from preoperative and post-operative surgical complications as follows:

- **Infection**. Obstructed bile is nearly always infected by aerobic gut organisms and surgical instrumentation may precipitate **ascending cholangitis**, if not already present, with the risk of sepsis syndrome and multiple organ dysfunction (see next bullet). Spillage of infected bile during operation causes peritoneal contamination and risks intraperitoneal or wound infection. Preoperative drainage of bile into the bowel by endoscopic sphincterotomy or stenting can prevent this. Prophylactic antibiotics against the usual gut flora should be used for the procedure
- **Endotoxaemia**. Endotoxins appear in the systemic circulation. These predispose to multiple organ dysfunction syndrome (MODS) by activating components of the inflammatory cascade and may precipitate a systemic inflammatory response. Renal function is particularly vulnerable if renal perfusion is already impaired. Renal failure following operation for obstructive jaundice is manifest as **hepatorenal syndrome**, but can occur in any patient with obstructive jaundice. Typical findings are oliguria and hyponatremia. Renal function can be protected by ensuring that the patient does not become dehydrated during any period of restriction of oral fluids. Intravenous fluids should be given overnight before an operation or procedure but may aggravate the hepatorenal syndrome. The patient should be catheterised and given prophylactic antibiotics
- **Hepatic impairment**. There is usually some degree of hepatic impairment due to biliary back pressure. This causes reduced hepatic metabolism of certain drugs and results in defective synthesis of clotting factors, even if vitamin K has been given. Patients with chronic parenchymal liver disease withstand the stresses of major abdominal surgery and anaesthesia poorly. Drugs excreted by the liver should be avoided
- **Malabsorption of fats**. Biliary obstruction leads to diminished absorption of fats, including vitamin K, a co-factor for prothrombin synthesis. This results in defective clotting. Parenteral vitamin K before operation usually improves the prothrombin ratio sufficiently to permit operation but needs to be given at least 24 hours beforehand. If this is not possible,

SUMMARY

Box 11.8 Special precautions to be taken when operating on a patient with obstructive jaundice

Note that most obstructive jaundice can now be relieved preoperatively by stone removal or stenting

Infected bile under pressure
- Use prophylactic antibiotics ± drainage preoperatively by endoscopic stenting or sphincterotomy

Risk of renal failure
- Ensure adequate hydration throughout—intravenous infusion overnight before operation, osmotic diuretics during operation
- Insert urinary catheter to monitor output

Impaired hepatic detoxification
- Give antibiotics to minimise endogenous endotoxin production
- Avoid drugs excreted by liver

Malabsorption of fat-soluble vitamins (causes impaired hepatic synthesis of clotting factors)
- Check clotting
- Give vitamin K intramuscularly for several days before operation

Thromboembolism
- Use prophylactic measures, e.g. low-dose subcutaneous heparin

fresh-frozen plasma is given perioperatively to correct the coagulopathy
- **Thromboembolism**. Paradoxically, considering the clotting deficiency, postoperative **deep vein thrombosis** is common in the jaundiced patient. Prophylactic measures should be taken to reduce this risk, e.g. low-dose subcutaneous heparin

ABDOMINAL MASS OR DISTENSION

An abdominal mass is sometimes discovered by the patient but more often on medical examination. An older patient with a definite palpable mass is likely to have a malignant tumour, but benign cysts, inflammatory masses, aneurysms or atypical hernias may be responsible. Occasionally masses have a 'medical' cause, e.g. hepatosplenomegaly of chronic lymphocytic leukaemia. Commonly, one of the 'five Fs'—fetus, faeces, flatus, fat or fluid—may masquerade as a 'surgical' mass or distension. These are common causes of embarrassment! An abdominal mass may be discovered without any related clinical features; usually however, the patient has gastrointestinal symptoms, anaemia or jaundice in addition. A careful history will often reveal useful clues as to the cause of the mass.

CLINICAL ASSESSMENT OF AN ABDOMINAL MASS

The location of the mass, its relations and mobility and its physical characteristics, such as size, shape and consistency, give valuable information about the organ of origin and the likely pathology. Incisional, umbilical and sometimes interstital (Spigelian) hernias (see Ch. 26, p. 348) may present as localised swellings but they usually shrink or reduce completely when the patient is supine or under anaesthesia. Unless the diagnosis of a hernia is considered, it may be overlooked. An incarcerated (irreducible but not obstructed) hernia is more appropriately considered a true 'mass'.

Mass in the right hypochondrium

A right hypochondrial mass is usually of hepatobiliary origin. If so, it will be continuous with the main bulk of the liver both to palpation and percussion. It will also descend on inspiration. The enlarging liver usually remains in contact with the anterior abdominal wall and is consequently dull to percussion. When the liver is diffusely enlarged, the inferior margin is regular and well defined and the consistency is usually normal. When infiltrated with primary or secondary cancer, the palpable liver may be hard and irregular or the liver may appear diffusely enlarged. Carcinoma of the gall bladder is indistinguishable from hepatic cancer on palpation. Rarely, a Riedel's lobe—a congenitally enlarged part of the right lobe—is mistaken for a pathological mass. Less commonly, a right hypochondrial mass is a diseased gall bladder. When a liver mass is suspected, other signs of liver disease should be sought. A mass continuous with the liver above and with a typical pear-shaped rounded outline is likely to be a mucocoele of the gall bladder. A more diffuse, tender mass may be an empyema of the gall bladder.

Epigastric mass

A mass in the epigastrium is usually due to a cancer of the stomach or transverse colon or sometimes omental secondaries from ovarian carcinoma (Fig. 11.10). Cancer involving the left lobe of the liver may also present in this way. These masses are usually hard and irregular and are mobile or fixed according to the degree of invasion. Occasionally an epigastric mass is an isolated enlargement of the left lobe of the liver or massive para-aortic lymph nodes due to lymphoma or testicular secondaries. A pulsatile epigastric mass is likely to be an abdominal aortic aneurysm.

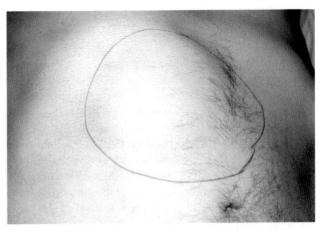

Fig. 11.10 Epigastric mass
This man of 44 presented having discovered an epigastric mass. It was asymptomatic. The margins of the mass are outlined on the skin. The mass moved downwards with respiration and proved to be a massive liver metastasis from a tiny pancreatic primary adenocarcinoma

Mass in the left hypochondrium

A cancer of the stomach or splenic flexure of the colon may present as a mass in the left hypochondrium. Tumour masses can usually be distinguished clinically from an enlarged spleen as the latter often has a discrete 'edge' and lies more posteriorly. The spleen also has a band of overlying resonance due to gas in bowel superficial to it. It is easier to palpate a spleen if the patient rolls towards the right side; the examiner then puts his or her left hand behind the patient's lower left ribs pulling the spleen towards the examining hand. The lower edge can be palpated when the organ moves downwards as the patient inspires. Note that a normal-sized spleen is rarely palpable.

Mass in the loin or flank

A mass in the loin or flank is likely to be of renal origin and can best be felt on **bimanual palpation**. This involves pushing the mass forward from behind with one hand so that it can be palpated anteriorly with the other. A renal mass will usually descend with inspiration since the kidneys lie just beneath the diaphragm. Very rarely, a hernia occurs in the lumbar region; this reduces spontaneously as the patient rolls over.

Mass in the left iliac fossa

Masses in the left iliac fossa usually arise from the sigmoid colon. A hard faecal mass may be mistaken for a cancer but it can often be indented like putty. A solid sigmoid mass is usually due to tumour or a complex diverticular inflammatory mass. Ovarian masses and sometimes eccentric bladder lesions may be palpable in either iliac fossa. These lesions, however, arise from out of the pelvis and can often be pushed up on to the abdominal examining hand by digital pressure in the rectum or vagina (bimanual palpation—most effectively performed under general anaesthesia). Note that a rectal examination is mandatory in a thorough abdominal examination.

Hernias in the groin are common (see Ch. 26) and may be chronically irreducible (incarcerated). Occasionally, an interstitial (Spigelian) hernia develops above the groin in either iliac fossa. This presents a somewhat confusing picture on examination by virtue of its site and because the peritoneal sac herniates between the muscle layers of the abdominal wall.

Suprapubic mass

Suprapubic masses usually arise from pelvic organs such as the bladder or uterus and its adnexae. A palpable bladder is most commonly due to chronic urinary retention and the patient should be catheterised and then examined again. A distended bladder is dull to percussion and disappears on catheterisation. Bladder enlargement is usually symmetrical and may extend above the umbilicus. The margins may be difficult to define accurately because of the bladder's soft consistency. Only massive bladder tumours are palpable and would be accompanied by urinary tract symptoms and urine abnormalities. Sometimes large bladder stones are palpable abdominally.

A uterus may be palpable abdominally when enlarged by pregnancy or fibroids. Bimanual examination involves digital examination of the vagina at the same time as palpation of the lower abdomen with the other hand. Ovarian tumours, particularly cysts, may become enormous and extend well up into the abdomen; again, bimanual examination (under general anaesthesia if necessary) helps to distinguish the origin.

Mass in the right iliac fossa

The right iliac fossa is a common site for an asymptomatic mass. It may be due to unresolved inflammation of the appendix which becomes surrounded by a mass of omentum and small bowel, giving rise to an 'appendix mass' (see Ch. 19). There is usually a recent history of right iliac fossa pain and fever. A carcinoma of the caecum may become very large without causing symptoms of obstruction because the caecum is large and distensible, and the faecal stream at this point is quite liquid. Thus, a caecal carcinoma often presents as an asymptomatic right iliac fossa mass; iron deficiency anaemia is often evident by this stage. Crohn's disease of the terminal ileum often presents with a tender mass, usually with typical symptoms of pain and diarrhoea.

Central abdominal mass

A central abdominal mass may originate in large or small bowel, as a result of malignant infiltration of the great omentum or from retroperitoneal structures such as lymph nodes, pancreas, connective tissues or the aorta. Retroperitoneal masses are only palpable if they are large. One of the most common central abdominal masses is an aneurysm of the abdominal aorta. Aneurysms usually arise just above the aortic bifurcation (at the umbilical level) which explains their central location in the upper part of the abdomen. The characteristic feature of an aneurysm is its **expansile pulsation**; other solid masses may transmit pulsation from large vessels nearby, but these masses are not expansile.

Several different types of hernia may present near the centre of the abdomen. Most common is an **incisional hernia** which protrudes through part or the whole of an abdominal wall incision. This may occur at any time after operation, from days to years later. It usually results from poor closure technique or postoperative infection. **Paraumbilical** or **umbilical hernias**, common in the obese, occur centrally and diagnosis is usually straightforward. **Divarication of the recti** (rectus abdominis muscles, not a true hernia) involves the recti being splayed apart, often as a result of pregnancy or obesity, leaving the central anterior abdominal wall devoid of muscular support. This condition is easily recognised because of its typical 'keel' shape and its symptomless nature; treatment is rarely necessary. Divarication and midline hernias can best be demonstrated when the abdominal muscles are contracted, e.g. the supine patient raises both heels from the bed.

Rectal mass and findings on rectal examination

Palpation of the normal rectum reveals the firm walls of the anal sphincter over the first 5 cm or so. Above that level, the rectal walls are soft and mobile. In the female, the uterine cervix is often felt anteriorly as a firm but localised mass. In the male, the normal prostate gland is felt near the tip of the finger anteriorly as a smooth, firm swelling about 2 cm in diameter with a midline groove between the lateral lobes. Enlargement of the prostate (usually benign) can be palpated, as can irregularity or nodularity which may represent carcinoma.

An abdominal or pelvic mass may be palpable solely on rectal (or vaginal) examination. The mass may be a rectal cancer or a cancer of the loop of sigmoid colon lying in the pelvic cavity; the latter is unlikely to be visible on sigmoidoscopy. Sometimes, secondary deposits from an impalpable tumour in the upper abdomen may seed the pelvic cavity. This may produce a palpable anterior lump known as **Blumer's shelf** or even a solid mass filling the pelvic cavity. The latter condition is known as a **frozen pelvis**. Frozen pelvis can also occur with endometriosis or local spread of a carcinoma of cervix or, rarely, prostate.

DIFFUSE ABDOMINAL DISTENSION

Diffuse distension of the abdomen is a separate problem from a solid but discrete abdominal mass.

Widespread peritoneal involvement with tumour secondaries may cause abdominal distension, particularly if there is also an accumulation of fluid (**ascites**). It is often difficult to recognise on abdominal examination but should be suspected if the patient has other symptoms suggestive of malignancy such as anorexia or marked weight loss. Typically there is a history of gastrointestinal or ovarian carcinoma, and a surgical scar may be obvious. Abdominal tuberculosis is an uncommon cause in developed countries but is common in the developing world.

Gas within the bowel is a common cause for long-standing and often intermittent abdominal distension. It usually occurs in healthy young adults, particularly women, in association with irritable bowel syndrome or air swallowing during hyperventilation. Women of reproductive age often complain of abdominal distension in the premenstrual phase which may be due to fluid retention. Chronic gaseous abdominal distension may also be found in elderly patients with partial volvulus of the sigmoid colon. A detailed history and examination will usually diagnose these problems and avoid unnecessary investigation.

Abdominal wall and intraperitoneal fat may give the impression of diffuse abdominal distension, especially if the patient has a lumbar lordosis. In the middle-aged and elderly, more sinister conditions should be excluded before fat is blamed. Gross faecal loading may also be responsible for diffuse abdominal distension. This is often seen in children with abdominal pain and sometimes in young adults with irritable bowel syndrome. Asymptomatic chronic constipation is very common in the elderly but if it becomes symptomatic with distension and pain it can also represent incomplete bowel obstruction due to diverticular disease or cancer. A faecal mass palpable through the thin abdominal wall of an elderly patient can give the impression of a sinister mass. This commonly leads to fruitless but unavoidable investigations.

ASCITES

Ascites is defined as a chronic accumulation of fluid within the abdominal cavity and has many causes, both malignant and non-malignant.

Sometimes in ovarian or colonic cancer, the peritoneum is seeded with tumour deposits which secrete a protein-rich fluid containing malignant cells. This **malignant ascites** may reach a volume of several litres. The peritoneum may be peppered with thousands of minute seedlings without a palpable mass or there may be several large masses hidden by the ascitic fluid. A rare cause of ascites is massive obstruction of abdominal lymphatic drainage. This is usually caused by malignant involvement of para-aortic lymph nodes with lymphoma or metastatic testicular malignancy. **Chylous ascites**, in which the ascitic fluid is milky-white, is rare and is due to proximal lymphatic obstruction and the presence of chylomicrons in the fluid originating from mesenteric lymphatics.

Ascites may also be caused by gross congestive cardiac failure, constrictive pericarditis, severe hypoalbuminaemia or portal venous obstruction, the last occurring in cirrhosis and occasionally with liver metastases. **Tuberculosis** can occasionally present as ascites; this form of tuberculosis is characterised by multiple tiny peritoneal tubercles, clinically indistinguishable from tumour secondaries. Tuberculosis must be considered in this situation and biopsies taken because the condition is usually curable, unlike its malignant counterpart.

Ascites can usually be recognised only when the volume exceeds 2 litres, but even then it is easily overlooked. Dullness to percussion in the flanks and suprapubic region with central resonance is suspicious of ascites and should be followed by an attempt to elicit a fluid thrill or 'shifting dullness' (see Fig. 11.11).

APPROACH TO INVESTIGATION OF AN ABDOMINAL MASS OR DISTENSION

History and examination

A thorough history will probably provide clues to the specific organ system involved. A history of intra-abdominal malignancy years before should be regarded with grave suspicion. The disease may have recurred or a new primary developed. This is especially common in large bowel cancer but uncommon once 5 years have elapsed since treatment.

General examination should seek systemic signs of disease (e.g. cachexia, anaemia and jaundice) or signs of malignant dissemination (e.g. supraclavicular lymphadenopathy in suspected stomach cancer). Abdominal and pelvic examination must be thorough and, if appropriate, proctoscopy and sigmoidoscopy should be performed.

Laboratory tests

Blood, urine and stool investigations will be performed as suggested by the history and examination, e.g. full blood count, function tests, dipstick urinalysis and faecal occult bloods.

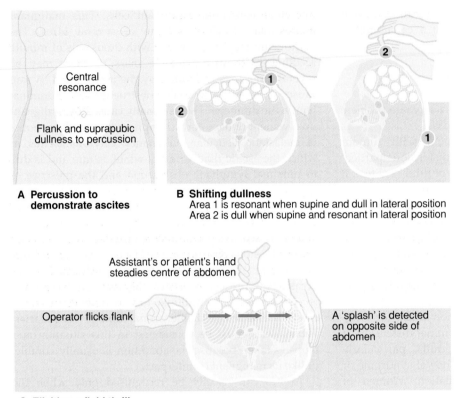

A **Percussion to demonstrate ascites**

B **Shifting dullness**
Area 1 is resonant when supine and dull in lateral position
Area 2 is dull when supine and resonant in lateral position

C **Eliciting a fluid thrill**

Fig. 11.11 Clinical signs of ascites

Radiology

A chest X-ray should be performed if malignancy is suspected. Ultrasonography or CT scanning (see Fig. 11.13) is useful for demonstrating the size and origin of a mass and one or other is often the first choice if pathology is suspected in the liver, biliary tree, pancreas, aorta or pelvic organs, or to confirm ascites. For pelvic masses, ultrasound is usually the investigation of first choice. CT scanning is most valuable in defining masses in the retroperitoneal area, e.g. pancreas, aorta or kidneys, but may be the investigation of choice for suspected large bowel cancer in frail patients. Ultrasound or CT scanning can be used to guide needle biopsy or aspiration cytology precisely and may avoid the need for a diagnostic laparotomy. Finally, contrast studies, e.g. barium meal, barium enema or intravenous urogram, may be indicated.

Endoscopy

Flexible endoscopic techniques such as gastroscopy or colonoscopy enable direct examination and biopsy of many gastrointestinal lesions. ERCP may be used to inject contrast material into the biliary and pancreatic duct systems if appropriate.

Other methods of tissue diagnosis

A tissue diagnosis should be obtained even if disseminated malignancy seems obvious. It can influence palliative and supportive treatment and, occasionally, an apparently hopeless case proves on histology to be treatable or even curable. Examples are tuberculosis, lymphoma or a germ cell tumour such as teratoma. Techniques of obtaining tissue for histology include needle or excision biopsy of enlarged cervical lymph nodes, and percutaneous biopsy of liver or an intra-abdominal mass (which may be guided by ultrasound or CT). Paracentesis abdominis (i.e. needle aspiration of ascitic fluid) is a safe and simple way of obtaining a specimen for cytology and micro-biology. Finally, when less invasive methods have failed to provide the necessary information, direct biopsy of tumour at diagnostic laparoscopy or open operation usually provides the definitive diagnosis.

Examination under anaesthesia, laparoscopy and exploratory laparotomy

Examination under anaesthesia (EUA) is sometimes necessary for estimating the mobility and spread of pelvic tumours. General anaesthesia with a muscle relaxant

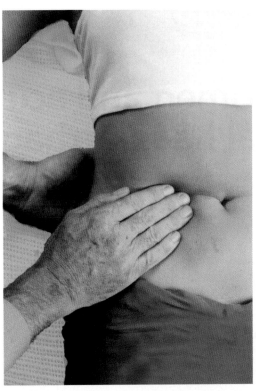

Fig. 11.12 Bimanual palpation of the abdomen
The posterior hand pushes forwards so that an enlarged viscus
(usually retroperitoneal e.g. kidney) or a mobile intra-abdominal mass
is pushed onto the anterior examining hand. Note that this is not
ballottment which involves short sharp palpation anteriorly thus
displacing ascites enabling a mass to bounce onto the examining hand.

allows thorough abdominal palpation and bimanual examination of the pelvis via rectum and vagina and the taking of biopsies. This may not be possible without anaesthesia because of tenderness or abdominal wall muscle tone. EUA is often combined with cystoscopy or other rigid endoscopies. Laparoscopy, widely used in gynaecology, is now a widely available diagnostic and therapeutic tool in general surgery. It allows direct inspection and biopsy of masses and visualisation of the extent of local spread governing resectability, as well as allowing a search for intra-abdominal metastases. Samples can be taken for cytology to demonstrate intraperitoneal spread. Special ultrasound probes may be applied directly to the liver and other organs where lesions are suspected which are too small to be detected by standard non-invasive ultrasonography. Diagnostic laparotomy, often necessary before the advent of modern imaging techniques, is now required only when less invasive procedures have failed to provide a clear diagnosis or when treatment to relieve symptoms such as bowel obstruction is urgently required.

(a)
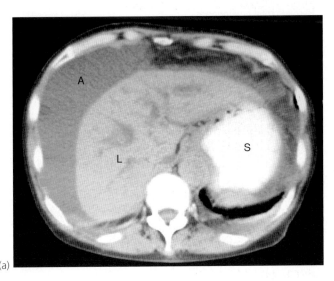

(b)
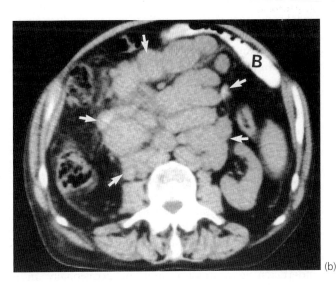

Fig. 11.13 CT scans showing gross ascites and enlarged lymph nodes
In **(a)** note the darker grey homogeneous shadow of fluid **A** around the liver **L** and the contrast in the stomach **S**. **(b)** Retroperitoneal mass of
lymph nodes due to lymphoma. This CT scan was taken to assess the stage of spread of a known lymphoma. This 40-year-old woman presented
with a large rubbery lymph node mass in her neck and was also found to have a large central abdominal mass. Abdominal CT scanning showed
an enormous mass of lymph nodes (arrowed). Small bowel **B** is seen anteriorly, enhanced by orally administered contrast material.

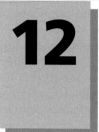

12 The acute abdomen and acute gastrointestinal haemorrhage

INTRODUCTION

The term **acute abdomen** is widely understood but is difficult to define precisely. Typically, the symptoms are of acute onset and strongly suggest an abdominal cause; abdominal pain is almost always a prominent feature. The illness is of such severity that admission to hospital appears necessary and operative surgery is a likely outcome. Many of the disorders causing an 'acute abdomen' are serious and potentially life-threatening unless treated promptly. On the other hand, simple and relatively trivial conditions such as constipation can produce acute and severe symptoms. These lesser diagnoses may only become apparent after a period of observation or after special investigations.

By the time of hospital admission, a patient with an 'acute abdomen' may have been managed conservatively at home for a day or two, during which the symptoms have either failed to settle or become progressively worse.

Major gastrointestinal haemorrhage is also a common reason for acute surgical referral, and is manifest by vomiting of blood (**haematemesis**) or rectal bleeding or passage of **melaena**. Many such patients are initially referred to a general (internal) physician or gastroenterologist, especially if the presumptive diagnosis is bleeding from a peptic ulcer or due to oesophageal varices. Management is usually conservative and may be undertaken in a medical unit, or occasionally in a combined gastroenterology/surgery unit.

Acute surgical emergencies constitute about 50% of all general surgical admissions (see Table 12.1). About half of these are for abdominal symptoms, predominantly pain, and half of this group resolve without operation. The rest undergo emergency surgery (e.g. for ruptured abdominal aortic aneurysm) or a scheduled surgical

Table 12.1 Composition of acute general surgical admissions in a typical district general hospital*

Reason for admission	Percentage of admissions
Non-specific abdominal pain, resolving without surgery	25%
Acute appendicitis	12%
Acute abdomen due to other causes	12%
Head injuries	20%
Abscesses	10%
Arterial emergencies	5%
Urological emergencies	5%
Hernia/scrotal emergencies	5%
Gastrointestinal haemorrhage	3%
Soft tissue wounds	2%
Burns	1%

*Without a separate head injury or urological emergency service

procedure during the same admission (e.g. cholecystectomy on the next available operating list), or are booked to have an operation later (e.g. interval appendicectomy for resolving appendix mass).

The common abdominal causes for emergency admission are summarised in Box 12.1. The list is not meant to be exhaustive and excludes obscure medical causes like acute intermittent porphyria or tabes dorsalis, as well as conditions mainly confined to infants and children (see Ch. 44).

BASIC PRINCIPLES OF MANAGING THE ACUTE ABDOMEN

In managing the acute abdomen, the first goal is to make a broad diagnosis which will help to decide whether an operation is necessary and how urgently it is required. Further detailed diagnostic information is obtained if possible, but the procedure performed often depends on what is found when the abdomen is opened.

Firstly, the basic pathophysiological phenomenon responsible for the patient's clinical state should be identified. Does the clinical picture suggest intestinal obstruction, bowel strangulation, peritonitis, intra-abdominal abscess, intra-abdominal bleeding or acute bowel ischaemia, or is it obviously gastrointestinal haemorrhage? More than one of these phenomena may occur at once. For example, strangulation is usually associated with signs of obstruction. Each of the main phenomena is described in detail in the following sections.

Once the main process has been diagnosed, a set of working probabilities as to the underlying cause can be put together from the clinical evidence.

Before operation, it is vital to **resuscitate** the patient and also to obtain basic haematological and biochemical measurements and to assess cardiorespiratory function.

INTESTINAL OBSTRUCTION

PATHOPHYSIOLOGY OF INTESTINAL OBSTRUCTION

Any part of the gastrointestinal tract may become obstructed and present as an acute abdomen. The causes are many and varied, as outlined in Box 12.2.

Obstruction leads to dilatation of bowel proximally and disrupts peristalsis. The manner of presentation depends on the level of obstruction within the gastrointestinal tract (i.e. stomach, proximal or distal small bowel or large bowel) and on the completeness of obstruction. The most acute presentation is upper small bowel obstruction which manifests within hours of onset. This is because the large volume of gastric and pancreaticobiliary secretions is prevented from moving

---

KEY POINTS

Box 12.1 Common causes of acute abdominal emergencies in adults

- **Non-specific abdominal pain which resolves without operation**
- **Acute appendicitis**
- **Acute biliary tract disorders—biliary colic, cholecystitis, occasionally ascending cholangitis**
- **Acute pancreatitis**
- **Acute manifestations of peptic ulcer disease— severe exacerbations of pain, haemorrhage, perforation, pyloric stenosis**
- **Acute diverticular disease—acute inflammation, abscess, haemorrhage, perforation, large bowel obstruction**
- **Strangulated hernias and other small bowel obstructions, e.g. bands or adhesions**
- **Colorectal carcinoma—large bowel obstruction, perforation**
- **Constipation**
- **Sigmoid volvulus**
- **Urinary tract infections**
- **Ureteric colic**
- **Acute urinary retention**
- **Leaking or ruptured abdominal aortic aneurysm**
- **Mesenteric arterial occlusion causing bowel ischaemia**
- **Abdominal trauma causing bleeding or perforation**
- **Gynaecological emergencies—ruptured ectopic pregnancy, torsion or bleeding of ovarian cyst, acute salpingitis**

KEY POINTS

Box 12.2 Mechanical causes of bowel obstruction

Adhesions or bands
- Resulting from previous surgery or intraperitoneal infection (rarely congenital bands)

Strangulated external hernias
- e.g. Femoral or inguinal hernias

Tumours
- e.g. Colonic carcinoma (particularly left-sided), gastric carcinoma near the pylorus, and tumours of small bowel (rare)

Volvulus of small bowel or large bowel
- A mobile or distended loop of bowel rotates causing obstruction at its neck

Inflammatory strictures
- e.g. Diverticular disease, Crohn's disease—obstruction usually incomplete

Bolus obstruction
- e.g. Impacted faeces (common), foreign bodies or solitary gallstones (rare), phytobezoar, i.e. a mass of impacted vegetable matter such as orange pith (very rare except after partial gastrectomy), trichobezoar (rare and found only in disturbed people who eat their own hair over a long period)

Internal hernias
- Causing bowel obstruction

Intussusception
- i.e. A segment of bowel becomes telescoped into the segment distal to it. Usually initiated by a mass in the bowel wall (e.g. enlargement of lymphatic tissue or tumour) which is dragged along by peristalsis; rare in adults but common in children

onwards, regurgitates into the stomach and is vomited. In contrast, distal large bowel obstruction is often much more chronic and may be present for a day or two before the patient seeks treatment.

SYMPTOMS OF INTESTINAL OBSTRUCTION

Symptoms and physical signs are summarised in Box 12.3, p. 180.

Vomiting

Obstruction of the bowel eventually leads to vomiting. The more proximal the obstruction, the earlier it develops. Vomiting can occur even if nothing is taken by mouth because saliva and other gastrointestinal secretions continue to be produced and enter the stomach. At least 10 litres of fluid are secreted into the gastrointestinal tract each day. The nature of the vomitus gives important clues to the level of obstruction. For example, vomiting of semi-digested food eaten a day or two previously strongly suggests gastric outlet obstruction, particularly if there is no bile present. Copious vomiting of bile-stained fluid suggests upper small bowel obstruction. If vomitus is thicker and foul-smelling (**faeculent**), a more distal obstruction is likely. This change to faeculent vomiting usually takes place gradually after about 24 hours of complete obstruction and is often an indication for urgent operation. The term faeculent vomiting is something of a misnomer as it comprises putrefying altered small bowel contents rather than faeces.

Pain

Fluid and swallowed air proximal to an obstruction, together with continuing peristalsis, cause pain. The general area of the pain gives a clue to the embryological origin of the affected bowel: upper, middle or lower abdominal pain originates in foregut, midgut or hindgut respectively. In obstruction, pain is not usually the most prominent symptom; it is of variable intensity, often quite mild, and usually colicky as peristalsis attempts to overcome the obstruction. In the small bowel, peristaltic action often increases for 24–48 hours and often fades after that.

Constipation

Distal to the obstruction, bowel gas is absorbed and propulsion of bowel contents is arrested. The resulting **absolute constipation** or **obstipation**, i.e. neither faeces nor flatus are passed rectally, is pathognomonic of bowel obstruction. The longer the duration of obstipation, the more important it becomes in the diagnosis of obstruction.

Effects of the competence of the ileocaecal valve

Symptoms develop more gradually in large bowel obstruction because of the large capacity of the colon and caecum and their absorptive activity. If the ileocaecal valve remains competent, backward flow of accumulating bowel contents is prevented; the thin-walled caecum progressively distends with swallowed air and eventually ruptures. The ileocaecal valve becomes incompetent in about half of large bowel obstructions, and this allows the small bowel to distend, delaying the onset of symptoms. If the ileocaecal valve remains competent, operation is clearly more urgent.

Incomplete obstruction

If the bowel is only partially obstructed, the clinical features are less clearly defined. Vomiting may be intermittent and bowel habit erratic. Chronic incomplete obstruction leads to gradual hypertrophy of the muscle of the bowel wall proximally. Peristaltic activity in this hypertrophic muscle is responsible for the bouts of colicky pain which are more prominent than those found in complete obstruction. The pain is often accompanied by **visible peristalsis**, which is the hallmark of incomplete obstruction. The most common cause is a slowly progressive obstructing colonic cancer. Note that incomplete obstruction should not be called subacute obstruction as the term is misleading.

PHYSICAL SIGNS OF INTESTINAL OBSTRUCTION

Vomiting, diminished fluid intake and sequestration of fluid in the small bowel commonly lead to **dehydration**. This is manifest clinically by extreme dryness of the mouth and characteristic loss of skin turgor and elasticity. Gas-filled loops of bowel proximal to the obstruction produce gaseous **abdominal distension**; the more distal the obstruction, the greater the distension. Episodes of **visible peristalsis** may be observed in thin patients in whom the obstruction is incomplete and of long duration. General examination may reveal signs of anaemia or lymphadenopathy attributable to the primary disorder.

The most striking feature on abdominal palpation is the lack of tenderness; the exception is when strangulation has occurred. Obstruction with tenderness must be diagnosed as strangulation, necessitating urgent operation after fluid resuscitation. An obstructing abdominal mass may be palpable if large. The groins must always be examined for hernias. An obstructed femoral hernia rarely causes local symptoms but instead produces symptoms and signs of small bowel obstruction. A strangulated femoral hernia is often no bigger than a large grape and is rarely red or tender; consequently, it is easily missed if not specifically sought. This is a clinical point of particular importance—an obstruction due to an irreducible hernia will not settle with the usual conservative treatment.

On percussion, the centre of the abdomen tends to be resonant and the periphery dull because bowel gas rises to the most elevated point; this may be difficult to distinguish from ascites.

Bowel sounds in obstruction are traditionally described as being loud and frequent, high-pitched and tinkling; nevertheless, in practice, obstructed bowel sounds may or may not be increased. They have an echoing, cavernous quality or can sound like the gentle lapping of water against a boat. This is due to fluid sloshing about in distended, gas-filled loops of bowel. A **succussion splash**, heard on gently shaking the patient's abdomen from side to side may add weight to the clinical diagnosis of obstruction.

INVESTIGATION OF SUSPECTED BOWEL OBSTRUCTION

The most useful investigation is a plain abdominal X-ray (see Fig.12.1). This is usually performed in both erect and supine positions, although the need for an erect film is doubted by some radiologists and clinicians. Bowel proximal to the obstruction is distended by gas. Bowel gas is absent beyond the obstruction but some rectal gas may be seen if a digital examination has been performed. The pattern and distribution of gas often indicates the approximate site of obstruction. Fluid levels may be seen in small bowel obstruction on an erect film. In some atypical cases, a small bowel series using orally administered water-soluble contrast may show a clearly defined obstruction. It will seldom diagnose the cause, but may demonstrate that the patient is obstructed.

When large bowel obstruction occurs at any point distal to the caecum and the ileocaecal valve remains competent, the caecum and ascending colon, being less muscular, take the brunt of the distension. When the radiological diameter of the caecum reaches 12 cm, it is considered to be in imminent danger of rupture, and therefore needs urgent operation. In large bowel obstruction of less acute onset, an unprepared barium enema is helpful to demonstrate the site and nature of the obstruction (including sigmoid volvulus) and to distinguish mechanical obstruction from pseudo-obstruction (see below).

ADYNAMIC BOWEL OBSTRUCTION

Temporary disruption of normal peristaltic activity without mechanical blockage causes adynamic bowel obstruction. Most commonly it occurs after abdominal surgery in which the bowel has been handled. Small bowel is particularly susceptible and the condition is known as **ileus** or **paralytic ileus**. Normal **postoperative ileus** should not persist for more than about 4 days. It is one of the reasons why fluids and solids are usually introduced gradually after abdominal surgery. Persisting postoperative 'ileus' is usually due to a complication of surgery such as anastomotic leakage or an intra-abdominal abscess, both of which have adverse local effects upon bowel wall function.

Occasionally, electrolyte disturbances like hypokalaemia or the use of anti-Parkinsonian drugs are responsible for adynamic obstruction. The condition is also common in patients admitted to intensive care, particularly the multiply-injured.

Pseudo-obstruction of the colon

A form of adynamic obstruction peculiar to the large bowel is called **pseudo-obstruction**, and is caused by a wide range of apparently unrelated conditions which compromise bowel peristalsis. These include retroperitoneal inflammation or haemorrhage, neurological illnesses, certain drugs (e.g. anticholinergics), pregnancy, orthopaedic injuries and surgery, particularly in the elderly, and prolonged recumbency.

Physical signs are similar to those of mechanical obstruction except that bowel sounds are not of the obstructed type or may be inaudible. The diagnosis of pseudo-obstruction is based on the clinical findings and confirmed if no mechanical obstruction is found on 'instant', i.e. unprepared, barium enema.

PRINCIPLES OF MANAGEMENT OF INTESTINAL OBSTRUCTION

Once intestinal obstruction has been recognised and the approximate level of obstruction identified, management proceeds as follows:

- Resuscitation is an essential first step (see Ch. 2, p. 29). Oral intake is discontinued and intravenous fluids are given, the volume and type of fluid depending on the state of hydration, the duration of the obstruction and serum electrolyte abnormalities. After prolonged vomiting, patients may be seriously depleted of fluid and electrolytes
- If the patient is vomiting or there is marked small bowel dilatation, a nasogastric tube is passed and the gastric contents are aspirated. This will control nausea and vomiting, remove swallowed air and reduce gaseous distension. Most importantly, it will minimise the risk of inhalation of gastric contents, particularly during induction of general anaesthesia
- At least two-thirds of uncomplicated cases of obstruction are due to adhesions and will usually

resolve with conservative measures. Those that resolve will not usually require operation later

- Large bowel obstruction due to faecal impaction can be relieved by enemas or manual removal of faeces
- Adynamic bowel obstruction in most cases eventually resolves with conservative measures and removal of any precipitating cause. Neostigmine is the treatment of choice for those failing to respond to conservative measures
- Operation may be required to relieve the obstruction. Provided strangulation can be excluded and the caecum is not dangerously distended, operation can safely be deferred for a day or two. Nevertheless, few obstructions that have not settled with 48 hours of adequate conservative treatment will resolve without intervention. This interval gives time for the patient to

be resuscitated and for any desirable investigations. The obstruction may settle during this period of conservative management, particularly if caused by adhesions from previous surgery

- At operation the cause of the obstruction is confirmed and dealt with appropriately (see Fig. 12.2)

BOWEL STRANGULATION

PATHOPHYSIOLOGY OF BOWEL STRANGULATION

Strangulation occurs when a segment of bowel becomes trapped so that its lumen becomes obstructed and its blood supply compromised. If unrelieved, this progresses to **infarction** and eventually perforation. Strangulation can occur when there is an external hernia, when loops

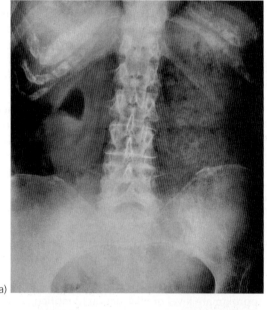

(a)

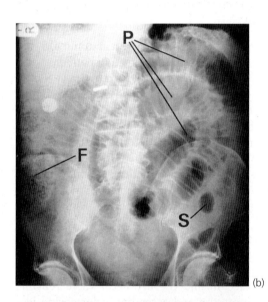

(b)

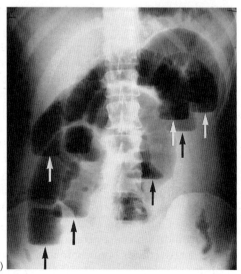

(c)

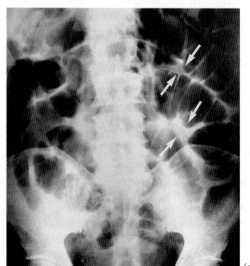

(d)

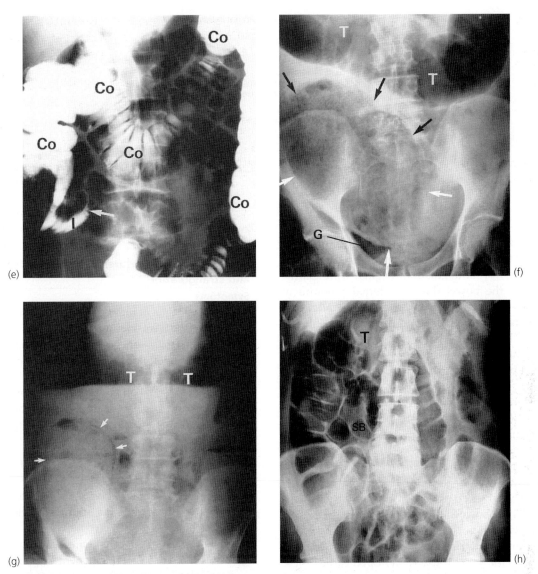

Fig. 12.1 Radiological appearances of obstructed bowel

(a) Plain abdominal film showing gastric outlet obstruction. The stomach is grossly distended with food, giving a typical mottled appearance over the whole left side of the abdomen. Bowel gas distal to the obstruction has been absorbed or expelled and so the rest of the abdomen is relatively gas-free. **(b)** Supine abdominal film showing mid small bowel obstruction. Dilated small bowel fills the upper left quadrant and centre of the abdomen, and can be identified by the plicae circulares (valvulae conniventes) **P** which extend across the whole width of the lumen. Distal small bowel is collapsed and is not seen on this film. The large bowel is also collapsed distal to the obstruction, with only a small amount of gas seen in the sigmoid colon **S**; there is faecal loading of the ascending colon **F**. Note also the metallic tip of the nasogastric tube and the incidental radiopaque gallstone. **(c)** Erect film from the same patient as in (b), showing multiple loops of dilated small bowel and multiple fluid levels (arrowed). **(d)** Supine abdominal X-ray in a middle-aged man with several days of small bowel obstruction due to adhesions. The abdomen is filled with grossly dilated small bowel loops. In addition, the small bowel wall is thickened, as shown by the apparent space between loops of bowel (arrowed); this is a characteristic feature of prolonged obstruction. **(e)** 'Instant' barium enema on the same patient as (d), showing contrast filling the normal colon **Co** and distal ileum **I** which abruptly terminates at the obstruction (arrowed). **(f)** Supine film showing gross caecal dilatation (outline arrowed) with loss of haustration. It can be deduced that the colon is obstructed near the splenic flexure because the transverse colon **T** is also dilated with gas whilst there is complete absence of colonic gas down the left side of the abdomen in the position of the descending and sigmoid colon. Gross caecal dilatation occurs in large bowel obstruction when the ileocaecal valve remains competent. In this patient, the caecum has perforated, as shown by the presence of gas **G** in the extra-peritoneal tissues. **(g)** Erect film of the same patient as in (f) showing gas in the caecal wall (arrowed); this indicates necrosis. Note also the long fluid level in the transverse colon **T**. This patient was an elderly man with an obstructing carcinoma at the splenic flexure. **(h)** Plain supine abdominal X-ray of another elderly man, also with an obstructing carcinoma at the splenic flexure. In this patient, the ileocaecal valve has become incompetent. Note the dilated transverse colon **T** and the multiple dilated loops of small bowel **SB** in the centre of the abdomen.

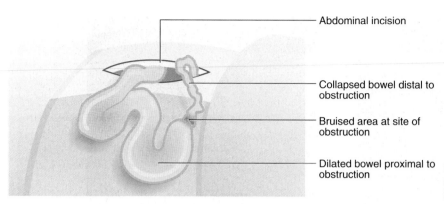

Abdominal incision

Collapsed bowel distal to
obstruction

Bruised area at site of
obstruction

Dilated bowel proximal to
obstruction

**Fig. 12.2 Findings at operation for
simple band obstruction of small
bowel**

of bowel become trapped within the abdominal cavity or when there is mass rotation of bowel (**volvulus**).

The process of strangulation begins with partial obstruction of the bowel due to external pressure or twisting. This leads to oedema of the bowel wall which aggravates the obstruction; venous return is initially obstructed. The closed loop of bowel becomes progressively dilated by gas from fermentation. The combination of gas pressure and venous back pressure progressively inhibits arterial inflow, causing ischaemia and then infarction.

Strangulation most commonly occurs when small bowel is caught within a hernia (inguinal, femoral, umbilical or incisional). The bowel undergoes necrosis and soon perforates within the hernial sac; this may be contained initially but generalised peritonitis usually ensues. Clinically, the patient first develops symptoms and signs of small bowel obstruction. A newly irreducible hernia can usually be found and this is likely to be tender and inflamed. However, a strangulated femoral hernia is a trap for the unwary. As indicated earlier, these are often deceptively small and non-tender and will be missed unless the groins are carefully examined.

Bowel may also become strangulated within the abdominal cavity if a loop becomes trapped by fibrous bands or adhesions or passes through an omental or mesenteric defect. Similarly, strangulation occurs if a large loop of bowel becomes twisted several times on its mesentery, a condition known as volvulus (see Ch. 22). Small bowel volvulus is rare but the sigmoid colon (or sometimes the caecum) is particularly susceptible to volvulus should it become excessively distended; this is most commonly seen in elderly patients with chronic constipation and in countries where the staple diet is extremely high in fibre.

SYMPTOMS AND SIGNS OF BOWEL STRANGULATION

Intra-abdominal strangulation causes the usual symptoms and signs of bowel obstruction (see Box 12.3) but these are accompanied by **abdominal tenderness** which is not

SUMMARY

**Box 12.3 Clinical features of bowel obstruction
and strangulation**

Symptoms
● Vomiting—time of onset and nature of the vomitus suggests the level of obstruction
● Abdominal pain—usually colicky in character, often mild in uncomplicated obstruction and more severe in strangulation
● Absolute constipation or obstipation (i.e. no flatus or faeces passed rectally)—pathognomonic of complete obstruction (but not present in partial obstruction)

Physical signs
● Dehydration—caused by vomiting, lack of fluid intake and fluid sequestration
● Abdominal distension—due to gas-filled loops of bowel. The more distal the obstruction, the greater the distension
● Visible peristalsis—uncommon finding; usually encountered in a very thin patient with prolonged distal small bowel obstruction which is incomplete
● Central resonance to percussion with dullness in the flanks—gas within dilated bowel loops rising to the uppermost point in the abdomen
● Abdominal tenderness—important feature distinguishing bowel strangulation from uncomplicated obstruction
● Abnormal bowel sounds—exaggerated, lapping, sloshing, perhaps high-pitched or tinkling. Bowel sounds are absent or normal in adynamic obstruction

a feature of uncomplicated bowel obstruction. The tenderness is probably due to distension of the closed loop. When compared with those with uncomplicated obstruction, patients with strangulation are systemically more unwell with a tachycardia and a leucocytosis. Pain increases over time and the pulse progressively rises. At this point, conservative treatment must be abandoned.

PRINCIPLES OF MANAGEMENT OF SUSPECTED BOWEL STRANGULATION

When strangulation is diagnosed or even suspected, operation must be performed urgently (after rapid fluid resuscitation) to try to prevent infarction and perforation (see Fig. 12.3). The patient is otherwise managed as for uncomplicated obstruction. Specific investigations are limited to plain abdominal X-ray in which a single dilated, gas-filled strangulated loop may be prominent. There are no other investigations to help diagnose bowel strangulation, which is a clinical diagnosis best confirmed at laparotomy.

PERITONITIS

PATHOPHYSIOLOGY AND CLINICAL FEATURES OF PERITONITIS

Peritonitis is defined as inflammation of the peritoneal cavity. This includes the serosal coverings of the bowel and mesentery, the omentum and the lining of the abdominal cavity. At the outset, peritoneal inflammation is often localised and the affected area contained by a wrapping of omentum, adjacent bowel and fibrinous adhesions. This may, however, be insufficient to prevent spread, and generalised peritonitis results. Sudden perforation of any viscus almost invariably leads to life-threatening generalised peritonitis.

Localised peritonitis occurs in the vicinity of any primary intra-abdominal inflammatory process. Appendicitis is a typical example. Once the parietal peritoneum becomes involved, pain becomes localised to the affected area and is exacerbated by movement of the abdominal musculature. The area is tender to palpation and there is contraction of the overlying abdominal wall muscles when examination is attempted. This sign is known as **guarding**. If the palpating hand is quickly removed, the sudden movement of the peritoneum causes intense pain which is described as **rebound tenderness**. However, this test is unkind and its diagnostic value overstated. Rebound tenderness is better elicited by gentle percussion and can often be inferred from the history. Hospital 'speed bumps' thus may perform an important diagnostic role! Rectal examination should always be performed as anterior tenderness can be a sign of pelvic peritonitis. Localised peritonitis is usually accompanied by mild systemic 'toxicity', i.e. low-grade fever, malaise, tachycardia and leucocytosis.

With **generalised peritonitis**, the patient is seriously ill. There is massive exudation of inflammatory fluid into the peritoneal cavity causing hypovolaemia. This is often compounded by toxaemia from absorbed products and sepsis if infection is present. The severity of the systemic illness depends on the cause of the peritonitis and is

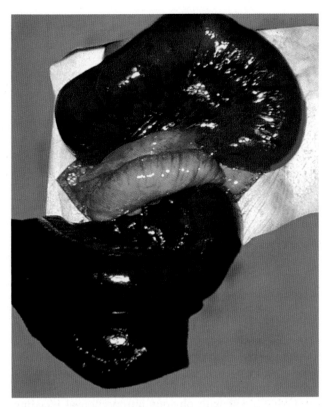

Fig. 12.3 Necrotic bowel after strangulation
This photograph, taken at operation for bowel obstruction, shows a dilated necrotic loop of small bowel which has strangulated after passing through a congenital defect in the sigmoid mesocolon. The bowel was on the point of perforation.

most severe when there is widespread contamination by faeces, pus or infected bile. Peritonitis is less severe when infection is absent (e.g. perforated duodenal ulcer in its early stages).

On examination in generalised peritonitis, the abdomen is rigid and tender and bowel sounds are absent because of peristaltic paralysis. Rectal examination provides a means of direct palpation of the pelvic peritoneum and will usually reveal anterior tenderness. This is a most important sign and is strong evidence of peritonitis.

There is no specific investigation which will confirm the diagnosis but plain abdominal X-ray may provide additional clues as to the cause. It is unkind and unnecessary, however, to subject a patient to abdominal X-rays if a decision has already been taken to perform an emergency laparotomy.

The causes of peritonitis are summarised in Box 12.4.

INTRA-ABDOMINAL HAEMORRHAGE

Blood may enter the abdominal cavity from a variety of sources including ruptured ectopic pregnancy, leaking aortic aneurysm or blunt trauma, especially to the liver and spleen. Blood in the abdominal cavity causes

> **KEY POINTS**
>
> **Box 12.4 Causes of peritonitis**
>
> **Localised peritonitis**
> - Transmural inflammation of bowel, e.g. appendicitis, Crohn's disease, diverticulitis
> - Transmural inflammation of other viscera, e.g. cholecystitis, salpingitis
>
> **Generalised peritonitis**
> - Irritation of the peritoneum by noxious materials, e.g. bile, stomach or small bowel contents (due to perforation), enzyme-containing exudates of acute pancreatis
> - Spreading intraperitoneal infection, e.g. rupture of intra-abdominal abscess or faecal contamination due to bowel perforation, trauma, surgical spillage or anastomotic leak

moderate peritoneal irritation and symptoms similar to peritonitis, but often more muted. Distinguishing between the two is usually not difficult because the history and other symptoms and signs give enough clues. In an unstable patient with obvious intraperitoneal bleeding, this is best diagnosed and managed at laparotomy. In the less urgent situation, intra-abdominal bleeding may be confirmed by computed tomography or ultrasound scan, or **peritoneal lavage** which involves instillation of saline via a peritoneal cannula; retrieval of blood-stained fluid is diagnostic.

PRINCIPLES OF MANAGEMENT OF PERITONITIS

Local peritonitis is treated according to the diagnosis. For example, appendicitis requires appendicectomy whilst acute diverticulitis and salpingitis are usually managed with antibiotics.

With generalised peritonitis, the patient is at risk of death from toxaemia or septic shock. As soon as the diagnosis is made, high doses of antibiotics are given intravenously. With the exception of acute pancreatitis, generalised peritonitis requires urgent laparotomy to discover the cause and to clear the contaminating material (**peritoneal toilet**).

INTRA-ABDOMINAL ABSCESS

PATHOPHYSIOLOGY AND CLINICAL FEATURES OF INTRA-ABDOMINAL ABSCESS

There are two common causes of intra-abdominal abscess. The first occurs after bowel perforation, when omentum and adjacent gut attempt to wall off the defect. The second is a complication of bowel surgery where

there has been localised faecal contamination or an anastomotic leak. Appendiceal perforation may cause a local abscess or one which tracks down into the pelvis. Diverticular disease often causes a **pericolic abscess** or **complex inflammatory mass**, particularly in the rectosigmoid area or pelvis. Less commonly, perforation of a colonic tumour results in a pericolic abscess. Gall bladder perforation is rare and occasionally results in a right-sided **subphrenic abscess**. Finally, perforation of an ulcer in the posterior wall of the stomach may produce a **lesser sac abscess**.

With intra-abdominal abscess, abdominal pain is usually continuous rather than colicky and tends to increase inexorably. Local bowel irritation may cause diarrhoea or adynamic obstruction. A swinging pyrexia (see Ch. 1) is an important sign which points to the diagnosis. There is usually a marked leucocytosis. The patient is otherwise relatively well, except with a post-operative abscess, where there is a degree of toxaemia or even septicaemia. There may be a palpable abdominal inflammatory mass which most commonly originates with appendicitis or acute diverticular disease. Rectal examination may reveal a hot, tender mass (a **pelvic abscess**), displacing the rectum backwards—a classic finding in the post-appendicectomy patient. These patients usually complain of diarrhoea due to inflammation close to the rectum.

Ultrasound of the abdomen and pelvis is most useful in demonstrating the site and size of an abscess and drainage may be possible under ultrasound control. CT scanning may also be useful. When an abscess is suspected but cannot be demonstrated, radioisotope scanning, using the patient's own radionuclide-labelled white cells may be helpful (see Fig. 12.4).

PRINCIPLES OF MANAGEMENT OF AN INTRA-ABDOMINAL ABSCESS

With a pelvic abscess in a patient who is otherwise well, there is usually no advantage in antibiotic treatment or attempting to drain the abscess because, given time, the abscess will usually drain spontaneously and safely into the rectum. Discharge of the abscess is recognised when the patient passes pus and blood per rectum; this is followed by resolution of the fever and healing.

Small subphrenic abscesses may also resolve without intervention but larger subphrenic abscesses can usually be drained percutaneously under ultrasound control. Many intra-abdominal abscesses can be successfully dealt with using percutaneous drainage, but these methods deal only with the abscess and not the underlying cause. Laparatomy may be required in some cases to deal with an intra-abdominal abscess, particularly if the underlying cause needs to be treated or if it is technically unsuitable for percutaneous drainage.

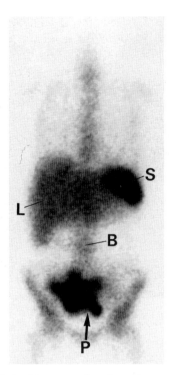

Fig. 12.4 Radioisotope scan showing a large pelvic abscess
Radionuclide scan of a 47-year-old woman who presented with lower abdominal tenderness and a swinging pyrexia. The patient's own leucocytes were labelled with a radionuclide. This scan shows a large pelvic abscess **P**, shown later to be due to diverticular perforation. Note also the radioisotope uptake by the spleen **S**, liver **L** and bone marrow **B**, which is a normal feature of such scans.

PERFORATION OF AN ABDOMINAL VISCUS

PATHOPHYSIOLOGY AND CLINICAL FEATURES OF PERFORATION

Disease in any hollow abdominal viscus may be complicated by perforation into the peritoneal cavity. The common sites of perforation are stomach and duodenum (from peptic ulcer), sigmoid colon (from diverticular disease) and the appendix (from acute appendicitis). The symptoms and signs of a perforated viscus depend on the nature of its contents, the volume of spillage and the effectiveness of the local defences.

A small perforation may be immediately walled off by omentum and nearby bowel, but a local abscess will then develop. In this case, symptoms and signs are often grumbling and rather non-specific at first but subsequently develop into those typical of an intra-abdominal abscess. A common example of this is appendicitis in adults. A small diverticular perforation without faecal spillage may cause localised peritonitis which may even resolve spontaneously. At the opposite extreme, a large colonic perforation due to a stercoral tear from severe constipation causes sudden overwhelming faecal peritonitis, which is

often fatal despite treatment. A perforated peptic ulcer causes marked abdominal signs of peritonitis but little initial systemic upset. This is because the fluid spilled is usually sterile. Acute cholecystitis sometimes perforates.

Perforation is essentially a clinical diagnosis but can usually be confirmed by the presence of free gas in the peritoneal cavity on plain X-ray. This can usually be seen as a radiolucent line beneath one or both hemidiaphragms on an erect chest film (see Fig. 12.5) or on a lateral decubitus film of the abdomen. Radiology does not always demonstrate free gas when there is a perforation; if X-rays fail to support the clinical diagnosis, action should be based on the clinical diagnosis. In the case of perforated appendicitis, free gas is very rarely seen. Large amounts of gas are typically seen with perforated duodenal ulcers and colonoscopic perforations. Less gas is seen with other colonic perforations.

PRINCIPLES OF MANAGEMENT OF PERFORATION

Perforation is a surgical emergency. Most cases require urgent laparotomy to repair the defect or resect the segment of diseased bowel. Duodenal ulcer perforations can be plugged with omentum or closed by suture. This may be accomplished at open surgery or laparoscopically. In large bowel perforations, a Hartmann's procedure, which leaves a temporary colostomy (see Ch. 20, p. 274), is frequently required because healing of an anastomosis may be impaired if there has been peritoneal contamination. Occasionally, conservative management is appropriate where there are few clinical signs: for example, perforation following colonoscopy. In the elderly, perforated duodenal ulcers may be managed conservatively using restriction of oral fluids, acid suppression and antibiotics; however, the outcome is unpredictable and the approach is not to be recommended if the patient is fit for surgery.

ACUTE BOWEL ISCHAEMIA

PATHOPHYSIOLOGY AND CLINICAL FEATURES OF INTESTINAL ISCHAEMIA

Occlusion of the **superior mesenteric artery** may lead to acute ischaemia of the primitive midgut-derived structures, i.e. jejunum, ileum and right colon (see Fig. 12.6). This causes massive infarction and later, fatal perforation. There are two fairly distinct types of acute superior mesenteric occlusion. The first is **embolism**, which originates from left atrial thrombus in atrial fibrillation or from left ventricular wall thrombus after recent myocardial infarction. Secondly, **thrombosis** of the artery may occur. This is usually a terminal event in gross low output cardiac failure or secondary to athero-

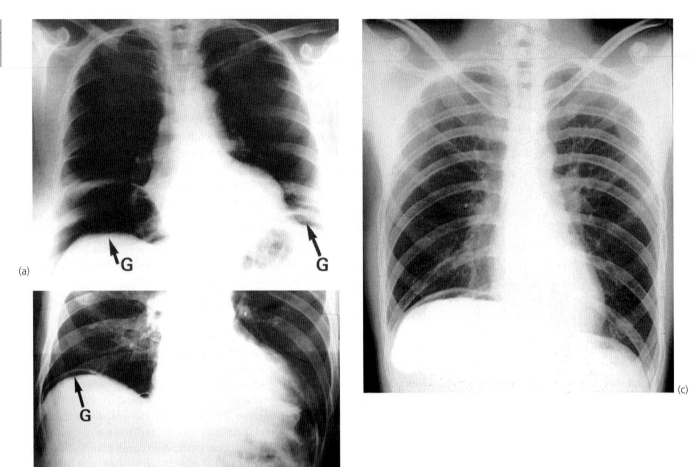

(a)

(b)

(c)

Fig. 12.5 Free perforation of an abdominal viscus shown on plain chest X-rays
(a) Erect chest X-ray from a man of 60 with a perforated sigmoid diverticulum who presented with a sudden onset of severe abdominal pain. The film shows large radiolucent gas shadows **G** under each hemidiaphragm. Fortunately in this case, no faeces entered the peritoneum and the patient did not suffer shock or peritonitis. **(b)** Similar view to (a) from a different patient, showing a smaller pneumoperitoneum **G** beneath the right hemidiaphragm. **(c)** Free gas under the diaphragm. This 22-year-old man presented with a 48-hour history of abdominal pain, initially central but latterly it had moved to the right iliac fossa (RIF). Clinically he had tenderness and rebound in the RIF. This erect chest X-ray shows free gas beneath both sides of the diaphragm indicating perforated bowel. Unusually, in this case it was due to a perforated appendicitis.

sclerotic stenosis; thrombosis takes place more readily if the mesenteric vessels are already atherosclerotic. The vulnerability of the superior mesenteric artery is poorly understood as is the sparing of the coeliac and inferior mesenteric territories. It probably relates to the nature of the collateral blood supply.

Acute bowel ischaemia can be a difficult diagnosis to make because of the lack of specific clinical features and diagnostic tests. The severity of abdominal symptoms and signs often gives no clue to the catastrophe within. There may be diffuse tenderness, abdominal distension and absent bowel sounds. Typically, there is a disproportionate degree of cardiovascular collapse or shock. Diagnosis depends therefore on clinical suspicion. In the late stages, gas may appear within the bowel wall and be visible on plain abdominal X-ray; by this time surgery is unlikely to be successful.

Some cases of intestinal infarction are due to **portal vein thrombosis**. The cause may be a prothrombotic disorder but is often idiopathic. In these patients, the infarction is often patchy and localised resections may allow some patients to survive.

PRINCIPLES OF MANAGEMENT OF INTESTINAL ISCHAEMIA

If intestinal ischaemia is suspected, laparotomy must be performed urgently unless it is clearly going to be fruitless. It is occasionally possible to restore the mesenteric arterial supply by embolectomy or vascular bypass before the bowel becomes necrotic. If the infarcted segment is not too extensive and the rest of the bowel looks healthy, resection gives a reasonable chance of recovery and an adequate amount of bowel to sustain

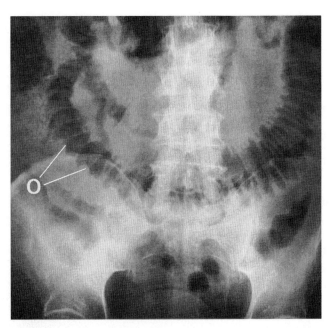

Fig. 12.6 Intestinal ischaemia
This 68-year-old woman with atrial fibrillation presented with collapse but only moderate abdominal pain. The patient had embolised her superior mesenteric artery (acute SMA occlusion) which supplies the embryological midgut-derived structures. The whole of her small bowel and the right half of her colon were necrotic but the left half of the colon was intact. This film shows the typical gross thickening of small bowel folds **O** caused by swelling from oedema and intramural haemorrhage.

nutrition. In nearly half the cases, however, the extent of necrosis is so great that resection is unrealistic and the patient should be allowed to die with as little interference as possible. In a few patients with arterial or venous infarction, resection and small bowel transplantation may be appropriate later.

Examination and investigation of the acute abdomen are summarised in Boxes 12.5 and 12.6.

SUMMARY

Box 12.5 Special points to note in examining a patient with an acute abdomen

General examination
- General demeanour, alertness and state of consciousness
- Posture and movement
- State of hydration, skin colour (anaemia or cyanosis), perfusion and sweating
- Temperature
- Pulse (rate, character and regularity)
- Blood pressure
- Respiratory pattern and rate, breath sounds on auscultation

Abdominal examination
- Inspection
  — distension, visible peristalsis, previous operation scars, obvious hernias, abdominal movement with respiration
  — always inspect the loins and back
- Palpation and percussion
  — tenderness, guarding, rigidity, rebound tenderness, pain on percussion
  — free fluid, succussion splash
  — groins, hernias and their reducibility, external genitalia
  — abdominal masses (including full bladder)
  — abnormal pulsation (aneurysm)
- Auscultation
  — bowel sounds, mesenteric arterial bruits
- Rectal examination (and vaginal examination if appropriate)
  — inspection of anal margin
  — peritoneal tenderness (unilateral tenderness may be an inflamed Fallopian tube)
  — lesions in the bowel wall, pelvic lesions
  — stool colour and consistency, blood
  — prostate size and consistency

MAJOR GASTROINTESTINAL HAEMORRHAGE

PATHOPHYSIOLOGY AND CLINICAL FEATURES OF GASTROINTESTINAL HAEMORRHAGE

Major gastrointestinal haemorrhage presents either as vomiting of blood or passage of frank or altered blood rectally. Vomited blood (**haematemesis**) may be fresh or partly digested. In the latter case, it is dark in colour and may have the typical appearance of 'coffee grounds'. Haematemesis usually indicates bleeding from the oesophagus or stomach but may indicate bleeding from the duodenum.

Blood loss beyond the duodenum will usually be passed rectally. The extent to which it is altered by digestion and the degree of mixing with the stool are useful indicators of its level of origin (described in Ch. 11, p. 151). Upper gastrointestinal bleeding is often manifest by **melaena**. This is the passage of loose, black, tarry stools with a characteristic foul smell. With upper gastrointestinal bleeding proximal to the duodeno-jejunal (DJ) flexure at the ligament of Treitz, hae-matemesis or melaena or both can occur. Haematemesis is more likely if the bleeding is rapid. The main causes of major gastrointestinal haemorrhage are summarised in Figure 12.7 and Table 12.2, p. 187.

KEY POINTS

Box 12.6 Investigation of the acute abdomen

Blood tests

- Haemoglobin
  - may be normal immediately after an acute bleed
  - low haemoglobin concentration may represent chronic anaemia due to occult blood loss rather than acute haemorrhage
- White blood count—leucocytosis is non-specific and rarely of much diagnostic value
- C-reactive protein
  - a non-specific indicator of inflammatory activation
  - confirms organic illness if elevated
- Plasma amylase—whenever pancreatitis cannot be excluded
- Urea and electrolytes—indicated in vomiting and diarrhoea, dehydration, poor urine output, diuretic therapy, urinary tract disease, known or suspected renal failure, pancreatitis and sepsis
- Glucose—for diabetics or those with glycosuria (beware of hyperglycaemia due to acute stress and steroid therapy)
- Blood group and ordering of blood for transfusion—for anaemic patients, major haemorrhage or when major surgery is contemplated
- Liver function tests and calcium estimation—for pancreatitis and acute biliary disease
- Clotting studies—for acute pancreatitis and septicaemia (disseminated intravascular coagulation), severe bleeding (consumption coagulopathy) or those with a history of bleeding disorders

Urine tests

- Ward ('stick') testing—for blood, protein, bile, glucose, nitrites and white cells
- Microscopy—for red and white blood cells, organisms
- Culture and sensitivity—suspected urinary tract infections
- Strain urine for stones—in ureteric colic

Radiology

- Chest X-ray
  - cardiovascular disease or abnormality, e.g. hypertension, cardiac failure
  - chest disease
  - suspected visceral perforation (gas under diaphragm)
- Plain abdominal X-rays (supine plus erect or decubitus)
  - bowel (gas pattern and dilatation, fluid levels, gas in the wall, faeces and faecoliths)
  - urinary tract (kidney size and position, calculi)
  - biliary tract (gallstones, gas in biliary tree in gallstone ileus)
  - aortic calcification (aneurysm)
  - psoas shadows (obscured by retroperitoneal inflammation or haemorrhage)
- Contrast radiology
  - 'instant' barium enema in colonic obstruction or acute colitis
  - emergency intravenous urography in ureteric colic

MANAGEMENT OF UPPER GASTROINTESTINAL HAEMORRHAGE

Initial management and resuscitation

Any patient presenting with severe upper gastrointestinal haemorrhage is at risk of death from hypovolaemic shock initially or as a result of rebleeding. Hospitals should ideally have clearly written and agreed protocols for combined medical and surgical management of upper gastrointestinal haemorrhage so that patients do not 'slip through the net' and perish by default. There is a very real danger of rebleeding in high-risk patients during a hospital stay (about 50%) and a combined management policy has been shown to reduce mortality for all cases of upper gastrointestinal haemorrhage from 10% to about 2%.

Clinical history, examination and investigation

More than two-thirds of patients presenting with upper gastrointestinal haemorrhage nowadays are over 60 years and one-third of these have a history of taking aspirin

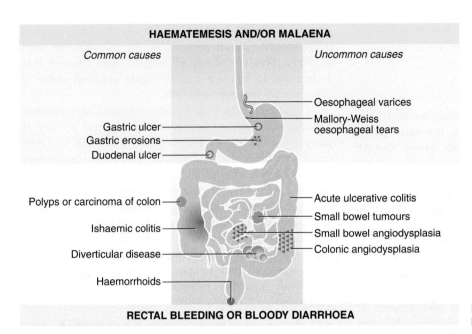

Fig. 12.7 **Causes of gastrointestinal haemorrhage**

Table 12.2 Causes of acute gastrointestinal haemorrhage

Pathology	Clinical features	Frequency
Oesophageal varices	Haematemesis and/or melaena	Uncommon
Mallory–Weiss oesophageal tears	Haematemesis or altered blood per rectum	Uncommon
Chronic gastric and duodenal ulcers, acute gastric ulcers or erosions	Haematemesis and/or melaena	Very common
Stress ulcers		Uncommon
Malignant small bowel tumours	Altered blood per rectum	Rare
Angiodysplasias of small bowel	Altered blood per rectum	Rare
Diverticular disease	Fresh rectal bleeding	Common
Ischaemic colitis	Abdominal pain then fairly fresh rectal bleeding	Fairly common
Angiodysplasias of colon	Pattern of bleeding depends on location within colon	Fairly common and increasingly recognised with the rise in colonoscopy
Acute or fulminant ulcerative colitis	Bloody diarrhoea	Uncommon
Haemorrhoids, rectal polyps and carcinomas	Fresh rectal bleeding but rarely in large quantities	Common

or other non-steroidal anti-inflammatory drugs. Other specific details of the history may be relevant. These include alcohol consumption, previous peptic ulceration or gastric surgery, or a history of cirrhosis and variceal haemorrhage.

Abdominal examination is usually unremarkable but general examination may show signs of chronic liver disease suggesting possible gastro-oesophageal varices. Rectal examination may reveal melaena stool or altered blood and this can be helpful if the history of haematemesis has not been substantiated, e.g. 'coffee-ground' vomit not seen by a doctor.

The volume of blood said to have been vomited or passed per rectum is unreliable as a measure of blood loss because a great deal may remain in the bowel. It is therefore essential initially to obtain good venous access and perform a full blood count, urea and electrolytes and prothrombin and liver function tests, to send blood for grouping and antibody screen (or cross-matching), and to order blood for transfusion in high-risk cases (see below). ECG and chest X-rays are useful in patients over 65 years or with cardiorespiratory disease. The patient should be made ready for theatre at a moment's notice, rather than laboratories being chased for results or blood for transfusion when the patient suddenly deteriorates!

Stratification of risk

Patients with acute upper gastrointestinal haemorrhage should be stratified clinically into a **low-risk group** (non-life-threatening) and a **high-risk group** (where continued bleeding or likely rebleeding is potentially life-threatening). This stratification is based on age, the presence of shock, the haemoglobin concentration and the presence of complicating disease (see Fig. 12.8). Stratification will determine the priorities of management and enable concentration of resources on those who really need it. Further risk factors may be found at endoscopy (see below).

It is vital that patients with signs of shock are monitored and resuscitated thoroughly; the rate and volume of intravenous fluid replacement (whether plasma expanders or blood) is adjusted against the responses of pulse rate, blood pressure, central venous pressure and hourly urine output.

Endoscopic management of acute upper gastrointestinal haemorrhage

Clinically high-risk patients should be assessed early by a surgical team, even if admitted under the care of a gastroenterologist or physician. Ideally, the same surgical team should remain responsible for that patient until recovery. This continuity of surgical care ensures that a decision to operate can be made without delay if conservative management fails.

All patients with upper gastrointestinal haemorrhage require endoscopy to determine the site and activity of bleeding, to diagnose oesophageal varices and to determine suitability for endoscopic treatment. Endoscopy also assists the surgeon in locating the source if surgery becomes necessary. Urgent endoscopy, within 12 hours of the first bleed, should be performed in clinically high-risk patients; all others should be endoscoped on the next available list, but ideally within 24 hours. This gives the best chance of locating the source of bleeding.

Unexpected endoscopic features may also place apparently low-risk patients in a high-risk category. These are:

● **Active spurting from an artery in an ulcer bed**. Endotherapy by gastroscopic injection of adrenaline or an adrenaline/sclerosant mixture should be attempted; there is a 25–40% rebleed rate necessitating surgery even in expert hands and the patient must be closely monitored

● **A visible elevated vessel or protruding adherent clot (Dieulafoy lesion)**. These lesions double the above risk of rebleeding. If the patient is also hypotensive, the risk of rebleeding is 80%

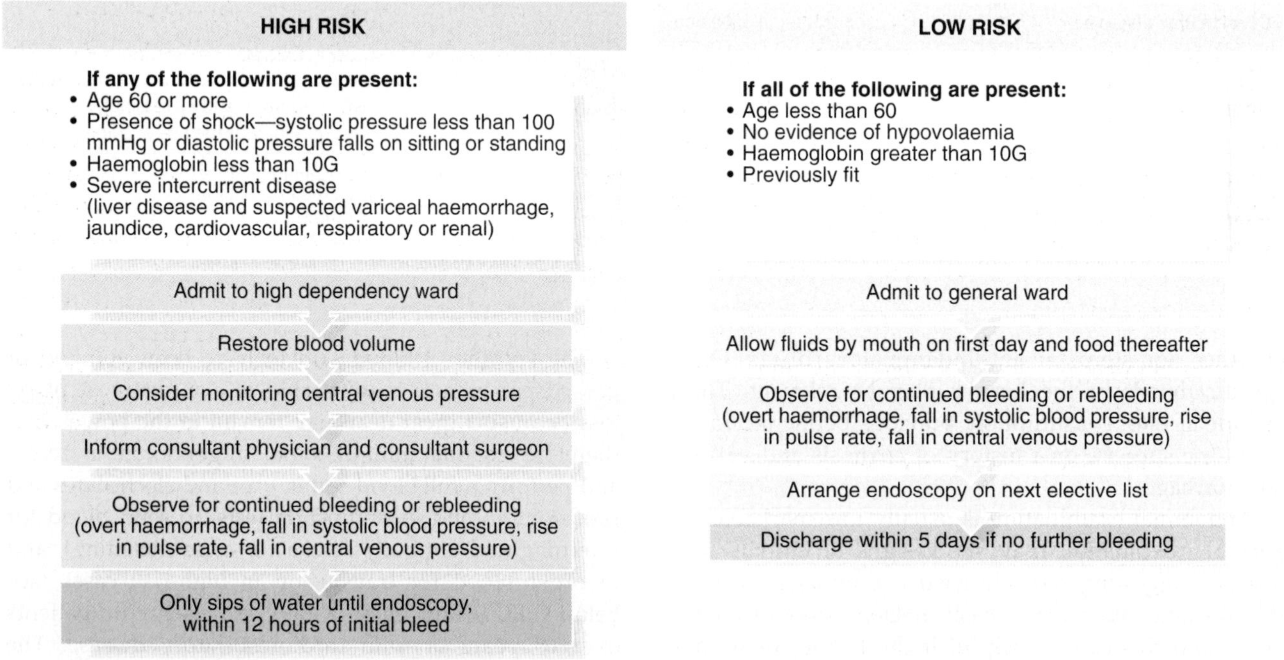

HIGH RISK

If any of the following are present:
• Age 60 or more
• Presence of shock—systolic pressure less than 100 mmHg or diastolic pressure falls on sitting or standing
• Haemoglobin less than 10G
• Severe intercurrent disease (liver disease and suspected variceal haemorrhage, jaundice, cardiovascular, respiratory or renal)

Admit to high dependency ward

Restore blood volume

Consider monitoring central venous pressure

Inform consultant physician and consultant surgeon

Observe for continued bleeding or rebleeding (overt haemorrhage, fall in systolic blood pressure, rise in pulse rate, fall in central venous pressure)

Only sips of water until endoscopy, within 12 hours of initial bleed

LOW RISK

If all of the following are present:
• Age less than 60
• No evidence of hypovolaemia
• Haemoglobin greater than 10G
• Previously fit

Admit to general ward

Allow fluids by mouth on first day and food thereafter

Observe for continued bleeding or rebleeding (overt haemorrhage, fall in systolic blood pressure, rise in pulse rate, fall in central venous pressure)

Arrange endoscopy on next elective list

Discharge within 5 days if no further bleeding

Fig. 12.8 Risk stratification in the management of acute upper gastrointestinal haemorrhage

● **Bleeding gastro-oesophageal varices**. Mortality is 30%. Immediate treatment is required with endoluminal rubber band ligation or injection sclerotherapy. Tamponade with special balloon catheters may also be necessary prior to endotherapy

Low-risk patients usually stop bleeding with conservative management after the initial haemorrhage that precipitated admission to hospital and are unlikely to rebleed. They may be given sips of water and acid suppression therapy (although there is little scientific evidence to support this practice), monitored by observation for rebleeding, pulse rate and blood pressure, and endoscoped on the next available list.

Surgical management

Immediate surgery is required for patients with exsanguinating haemorrhage or those unable to be stabilised during initial resuscitation. Even in the most acute case of upper gastrointestinal haemorrhage, gastroscopy can usually be performed on the operating table before operation. The common causes, duodenal or gastric ulceration, should be easily identifiable by gastroscopy (although these could be found at operation without this assistance) but the real value of gastroscopy is the ability to diagnose unusual sources of bleeding, most of which present particular operative problems. Thus, oesophageal ulceration or a Mallory–Weiss tear (see Ch. 15) may be discovered, and the surgeon can avoid operating on unsuspected variceal haemorrhage. Even in patients with known varices, endoscopy is essential, as blood loss will be from a different lesion in 50% of cases, e.g. peptic ulcer, gastric erosions. Occasionally blood loss is so rapid that an unguided laparotomy must be performed immediately to staunch the flow.

A policy of early surgery for patients over 60 has been shown to reduce mortality. Urgent surgery is also required for patients defined clinically or endoscopically as being 'high-risk' and who suffer one rebleed, or for any patient who suffers two rebleeds. Surgical procedures depend on the source of haemorrhage but there is a trend towards less radical procedures with improved postoperative medical management of peptic ulcer disease. Bleeding is arrested with under-running sutures after gastrotomy or duodenotomy. Gastric ulcers should be biopsied in case of malignancy but gastrectomy or vagotomy and pyloroplasty are rarely necessary (see

Ch. 14). Postoperative anti-*Helicobacter* therapy is of course essential but is often overlooked.

MORE DISTAL GI HAEMORRHAGE

More distal gastrointestinal bleeding is usually not investigated immediately to find the site but is managed conservatively anticipating spontaneous cessation. Around 80% will settle without transfusion, and the majority of the remaining 20% will settle with transfusion alone. If bleeding continues, it is an important principle that the source of bleeding should be localised by investigation so that appropriate treatment can be targeted accurately. 'Blind' laparotomy is often unsatisfactory because the cause may need non-surgical treatment or the source of bleeding may be difficult or impossible to find.

Blood loss from diverticular disease and ischaemic colitis is usually self-limiting. Several small bleeds may occur over a few days but the volume lost is usually small and hypovolaemia is rare. Typically the presentation is late and the bleeding has often stopped, with blood per rectum the only trace.

Investigation involves colonoscopy when bleeding has stopped, as the procedure is dangerous whilst there is limited vision. Sigmoidoscopy and barium enema are alternatives, but bleeding usually arises from the mucosa and this is not well seen radiologically. Occasionally an unsuspected carcinoma or polyp is discovered.

In ulcerative colitis, the diagnosis is evident from the other symptoms and signs, and management depends on the success of medical treatment (see Ch. 21). Persisting large bowel haemorrhage which is less rapid but recurrent is usually due to **angiodysplasias** (see Ch. 20, p. 274). Colonoscopy can be both diagnostic and therapeutic. If this is negative, impossible or unsatisfactory, radioisotope scanning using the patient's own labelled red cells or highly selective arteriography may be used to localise the source of bleeding at least to a general area of bowel (see Fig. 12.9). At laparotomy the whole bowel can be examined and any suspect area resected if appropriate. As a last resort, a colonoscope inserted through an incision in the bowel wall can be used to examine the whole colon and small bowel for bleeding sites. This may be the only means of diagnosing small bowel angiodysplasia. Occasionally, therapeutic embolisation of localised bleeding lesions using selective angiography is employed.

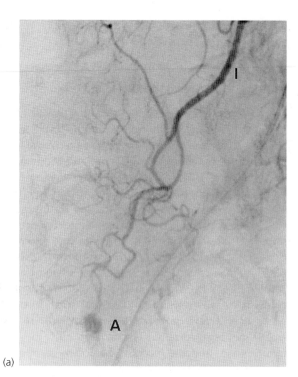

(a)

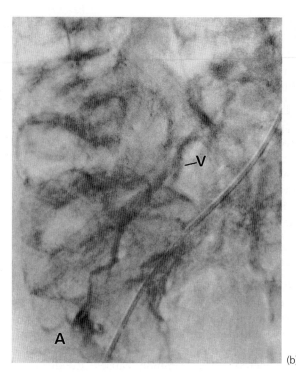

(b)

Fig. 12.9 Angiogram showing angiodysplasia of caecum

This man of 70 had been admitted to hospital on 12 occasions for rectal bleeding and chronic anaemia and had received 55 units of blood transfusion in all. On the last admission, this superior mesenteric arteriogram was performed, revealing the source of blood loss. **(a)** Subtraction film showing the arterial phase; the ileocolic artery **I** feeds a knot of abnormal blood vessels, an angiodysplasia **A**, at the lower pole of the caecum; this was responsible for the bleeding. **(b)** Subtraction film of the venous phase; the angiodysplasia **A** is still visible and there is early filling of a large draining vein **V**. These appearances are typical of angiodysplasia; the caecum is the most common site of occurrence. The lesion was resected by right hemicolectomy.

13 Gallstone diseases and related disorders

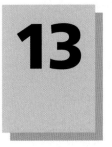

INTRODUCTION

Gallstones and related disorders account for all but a small proportion of biliary tract disease. The most important of the remainder, cholangiocarcinoma and sclerosing cholangitis, are discussed in Chapter 17. Gallstone disease is also known as **cholelithiasis**. When stones are present in the bile ducts, this is known as **choledocholithiasis**.

Most gallstone-related disease presents with pain, located typically in the epigastrium or right hypochondrium (upper quadrant). The character of the pain varies with the diagnosis; in most cases, it is acute and intermittent. The severity ranges from very severe and requiring hospital admission to moderately severe and managed at home. For the less severe group, gallstone disease tends to be investigated from the outpatient clinic. Less commonly, gallstone disease presents as **jaundice** caused by a stone passing into and obstructing the common bile duct.

Non-acute upper abdominal pain is a common cause of surgical referral, accounting for up to 7% of outpatient referrals in a typical district general hospital. Of these, about half will be diagnosed as having gallstone disease. Furthermore, about 25% of elective abdominal operations on adults in district general hospitals are performed for gall bladder disease. As gall bladder surgery is fraught with potentially serious complications, there is considerable scope for the development of effective preventative measures, safer surgical techniques and better non-surgical methods of managing gallstone disease.

STRUCTURE AND FUNCTION OF THE BILIARY SYSTEM

Bile collects in the canaliculi between hepatocytes and drains via collecting ducts within the portal triads into a system of ducts within the liver. These progressively increase in diameter until they become the **right** and **left hepatic ducts** which fuse to form the **common hepatic duct** 3–4 cm outside the liver; this is joined further down by the **cystic duct** to become the **common bile duct** (see Fig. 13.1). The common bile duct is 4–5 cm long and passes down behind the duodenum close to the head of the pancreas to drain via the **ampulla of Vater** into the second part of the duodenum. Reflux of duodenal contents is prevented by the **sphincter of Oddi**. In most cases, the **main pancreatic duct** joins the common bile duct at the ampulla although it may enter the duodenum independently.

The **gall bladder** is a muscular sac lined by a mucosa characterised by a single, highly folded layer of tall columnar epithelial cells. The lining epithelium is supported by loose connective tissue which contains numerous blood vessels and lymphatics. Mucus-secreting

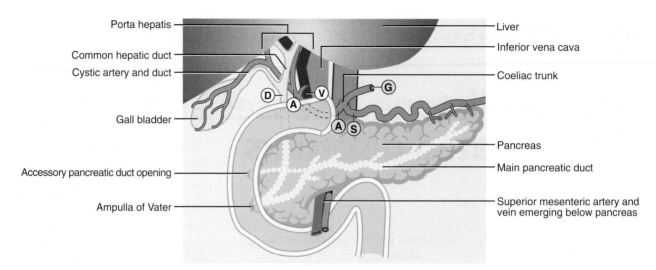

Fig. 13.1 Surgical anatomy of the gall bladder, biliary tract and pancreas
The coeliac trunk (the foregut artery) arises from the aorta and divides into the hepatic artery **A**, the splenic artery **S** and the left gastric artery **G**. The porta hepatis consists of the hepatic artery **A**, the extrahepatic bile ducts and the portal vein **V**. The hepatic artery divides into right and left branches. The extrahepatic bile ducts consist of the right and left hepatic ducts which join to form the common hepatic duct; in turn this is joined by the cystic duct to form the common bile duct **D**.

glands are found at the neck of the gall bladder but are absent from the body and fundus. The proximal part of the duct is disposed into a spiral arrangement called the **spiral valve**, the function of which is not well understood. The gall bladder lies in a variable depression in the under-surface of the right hepatic lobe and is covered by the same peritoneal covering as the liver. The common bile duct is a fibrous tissue tube lined by a simple, tall columnar epithelium. It is normally up to 0.6 cm in diameter which can be measured on ultrasound scanning.

Bile is made continuously by the liver and passes along the biliary tract to the gall bladder where it is stored. Bile is concentrated by as much as 10 times in the gall bladder by active mucosal reabsorption of water. Lipid-rich food passing from stomach to duodenum promotes secretion of the hormone **cholecystokinin-pancreozymin** (CCK) by endocrine cells of the duodenal mucosa. This hormone stimulates contraction of the gall bladder, squeezing bile into the duodenum. Bile salts (acids) act as emulsifying agents and facilitate hydrolysis of dietary lipids by pancreatic lipases. If bile fails to reach the duodenum because of biliary tract obstruction, lipids are neither digested nor absorbed, resulting in the passage of loose foul-smelling fatty stools (**steatorrhoea**). Furthermore, the fat-soluble vitamins (A, D, E and K) are not absorbed. The lack of vitamin K soon leads to inadequate prothrombin synthesis and hence defective clotting; this may pose problems if surgery is necessary in a patient with obstructive jaundice.

PATHOPHYSIOLOGY OF THE BILIARY SYSTEM

GALLSTONE COMPOSITION

In developed countries, most gallstones contain a predominance of cholesterol mixed with some **bile pigment** (calcium bilirubinate) and other **calcium salts**. A small proportion are virtually 'pure' cholesterol stones ('**cholesterol solitaire**'). In Asia, most gallstones are composed of bile pigment alone. The composition and pathogenesis of the various types of gallstone are summarised in Table 13.1, and some examples are illustrated in Figure 13.2.

The physical structure of mixed gallstones gives an insight into the time sequence of their formation. There is usually a small core of organic material which often contains bacteria. The main part of the stone is made up of concentric layers, which reveals that the stone does not form in a single episode but by a series of discrete precipitation events. Furthermore, there are often several 'families' of gallstones, each of a different size, found in the same gall bladder. This suggests that each family began at a different time, presumably due to a transient change in local conditions. All families then build up by lamination at the same rate, leading to the variety of different sizes. Radioisotope dating studies have shown that the average gallstone is 11 years old when it is removed!

The full story of how the common cholesterol-predominant (mixed) stones are formed has not yet been elucidated but several clues are available. The main

Table 13.1 Composition and pathogenesis of gallstones

Chemical composition	Pathogenesis	Morphology
Mixed stones (75–90% of all stones) Cholesterol is the predominant constituent. Heterogenous mixture of cholesterol, bile pigments and calcium salts in a 'core' and laminated structure	Combination of: • Abnormalities of bile constituents • Bile stasis • Infection	Multiple stones, several generations of different sizes often found together. Stones may be hard and faceted (where they have developed in contact) or irregular, 'mulberry'-shaped and softer. Colours range from near-white through yellow and green to black. Most are radiolucent but 10% are radiopaque
Cholesterol stones (up to 10% of all stones)	As for mixed stones	Large, smooth, egg- or barrel-shaped and usually solitary ('cholesterol solitaire'). Yellowish. Up to 4 cm diameter and may fill the gall bladder. Radiolucent
Pigment stones (uncommon in developed countries, common in Asia) Calcium bilirubinate	Excess bilirubin excretion due to haemolytic disorders, e.g. haemolytic anaemias, infections, malaria, leukaemias	Multiple, jet-black, shiny 'jack' stones; 0.5–1 cm diameter. Usually of uniform size and often friable
Calcium carbonate stones (rare)	Excess calcium excretion in bile	Greyish faceted stones. Radiopaque

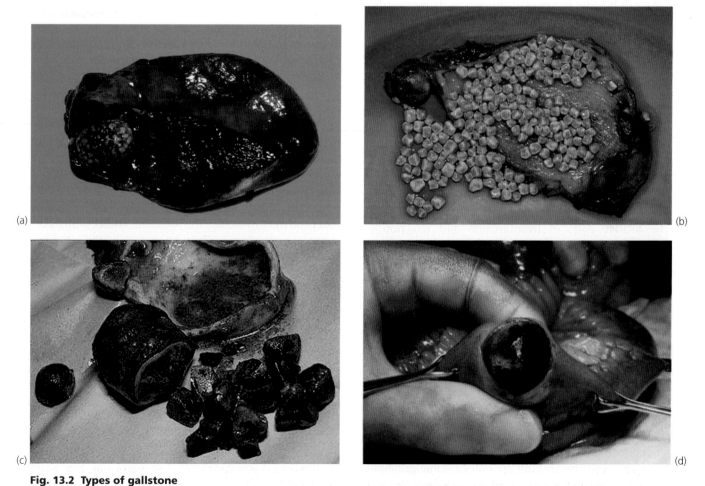

(a)
(b)
(c)
(d)

Fig. 13.2 Types of gallstone
(a) Thick-walled chronically inflamed gall bladder found to be obstructed at its neck by a single stone. Note the stone is an aggregate of many smaller stones. **(b)** Multiple small gallstones in the gallbladder, all of much the same 'generation'. **(c)** Gallbladder containing one huge stone and multiple smaller stones. These stones all fitted together with adjoining facets. **(d)** 'Cholesterol solitaire' which had caused **gallstone ileus** by obstructing the terminal ileum. The photograph shows it being removed from the distal ileum at operation.

factors are changes in concentration of the different constituents of bile, biliary stasis and infection. It is likely that several subtle abnormalities combine to bring about precipitation of bile constituents.

Bile salts and lecithin are responsible for maintaining cholesterol in a stable micelle formation. The normal micellar structure of bile supports a greater concentration of cholesterol than could normally be held in solution and it is therefore inherently unstable. An excess of cholesterol in relation to bile salts and lecithin is probably one of the main factors in stone formation. This is supported by the observation that patients in whom the terminal ileum has been resected or who have chronic distal ileal disease have a threefold risk of developing cholesterol-rich stones. The terminal ileum is the main site for reabsorption of bile salts. When this is removed or diseased, reabsorption falls off, leading to loss of bile salts via the bowel and a consequent reduction in the bile salt pool. Bile salts are then insufficient to maintain the micellar structure of cholesterol suspension.

Precipitation is enhanced by biliary stasis. This occurs if the gall bladder becomes obstructed or its contractility becomes defective. It is not known whether obstruction of the gall bladder outlet is a primary event in the formation of stones but it is believed to play a part in their continued accretion. Obstruction could be caused by dysfunction of the spiral valve in the cystic duct, by reflux of duodenal contents (which may be infected) or by small stones already formed. The muscular gall bladder wall is damaged by longstanding inflammation or infection which interferes with its ability to empty. Pregnancy is a predisposing factor.

THE ROLE OF INFLAMMATION AND INFECTION

The relative roles of inflammation and infection in gallstone formation are still in doubt, but probably both play a part. Abnormalities of bile composition may cause chemical inflammation of the gall bladder, resulting in inflammatory exudation and perhaps accumulation of inflammatory debris. Infection probably plays an important part in the pathogenesis of gallstones. Bacteria usually form the organic nidus upon which gallstones are built; they enter the gall bladder intermittently by reflux from the duodenum or via the bloodstream. This process is probably normal in itself but becomes pathological if the bacteria are not flushed out, as when the gall bladder does not adequately empty. Once stones are formed, episodic bacterial ingress could be responsible for periods of precipitation in which layers of the laminated structure are built up. Indeed, some gallstones continue to harbour bacteria so the process becomes self-perpetuating. In support of this is the fact that faecal organisms can be cultured from at least 25% of cholecystectomy specimens.

THE ROLE OF CHRONIC OBSTRUCTION

Transient obstruction of the gall bladder by stone may cause episodes of acute pain (**biliary colic**). If the obstruction persists, the gall bladder becomes chemically inflamed causing **acute cholecystitis**. If obstruction does not resolve by itself and the contents do not become infected, the gall bladder becomes distended with mucus; this is known as a **mucocoele**, and is often palpable and tender. If the contents become infected, an abscess develops within the gall bladder and this is known as an **empyema of the gall bladder**.

The majority of gall bladders removed for chronic pain show a range of histological features more in keeping with a **chronic obstructive aetiology** than an infective one. These features include intact but often atrophic mucosa, submucosal and subserosal fibrosis, hypertrophy of the muscular wall, and mucosal diverticula extending into the muscular layer (known as **Rokitansky–Aschoff sinuses**). Evidence of active or previous infection is uncommon. Inflammatory infiltrates are mainly associated with traumatic gallstone erosion of the mucosa or intrusion of inspissated bile into the gall bladder wall, particularly around the mucosal diverticula. In some cases the gall bladder is so grossly scarred, distorted or contracted that its absorptive and contractile functions have been completely destroyed.

OTHER PATHOLOGICAL MECHANISMS

In about 10% of patients with symptoms typical of gall bladder disease, no stone can be demonstrated during investigation or at operation. In some of these cases, a stone may have passed out of the duct system into the bowel. In other cases, chronic inflammation occurs independently of stones, the so-called '**cholecystitis sans stones**'; again, chronic obstruction may be the aetiology. Finally, the terms '**biliary dyskinesia**' and '**cystic duct syndrome**' are used to explain the situation where patients have typical symptoms of gall bladder disease but essentially normal standard investigations. When biliary manometry is used, many of these patients are shown to have an abnormally high pressure in the sphincter of Oddi. Confirming this diagnosis is difficult but a fair proportion of patients suspected of this are cured by endoscopic sphincterotomy or surgical sphincteroplasty.

EPIDEMIOLOGY OF GALLSTONES

In developed countries, at least 10% of the adult population probably develop gallstones during their lifetime although most remain asymptomatic. Gallstones are rare before adulthood and increase in prevalence with age. Women are affected four times as often as men and it appears that pregnancy is a very important predisposing factors; obesity and diabetes may also play a part. The typical patient is said to be a 'fair fat fertile female of forty', but many gallstone patients do not fit this description! Gallstone disease is rare in the rural communities of developing countries but is increasing with urbanisation. Western-style processed foods, high in fats and refined carbohydrates but poor in fibre, may be responsible. Their contribution to gall bladder disease would be compatible with the theory that changes in the composition of bile are the most important factors in stone pathogenesis.

INVESTIGATION OF GALL BLADDER PATHOLOGY

When gallstone disease is suspected, investigation has the following objectives:

- Exclude haematological, liver function and other systemic abnormalities
- Establish whether gallstones are present in the gall bladder and/or common duct and whether the gall bladder wall is abnormally thickened
- Assess the integrity of the bile duct system and the pancreatic duct (if there is any suggestion of obstruction)

BLOOD TESTS FOR HAEMATOLOGICAL AND LIVER ABNORMALITIES

In many straightforward cases, no blood tests are necessary except to exclude anaemia in susceptible groups such as women of child-bearing age. **Haemolytic disorders** such as hereditary spherocytosis, thalassaemia and sickle cell trait should be considered as they may predispose to pigment stones. Liver function tests are indicated if there is any suggestion of jaundice or other liver abnormality. Finally, blood cultures to exclude systemic infection may be appropriate in seriously ill patients.

INVESTIGATION OF GALL BLADDER PATHOLOGY

Investigation for gall bladder disease aims to demonstrate the presence of stones and signs of chronic gall bladder inflammation. Ultrasonography is the mainstay of investigation but cholecystography is occasionally employed.

Ultrasonography

Ultrasonography (see Fig. 13.3) is reliable for identifying stones in the gall bladder and increased gall bladder wall thickness (caused by inflammation or fibrosis). Ultrasound provides a simple and accurate means of demonstrating **dilatation of the common duct system**, which often indicates distal duct obstruction. Unfortunately, it is unreliable for identifying bile duct stones directly, particularly at the lower end. Ultrasound has the great advantage of being suitable for the seriously ill or jaundiced patient.

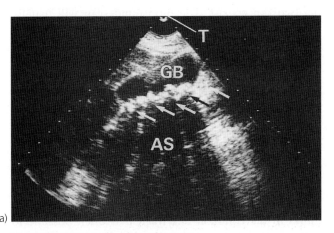
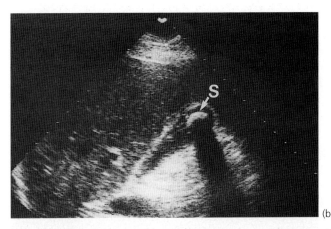

(a)   (b)

Fig. 13.3 Biliary ultrasound scans
(a) Longitudinal scan of gall bladder in a 46-year-old woman who complained of intermittent attacks of right upper quadrant pain. The scan shows the outline of the gall bladder **GB** and a layer of gallstones (arrowed) along its posterior wall. The stones each cast a clear acoustic shadow **AS** beyond them. Note that these shadows can be projected back to the transducer **T**. **(b)** Longitudinal scan of the gall bladder in a 37-year-old woman showing a single large stone **S** in the fundus. Note that only the anterior surface of the stone is seen (as an arc) because all sound waves are reflected from it, casting a dense acoustic shadow beyond. Note that ultrasound is a poor method of demonstrating stones at the lower end of the common bile duct because the image tends to be obscured by overlying duodenal gas.

Oral cholecystography

Oral cholecystography, once the mainstay of investigation, has now largely been superseded by ultrasonography. It provides a different perspective by showing gall bladder function and only incidentally revealing stones. It involves ingestion of contrast medium which is absorbed, excreted by the liver and then radiographically demonstrated in the extrahepatic biliary system. A plain radiograph of the biliary area (**control film**) may demonstrate stones, although only about 10% of all stones are radiopaque (see Fig. 13.4). It may occasionally show **calcification** in the pancreas (indicating previous pancreatitis), or a gall bladder outlined by calcification ('**porcelain gall bladder**').

If the concentrating function of the gall bladder is normal, the gall bladder will be visible as a radiopaque viscus in which negative shadows of stones may be seen as **filling defects**. A non-opacifying gall bladder may be diseased. Oral cholecystography is of no value in jaundice, hepatic failure, intestinal malabsorption and vomiting and is rarely indicated in acute gall bladder disease because the gall bladder is usually obstructed.

INVESTIGATION OF THE BILIARY DUCT SYSTEM

See Figure 13.5.

The non-jaundiced patient

Patients with gallstones but no history of obstructive jaundice do not require preoperative investigation for duct stones. If open cholecystectomy is performed, **operative cholangiography** (also known as peroperative

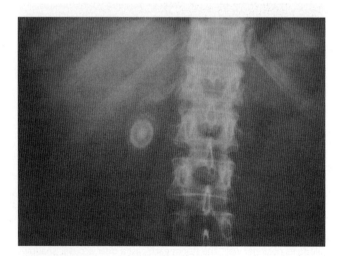

Fig. 13.4 X-ray of radiopaque gallstone
Plain abdominal X-ray showing large radiopaque gallstone in the right upper quadrant. Note that the stone is obviously laminated, having built up in layers over many years

cholangiography) is carried out routinely but is less often employed at laparoscopic cholecystectomy, p. 205. At open operation, the bile duct system is outlined by passing a cannula through the cystic duct into the common bile duct and injecting radiopaque contrast material. This fills the biliary tree and should flow into the duodenum. X-rays or fluoroscopic imaging are then used to demonstrate the duct morphology and any abnormalities such as duct dilatation, filling defects caused by stone or distortion of the tapering lower end of the common duct, as well as obstruction of flow into the duodenum. If cholangiography shows a stone or stones, the duct is usually explored as described on page 203.

A different problem is the patient with a history of **transient jaundice** possibly attributable to stones. Most cases will have either operative cholangiography at open cholecystectomy or preoperative endoscopic retrograde cholangio-pancreatography (ERCP), described in Chapter 6, p. 65. Intravenous cholangiography is sometimes employed but it gives poor definition and may cause unpleasant side effects like nausea or even anaphylaxis.

The jaundiced patient

When obstructive jaundice has been diagnosed, it is important to distinguish between stone and tumour in order to plan appropriate management.

Ultrasonography is usually the initial investigation. This shows the extent of dilatation of both intrahepatic and extrahepatic ducts and may even show a stone lodged at the lower end of the duct. If stones are demonstrated in the gall bladder, this adds weight to the impression that stones are blocking the duct rather than tumour, but the two can coexist. The ultrasound scan will usually demonstrate a carcinoma of the pancreatic head or enlarged lymph nodes in the porta hepatis; either may cause extrahepatic biliary obstruction.

Ultrasound may make the diagnosis, but if more detailed information is required, biliary tract morphology can be outlined by direct injection of contrast. There are two methods: ERCP and percutaneous transhepatic cholangiography. When available, **ERCP** is the more useful and less invasive investigation; it avoids needle injection into the liver and also allows the ampullary region to be inspected for tumour. Furthermore, the pancreatic duct may be outlined if required. If stones are found in the common bile duct, it is often possible to perform immediate **endoscopic sphincterotomy**, releasing the stones, thus diagnosing and relieving the jaundice in one procedure. This may be life-saving for the patient with ascending cholangitis and is the treatment of choice on its own for the patient who is a poor risk for laparotomy.

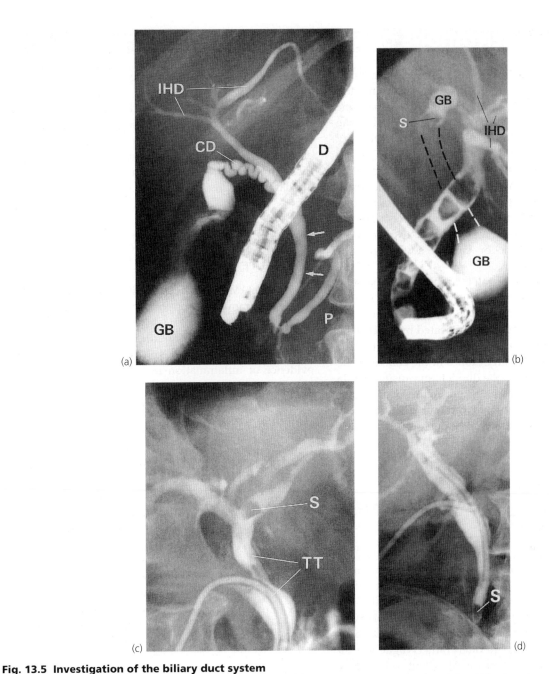

Fig. 13.5 Investigation of the biliary duct system
(a) Normal ERCP showing duodenoscope **D** in the second part of the duodenum. Contrast has been injected first into the pancreatic duct **P** and then into the common bile duct (arrowed). Note also the cystic duct **CD**, gall bladder **GB** and intrahepatic bile ducts **IHD**.
(b) Endoscopic retrograde cholangiogram in a woman of 77 who presented with mild epigastric pain and obstructive jaundice. The film shows multiple large stones in the common bile duct, represented by filling defects. The common bile duct is moderately dilated, but the intrahepatic ducts **IHD** are not. The fundus and neck of the gall bladder **GB** are shown, but the body is empty of contrast (dotted lines). There is a stone **S** near the neck of the gall bladder. **(c)** and **(d)** Postoperative T-tube cholangiogram films taken (routinely) 7 days after a cholecystectomy and removal of stones from the common bile duct. The films show the T-tube **TT** in situ. In (c), a stone **S** can be seen in the left hepatic duct, and in (d), another stone **S** can be seen at the lower end of the common bile duct. Both stones were successfully retrieved percutaneously 6 weeks later. The T-tube was removed and steerable grasping forceps passed into the biliary system through the skin defect. Each stone was then grasped and drawn to the surface along the track.

Percutaneous transhepatic cholangiography is used if ERCP is unavailable or unsuccessful. It involves inserting a long, fine (22 gauge) needle through the skin into one of the dilated intrahepatic ducts under radiological control. Contrast medium is then injected. An obstructing stone produces a characteristic rounded filling defect (Fig. 13.6d), as opposed to the tapering stricture typical of tumour.

CLINICAL PRESENTATIONS OF GALLSTONE DISEASE

The names attached to the various clinical syndromes associated with gallstones are somewhat confusing and at best imprecise. This is partly because more than one pathological process may occur at once; hence the true diagnosis can often be made only in the histopathology laboratory.

In the past, gallstones have been blamed for causing chronic, low-grade symptoms, and labelled **chronic cholecystitis** or **flatulent dyspepsia**. In fact chronic low-grade obstructive gall bladder disease probably does not exist and the symptoms can usually be explained by irritable bowel syndrome or chronic aerophagia (air swallowing).

Severe pain occurs if the gall bladder becomes acutely obstructed, even transiently. This is known as **biliary colic**. Acute inflammation of the gall bladder is known as **acute cholecystitis**. It may be complicated by **mucocoele of the gall bladder**, abscess formation (**empyema**) or free **perforation**. Rarely, large stones in the common bile duct ulcerate through into the duodenum causing **fistula** formation and sometimes **gallstone ileus**. Finally, gallstones probably predispose to **carcinoma** in the very long term. The spectrum of clinical disorders associated with gallstones is summarised in Figure 13.6.

CHRONIC SYMPTOMS SUGGESTIVE OF GALL BLADDER DISEASE

CLINICAL FEATURES

Many patients are referred with a long history of almost daily pain which is poorly localised in the right upper quadrant or epigastrium. It is often accompanied by nausea or even vomiting. The pain may be exacerbated by large or fatty meals and may radiate around towards the back. The symptoms are often rather vague and ill defined; this probably explains why patients often delay consulting a doctor. Examination rarely reveals more than vague upper abdominal tenderness.

MANAGEMENT

Most of these patients turn out not to have gallstones on ultrasonography. The most frequent diagnosis is irritable bowel syndrome but the differential diagnosis includes peptic ulcer disease, urinary tract infection and chronic constipation. Note that even if a patient has upper abdominal symptoms and demonstrable gallstones, this does not prove the one is caused by the other. Asymptomatic gallstones are a common enough incidental finding and it sometimes takes fine clinical judgement to decide whether cholecystectomy is likely to cure the symptoms.

When symptoms are characteristic of gall bladder disease, no special investigations other than ultrasonography are required. When the symptoms are less clear-cut, a more extensive search is necessary, perhaps including upper gastrointestinal endoscopy, plasma amylase and ECG.

BILIARY COLIC

CLINICAL FEATURES

Intermittent cystic duct obstruction by stone is probably the most common reason for symptoms from gallstones. Typically, patients are female and chiefly fall into two groups: the young or middle-aged, often overweight woman, where there is likely to be little histological evidence of inflammation in the gall bladder, and the elderly woman in whom the gall bladder is grossly thickened, chronically inflamed and shrunken. The same conditions arise less frequently in males.

Biliary colic describes the symptom complex arising from sudden and complete obstruction of the cystic duct or common bile duct by stone. The pain produced is severe, typically rising to a plateau over a few minutes, then continuing unrelentingly. The patient writhes in agony until the pain resolves spontaneously after several hours or after opiate analgesia. A bout of vomiting often heralds the end of the attack and the patient feels exhausted and sore for the next day or so. There is commonly a history of previous similar episodes. On examination, there are few positive findings. There is no fever but there may be some local tenderness due to gall bladder distension. If the attack does not settle within 24 hours, acute cholecystitis is a more likely diagnosis.

MANAGEMENT

Most cases of biliary colic can safely be managed at home if the diagnosis is recognised. Pain relief usually requires only one injection of an opiate and the attack then passes. Severe attacks of biliary colic usually lead to emergency hospital admission since the differential diagnosis includes other conditions which may require urgent operation, e.g. perforated peptic ulcer. A presumptive diagnosis can be made on clinical grounds but ultrasound is important in making a definitive diagnosis. Ultrasound examination should be performed as soon as possible, since early diagnosis may save several unnecessary days in hospital. In acute gallstone disease, cholecystectomy scheduled for the next available list is

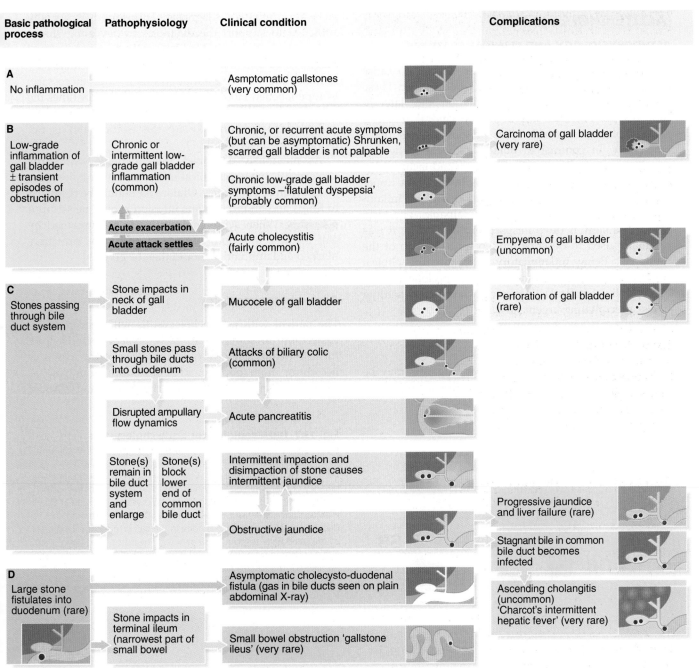

Basic pathological process	Pathophysiology	Clinical condition	Complications

A
No inflammation — Asmptomatic gallstones (very common)

B
Low-grade inflammation of gall bladder ± transient episodes of obstruction

Chronic or intermittent low-grade gall bladder inflammation (common)

Chronic, or recurrent acute symptoms (but can be asymptomatic) Shrunken, scarred gall bladder is not palpable — Carcinoma of gall bladder (very rare)

Chronic low-grade gall bladder symptoms –'flatulent dyspepsia' (probably common)

Acute exacerbation
Acute attack settles

Acute cholecystitis (fairly common) — Empyema of gall bladder (uncommon)

C
Stones passing through bile duct system

Stone impacts in neck of gall bladder — Mucocele of gall bladder — Perforation of gall bladder (rare)

Small stones pass through bile ducts into duodenum — Attacks of biliary colic (common)

Disrupted ampullary flow dynamics — Acute pancreatitis

Stone(s) remain in bile duct system and enlarge | Stone(s) block lower end of common bile duct

Intermittent impaction and disimpaction of stone causes intermittent jaundice

Obstructive jaundice — Progressive jaundice and liver failure (rare)

Stagnant bile in common bile duct becomes infected

D
Large stone fistulates into duodenum (rare)

Asymptomatic cholecysto-duodenal fistula (gas in bile ducts seen on plain abdominal X-ray)

Ascending cholangitis (uncommon) 'Charcot's intermittent hepatic fever' (very rare)

Stone impacts in terminal ileum (narrowest part of small bowel — Small bowel obstruction 'gallstone ileus' (very rare)

Fig. 13.6 Clinical consequences of gallstones

preferred by many surgeons but others perform the operation electively at a later date. Early operation appears to be the better option, reducing the risk of the complications of gallstones. If a mucocoele of the gall bladder is found, the attack is likely to persist and there is a high risk of an **empyema of the gall bladder** developing. In this case, cholecystectomy often becomes necessary during the current admission.

Cholecystectomy is the definitive treatment for biliary colic. Patients are frequently put on a low-fat diet initially or while awaiting operation; this often relieves

symptoms, presumably by removing a stimulus to gall bladder contraction. It also facilitates weight loss, if appropriate.

In younger patients, cholecystectomy is usually straightforward. The gall bladder is usually found to contain stones or thick dark biliary sludge and its wall is often thin, although it may be inflamed. Occasionally a **mucocoele** is found. In a few patients, the gall bladder is thickened and scarred and technically more difficult to remove. Techniques of cholecystectomy are discussed on pages 203–207.

ACUTE CHOLECYSTITIS

PATHOPHYSIOLOGY AND CLINICAL FEATURES

Several factors contribute in varying degrees to cause acute inflammation in an obstructed gall bladder. These include physical and chemical irritation and, later in the episode, bacterial infection. The clinical result is acute cholecystitis which often presents as a surgical emergency. In contrast to biliary colic, the patient is usually systemically unwell with fever and tachycardia. On examination there is tenderness in the right upper quadrant, more marked on inspiration, and an inflammatory gall bladder mass may be palpable. The term **'Murphy's sign'** is often misused in this context; it was originally used to describe tenderness at the tip of the ninth rib. Being inflammatory in origin, the clinical course of acute cholecystitis is more prolonged than biliary colic, usually lasting several days before settling or else precipitating urgent surgery.

MANAGEMENT

As with biliary colic, a presumptive diagnosis may be made on clinical grounds, but it is worthwhile obtaining an early definitive diagnosis. Ultrasound is usually sufficient to support the diagnosis by revealing stones and a thickened gall bladder wall. A more positive diagnosis of gall bladder obstruction can be made by radionuclide scanning although this is rarely necessary; isotope-labelled HIDA is excreted in bile and outlines the normal gall bladder and bile duct system. An obstructed gall bladder fails to take up the isotope and is not demonstrated (see Fig. 13.7).

As previously described, most patients with acute cholecystitis have a chemical inflammation and therefore do not require antibiotics. Oral intake should be restricted to fluids and an intravenous infusion should be set up if necessary. When acute cholecystitis is accompanied by gall bladder infection, symptoms and signs are more marked and antibiotics should then be given.

Acute cholecystectomy

The patient with acute cholecystitis will need a cholecystectomy at some stage. Early cholecystectomy, performed within a few days of the onset of the attack, is becoming more popular. The procedure is as safe as elective surgery, convenient for the patient and efficient

Fig. 13.7 HIDA scanning for acute cholecystitis
(a) Normal HIDA scan. This scan was taken 30 minutes after ingestion of the radioisotope. Radioactivity has been detected in the liver **L**, gall bladder **GB**, common bile duct **C** and small bowel **SB**, demonstrating patency of the whole biliary system. **(b)** HIDA scan in a patient with symptoms and signs suggesting acute cholecystitis. This scan at 30 minutes shows contrast in the liver and a little in the common bile duct and small bowel; there is none in the gall bladder. **(c)** HIDA scan of the same patient taken at 60 minutes. The isotope has now virtually cleared from the liver and is seen in small bowel. There is still no filling of the gall bladder, which must therefore be obstructed, confirming the diagnosis of acute cholecystitis.

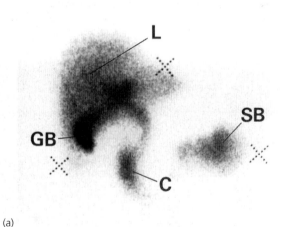

(a)

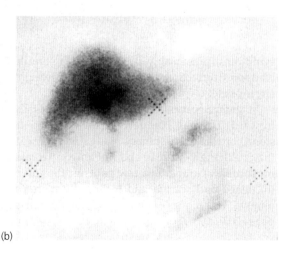

(b)

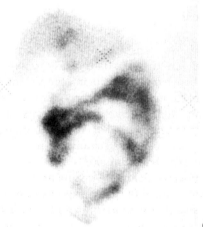

(c)

in terms of hospital bed usage. The alternative policy of conservative management is to discharge the patient after the acute attack resolves and readmit the patient for elective cholecystectomy after about 6 weeks, by which time the inflammation has usually settled. However, in the mean time, there is a risk of further acute attacks or some other manifestation of gallstone disease such as acute pancreatitis. Even if delayed cholecystectomy is preferred, the acute attack may not settle, necessitating cholecystectomy on the same admission.

When operation is performed during the acute illness, the gall bladder is found to be obstructed and tense. The serosal surface is oedematous and inflamed with petechial haemorrhages or even purulent exudate and there are fibrinous adhesions to nearby structures. The gall bladder neck or cystic duct is blocked by an impacted stone and the gall bladder is usually found to contain further stones or sludge mixed with inflammatory exudate. Bowel organisms can be cultured from the contents in about 70% of cases.

In older patients, the operation is often much more difficult; the gall bladder may be grossly inflamed, thickened and scarred and has to be patiently dissected out of the liver bed. Great care must be taken to avoid damaging the bile ducts. The gall bladder often contains several stones and may be filled with pus. A culture swab should be taken from within the gall bladder at operation as any postoperative infective complications are likely to involve the same organisms.

Empyema of the gall bladder

In a more extreme clinical variant, the gall bladder becomes distended with pus. The condition, known as an empyema, represents an abscess of the gall bladder. As with abscesses elsewhere, a swinging pyrexia is often found. Sometimes part of the gall bladder wall becomes necrotic, leading to perforation. This may be walled off by adjacent omentum, resulting in localised abscess formation and a palpable gall bladder mass. Occasionally perforation leads to a subphrenic abscess or generalised peritonitis. **Gangrenous cholecystitis** and perforation are rare because the gall bladder has a rich blood supply from its hepatic bed as well as from the cystic artery. These patients require surgery without delay.

CHOLECYSTO-DUODENAL FISTULA AND GALLSTONE ILEUS

These uncommon complications of gallstones result from the inflamed gall bladder becoming adherent to the adjacent duodenum and a stone ulcerating through the wall to form a cholecysto-duodenal fistula. The fistula decompresses the obstructed gall bladder and allows stones to pass into the bowel and gas to enter the biliary tree. As such, the condition is usually harmless and unsuspected. It may be diagnosed on plain abdominal X-ray by the presence of gas outlining the biliary tree. Sometimes it is discovered at operation.

Occasionally, a solitary cholesterol stone passing into the bowel is so large that, after traversing the small bowel, it impacts in the narrowest part, the distal ileum, causing gallstone ileus. This occurs in the elderly and presents as an unexplained intermittent and sometimes incomplete small bowel obstruction. Unfortunately, the diagnosis is often difficult to make and the delay is detrimental to the patient. Diagnosis can be confidently made if gas is recognised in the biliary tree on a plain abdominal X-ray of an elderly patient with distal small bowel obstruction (see Fig. 13.8). Barium follow-through will demonstrate the small bowel obstruction.

CARCINOMA OF THE GALL BLADDER

Chronic irritation by stone over a long period is believed to predispose to **adenocarcinoma of the gall bladder**. This condition is rare and only found in the elderly. The presenting symptoms are similar to chronic inflammatory gall bladder disease. Jaundice may develop if the tumour obstructs the bile ducts. Carcinoma of the gall bladder is

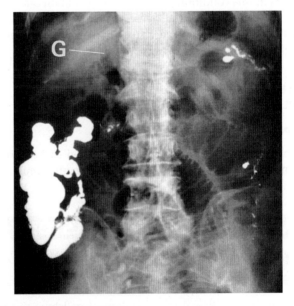

Fig. 13.8 Gallstone ileus
This 78–year-old woman presented with a gradual onset of small bowel obstruction. A large cholesterol solitaire stone had ulcerated from the gall bladder into the duodenum, travelled down the small bowel and finally impacted in the distal ileum causing complete obstruction. This plain supine abdominal X-ray shows residual barium from a barium enema performed 2 weeks previously. There is widespread small bowel dilatation. The diagnostic feature is the presence of gas **G** in the biliary tree (in this case, the common bile duct and cystic duct).

usually an unexpected finding at cholecystectomy for stones and is usually incurable by the time of detection.

The possibility of malignant transformation is one argument in favour of removing a chronically inflamed gall bladder, even if symptoms are not severe.

BILE DUCT STONES

PATHOPHYSIOLOGY

Bile duct stones nearly always originate in the gall bladder and pass through the cystic duct. Most stones are small enough to pass out of the biliary system into the duodenum but may cause biliary colic or mild jaundice during transit. This explains many of the symptoms of recurrent gallstone-related disease.

Initially, stones in the bile ducts are small and enlarge progressively in situ. This is evident from the occasional finding of multiple faceted gallstones fitting neatly together in the common duct which could only have formed within the duct. The common bile duct is narrowest at its lower end and stones too large to pass out tend to lodge at this point. A stone here either becomes impacted, causing **progressive jaundice**, or acts as a ball-valve, causing **intermittent jaundice**. Obstruction results in gradual dilatation of the biliary tree; if dilatation is long-standing it does not regress even after the obstruction is removed and may lead to stagnation of bile and further stone formation. Note that the gall bladder rarely distends in this condition even when the common bile duct is completely obstructed. This is because of the inflammatory fibrosis or mural hypertrophy caused by gall-stones (Courvoisier's law—see Ch. 11, p. 151).

CLINICAL PRESENTATIONS OF STONES IN THE BILIARY TRACT

Obstructive jaundice

Stones in the common bile duct, as stated earlier, are a common cause of obstructive jaundice and must be considered in the differential diagnosis; details are given in Chapter 11.

Asymptomatic duct stones

Any patient with gallstones may have duct stones. Therefore, at open cholecystectomy, it is standard practice to investigate the biliary tree by operative cholangiography and to remove any stones by exploration of the common bile duct (see p. 203). This avoids the need for a subsequent procedure. Some surgeons perform cholangiography at laparoscopic cholecystectomy but others do not.

Acute pancreatitis

Stones passing through or lying near the ampulla of Vater may interfere with drainage of pancreatic enzymes into the duodenum. Bile reflux into the main pancreatic duct may cause acute pancreatitis (see Ch. 18).

Ascending cholangitis

Bile stasis in the common duct occurs with chronic obstruction and dilatation and predisposes to bacterial infection. The infection then extends proximally to involve the intrahepatic duct system. The condition is known as ascending cholangitis and is characterised by intermittent attacks of pain, swinging pyrexia and jaundice. This triad is also referred to as **Charcot's intermittent hepatic fever** and is often accompanied by marked weight loss. Ascending cholangitis is a serious condition and may culminate in life-threatening **acute suppurative cholangitis**. The bile duct must be drained urgently, either by surgical operation or preferably by endoscopic sphincterotomy.

Ascending cholangitis more commonly develops as a late complication of biliary tract surgery, particularly bypass operations.

MANAGEMENT OF GALLSTONE DISEASE

NON-SURGICAL TREATMENT OF GALLSTONES

Whatever the clinical manifestation of gallstone-related disease, most cases are treated surgically. A small proportion, however, are suitable for oral drug therapy. **Chenodeoxycholic acid** (a bile acid) and related drugs increase the bile salt pool and inhibit hepatic cholesterol secretion. When administered over a long period, these drugs cause slow dissolution of cholesterol stones.

Unfortunately, the drugs have several disadvantages apart from their very slow action. Only cholesterol-predominant stones can be dissolved and even if this treatment is successful, there is a high rate of stone recurrence; there are frequent drug side effects such as severe diarrhoea and hepatic damage. Thus, drug therapy has largely gone out of favour and should only be considered in young patients with small radiolucent stones in a gall bladder which concentrates contrast and contracts in response to a fatty meal.

There was a vogue for gallstone destruction using **extra-corporeal shock wave lithotripsy** as for urological stones (see Ch. 31). However, the results were disappointing. There are problems in passing shattered stone debris through the narrow cystic duct, and further stones are likely to be formed if the gall bladder itself is diseased and any underlying metabolic predisposing factors remain unchanged.

SURGICAL MANAGEMENT OF GALLSTONES

INDICATIONS FOR SURGERY AND PREPARATION OF THE PATIENT

There are two main indications for cholecystectomy:

- Symptomatic gallstone disease
- Asymptomatic gallstones when there is a reasonable likelihood of future symptoms or complications

In most cases high-quality biliary ultrasound is the only imaging study required. This demonstrates gall bladder disease and gallstones and the diameter of the intrahepatic and extrahepatic bile ducts. Information from ultrasound about gall bladder wall thickness or the number and size of stones has not proved useful in predicting the feasibility of laparoscopic surgery. If there are stones in the duct system, common duct exploration is added to open cholecystectomy or else stones are extracted at ERCP.

Any jaundiced patient is at particular risk during surgery because of infection, hepatic impairment, defective clotting, acute renal failure and venous thrombosis and it is preferable to relieve obstructive jaundice prior to surgery by endoscopic sphincterotomy and stone extraction or bile duct stenting.

CHOLECYSTECTOMY—OPEN VERSUS LAPAROSCOPIC SURGERY

The traditional method of cholecystectomy is by open operation at laparotomy. Laparoscopic cholecystectomy has rapidly increased in popularity in recent years and is already the standard method of treating gallstones in many centres where expertise is available. However, public awareness of catastrophic complications (which often, but by no means always, occur early in a surgeon's experience) has meant that questions are often asked about the appropriateness and safety of laparoscopic surgery. Some centres perform open cholecystectomy through small incisions, 7–10 cm long, the so-called **mini-cholecystectomy** (see Fig. 13.9), and randomised studies have shown that recovery is similar to laparoscopic cholecystectomy. Despite this, it is likely that laparoscopic cholecystectomy will become the standard method, given improved training, greater experience and close audit of outcomes. All surgeons performing this operation must, however, be able to perform an open operation to cope with complications or particular difficulties arising during a laparoscopic operation which oblige conversion to an open operation.

OPEN CHOLECYSTECTOMY AND OPERATIONS ON THE COMMON DUCT

The main choice of incisions for biliary surgery are illustrated in Figure 13.9 and the main steps in cholecystectomy are shown in Figure 13.10. Students and junior surgical staff should be familiar with these if they are to assist at operation as well as appreciate the potential for operative complications.

Exploration of the common bile duct

If stones are known to be present in the bile ducts by preoperative ERCP or operative cholangiography, the

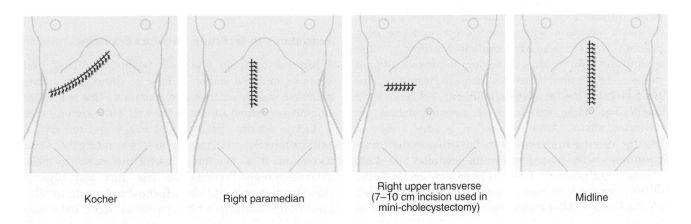

| Kocher | Right paramedian | Right upper transverse (7–10 cm incision used in mini-cholecystectomy) | Midline |

Fig. 13.9 Incisions for biliary surgery

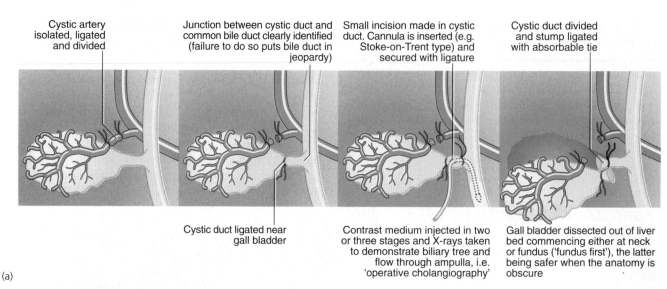

Cystic artery isolated, ligated and divided

Junction between cystic duct and common bile duct clearly identified (failure to do so puts bile duct in jeopardy)

Small incision made in cystic duct. Cannula is inserted (e.g. Stoke-on-Trent type) and secured with ligature

Cystic duct divided and stump ligated with absorbable tie

Cystic duct ligated near gall bladder

Contrast medium injected in two or three stages and X-rays taken to demonstrate biliary tree and flow through ampulla, i.e. 'operative cholangiography'

Gall bladder dissected out of liver bed commencing either at neck or fundus ('fundus first'), the latter being safer when the anatomy is obscure

(a)

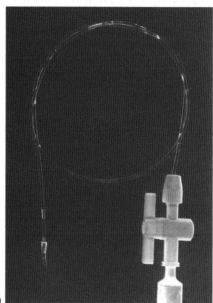

(b)

Fig. 13.10 Cholecystectomy
(a) Principal steps in cholecystectomy. **(b)** Cannula for operative cholangiography.

common duct is explored. The duct is opened through a longitudinal incision and stones are retrieved, often with some difficulty, by a combination of manipulation, irrigation, grasping with stone forceps and use of a balloon catheter. **Operative choledochoscopy** is often used to check for residual stones and to remove difficult stones. The flexible fibreoptic choledochoscope gives good visibility and manoeuvrability but, unlike its rigid counterpart, lacks the range of instrumentation for retrieving stones. After exploration, a latex T-tube is usually inserted to drain bile to the exterior, the transverse limb being placed within the common bile duct. The main purpose of a T-tube is to provide access to the biliary tree for a further cholangiogram about 1 week after operation (**T-tube cholangiography,** see Fig. 13.11). This is to ensure that no stones remain. If no stones are found on surgical exploration or if the surgeon is

satisfied that no stones remain, the common bile duct can be closed without T-tube drainage.

Procedures to facilitate bile duct drainage

When the common bile duct is grossly dilated and contains multiple stones, it may be difficult to ensure complete stone clearance at exploration. This is because fragments of stone adhere to the wall. Furthermore, such a duct is usually stretched and baggy and remains so postoperatively, predisposing to stasis and further stone formation. It is therefore a useful precaution to make an anastomosis between the bile duct and adjacent duodenum known as a **choledocho-duodenostomy**. This ensures bile drainage even if stones or debris have been left behind. The anastomosis must be wide or it will predispose to ascending cholangitis.

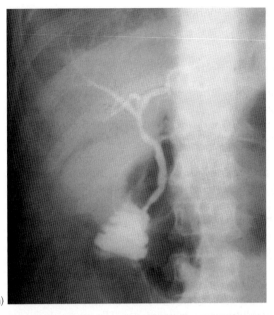
(a)

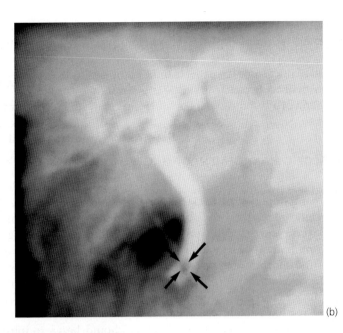
(b)

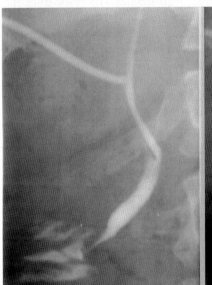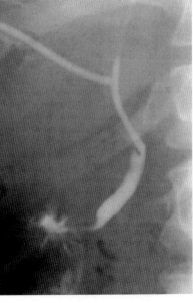
(c)

Fig. 13.11 Operative cholangiogram and T-tube and cholangiogram
(a) Normal operative cholangiogram. The bile ducts are not dilated, the hepatic ducts fill and contrast flows easily into the duodenum. There are no filling defects in the duct and the duct tapers normally at its lower end. **(b)** Operative cholangiogram showing stone at lower end. This poorer quality image was seen better on the screen of the image intensifier used in the operating theatre. A filling defect (arrowed) is seen towards the lower end of the common bile duct representing a stone. This was removed at operation via a choledochotomy. A T-tube was placed into the bile duct, draining to the exterior. (c) T-tube cholangiogram. This series was taken 10 days after operation. The tube can be seen in situ and there is no evidence of retained stones (contrast Fig. 13.5 earlier). The tube was therefore removed.

An alternative operation, **transduodenal sphinctero-plasty**, involves opening the second part of the duodenum and splitting the sphincter of Oddi by a large longitudinal incision. The mucosal edges are then sutured in apposition to minimise stricture formation. This operation may also be used to remove a firmly impacted stone from the lower end of the common duct. After any operation in which bile ducts are opened, an abdominal drain should be placed nearby to minimise the hazards of any biliary leakage. Few of these operations are performed nowadays as these patients are often better and more safely managed by endoscopic sphincterotomy.

ENDOSCOPIC MANAGEMENT OF BILE DUCT STONES

With the widespread availability of ERCP and endoscopic sphincterotomy, stones in the common duct can often be retrieved without an open operation. This technique represents a real advance in the management of duct stones over the earlier need for open surgery. **Endoscopic sphincterotomy** may be employed in the following circumstances:

● Urgent drainage of the bile duct in obstructive jaundice complicated by cholangitis. Definitive surgery can thus be deferred until the risks of infection have been overcome

- Retrieval of stones missed at operation. This avoids a difficult and hazardous operation to explore or re-explore the duct
- Removal of duct stones in patients unfit for operation
- Some cases of acute pancreatitis due to gallstones
- Preparation of a jaundiced patient for elective gall bladder surgery

LAPAROSCOPIC MANAGEMENT OF GALL BLADDER DISEASE

Absolute contraindications to laparoscopic cholecyst-ectomy include generalised abdominal infection, the late stages of pregnancy and major bleeding disorders. Relative contraindications for less experienced surgical teams include morbid obesity, acute cholecystitis, un-treated bile duct stones including obstructive jaundice, acute gallstone pancreatitis, previous abdominal surgery (adhesions) and intra-abdominal malignancy.

Patients undergoing laparoscopic surgery should be prepared for and have consented to open surgery in case conversion proves necessary. In most centres, 5–10% of elective patients require conversion. If bile duct stones are suspected, a preoperative ERCP (or equivalent magnetic resonance investigation) is advisable and stone extraction is carried out if necessary as laparoscopic exploration of the bile duct has not yet proved its value. With experience, at least 95% of stones can be success-fully extracted by endotherapy. Some surgeons favour operative cholangiography in every case to give a 'road map' of the duct anatomy, to exclude bile duct stones and to provide experience for when cholangiography is essential.

Operative technique

A common operating theatre set-up for laparoscopic cholecystectomy is shown in Figure 13.12. The patient is anaesthetised and prepared as for open cholecyst-ectomy but with the addition of a nasogastric tube and a urinary catheter; this decompresses the stomach and bladder respectively and minimises the risk of trocar injury. A pneumoperitoneum is established via an open Hassan procedure (a safer technique, gradually super-seding the subumbilical Verress needle) using an auto-matic gas insufflator. A 10 mm cannula is then placed for a video laparoscope. The abdominal cavity is inspected for other pathology and the feasibility of endoscopic cholecystectomy is then determined.

Three additional abdominal punctures are usually made to introduce operating instruments. The cystic duct and artery are identified and an operative cholangiogram per-formed if desired via the most lateral cannula or percu-taneously through the abdominal wall. It is extremely important to be certain of the ductal anatomy before cutting anything because of the lack of depth perception, the distortion introduced by retraction of the gall bladder and the limitations of the two-dimensional imaging system.

The cystic duct is doubly ligated with metal clips or ligatures, the gall bladder is dissected from the liver bed using diathermy or laser probes; haemostasis is secured.

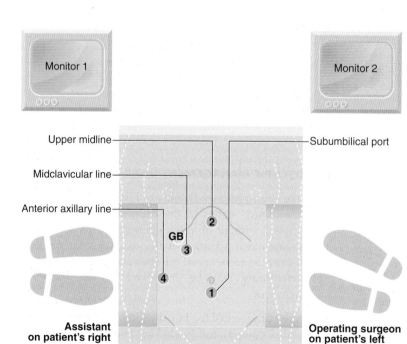

Fig. 13.12 Operating theatre arrangement for laparoscopic cholecystectomy
A common arrangement of the various operating ports (numbered 1–4) is shown. The subumbilical port **(1)** is usually placed with the Hassan open technique to take a 10 mm video laparoscope. A Verress needle is still sometimes used for initial gas insufflation. At the upper midline port **(2)** a 10 mm trocar is placed 5 cm below the xiphoid under video vision to the right of the falciform ligament. This is used to introduce operating instrument—curved dissectors, clip applier, and suction and irrigation tubes. At the midclavicular **(3)** and anterior axillary **(4)** lines, 5 mm trocars give access for grasping forceps, which are used to retract the gall bladder.

The now free gall bladder is usually removed via the umbilical port. To achieve this, the laparoscope is moved to the upper midline port and forceps inserted through the umbilical cannula. The neck of the gall bladder is grasped and pulled into the cannula and the entire cannula and gall bladder neck withdrawn through the abdominal wall. If large stones prevent its passage, the incision is enlarged. The umbilical fascial defect should be sutured to prevent herniation but the upper midline puncture is usually left unsutured along with the lateral punctures. The nasogastric tube and urinary catheter are removed before the patient leaves theatre.

RESULTS OF LAPAROSCOPIC CHOLECYSTECTOMY

Most patients are able to walk and tolerate food within 6 hours of operation and up to 80% can be discharged within 24 hours. The time to return to work and other normal activities appears to be reduced compared with open cholecystectomy.

The risk of bile duct injuries is undoubtedly related to the experience of the operating team but overall it is twice as high in laparoscopic as in open surgery. Bile duct injuries probably occur in 0.3–1% of patients. The consequences of bile duct injury can be catastrophic; patients have died with multi-organ failure resulting from unrecognised biliary peritonitis whilst others have

required open operations to repair bile ducts and have risked the consequences of long-term bile duct strictures. Other potential complications are listed in Table 13.2.

COMPLICATIONS OF BILIARY SURGERY

The particular complications of laparoscopic cholecystectomy are listed in Table 13.2. General complications of cholecystectomy are described below.

The retained stone

Despite considerable care at exploration of the common duct at open surgery, stones occasionally remain in the duct system after operation and are revealed by postoperative T-tube cholangiography. Until two decades ago, there were only two courses of remedial action. The first, attempting to flush the stone into the duodenum by irrigating the T-tube with heparin, saline or bile acids, was rarely successful. The second choice was a further laparotomy. Reoperation was technically difficult and carried a greatly increased risk of morbidity and mortality. Retained stones are usually retrieved now by ERCP and sphincterotomy although it is possible to retrieve retained stones percutaneously via a mature T-tube track using steerable grasping forceps or a Dormia basket.

Retained stones sometimes make themselves known many years later, when, having enlarged, they cause pain or obstructive jaundice. This possibility should be considered if a patient with previous biliary tract surgery develops typical pain or obstructive jaundice.

Biliary peritonitis

Bile leaking into the peritoneal cavity is irritant and causes a chemical peritonitis. If the bile is infected, it causes generalised peritonitis and sepsis with a high risk of fatality. Bile tends to leak through suture lines because of its detergent action. Therefore, whenever the duct system has been opened, a drain should be left in the vicinity for at least 5 days. Small leaks after bile operations usually settle spontaneously but if biliary peritonitis develops, the area must be drained percutaneously or, more often, re-explored urgently and drained under intravenous antibiotic cover.

Bile duct damage

The bile ducts can easily be damaged at cholecystectomy or common duct exploration unless their anatomy, which is commonly aberrant, is carefully displayed. The most serious error is unrecognised transsection or ligation of the common duct. This presents as a major biliary leak or increasing jaundice; urgent re-exploration is mandatory. Lesser degrees of bile duct damage from

Table 13.2 Potential complications of laparoscopic cholecystectomy

Stage of procedure	Complication
Placement of insufflation needle or trocar	
During operation	Injuries to bowel
	Injuries to blood vessels, e.g. iliac artery
	Diaphragmatic injury with tension pneumothorax
Postoperative	Bleeding from trocar insertion sites
	Subcutaneous emphysema
Late	Herniation through trocar entry points and bowel strangulation
Trauma to biliary system	
During operation	Injuries to common bile ducts and hepatic ducts
	Bleeding from cystic or right hepatic artery
	Gall bladder perforation with spillage of bile and stones
Postoperative	Bleeding and bile leakage from liver bed
	Bile leakage from cystic duct remnant
	Retained bile duct stones
Other complications	Bowel damage by diathermy or laser
	Postoperative shoulder tip pain

crushing or a careless ligature will heal but eventually result in a fibrotic stricture. This presents much later with obstruction. Regardless of how the bile ducts are damaged, complex reconstructive surgery is usually required, although endoscopic placement of a long-term stent allows rescue of some strictured ducts without operation. In the long term, stents inevitably become blocked and have to be replaced every 3–6 months.

Haemorrhage

The cystic and hepatic arteries and the vascular liver bed are vulnerable to operative trauma and bleed profusely. Removing a grossly inflamed or fibrotic gall bladder is particularly hazardous. Manoeuvres to control haemorrhage may damage other structures, passing unnoticed at the time; this is a common cause of bile duct trauma.

Hazards of pre-existing jaundice

These are discussed under 'Obstructive jaundice' in Chapter 11 (p. 161).

Ascending cholangitis and other infections

Ascending cholangitis can be a late complication of biliary surgery where an anastomosis has been formed between bile ducts and bowel. Reflux of intestinal contents and organisms takes place continually in such cases but active infection only occurs when bile stagnates in the duct system because of inadequate drainage. Usually the diameter of the anastomosis has shrunk to a point when it no longer drains adequately. Ascending cholangitis may also occur early after common duct exploration for jaundice, since bile in this situation is nearly always infected. Prophylactic antibiotics should always be used when operating on jaundiced patients with duct obstruction to minimise this complication.

Another early complication of biliary surgery is a **subphrenic abscess**. This must be considered if the patient develops an unexplained swinging fever a few days after operation. Diagnosis may be elusive and is best made by ultrasound. Treatment is by percutaneous needle drainage under ultrasound guidance or occasionally by open operation.

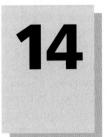

14 Peptic ulceration and related disorders

INTRODUCTION

Peptic ulcer disease encompasses disorders of the oesophagus, stomach and duodenum. The conditions share the symptom of epigastric pain and all have the common aetiology of mucosal inflammation associated, to a greater or lesser extent, with gastric acid-pepsin secretions. Recent work has demonstrated that perhaps the most important aetiological factor in gastric and duodenal ulcer disease is chronic mucosal infection with the bacterium *Helicobacter pylori*. Peptic disorders, together with gallstone disease, are the most common causes of organic upper abdominal pain.

With the advent of highly effective pharmacological agents to block acid secretion and more reliable diagnostic and treatment monitoring techniques such as flexible endoscopy, the use of surgery in peptic ulcer disease has declined by over 90% in the last 25 years. More recently, antibiotic and other treatments against *H. pylori* promise even greater reductions and perhaps permanent cure for many peptic ulcer disorders. Most patients with suspected peptic ulcer disease are treated empirically by family practitioners; the rest are largely managed by gastroenterologists. Only a minority present to surgeons because of failed medical treatment. Rates of emergency complications such as perforation and haemorrhage have remained more static but peptic pyloric stenosis has markedly declined as chronic ulceration has become less common. Nevertheless, because of the diagnostic difficulties posed by upper abdominal symptoms, surgeons still manage many patients who turn out to have peptic disorders.

PATHOPHYSIOLOGY AND EPIDEMIOLOGY OF PEPTIC DISORDERS

PATHOPHYSIOLOGY OF PEPTIC ULCERATION

Inflammation, probably initiated by *H. pylori* infection and sustained by the combined effect of gastric acid and pepsin upon the mucosa, is probably the cause of all peptic disorders of the upper gastrointestinal tract other than reflux oesophagitis. *H. pylori* is a Gram-negative microaerophilic spiral bacterium which has the ability to colonise the gastric mucosa over a very long period. In many cases, infection appears to have been acquired in childhood and there is often an association with poor living conditions in early life. Normally, a dynamic balance is maintained between the inherent protective characteristics of the mucosa (the mucosal barrier) and the irritant effects of acid-pepsin secretions. The delicate balance between secretion and protection may be disrupted by diminution of mucosal resistance or excessive acid-pepsin secretion or a combination of both. In some cases, the mucosal surface may become eroded by the direct action of some external agent, e.g. strong alcohol. Whatever the aetiology, the range of pathological outcomes is similar and is summarised in Figure 14.1. If, at any stage, the balance of resistance over attack is restored, the process is halted and the tissue repaired. This explains the chronic and remittent nature of peptic ulcer disease.

OUTCOMES OF BREACHES OF THE MUCOSAL BARRIER

When the protective mucosal barrier is breached, the delicate underlying connective tissue is exposed to acid-pepsin attack, exciting an acute inflammatory response. If the protective balance is restored at this early stage, the inflammation will resolve and the epithelium regenerates. Little if any residual damage will result. If, however, the healing balance is not restored, continued acid-pepsin attack on the unprotected submucosa leads to an **acute peptic ulcer**. This tends to become progressively larger and deeper.

From here, there are several possible outcomes. Sometimes the ulcerative process continues virtually

unchecked through the full thickness of the gut wall. The ulcer perforates and intestinal contents escape into the peritoneal cavity resulting in peritonitis. More often, the layer of necrotic slough and acutely inflamed underlying tissue in the ulcer base temporarily resist acid-pepsin attack. This allows granulation tissue to form which initiates the process of fibrous repair. If, for example, acid-reducing drugs are used, the ulcer may heal, leaving a small scar with normal overlying mucosa. Usually, however, a tenuous balance is established between resistance and attack, matched by an unstable equilibrium between the rate of repair and the rate of tissue destruction. A **chronic peptic ulcer** then results which may persist for many years, its size and symptoms varying as mucosal resistance and exacerbating factors fluctuate.

If local or systemic factors change and swing the balance in favour of repair, the lesion may heal completely. On the mucosal surface, the healed ulcer site is usually puckered by scar contraction in the muscular wall. Externally, the serosa is thickened and may adhere to adjacent structures. If scarring occurs in a narrow part of the tract, i.e. the lower oesophagus or pyloric region, the lumen may become even narrower to produce a stricture, and subsequent acute mucosal inflammation and swelling may then precipitate obstruction. If healing does not occur at all, a chronic ulcer may slowly enlarge and

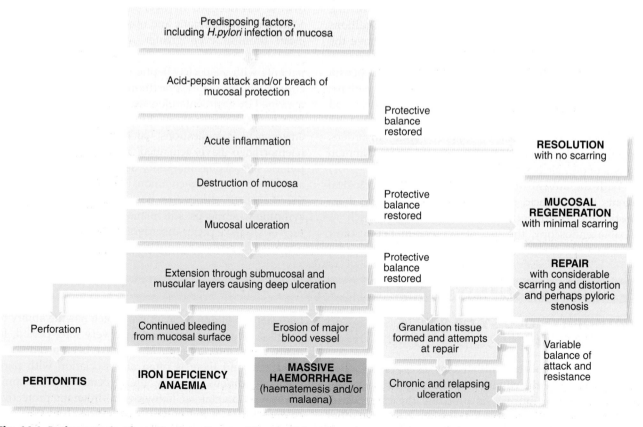

Fig. 14.1 Pathogenesis of peptic ulceration and its possible outcomes

deepen. Continual bleeding from the ulcer may cause anaemia (p. 160) or ulceration may erode into a large blood vessel causing major haemorrhage (see Fig. 14.2), or perforate into the peritoneal cavity.

EPIDEMIOLOGY AND AETIOLOGY OF PEPTIC ULCER DISEASE

THE SIZE OF THE PROBLEM

Chronic peptic disease is very common in developed countries, affecting around 10% of the population at some time in their lives. Duodenal ulcer seems to have a natural history characterised by recurrent attacks over 5–10 years then a gradual spontaneous remission. About 15% of patients have severe symptoms and aggressive disease. Peptic ulceration is quite rare in developing rural communities which may suggest stress or other factors associated with modern life as additional factors in the disease. In many sufferers, symptoms are trivial or sporadic and settle either spontaneously or with the help of antacids. Medical advice may never be sought.

SITES OF PEPTIC ULCERATION (see Fig. 14.3)

Stomach and duodenum

Around 98% of all chronic peptic ulcers occur in either the duodenum or stomach, and sometimes both at the

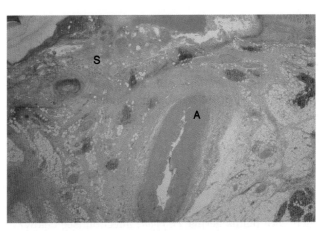

Fig. 14.2 Bleeding gastric ulcer—histopathology
Post-mortem specimen showing the base of a bleeding duodenal ulcer. The inflammatory process has destroyed the mucosa, submucosa and most of the muscle wall, these being replaced by ulcer slough **S**. The ulcer has eroded into a medium-sized artery **A**. The patient died from massive haemorrhage.

same time. The most common sites are in the **first part of the duodenum** (duodenal bulb) or the **gastric antrum**, particularly along the lesser curve. A chronic **stomal ulcer** may also appear at the margin of a surgically created communication between stomach and intestine (gastroenterostomy).

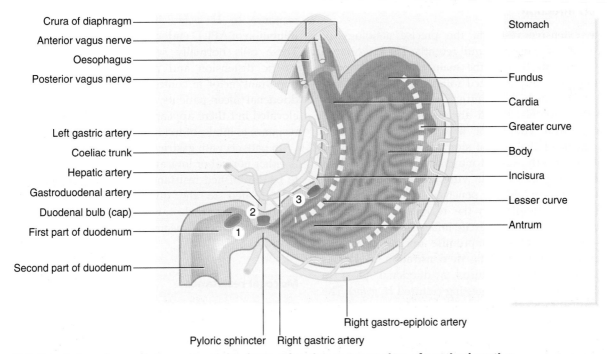

Fig. 14.3 Surgical anatomy of stomach and duodenum showing common sites of peptic ulceration
Acid secretion by the gastric mucosa is controlled by two mechanisms: **(a)** the vagus nerve stimulates acid secretion by the parietal cells (cholinergic stimulation) and **(b)** gastrin (produced by the APUD cells in the antrum) promotes secretion of acid and pepsin by the parietal and peptic cells of the fundus and body. The second is mediated via H_2 receptors. **(1)** marks the common site for duodenal ulcers which may be anterior or posterior; **(2)** the site of pyloric channel ulcers; and **(3)** the common site of lesser curve gastric ulcers.

In the rare **Zollinger–Ellison syndrome**, a gastrin-secreting tumour of pancreatic origin overstimulates acid-pepsin production and causes severe and widespread peptic ulceration. The ulcers commonly involve stomach and duodenum and extend into the second part of the duodenum or even further distally.

Oesophagus

Peptic inflammation and superficial ulceration may involve the lower oesophagus and it is almost always secondary to acid-pepsin reflux, which is often associated with hiatus hernia. *H. pylori* infection (see below) is probably not an important factor here. Reflux causes intermittent destruction of the lower oesophageal mucosa by acid or bile or both, causing **linear ulceration** and prompting vigorous attempts at healing. One outcome is replacement of the normal squamous epithelium with metaplastic columnar mucosa. This is known as **Barrett's oesophagus** and is the only known predisposing factor for adenocarcinoma of the lower oesophagus, a condition that has increased by 70% over the last 20 years (see Ch. 15, p. 231). Chronic peptic ulcers, similar to gastro-duodenal ulcers, may also develop at the lower end of the oesophagus.

AETIOLOGICAL FACTORS IN PEPTIC DISEASE

H. pylori infection

Despite extensive research, the precise aetiology of peptic ulcers was obscure until recently. The importance of *H. pylori* infection as the main initiating factor is becoming gradually accepted following the pioneering work of Dr Mitchell in Perth, Australia, in the early 1980s. Prior to this, it had always been believed that microorganisms could not live in the highly acid environment of the normal stomach. However, gastric biopsies frequently showed intramucosal bacteria, which were eventually cultured in vitro. These spiral-shaped organisms appear able to penetrate protective surface mucus and accumulate in the region of intercellular junctions. There they may excite inflammation, stimulate excess acid-pepsin or compromise normal protective mechanisms. In a dramatic demonstration of Koch's postulates, Mitchell produced a duodenal ulcer in himself, a few days after ingesting cultured *H. pylori*. The ulcer proved to be *H. pylori*-positive on biopsy and was cured by anti-*Helicobacter* antibiotic therapy.

The jigsaw began to fit together when it was found that peptic ulcers could regularly be successfully treated with a combination of bismuth and antibiotics. Later work showed that *H. pylori* infection in duodenal ulcer patients was associated with a sixfold increase in gastric

acid production which remitted when the infection was eliminated. There is now evidence that *H. pylori* is carcinogenic, initiating certain types of gastric lymphoma and some cases of gastric cancer. The broad picture is now apparent; *H. pylori* causes a chronic infection with complications that include gastric and duodenal ulcer, gastric mucosa-associated lymphoma and gastric cancer. Only 2–3% of patients with duodenal or gastric ulcers are *H. pylori*-negative. Tests for *H. pylori* infection include serum **anti-*H. pylori*** IgG, direct tests on gastric biopsies for urease produced by the organism, hydrogen breath tests and histological examination of biopsy specimens.

Further details of this fascinating story remain to be worked out; for example, why not all patients with *H. pylori* infection develop upper gastrointestinal lesions, and why not all patients with gastric cancer have been exposed to *H. pylori*.

Acid-pepsin production

Parietal cells secrete acid in direct or indirect response to acetylcholine, gastrin and histamine. It is likely that the common mediator is histamine. The final common pathway for hydrogen ion secretion is via activation of a specific enzyme, H^+/K^+ ATPase, which exchanges hydrogen ions generated in the parietal cell for potassium ions in the gastric lumen. In **duodenal ulceration**, the fundamental abnormality appears to be excessive production of acid-pepsin by the stomach, both basal (i.e. overnight) and stimulated. This may be a defensive response to *H. pylori* infection mediated via a de-inhibition of APUD endocrine cells of the gastric antrum. These cells normally secrete **gastrin** in response to gastric distension and protein ingestion and are an important factor in controlling acid-pepsin secretion. In duodenal ulcer patients, resting gastrin levels are not elevated but there appears to be an exaggerated gastrin response to intake of food.

In patients with **gastric ulcers**, measured acid secretion is either normal or low, and the essential problem seems to be diminished resistance to acid-pepsin attack, probably related to the quantity or quality of mucus produced. Nevertheless, reduction of acid production by medical or surgical means is effective in healing gastric ulcers.

Mucosal resistance

There are several mechanisms which protect the upper gastrointestinal mucosa against autodigestion. Somatostatin and prostaglandins are inhibitors of parietal cell secretion and the latter have other cytoprotective properties. Two forms of mucus, soluble and insoluble, are secreted continuously by gastric and duodenal mucosa; they contain bicarbonate and together maintain the cell surface pH at neutrality. Mucosal blood flow probably plays an important part by removing hydrogen ions which back-diffuse into the cells.

With increasing age, there is reduced turnover of surface cells and generalised mild mucosal atrophy, which might explain why the incidence of gastric ulcers rises with age. Non-steroidal anti-inflammatory drugs (NSAIDs) prescribed for arthritic disorders are commonly and increasingly identified as the causative factor for acute presentations of peptic ulceration. NSAIDs probably have their greatest effect systemically via their blocking effects on prostaglandin production which has several cytoprotective properties. Indeed, in elderly patients presenting with upper gastrointestinal bleeding or perforation, ulceration may occur after only a few tablets have been taken, or at any stage during a long period of medication. This risk is not diminished by enteric-coated preparations, nor by administration by routes other than orally. The risk of NSAID-induced ulceration increases steeply in later life. All of these drugs have been incriminated and their power to provoke peptic ulceration is in direct proportion to their effectiveness at relieving arthritic symptoms. A history of 'indigestion' in patients taking NSAIDs must be taken seriously.

Other mucosal irritants

Alcohol, aspirin and other NSAIDs are all known to induce acute mucosal inflammation directly (**acute gastritis**). In a susceptible individual, the inflammation may persist, resulting in chronic ulceration. Prolonged heavy alcohol intake is also a recognised risk factor. Reflux of pancreatic digestive enzymes back through the pylorus may also play a part, and is probably caused by defective pyloric closure. Another possible factor is antral stasis (perhaps also caused by abnormal pyloric function), leading to increased gastrin secretion. The area of the junction between parietal and antral cells on the lesser curvature of the stomach has been noted to be particularly vulnerable to gastric ulceration, although the reason is not understood.

Smoking

Cigarette smoking is twice as common in patients with chronic peptic ulcer disease as in the general population. Its pathogenic role is attributed to increased vagal activity, and its effect on producing relative gastric mucosal ischaemia. Cessation of smoking, however, greatly assists in the healing of peptic ulcers.

INVESTIGATION AND CLINICAL FEATURES OF PEPTIC DISORDERS

INVESTIGATION OF SUSPECTED PEPTIC ULCER DISEASE

The diagnosis and management of peptic disorders relies mainly on flexible endoscopy which revolutionised the process after its introduction in the late 1960s. Barium meal contrast radiography has largely been superseded for this purpose.

ENDOSCOPY

Oesophago-gastro-duodenoscopy, also known as OGD or gastroscopy, involves visual examination of the mucosa using a steerable, flexible endoscope. Gastroscopy enables direct and comprehensive examination of the whole area of the upper gastrointestinal tract which is prone to peptic ulcer disease.

In peptic ulcer disease, gastroscopy has definite advantages over contrast radiography, which by its nature can only demonstrate substantial structural abnormalities and then only as two-dimensional images. Shallow mucosal abnormalities such as superficial ulceration or vascular malformations are invisible on barium meal but can be directly inspected and diagnosed from their endoscopic appearance. Distortion resulting from

previous disease or surgery often interferes with radiological interpretation. This too can usually be overcome by endoscopic inspection.

Benign gastric or oesophageal ulceration can be reliably distinguished from malignancy if endoscopic biopsies are taken from several places around the ulcer edge. In patients with peptic disorders, biopsies of distal gastric mucosa are now taken routinely to investigate *H. pylori* infection.

In acute upper gastrointestinal haemorrhage, gastroscopy is almost mandatory, as described in Chapter 12, p. 185. Gastroscopy can identify the site of the bleeding and is particularly useful if gastro-oesophageal varices are suspected to be the source of bleeding. Gastroscopy also allows recognition of features which can help stratify patients into low or high risk of rebleeding and provides an important means of treating bleeding sites by injection of vasoconstrictors or sclerosants.

CONTRAST RADIOLOGY

Contrast radiography of the upper gastrointestinal tract involves the patient swallowing barium suspension (**barium meal**). Its passage is followed through the upper gastrointestinal tract by fluoroscopic imaging, with points of special diagnostic importance recorded on film or electronically. During the investigation, the patient is tilted and rolled in various directions to demonstrate the whole region of interest. Effervescent tablets are given to produce gaseous distension of the stomach and duodenum and spread the contrast in a thin, even layer over the mucosal surface. This standard **double contrast technique** improves the imaging of mucosal detail, particularly when the duodenum is relaxed by giving intravenous anticholinergic drugs such as hyoscine butylbromide.

PRESENTING FEATURES OF PEPTIC ULCER DISEASE

The various ways in which peptic inflammation affects the oesophagus, stomach and duodenum are summarised in Table 14.1.

Epigastric pain (usually described as 'boring', 'gnawing' or 'burning') is the principal presenting symptom and is common to peptic disorders whatever the site. Pain is often accompanied by other forms of discomfort, often

Table 14.1 Clinical consequences of peptic ulcer disease in different anatomical sites

Pathological process	Clinical lesion	Symptoms
Oesophagus		
Transient acid-pepsin reflux	Mild reversible acute inflammation, i.e. transient oesophagitis	Burning retrosternal pain (i.e. 'heartburn')
Recurrent acid-pepsin reflux or failure of oesophagus to expel acid by peristalsis (often found in hiatus hernia)	Episodes of acute inflammation, i.e. reflux oesophagitis—probably reversible with no scarring. Chronic low-grade blood loss	Recurrent epigastric and retrosternal pain. Chronic iron deficiency anaemia may occur
Persistent severe reflux	Continuous severe inflammation with superficial ulceration. May lead to chronic ulceration and/or stricture	Severe retrosternal pain, dysphagia and sometimes recurrent small haematemeses
Stomach		
Acute gastric irritation, e.g. by NSAIDs or alcohol	Acute (reversible) mucosal inflammation, i.e. acute gastritis or erosive/haemorrhagic gastritis	Epigastric pain, vomiting, acute upper gastrointestinal bleeding
Acute reduction in mucosal resistance provoked by visceral ischaemia or the systemic inflammatory response syndrome (usually in intensive therapy unit patients or after burns)	Widespread superficial gastric ulceration	May bleed uncontrollably or perforate
Chronic *H. pylori* infection, probably with longstanding diminished resistance to acid-pepsin attack, with or without extrinsic irritation	Chronic or recurrent gastric ulceration	Epigastric pain—characteristically exacerbated by food (especially if acid or spicy), anorexia and weight loss. Symptoms of chronic anaemia
Duodenum		
Episodic acid-pepsin attack	Acute (reversible) mucosal inflammation, i.e. duodenitis	Episodic epigastric pain
Chronic *H. pylori* infection, probably with persistent acid-pepsin attack	Duodenal ulceration (may involve pyloric canal)	Epigastric pain —typically relieved by food and occurring several hours after food, especially at night
Pre-existing duodenal scarring causing pyloric stenosis with superadded acute inflammation and mucosal swelling	Complete pyloric obstruction	Symptoms of chronic anaemia. Severe vomiting, dehydration, shock, gross electrolyte disturbance (hypochloraemic alkalosis)
Both stomach and duodenum		
Periodic loss of protective equilibrium	Recurrent ulceration	Intermittent symptomatic episodes
Erosion of a major vessel in ulcer floor	Severe haemorrhage	Massive haematemesis or melaena
Unchecked ulceration	Perforation and peritonitis	Acute severe abdominal pain and shock

described by the patient as 'indigestion' or 'dyspepsia'. A more specific description may suggest particular diagnostic entities. Retrosternal pain ('heartburn') suggests reflux oesophagitis, whereas bitter regurgitation ('waterbrash') is characteristic of both oesophageal reflux and duodenal ulceration. Nausea or vomiting, anorexia (loss of appetite) and abdominal fullness or bloating are common in gastric ulcer and pyloric stenosis, but may also occur in a variety of other upper gastrointestinal disorders, e.g. gallstone disease and irritable bowel syndrome.

The relationship of symptoms to food intake may help to distinguish gastric from duodenal ulceration; gastric ulcer pain is typically exacerbated by food and duodenal ulcer pain relieved by it.

Untreated peptic disorders are by nature protracted, with exacerbations and remissions over weeks or months. Symptoms tend to follow the disease activity and often wax and wane over many years before finally remitting.

Peptic ulcers may be virtually asymptomatic, particularly those caused by NSAIDs. Recognition then depends on acute presentation with bleeding or perforation or on investigation of iron deficiency anaemia. Asymptomatic peptic ulceration should always be suspected if there is no obvious cause for anaemia.

NON-ACUTE CLINICAL PRESENTATIONS OF PEPTIC ULCER DISEASE

PEPTIC DISORDERS OF THE OESOPHAGUS

Reflux of gastric contents is associated with all peptic disorders of the oesophagus. These range from mild reversible inflammation, through moderate acute inflammation with superficial ulceration (**reflux oesophagitis**), to severe persistent inflammation. The latter may lead to **fibrotic scarring and stenosis** (see Fig. 14.4) and sometimes **chronic peptic ulceration**. In many patients, reflux is associated with hiatus hernia (see Ch. 15, p. 230) but in the remainder, the mechanism of the damaging reflux is poorly understood.

Barium meal examination is often more useful than gastroscopy for demonstrating strictures, hiatus hernia or the existence of gross reflux and the relationship of abnormalities to the level of the diaphragm; both investigations are usually necessary.

On gastroscopy, reflux oesophagitis is characterised by mucosal reddening and in more severe cases, by typical linear superficial ulceration (see Fig. 14.5). Peptic strictures occur only in the last few centimetres of the distal oesophagus and are recognised if the lumen is found to be too narrow to allow the endoscope to pass. The stricture is usually located just above the oesophago-gastric junction, which often lies above the diaphragm because of inflammatory shortening of the oesophagus. The normal oesophago-gastric junction is about 40 cm from the incisor teeth when seen on endoscopy. The mucosa near the stricture varies in the amount of inflammation and ulceration present. Specialised intestinal metaplasia, dysplasia and carcinoma must be excluded by biopsies because the visual appearances may not be characteristic. Occasionally, a deep chronic ulcer occurs in the lower oesophagus; this looks and behaves like a gastric or duodenal ulcer. When squamous oesophageal epithelium is repeatedly damaged by reflux, it may be replaced by metaplastic columnar epithelium. This is known as **Barrett's oesophagus** and there is strong evidence that it predisposes to malignant change. If found, it should be biopsied to exclude dysplasia. When dysplasia is severe, there is about a 1% annual risk of malignant change and continued surveillance or surgery is needed.

PEPTIC DISORDERS OF THE STOMACH

Peptic disorders of the stomach range from mild inflammation (**gastritis**) to **chronic gastric ulcers**, and most often occur in the antral region and along the lesser curve beyond the incisura.

Chronic gastric ulcers must be distinguished from malignant ulcers. The site may aid recognition of a benign ulcer, but carcinoma may occur in any part of the stomach, although the region of the gastro-oesophageal junction is now the most common site of gastric carcinoma. Malignancy can only be excluded by histological examination of multiple representative biopsies taken from around the ulcer circumference (not the base) or by examining the whole ulcer in a resection specimen. In most cases, carcinoma probably arises de novo but occasionally a benign ulcer may undergo malignant transformation.

GASTRITIS

Gastritis can only be proved by endoscopy and appears as widespread reddening of the mucosa. The inflamed mucosa is often awash with bile, and the condition is sometimes referred to as 'biliary gastritis' on the assumption that it is caused by the irritant effect of biliary and pancreatic secretions. Acute gastritis, often caused by alcohol (chronic alcoholism or single alcoholic binges) or aspirin ingestion, can cause symptoms of sufficient severity to warrant gastroscopy. The mucosa often exhibits patchy shallow ulceration (erosive gastritis) and is friable and easily traumatised, causing bleeding.

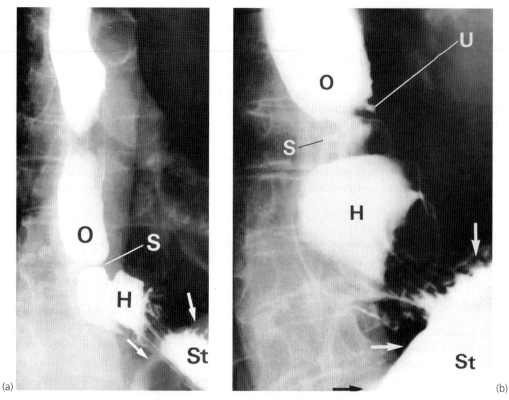

(a)   (b)

Fig. 14.4 Peptic stricture of the oesophagus
(a) A barium swallow in a 60-year-old woman who complained of burning retrosternal pain when lying flat (present for several years) and the recent onset of pain and difficulty when swallowing solid foods. The X-rays show the lower end of the oesophagus **O** and stomach **St**, part of which lies above the level of the diaphragm (position arrowed), forming a sliding hiatus hernia **H**. There is a tight stenosis in the last 2 cm of the oesophagus due to a peptic stricture **S**. **(b)** At greater magnification, barium can be seen filling the crater of a chronic peptic ulcer **U** immediately above the stricture.

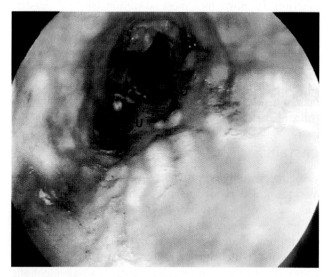

Fig. 14.5 Reflux oesophagitis
Gastroscopic view of the lower end of the oesophagus in a woman of 62 with a long history of reflux. Note the patchy ulceration **U** and the irregular fibrotic cardia caused by recurrent ulceration and attempts at healing. Further scarring may cause stricture formation.

STRESS ULCERS

Acute 'stress' ulcers are single or multiple small discrete superficial lesions that may develop rapidly in seriously ill patients. This condition may be a complication of extensive burns, systemic sepsis (possibly via visceral hypoperfusion), multiple trauma, major head injuries, uraemia or terminal illness. Stress ulcers typically present with haemorrhage (**haemorrhagic gastritis**) which is sometimes catastrophic, and occasionally with perforation. There is minimal mucosal inflammation around the ulcers and the aetiology may be primarily mucosal ischaemia rather than peptic. The risk of this life-threatening complication can be minimised in vulnerable patients by prophylactic treatment with mucosal protective agents, e.g. sucralfate.

CHRONIC GASTRIC ULCERATION

Chronic gastric ulcers vary greatly in size but the majority are small (less than 2 cm in diameter). **Giant ulcers** (up to 10 cm) are occasionally seen in the elderly; if posteriorly situated, they may erode through the stomach wall, obliterating the lesser sac and adhering to the surface of the pancreas (Fig. 14.7b). In these cases, the ulcer base or floor is composed of pancreatic tissue and catastrophic haemorrhage may occur. Often symptoms prior to the acute event are minimal.

Benign gastric ulcers are typically regular in outline with a base consisting of white fibrinous slough. The ulcer gives the impression of having been punched out of the gastric wall, and there is no heaping-up of the mucosal margin as seen in malignant ulcers. The surrounding mucosa is surprisingly normal, although there may be radiating folds resulting from fibrotic contractures. The typical endoscopic appearance of a gastric ulcer is shown in Figure 14.6(a) and the barium meal appearance in Figure 14.7.

Peptic disorders of the stomach typically cause severe, often disabling, epigastric pain which tends to be exacerbated by food, especially if acidic or spicy. The pain may be so severe that patients lose weight and develop a fear of food. Symptoms tend to persist for weeks or months, fluctuating in intensity and then disappearing completely, only to recur weeks or months later. Symptoms are a poor guide to disease activity or response to treatment. Indeed, major ulcers may be silent. Both can be monitored only by repeated gastroscopy until healing. A rare complication of peptic disease is perforation of a gastric ulcer into the transverse colon. The resulting gastro-colic fistula causes true faecal vomiting.

PEPTIC DISORDERS OF THE DUODENUM

DUODENITIS

Duodenitis, a non-ulcerative form of duodenal inflammation, has a similar endoscopic appearance to gastritis. It is commonly discovered in patients suspected of having duodenal ulceration, and probably represents a mild form of peptic disease.

CHRONIC DUODENAL ULCERATION

Chronic duodenal ulcers almost exclusively occur in the pyloric channel and the first part of the duodenum. The latter area is known endoscopically as the 'duodenal bulb' and radiologically as the 'duodenal cap'. On endo-

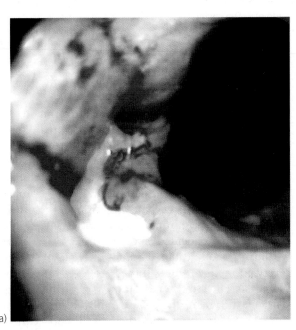

(a)

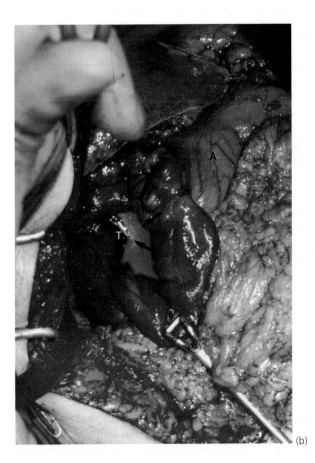

(b)

Fig. 14.6 Peptic ulcers
(a) Lesser curve benign gastric ulcer as seen through a gastroscope. At the original examination, the ulcer could be viewed from several directions and biopsies taken of the edge to exclude malignancy.
(b) Photograph taken at emergency laparotomy for bleeding duodenal ulcer. The gastric antrum is seen at **A**; the pylorus has been opened longitudinally and a deep chronic posterior ulcer crater is identified (arrowed). Thrombus **T** overlying an eroded artery is visible (Dieu-la-foy lesion). A bleeding artery in the ulcer crater was under-run with sutures to arrest the haemorrhage.

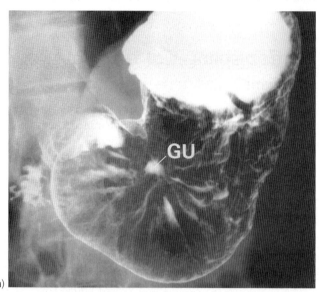

(a)

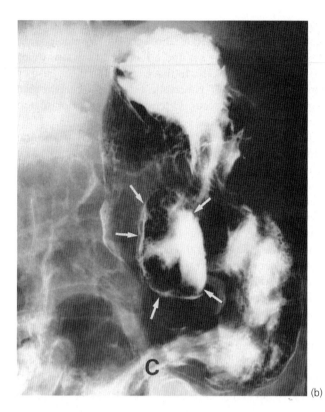

(b)

Fig. 14.7 Chronic gastric ulcer
(a) Double contrast barium meal in a 54-year-old man with a 6-month history of epigastric pain after meals. A gastric ulcer crater **GU** containing barium is seen on the lesser curve. Abnormal folds of gastric mucosa radiate out from the ulcer. Endoscopy and biopsy are indicated to exclude malignancy. **(b)** Barium meal in an 88-year-old woman who suffered a haematemesis. The patient had been taking non-steroidal anti-inflammatory drugs for several months. The X-ray shows a giant gastric ulcer (outline arrowed) on the lesser curve, partly filled with barium.

scopy, duodenal ulcers have a range of appearances similar to chronic gastric ulcers. There is usually a single ulcer but two or more ulcers at one time are common ('kissing ulcers'). Malignancy is very rare in the duodenal bulb, so biopsy of the ulcer for this purpose is seldom necessary; biopsy of the gastric antrum for confirmation of *H. pylori* infections is, however, indicated. The radiological characteristics of duodenal ulcers are shown in Figure 14.8.

Duodenal ulcer symptoms follow the same general pattern as for gastric ulcer but with important exceptions. The pain tends to appear several hours after a meal ('hunger pain') and is relieved by eating. A typical history includes episodic early morning waking (often around 2 a.m.) with epigastric pain; this pain is relieved by drinking milk and eating bland foods. Consequently, patients tend to gain weight from the increased intake of food and milk. This is in contrast to the weight loss often associated with gastric ulcer. Symptoms in duodenal ulcer are more useful as a guide to disease activity and response to treatment than in gastric ulcer; this, and together with the rare association with malignancy, removes the need for regular gastroscopic follow-up in most cases of duodenal ulcer.

NON-ULCER DYSPEPSIA

This condition is by far the most common set of symptoms in patients with upper abdominal pain. The cause is unknown and the diagnosis is made by excluding peptic ulcer disease and other organic diseases on the basis of a very long history, atypical symptoms and, if appropriate, negative gastroscopy. There is probably a range of causative mechanisms, from 'excess acid' to irritable bowel syndrome. Treatment is generally supportive. Some patients respond to mild antacids, others to dietary modification and yet others to changes in lifestyle to reduce stress. If they are *H. pylori*-positive on biopsy or other test, eradication is probably indicated, particularly where there is a family history of gastric carcinoma. Unfortunately, there is a poor correlation between elimination of infection and relief of symptoms.

MANAGEMENT OF CHRONIC PEPTIC ULCER DISEASE

Both the nature and the management of peptic ulcer disease have undergone extraordinary changes over the

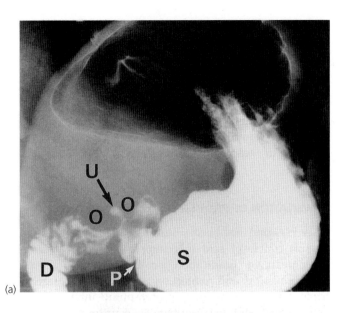
(a)

Fig. 14.8 Chronic duodenal ulceration

Barium meal examinations; stomach marked **S**, duodenum **D** and pylorus **P** in **(a)** and **(b)**. **(a)** A 35-year-old man complaining of epigastric pain at night and before meals. The X-ray shows a deep chronic duodenal ulcer **U** with contrast filling the ulcer crater; on either side are large areas free of contrast **O** caused by a ring of oedematous duodenal mucosa surrounding the ulcer. **(b)** Two contrast-filled duodenal ulcers **U** in a 50-year-old male who smoked heavily. Note the otherwise normal duodenal appearance. **(c)** Endoscopic view of lesser curve gastric ulcer. This ulcer has probably only been present for about 4 months. It does not show surrounding scarring and distortion of the gastric wall that would be characteristic of long standing ulcers.

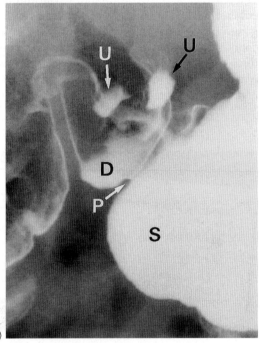
(b)

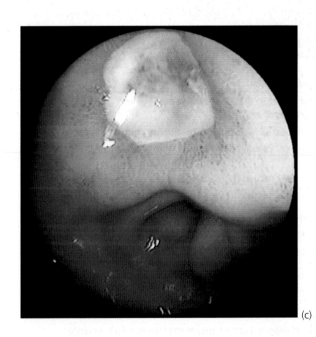
(c)

past four decades. The aim of treatment has always been to heal the ulcer with the minimum harm or inconvenience to the patient and with the lowest risk of recurrence. Several decades ago, medical management was relatively ineffective and was largely confined to antacid drugs, bland diets and bed rest. The only definitive treatment was major surgery and it was widely employed, often after a long period of chronic symptoms. Surgery was deferred as long as possible in the hope of spontaneous remission, and patients often had to 'earn' their operations by years of suffering! Partial gastrectomy offered the best cure rate and was

thus the most common operation despite its mortality of 2–10% and its serious long-term complication rate. Later, various versions of vagotomy were shown to be almost equally effective, but with fewer complications.

The principles of modern management of peptic disorders are summarised in Box 14.1.

CONTROL OF PREDISPOSING OR AGGRAVATING CAUSES

The patient's history may reveal adverse factors which can be easily eliminated. These are summarised at the start of Box 14.1. Radical dietary modification is unnecessary; patients should merely be advised to avoid food which they find aggravates the symptoms. Spicy or acidic foods are often blamed.

Aspirin and other NSAIDs should be avoided, although this is often difficult in patients with arthritic disorders; the detrimental effect of these drugs is greatest in the elderly, the main sufferers from arthritis. The ulcerogenic effect of these drugs is directly proportional to their effectiveness and relates largely to their systemic anti-cyclo-oxygenase activity. There is therefore little to be gained from changing drugs within the group or by using them in enteric-coated or suppository form. If NSAIDs cannot be avoided in patients with a predisposition to peptic ulceration, concurrent use of cytoprotective drugs may be indicated.

Recently introduced specific **cyclo-oxygenase 2 inhibitors (COX-2)** hold out a better hope of avoiding adverse NSAID effects on the upper gastrointestinal tract. COX-1 is an enzyme present throughout the body that initiates the production of prostaglandins, key mediators in both health and disease. COX-2, on the other hand, is an inducible form of the enzyme present at very low levels in normal tissues; in disease, it stimulates production of prostaglandins that mediate inflammation and pain.

Patients with oesophageal reflux, especially if associated with hiatus hernia, can minimise the damage by simple mechanical measures such as losing weight, elevating the head end of the bed and avoiding stooping.

ELIMINATION OF PROVEN *H. PYLORI* INFECTION

Once *H. pylori* has been confirmed, treatment involves a short course of acid inhibition combined with antibiotic treatment. Eradication usually produces long-term ulcer remission, and reinfection with *H. pylori* is rare. A triple regimen including a proton-pump inhibitor (e.g. omeprazole) and two antibiotics (clarithromycin plus either amoxycillin or metronidazole) given for 1 week gives *Helicobacter* elimination in over 90%. Longer courses give potentially higher elimination rates but produce more side effects and lower compliance. Confirmation of eradication can be achieved by re-endoscopy and rapid urease testing, or by breath-hydrogen analysis.

SUMMARY

Box 14.1 Principles of management of peptic disorders

Control of predisposing or aggravating causes
- Modify diet, reduce alcohol intake, cease smoking, avoid irritant and ulcer-provoking drugs (aspirin and other NSAIDs), avoid stress, reduce oesophageal reflux by losing weight and attention to posture

Elimination of proven *H. pylori* infection
- Triple therapy with anti-acid, bismuth and antibiotic combinations

Diminishing of irritant effects of acid-pepsin
- Simple antacid drugs, alginate preparations, liquorice derivatives, bismuth preparations

Administration of mucosal protective agents
- Sucralfate

Reduction of acid secretion
- H_2-receptor-blocking drugs (cimetidine, ranitidine), proton pump inhibitors (PPIs, e.g. omeprazole), surgical vagotomy (rarely employed nowadays)

Surgical removal of intractable ulcers and gastrin-secreting tissue
- Partial gastrectomy

Correction of secondary anatomical problems
- Dilatation of oesophageal strictures, operations for pyloric stenosis

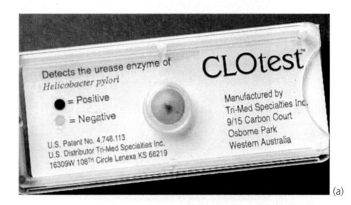

(a)

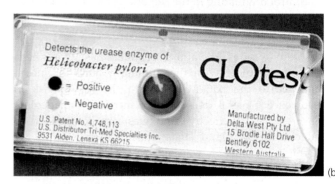

(b)

Fig. 14.9 Proprietary urease testing kit for *H. pylori*
Biopsies of gastric or duodenal mucosa are placed in the well and the result read after a set period. A positive results is indicated by the colour change seen here in **(b)**.

DIMINISHING OF IRRITANT EFFECTS OF ACID-PEPSIN

An array of proprietary antacid preparations is available over the counter and on prescription. When used assiduously, they promote ulcer healing almost as effectively as any other drug, although more slowly. The main active ingredients are few. **Sodium bicarbonate** offers rapid but temporary relief of symptoms, while **magnesium trisilicate** or **aluminium hydroxide** promotes ulcer healing. Some of these agents, however, interfere with proton pump inhibitors. **Colloidal bismuth compounds** have been in use for many years. They have an antacid action and have been found to be active against *H. pylori*.

Alginate preparations form a foamy layer on the surface of gastric contents, coating the upper stomach and lower oesophagus and protecting it from oesophageal reflux.

ADMINISTRATION OF MUCOSAL PROTECTIVE AGENTS

Sucralfate is a complex of aluminium hydroxide and sulphated sucrose that is minimally absorbed from the gastrointestinal tract. It is believed to act by binding to denuded areas of mucosa and protecting them from acid-pepsin attack. It has been shown to be as effective as H_2-blockers in providing symptom relief and healing when given in the dose of 2 g twice daily. It does not interfere with other drugs and is safe in pregnancy. It is also effective for preventing stress ulcers in seriously ill patients.

REDUCTION OF ACID SECRETION

Acid secretion by the gastric mucosa is normally controlled by two mechanisms:

- Direct cholinergic stimulation of parietal cells mediated via the **vagus nerve**. This is under reflex control originating in the cerebral cortex triggered by the sight and taste of food
- Gastrin is secreted by APUD cells in the gastric antrum and promotes acid secretion via histamine released from mast cells in the vicinity of the parietal cells. The histamine receptors on the parietal cells are distinct from those elsewhere in the body and are designated as **type 2 (H_2) receptors**; these receptors are not blocked by standard 'antihistamine' drugs such as chlorpheniramine. Gastrin secretion is partly controlled by the vagus and partly by local (vagally independent) reflexes initiated by gastric distension and the presence of food or alcohol in the stomach

From this, two practical methods have been found to reduce acid secretion: drugs which selectively block H_2-receptors or the proton pump mechanism (described earlier), and surgical division of the vagus nerve.

H_2-receptor blockade and proton pump antagonists

H_2-receptor blocking drugs were developed in the 1970s and were the first 'medical' revolution in the management of peptic disorders as sole therapy. **Cimetidine** was alone in the market for several years but was joined by **ranitidine**, which has a few minor advantages but is no more effective for healing ulcers. H_2-receptor antagonists are highly effective in reducing gastric acid secretion. Symptomatic response is rapid, usually within a day or two, and healing follows within a few weeks in 70–90% of cases. Recurrence rates, however, are high, with 50–75% recurring within 2 years even with maintenance therapy.

A newer group of drugs, the substituted **benzimidazoles**, are extremely potent and reduce acid production to near-zero by direct inhibition of the proton pump. **Omeprazole** is the best known member of this group and is often employed for oesophagitis, recurrent ulcers and Zollinger–Ellison syndrome. Where *H. pylori* infection is present, the use of these drugs alone is not recommended as the recurrence rate is unacceptably high.

Vagotomy

Vagotomy was first performed in the 1920s and popularised by Dragstedt from 1943. It gradually superseded classic partial gastrectomy as the surgical treatment of choice for chronic duodenal ulcer. The various vagotomy operations illustrated in Figure 14.10 are now only of historical interest. The simplest involved dividing the anterior and posterior vagal trunks close to the abdominal oesophagus just below the diaphragm (**truncal vagotomy**). The operation is effective in promoting ulcer healing but paralyses gastric motility and slows pyloric emptying. A surgical **drainage procedure**, usually **pyloroplasty** ('V & P'), less commonly **gastro-jejunostomy**, was therefore a necessary part of the operation.

Attempts to reduce the gastric emptying complications of truncal vagotomy led to operations designed to preserve the innervation of the distal antrum and pylorus whilst denervating the proximal acid-secreting portion of the stomach. **Highly selective vagotomy** preserves the nerves of Latarjet and avoids the need for a gastric drainage procedure. Early postoperative side effects are fewer but ulcer recurrence rate is higher than for truncal vagotomy.

All surgical treatments for duodenal ulcer were eclipsed by the introduction of the H_2-blockers and the operate rate is now only 1% of that of four decades ago. The vagotomies are now occasionally employed for chronic symptomatic duodenal ulceration that recurs after effective elimination therapy; most are performed laparoscopically.

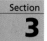

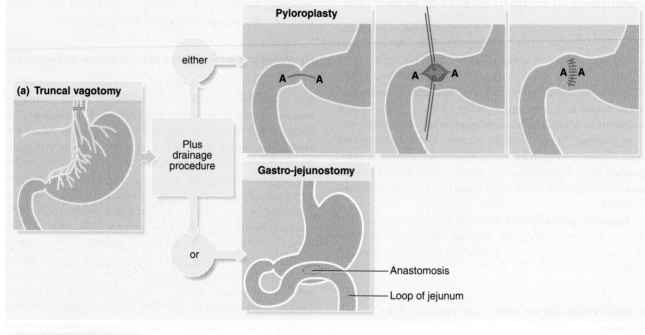

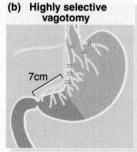

Fig. 14.10 The vagotomies and gastric drainage procedures (rarely performed nowadays but of historical interest)
(a) Truncal vagotomy is followed by a drainage procedure, either pyloroplasty (Heinecke–Mikulicz is illustrated) or gastro-jejunostomy. In gastro-jejunostomy an anastomosis is created to the most dependent part of the stomach; a short efferent loop of jejunum is brought up either in front of the transverse colon and sutured to the anterior wall of the stomach (antecolic), or behind the transverse colon via an incision in the mesentery and sutured to the posterior wall of the stomach (retrocolic). **(b)** Highly selective vagotomy does not require a drainage procedure. Only the parietal cell mass is denervated, preserving the innervation of the pylorus and antrum plus the rest of the abdominal viscera.

SURGICAL REMOVAL OF INTRACTABLE ULCERS AND GASTRIN-SECRETING TISSUE

Partial gastrectomy was occasionally used for patients where medical management had failed to heal a benign gastric ulcer or to treat repeated recurrences. The operation had the dual role of removing the ulcer and the gastrin-secreting mucosa. The classic gastrectomy for chronic gastric ulcer was known as the **Billroth I** type (Billroth, 1881) and involved removing the distal two-thirds of the stomach. The gastric remnant was then anastomosed to the first part of the duodenum (see Fig. 14.11).

The standard partial gastrectomy for duodenal ulcers was a **Polya-type gastrectomy**, also involving resection of the distal two-thirds of the stomach but anastomosing the cut end of the stomach to the side of a loop of proximal jejunum (gastro-jejunostomy). The cut end of the duodenum (duodenal stump) was closed and the ulcer left in situ to heal (see Fig. 14.10). Numerous variations on gastrectomy have been described over the years and many still carry their authors' names, e.g. Polya (1911), Finsterer (1909), Billroth II (1881), Hofmeister (1908), Balfour (1934). The use of eponymous titles to describe particular operations has become somewhat confused but the essential difference is whether the gastric remnant is anastomosed to the duodenum (Billroth I-type) or to a jejunal loop (Polya-type).

In general, partial gastrectomy was highly effective in relieving symptoms and preventing recurrence of peptic disease but long-term side effects were a serious problem affecting 30–40% of patients.

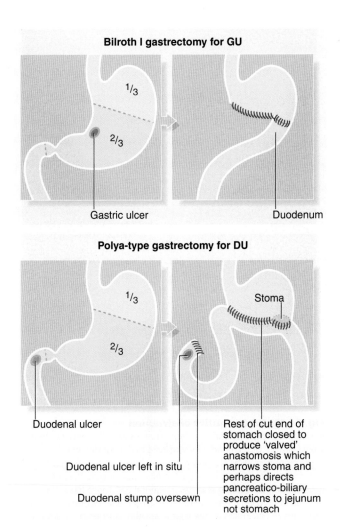

Bilroth I gastrectomy for GU

1/3

2/3

Gastric ulcer

Duodenum

Polya-type gastrectomy for DU

1/3

Stoma

2/3

Duodenal ulcer

Duodenal ulcer left in situ

Duodenal stump oversewn

Rest of cut end of stomach closed to produce 'valved' anastomosis which narrows stoma and perhaps directs pancreatico-biliary secretions to jejunum not stomach

Fig. 14.11 Types of partial gastrectomy formerly performed for peptic ulcer disease

KEY POINTS

Box 14.2 Side effects of partial gastrectomy

- Inability to eat normal-sized meals due to reduced gastric capacity
- 'Dumping' due to rapid emptying of stomach contents—common but most patients adapt with time
- Episodic bilious vomiting due to reflux of bile into stomach via the anastomosis
- Tendency to bolus obstruction of the gastric outlet stoma
- Weight loss due to a combination of above factors and malabsorption—especially common in women
- Vitamin B_{12} deficiency due to loss of gastric intrinsic factor; may presents as macrocytic anaemia or subacute combined degeneration of the spinal cord—potentially catastrophic, occurring many years after operation and preventable by regular vitamin B_{12} (hydroxycobalamin) injections
- Iron deficiency anaemia due to reduced iron absorption—common but easily prevented by taking iron tablets, e.g. once weekly
- Malignant change in gastric remnant possibly due to bacterial production of carcinogens—rare

Complications and side effects of partial gastrectomy

Partial gastrectomy is a major operative procedure yet recovery tends to be surprisingly straightforward. A small proportion of patients develop serious complications such as duodenal stump leakage and anastomotic breakdown. However, the main complications of partial gastrectomy occur in the long term and may not become manifest for years (see Box 14.2). Recurrent ulceration after partial gastrectomy was rare and occurred in the gastric remnant or at the stomal margin. The usual reason was that insufficient stomach had been removed but occasionally malignant change was responsible (3% risk over 15 years). Abnormally high acid production was another cause, sometimes due to Zollinger–Ellison syndrome or hyperparathyroidism.

CORRECTION OF SECONDARY ANATOMICAL PROBLEMS

The main anatomical problems secondary to peptic disease are oesophageal stricture (p. 232) and pyloric stenosis (p. 225).

Oesophageal strictures can usually be managed by periodic dilatation and medical or surgical treatment of the underlying cause. With the patient sedated intravenously, a guide-wire is inserted across the stricture endoscopically, and then metal or plastic dilators are inserted over it. Occasionally, reflux continues to cause damage and stricturing; it may then become necessary to perform anti-reflux surgery.

EMERGENCY PRESENTATIONS OF PEPTIC ULCER DISEASE

The emergency presentations of peptic ulcer disease are acute haemorrhage, perforation and, much less commonly, pyloric stenosis. Peptic ulcer disease was responsible for much major emergency abdominal surgery until the early 1970s. Since then there has been a remarkable reduction in emergency presentations of peptic ulcer and emergency surgery is now a rarity except in elderly patients taking NSAIDs for arthritic symptoms. This change was well under way before the introduction of effective modern drug therapy and can probably be attributed to the progressive improvement in living standards following World War II.

HAEMORRHAGE FROM A PEPTIC ULCER

Acute bleeding from a peptic ulcer presents with haematemesis or melaena or both. Management is discussed in detail in Chapter 12, p. 185.

PERFORATION OF A PEPTIC ULCER

Perforation of a gastric or duodenal ulcer into the peritoneal cavity causes peritonitis. Until about 25 years ago, these perforations were a common cause of an acute abdomen but the incidence has fallen in parallel with the general decline in peptic ulcer disease. Nowadays, as with haemorrhage, perforations of peptic ulcers occur most commonly in elderly patients taking NSAIDs. Occasionally, a younger patient presents with a perforated duodenal ulcer without an obvious predisposing cause.

Duodenal ulcer perforations are two or three times more common than gastric ulcer perforations. The perforation typically occurs on the anterior surface of the duodenal bulb just beyond the pylorus. There is often a short history of NSAID ingestion, but a long history of taking such drugs does not rule them out as an aetiological factor. About half the patients with a peptic ulcer perforation have had recent ulcer symptoms but the other half are asymptomatic.

Gastric ulcer perforations are uncommon and occur only in the elderly. About a third of these are due to perforation of a gastric carcinoma but present in the same way as a perforated peptic ulcer. This explains why the standard surgical treatment for gastric perforation includes excision or extensive biopsy of the ulcer. Oesophageal peptic ulcers occur much less commonly and perforate even more rarely.

CLINICAL PRESENTATION OF PERFORATED PEPTIC ULCER

Perforation of a gastric or duodenal ulcer usually presents as a sudden onset of epigastric pain, rapidly spreading to the whole abdomen. The pain is continuous and is aggravated by moving about. Paradoxically, there may be vomiting of brownish or even blood-stained fluid. On examination, the patient is in obvious pain but is not shocked or toxic.

There is generalised involuntary abdominal guarding,

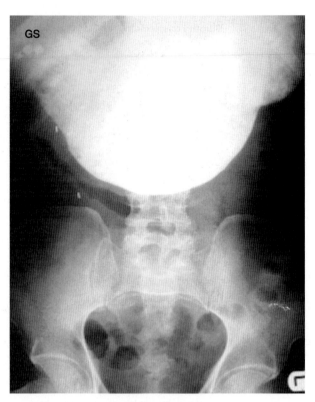

GS

Fig. 14.12 Gastric outlet obstruction
Barium meal examination in a woman of 78 who presented with two weeks history of vomiting. She was grossly dehydrated with a hypochloraemic alkalosis. She was resuscitated and a nasogastric tube passed. This film shows huge gastric dilatation and no flow of barium beyond the pylorus. She also has incidental gallstones **(GS)**. The obstruction proved to be due to chronic duodenal ulceration, but a diagnosis of carcinoma of the gastric antrum must be considered in such a patient.

which in younger patients is so tense as to be described as **'board-like rigidity'**. There is also generalised abdominal tenderness but this may only be detectable on firm palpation because of muscle spasm of the abdominal wall. After several hours, abdominal wall rigidity tends to relax although tenderness remains. In older patients, rigidity is less marked because of a lack of muscle bulk. Peptic ulcer perforation initially causes a chemical, as opposed to bacterial, peritonitis, unlike more distal bowel perforations. This explains the lack of general toxicity in the early stages. If untreated for more than 24 hours, secondary infection may take place and systemic signs appear.

If posterior wall gastric ulcers perforate, they leak gastric contents into the lesser sac, which tends to confine the peritonitis. These patients thus present with more muted symptoms.

DIAGNOSIS OF PERFORATED PEPTIC ULCER

Diagnosis of an upper gastrointestinal perforation can usually be made from the symptoms and signs alone. A plain erect radiograph of the upper abdomen will often reveal gas under the diaphragm, confirming the perforation of a hollow viscus but not its origin. This radiographic evidence of perforation, however, is not always present. If perforation is suspected but the signs are equivocal, an abdominal radiograph may be taken after the patient has swallowed 25 ml of water-soluble contrast; this may confirm the leakage. Diagnostic gastroscopy is contraindicated because the stomach must be inflated during this examination and air and gastric contents would erupt into the peritoneal cavity.

SURGICAL MANAGEMENT OF PEPTIC PERFORATION

Emergency surgery is indicated in nearly all cases of upper gastrointestinal perforation. The patient is first resuscitated and a nasogastric tube inserted. The operation is most commonly performed at laparotomy, but there is increasing interest in a laparoscopic approach for duodenal ulcer perforation. The principles are similar in either case. At surgery, the abdomen is inspected and the diagnosis confirmed. 'Peritoneal toilet' is performed to remove fluid and food contaminating the peritoneal cavity. A perforated duodenal ulcer is usually obvious as a punched-out hole near the pylorus. An anterior gastric perforation is also obvious, but a posterior gastric ulcer is not visible unless the lesser sac is opened, usually along the greater curve.

In duodenal perforation, simple closure of the perforation is the treatment of choice, usually performing biopsies for *H. pylori* testing. This should be followed later by *Helicobacter* eradication therapy.

In perforated gastric ulcer, the classic operation was Billroth I gastrectomy, including the whole ulcer in the resection. However, local excision of the ulcer and simple closure are increasingly employed, provided the ulcer is believed to be benign. In any case, the ulcer edge must be biopsied is several places to be sure.

CONSERVATIVE MANAGEMENT OF PERFORATED DUODENAL ULCER

If an elderly, unfit patient presents late with a perforated duodenal ulcer, many surgeons treat this conservatively. This involves nasogastric aspiration, intravenous fluids, gastric acid suppression and antibiotics. Many of these patients recover satisfactorily but might have succumbed with major surgery.

PYLORIC STENOSIS

The pyloric canal and the immediate pre-pyloric area are common sites of chronic ulceration. Ulcers in this area are probably aetiologically related more closely to duodenal than gastric ulcers and should be managed accordingly. There may be typical symptoms of chronic duodenal ulcer or the presentation may be with pyloric stenosis and a minimal history of ulcer pain. Chronic ulceration near the pylorus causes fibrosis which may progress to stricture formation. In the early stages, this leads to partial gastric outlet obstruction. An acute exacerbation of the ulcer leads to mucosal swelling and pyloric sphincter spasm which then precipitates complete luminal obstruction.

CLINICAL FEATURES OF PYLORIC STENOSIS

These patients rarely give any recent history of peptic ulcer pain but tend to present with a short history (a few weeks at most) of episodic and sometime projectile vomiting. This is unrelated to eating, and the vomitus typically contains foul-smelling semi-digested food eaten a day or more previously. It does not contain bile. Often patients do not seek medical advice until they have become severely dehydrated with gross electrolyte disturbance.

On clinical examination, undernourishment, dehydration, constipation, weakness and weight loss may dominate the picture. Because the stomach is full of residual fluid and food, shaking the patient's abdomen from side to side produces an audible **succussion splash**. Gastric peristalsis may be visible in longstanding cases and a dilated stomach full of residual food may be palpable. On plain abdominal X-ray, it may be possible to see the grossly dilated stomach filled with mottled food material.

Several gastric washouts using a large-bore oral tube will be necessary to clear the gastric residue before endoscopy or barium meal is attempted.

Nowadays, distal gastric cancer is a more common cause of gastric outlet obstruction. With cancer, the obstruction rarely resolves with conservative treatment whereas benign stenoses usually do.

The differential diagnosis of gastric outflow obstruction also includes carcinoma of the head of the pancreas (with or without obstructive jaundice) and, rarely, chronic pancreatitis.

BIOCHEMICAL ABNORMALITIES IN PYLORIC STENOSIS

The biochemical disturbances in these patients are complex and depend on the volume and composition of fluid lost by vomiting and on the body's compensatory mechanisms. Hydrogen and chloride are the principal ions lost in the vomitus. In response, the kidney conserves hydrogen ions by exchanging them for sodium ions (and some potassium ions), which are necessarily lost in the urine. The kidney also conserves chloride ions by exchanging them for bicarbonate ions. The net result may be a profound depletion of total body sodium (which is not accurately reflected in the plasma sodium level), profound hypochloraemia and profound metabolic alkalosis (**hypochloraemic alkalosis**). The plasma urea level is often high as a result of dehydration. Finally, the proportion of ionised calcium in the serum may fall as a result of the alkalosis, inducing tetany.

MANAGEMENT OF PYLORIC STENOSIS

The first management priority in gastric outlet obstruction is resuscitation. Fluid and electrolyte deficiencies are corrected by infusion of physiological saline with added potassium chloride. The volume required often amounts to 10 litres or more. Rehydration will usually return the blood urea level to normal but may unmask an anaemia serious enough to require blood transfusion.

Often the obstruction has a significant inflammatory element, and acid suppression and *Helicobacter* eradication will produce a significant clinical response. If these fail, or malignancy is suspected, endoscopy should be repeated. Operative treatment may then become necessary.

15 Disorders of the oesophagus

INTRODUCTION

Diseases of the oesophagus form a small but significant part of the workload of some general surgeons but the majority of oesophageal surgery is performed in specialised units. Most cases are managed by medical gastroenterologists except those likely to require surgery, when close collaboration between medical and surgical specialists is needed.

Difficulty in swallowing, **dysphagia**, is the most common presenting symptom. **Reflux oesophagitis** and other peptic disorders of the lower oesophagus (often associated with hiatus hernia) and **oesophageal carcinomas** are the main conditions encountered. **Achalasia** and **pharyngeal pouch** are occasionally seen; **oesophageal web** (as in Plummer–Vinson syndrome) and **leiomyoma** (see Ch. 16, p. 242) are extremely rare.

Oesophageal varices secondary to cirrhosis usually present as massive haematemesis. Surgical treatment is seldom required; most acute cases are now managed with non-surgical therapy.

CARCINOMA OF THE OESOPHAGUS

PATHOLOGY AND CLINICAL FEATURES OF OESOPHAGEAL CARCINOMA

The oesophagus is lined by stratified squamous epithelium and thus the majority of oesophageal malignancies are **squamous carcinomas**. The rest are **adenocarcinomas**, probably derived from metaplastic intestinal mucosa, i.e. Barrett's oesophagus (see p. 231), and occur in the lower third of the oesophagus. Tumours at the gastro-oesophageal junction originate from three areas: the distal oesophagus, the cardia of the stomach or the subcardial gastric wall. Both squamous and adenocarcinomatous forms are usually only moderately differentiated and behave aggressively.

Oesophageal cancers may fungate into the lumen but more often infiltrate diffusely along and around the oesophageal wall. Once through the wall, the tumour invades surrounding mediastinal organs.

Difficulty in swallowing (dysphagia) is the classic symptom, but it tends to develop insidiously. Patients initially have trouble with solids but they tend to compensate (liquidising their food, for example) before seeking medical advice. Later they have trouble swallowing liquids. By the time a patient presents with dysphagia, the tumour is often incurable and lymphatic spread to mediastinal nodes has already occurred. Sometimes, involvement of other mediastinal organs, e.g. recurrent laryngeal nerve invasion or an oesophago-tracheal fistula, produces the first symptoms. Low oesophageal lesions tend to metastasise to upper abdominal nodes and the liver.

EPIDEMIOLOGY AND AETIOLOGY OF OESOPHAGEAL CARCINOMA

The incidence of oesophageal cancer in Western countries is relatively low compared with carcinoma of the colon and stomach. It accounts for about 5% of all deaths from cancer, with males and females equally at risk. The disease is usually advanced by the time of presentation, hence the mortality rate is appalling, with 75% dying within a year of presentation and only 6% surviving 5 years (see Fig. 15.1).

Oesophageal carcinoma is uncommon before the age of 50 years. At least 50% of tumours occur in the lower third of the oesophagus and only about 15% in the upper third. Heavy alcohol intake is associated with at least a 20 times greater risk and smokers have at least five times

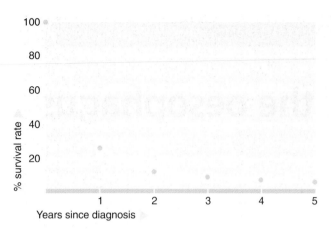

Fig. 15.1 Survival after diagnosis of oesophageal carcinoma

the risk of non-smokers; however, these risk factors classically predispose only to squamous cell carcinoma.

Since 1980 there has been a 70% increase in the proportion of adenocarcinomas relative to squamous cell carcinomas in many Western countries. The reason is not clear, but may be related to the widespread use of acid-suppressing medication and possibly to alterations in diet. There appears to be no familial predisposition but people with structural and functional disorders, such as peptic oesophagitis and stricture, achalasia, oesophageal web or pharyngeal pouch, are all at considerably greater risk of the disease. Most women who develop upper third lesions have a pre-existing oesophageal web or pharyngeal pouch, both in themselves very rare.

Areas of exceptionally high incidence have been reported in China, elsewhere in the Far East and around the Caspian Sea. There is some evidence that a fungus which grows on food grain may be responsible. This epidemiological pattern suggests that chronic local tissue irritation is an important aetiological factor, with different factors predisposing to the two main histological types.

INVESTIGATION OF SUSPECTED OESOPHAGEAL CARCINOMA

Dysphagia or pain on swallowing (**odynophagia**) in a middle-aged or elderly patient demands investigation in order to exclude carcinoma. General physical examination is usually unrewarding except in very advanced disease when there may be signs of **wasting, hepatomegaly** due to metastases, a **Virchow's node** in the left supraclavicular fossa or sometimes **hoarseness** as a result of recurrent laryngeal nerve involvement.

Direct inspection is necessary using a flexible endoscope. Biopsies are taken of any suspicious areas. In addition some surgeons advocate contrast radiography (see Fig. 15.2b); this will localise the tumour and, if the

lesion cannot be traversed at endoscopy, will show if the proximal stomach is suitable to use as a surgical conduit.

Staging the tumour

Once carcinoma of the oesophagus is diagnosed, it is important to establish the extent of local invasion and discover whether metastasis to thoracic or abdominal lymph nodes or the liver has occurred; this will determine whether potentially curative or palliative treatment is offered. CT scanning is the principal investigation but it frequently understages the disease. **Staging laparoscopy** can show peritoneal or visceral metastases not seen on CT scan; some units employ staging **thoracoscopy** to assess the pleural cavity for the same reasons. **Endoscopic ultrasound** helps to delineate the tumour and can often show locally involved lymph nodes. As the number of involved nodes increases, the chance of surgical cure diminishes.

MANAGEMENT OF CARCINOMA OF THE OESOPHAGUS

The ideal treatment would be to eliminate the cancer. In practice, this can rarely be achieved because of overt or occult spread. Even if cure is impossible, oesophageal obstruction must be relieved to allow the patient to eat and to prevent the appalling consequence of complete obstruction, i.e. inability to swallow even saliva.

Resection of the tumour is mainly employed only when the aim is cure. For incurable patients with dysphagia, palliative procedures to restore swallowing can be effective and are certainly preferable to major surgery, particularly if life expectancy is short.

Radiotherapy has a role in some patients with carcinoma of the oesophagus. It can be given alone or in combination with chemotherapy (chemoradiotherapy) before surgery (**neo-adjuvant therapy**) in an attempt to shrink or downstage the tumour. Alternatively, it may be given as the sole form of treatment. Intubation of the tumour may be needed before radiotherapy in the short term to avoid total obstruction as a result of swelling. Results of radiotherapy as sole therapy are often disappointing because of adverse local effects. Radiotherapy thus tends to be reserved for palliation.

The choice of treatment depends on the patient's fitness and the stage of the disease. Comorbidity due to the adverse effects of alcohol and cigarettes may influence the decision, e.g. chronic lung disease, cirrhosis. Cardiac fitness is assessed clinically and by electrocardiography (ECG) and sometimes echocardiography. In addition, spirometry and blood gases should be performed to assess the patient's fitness for thoracotomy. If the FEV_1 is less than 2 L, single lung ventilation used during thoracotomy is unlikely to be tolerated. A preoperative staging work-up usually includes CT scanning of chest

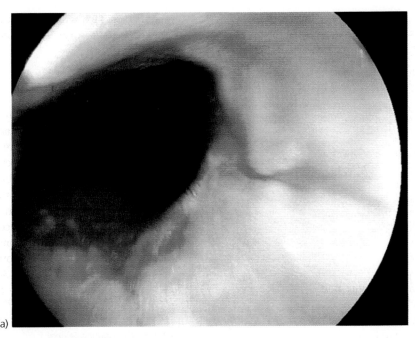

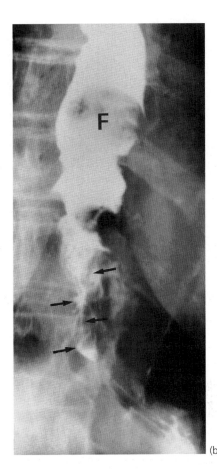

(a)

(b)

Fig. 15.2 Barrett's oesophagus and oesophageal carcinoma
(a) Endoscopic view of Barrett's oesophagus demonstrating linear ulceration and deeper red mucosa with chronic ulceration at the oesophago-gastric junction. Diagnosis is confirmed on biopsy. This condition is premalignant. **(b)** Barium swallow in an elderly man who presented with almost complete dysphagia. The film shows the lower end of the oesophagus which has an irregular narrowing of the lumen (arrowed). This appearance did not alter in several views of the same area and is characteristic of malignancy. Nevertheless, endoscopy is usually performed to obtain histological confirmation by means of biopsies. The oesophagus above is moderately dilated and contains a bolus of food **F** which cannot pass onwards.

and abdomen and laparoscopy, with endoscopic ultrasound if available.

Surgery

Once a decision has been made to undertake surgery, the choice of operation depends on the level of the lesion. In general, the aim is to remove the tumour with an appropriate safety margin, to perform a two-field lymphadenectomy (removing mediastinal and abdominal lymph nodes) and to achieve a leak-free anastomosis.

Lesions above the carina (the tracheal bifurcation) are usually dealt with by a three-stage **oesophagectomy** known as the **McKeown operation**, with all stages performed at the same operation. The first stage is to mobilise the tumour and the oesophagus via a right thoracotomy with the patient in the left lateral position. The second stage involves rolling the patient into a supine position and performing a laparotomy to allow the stomach to be mobilised and fashioned into a conduit. A third incision is then made in the neck through which oesophagus and tumour are delivered and the gastric conduit is anastomosed to the cervical oesophagus. A cervical anastomosis is safer than an intrathoracic one, as the consequences of anastomotic leakage would be less devastating.

If the tumour arises lower in the oesophagus, a two-stage **Ivor Lewis operation** is usually performed. The abdomen is opened first, and the stomach mobilised and fashioned into a conduit. The patient is then turned into a left lateral position and the right chest opened, the oesophagus mobilised and the tumour and lymph nodes excised. Finally the gastric conduit is drawn up into the chest and anastomosed to the proximal oesophageal remnant. If this is impossible, a loop of jejunum or a single end of jejunum (roux-en-Y) is drawn up and used to make the connection (see Fig. 15.3). Controversy exists about whether extending lymphadenectomy into the neck, so-called 'three-field lymphadenectomy', is beneficial. The procedure increases the operative risks and only appears to benefit a subgroup with proximal tumours and fewer than five nodes involved.

An operation that has gained some popularity is **transhiatal oesophagectomy**. A thoracotomy is avoided by mobilising the oesophagus and the cancer by blunt dissection from the abdomen via the diaphragmatic hiatus and via a neck incision, performing the anastomosis after resection in the neck. However, interest is waning mainly because of concerns that the safety margins of excision may be insufficient for potential cure and adequate lymphadenectomy is impossible in the chest. There is also an increased risk of damaging veins

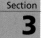

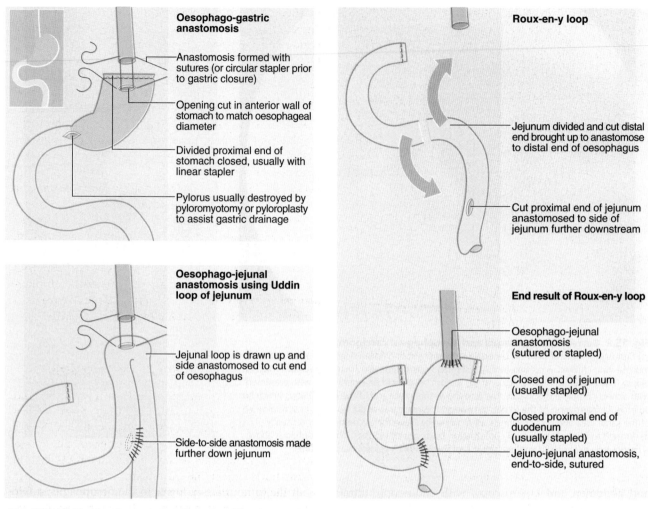

Fig. 15.3 Methods of reconstruction after distal oesophagectomy and partial or total gastrectomy

in the chest during dissection (particularly the azygos vein) and causing catastrophic haemorrhage.

Techniques involving combined laparoscopic and thoracoscopic oesophagectomy are being evaluated but their role is still controversial. They may be best suited to early or in situ lesions.

Oesophagectomy is always a major undertaking and carries the potentially fatal risk of anastomotic breakdown. This may lead to mediastinitis, lung abscess or oesophago-pleural fistula. Patients should be made aware of the risks in relation to the benefits as well as the expected prolonged convalescent period and long-term morbidity. Problems include dysphagia, small capacity for food (early satiety), and reflux.

Inoperable lesions

If operation is inappropriate, oesophageal patency can often be restored by palliative ablation of tumour with absolute alcohol injections or by cutting a pathway

through the tumour with laser therapy via a gastroscope. Both of these treatments can be repeated as the tumour regrows. Alternatively, the oesophagus can be intubated by inserting a cloth-covered metal stent (see Fig. 15.4) or a permanent reinforced rubber or plastic tube through the lesion. This is usually done under intravenous sedation using the endoscopic technique of **pulsion intubation**, after dilatation. These tubes relieve symptoms, but food has to be liquidised and the tube kept 'clean' by taking fizzy drinks after eating.

HIATUS HERNIA AND REFLUX OESOPHAGITIS

PATHOPHYSIOLOGY

The oesophagus is essentially a tube of smooth muscle conveying food to the stomach by peristalsis. At the lower end of the oesophagus there is a tonically active

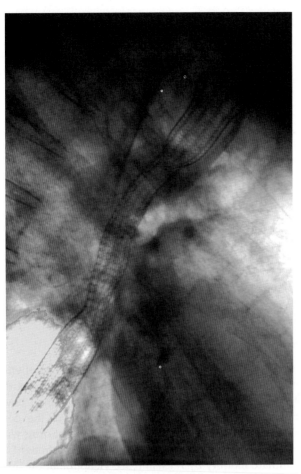

Fig. 15.4 Intubation of oesophageal cancer: cloth-covered metal stent in situ
This 70-year-old man presented with inoperable carcinoma of the middle third of the oesophagus. The malignant stricture was dilated via a flexible gastroscope and a Dacron-covered metal stent inserted to keep the stricture open as a palliative measure. This lateral chest X-ray shows the stent in situ.

sphincter mechanism. Its activity coordinates with peristalsis, relaxing to allow food to enter the stomach. The sphincter mechanism prevents reflux of stomach contents into the oesophagus. After passing through the diaphragm, the oesophagus continues for about 2 cm within the abdomen before joining the stomach. The sphincter mechanism is not completely understood but it probably involves several components: a functional (but not anatomical) sphincter of the oesophageal wall (immediately above the diaphragm) and the smooth muscle at the gastric cardia. This is reinforced by contraction of the diaphragmatic crura, by the acute angle at which the oesophagus enters the stomach and by the 'flutter valve' effect of intra-abdominal pressure on the abdominal portion of the oesophagus causing collapse of the lumen.

Hiatus hernia is an abnormality which occurs when the proximal part of the stomach passes through the diaphragmatic hiatus into the chest (see Fig. 15.5). Around 90% of hiatus hernias are of the **sliding type**, in which the gastro-oesophageal junction is drawn up into the chest and a segment of stomach becomes constricted at the diaphragmatic hiatus. The hernia tends to slide up into the chest with each peristaltic contraction. These hernias may reach a huge size. In the other 10% of cases, the gastro-oesophageal junction remains below the diaphragm and a bulge of stomach herniates through the hiatus beside the oesophagus. These are described as **para-oesophageal** or **rolling hiatus hernias** and are usually small (see Fig. 15.5). In sliding hiatus hernia, the lower oesophageal sphincter mechanism often becomes defective, causing reflux of acid-peptic stomach contents into the oesophagus. This is not a problem with rolling hiatus hernias.

Hiatus hernia in adults is commonly associated with smoking and obesity. Perhaps the pressure of intra-abdominal fat is contributory. Hiatus hernia can also be a congenital abnormality presenting in early infancy.

CLINICAL FEATURES OF REFLUX OESOPHAGITIS

Hiatus hernia is common, especially in women, and becomes more common with advancing years. Only a small proportion of patients with a hiatus hernia experience symptoms of **acid-peptic reflux**, i.e. 'heartburn', and reflux can occur without a hiatus hernia. Research has shown that the adverse effects of reflux are more likely to affect patients with impaired peristaltic 'clearing' of gastric contents from the lower oesophagus. Reflux causes acute inflammation (**oesophagitis**). This is experienced as burning retrosternal pain (**heartburn**), bitter-tasting regurgitation or other forms of 'indigestion'. Symptoms are typically worse at night when the patient lies flat in bed or on bending forward during the day.

If reflux is severe and persistent, mucosal destruction is recurrent and inflammation becomes chronic. Progressive scarring leads to fibrosis of the wall and this may lead to narrowing (stricture) of the lumen and the symptom of dysphagia. Longstanding oesophageal reflux predisposes to the development of **Barrett's oesophagus** with normal squamous oesophageal epithelium replaced by metaplastic columnar mucosa. Barrett's oesophagus is the only known predisposing factor for adenocarcinoma of the lower oesophagus, a condition that has increased by 70% in developed countries since 1980. Histologically, biopsy may reveal **specialised intestinal metaplasia** (SIM) or **severe dysplasia,** both of which are markers for malignant change, supporting the metaplasia/dysplasia/carcinoma model for the evolution of lower oesophageal cancer.

Occasionally, oesophageal reflux symptoms are severe and acute, causing chest pain which may easily be

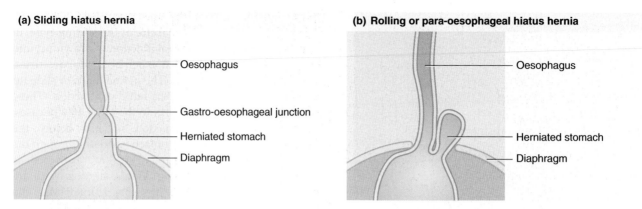

(a) Sliding hiatus hernia

Oesophagus

Gastro-oesophageal junction

Herniated stomach

Diaphragm

(b) Rolling or para-oesophageal hiatus hernia

Oesophagus

Herniated stomach

Diaphragm

Fig. 15.5 Types of hiatus hernia
(a) Sliding hiatus hernia, which is common. This type disrupts the physiological anti-reflux mechanism. **(b)** Rolling or para-oesophageal hiatus hernia, which is rare. The anti-reflux mechanism is usually left intact.

mistaken for angina or even myocardial infarction. There is often an element of **oesophageal spasm** which, like angina, is relieved by glyceryl trinitrate and similar drugs. This may confuse the diagnosis.

In general, hiatus hernia and reflux can be demonstrated by barium swallow examination (see Fig. 15.6) but assessment of mucosal inflammation requires endoscopy and biopsy. The latter is important to exclude carcinoma, especially if dysphagia is experienced. In specialised units, physiological pressure and pH studies are often used to help determine which patients are likely to benefit from surgery.

MANAGEMENT OF HIATUS HERNIA AND REFLUX OESOPHAGITIS

Nearly all patients can be managed conservatively with surgery reserved for intractable cases. Treatment is aimed at reducing acid-pepsin activity and preventing reflux.

Reducing reflux

Weight reduction, where appropriate, is the most effective long-term anti-reflux measure. Changes in the diet will often of themselves improve symptoms of reflux. For example, alcohol causes the sphincter to relax and many medical students can personally vouch for the combined effect of beer and spicy food. Other foods that may precipitate reflux are coffee, tea and chocolate. Reflux can be reduced substantially by taking smaller, more frequent and drier meals, by using blocks to elevate the head of the bed at night and by sleeping on more pillows in an upright position. Smoking induces sphincter relaxation and quitting often reduces reflux dramatically. **Alginate drugs**, available in liquid or chewable tablet form, produce a foamy surface layer on the stomach contents and are said to coat the lower

oesophagus, protecting it from the effects of reflux. These drugs are most effective if taken soon after food.

Prokinetic agents

Drugs which stimulate motility can have a useful effect in reflux. **Metoclopramide** is a dopamine antagonist that stimulates gastric emptying and increases small bowel transit as well as enhancing contraction of the oesophageal sphincter. **Cisapride** is a more recent drug without dopamine antagonist action; it is thought to stimulate motility by releasing acetylcholine in the intestinal wall. This drug is helpful in oesophageal reflux, gastric stasis and some cases of non-ulcer dyspepsia.

Reducing acid-pepsin production

Reducing acid-pepsin attack is probably the mainstay of treatment for reflux disease. It is accomplished as for chronic peptic ulcer disease (see Ch. 14). Simple antacid drugs and H_2-receptor antagonists are sometimes effective but in severe cases they are inadequate, and **omeprazole** or another proton pump inhibitor (PPI), is the drug of choice. Drugs and food that irritate the lower oesophagus should be avoided.

Management of strictures

Inflammatory fibrous strictures used to be regularly dilated with gum-elastic **bougies** of progressively increasing size under general anaesthesia via a rigid oesophagoscope. Nowadays, dilatation is usually performed under intravenous sedation using flexible gastroscopy. A flexible guide-wire is first positioned across the stricture via the endoscope and graded metal or plastic dilators passed over the wire to dilate the stricture. If the stricture recurs and causes dysphagia despite suitable conservative treatment for reflux, an anti-reflux operation may be indicated.

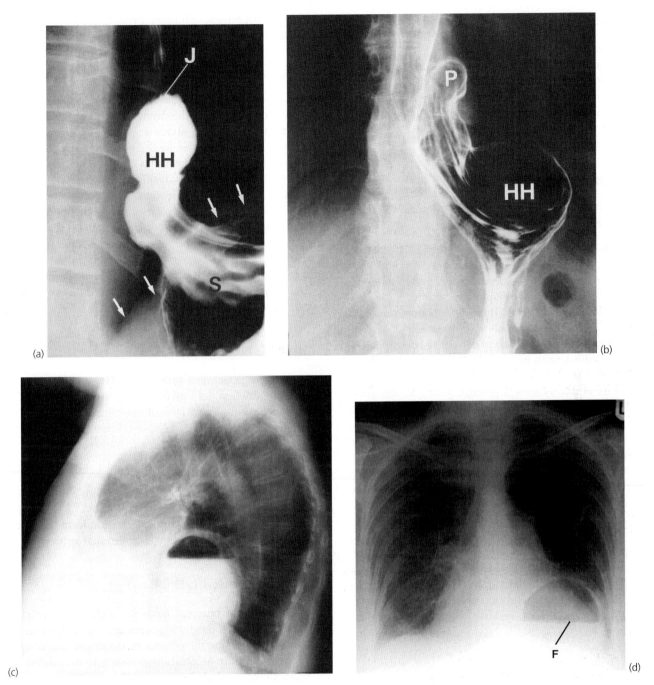

Fig. 15.6 Hiatus hernia
(a) Sliding hiatus hernia in a 63-year-old woman. The hiatus hernia is marked **HH**, the stomach **S** and the oesophago-gastric junction **J**; the position of the diaphragm is arrowed. (b) and (c) Large incarcerated (irreducible) sliding hiatus hernia in an elderly woman with few symptoms. Note there is also a small para-oesophageal 'rolling' hiatus hernia **P**. The lateral film (b) shows the hernia containing barium and a fluid level. (d) Plain chest X-ray of the same patient showing a fluid level **F** strongly suggestive of a hiatus hernia.

This usually allows healing of mucosal damage and may prevent further stricture formation.

Surgery for hiatus hernia and reflux oesophagitis

Surgery is reserved for intractable symptoms, recurrent stricture and chronic peptic ulceration, particularly with Barrett's oesophagus (having excluded a high risk of malignancy by biopsy), which fail to respond to PPI therapy. The traditional operations for formal repair of hiatus hernia, performed via chest or abdomen (e.g. Belsey Mark IV), have largely been superseded by **Nissen fundoplication**. This abdominal (or thoracic) operation involves dissection of the gastro-oesophageal junction at

233

the hiatus and wrapping the gastric fundus around the intra-abdominal portion of the oesophagus to re-create a flutter valve.

In experienced hands, laparoscopic Nissen fundoplication is the operation of choice and allows the patient a rapid return to normal levels of activity. Clinical trials have shown the laparoscopic approach to give comparable results to open fundoplication.

ACHALASIA

PATHOPHYSIOLOGY AND CLINICAL PRESENTATION OF ACHALASIA

Achalasia is an uncommon disorder of oesophageal motility. Normal peristalsis is disrupted throughout the oesophagus, causing uncoordinated and inadequate relaxation of the lower oesophageal sphincter.

In pathological terms, there is a poorly understood neurological defect involving Auerbach's myenteric (parasympathetic) plexus. The entire oesophagus is affected rather than just the cardia, as the obsolete term 'achalasia of the cardia' would imply. The condition presents in two main age groups, young adults and the elderly. In the latter, the cause may be a central rather than a local neurological defect. Achalasia, as with any structural abnormality of the oesophagus, predisposes to carcinoma.

Clinically, the cardiac sphincter becomes constricted and the proximal oesophagus dilates with accumulated fluid and solids. Difficulty in swallowing fluids is the usual presenting symptom. Solids tend to sink to the lower end of the dilated oesophagus, whereas fluids spill over into the trachea causing **spluttering dysphagia** (see Ch. 11) and coughing, particularly at night. Vomiting and retrosternal pain may occur in more severe cases. The degree of dysphagia tends to vary and probably depends on the amount of food residue in the oesophagus at the time.

INVESTIGATION OF SUSPECTED ACHALASIA

Chest X-ray may demonstrate the mediastinal shadow widened by a dilated oesophagus, and sometimes a fluid level is visible in the oesophagus behind the heart. Barium swallow examination reveals gross dilatation of the oesophagus with a tapering constriction at the lower end. The constriction barely allows contrast to pass into the stomach (see Fig. 15.7). Under fluoroscopic screening, uncoordinated purposeless peristaltic waves can often be seen; these are described as **'tertiary contractions'** and are distinct from the normal co-ordinated pattern of primary and secondary contractions. Oesophageal manometry is the cardinal test for achalasia and demonstrates excessive

lower oesophageal sphincter pressure that fails to relax on swallowing.

MANAGEMENT OF ACHALASIA

The condition is, by its nature, incurable, and treatment is directed at relieving the distal obstruction. The standard operation is via the abdomen, and involves a longitudinal incision of the lower oesophageal and upper gastric muscle wall until the mucosa bulges through (**Heller's cardiomyotomy**); this is best combined with a partial Nissen fundoplication to combat the almost inevitable reflux it will cause. The operation can be performed open or laparoscopically. Balloon dilatation is sometimes used as an alternative to operation and results appear to be virtually as good in experienced hands. Patients with achalasia should be followed up and periodically endoscoped to exclude developing carcinoma (see Fig. 15.8).

PHARYNGEAL POUCH

Pharyngeal pouch is a rare cause of dysphagia. It arises at the junction of pharynx and oesophagus, and probably results from lack of coordination between the inferior constrictor muscle and cricopharyngeus during swallowing. The result is a progressive mucosal outpouching between the two muscles. The condition is best diagnosed by barium swallow (see Fig. 15.9). Endoscopy should be avoided in patients with 'high' dysphagia as a pharyngeal pouch is easily perforated. Treatment of pharyngeal pouch is by surgical excision from the side of the neck, or via a completely endoluminal approach.

OESOPHAGEAL WEB

Circumferential mucosal folds (or webs) may occur in the oesophagus producing annular narrowing of the lumen and causing dysphagia. In the upper oesophagus, they are found in association with severe iron deficiency anaemia, particularly in women. The triad of dysphagia, anaemia and atrophic glossitis is known as **Plummer–Vinson** or **Patterson–Kelly syndrome**.

GASTRO-OESOPHAGEAL VARICES

PATHOPHYSIOLOGY OF GASTRO-OESOPHAGEAL VARICES

Gastro-oesophageal varices result from **portal venous hypertension**. The most common cause is cirrhosis of the liver, usually associated with alcohol abuse. Less common causes include portal vein thrombosis, hepatic vein thrombosis (**Budd–Chiari syndrome**) and schistosomiasis.

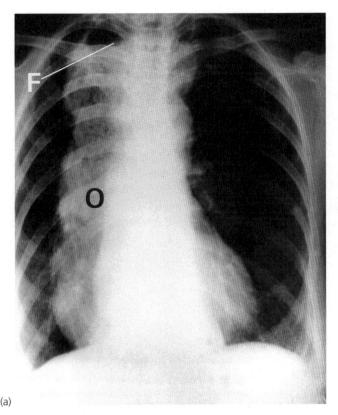

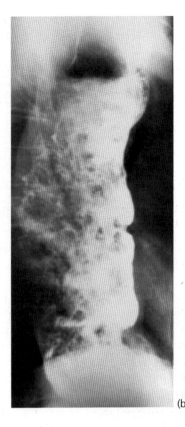

(a)

(b)

Fig. 15.7 Late-stage achalasia in a 60-year-old man
(a) The chest X-ray shows gross mediastinal widening caused by a massively dilated oesophagus **O** filled with food debris. Note the mottled appearance of the oesophagus and the fluid level **F** at its upper end. Note also the absence of a gastric air bubble below the diaphragm. This is characteristic of achalasia. **(b)** Barium swallow in the same patient. This confirms the findings on the chest X-ray.

As resistance to flow and pressure rises in the portal venous system, abnormal venous communications develop between the peripheral part of the portal system and the systemic venous circulation. This is known as **portal-systemic shunting**. Multiple large veins appear in the peritoneal cavity and retroperitoneal area, making any form of abdominal surgery hazardous. Large submucosal veins also appear at the lower end of the oesophagus and gastric fundus and these are known as **gastro-oesophageal varices** (see Fig. 15.10). These varices can produce massive gastrointestinal haemorrhage, possibly related to rises in intravariceal pressure. Up to 40% of cirrhotic patients suffer variceal haemorrhage at some stage.

A further result of portal hypertension is splenic enlargement. This may cause the effects of **hypersplenism**, namely anaemia, thrombocytopenia and leucopenia. Patients in late stages of cirrhosis also develop **ascites**.

If massive portal-systemic shunting occurs either spontaneously or as a result of a surgically created shunt to treat portal hypertension, **portal-systemic encephalopathy** may develop. This is due to toxic substances absorbed from the intestine such as ammonia passing directly into the systemic circulation without first traversing the liver where they would normally be detoxified.

ELECTIVE MANAGEMENT OF GASTRO-OESOPHAGEAL VARICES

Gastro-oesophageal varices are not usually treated unless they have bled. Occasionally, elective treatment is carried out in high-risk cases where haemorrhage is considered highly likely; with the improving efficacy of banding and sclerotherapy, some clinicians believe that lower-risk asymptomatic varices should be treated electively. After recovery from an acute bleed, however, varices should be treated at regular intervals by banding or injection sclerotherapy until they are eliminated.

MANAGEMENT OF BLEEDING GASTRO-OESOPHAGEAL VARICES

Diagnosis and resuscitation

When a patient with known cirrhosis or varices presents with massive upper gastrointestinal haemorrhage, the first priority is resuscitation. Following this, the source of

235

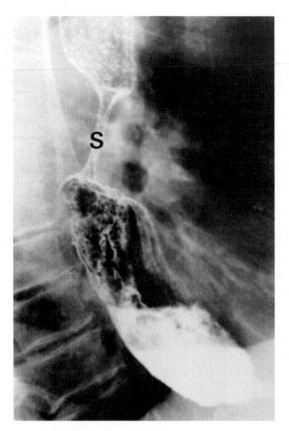

Fig. 15.8 Oesophageal carcinoma secondary to achalasia
Malignant stricture **S** in the middle third of the oesophagus in a 60-year-old woman with achalasia of long standing. She had a Heller's myotomy at the age of 26. Note that this surgery does not alter the predisposition to carcinoma.

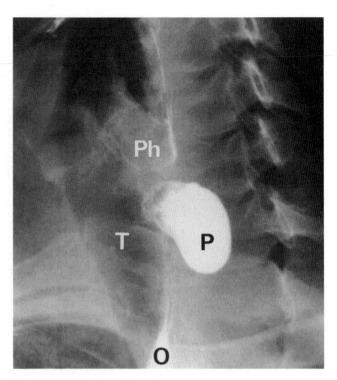

Fig. 15.9 Pharyngeal pouch
Lateral view during barium swallow examination in a 41-year-old man complaining of mild dysphagia; the X-ray shows a contrast-filled pouch **P** extending from the pharynx **Ph**. Note the gas-filled trachea **T** lying anteriorly. **O** = oesophagus.

haemorrhage is sought by endoscopy. In fact only about half of these patients will be bleeding from oesophageal varices. The rest will have bleeding gastric varices, gastric erosions or Mallory–Weiss tears of the lower oesophagus. In this last condition, arterial bleeding is the cause and it does not respond to measures designed to treat bleeding varices. Occasionally bleeding duodenal or gastric ulcers are found. The management of the patient varies according to the diagnosis. Whatever treatment is undertaken, it must be remembered that cirrhotic patients often have defective clotting. It is prudent to perform clotting studies and give specific corrective factors.

Treatment

If bleeding is from varices, the mainstay of initial treatment is an **octreotide infusion**. More than 75% of patients initially respond to this therapy. Meanwhile, resuscitation continues with blood volume replacement, fresh-frozen plasma and platelets. Excess water and sodium should be avoided as this rapidly migrates into the peritoneal cavity as ascites. Hepatic encephalopathy should be anticipated as a result of the protein load of

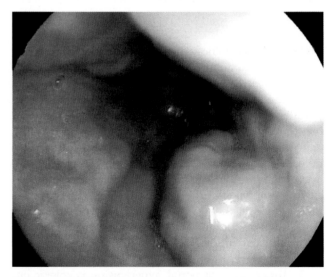

Fig. 15.10 Endoscopic view of oesophageal varices
This man of 63 was known to have alcoholic cirrhosis and had suffered one acute GI haemorrhage, treated successfully by injection of bleeding varices. The bulging blue masses can be seen protruding into the oesophageal lumen.

blood in the bowel and oral neomycin or lactulose administered. Delirium tremens may also require treatment if the patient is an alcoholic.

In patients not responding to octreotide, an attempt is made to apply tamponade. After endotracheal intubation to protect the airway, a special tube is passed through the mouth into the stomach and a balloon inflated. Traction is exerted on the upper end for up to 4 hours to arrest the haemorrhage. Several varieties of tube are in use: the **Sengstaken–Blakemore tube** has separate intragastric and oesophageal balloons and depends for its action upon physiological arrest of bleeding. Most cases cease bleeding with inflation of the gastric balloon alone and traction. The **Linton balloon** is an alternative comprising a single large intragastric balloon (300–600 ml) which allows simultaneous endoscopy and rubber banding or injection sclerotherapy of varices.

Operative surgery for oesophageal varices has dwindled in recent years because of the effectiveness of injection sclerotherapy. Now that the problem of variceal haemorrhage can be overcome, the mortality in these patients is related to the progression of the underlying cirrhosis.

If variceal haemorrhage continues despite effective conservative therapy, transjugular intrahepatic portosystemic stenting is used (**TIPS**). This involves cannulating the internal jugular vein and placing an angiography catheter first within the intra-hepatic vena cava. Using combined fluoroscopy and ultrasound, the catheter is guided into the portal system within the liver. Then an expanding metal stent is placed to connect the intra-hepatic portal system to the vena cava.

As a last resort, emergency surgical treatment is performed but all operations carry a high mortality in such seriously ill patients. The simplest operation is **transgastric oesophageal stapling**. A circular stapler is passed into the oesophagus via a gastrotomy, a ligature tied around the oesophagus between the staples and the anvil, and the gun fired. This places two rows of staples through the full thickness of the oesophageal wall, disconnecting the longitudinal veins. However, this is not effective for bleeding gastric varices.

Emergency **portal-systemic shunting** is occasionally used but carries a risk of portal-systemic encephalopathy although it reliably arrests haemorrhage. Shunting operations are still sometimes used following recovery from acute haemorrhage but many doctors believe that repeated rubber banding or injection sclerotherapy via a flexible endoscope is the best prophylaxis against further haemorrhage.

All types of surgical portal-systemic shunts carry a risk of **encephalopathy**, although shunt design has been modified to minimise this risk. The original operation was **portacaval shunting**, in which the main portal vein is anastomosed to the inferior vena cava. Later variations include **mesocaval shunting** in which the superior mesenteric vein is connected to the inferior vena cava via an interposition graft, and **lienorenal shunting** (the **Warren shunt**) in which the splenic vein is anastomosed to the left renal vein. The last is said to cause the lowest incidence of encephalopathy but is also the least effective for decompressing the portal venous pressure.

Operative risk has been calculated using **Child's criteria**, shown in Table 15.1.

Table 15.1 Child's criteria for assessing operative risk in portal hypertension

Risk factor	Score points		
	1	2	3
Encephalopathy	None	Minimal	Marked
Ascites	None	Slight	Moderate
Bilirubin (micromoles/L)	< 35	36–50	> 50
Albumin (g/L)	> 35	28–35	< 28
Prothrombin ratio	< 1.4	1.4–2.0	> 2.0

Each criterion is scored and the total added:
Child's grade A (good risk) scores 5–6
         grade B (moderate risk) scores 7–9
         grade C (bad risk) scores 10–15

16 | Tumours of the stomach and small intestine

INTRODUCTION

Benign tumours occasionally occur in the stomach but most gastric tumours are malignant. The great majority are adenocarcinomas, whilst lymphomas and the occasional carcinoid tumour or sarcoma make up the remainder. True adenomatous **gastric polyps** are rare; most gastric polypoid lesions are small benign hyperplastic nodules.

Tumours of the small bowel are rare. Of the malignant tumours, lymphomas and leiomyosarcomas are much more common than adenocarcinomas. **Peutz–Jeghers syndrome** is a rare inherited disorder characterised by multiple benign polyps in the small bowel and peri-oral pigmentation. It is most commonly encountered at student examinations!

CARCINOMA OF STOMACH

PATHOLOGY OF GASTRIC CARCINOMA

Gastric carcinomas are almost exclusively adenocarcinomas. Two distinct histopathological groups are recognised, each with its unique epidemiological associations.

The **intestinal type** has histological features similar to intestinal epithelium. Cells grow in clumps and there is a marked inflammatory infiltrate. Variations in the incidence of this type of tumour explain the regional variations in incidence of gastric cancer described below. Furthermore, the decline in incidence of gastric cancer in the developed world is almost exclusively a decline of the intestinal type of cancer. These factors suggest that environmental factors have a great influence on the development of intestinal-type gastric cancer.

The second histological type of gastric adenocarcinoma is the **diffuse type**. Here the cells are singular,

often arranged in files, and surrounded by a marked stromal reaction. The tumour cells have large intracellular mucin droplets which displace the nuclei peripherally giving the characteristic **signet ring appearance**.

Gastric carcinomas may develop in three morphological forms; the first two largely represent the intestinal histological type and the third the diffuse type. The first two have a somewhat better prognosis than diffuse-type infiltrating cancers:

- **Fungating tumours**. These are polypoid and may grow to a huge size (see Fig. 16.3)
- **Malignant ulcers**. These lesions probably result from necrosis in the centre of broad-based solid tumours. Malignant ulcers are often larger than peptic ulcers (except for the giant benign ulcer of the elderly) with a heaped-up indurated (hardened) margin. There is no surrounding mucosal puckering typical of inflammatory scarring
- **Infiltrating carcinomas**. This form of gastric cancer spreads widely beneath the mucosa and diffusely invades the muscular wall. This causes marked wall thickening and rigidity and the whole stomach contracts to a very small capacity. The condition is known as **linitis plastica** and its appearance is likened to a 'leather bottle'. Linitis plastica affects a slightly younger age group and has a very poor prognosis. Diagnosis may be delayed because the endoscopic changes are often subtle, and biopsies of the mucosa may not show tumour

'Early gastric cancer' is defined as cancer limited to the mucosa and submucosa of the stomach. This is rarely detected in patients with symptoms, but is found more commonly with endoscopic screening programmes or incidentally. Results of surgery in this group are excellent, with about a 90% cure rate.

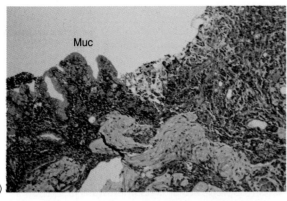
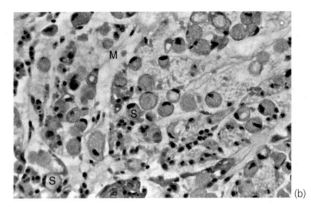

Fig. 16.1 Carcinoma of the stomach—histopathology
(a) Typical gastric carcinoma originating within the stomach mucosa **Muc**. The tumour consists of a mass of signet ring cells and extracellular mucin. **(b)** High-power view showing numerous signet ring cells **S**. This appearance is due to the presence of intracellular mucin **M**.

EPIDEMIOLOGY OF GASTRIC CARCINOMA

Gastric cancer is the second most common cancer in the world, surpassed only by lung cancer. Cancer of the stomach is rare before the age of 50 and increases in frequency thereafter. Males have one and a half times the risk of females, and the disease is more common in lower socio-economic groups. Costa Rica has the highest death rate from the disease in men, with an age-adjusted death rate of 70 per 100 000. Japan and Chile follow close behind but the offspring of Japanese immigrants to America appear to carry the same risk as other Americans. In much of the Western world, the incidence and death rates have steadily decreased in recent years. In the USA, the mortality rate for men has fallen from 10 per 100 000 per annum in 1980 to 7.4 in 1991 and for women from 5 to 3.4. The epidemiology of gastric carcinoma gives tantalising clues as to the causes of the disease. The vast variation in incidence of intestinal-type gastric cancer between different countries and the fact that this type is more prominent in lower socio-economic groups suggest that environmental factors play an important part. It is likely that there is no single aetiological factor but rather a combination of co-factors which together bring about malignant change.

Japan plays a leading role in research into early detection and management of gastric cancer, reflecting the high incidence of this disease in that country.

AETIOLOGY OF GASTRIC CARCINOMA AND PREMALIGNANT CONDITIONS

Atrophic gastritis

Multifocal atrophic gastritis (type B) has often been incriminated as a pre-existing condition in intestinal-type gastric cancer, which may represent the end point of

a sequence running between superficial gastritis, atrophic gastritis, intestinal and colonic metaplasia, dysplasia and cancer. Multifocal atrophic gastritis is the result of chronic inflammation and appears first on the lesser curve of the stomach. Other risk factors such as diet and *Helicobacter pylori* infection may initiate atrophic gastritis and act through the same pathway. The **diffuse corporeal type of gastritis (type A)** which occurs in pernicious anaemia is a much weaker aetiological factor. Patients with this have a three- to six-fold increase in risk of developing gastric cancer, but the absolute risk remains low.

Helicobacter pylori infection

In recent years, chronic infection with *H. pylori* has become a prime suspect for initiating gastric cancer, as it is for peptic ulceration. *H. pylori* has the ability to colonise gastric mucosa chronically, and infection has been strongly linked with chronic gastritis which may progress over many years to atrophic gastritis type B. *H. pylori* infection is the main carcinogen leading to gastric cancer of the intestinal type; in one series *H. pylori* was found histologically in 90% of intestinal-type cancers, whilst only 30% of the diffuse type had evidence of infection. Elevated levels of IgG antibody to *H. pylori* have been found in gastric cancer patients compared with controls, with odds ratios of between 4 and 6 in favour of an association. The risk progressively increases with increasing antibody levels. Nevertheless, more than 60% of controls without gastric cancer demonstrate elevated antibodies. As mentioned on page 243, *H. pylori* also appears likely to be involved in gastric lymphoma of the mucosa-associated lymphoid tissue (MALT) type.

The carcinogenic mechanism of *H. pylori* is debated but probably involves altering the gastric acid/pepsin milieu, increasing cell turnover and enhancing gastric

239

mucosal susceptibility to ingested carcinogens. *H. pylori* appears to play a major but far from exclusive role.

Other factors

Dietary factors have been shown to influence the incidence of gastric cancer, in particular excess intake of salt and nitroso compounds, and a low ascorbic acid intake. In this respect, diets high in dried and salted fish, and salt- and smoke-cured meats appear to pose a particular risk.

CLINICAL FEATURES OF GASTRIC CARCINOMA

Symptoms are minimal until late in the course of the disease and patients most commonly present with advanced local and metastatic disease. However, retrospective review of the records of patients with early gastric cancer has shown that a high proportion have some pre-existing upper gastrointestinal symptoms, most often dyspepsia and epigastric pain with food. In advanced disease, 40% may be asymptomatic, but up to half have pain, nausea, vomiting, anorexia or a feeling of fullness after small meals (**early satiety**). Vomiting occurs if the gastric outlet becomes obstructed; this is more common with tumours of the antrum. Overall, one-third have cachexia (severe weight loss and wasting). This, in combination with an epigastric mass, renders, the possibility of surgical cure remote. Anaemia resulting from chronic occult blood loss is common and one-third have positive stool tests for occult blood.

Severe weight loss usually indicates metastatic disease and may be its only manifestation; indeed, dramatic weight loss in the absence of other symptoms should alert the clinician to possible gastric carcinoma. Virtually 70% of gastric cancer patients present with advanced local disease (stage T_3) of whom more than half have extensive nodal spread and half have distant metastases. Patients are now tending to present earlier, perhaps because persistent indigestion and upper gastrointestinal symptoms tend nowadays to be more effectively investigated than hitherto.

The presenting features of gastric carcinoma are summarised in Box 16.1.

INVESTIGATION OF GASTRIC CARCINOMA

Tumour staging

Invasive cancer progresses to involve submucosal lymphatics. The depth of tumour penetration correlates directly with the incidence of nodal metastases. The TNM system is the most widely used staging system and is now agreed internationally. Japanese nomenclature has designated lymph nodes draining the stomach by

> **SUMMARY**
>
> **Box 16.1 Presenting features of gastric carcinoma**
> - Often asymptomatic until a late stage
> - Epigastric pain and dyspepsia
> - Marked weight loss (cachexia)
> - Iron deficiency anaemia
> - Nausea and vomiting
> - Anorexia and early satiety
> - Feeling of abdominal fullness or discomfort, often after only small meals
> - Epigastric mass
> - Left supraclavicular mass (metastasis in Virchow's node)
> - Obstructive jaundice (metastases in the porta hepatis)
> - Pelvic mass

stations numbered 1–16. Perigastric stations 1–6 are considered N_1, whilst other more distant stations denote N_2, N_3 or M_1. These stations are important when more radical R1 or R2 gastrectomies, pioneered by the Japanese, are performed and provide useful prognostic information. The results of surgical treatment correlate directly with the TNM stage.

Metastatic spread initially involves local lymph nodes in the coeliac axis and periduodenal area. Later secondary nodes in the para-aortic area, splenic hilum and porta hepatis become involved, the latter sometimes causing obstructive jaundice. Classically, left supraclavicular (**Virchow's**) nodes may become invaded via the thoracic duct and give rise to a palpable mass (**Troisier's sign**). These nodes are palpable in a small proportion of cases at initial presentation. **Hepatic metastasis** via haematogenous spread is also a common initial finding. Widespread metastasis to lungs, brain and bone may also occur. Gastric carcinoma sometimes spreads across the peritoneal cavity, particularly to the surface of the ovaries (**Krukenberg tumour**) or the pouch of Douglas. In either case, a mass is often palpable on rectal examination. Direct spread into the transverse colon is not unusual in neglected cases and sometimes results in **gastro-colic fistula** formation.

Investigative procedures

Endoscopy alone is now the preferred investigation for suspected carcinoma of the stomach. **Barium meal** held this position for many years but it is often difficult to differentiate between gastric ulcer and carcinoma radiologically, even on double contrast studies. The typical radiological appearances of gastric malignancies are shown in Figure 16.2.

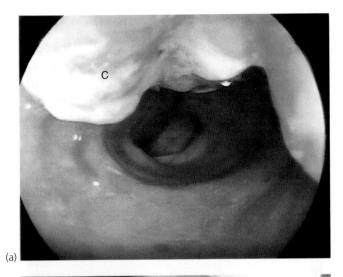

(a)

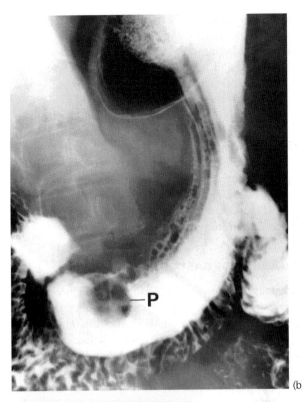

(b)

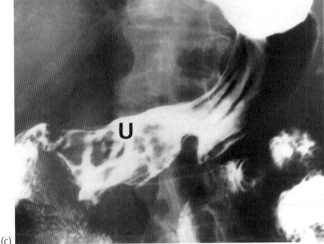

(c)

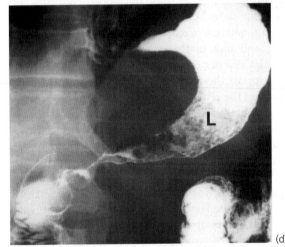

(d)

Fig. 16.2 Endoscopy and barium meals showing carcinoma of the stomach

(a) Gastroscopic view of large fungating carcinoma of stomach in the prepyloric region **C**. This corresponds to the barium meal examination in **(b)**. Diagnosis was confirmed by endoscopic biopsy. **(c)** Ulcerating carcinoma of stomach **U** in a 55-year-old man presenting with weight loss. **(d)** Linitis plastica-type carcinoma of the stomach **L**. Note the shrunken appearance of the whole stomach caused by widespread submucosal invasion of the tumour. Endoscopic biopsy may not give the correct diagnosis because the mucosa is often intact. This 60-year-old woman presented with anorexia. She had a total gastrectomy but died 5 months later of widespread metastases.

Endoscopy and biopsy are essential if there is any doubt about the diagnosis on radiological grounds. Diagnostic accuracy is greatest with exophytic lesions (90%) and lower for infiltrating lesions (50%). Diagnostic accuracy increases as more biopsies taken, and there should be little hesitation to re-biopsy suspicious lesions to obtain a representative sample. Carcinomas can arise in any part of the stomach, including the lesser curve, whereas benign gastric ulcers are usually found on the lesser curve or prepyloric area. The site of a lesion may therefore be of diagnostic significance.

In areas of high incidence, **endoscopic screening** is a popular and effective method of detecting early disease. It is widely employed in Japan and the result has been that over 40% of cancers operated upon have been discovered in a pre-symptomatic stage by this method, and can truly be defined as 'early gastric cancer'. About 90% of these patients have potentially curative operations.

241

Ultrasonography via a flexible endoscope is not yet widely available, but in pilot studies is proving highly accurate in predicting the depth of penetration of small gastric cancers, and hence the 'T' (tumour) stage. Local nodal spread and left hepatic lobe metastases are also detectable by this method.

CT scanning is used most widely for staging purposes before embarking upon surgery. This investigation is useful for showing local tumour invasion, lymph node involvement and hepatic metastases but remains relatively insensitive. **Laparoscopy** has proved to be more accurate for staging than CT alone; when disseminated disease is found on laparoscopy, the patient may be saved an inappropriate laparotomy.

MANAGEMENT OF GASTRIC CARCINOMA

Metastasis in gastric cancer tends to be early, occult and widespread. Therefore, **radical surgery** offers the only prospect of cure even when the tumour is small. The cure rate is determined by the stage of the disease at presentation. In Western countries, early gastric cancer is usually discovered only fortuitously—for example,when a patient is gastroscoped for dyspepsia. This situation is improving, however, in some developed countries. In one American series, only 15% of gastric cancers were considered unsuitable for operation at the time of initial diagnosis, and half of the operations were performed with the aim of cure. In gastric cancer, survival results strongly support the view that early detection dramatically increases the chance of curative surgery.

Even if the disease has progressed to local lymph nodes, radical gastrectomy may be curative. In early gastric cancer, confined to the mucosa and submucosa, 5-year survival approaches 90%, and with only local nodal involvement, about 50%; with more extensive spread, 5-year survival rates fall to only 5%. Palliative gastrectomy is often indicated to treat local problems such as blood loss or obstruction.

Japanese surgeons have developed radical gastrectomies (known as R1 and R2 gastrectomies) which include subtotal or total gastrectomy combined with removal of the local nodal fields in R1 and the secondary nodal fields as well in R2. With these procedures, much-improved 5-year survival rates have been achieved and local recurrences almost eliminated. This experience was not immediately seen in Western studies, where higher complication rates were evident.

The decision to attempt removal of a gastric cancer depends on the general fitness of the patient as well as the stage of the tumour. It is kindest to treat patients with advanced cancer symptomatically and perform palliative surgical bypass procedures or local resections only if symptomatic. Patients with obviously incurable tumours may have very few symptoms and their quality of life

may only be diminished by surgery. In other cases, tumour bleeding, necrosis or encroachment on the gastric lumen results in distressing symptoms of nausea, anorexia, vomiting (sometimes complete gastric outlet obstruction) or symptoms of anaemia. These symptoms can be greatly relieved by palliative gastrectomy. Afterwards, patients survive about 12 months on average, compared with about 3 months without operation. Gastric outlet obstruction may be relieved by placement of a self-expanding intraluminal stent.

There is increasing interest in preoperative treatment of some gastric cancers with chemo-radiotherapy. A long-held belief that there is little benefit in postoperative chemo-radiotherapy is being reconsidered with the development of newer agents and modified regimens.

GASTRIC POLYPS

Gastric polyps are mostly small benign hyperplastic nodules of the gastric mucosa. They may be single or multiple and occur anywhere in the stomach. They are all less than 1.5 cm in diameter and can confidently be observed as they almost never become malignant.

Genuine **adenomatous polyps** are rare. These are true neoplasms with histological and morphological forms similar to adenomatous polyps of the large intestine (see Ch. 20, p. 274). Adenomas are usually single, large and asymptomatic. Most are found incidentally on radiological or endoscopic examination. Up to 40% of adenomatous gastric polyps show histological features of malignancy. Treatment is by endoscopic excision biopsy and regular endoscopy is arranged to monitor recurrence or the appearance of new lesions.

LEIOMYOMAS

Leiomyomas are benign tumours of smooth muscle and may arise anywhere in the muscular wall of the gastrointestinal tract. They are especially common in the stomach and small bowel. These lesions are usually only a few centimetres in diameter and are discovered incidentally on endoscopy or barium examinations. Occasionally, larger lesions are found to be the cause of acute or chronic gastrointestinal blood loss or intermittent gastric outlet obstruction by impacting in or through the pylorus. Morphologically, leiomyomas are sessile or pedunculated lesions covered by normal mucosa. This may ulcerate, causing insidious blood loss and anaemia (see Fig. 16.3). Major haemorrhage sometimes occurs, presenting as haematemesis or melaena.

Leiomyosarcomas (see Fig. 16.4), the malignant counterpart of leiomyomas, are rare and present with similar symptoms or as an abdominal mass. Leiomyosarcomas

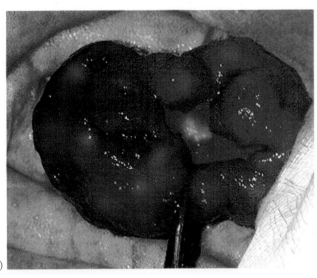

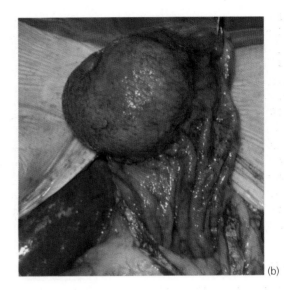

(a) (b)

Fig. 16.3 Gastric leiomyoma
(a) This 64-year-old woman presented with recurrent iron deficiency anaemia. A large ulcerated polyp had been seen at endoscopy. Here, the stomach has been opened at laparotomy and the polyp is held up in the surgeon's hand. Deep peptic ulcers can be seen on its surface. Histologically, it proved to be a benign leiomyoma. **(b)** Another benign gastric leiomyoma which had become impacted in the pylorus causing gastric outlet obstruction. It was delivered through the gastrotomy, excised and the defect closed with sutures.

spread locally and tend to metastasise early via the bloodstream. Treatment involves resection of the primary lesion plus palliative chemotherapy if metastasis has occurred.

LYMPHOMAS

PATHOLOGY AND CLINICAL FEATURES OF LYMPHOMAS

Primary lymphomas may arise in the stomach or small bowel. In the stomach, they constitute about 10% of malignancies. As with peptic ulcer and gastric adeno-carcinoma, *H. pylori* infection is an important initiating factor. In the small bowel, the lymphoid tissue may become secondarily involved in non-Hodgkin lymphomas.

In the stomach, lymphomas become extensive, either projecting into the lumen as a bulky ulcerating mass or, more often, diffusely infiltrating the stomach wall. They closely resemble gastric carcinoma in symptoms and endoscopic appearance but it is important to make the distinction because the prognosis of treated lymphoma (usually with chemotherapy or radiotherapy) is much better than adenocarcinoma. Biopsy is the only reliable means of diagnosis. In contrast to gastric carcinoma, lymphomas have a tendency to occur in children and young adults. Low-grade lymphoma has been reported to resolve following *Helicobacter* eradication.

In the small intestine, lymphomas also produce bulky lesions which may obstruct, ulcerate, bleed or even perforate. Occasionally, a lymphoma provides the focus for an intussusception (see Fig. 16.5 and also Fig. 44.9,

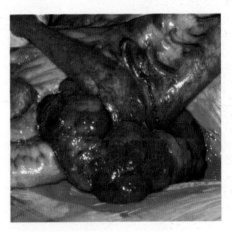

Fig. 16.4 Leiomyosarcoma of the jejunum
This operative specimen shows a large fleshy lesion on the outer surface of the upper jejunum. The patient was a 33-year-old woman who presented with iron deficiency anaemia refractory to oral iron. An abnormality was finally seen on a barium small bowel study after many fruitless investigations. This tumour was histologically well differentiated and amenable to resection; after 5 years, there was no recurrence.

p. 598). Small bowel lymphoma may be a complication of coeliac disease but this is very rare.

MANAGEMENT OF LYMPHOMAS

In both stomach and small intestine, investigation involves barium studies and endoscopic biopsy, but only laparotomy or laparoscopy and biopsy can distinguish primary lymphomas from secondary carcinoma. Primary

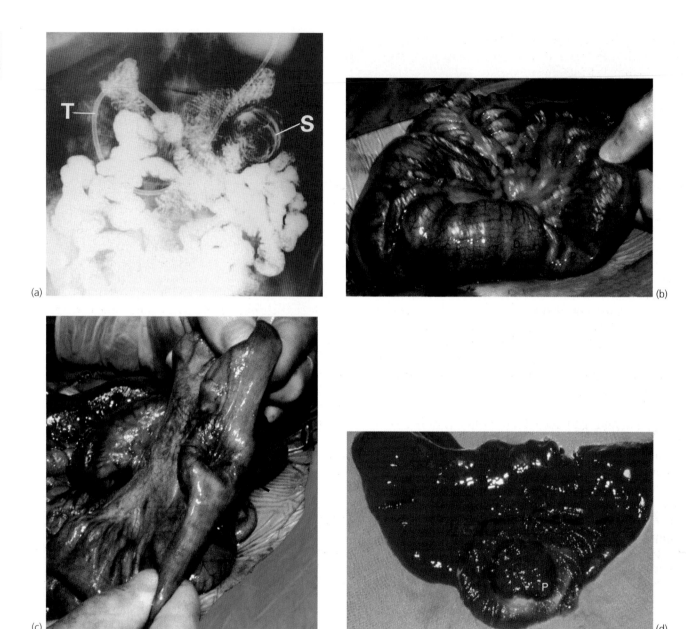

Fig. 16.5 Intussescepting tumours of small bowel
(a) This 35-year-old woman suffered several self-limiting episodes of small bowel obstruction. During one of those episodes this small bowel barium enema was performed by placing the tip of a nasojejunal tube **T** just distal to the duodeno-jejunal flexure and instilling barium. A small bowel intussusception is demonstrated by the 'coiled spring' sign **S**, due to the presence of barium between the telescoping layers of bowel. At surgery, a leiomyoma was found to be responsible. **(b)–(d)** This 22-year-old man presented with small bowel obstruction. At laparotomy, the obstruction was found to be caused by an ileo-ileal intussusception. In this set of operative photographs (b) shows how the proximal ileum **P** had intussuscepted into the distal ileum **D**. When this was reduced (c), an abnormality of the bowel wall could be seen to have formed the apex of the intussuscipiens (arrowed). In (d), a polypoid tumour **P** can be seen on the luminal surface, which proved histologically to be a lymphoma.

lymphomas are often discrete and bulky lesions which may be amenable to surgical excision. Subsequent radiotherapy or chemotherapy or both may be necessary. Treatment gives a 5-year survival rate of around 50%. Radiotherapy alone can succeed in treating some primary gastric lymphomas, emphasising the importance of a tissue diagnosis before surgery is embarked upon.

CARCINOID TUMOURS

PATHOLOGY OF CARCINOID TUMOURS

Carcinoid tumours probably arise from APUD cells of the gastrointestinal endocrine system. Thus, they can arise anywhere in the gastrointestinal tract or in tissues embryologically derived from it, including the pancreas and biliary system. More than 50% of carcinoid tumours are found in the appendix, and most of the remainder occur in the small intestine.

CLINICAL PRESENTATION OF CARCINOID TUMOURS

Appendiceal carcinoid tumours are usually discovered incidentally in appendicectomy specimens and virtually always remain small and benign (Fig. 16.6). In contrast, carcinoid tumours elsewhere in the bowel spread locally in the bowel and mesentery, later becoming disseminated to the liver and other sites. The bowel lesions usually present with symptoms of partial or complete obstruction.

Carcinoid tumours secrete a variety of catecholamines, including **serotonin**. When there is a large volume of tumour, usually in the form of liver metastases, enough catecholamines are secreted to cause the **carcinoid syndrome**. This is characterised by an array of clinical phenomena including transient 'hot flushes', hypotension, asthma and diarrhoea. A metabolite of serotonin, **5-hydroxy-indoleacetic acid** (5-HIAA), can be measured in the urine as a diagnostic test.

MANAGEMENT OF CARCINOID TUMOURS

Treatment usually involves resection of the primary lesion along with the local lymph nodes. Appendiceal carcinoid present at the tip and less than 2 cm in diameter can be treated by appendicectomy alone. Metastatic disease progresses very slowly and is not curable by radiotherapy or chemotherapy. It does respond well to surgery, and in the typically young patient, a more radical approach can be advocated than for other intra-abdominal malignancies.

The full carcinoid syndrome is associated with hepatic tumour outside the portal circulation which is usually of large volume and not amenable to surgical or other cure. It is uncommon and symptoms can be controlled with the help of drugs such as **octreotide**, a somatostatin analogue. Radiotherapy is useful if pain is caused by massive liver enlargement and may induce some shrinkage.

OTHER TUMOURS OF THE SMALL INTESTINE

Other small bowel tumours include **solitary benign angiomas**. These are usually found incidentally at operation or autopsy but sometimes present with intussusception or chronic haemorrhage.

Adenocarcinomas do occur in the small intestine (especially in the duodenum) but are rare compared with their incidence in stomach and large bowel. Adenocarcinomas present with symptoms of bowel obstruction, biliary obstruction when in the periampullary region, bleeding or metastases. Barium follow-through examination for chronic symptoms may demonstrate the lesion, but more commonly it is found and resected at laparotomy for acute obstruction, only being categorised later by histological examination. In many patients, spread has already occurred to regional lymph nodes or the liver by the time of presentation.

PEUTZ–JEGHERS SYNDROME

Peutz–Jeghers syndrome is a rare inherited **autosomal dominant disorder** in which multiple small benign polypoid lesions develop diffusely throughout the

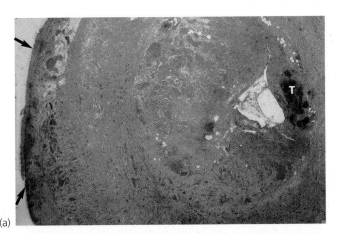
(a)

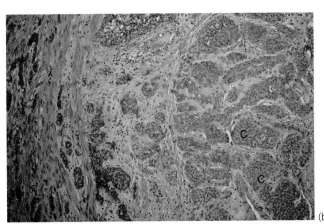
(b)

Fig. 16.6 Carcinoid tumour in the appendix—histopathology
(a) Incidental finding of carcinoid tumour **T** in appendix removed for appendicitis. Tumour extends to the serosal surface **arrowed**. **(b)** High-power view showing close-packed neoplastic carcinoid cells **C**. These typically stain positive with silver stains, such as Grimelius, as well as with immunohistochemical techniques for neuroendocrine markers.

gastrointestinal tract. These are accompanied by characteristic mucocutaneous melanin pigmentation of the lips, gums, hands and feet. The bowel lesions represent hamartomatous malformations of mucosa, submucosa and smooth muscle rather than true adenomas. They may cause chronic intestinal blood loss or present with intestinal obstruction due to intussusception. Malignant transformation does not occur. This condition should not be confused with **familial adenomatous polyposis coli** (FAP) characterised by multiple adenomatous colonic polyps which almost invariably undergo malignant change (see Ch. 20).

17 | Tumours of the pancreas and hepatobiliary system

INTRODUCTION

Adenocarcinoma derived from ductal cells of the exocrine pancreas makes up more than 90% of pancreatic cancers; these have the worst 5-year survival of all gastrointestinal malignancies with only about 5% of patients surviving 5 years. Much less commonly, tumours arise from **exocrine acinar cells** (2%) or from **endocrine islet cells**. Most endocrine tumours become manifest because of the effects of their excess hormone secretion, e.g. insulin, glucagon, gastrin. Around 90% of insulinomas are benign but most of the others are malignant, although survival in such cases is often prolonged.

Intractable abdominal pain, marked weight loss and obstructive jaundice caused by compression of the common bile duct are the most common presenting features of non-endocrine pancreatic adenocarcinoma. In jaundiced patients, pain often develops at a later stage. Obstructive jaundice is also a frequent presentation of the less common primary cholangiocarcinomas of the biliary tree and adenocarcinomas of the ampulla of Vater and the duodenum ('**periampullary carcinomas**').

Sclerosing cholangitis, a rare non-malignant condition, has a similar mode of presentation, and is thus included in this chapter. In contrast, the uncommon **carcinoma of the gall bladder** does not usually present with jaundice.

Primary liver tumours are rare in developed countries but relatively common in some developing countries where hepatitis B and C are the main predisposing factors. **Secondary liver tumours** are common everywhere.

CARCINOMA OF THE PANCREAS

PATHOLOGY

Histologically, carcinoma of the pancreas is usually an adenocarcinoma arising from cells lining the duct system.

About 70% of tumours arise in the head of the gland (the largest part) and the remaining 30% in the body or tail. The tumours tend to form a well-differentiated ductular pattern but the sheets of cells between the ducts often have a more anaplastic appearance. Despite the organised histological pattern, carcinoma of the pancreas is a highly malignant tumour. It metastasises early to local lymph nodes (including nodes in the porta hepatis), to the peritoneum and to the liver via the portal vein (see Fig. 17.1). By the time pancreatic carcinoma presents, the tumour has already disseminated in nearly all cases and the prognosis is poor.

Carcinoma of the pancreas is extremely rare under the age of 50 years and presents at a mean age of 65. Males are affected about 1.5–2 times as often as women. Pancreatic carcinoma ranks third in incidence among gastrointestinal carcinomas after cancer of the large bowel and stomach. Nevertheless, it is relatively uncommon in absolute numbers and is responsible for about 6500 deaths annually in the UK. Its incidence is only half that of gastric carcinoma and it represents only about 3% of all malignancies. Risk factors include cigarette smoking (2–3 times the risk and presenting 15 years earlier) and previous resectional gastric surgery (2–5 times the risk). Ingested nitrosamines and N-nitroso compounds are probably the common factors. Having risen for many years, the incidence of pancreatic cancer in developed countries is now stable.

CLINICAL FEATURES OF PANCREATIC CARCINOMA

There are no suitable screening tests and so pancreatic cancer nearly always presents with symptoms. The main presenting symptoms are substantial weight loss (80%), abdominal pain (60%) and obstructive jaundice (50%). Ascites and an abdominal mass are uncommon. The

247

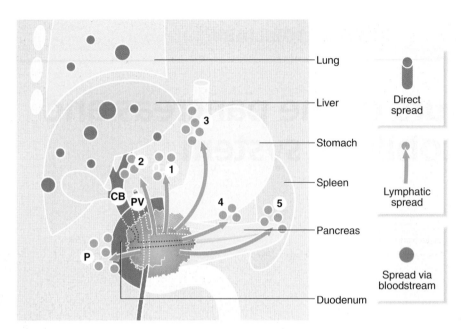

Lung

Liver

Stomach

Spleen

Pancreas

Duodenum

Direct spread

Lymphatic spread

Spread via bloodstream

Fig. 17.1 Spread of carcinoma of the pancreas
Direct spread may involve the common bile duct **CB**, the duodenum and the portal vein **PV**. Lymphatic spread may reach the paraduodenal peritoneum **P** and the nodes of the coeliac axis **1**, the porta hepatis **2**, the lesser and greater curves of the stomach **3, 4** and the hilum of the spleen **4**. Spread may also occur via the bloodstream to the liver, lungs etc.

presenting features of pancreatic carcinoma are shown in Box 17.1.

Pain and other abdominal symptoms and signs

The **pain** of pancreatic carcinoma is severe and continuous and is typically described as 'deep' and 'gnawing'; it may drive patients to contemplate suicide. The pain tends to be nocturnal and poorly relieved by analgesics but may be alleviated somewhat by leaning forwards from a sitting position ('the pancreatic position'). This severe pain often represents locally advanced disease. There are often ill-defined **dyspeptic symptoms** like anorexia, nausea or sporadic vomiting. **Weight loss** may be dramatic even

> **SUMMARY**
>
> **Box 17.1 Presenting features of pancreatic carcinoma**
>
> **Common presenting features**
> - Substantial weight loss (about 80% of cases)
> - Abdominal pain (about 60%)
> - Obstructive jaundice, often without pain (about 50%)
>
> **Less common presenting features**
> - Acute pancreatitis (rare)
> - Diabetes mellitus (preceding or following diagnosis)
> - Gastric outlet obstruction (due to external compression)
> - Thrombophlebitis migrans (recurrent superficial venous thromboses)
> - Pancreatic steatorrhoea (due to pancreatic duct obstruction)

without liver metastases, and is much greater than could be explained by anorexia alone.

Obstructive jaundice

Jaundice, often without pain, develops insidiously over several weeks, during which time the patient gradually assumes a deep greenish-yellow hue. Surprisingly, pruritus and other distressing symptoms are uncommon. Obstructive jaundice is usually caused by compression of the common bile duct where it lies in contact with the head of the pancreas. Thus, the proximal bile duct system including the gall bladder becomes dilated. The gall bladder often becomes palpable (**Courvoisier's law**, see Ch. 11, p. 163). Bile duct obstruction may also be caused by metastatic lymph nodes in the porta hepatis. Liver metastases alone rarely cause jaundice. Note that carcinoma of the pancreas and other obstructing tumours of the biliary tree typically produce an unremitting, painless and progressively deepening jaundice, whereas the jaundice of gallstone disease tends not to be as profound. It also tends to fluctuate in intensity and there is usually a typical history of biliary pain.

APPROACH TO INVESTIGATION OF SUSPECTED PANCREATIC CARCINOMA

The patient presenting with obstructive jaundice should be investigated as described in Chapter 11. Ultrasound is used to look for masses in the pancreas and liver, dilated bile ducts and stones. This is usually followed by endoscopic retrograde cholangio-pancreatography, or ERCP (see Fig. 17.2b) both to inspect the ampulla of

Vater and to demonstrate the anatomy of the biliary and pancreatic ducts; sites of obstruction are identified by injecting contrast.

When pancreatic cancer is suspected in a non-jaundiced patient and no clear causative factor has yet been seen, abdominal CT scanning may be indicated (see Fig. 17.2c and d). CT scanning is a more reliable method of

diagnosing pancreatic cancers than ultrasound, but tumours smaller than 2 cm may not be detected. CT scanning also demonstrates metastatic deposits in the porta hepatis or liver parenchyma and gives an idea of the extent of local invasion into the retroperitoneal area and portal vein; this can help the surgeon decide whether the lesion might be resectable. CT scanning

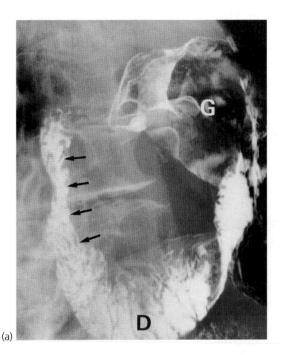

(a)

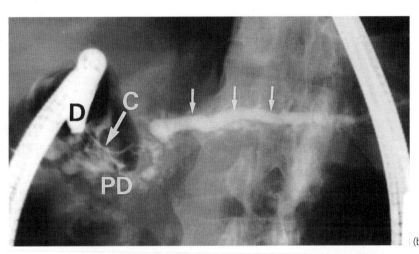

(b)

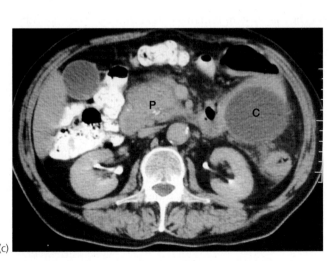

(c)

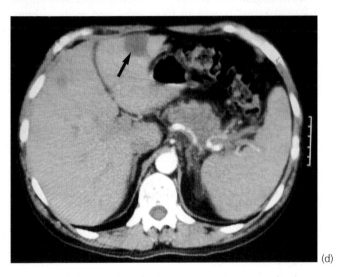

(d)

Fig. 17.2 Carcinoma of the head of the pancreas
(a) This 77-year-old man presented with 4 weeks of painless obstructive jaundice. This barium meal shows the gastric antrum **G** and duodenum. The duodenal loop **D** is grossly distended by the obstructing effect of the head of the pancreas. The medial wall of the second part of the duodenum (arrowed) is compressed and distorted by the tumour. **(b)** Endoscopic retrograde pancreatogram in a jaundiced patient with carcinoma of the head of the pancreas. The tip of the duodenoscope **D** lies opposite the ampulla of Vater, into which a catheter **C** has been passed. The distal pancreatic duct is dilated (arrowed) and the proximal duct **PD** is compressed and distorted by the tumour. **(c)** CT scan showing enlargement of the head of the pancreas **P** most suspicious of carcinoma. The dark circular lesion within the tail of the pancreas is a secondary cyst or pseudocyst **C**. **(d)** CT scan further cephalad (towards the head) of the same patient showing one obvious low-attenuation lesion in the liver consistent with a metastasis (arrowed). The diagnosis of carcinoma of the pancreas was confirmed on percutaneous biopsy of the pancreatic lesion. Thus this 54-year-old man had inoperable disease. Unfortunately, this is all too common a presentation.

alone, however, often understages the disease. Pancreatic masses can be biopsied percutaneously using ultrasound or CT control to confirm malignancy and cell type, although this is not favoured in many centres.

Staging of pancreatic cancer is vital if resection is contemplated as the results in disease that has metastasised are abysmal. Various methods have been employed but many specialist centres depend on CT and staging laparoscopy. Laparoscopy allows more precise staging as small peritoneal seedlings can be visualised (and biopsied) and cytology of peritoneal fluid performed. Laparoscopic ultrasound is finding favour to assess possible portal vein invasion and to seek microscopic liver metastases.

MANAGEMENT OF PANCREATIC CARCINOMA

Most patients with pancreatic cancer present at an incurable stage with local invasion or metastases. Only about 20% have apparently localised disease with a potential for cure by resection. **Whipple's operation** (pancreatico-duodenectomy, see Fig. 17.5, p. 253) is the standard procedure for the rare instances when resection of carcinoma of the head of the pancreas is indicated. It is a major undertaking with high operative morbidity and mortality. Even in specialist centres, operative mortality is about 5% and 5-year survival about 20%.

The main indication for pancreatico-duodenectomy is a periampullary lesion. External beam radiotherapy and 5-fluorouracil (5-FU) chemotherapy after operation extend mean survival from 6 to 10 months, and trials of intra-operative radiotherapy appear to increase this slightly. Thus, for most patients, any treatment must be regarded as palliative at best.

Cystic neoplasms of the pancreas are sometimes discovered incidentally on CT scanning or ultrasonography. The most common are mucinous cystadenomas and cystadenocarcinomas. As all probably have a malignant potential and are largely curable if treated early, radical resection is the treatment of choice.

Palliation

Palliation takes several forms. If there is obvious widespread disease, the patient should be allowed to die with minimal surgical interference. Adequate analgesia is essential and severe pain can be effectively relieved by permanent **blockade of the coeliac ganglion**, which is performed percutaneously or thoracoscopically. If obstructive jaundice is the dominant feature, this can usually be relieved by inserting a biliary stent (**endoprosthesis**) into the compressed bile duct at ERCP or via a percutaneous transhepatic route; techniques are illustrated in Figure 17.3. Bypass can be achieved surgically at laparotomy or laparoscopically. Options include both biliary bypass and enteric bypass. The standard palliative operation of triple bypass (cholecysto-jejunostomy, gastro-jejunostomy and an anastomosis between the loops of small bowel attached to the gall bladder) has largely fallen out of favour because of the success of biliary stenting and the short lifespan of such patients (see Fig. 17.3).

BILIARY AND PERIAMPULLARY TUMOURS

Adenocarcinomas originating from the epithelium lining the biliary duct system are known as **cholangiocarcinomas**. They may develop anywhere in the intrahepatic or extrahepatic duct system. The less common intrahepatic cholangiocarcinomas tend to invade the liver parenchyma, presenting in a manner similar to primary hepatocellular carcinomas. Since most of the bile system remains patent in these cases, jaundice is rare. In contrast, extrahepatic cholangiocarcinomas tend to obstruct bile drainage. They present with painless progressive jaundice in the same way as carcinoma of the pancreatic head. Unlike pancreatic cancer, cholangiocarcinomas are slow-growing and metastasise late so that complete resection is often possible. Cholangiocarcinomas have a dense fibrous stroma and tend to grow along the duct system rather than producing a focal proliferative lesion. The resulting smooth elongated stricture can be demonstrated by ERCP, MRCP (see p. 50) or transhepatic cholangiography (see Fig. 17.4). Histological proof of malignancy may be difficult to obtain owing to the fibrous nature of the tumour.

Fig. 17.3 Palliative procedures for obstructive jaundice caused by carcinoma of the head of the pancreas or a periampullary tumour
(a) Obstruction of the common bile duct and duodenum. Carcinoma of the pancreatic head obstructs the lower end of the common bile duct and potentially the duodenum, i.e. the gastric outlet. **(b)** Endoscopic stent placement. The sphincter of Oddi may require a preliminary endoscopic sphincterotomy prior to intubation. A self-retaining plastic stent, placed endoscopically or percutaneously, lies in situ across the biliary stricture. Note the 'pig-tail' ends of this type of stent which curl up when the wire is removed, retaining the stent in the correct position. **(c)** Triple bypass operation, rarely performed nowadays because of the efficacy of endoscopic stenting and the short life expectancy of patients with pancreatic cancer.

(a) Anatomy of obstruction of the common bile duct and duodenum

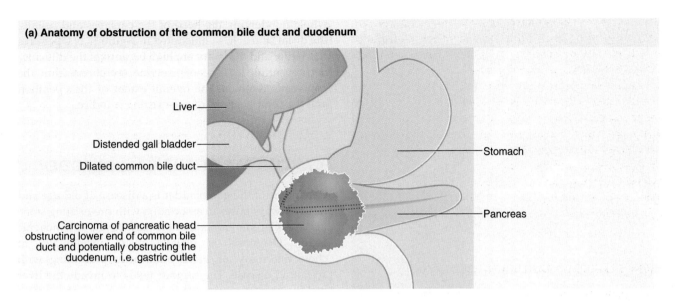

Liver

Distended gall bladder

Dilated common bile duct

Stomach

Pancreas

Carcinoma of pancreatic head
obstructing lower end of common bile
duct and potentially obstructing the
duodenum, i.e. gastric outlet

(b) Endoscopic stent placement

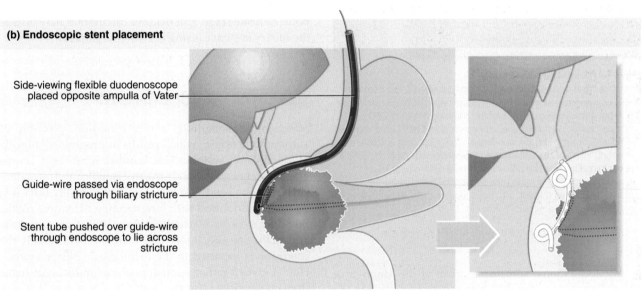

Side-viewing flexible duodenoscope
placed opposite ampulla of Vater

Guide-wire passed via endoscope
through biliary stricture

Stent tube pushed over guide-wire
through endoscope to lie across
stricture

(c) Triple bypass operation

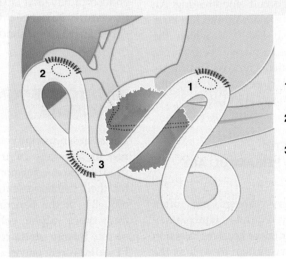

1 Gastro-jejunostomy to bypass
   duodenal obstruction

2 Cholecysto-jejunostomy to bypass
   obstructed common bile duct

3 Jejuno-jejunostomy to divert food
   away from biliary tract

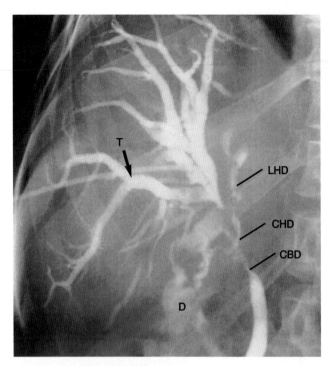

Fig. 17.4 Cholangiocarcinoma
Percutaneous transhepatic cholangiogram in a 66-year-old man with painless progressive jaundice from an inoperable cholangiocarcinoma; this X-ray shows a long stricture of the common bile duct **CBD**, common hepatic duct **CHD** and left hepatic duct **LHD**. Some contrast has flowed through into the duodenum. The cystic duct is obliterated, preventing filling of the gall bladder. A percutaneous drainage tube **T** has been inserted into the right hepatic duct system prior to an attempt to place a stent across the stricture by the same route. Some contrast has flowed through into the duodenum **(D)**. Nowadays, most stents are placed endoscopically (see Fig. 17.3).

Adenocarcinoma sometimes arises at the ampulla of Vater, forming a polypoid lesion which projects into the duodenum and obstructs biliary drainage causing jaundice. These tumours are friable and tend to bleed insidiously, giving a positive result on faecal occult blood testing. An association with intestinal polyposis syndromes has been described. Diagnosis is made at ERCP at which the tumour is visible and accessible to biopsy. Very rarely, adenocarcinoma arises in the duodenal mucosa and causes obstructive jaundice if situated close to the ampulla. Again, the lesion is readily diagnosed at ERCP.

MANAGEMENT OF EXTRAHEPATIC CHOLANGIOCARCINOMA AND PERIAMPULLARY CARCINOMA

Extrahepatic and periampullary cancers are often amenable to curative resection by Whipple's pancreatico-duodenectomy. This extensive procedure involves resection of most of the extrahepatic biliary system as well as the whole duodenum, the head of the pancreas and usually the distal stomach, as illustrated in Figure 17.5. Operative morbidity and mortality are high because of the difficulty of preventing leakage of exocrine secretions from the pancreatic remnant, the overall extent of the operation and the complications of pre-existing jaundice.

CARCINOMA OF THE GALL BLADDER

Carcinoma of the gall bladder is a disease of old age and nearly always arises in association with pre-existing stone disease. Chronic inflammation may be the carcinogenic factor. Diagnosis is usually made incidentally at cholecystectomy, or more often after presenting with advanced disease. The tumour tends to invade the liver bed by direct venous and lymphatic spread at an early stage making resection impracticable and the prognosis poor. At a late stage, gall bladder carcinomas may invade the biliary system causing obstructive jaundice.

SCLEROSING CHOLANGITIS

Sclerosing cholangitis is a rare condition, probably of autoimmune origin, which results in progressive fibrosis of the biliary system. The luminal narrowing causes gradual and progressive obstructive jaundice and secondary cirrhosis. The condition may arise sporadically but often occurs in association with longstanding ulcerative colitis. Bile duct stenosis is usually diffuse with a characteristic appearance on ERCP (see Fig. 17.6), but occasionally the condition is localised to the extrahepatic biliary system. Here it gives a radiological appearance indistinguishable from cholangiocarcinoma.

In the case of localised obstruction, an indwelling plastic stent may be passed through the stricture, either endoscopically or at laparotomy. More extensive intubation procedures have been devised for diffuse disease but life expectancy is only about 5–10 years.

ENDOCRINE TUMOURS OF THE PANCREAS

The neuroendocrine cells of the islets of Langerhans give rise to a variety of uncommon tumours which often produce excess hormone secretions that are responsible for their usual presenting features. The islets make up only 2% of the pancreatic mass and comprise cells of four types; **alpha cells** secrete glucagon, **beta cells** secrete insulin, **delta cells** secrete somatostatin and **F** or **PP cells** secrete pancreatic polypeptide.

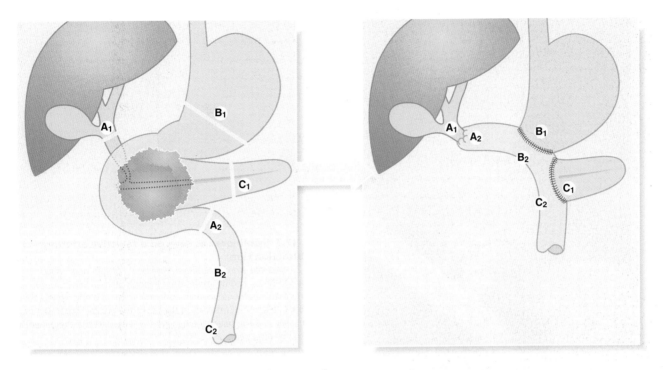

Fig. 17.5 Whipple's operation (pancreatico-duodenectomy)
(a) Structures are divided at the lines A, B and C. **(b)** The distal half of the stomach, the entire duodenal loop, the head and body of the pancreas and the lower end of the common bile duct are all removed, then reconstruction performed with anastomoses between A_1 and A_2, B_1 and B_2 and C_1 and C_2.

INSULINOMAS AND GLUCAGONOMAS

The most common endocrine tumours of the pancreas are **insulinomas** derived from beta cells. Nevertheless these occur in only 17 per 10 million people per annum. The main symptoms are cerebral disturbances caused by attacks of hypoglycaemia, particularly when fasting or exercising. The attacks are relieved by oral or intravenous glucose. About 90% of insulinomas are single and 90% are benign and amenable to curative resection. They occur with equal frequency in the head, body and tail of the pancreas. Histology almost always appears benign and malignancy is only diagnosed by the appearance of metastases. The diagnosis is usually made after metabolic investigation for bizarre 'funny turns'. Once hyper-insulinism has been confirmed, CT scanning and selective pancreatic arteriography (see Fig. 17.7) are used to identify the site of the lesion.

Alpha cells may give rise to **glucagonomas** which are very rare and present with diabetes mellitus and a characteristic skin rash known as **migratory necrolytic erythema**.

ZOLLINGER–ELLISON SYNDROME

Gastrin-secreting tumours (**gastrinomas**) arise in the islets of Langerhans or in the duodenal wall in 10 per 10 million people per annum. About 25% develop in patients with MEN 1, described below. Gastrinomas give rise to severe and intractable peptic ulceration and diarrhoea. This condition is known as Zollinger–Ellison syndrome.

Diagnosis is made by demonstrating persistently high serum gastrin levels. The tumour is localised by CT scanning and selective pancreatic angiography. Many of the lesions are too small to be demonstrated by either method and their location can only be established at laparotomy using intraoperative ultrasonography. About 60% of gastrinomas are classified as malignant but they grow slowly and metastasise late. Thus, excision is often curative. In patients where the primary tumour is inoperable, palliation with **omeprazole** often prevents peptic ulcer symptoms and complications.

MULTIPLE ENDOCRINE NEOPLASIA SYNDROMES (MEN)

Pancreatic neuroendocrine cell tumours sometimes form part of a multiple endocrine neoplasia syndrome (MEN) of which two types are recognised:

● MEN I—islet cell tumours, pituitary adenomas and parathyroid hyperplasia
● MEN II—medullary carcinoma of the thyroid, phaeochromocytoma and parathyroid adenoma

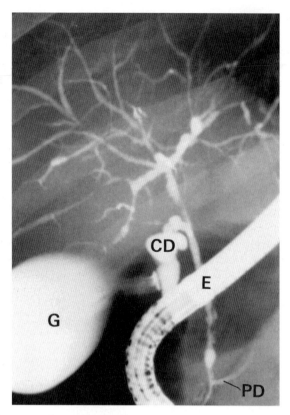

Fig. 17.6 Sclerosing cholangitis
ERCP in a 52-year-old man with longstanding ulcerative colitis who developed painless jaundice. There is widespread irregular narrowing of both the intrahepatic and extrahepatic bile ducts typical of sclerosing cholangitis. Note the endoscope **E**, the normal gall bladder **G** and the cystic duct **CD** filling with contrast. The proximal part of the pancreatic duct **PD** also contains contrast.

PRIMARY TUMOURS OF THE LIVER

Primary tumours of the liver are uncommon in developed countries and the majority are **hepatocellular carcinomas** derived from hepatocytes. A small minority of primary liver tumours are **haemangiomas** derived from the vascular system; these benign neoplasms are a separate pathological entity from the common congenital vascular hamartomas of the liver.

HEPATOCELLULAR CARCINOMA

Hepatocellular carcinomas (also known as **hepatomas**) are malignant, slow-growing tumours which often arise multicentrically throughout the liver. It is of great interest that an aetiological factor can be identified in nearly all cases; factors include pre-existing infection with hepatitis B and particularly hepatitis C, alcoholic cirrhosis, haemochromatosis and chronic active hepatitis. In 80% of cases, there is some form of pre-existing cirrhosis. **Alcoholic cirrhosis** is the most common aetiological factor in

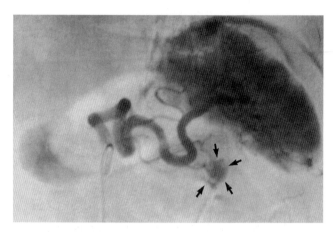

Fig. 17.7 Insulinoma as seen on a selective arteriogram (subtraction film)
This 31-year-old woman suffered from bouts of faintness which proved to be caused by intermittent hypoglycaemia. Selective splenic arteriography demonstrated an abnormal mass of blood vessels about 1.5 cm in diameter (arrowed) in the tail of the pancreas representing an insulinoma. The tail of the pancreas was excised and the patient's symptoms disappeared.

developed countries; indeed, hepatoma occurs in about 25% of patients with cirrhosis of more than 5 years' standing. The risk in patients with **haemochromatosis** and **chronic active hepatitis** is even higher. Although uncommon in developed countries, hepatocellular carcinoma is one of the most common cancers in parts of Africa. Here the most common cause is cirrhosis resulting from hepatitis B or C but a variety of environmental carcinogens have been implicated; these include **aflatoxin**, a toxin produced by a species of *Aspergillus* which grows on stored grains and peanuts. Various **parasitic infestations**, e.g. schistosomiasis, *Echinococcus* (tapeworm) and *Clonorchis sinensis* (liver fluke), also predispose to hepatocellular carcinoma. In developed countries, the peak incidence of hepatocellular carcinoma is between the ages of 40 and 60, but in those developing countries where the disease is common, most cases occur between 20 and 40 years of age.

Clinical features and management of hepatocellular carcinoma

The presenting features of hepatocellular carcinoma are anorexia, weight loss, abdominal pain and distension. These are often associated with stigmata of cirrhosis. On examination, a liver mass is usually palpable. Ultrasound or CT scanning or laparoscopy can be used to establish the size and position of the liver mass or masses and to guide needle biopsy.

By the time it is diagnosed, hepatocellular carcinoma is usually widespread within the liver and the only surgical option would be liver transplantation. Unfortunately, recurrence has proved inevitable after transplantation and this has now been abandoned. Isolated lesions are occasionally amenable to segmental resection but again recurrence is likely. Recurrence is due to the multicentric origin of the tumour, although this does not explain recurrence after transplantation. Embolisation or local administration of cytotoxic drugs via an intra-arterial cannula is sometimes attempted by way of palliation but complication rates are high and efficacy is unproven.

SECONDARY LIVER TUMOURS

Secondary tumours in the liver are extremely common. These arise from a wide variety of primary sources, especially the stomach, pancreas, large bowel, breast and bronchus. Liver metastases are usually asymptomatic but as the liver parenchyma is progressively destroyed, the patient begins to feel unwell with anorexia and weight loss. Jaundice is unusual and tends to appear only at a terminal stage of the illness. Jaundice results from a combination of compressive obstruction of the intrahepatic biliary system and gross loss of parenchyma so that bile pigments cannot be excreted. Consequently, the biochemical picture tends to be that of a mixed hepatitic and obstructive pattern.

Depending on the source, the presence of liver metastases usually indicates incurable disease. Isolated metastases, however, especially of colonic or renal origin, can sometimes be removed by segmental resection with about a 35% chance of 5-year disease-free survival; repeat resection of recurrences has also been described. If liver metastases are responsible for pain, systemic chemotherapy may retard their growth and suppress symptoms. Large metastases causing intractable pain can be controlled by several different physical methods including local cryotherapy, microwave and thermal ablation, percutaneous alcohol injection and palliative radiotherapy.

18 Pancreatitis

INTRODUCTION

Pancreatitis is an inflammatory disorder of the pancreas that is characterised by abdominal pain. Most cases present in an acute form known as **acute pancreatitis**. Attacks range in severity from mild to life-threatening. Some patients suffer recurrent acute attacks (**acute relapsing pancreatitis**) and a small proportion appear to suffer a persistent form known as **chronic pancreatitis**; this is often associated with high alcohol intake.

ACUTE PANCREATITIS

AETIOLOGY AND EPIDEMIOLOGY OF ACUTE PANCREATITIS

Gallstones and alcoholism together account for about 80% of acute pancreatitis world-wide. These and the other main causes of acute pancreatitis are listed in Box 18.1. Opie first pointed out the relationship between gallstones and pancreatitis in 1901 based on autopsy evidence. Later it became apparent that stone obstruction of the ampulla of Vater allowed bile to reflux into the pancreatic duct, thus activating enzymes within the gland. Small gallstones may cause transient obstruction as they pass through the ampulla or larger stones may impact at the lower end of the common bile duct. Beyond this, the precise mechanism of gallstone pancreatitis remains obscure even today.

The proportion of acute pancreatitis caused by alcoholism varies from country to country; about two-thirds of patients in the UK have a gallstone aetiology whereas about two-thirds have an alcoholic aetiology in parts of the USA and continental Europe. Longstanding high alcohol intake for at least 2 years is usually required to cause alcoholic pancreatitis; the mean daily alcohol intake in the subjects of one study was 140 g compared with 40 g in controls. Occasionally acute pancreatitis can result from a single session of heavy drinking—students finishing exams beware! In most cases of acute pancreatitis the initiating factor is some form of pancreatic duct obstruction. This is most often due to gallstones, but chronic alcoholic pancreatitis may also have an obstructive element.

In developed countries, the annual incidence of acute pancreatitis requiring hospital admission is about 1:2000 population and the mortality is about 2%. About 15% fall into the clinical category of **severe pancreatitis**. Women are affected more than men, but men are more likely to suffer recurrent attacks. Most patients are over 45 years of age and the peak incidence is between 50 and 60 years. The incidence appears to have risen by a factor of 10 over the last 40 years with only part of this due to improved diagnosis. The other causative factors are unknown.

PATHOPHYSIOLOGY OF ACUTE PANCREATITIS

Acute pancreatitis is characterised by the sudden onset of diffuse inflammation of the pancreas. A range of diverse factors initiate disturbances of cellular metabolism, chiefly revolving around membrane stability. This leads to inappropriate activation of zymogens within the pancreas. Activation of trypsin is probably the key initiating event and this overwhelms intrinsic antitrypsin activity, leading to **interstitial oedematous** pancreatitis. Fortunately, the extent and severity of inflammation remain mild and

Box 18.1 Aetiology of acute pancreatitis

Obstruction

- Gallstones—30–70% of cases
- Congenital abnormalities: pancreas divisum with accessory duct obstruction; choledochocoele; duodenal diverticula—5%
- Ampullary or pancreatic tumours—3%
- Abnormally high pressure in the sphincter of Oddi (above 40 mmHg)—1–2%
- Ascariasis (second most common cause in endemic areas, e.g. Kashmir)

Drugs and toxins

- Alcoholism—30–70% of cases
- Drugs: azathioprine and 6-mercaptopurine, antibacterials such as metronidazole and tetracycline, H_2 blockers and many other classes of drug—1–2%

Iatrogenic and traumatic causes

- Following endoscopic retrograde cholangio-pancreatography (ERCP) or endoscopic sphincterotomy (2–6% of patients having the procedure)
- Following cardiopulmonary bypass (0.5–5% of patients having bypass)
- Blunt pancreatic trauma usually due to motor vehicle accidents (very rare)

Metabolic causes

- Hypertriglyceridaemia (> 11 mmol/L)—2%
- Hypercalcaemia—rare

Infection

- AIDS: secondary infection with cytomegalovirus and others—incidence about 10% in AIDS patients
- Other viruses: mumps, chickenpox, Coxsackie viruses, hepatitis A, B and C (very rare)

Idiopathic pancreatitis

- About 10% have no definable cause after diagnostic evaluation including ERCP; research studies show about two-thirds of 'idiopathic' cases have microlithiasis

mesentery, representing areas of **fat saponification** ('fat necrosis'). If saponification is extensive, calcium becomes sequestered in areas of fat necrosis and this has been incriminated in the fall in blood calcium level characteristic of more severe acute pancreatitis.

As severity increases, trypsin and other enzymes cause more extensive local damage as well as activation of complement and kinin systems leading to the development of the systemic inflammatory response syndrome (SIRS). Manifestations include shock, acute respiratory distress syndrome (ARDS), renal failure and disseminated intravascular coagulation (see Ch. 2). At this stage, **acute peripancreatic fluid collections** become detectable on CT scanning. Severe pancreatitis is associated with **pancreatic necrosis**. An element of ischaemia within the gland and an associated reperfusion injury have been incriminated in transforming acute oedematous pancreatitis into this necrotising disease. Complications are common in this group and mortality is up to 10%.

A substantial proportion of patients with pancreatic necrosis develop **infected necrotising pancreatitis**, usually with Gram-negative organisms translocated from the bowel. This occurs within 2 weeks of the onset and greatly increases mortality. Diagnosis of this crucial development can be difficult to make. **Pancreatic abscess formation** is a different phenomenon developing later and having a somewhat better prognosis.

At autopsy in patients dying of acute necrotising pancreatitis, the peritoneal cavity is filled with a dark, blood-stained inflammatory exudate containing fine lipid droplets leading to the term **acute haemorrhagic pancreatitis** being employed. The peritoneal surface is grossly inflamed and semi-digested and all that is left of the pancreas is a necrotic mass.

CLINICAL FEATURES OF ACUTE PANCREATITIS

Acute pancreatitis presents as an acute abdomen. Pain begins suddenly and is severe and continuous from the outset. Initially it is poorly localised in the upper abdomen and is often described by the patient as 'going through to the back'. As the peritoneal cavity becomes involved over the next few hours, the pain spreads throughout the abdomen and may be referred to the shoulder tips if the diaphragmatic peritoneum becomes inflamed. Relentless vomiting is an early feature. In the early stages, the patient is restless and constantly changes posture in the search for a comfortable position. Pain is most often relieved by leaning forward in the so-called '**pancreatic position**'. With the onset of peritonitis, movement becomes increasingly painful and the patient tends to lie still. The clinical signs depend on the severity of the inflammatory process and the stage to which it has progressed.

self-limiting in most patients and any systemic effects are mild. In the least severe cases, there is minimal peritoneal exudation and no pancreatic changes are detectable on contrast-enhanced CT scanning. In more severe disease, the pancreas becomes swollen and oedematous but remains viable. If laparotomy is inadvertently performed at this stage, clear, non-infected peritoneal fluid can be seen with whitish patches on the great omentum and

Clinical classification

The initial clinical picture cannot be relied upon to predict which patients are likely to deteriorate. Only a small proportion eventually suffer necrotising pancreatitis but a case of mild pancreatitis can rapidly deteriorate to 'death's door'. To provide early warning of severity, each patient with acute pancreatitis is placed into one of two categories, **mild** or **severe**. This provides an early indicator of prognosis and is central to the generation of a management strategy. Categorisation is based on carefully tested scoring systems originally developed by Ranson (see Box 18.2) or by Imrie (Glasgow criteria—see Table 18.1). If three or more of the factors listed are present, the patient is diagnosed as having severe pancreatitis and should be admitted to an intensive care or high-dependency unit for careful monitoring. The more adverse factors present, the worse the prognosis. Even if a patient is initially placed in the mild group, continued observation is essential as a shift to severe pancreatitis can occur at any time.

Mild acute pancreatitis

Mild attacks are common. The patient looks generally well with minimal systemic features. Nevertheless, there is often considerable pain. The abdomen is usually distended and diffusely tender but with little guarding. Bowel sounds are absent as a result of inflammatory ileus and rectal examination is normal. The patient may be mildly jaundiced as a result of periampullary oedema. The differential diagnosis in this situation includes biliary colic, acute cholecystitis, an acute exacerbation of a peptic ulcer or even a small perforation of a peptic ulcer. Lower lobe pneumonia or an inferior myocardial infarction may sometimes present in this way. Sometimes the diagnosis is made when the serum amylase is found to be unexpectedly elevated (see below).

Severe acute pancreatitis

In a severe attack the patient looks apathetic, grey and shocked and there are typical abdominal signs of generalised peritonitis, i.e. extreme tenderness, guarding and rigidity. In this case, the differential diagnosis includes other major abdominal catastrophes, especially faecal peritonitis from perforated large bowel and concealed haemorrhage from a leaking aortic aneurysm. Massive bowel infarction due to arterial occlusion may present in this way but the abdominal signs are often less marked. An important early and dangerous complication of severe acute pancreatitis is **ARDS**.

The clinical features of acute pancreatitis are summarised in Box 18.3.

KEY POINTS

Box 18.2 Criteria for early identification of severe pancreatitis (after Ranson)

'Severe pancreatitis': high risk of major complications or death defined by the presence of three or more of the following features:

On admission
- Age over 55 years (non-gallstone pancreatitis) or 70 years (gallstone pancreatitis)
- Leucocyte count greater than $16\,000 \times 10^9$/L
- Blood glucose greater than 10 mmol/L in a patient who is not diabetic
- Lactate dehydrogenase (LDH) greater than 350 i.u./L
- SGOT > 100 u/L

During the next 48 hours
- Haematocrit increase of more than 10%
- Serum urea increase of more than 10 mmol/L despite adequate i.v. therapy
- Hypocalcaemia (corrected serum Ca < 2.0 mmol/L)
- Low arterial pO_2 (< 8 kPa or 60 mmHg)
- Metabolic acidosis (base deficit more than 4 mEq/L)
- Estimated fluid sequestration more than 6 L

Table 18.1 A mnemonic ('PANCREAS') for remembering a modified Glasgow scoring system of severity prediction in acute pancreatitis

Mnemonic letter	Criterion	Positive when
P	PaO₂	< 8 kPA or 60 mmHg
A	Age	> 55 years (non-gallstone pancreatitis) or > 70 (gallstone)
N	Neutrophil count	> 16 × 10⁹/L
C	Calcium (blood)	< 2 mmol/L
R	Raised plasma urea	raised by > 10 mmol/L
E	Enzyme (plasma lactate dehydrogenase, LDH)	> 350 i.u./L
A	Albumin (plasma)	< 32 g/L
S	Sugar (plasma glucose)	> 10 mmol/L

After E M Moore, with permission

INVESTIGATION OF SUSPECTED PANCREATITIS

Acute pancreatitis must be excluded in any adult presenting with acute abdominal pain, and in any child with peritonitis not readily attributable to appendicitis.

SUMMARY

Box 18.3 Clinical features of acute pancreatitis

Mild attack
- Acute abdominal pain
- Minimal or rapidly resolving abdominal signs, e.g. abdominal distension, some abdominal tenderness and guarding, absent bowel sounds
- Minimal systemic illness
- Moderate tachycardia

Severe attack
- Severe acute abdominal pain
- Severe toxaemia and shock
- Generalised peritonitis (diffuse abdominal tenderness, guarding, rigidity, absent bowel sounds)
- Acute respiratory distress syndrome (may develop during the first few days)

Plasma amylase

Amylase is one of the enzymes absorbed into the circulation in pancreatitis; **plasma amylase** measurement is simple to perform in the laboratory and provides a generally reliable diagnostic test. A plasma amylase level above 1200 i.u./ml is usually regarded as diagnostic of acute pancreatitis but amylase levels are often lower in alcoholic pancreatitis, particularly in recurrent attacks. Any upper abdominal inflammatory condition close to the pancreas (e.g. cholecystitis, perforated peptic ulcer or strangulated bowel) may cause a moderate rise in plasma amylase, although this rarely reaches 1000 i.u./ml. Most other enzyme estimations have not proved more sensitive or specific although **serum lipase** estimation may be useful in difficult or late-presenting cases.

Plasma amylase levels rise rapidly at the outset of an attack of pancreatitis and levels of 10 000 i.u./ml or more may be recorded on admission to hospital. The peak amylase level is not an indicator of the severity of the pancreatitis nor of the likelihood of subsequent complications. However, persistently raised levels over several days warn of developing complications. False negative amylase results may occur in lipaemic serum. In this case, true results can be obtained on diluted specimens.

Alanine aminotransferase (ALT) levels elevated to more than three times normal are said to be highly specific for gallstone pancreatitis.

Imaging

Plain X-rays of chest (erect) to look for free gas under the diaphragm, and abdomen (supine) are usually performed during the initial investigation. Abdominal X-ray may show a 'ground-glass' appearance if peritoneal exudate is present. Bowel gas tends to be absent except perhaps for a 'sentinel loop' of dilated adynamic small bowel in the centre of the abdomen. These signs are often absent in pancreatitis and even if present, are not diagnostic. Rarely, radiopaque gallstones are visible.

An ultrasound scan of the biliary tree is essential if a good-quality examination has not been performed recently; a delay of 48–72 hours may improve the image quality and a decision to perform therapeutic ERCP may render urgent scanning unnecessary. In either case, the goal is to look for small calculi in the gall bladder or bile ducts which are typically responsible for gallstone pancreatitis. If no definite cause for the pancreatitis is found, ultrasound examination should be performed following recovery from the attack.

Endoscopy

In patients where a cause for pancreatitis is not evident from the history or initial imaging studies, **ERCP** can have an important diagnostic role. A cause can be found in up to 50% of this group of patients, e.g. small pancreatic or periampullary tumours, pancreatic duct stricture, gallstones, pancreas divisum or hypertensive sphincter of Oddi.

A **peritoneal tap** (abdominal paracentesis) or **laparoscopy** may be useful in patients with severe abdominal signs without a firm diagnosis of pancreatitis. Clear fluid is obtained in mild pancreatitis and dark ('prune juice'), sterile fluid in severe necrotising pancreatitis. If foul-smelling fluid containing bacteria is found, the alternative diagnosis of intestinal perforation is likely.

MANAGEMENT OF ACUTE PANCREATITIS

Mild attacks

Mild attacks require no further emergency investigation and are managed by fluid resuscitation and analgesia. Recovery is usually rapid. The withholding of oral intake was originally designed to 'rest' the pancreas, but this belief is not held as firmly as it once was. Subsequent management is aimed at treating predisposing factors. Gallstones should be sought by ultrasonography. Ductal stones should be removed endoscopically before discharge from hospital. Cholecystectomy should be performed early in the recovery period. Alcohol abuse must be discouraged.

Even when pancreatitis is more severe, supportive measures (including careful intravenous fluid resuscitation) are still the mainstay of treatment. A nasogastric tube is usually passed to aspirate the stomach and adds to the patient's comfort and safety if gastroparesis causes troublesome vomiting. Controversially, early oral feeding or feeding via a tube has been reported in some series to decrease morbidity significantly. Prophylactic parenteral antibiotics (e.g. a cephalosporin or imipenem) may be administered, although any role for infection in mild pancreatitis is controversial.

Plasma amylase is measured daily to chart the progress of the disease; as the inflammation begins to resolve, the amylase levels fall accordingly. If the level remains elevated beyond a week, complications such as pancreatic infection, abscess or pseudocyst may be responsible. Biochemical estimations, particularly liver transaminases and bilirubin, are charted regularly chiefly looking for evidence of biliary obstruction; renal function tests are performed to seek evidence of acute renal failure.

Severe attacks

A severe attack is defined by reference to a list of criteria which should be evaluated on admission and over the next 48 hours (see Box 18.2, p. 258). Patients with severe pancreatitis may die early because of profound systemic toxaemia and **multiple organ dysfunction syndrome (MODS—see Ch. 2).** ARDS develops rapidly with little warning but a deteriorating arterial pO_2 may herald its onset. This is an indication for urgent ventilatory support before the condition becomes established.

Gross fluid and electrolyte disturbances and hypocalcaemia are also likely to occur. Fluid balance in the shocked patient is complicated by massive losses of protein-rich fluid into the peritoneal cavity and interstitially ('third space'). This sequestration of fluid needs to be countered by large amounts of colloid and crystalloid solutions, carefully monitored by measuring central venous pressure and hourly urine output. Any patient recognised to have severe pancreatitis or anyone with acute pancreatitis, however mild, with signs of serious deterioration should be admitted to an intensive care unit without delay for close monitoring and early treatment of cardiovascular, pulmonary, renal and septic complications. Box 18.4 lists recommended investigations to guide management.

Peritoneal lavage, using up to 48 L of lavage fluid per 24 hours, has been employed in severe cases in an attempt to reduce systemic absorption of enzymes and other toxins. Results, however, are mixed and the procedure is not generally recommended.

Endoscopy and surgery in acute pancreatitis

Trials of early endoscopic removal of causative bile duct stones suggest the infection rate is lower and overall morbidity reduced. However, this is a technically demanding procedure, and there is a risk of worsening the attack. The patients who benefit the most are those with fairly sever gallstone pancreatitis with progressive biochemical abnormalities. If a stone is impacted at the lower end of the common duct, preventing resolution of acute pancreatitis, early stone removal is sometimes necessary. In most cases, endoscopic sphincterotomy or biliary tract surgery for stones is performed after recovery.

The role of surgery during the acute attack continues to be uncertain but, for most patients, surgery does not improve results and often adversely affects recovery. However, deferring cholecystectomy until months after the acute attack increases the risk of a second attack. Some surgeons offer laparoscopic cholecystectomy with operative cholangiography before discharge but most prefer to operate after about 4 weeks.

In the small group of critically ill patients with infected necrotic tissue and infected peripancreatic fluid collections, there is evidence that surgical debridement improves survival.

The principles of management of acute pancreatitis are summarised in Box 18.5.

COMPLICATIONS OF ACUTE PANCREATITIS

Mortality

About 15% of patients admitted to hospital with acute pancreatitis have severe disease with potential complications. In this group, mortality is 8–10%, i.e. 2% of all

---

KEY POINTS

Box 18.4 Recommended daily investigations in severe acute pancreatitis

- Haemoglobin estimation and white cell count
- Arterial blood gas estimations
- Blood sugar
- Plasma electrolytes, creatinine and urea
- 'Liver function tests' (i.e. bilirubin, alkaline phosphatase, lactate dehydrogenase (LDH), transaminases, serum proteins)
- Plasma calcium and phosphate

SUMMARY

Box 18.5 Principles of management of acute pancreatitis

(Treatments added according to severity of attack)
- 'Nil by mouth', nasogastric tube and gastric aspiration
- Resuscitation with intravenous fluids; antibiotics
- Intensive care:
  — fluid and electrolyte management
  — treatment of hypocalcaemia
  — ventilatory support
- Laparotomy and pancreatic necrosectomy

cases. Obese patients have a much higher mortality. About half of these die within the first week, usually of ARDS and pulmonary failure. The other early life-threatening complications mainly involve **multiple organ dysfunction**: cardiovascular collapse resulting from fluid shifts, pulmonary failure from ARDS, and renal failure from hypotension. Septic complications are the usual cause of death after the first week.

Pancreatic necrosis and infection

During the first 2 weeks, **pancreatic and peripancreatic necrosis** may manifest in cases of severe pancreatitis (see Figure 18.1). Necrosis is identified using intravenous contrast-enhanced CT scanning in which the necrotic pancreas does not opacify, having lost its blood supply. Infection of devitalised pancreatic and peripancreatic tissues occurs in about one-third of patients with severe pancreatitis despite prophylactic antibiotics, and is often lethal. With infection, the pancreatitis fails to resolve and signs of SIRS appear. Infection can be confirmed only by percutaneous aspiration under CT guidance. In proven infected cases, operative debridement and drainage may be necessary, along with aggressive supportive measures.

Fluid collections around the pancreas

During the initial attack, **acute fluid collections** may develop around the gland. Most of these resolve spontaneously. After the initial period, **pseudocysts** appear within the lesser sac in 1–8% of cases; these are less likely to resolve spontaneously. Later in the course of the disease, a pancreatic abscess may develop. These occur in 1–4% of cases. An abscess represents a well-localised collection of pus within the gland and contrasts with the infected necrotising pancreatitis which appears earlier and is not localised.

Pancreatic pseudocyst

A pancreatic pseudocyst is a collection of pancreatic enzymes, inflammatory fluid and necrotic debris encapsulated within the lesser sac. It is not a true cyst (i.e. there is no epithelial lining) although the surrounding tissues become thickened by the inflammatory response. Pseudocysts may occur after even a moderate attack of pancreatitis and sometimes reach the size of a football!

Clinically, the acute attack fails to resolve completely; at the end of the second week, the serum amylase remains elevated and normal bowel peristalsis has not returned. An upper abdominal mass may be palpable. If a pseudocyst is suspected, CT scanning is the investigation of choice (see Fig. 18.2).

Management varies according to the size of the cyst. Larger cysts, especially those larger than 10 cm, are unlikely to resolve. Those around 6 cm can be safely observed for up to 6 months, provided they are typical on CT scanning and asymptomatic. If they have failed to resolve by then, operative intervention should be considered. CT-guided percutaneous drainage seems attractive, but the relapse rate is high. Operative intervention by laparoscopy or an open approach involves 'marsupialising' the pseudocyst into the posterior wall of the stomach. This can be performed after about 6 weeks, when the wall of the pseudocyst has 'matured' enough to hold sutures.

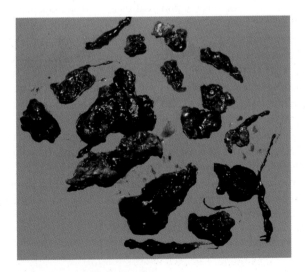

Fig. 18.1 Pancreatic necrosis
Necrotic pancreas removed 16 days after a severe attack of pancreatitis complicated by peripancreatic infection. The patient made a slow recovery but became diabetic in the convalsescent period.

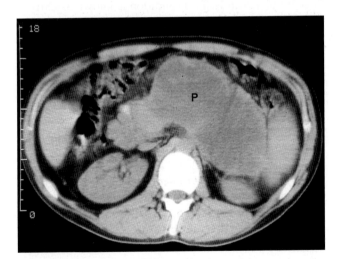

Fig. 18.2 Pancreatic pseudocyst
This 57-year-old man was admitted to hospital with an acute abdomen 3 weeks before this scan. He was found to have acute pancreatitis due to gallstones. The symptoms and signs of pancreatitis smouldered on and the plasma amylase failed to return to normal. This CT scan of his upper abdomen shows the cause of the persistent pancreatitis, a pseudocyst arising from the tail of the pancreas **P**.

Pancreatic abscess

Some patients remain systemically well despite pancreatic necrosis. The illness may grumble on for several weeks with a high swinging fever indicating the presence of an abscess. By now the necrotic pancreas is likely to have formed a discrete red-grey mass lying free within the pancreatic bed surrounded by pus, which may extend widely in the retroperitoneal tissues. Operation is required to remove the necrotic tissue and drain the abscesses.

Late complications of acute pancreatitis

Diabetes mellitus, and intestinal malabsorption due to loss of pancreatic secretions sometimes occur after severe attacks, but it is surprising how uncommon these are considering the extent of pancreatic damage that occurs.

RECURRENT, RELAPSING AND CHRONIC PANCREATITIS

RECURRENT ACUTE PANCREATITIS

Some patients suffer recurrent attacks of acute pancreatitis, usually resulting from either alcohol abuse or gallstone disease. The first and second attacks may be severe, but attacks after that almost never produce lethal complications. The patient is entirely well between attacks. In different patients, the attacks vary in severity but are rarely extreme. This condition is often described as 'chronic relapsing pancreatitis' but both types are better described as recurrent acute pancreatitis.

CHRONIC PANCREATITIS

Other patients suffer persistent and severe upper abdominal pain, similar in character to a prolonged attack of acute pancreatitis. This condition is known as chronic pancreatitis. These patients do not develop the other clinical features of acute pancreatitis and may not develop hyperamylasaemia. The pain is so severe and so persistent as to drive some patients to suicide. Carcinoma of the pancreas and chronic pancreatic inflammation should both be considered in patients with this pattern of pain. Inflammatory swelling of the pancreatic head occasionally causes obstructive jaundice but carcinoma in this position is a far more common cause.

Despite the pain, there are usually no abnormal abdominal signs. The serum amylase may be moderately elevated on occasion; the diagnosis of chronic pancreatitis may, however, be missed if raised serum amylase levels are not detected. This may be because tests are not done at an appropriate time or the patient is unfortunate enough never to have elevated levels. There is a danger that these patients may be dismissed as suffering from psychosomatic pain.

Ultrasound or CT scans may show glandular swelling (sometimes difficult to differentiate from pancreatic carcinoma) and a dilated pancreatic duct. If ERCP is performed, the pancreatic duct system may look normal or else may be distorted and irregular in calibre, confirming chronic inflammation and fibrosis (see Fig. 18.3). Sometimes pancreatic duct stones are demonstrated.

Chronic pancreatitis may cause years of misery, perhaps eventually 'burning out' as the gland atrophies completely. It is important to make the diagnosis in good time so that pain can be relieved. In the long term, malabsorption or diabetes are more likely to develop than after acute pancreatitis.

Pancreatic calcification seen on abdominal X-rays is diagnostic of chronic pancreatitis but is a rare finding and is sometimes found in asymptomatic patients (see Fig. 18.4). X-rays are therefore of little clinical value.

Treatment of chronic pancreatitis is far from satisfactory. Surgery is only useful if structural abnormalities can be found. Surgical procedures include removal of pancreatic duct stones, partial pancreatectomy of the body and tail for duct stenosis, sphincteroplasty of the pancreatic duct opening, or occasionally complete pancreatectomy. Chemical coeliac ganglion blockade provides useful (and often permanent) pain relief, but does nothing to prevent inflammation. If there are multiple duct strictures, the pancreatic duct can be surgically split along its whole length and a loop of jejunum sutured to the gland to allow unrestricted drainage. Interventional endoscopy can be employed for dilatation and stenting of pancreatic duct strictures.

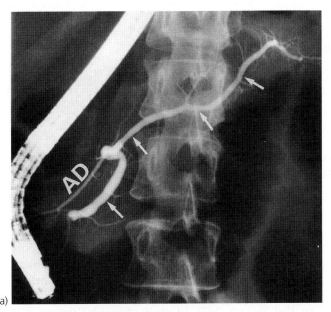

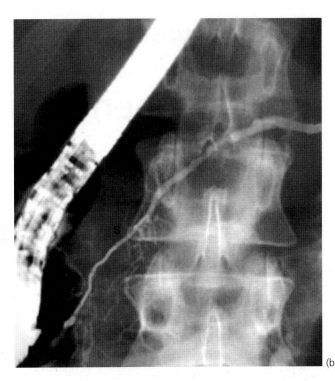

(a)

(b)

Fig. 18.3 Retrograde pancreatography
These films were both obtained by injecting contrast into the pancreatic duct using a flexible duodenoscope. **(a)** This pancreatogram is normal. The main duct (arrowed) narrows regularly towards the tail of the pancreas and there are no strictures or dilatations along its length. The accessory pancreatic duct **AD** also fills in this patient. **(b)** This pancreatogram is from a man of 26 with a history of severe upper abdominal pain. There is a long stricture of the main duct **S** of unknown origin. Typical changes of chronic pancreatitis, i.e. irregularity of the wall with dilatations and poor filling of small ducts, are seen in the duct distal to the stricture.

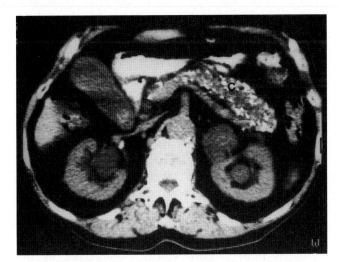

Fig. 18.4 Pancreatic calcification in chronic pancreatitis
This obese 55-year-old man had a long history of severe abdominal pain and alcohol abuse. Pancreatic calcification was not visible on a plain abdominal X-ray but extensive calcification is clearly seen on this CT scan.

19 Appendicitis

INTRODUCTION

Acute appendicitis is the most common cause of intra-abdominal infection in developed countries and appendicectomy is the most common emergency surgical operation. In the UK, 1.9 females per thousand have the operation each year compared with 1.5 males, and 1 in about 6 or 7 people eventually undergo the operation. Surprisingly, the incidence of appendicitis fell by about 50% between the 1960s and the 1980s.

Appendicitis can occur at any age but is most common below 40 years, especially between the ages of 8 and 14. It is very rare below the age of 2. Appendicitis is rare in rural parts of developing countries, but in the cities the incidence approaches that of the West. This different susceptibility in people of similar ethnic origin is probably related to a much reduced intake of dietary fibre in city-dwellers.

Acute appendicitis should be in the differential diagnosis of all patients presenting to hospital with abdominal pain. Even previous appendicectomy does not absolutely rule out the diagnosis. Despite lay impressions, a positive diagnosis is often difficult to make and this is partly because of the wide range of differential diagnoses. Sometimes a non-inflamed appendix is found at operation. The fact is that there is no definitive test for the confirmation or exclusion of appendicitis and thus a proportion of unnecessary appendicectomy operations is unavoidable. Diagnostic laparoscopy can improve diagnostic accuracy, particularly in young women, and can also be used therapeutically to remove an inflamed appendix.

ANATOMY OF THE APPENDIX

The appendix is a blind-ending tube arising from the caecum at the meeting point of the three taeniae coli, just distal to the ileo-caecal junction. The base of the appendix thus lies in the right iliac fossa, close to **McBurney's point**. This is two-thirds of the way along a line drawn from the umbilicus to the anterior superior iliac spine (see Fig. 19.7, p. 272). In most cases, the appendix is mobile within the peritoneal cavity, suspended by its mesentery (**meso-appendix**) with the appendicular artery in its free edge. This is effectively an end-artery, with anastomotic connections only proximally.

The appendix has been described as lying in several 'classic' sites, but apart from the true retrocaecal appendix, the organ probably floats in a broad arc about its base (see Fig. 19.1). Only inflammation will fix it in a particular place. Its position will then determine the clinical presentation of the disease. In about 30% of appendicectomies, the appendix lies over the brim of the pelvis ('**pelvic appendix**'). This is adjacent to the bladder and rectum in males and to the uterus, Fallopian tubes and bladder in females. In some cases, the appendix lies retroperitoneally behind the caecum and is often plastered to it by fibrous bands. Thus, an inflamed retrocaecal appendix may irritate the right ureter and psoas muscle, and may even lie high enough to simulate gall-bladder pain.

Histologically, the appendix has the same basic structure as the large intestine. Its glandular mucosa is separated from a loose vascular submucosa by the delicate muscularis mucosa. External to the submucosa is the main muscular wall. The appendix is covered by a serosal layer (the visceral layer of peritoneum) which contains the large blood vessels and becomes continuous with the serosa of the mesoappendix. When the appendix lies retroperitoneally, there is no serosal covering. A prominent feature of the appendix is its collections of lymphoid tissue in the lamina propria. This lymphoid tissue often has germinal centres and is prominent in childhood but diminishes with increasing age.

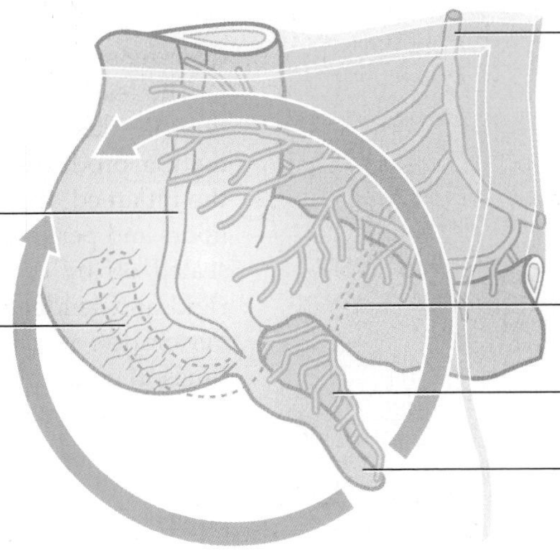

Fig. 19.1 Surgical anatomy of the appendix
The appendix can be positioned anywhere on the circumference shown by the arrowed arc.

The mucosa contains a large number of cells of the gastrointestinal endocrine system (APUD system). These secrete mainly serotonin and were formerly known as **argentaffin cells**. Carcinoid tumours commonly occur in the appendix and arise from these cells.

PATHOPHYSIOLOGY OF APPENDICITIS

Appendicitis is probably initiated by obstruction of the lumen by impacted faeces or a faecolith. This explanation fits with the epidemiological observation that appendicitis is associated with a low dietary fibre intake.

In the early stages of appendicitis, the mucosa becomes inflamed first. This inflammation eventually extends through the submucosa to involve the muscular and serosal (peritoneal) layers. A fibrinopurulent exudate forms on the serosal surface and extends to any adjacent peritoneal surface, e.g. bowel or abdominal wall, causing a localised peritonitis.

By this stage the necrotic glandular mucosa sloughs into the lumen, which becomes distended with pus. Finally, the end-arteries supplying the appendix become thrombosed and the infarcted appendix becomes necrotic or **gangrenous**. This usually occurs at the distal end and the appendix begins to disintegrate. Perforation soon follows and faecally contaminated appendiceal contents spread into the peritoneal cavity. If the spilled contents are enveloped by omentum or adherent small bowel, a localised abscess results; otherwise spreading peritonitis develops. The evolution of acute appendicitis is illustrated histologically in Figure 19.2.

CLINICAL FEATURES OF APPENDICITIS

The pathophysiological evolution of appendicitis and the corresponding symptoms and signs are illustrated in Figure 19.3.

CLASSIC APPENDICITIS

Acute appendicitis classically begins with poorly localised, colicky central abdominal visceral pain; this results from smooth muscle spasm as a reaction to appendiceal obstruction. Anorexia and vomiting often accompany the pain at this stage.

As inflammation advances over the ensuing 12–24 hours, it progresses through the appendiceal wall to involve the parietal peritoneum (which is innervated somatically). At this stage the pain typically becomes localised to the right iliac fossa. Signs of local peritonitis, i.e. tenderness and guarding, can be elicited at this stage. This classic picture is seen in less than half of all cases, largely because the localising symptoms and signs vary with the anatomical relations of the inflamed appendix.

OTHER PRESENTATIONS OF ACUTE APPENDICITIS

If the appendix lies in the pelvis near the rectum, it may cause local irritation and diarrhoea. If it lies near the bladder or ureter, inflammation may cause urinary symptoms of frequency, dysuria and (microscopic) pyuria. These may readily be mistaken for urinary tract infection. An inflamed retrocaecal appendix produces none of the usual localising symptoms or signs, but may irritate the psoas muscle causing involuntary right hip

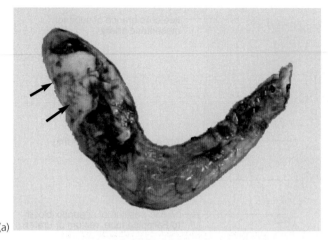

(a)

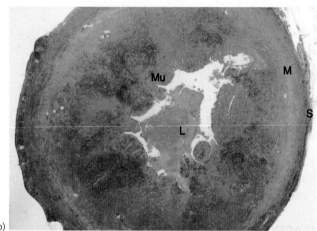

(b)

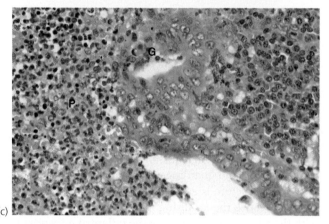

(c)

Fig. 19.2 Acute appendicitis
(a) Macroscopic photograph showing acutely inflamed appendix. The distended tip shows a purulent exudate on the serosal surface (arrowed). **(b)** Microscopy showing mucosal ulceration **Mu** with acute inflammatory cells within the lumen **L**. Inflammation extends through the muscle wall **M** to the serosal surface **S**. **(c)** High-power view showing acute inflammatory cells, mostly polymorphs **P**, destroying glands **G**.

flexion and pain on extension. A high retrocaecal appendix may cause pain and tenderness below the right costal margin. An inflamed appendix near the Fallopian tube

causes pelvic pain suggestive of an acute gynaecological disorder such as salpingitis or torsion of an ovarian cyst.

The early phase of poorly localised visceral pain typically lasts for a few hours until peritoneal inflammation produces somatic localising signs. If untreated, the inflamed appendix becomes gangrenous after 12–24 hours and perforates, causing spreading peritonitis unless sealed off by omentum. The whole abdomen becomes rigid and tender and there is marked systemic toxicity. Perforation is particularly common in children. Sometimes, the pathological sequence is extremely rapid and the patient presents with sudden peritonitis.

In older patients, a gangrenous or perforated appendix tends to be contained by omentum or loops of small bowel. This results in a palpable **appendix mass**. This may contain free pus and is then known as an appendiceal abscess. As with any significant abscess, there is a tachycardia and swinging pyrexia. An appendix mass usually resolves spontaneously over 2–6 weeks. In the elderly, a delayed diagnosis may prouce an appendix abscess walled off by loops of small bowel. There may be no palpable mass and the symptoms and signs may not be recognisable as appendicitis. These include non-specific abdominal pain and features of small bowel obstruction due to localised paralytic ileus. Occasionally, appendicitis may present in a most unusual way. Examples include discharge of an appendix abscess into the Fallopian tube presenting as a purulent vaginal discharge, and inflammation of an appendix lying in an inguinal hernia presenting as an abscess in the groin.

MAKING THE DIAGNOSIS OF APPENDICITIS

Acute appendicitis is a clinical diagnosis, relying almost entirely on the history and physical examination. Investigations are only useful in excluding other differential diagnoses. If possible, the diagnosis should be made and the appendix removed before it becomes gangrenous and perforates. On the other hand, unnecessary appendicectomies must be kept to a minimum.

Diagnosis of acute appendicitis poses little difficulty if the patient exhibits the classic symptoms and signs summarised in Box 19.1. The problem in appendicitis occurs when the symptoms and signs are not typical. The patient may present at a very early stage, or the signs may have some other pathological cause. At least two out of every three children admitted to hospital with suspected appendicitis do not have the condition.

If the evidence for acute appendicitis is insufficient and no other diagnosis can be made, the patient should be kept under observation, admitted to hospital if necessary and re-examined periodically. Eventually, the symptoms settle or the diagnosis becomes clear.

PATHOLOGICAL SEQUENCE

CLINICAL MANIFESTATIONS

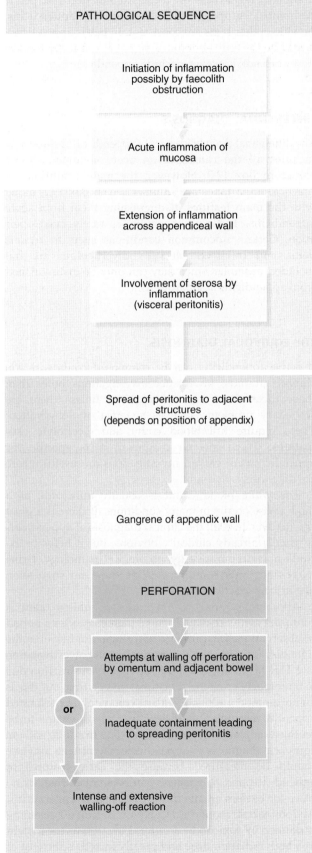

Initiation of inflammation
possibly by faecolith
obstruction

Acute inflammation of
mucosa

Extension of inflammation
across appendiceal wall

Involvement of serosa by
inflammation
(visceral peritonitis)

Spread of peritonitis to adjacent
structures
(depends on position of appendix)

Gangrene of appendix wall

PERFORATION

Attempts at walling off perforation
by omentum and adjacent bowel

or

Inadequate containment leading
to spreading peritonitis

Intense and extensive
walling-off reaction

Poorly localised colicky central abdominal pain

Continuous central abdominal pain often
associated with nausea and vomiting
(due to autonomic stimulation)

Localisation of symptoms and signs as parietal
peritoneum becomes involved
(somatic innervation)

Classically:
tenderness, rebound and guarding in the right
iliac fossa

Moderate fever, facial flush and tachycardia

Tenderness extends to
whole abdomen with
increasing rigidity and
more pronounced systemic
features of toxicity,
i.e. an increasingly ill,
apathetic patient with
dehydration

or

Formation of 'appendix mass'
with gradual recovery

Fig. 19.3 Pathophysiology and clinical manifestations of acute appendicitis

SUMMARY

Box 19.1 Cardinal features of acute appendicitis

- Abdominal pain for less than 72 hours
- Vomiting 1–3 times
- Facial flush
- Tenderness concentrated on the right iliac fossa
- Anterior tenderness on rectal examination
- Fever between 37.3 and 38.5°C
- No evidence of urinary tract infection on urine microscopy

SPECIAL POINTS IN THE HISTORY AND EXAMINATION

Acute appendicitis typically runs a short course, between a few hours and about 3 days. If symptoms have been present for longer, appendicitis is unlikely unless an 'appendix mass' has developed. A recent or current sore throat or viral-type illness, particularly in children, favours the diagnosis of **mesenteric adenitis** (inflammation of the mesenteric lymph nodes analogous to viral tonsillitis). Urinary symptoms suggest **urinary tract infection** but may also occur with pelvic appendicitis.

The patient with appendicitis is typically quiet, apathetic and flushed; the lively child doing jigsaw puzzles almost never has appendicitis! Oral foetor may be present but is not a reliable sign of appendicitis. Cervical lymphadenopathy tends to suggest a viral origin for the abdominal pain. Mild tachycardia and pyrexia are typical of appendicitis but a temperature much over 38°C makes the diagnosis of acute viral illness or urinary tract infection more likely.

Signs of peritoneal inflammation in the right iliac fossa are often absent in the early stages of the illness. The patient should be asked to cough, blow the abdominal wall out and draw it in; all of these cause pain if the parietal peritoneum is inflamed. In children, it may be difficult to interpret apparent tenderness, especially if the child cries and refuses to cooperate. This can usually be overcome by distracting the child's attention whilst palpating the abdomen through the bedclothes or even with the child's own hand under the examiner's hand. Several signs (e.g. Rovsing's sign—pressure in the left iliac fossa causing pain in the right iliac fossa) have been described which are said to point to the diagnosis of appendicitis but these are all unreliable. One useful test is to ask the child to stand, then to hop on the right leg. If this can be achieved, there is unlikely to be any significant peritoneal inflammation.

Rebound tenderness can best be demonstrated by gentle percussion of the right iliac fossa. Pain on percussion is a reliable sign of local peritonitis. Anterior peritoneal tenderness on rectal examination (i.e. pelvic peritonitis) supports the diagnosis of appendicitis, provided other signs are consistent. In pelvic appendicitis, it may be the only abdominal sign. Lack of rectal tenderness does not, however, exclude appendicitis.

DIFFERENTIAL DIAGNOSIS

The differential diagnosis of acute appendicitis theoretically includes all the causes of an acute abdomen shown earlier in Box 12.2. However, the main conditions of practical importance are summarised in Box 19.2, along with the main features distinguishing them from acute appendicitis. These other conditions rarely need operation. Certain uncommon conditions such as *Yersinia* ileitis and inflamed Meckel's diverticulum are not included in the list since they can only be distinguished from appendicitis at laparotomy.

THE EQUIVOCAL DIAGNOSIS

If acute appendicitis can be diagnosed confidently on clinical grounds, no further investigations other than those dictated by age are required unless there are secondary problems such as anaemia or dehydration. These require full blood count and electrolyte estimations. There are no diagnostic tests specific for appendicitis but certain investigations are useful where the diagnosis is in doubt.

The white blood count is usually unhelpful, as a modest rise occurs in many conditions. If there is a great rise (to over 16 000), the clinical diagnosis of appendicitis is usually already clinically obvious, but it helps to exclude non-suppurative gynaecological pathology. Urine microscopy must be performed if there is any suggestion of a urinary tract infection.

Abdominal X-rays are not needed unless there is confusing evidence of abdominal pathology after a period of observation. The presence of a single fluid level in the right iliac fossa or even widespread small bowel dilatation (see Fig. 19.5a) suggests local adynamic obstruction due to appendicitis causing functional obstruction, but this is an uncommon finding. Even less commonly, a perforated appendix may allow sufficient free gas to escape to be revealed on plain X-rays (see Fig. 19.5b). In adults with an equivocal diagnosis of appendicitis, the plasma amylase should be measured because the early features of appendicitis and pancreatitis can be similar. There is no place for barium enema in the diagnosis of appendicitis. Abdominal ultrasound is largely unhelpful. CT scanning is claimed by some to be accurate but submits the patient to a high radiation dose and greatly increases the cost of investigation.

KEY POINTS

Box 19.2 Main differential diagnoses of acute appendicitis

Urinary tract infection (cystitis or pyelonephritis)
● Unlikely if nitrites are absent from dipstick testing of the urine and can be excluded if there are not significant numbers of white blood cells or bacteria on urine microscopy

Mesenteric adenitis
● Inflammation and enlargement of the abdominal lymph nodes, probably viral in origin, and often associated with an upper respiratory infection or sore throat.
● Symptoms and signs may be similar to those of early appendicitis but without rectal tenderness
● Fever is typically higher than in appendicitis (i.e. greater than 38.5°C) and settles rapidly
● A firm diagnosis can only be made at laparotomy or laparoscopy

Constipation
● May cause colicky abdominal pain and iliac fossa tenderness
● There is no fever and the rectum is loaded with faeces

Gynaecological disorders
● The pain of ovulation about 14 days after the last menstrual period (**mittelschmerz**) may cause right iliac fossa pain. There is often a history of similar pain in the past. There are no signs of infection and the pain settles quickly
● Salpingitis (most comonly Chlamydial) causes lower abdominal pain, often with a vaginal discharge. Digital vaginal examination typically reveals adnexal tenderness, and moving the cervix from side to side induces pain ('cervical excitation')
● Torsion of, or haemorrhage into a right ovarian cyst may produce symptoms like appendicitis, but there is no fever. A tender mobile mass may be palpable in the right suprapubic region or on vaginal examination. This diagnosis can be confirmed with ultrasound

Perforation of another abdominal viscus
● A perforated Meckel's diverticulum (see Fig. 19.4) may present exactly like appendicitis
● Necrotic small bowel from strangulation usually presents with intestinal obstruction

Acute pancreatitis
● Pain is predominantly central
● If there is tenderness in the right iliac fossa, it will also be present in the epigastrium
● If in doubt, the serum amylase should be measured

Non-specific abdominal upset
● Vague abdominal pain and tenderness which may be associated with vomiting and diarrhoea
● Usually improves steadily during a period of observation

PROBLEMS IN DIAGNOSIS OF APPENDICITIS

THE VERY YOUNG

Appendicitis is rarely seen below 2 years of age, but when it does occur, the 'typical' abdominal symptoms and signs are obscure or absent. An infant or toddler may display signs of sepsis without revealing the abdominal origin. Abdominal X-rays may demonstrate dilated loops of bowel and fluid levels. Generalised peritonitis supervenes rapidly in this age group because the abdominal defence mechanisms, in particular the 'wrapping' effect of the greater omentum, are rudimentary. Laparotomy is usually indicated in an ill infant with abdominal signs.

THE ELDERLY

Appendicitis tends to develop more slowly in the elderly. The appendix wall becomes fibrotic with age and the area is more readily walled off by omentum and adherent small bowel. Many cases probably resolve spontaneously. In those who reach hospital, the history is often as long as 1 week. Symptoms and signs of obstruction may be present. These include vomiting, colicky abdominal pain and obstructed bowel sounds. A mass may be palpable if the patient is relaxed and not too tender but can often be palpated only under general anaesthesia. Abdominal X-rays may reveal fluid levels in the right iliac fossa.

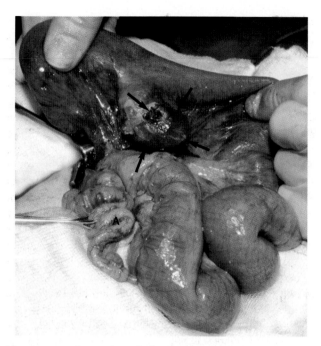

Fig. 19.4 Perforated Meckel's diverticulum
This man of 28 presented with a typical history and clinical findings of acute appendicitis. However, at operation he was found to have a normal appendix but a perforated Meckel's diverticulum (arrowed). The diverticulum was resected and the appendix also removed to prevent future confusion and the patient made a good recovery. On histological examination, the Meckel's was found to contain gastric mucosa.

PREGNANCY

Appendicitis occurs at least as often during pregnancy as at other times but the diagnosis can be difficult. The appendix is displaced upwards by the enlarging uterus so that abdominal pain and tenderness are in a much higher position than usual. Diagnosis and management of the pregnant patient must be shared with an obstetrician. Laparoscopy may be indicated if the diagnosis is in doubt, but this becomes technically difficult beyond 26 weeks. Mortality from appendicitis for both mother and fetus rises as the pregnancy progresses; this is as high as 9% for the mother and 20% for the fetus in the third trimester.

THE 'GRUMBLING' APPENDIX

Recurrent bouts of right iliac fossa pain occur in some children and are often labelled as 'grumbling appendix'. Appendicular pathology is probably the cause in very few of these cases. Persistent chronic inflammation of the appendix probably does not occur, but recurrent bouts of appendicular colic or low-grade acute appendicitis undoubtedly do. These children may have several abortive admissions for abdominal pain and it may eventually be justifiable to remove the appendix to allay parental

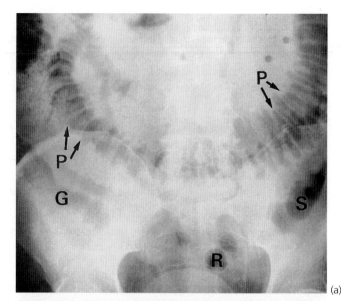

(a)

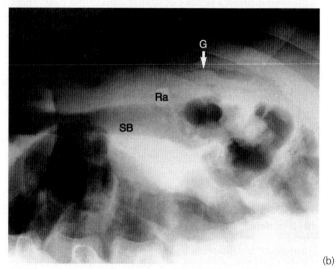

(b)

Fig. 19.5 Perforated gangrenous sub-hepatic appendix
This 12-year-old boy presented with 2 days' abdominal pain and vomiting. On examination, there was tenderness in the right side of the abdomen. There was also abdominal distension resonant to percussion and obstructed bowel sounds, which indicated possible small bowel obstruction. **(a)** Supine plain abdominal film showing grossly dilated small bowel filling the centre of the abdomen. The plicae semilunares **P** can be seen to cross the lumen completely, characterising dilated small bowel. There is a little gas in the rectum **R** and sigmoid colon **S**. These signs are diagnostic of small bowel obstruction. There is some free gas **G** visible in the right iliac fossa suggesting perforation. **(b)** A lateral decubitus plain abdominal film (right-side upwards) in another similar patient shows a featureless loop of small bowel **SB**, which is adynamic due to nearby inflammation. The radio-opacity **Ra** is a faecolith in the appendix (appendolith) and the linear radiolucency **G** is free gas under a Riedel's lobe of the liver. At operation, the appendix was found to be gangrenous and perforated, but was lying in a high position close to the liver.

anxiety. A non-inflamed appendix containing a faecolith or threadworms (assumed to have caused the pain) is often found.

The management of suspected appendicitis is summarised in Figure 19.6.

APPENDICECTOMY

The annual death rate from appendicitis has fallen dramatically since 1960. In 1934 there were 3193 deaths from appendicitis in the UK, whereas in 1982 there were 110 deaths. The improvement results from several factors including better general nutrition, earlier presentation, better preoperative preparation and better anaesthesia. Deaths that now occur are usually due to dehydration and electrolyte changes which are unrecognised or ineffectively treated before surgery. Infective complications of appendicitis have dramatically fallen since the 1970s because of the widespread use of prophylactic antibacterial agents.

ANTIBIOTIC PROPHYLAXIS

In appendicitis, most intra-abdominal infective complications and wound infections occur in perforated or gangrenous appendicitis. The majority of the infecting organisms are anaerobic and the infections can largely be prevented by prophylactic metronidazole. Rectal suppositories are just as effective as intravenous metronidazole and are cheaper but need to be given 2 hours before operation. Aerobic organisms are involved in a smaller number of cases and some surgeons therefore advocate additional prophylaxis with an antibiotic such as a first- or second-generation cephalosporin.

TECHNIQUE OF APPENDICECTOMY

The principal steps in appendicectomy are illustrated in Figure 19.7 and should be understood by any doctor called upon to assist in the operation. Increasingly, laparotomy is being replaced by laparoscopic diagnosis and surgery but the principles are similar.

A low skin crease incision (**Lanz**) rather than the higher and more oblique one centred on McBurney's point is now favoured as it gives a better cosmetic result. The superficial fascia (well marked in children) is then incised and the three musculo-aponeurotic layers of the abdominal wall are split along the line of their fibres. This produces the '**gridiron**' incision, described as such because the fibres of external oblique and internal oblique run at right angles to each other. The peritoneum is then lifted and opened and may reveal pus or mucopurulent watery fluid; a swab of this is taken for microscopy and culture. The appendix is located digitally and delivered into the wound; further exploration may be needed if it does not lie in the immediate vicinity. A retrocaecal appendix will require mobilisation of the caecum by dividing the peritoneum along its lateral side.

Once the appendix has been delivered into the wound, its blood supply in the meso-appendix is divided between clips and ligated. The appendix base is crushed with a haemostat which is then reapplied more distally. An absorbable ligature is then tied around the crushed area. After this preparation, the appendix is then excised. A 'purse-string' suture is usually placed in the caecum near the appendix base, the appendix is inverted and the suture tied. If the appendix was perforated or gangrenous, or if pus was found, thorough peritoneal toilet is performed. A sump sucker is guided down into the pelvis with a finger to suck out any fluid, and the area is then gently swabbed out with gauze to remove any adherent infected material. Any pus or faecolith left in the pelvis predisposes to subsequent pelvic abscess.

The peritoneum, internal oblique and external oblique are each closed with two or three absorbable sutures. Drainage is not usually recommended unless there is a thick-walled abscess cavity which will not collapse.

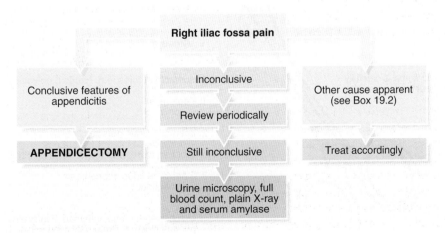

Fig. 19.6 Summary—management of suspected appendicitis

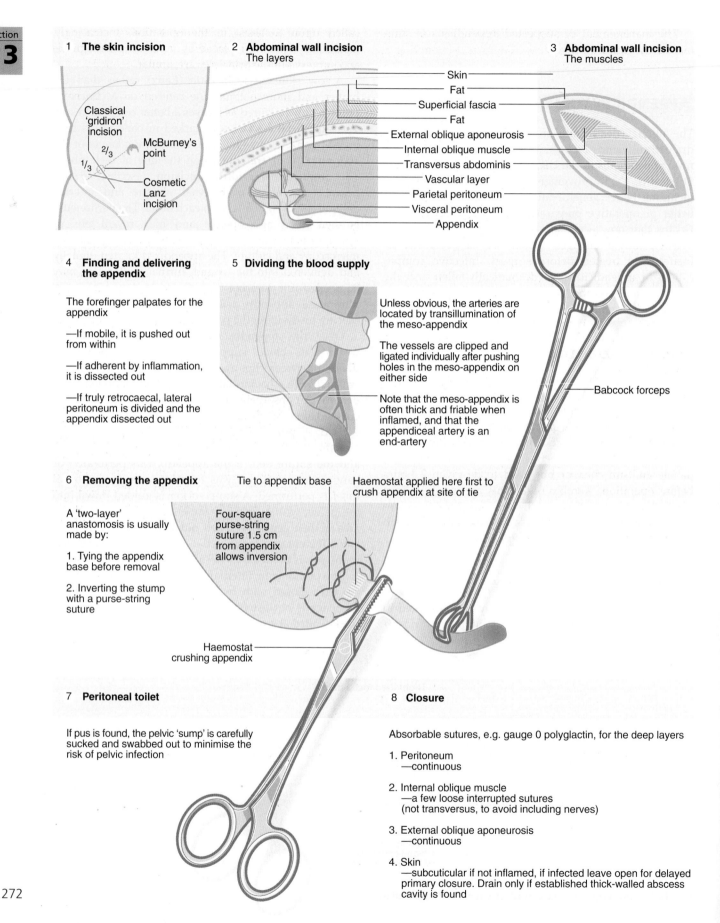

1 The skin incision

Classical 'gridiron' incision

McBurney's point

2/3

1/3

Cosmetic Lanz incision

2 Abdominal wall incision
The layers

Skin
Fat
Superficial fascia
Fat
External oblique aponeurosis
Internal oblique muscle
Transversus abdominis
Vascular layer
Parietal peritoneum
Visceral peritoneum
Appendix

3 Abdominal wall incision
The muscles

4 Finding and delivering the appendix

The forefinger palpates for the appendix

—If mobile, it is pushed out from within

—If adherent by inflammation, it is dissected out

—If truly retrocaecal, lateral peritoneum is divided and the appendix dissected out

5 Dividing the blood supply

Unless obvious, the arteries are located by transillumination of the meso-appendix

The vessels are clipped and ligated individually after pushing holes in the meso-appendix on either side

Note that the meso-appendix is often thick and friable when inflamed, and that the appendiceal artery is an end-artery

Babcock forceps

6 Removing the appendix

A 'two-layer' anastomosis is usually made by:

1. Tying the appendix base before removal

2. Inverting the stump with a purse-string suture

Tie to appendix base

Four-square purse-string suture 1.5 cm from appendix allows inversion

Haemostat applied here first to crush appendix at site of tie

Haemostat crushing appendix

7 Peritoneal toilet

If pus is found, the pelvic 'sump' is carefully sucked and swabbed out to minimise the risk of pelvic infection

8 Closure

Absorbable sutures, e.g. gauge 0 polyglactin, for the deep layers

1. Peritoneum
   —continuous

2. Internal oblique muscle
   —a few loose interrupted sutures
   (not transversus, to avoid including nerves)

3. External oblique aponeurosis
   —continuous

4. Skin
   —subcuticular if not inflamed, if infected leave open for delayed primary closure. Drain only if established thick-walled abscess cavity is found

Fig. 19.7 Appendicectomy—operative technique

After operation, oral fluids followed by solids are gradually increased over a few days unless vomiting or other complications occur.

Laparoscopic appendicectomy

Laparoscopy allows the appendix to be found wherever it may lie. The principles and techniques are similar to the open operation; the appendix can be visualised and appendicectomy performed if it is abnormal. Laparoscopic removal gives a lower wound infection rate and may allow an earlier return to normal activities. However, it is a more technically demanding operation.

THE 'LILY-WHITE' APPENDIX

If the appendix is found not to be inflamed at open operation (colloquially termed 'lily-white'), it should always be removed because an appendicectomy scar would lead doctors in future to assume that the appendix has been removed. The abdomen is explored as allowed by the incision to search for a cause for the symptoms:

- **Mesenteric lymph nodes** in children may be grossly enlarged by mesenteric adenitis—this is probably viral in origin
- **The terminal ileum** may be thickened and reddened by Crohn's disease or by *Yersinia* ileitis—the appendix is removed but the bowel is left alone. If possible, an enlarged mesenteric node is removed for histological examination

- **An inflamed Meckel's diverticulum** may be found within 30 cm of the ileocaecal valve—if inflamed, this is removed but a wide-mouthed non-inflamed diverticulum is usually left alone
- **Both ovaries can usually be palpated**—ovaries may be twisted, inflamed or enlarged or an inflamed Fallopian tube may be seen
- **Cholecystitis, hydronephrosis or a leaking aneurysm**—these are rarely found

THE APPENDIX MASS

A vigorous response to appendicitis may result in a mass in the right iliac fossa, often with fever. Usually the patient has few systemic symptoms or signs of ill health. A conservative regime followed by interval appendicectomy 6 weeks later (**Ochsner–Sherren regimen**) was advocated in pre-antibiotic days but is now less favoured. Early operation under antibiotic cover is now performed more frequently.

YERSINIA ILEITIS

Acute inflammation of the ileum by the organism *Yersinia pseudotuberculosis* is an uncommon cause of right iliac fossa pain which is clinically identical to acute appendicitis. The diagnosis is made at operation, when the terminal ileum is seen to be bright red and thickened by the inflammatory process. Sometimes the appearance may be difficult to distinguish from Crohn's disease. *Yersinia* ileitis is a self-limiting condition and requires no treatment.

20 Colorectal polyps and carcinoma

INTRODUCTION

Cancer of the colon and rectum is the third most common malignancy in both men and women in Western countries. It is less common in the developing world, but is still the fourth most common newly diagnosed cancer in the world. Most colorectal cancers originate in the glandular mucosa and are therefore **adenocarcinomas**. Familial adenomatous polyposis is a rare autosomal dominant disorder which invariably predisposes to adenocarcinomas of the colon (often multiple) from the late teenage years. Other forms of malignancy in the large bowel such as **carcinoid tumour** or **lymphoma** are rare. Squamous (epidermoid) carcinomas occur in the anus or anal canal skin (see Ch. 23) but these make up only about 1% of large bowel cancers and are not usually difficult to distinguish clinically from rectal tumours.

The term **polyp** can cause more confusion than understanding. The term is a morphological one and is used to describe any localised lesion protruding from the bowel wall into the lumen; it does not imply any specific pathology. This conforms with the use of the term elsewhere in the body, e.g. nasal polyps (usually allergic in origin), endometrial polyps (hyperplastic), polyps of Peutz–Jeghers syndrome (hamartomatous).

Colonic angiodysplasias are covered in this chapter as they can also present with large bowel bleeding and are often part of a differential diagnosis with polyps and carcinoma.

The common complications of large bowel surgery are described in this chapter and finally, the different types of intestinal stoma and their indication are outlined.

COLORECTAL POLYPS

Polyps are a common finding in the large bowel. Their great importance is in relation to malignant change. Most colorectal polyps are **adenomas** (i.e. benign neoplasms) and all of these have the potential for malignant change. Not all adenomas are polypoid, however. **Flat adenomas** are fairly common in the Far East and occasionally occur in developed countries. These can be very small and are often found as slight depressions in the colonic wall. Recognition requires special dye-spray techniques at colonoscopy. A polyp may already have undergone malignant change, yet still be at an early and potentially curable stage. Thus for practical purposes, almost any colorectal polyp must be considered adenomatous and malignant or premalignant until proved otherwise on histology. Hence the terminological difficulty of calling these lesions polyps, which might be taken to imply that they are all benign.

A simple pathological classification of large bowel polyps is shown in Box 20.1.

ADENOMATOUS POLYPS (ADENOMAS)

Malignant potential

Adenomas are clinically important because they undergo **malignant change**. The degree of epithelial dysplasia in adenomatous polyps is highly variable. In benign lesions and carcinoma in situ, the abnormality is, by definition, confined to the epithelium. Early malignant change is represented by invasion of tumour cells through the epithelial basement membrane, from where progression occurs through the muscularis mucosa and into the sub-mucosa. In apparently benign lesions, there may be discrete areas of frank malignancy and thorough histological examination is needed if these are not to be overlooked. With pedunculated lesions removed by colonoscopic snaring, it is crucial to establish whether there is invasion of the stalk as this will determine whether further treatment is required.

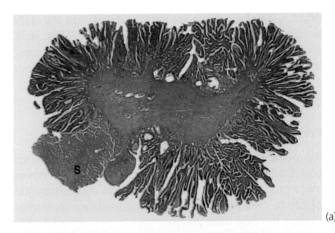

(a)

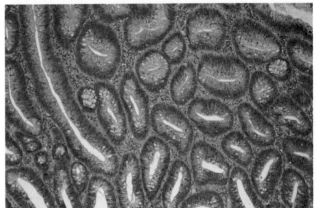

(b)

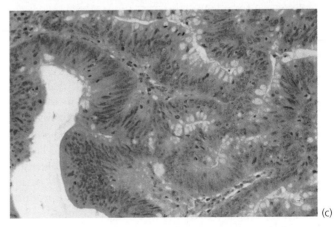

(c)

Fig. 20.1 Adenomatous colonic polyps—histopathology
(a) Adenomatous polyp having mainly villous glandular architecture. The example shown has a well-defined stalk **S**, although this is more typical of tubular or tubulovillous polyps, villous adenoma often having a broad base. **(b)** Early malignant change in a tubulo-villous adenomatous polyp showing carcinoma breaching the muscularis mucosae and invading the stalk. **(c)** High-power view showing high-grade dysplasia. Diagnosis of malignancy, however requires examination of multiple histological sections for invasion of the muscularis mucosae.

Box 20.1 Pathological classification of colorectal polyps and adenomas

Neoplasms
● Adenomas—very common, all potentially malignant; these include villous, tubular and tubulo-villous types
● Early carcinomas—common
● Lymphomas—rare
● Leiomyomas and leiomyosarcomas—rare
● Lipomas and liposarcomas—rare
● Carcinoid tumours—rare

Hyperplasias
● Metaplastic mucosal polyps—common
● Lymphoid aggregations—common in young children

Hamartomas
● Angiomas (related to angiodysplasias)—uncommon
● Juvenile polyps—uncommon, found only in children; no malignant potential

Inflammatory polyps
● 'Pseudopolyps' of severe ulcerative colitis

Adenomas have two basic morphological forms, globular **pedunculated** polyps with stalks of variable length, and broad-based (**sessile**) lesions. The flat adenoma is a variant of the sessile lesion.

Histologically, three patterns of growth are recognised: tubular adenomas, villous adenomas and tubulo-villous adenomas (see Fig. 20.1).

Tubular adenomas

These are small pedunculated or sessile lesions in which the adenoma cells retain a tubular form similar to normal colonic mucosa. Tubular adenomas have the least potential for malignant transformation. The exception is when multiple tubular adenomas occur throughout the large bowel in the rare disorder of **familial adenomatous polyposis** (FAP). In this inherited condition there is a very high risk of early malignant transformation (see p. 285).

Villous adenomas

Villous adenomas are usually sessile and frond-like (papilliferous) lesions which tend to secrete mucus. This may be so copious as to be the main presenting complaint. Occasionally, symptomatic hypokalaemia may develop because so much potassium-containing mucus is lost. The epithelial component of villous adenoma is more dysplastic than that of tubular adenoma and there is a greater potential for malignant change; as with tubulo-villous adenomas, the malignant potential is proportional to the size.

Tubulo-villous adenomas

Histologically, these lesions are intermediate between tubular and villous adenomas and comprise the majority of colonic polyps. Most are pedunculated, and the stalk is covered with normal colonic epithelium. The stalk probably develops by the action of peristalsis dragging the tumour mass distally and varies in length from about 0.5 to 10 cm.

Presentation of colorectal adenomatous polyps

Adenomatous polyps may occur in any part of the large bowel, although three-quarters of them arise in the rectum and sigmoid colon. This exactly parallels the distribution of carcinomas and provides strong evidence that most cancers develop from polyps.

As a general rule, the larger the lesion, the more likely it is to be malignant—only 1% of polyps smaller than 1 cm in diameter are malignant whereas about half of those larger than 2.5 cm are malignant.

Adenomas and especially villous adenomas often arise singly but multiple polyps are present in more than 20% of patients with colonic polyps; these multiple polyps are most often tubulo-villous. Patients with frank carcinoma are often found to have coexisting benign adenomas (synchronous) and these may become malignant later if not removed (see Fig. 20.2). This explains why the whole colon should be examined before colectomy wherever possible, preferably by colonoscopy, and why long-term follow-up after treatment of large bowel cancer should include regular colonoscopy.

SYMPTOMS AND SIGNS OF COLORECTAL POLYPS

Many polyps cause no symptoms, at least in their early stages, and remain undiagnosed or are found incidentally on colonoscopy or barium enema examination. Screening aims to detect these (as well as invasive cancers) so they can be removed before they undergo malignant change. Symptomatic polyps present typically with **rectal bleeding** and sometimes iron deficiency **anaemia** due to occult blood loss. Distal lesions may occasionally produce **tenesmus** or they may **prolapse** through the anus.

DIAGNOSIS AND MANAGEMENT OF COLORECTAL POLYPS

Diagnosis may be made at sigmoidoscopy (rectoscopy) with nearly half of all polyps lying within reach of the 25 cm rigid instrument. Flexible sigmoidoscopy has a greater range and enables the area at greatest risk of adenoma/carcinoma to be fully examined, namely the rectum and left side of colon as far as the splenic flexure. Flexible sigmoidoscopy is becoming popular because the examination can be performed in the outpatient clinic with minimal bowel preparation and any polyps can be

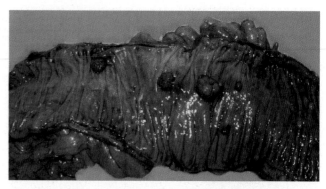

Fig. 20.2 Multiple colonic adenomatous polyps
This length of opened descending colon is from a 64-year-old man who presented with an invasive carcinoma of the rectum (not shown here). Several adenomatous polyps of various sizes can be seen in this part of the bowel; the larger polyps have greater malignant potential.

removed at the same time by diathermy snare ('excision biopsy'). If adenomatous polyps are discovered, the rest of the large bowel must be examined by colonoscopy and any more polyps removed for histological examination as described below.

For examining the transverse and right side of the colon, barium enema examination reveals most polyps of significant size, and is often the first choice, particularly if symptoms include change of bowel habit (see Fig. 20.3). Colonoscopy is a better diagnostic alternative for patients presenting with rectal bleeding considered to arise above the anal canal as it allows direct visual inspection for polyps and carcinomas as well as biopsy of suspicious lesions. It can also demonstrate small lesions likely to be missed on barium examination. Colonoscopy also enables polyps to be excised by snare or diathermy at the same time. In addition it is a more complete examination for follow-up after colectomy or polyp removal. However, it should be noted that colonoscopy carries a 1–2 per 1000 risk of perforation or haemorrhage.

Both barium enema and colonoscopy are operator-dependent and it may be technically difficult to demonstrate the whole colon in sufficient detail to show small lesions; the caecum is particularly difficult to see well. If a barium enema demonstrates polyps or is technically unsatisfactory, colonoscopy should then be performed. Sessile adenomas in any location can be difficult to recognise even on colonoscopy and these potientially malignant lesions can thereby be missed.

At colonoscopy, polyps can be excised using a diathermy snare passed around the stalk or sessile base (see Fig. 20.4). Pedunculated lesions less than 2 cm in diameter can usually be removed with ease but larger ones or sessile lesions may require snaring in several pieces. Histology is mandatory to establish whether the lesion is malignant and whether it has been completely removed. If a malignant polyp has been incompletely

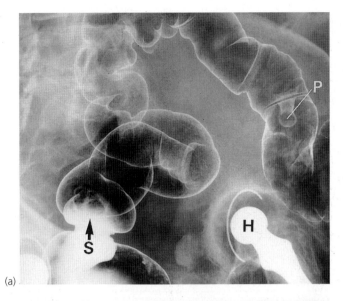

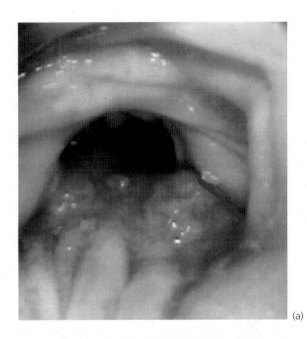

(a)

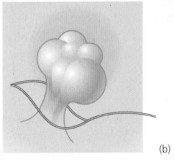

(b)

Fig. 20.4 Colonoscopic snaring of a polyp
(a) A 2 cm polyp on a long stalk in the sigmoid colon. **(b)** The snare loop is tightened around the stalk of the polyp before applying diathermy current to remove it and coagulate the blood vessels in the stalk.

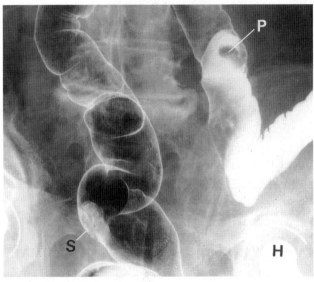

(b)

Fig. 20.3 Colorectal polyps
This 65-year-old man presented with rectal bleeding. On sigmoidoscopy, a large polypoid lesion was seen in the upper rectum. The X-rays show two views of the rectum and sigmoid colon during a barium enema (note the hip prosthesis **H**). Both views show the sessile rectal lesion **S**, which was visible at sigmoidoscopy. In addition, a pedunculated polyp **P** was found in the sigmoid colon. No other polyps were demonstrated in the large bowel. Sigmoidoscopic biopsies showed no malignancy, but the lesions looked suspicious and were removed by surgically resecting the upper rectum and sigmoid colon. Histology showed the rectal lesion was an adenoma, but it was found to have early invasive carcinoma in one area. The sigmoid polyp proved to be a benign tubulo-villous adenoma. **(a)** Single contrast. **(b)** Double contrast—note the difference in appearance of the pedunculated polyp from **(a)**.

removed, then bowel resection is required. After removal of dysplastic or frankly malignant polyps, patients should be scheduled for colonoscopy after 1 year and then again every 3–5 years.

ADENOCARCINOMA OF COLON AND RECTUM

EPIDEMIOLOGY OF COLORECTAL CARCINOMA

As shown in Table 20.1, colorectal cancer is the third most common cause of death from cancer in the developed world; if is responsible for about 26 000 deaths in the UK every year. Almost one-third arise in the rectum. In industrialised countries approximately one person in 25 will develop this cancer in their lifetime. The disease is rare before the age of 50 (except in familial adenomatous polyposis, FAP—see p. 285) but common after the age of 60. There is little difference in incidence between the sexes. First-degree relatives (i.e. siblings and children) of patients with colorectal cancer (excluding FAP) have an increased risk of developing this malignancy if the affected relative was under 50 at the time of diagnosis or

Table 20.1 Death rates from colorectal cancer compared with other malignancies (UK 1997)

Males	Annual no. of deaths	Rate/million population	Percentage of male cancer deaths	Females	Annual no. of deaths	Rate/million population	Percentage of female cancer deaths
1 Lung	22 000	760	28.6	1 Breast	13 400	446	17.4
2 Prostate	9500	326	12.3	2 Lung	12 800	427	16.6
3 Colon and rectum	9000	308	11.7	3 Colon and rectum	8400	280	10.9
4 Stomach and oesophagus	8500	299	11.0	4 Stomach and oesophagus	5600	185	7.3
5 Leukaemias, lymphomas and myeloma	5600	195	7.3	5 Leukaemias, lymphomas and mylemoa	5000	170	6.5
6 Kidney and bladder	5200	179	6.8	6 Ovary	4500	150	5.8
7 Pancreas	3000	108	3.9	7 Pancreas	3400	112	4.4
8 Brain	1800	63	2.3	8 Kidney and bladder	3000	99	3.9
9 Liver	1300	45	1.7	9 Uterus and cervix	1800	50	2.3
10 Malignant melanoma	760	26	1.0	10 Brain	1300	45	1.7
All others	10 344		13.4	All others	17 800		23.1
All cancers	77 000		100.0	All cancers	77 000		100.0

if more than one such relative was affected at any age. In some countries, screening is recommended for these relatives every 3–5 years using colonoscopy, with faecal occult blood testing in the intervening years. Screening should commence at age 50, or 10 years before the age at which the affected member developed the cancer. Where screening is not recommended or available, relatives should be made aware of their greater risk and advised to be particularly vigilant in acting upon possible early presenting symptoms.

Most colorectal carcinomas are now known to arise in pre-existing adenomas. This adenoma–carcinoma sequence is of crucial importance in the prevention of colorectal cancer because recognising and treating adenomas before invasive cancer develops is curative. A small proportion are secondary to malignant change in familial adenomatous polyposis or longstanding ulcerative colitis (see Ch. 21). Colorectal cancer is a disease of developed countries, almost unknown in rural Third World communities, strongly suggesting an environmental factor in the aetiology. This was first highlighted by Denis Burkitt in the early 1970s and led to the belief that the Western low-fibre, high-fat diet is in some way responsible. It is well established that the Western diet results in a much slower whole-gut transit time and it may be that carcinogens in the stool thereby maintain contact with the bowel mucosa for longer. Low-fibre diets are usually low in fruit and raw vegetables and consequently low in **antioxidants** which are thought to have a protective role in colorectal cancer. Recent studies have shown a reduction in colorectal cancer in people taking a small daily dose of aspirin (75–150 mg) as prophylaxis against cardiovascular disease. This may also be due to its antioxidant action.

PATHOPHYSIOLOGY OF COLORECTAL CARCINOMA

Colorectal carcinomas exhibit a wide range of differentiation which broadly correlates with their clinical behaviour and prognosis. Most carcinomas are initially **exophytic** (i.e. protruding into the lumen) and later ulcerate and progressively invade the muscular bowel wall (see Fig. 20.5). Eventually, the tumour involves the serosa and surrounding structures. Stromal fibrosis may cause luminal narrowing, which is responsible for the common acute presentation of large bowel obstruction.

Large bowel carcinomas metastasise mainly via lymphatics and the bloodstream. Lymphatic spread is sequential, first to mesenteric nodes and then to para-aortic nodes. Occasionally lymph node involvement is directly responsible for the clinical presentation. For example, para-aortic nodes may present as a palpable mass or cause duodenal obstruction. Other enlarged nodes may compress the bile ducts in the porta hepatis causing jaundice.

Haematogenous spread is predominantly to the liver and usually occurs later than lymphatic spread; therefore

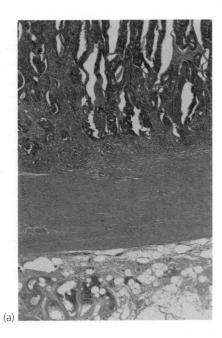

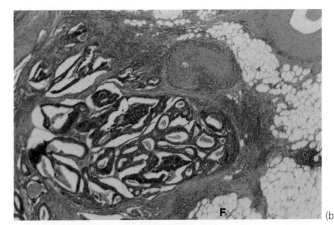

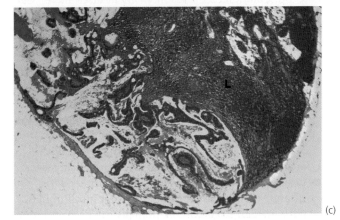

Fig. 20.5 Colorectal carcinoma—histopathology

(a) Invasive carcinoma arising in a tubulovillous adenoma **(b)** Carcinoma has invaded through the entire thickness of the colonic muscular wall to reach fat **F**, but has not spread to lymph nodes, making this a Dukes' B carcinoma **(c)** Mesenteric lymph node in which lymphoid tissue **L** has been partly replaced by carcinoma.

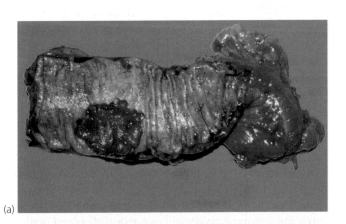

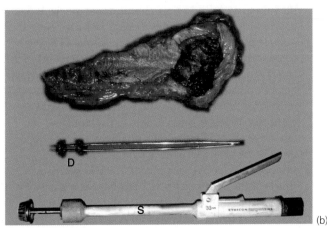

Fig. 20.6 Cancers of the colon and rectum

(a) Ulcer cancer of sigmoid colon. This 52-year-old man presented with 3-months' history of rectal bleeding. This ulcer was seen and biopsied on colonoscopy and resected soon afterwards without a colostomy. **(b)** Annular carcinoma of rectum in a 68-year-old woman who presented with large bowel obstruction. A low anterior resection was performed with a covering loop ileostomy. The bowel was rejoined using the circular stapler **S**. Two complete 'doughnuts' of tissue **D** indicate successful firing of the stapler. **(c)** Synchronous cancers of the transverse colon. This elderly man presented with a change in bowel habit, with constipation and overflow diarrhoea. Preoperative barium enema examination revealed two cancers that were resected at operation and the ends anastomosed.

279

a patient with only early lymph node involvement at the time of presentation has a better chance of avoiding liver metastases. Despite this, hepatic involvement often occurs without evidence of lymphatic spread. The effects of liver secondaries often cause death even after an apparently successful resection of the primary cancer. Haematogenous spread to other sites such as lung or bone is uncommon, as are systemic manifestations. By the time of diagnosis, as many as 25% of patients with colorectal cancer already have widespread metastases.

PRESENTATION OF LARGE BOWEL CARCINOMA

Late presentations as a result of metastases have been discussed in the last paragraph. For local disease, the mode of growth and clinical presentation of large bowel cancer depend to some extent on the site of the lesion:

- The right colon is larger in diameter than the left colon and the faecal stream more fluid. Therefore tumours of the right colon rarely cause obstruction unless the ileo-caecal valve is involved. Occult bleeding from the tumour surface commonly causes iron deficiency anaemia and these patients typically present with anaemia and a palpable mass in the right iliac fossa
- Lesions elsewhere in the colon or rectum tend to ulcerate earlier, perhaps due to greater intraluminal pressure and stool trauma. In many cases, the tumour progressively encircles the bowel wall, encroaching on the lumen and producing an **annular stenosis**. It has been estimated that it takes a year to involve each quarter of the bowel circumference. The stool in the left colon is more solid than on the right. Consequently, left-sided cancers usually present with a change in bowel habit or precipitate an emergency admission to hospital with large bowel obstruction; this may be partial or complete. Blood is often visible in the stool and the character of the blood and its mixing with stool depend on how far proximally the lesion is from the anus
- Lesions (carcinomas or polyps) in the lower two-thirds of the rectum may be perceived as a mass of faeces. This stimulates a persistent defaecation response causing the symptom of **tenesmus**
- A cancer eroding through the bowel wall may stimulate a vigorous local inflammatory process resulting in a **pericolic abscess**. This occurs in the recto-sigmoid area and usually presents with left iliac fossa pain and tenderness and a swinging fever. Differential diagnosis is acute diverticulitis or a diverticular abscess
- A carcinoma anywhere in the colon (but rarely in the rectum) may perforate and present as an acute abdomen with peritonitis. Occasionally a malignant fistula occurs into stomach, bladder, uterus or vagina or to the skin

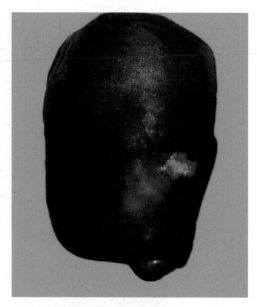

Fig. 20.7 Right hepatectomy specimen
This 49-year-old man presented with a 9-month history of rectal bleeding, found to be due to a sigmoid colon carcinoma. This was resected but two years later he was found to have a single metastasis in the right lobe of the liver seen here. No other metastases were found so he underwent a resection of the right lobe of the liver. Three years later, he returned with a paraduodenal mass and widespread peritoneal metastases, from which he died.

CLINICAL SIGNS IN SUSPECTED COLORECTAL CARCINOMA

The symptoms and signs of colorectal cancer are illustrated in Figure 20.8. Abdominal examination may reveal a colonic mass, liver enlargement due to metastases or ascites. All of these signs represent late and often incurable disease; the majority of patients have no abnormal abdominal symptoms. Rectal examination is mandatory as many carcinomas occur in the lowest 12 cm of the large bowel and can be reached with an examining finger. In addition, local tumour spread into the pouch of Douglas may be palpable through the rectal wall anteriorly. The degree of fixation of a rectal tumour to surrounding structures can also be evaluated digitally and this gives some indication of potential operative difficulty. Finally, the glove should be inspected for blood and mucus and stool colour and consistency. General examination may show other features suggesting disseminated malignant disease, e.g. anaemia, obvious weight loss, supraclavicular node enlargement.

INVESTIGATION OF SUSPECTED COLORECTAL CARCINOMA

Proctoscopy and rigid or flexible sigmoidoscopy are performed at the initial consultation. Proctoscopy may show

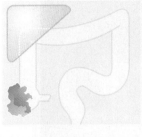

Effects of primary cancer

Symptomless anaemia
Mass in right iliac fossa
Diarrhoea

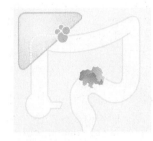

Due to secondary deposits

Obstructive jaundice
(node compression of porta
hepatis)

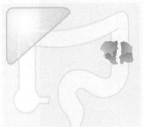

Rectal blood loss
Change in bowel habit
Colicky pain/obstruction
Mucus with stool
Internal fistula
Perforation/peritonitis

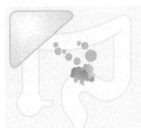

Retroperitoneal lymph node
involvement causing:
    Ureteric obstruction
    Duodenal obstruction

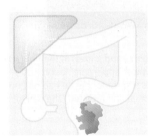

Tenesmus/Bleeding/Mucus
Diarrhoea (Fluid depletion)
Hypokalaemia
Local pain due to infiltration of
sacral plexus

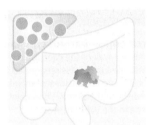

Systemic effects

Widespread liver and/or other
metastases causing:
    Malaise
    Anorexia
    Weight loss

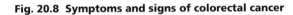

Fig. 20.8 Symptoms and signs of colorectal cancer

local causes for rectal bleeding such as haemorrhoids. About 50% of colorectal cancers lie within reach of a rigid sigmoidoscope and 75% within reach of a flexible sigmoidoscope; in either case, lesions can be biopsied. A barium enema or colonoscopy should be arranged, even if a tumour has been identified at sigmoidoscopy (see Fig. 20.9). This is because synchronous tumours or potentially malignant adenomatous polyps may also be present. Colonoscopy may be employed to obtain a histological diagnosis of more proximal lesions found on barium enema if the diagnosis is in doubt. Ultrasound or CT scanning of the liver is often performed to seek metastases, but in the absence of clinical suspicion the chance of finding metastases is low and, even if found, they are unlikely to affect the early management. Higher-resolution CT scanning with contrast enhancement is making progress as a first-line examination of the large bowel. Finally, if there is a risk of ureteric involvement by local spread, intravenous urography can be a useful preoperative investigation.

Many patients, especially the elderly, present as emergencies with complete large bowel obstruction, often at the sigmoid colon or recto-sigmoid junction. This typically takes several days to develop. Plain abdominal X-rays often show large bowel dilated by gas down to the level of obstruction and empty of gas beyond it. Sigmoidoscopy may confirm the diagnosis of carcinoma; if not, an 'instant' barium enema (i.e. without bowel preparation) will usually do so, and will exclude pseudo-obstruction.

MANAGEMENT OF COLORECTAL CARCINOMA

Surgical resection is the main treatment for colorectal carcinoma. Adjuvant radiotherapy and chemotherapy are sometimes used but the indications are as yet uncertain. For small tumours localised to the bowel wall, resection offers an excellent chance of complete cure. The cure rate falls markedly with invasion through the bowel wall but cures can still be achieved. Even in very extensive tumours, palliative resection is usually still worth while to relieve obstruction or prevent continuing blood loss.

Staging of colorectal carcinoma

Staging of colorectal cancers largely depends on the findings at laparotomy and histological examination of the resected specimen. Several staging systems have been proposed but the most widely used one is still

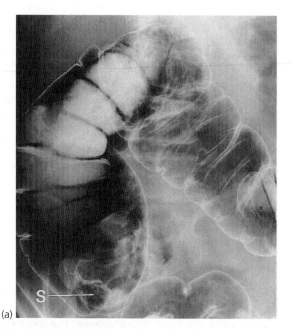

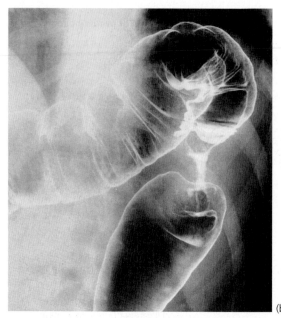

(a)   (b)

Fig. 20.9 Caecal and colonic carcinomas—barium enema examinations
(a) Polypoid carcinoma arising on the medial wall of the caecum in a 73-year-old man with an iron deficiency anaemia and a mass in the right iliac fossa. Note the lesion is growing out into the lumen; it is recognised by the overlapping double shadows **S**. **(b)** Typical 'apple-core' lesion just distal to the splenic flexure of a man of 39 who complained of rectal bleeding. With this degree of stenosis, it was surprising that he had had no change in bowel habit. Acute obstruction would probably soon have occurred if the tumour had not been recognised and resected. The patient is unusually young for colorectal carcinoma in the Western world.

based on **Dukes' classification**. Dukes was a pathologist and staged tumours based on the specimens he received. His classification was first described for rectal carcinomas and later for colonic carcinomas and is outlined in Box 20.2. Staging of colorectal carcinoma seldom influences treatment but it does give an estimate of the statistical probability of cure and likelihood of surviving 5 years. In fact, survival is largely determined by the presence or absence of liver metastases. Indeed, small metastases impalpable at operation can be detected most sensitively by intraoperative ultrasonography, placing the probe directly on the liver surface. Intraoperative ultrasound is not yet widely available so conventional ultrasound or CT scanning is often used to provide this prognostic information.

Approximately half of all patients with colorectal cancer are incurable at presentation; all of these die within 5 years. Of the other half that undergo radical surgery with the aim of cure, 50% are alive and well 5 years later. Very few patients surviving 5 years die later of recurrent disease.

Operations for colorectal cancer

The principles of colorectal tumour resection are as follows:

- Operative access is achieved by laparotomy, usually via a long midline incision. In specialist units, laparoscopic or laparoscopic-assisted surgery is sometimes employed
- The affected segment of bowel is removed with a margin of normal bowel. A minimum of 5 cm clear each side of the tumour removes local lymphatics likely to be involved. Rectal cancers are a special case. They require excision of the tumour and an intact envelope of fat around it (**the mesorectum**) to a distance of 5 cm below the primary tumour. This allows the anal sphincter to be preserved in many patients, provided the lower edge of the tumour is 8 cm or more from the anal verge
- The precise lines of resection are determined by the distribution of mesenteric blood vessels. There must be a good blood supply to the cut ends of bowel to ensure healing. Some surgeons first perform proximal ligation of the venous drainage, in an attempt to minimise the risk of tumour embolisation from handling during resection. Recent advances in tumour biology suggest that this is likely to be ineffective since cancers embolise continually and whether or not metastases form depends on the interaction between 'seed' and 'soil'
- The primary lesion plus a safety margin is resected en bloc with a wedge-shaped section of mesentery and its contained lymph nodes to remove the primary field of lymphatic drainage. If there are other obvious lymph node metastases, these are usually included in the resection specimen

● In most cases, the cut ends of bowel can be rejoined at the same operation without the need for a temporary or permanent colostomy. The indications for stomas, and their types and management are described on

pages 286–290.) The method used depends on the site of the anastomosis and whether there is much disparity in diameter between the ends to be joined. Standard operations vary with the site of the tumour, and each is modified according to the operative findings. Details of technique vary from surgeon to surgeon, but an outline of standard operations is given in Figure 20.10. The technique of right hemicolectomy is illustrated in Figure 20.11 and methods of large bowel anastomosis in Figure 20.12. Methods of matching the diameter of the bowel ends are illustrated in Figure 20.13.

KEY POINTS

Box 20.2 Staging and survival rates from treated colorectal carcinoma based on Dukes' classification

Dukes' A
● Tumour confined to the bowel wall with no extension into the extrarectal or extracolic tissues and no lymph node metastases—75% 5-year survival

Dukes' B
● Tumour spread through the muscularis propria (i.e. the bowel wall) into the extrarectal or extracolic tissues by direct continuity but without lymph node metastases—55% 5-year survival

Dukes' C
● Lymph node metastases are present. This category is subdivided into:
  C1: — only a few nodes are involved near the primary growth, leaving proximal nodes free from metastases—40% 5-year survival
  C2: — there is a continuous string of involved lymph nodes up to the proximal limit of resection—20% 5-year survival

Stage D
● This is a later addition to Dukes' staging, based on clinical rather than pathological evidence. These patients are found at operation to have distant metastases or such extensive local or nodal spread that the lesion is surgically incurable whatever the pathological staging

The role of adjuvant radiotherapy and chemotherapy

The use of adjuvant radiotherapy and chemotherapy in colorectal cancer is becoming clearer as the results of clinical trials emerge. Radiotherapy can be used preoperatively to shrink a large or tethered tumour to make it operable or to enable the anal sphincter to be preserved (**downstaging**); short, sharp courses of treatment immediately prior to surgery may be beneficial in terms of reducing local recurrence where tumours extend through the rectal wall. Radiotherapy after surgery is probably less effective and risks radiation damage to small bowel now lying in the pelvis.

As regards chemotherapy, **5-fluorouracil (5-FU)** is the chief adjuvant agent and it is often given in combination with its biomodulator, **folinic acid**. Several clinical trials have shown an increase in time before recurrence in Dukes' C cases but no convincing prolongation of survival. There may be a benefit in combining preoperative radiotherapy with postoperative chemotherapy in certain locally advanced cases but conclusive evidence of its value is lacking.

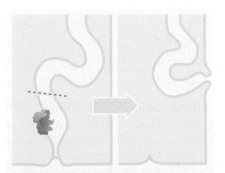

Abdominoperineal resection of rectum

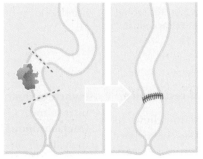

Anterior resection of rectum

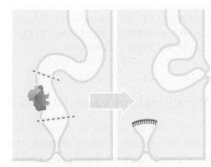

Hartmann's operation

Fig. 20.10 Standard operations for rectal cancer
Hartmann's procedure is described on p. 288 and 289.

1   Divide lateral peritoneum

2   Reflect ascending colon forwards on its mesentery, identifying and preserving ureter and retroperitoneal duodenum

3   Select points at which to divide bowel, retaining as much ileum as possible; ensure good blood supply to colon by transilluminating mesocolon, aiming to retain a good vessel close to line of section

4   Divide greater omentum

5   Ligate and divide vessels of mesentery

6   Anastomose cut ends of ileum and colon

7   Repair defect in mesentery

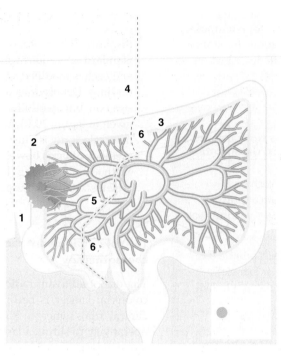

Fig. 20.11 Principles of right hemicolectomy

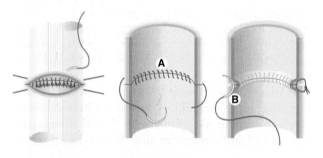

(a) **Single-layer anastomosis**   (b) Two-layer anastomosis

Fig. 20.12 Standard methods of bowel anastomosis
(a) A single-layer anastomosis uses interrupted absorbable sutures. It is a standard method of anastomosis for all types of bowel. The posterior layer can be placed from inside the bowel. Sutures usually include only the muscle wall and submucosa. **(b)** A two-layer anastomosis is sometimes used for small bowel but is rarely used for large bowel. It is unsuitable for the rectum and oesophagus. The first layer **A** is an 'all-coats' suture and it is usually continuous. The second layer **B** is an inverting layer including only the sero-muscular coat; it may be continuous or interrupted.

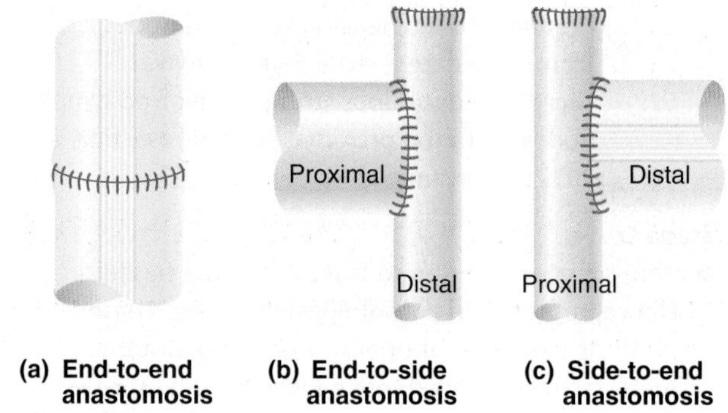

(a) **End-to-end anastomosis**   (b) **End-to-side anastomosis**   (c) **Side-to-end anastomosis**

Fig. 20.13 Methods of matching the diameter of the bowel ends to effect a safe anastomosis
(a) An end-to-end anastomosis is used when bowel ends are of similar diameter. **(b)** An end-to-side anastomosis is used where the proximal end is greater in diameter than the distal end, e.g. in small bowel obstruction. **(c)** A side-to-end anastomosis is used where the distal end is greater in diameter than the proximal end, e.g. in right hemicolectomy.

Management of advanced disease and recurrence

The primary tumour is usually resected to relieve its local effects even when distant metastases have been diagnosed. Most of these patients die within 1 or 2 years, and only about 1 in 10 survives 2 or 3 years; none survives 5 years.

The liver is the most common site of distant metastasis. Liver metastases may be discovered at operation (**synchronous**) or appear later on surveillance with ultrasound, CT or blood tumour marker estimation (**metachronous**). In most cases, there are multiple liver metastases in both lobes by the time of diagnosis. Occasionally there may be one or two metastases confined to a resectable anatomical lobe. These may be excised locally, or the affected segment of liver removed by partial hepatectomy. About 20% of these patients survive

5 years. Liver resections for metastases are rarely performed, however, because few patients fulfil the criteria for operation just described.

Patients with liver metastases seldom become jaundiced, since this only occurs when the parenchyma is almost completely destroyed or major bile ducts are compressed. This is usually a late event and treatment is rarely worth while unless gallstones are found to be the cause. Colorectal tumours sometimes metastasise to bone, particularly the lumbar spine, and painful lesions may be palliated by radiotherapy.

Metastatic colorectal carcinomas are relatively unresponsive to current chemotherapeutic regimens. Occasionally 5-fluorouracil is given by direct infusion into the liver to control painful liver metastases. Colorectal carcinomas do respond to radiotherapy but its application is limited by the difficulty of directing the radiation beam at the tumour without damaging surrounding bowel. Radiotherapy is a useful palliative treatment for recurrent pelvic cancer following removal of the rectum. Pelvic recurrence used to be a common problem before the importance of mesorectal excision was realised; it causes intractable perineal pain. Occasionally a fungating mass grows in the anal region or buttocks and this very distressing complication may also be palliated with radiotherapy.

FAMILIAL ADENOMATOUS POLYPOSIS

Familial adenomatous polyposis is a rare **autosomal dominant disorder** caused by a deletion in the long arm of chromosome 5. It has a high degree of penetrance and is characterised by multiple tubular adenomatous polyps throughout the colon and rectum; there are often polyps in the proximal small bowel. The polyps first develop in adolescence and are usually asymptomatic but may present with rectal bleeding or change in bowel habit. The polyps are initially benign but malignant change almost inevitably occurs in early adulthood, often in more than one polyp at the same time.

Patients presenting with this condition should have their close relatives screened, in adolescence if possible, by retinal examination for hypertrophy of pigment epithelium (present in 95%), colonoscopy and DNA studies. Once familial polyposis coli has been diagnosed, the whole colorectal mucosa should be removed. **Pan-proctocolectomy** with ileostomy is the standard treatment. A popular alternative to ileostomy is the creation in the pelvis of a pouch or reservoir of ileum which is connected to the anus. The anal sphincter mechanism is preserved so that the patient is usually continent and can control evacuation. As in pan-proctocolectomy, all mucosa at risk of malignant change is removed.

COMPLICATIONS OF LARGE BOWEL SURGERY

Infection arising from faecal contamination is the main early complication of large bowel surgery. This carries a high risk of systemic sepsis and multi-organ dysfunction syndrome. Contamination may result from perforation prior to operation, inadvertent faecal spillage during the operation, or anastomotic leakage or breakdown post-operatively. Three main types of infection occur: wound infection and dehiscence, intraperitoneal abscesses and generalised peritonitis. Large bowel surgery has always been associated with a high risk of infective complications, particularly in emergency operations; these are dramatically reduced by the use of prophylactic antibiotics and pre-operative bowel cleansing techniques.

The complications of large bowel surgery are summarised in Box 20.3.

BOWEL CLEANSING TECHNIQUES PRIOR TO SURGERY

The objective is to clear the bowel of faecal material and to reduce the load of bacterial flora. This is achieved by a combination of the following procedures:

- **Withdrawal of solid foods**. The patient may be limited to fluids or a low-fibre diet for a few days before operation
- **Purgation**. This is usually with stimulant laxatives (e.g. sodium picosulphate) or sometimes osmotic laxatives (e.g. magnesium sulphate mixture, mannitol). If mannitol is used, non-absorbed oral

---

SUMMARY

Box 20.3 Complications of large bowel surgery

Early complications
- Wound infections—abscess and cellulitis
- Intra-abdominal abscess—at site of surgery, pelvic or subphrenic
- Anastomotic leak or breakdown
- Systemic sepsis and multi-organ dysfunction syndrome
- Inadvertent damage to other organs, e.g. ureters, bladder, duodenum or spleen
- Stoma problems—sloughing or retraction

Later complications
- Diarrhoea—due to short bowel
- Division of pelvic parasympathetic nerves—causes impotence
- Small bowel obstruction—due to pelvic peritoneal adhesions or tangling of small bowel with colostomy or ileostomy, or later as a complication of radiotherapy causing small bowel damage

antibacterial agents like neomycin must be used to prevent bacterial fermentation and formation of potentially explosive gas within the bowel

● **Enemas and distal bowel washouts**. For incomplete obstruction, purgation must be used with great care to avoid precipitating acute obstruction. When there is complete obstruction, distal washouts and enemas only can be given preoperatively. In these cases, it is possible to clear the proximal colon of faeces by an 'on-table washout' during the operation, once the tumour has been resected. This involves inserting a Foley catheter through the wall of the caecum (usually through the appendix stump) which is used to irrigate 2–3 L of warm saline into the colon. This is drained via a large-bore tube connected to the distal end of the colon into a bucket. In some cases, this allows a primary anastomosis to be performed safely.

PERIOPERATIVE PROPHYLACTIC ANTIBIOTICS

A variety of faecal commensals and other organisms cause abdominal infections after large bowel surgery. These include *Escherichia coli* and other enterobacteriaceae (Gram-negative aerobes), *Bacteroides* and related organisms (Gram-negative anaerobic rods), *Staph. aureus* (Gram-positive aerobic cocci), *Enterococcus faecalis* (Gram-positive anaerobic cocci) and the clostridia (Gram-positive anaerobic rods). An antibiotic combination for prophylaxis is chosen to cover the main organisms, and popular regimens are shown in Box 20.4. It is important to achieve high circulating blood levels at the time of operation, so the first dose is usually given at anaesthetic induction or with the premedication.

COLONIC ANGIODYSPLASIAS

Colonic angiodysplasias have only been recognised as a common cause of acute or chronic rectal bleeding and

> **KEY POINTS**
>
> **Box 20.4 Prophylactic antibiotic regimens for large bowel surgery, started intravenously at induction of anaesthesia**
>
> **Standard regimen**
> Gentamicin 120 mg plus benzylpenicillin 1.2 g plus metronidazole 500 mg
>
> **If minor penicillin allergy (rash)**
> Cephalosporin (e.g. cefotaxime 1 g) plus metronidazole 500 mg i.v.
>
> **If major penicillin allergy (anaphylaxis or angio-oedema)**
> Ciprofloxacin 200 mg plus metronidazole 500 mg

iron deficiency anaemia since the mid-1970s. They are tiny hamartomatous vascular lesions in the colonic wall and produce bleeding out of proportion to their size (see Fig. 20.14). Their origin is unknown but since they occur later in life, they are more likely to be acquired and degenerative than congenital.

If bleeding is acute and is occurring rapidly, selective mesenteric arteriography may demonstrate the source of bleeding. In chronic or recurrent haemorrhage, the lesions can be visualised by colonoscopy but are invisible on barium enema. This underlines the importance of thorough colonoscopy in patients with unexplained gastrointestinal blood loss. The lesions can often be treated by electrical coagulation via the colonoscope. If unsuccessful, the affected segment is resected. Similar lesions occur more rarely in the small bowel and bleed in the same way.

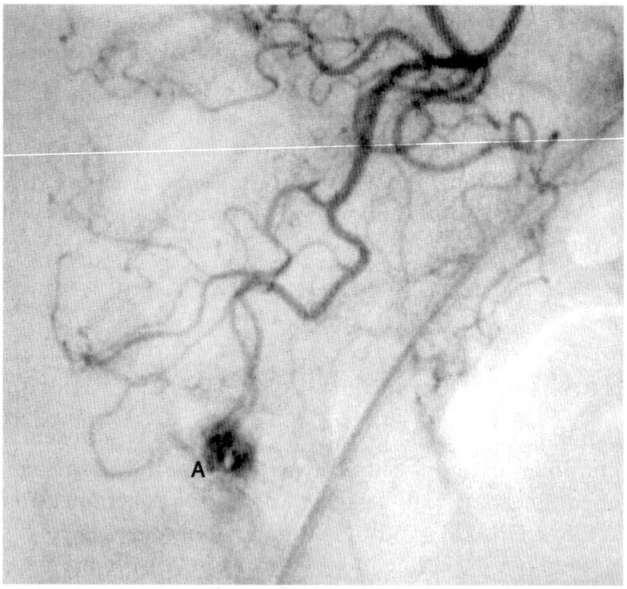

Fig. 20.14 Caecal angiodysplasia
This 66-year-old man had been admitted to hospital on 12 occasions for rectal bleeding or anaemia and received a total of 77 units of blood by transfusion. This selective arteriogram was performed on the most recent admission, and shows an abnormal mass of blood vessels **A** in the caecum typical of angiodysplasia. This part of the bowel was resected and the patient had not re-bled 3 years later.

STOMAS

INDICATIONS AND GENERAL PRINCIPLES

It is often necessary to divert the faecal stream to the anterior abdominal wall via a stoma. The effluent is collected in a removable plastic bag attached by adhesive to the abdominal skin. Stomas are named according to the part of the bowel opening on to the abdominal wall, i.e. **ileostomy** or **colostomy**. The more distal the location of the original lesion, the more likely a stoma will be required. The majority of stomas are performed in cancer surgery, although they are sometimes necessary in inflammatory bowel disease and diverticular disease, and at emergency operations for large bowel perforation or obstruction. The indications for stomas and the principles of stoma design and aftercare are similar for all these conditions.

Stomas may be permanent or temporary. Wherever possible, the need for a stoma should be anticipated before operation and discussed with the patient. This is done to ensure that informed consent is obtained and to prepare the patient for what is often perceived as a 'fate worse than death'. Specialised **stoma nurses** are employed to assist in planning and aftercare. They counsel the patient before operation, when he/she is encouraged to try out a dummy appliance and talk to other stoma patients. The stoma nurse will also identify and mark the most suitable and comfortable site for the stoma appliance. This takes into account the patient's occupation and leisure activities, clothing and ability for self-care.

Permanent stomas

These are necessary when there is no distal bowel segment remaining after resection or when for some reason the bowel cannot be rejoined. A colostomy is required after **abdomino-perineal resection** of a low rectal or anal canal tumour. An ileostomy (Fig. 20.15) is required after excision of the whole colon and rectum (pan-proctocolectomy) unless a pelvic reservoir (pouch) is constructed. The usual indications are inflammatory bowel disease or familial adenomatous polyposis.

Permanent stomas must be carefully sited to facilitate long-term management. They are usually below the belt line. Permanent colostomies are usually fashioned in the left iliac fossa and ileostomies in the right iliac fossa.

Temporary stomas

A stoma is often required temporarily to divert the faecal stream away from a more distal part of the bowel. When the distal bowel problem has resolved, the colostomy can be closed.

Firstly, a colostomy may be created as an emergency measure to relieve complete distal large bowel obstruction causing proximal dilatation. A particular application is when the ileo-caecal valve has remained competent, resulting in extreme caecal dilatation and imminent rupture. The obstructing lesion may be removed at the same operation or later as a scheduled procedure.

Secondly, a 'defunctioning' stoma (ileostomy or colostomy) may be used to protect a more distal anastomosis that is at particular risk of leakage or breakdown. Common examples are a technically difficult low anastomosis (flatus and faeces may leak from the anastomosis), an anastomosis performed after resection of an obstructing lesion (distension may compromise the blood supply), emergency resection involving unprepared bowel (solid faeces in the lumen) or elective surgery where the bowel has not been adequately cleared of faeces.

Thirdly, a temporary colostomy may be used to 'rest' a more distal segment of bowel involved in an inflammatory process such as a pericolic abscess, a complex anorectal fistula, acute Crohn's disease or a colo-vesical or colo-vaginal fistula.

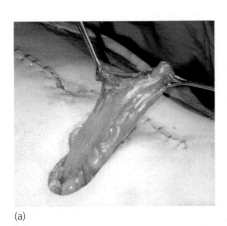
(a)

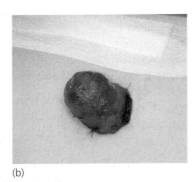
(b)

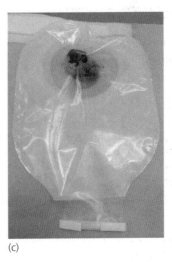
(c)

Fig. 20.15 End ileostomy
This man of 45 had suffered remittent ulcerative colitis for 12 years which could only be managed with high doses of steroids. He underwent subtotal colectomy and formation of this end ileostomy. Later, he will be considered for a pouch reconstruction. **(a)** Formation of ileostomy. The end of the ileum is brought to the surface via an opening made in the right iliac fossa at a point predetermined by the stoma therapist. **(b)** The end of the ileum has been turned back on itself like a cuff to form a spout or Brooks ileostomy. **(c)** The stoma bag placed in the operating theatre.

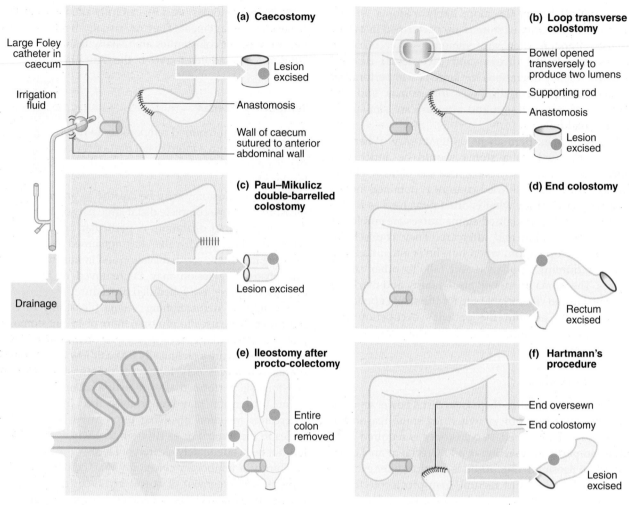

Fig. 20.16 Principal types of ileostomy and colostomy
(a) Caecostomy is temporary. **(b)** Loop transverse colostomy is usually temporary, and is used to defunction the distal bowel. **(c)** Paul–Mikulicz double-barrelled colostomy is usually temporary. There is no anastomosis within the abdominal cavity. **(d)** End colostomy is usually permanent. **(e)** Ileostomy after procto-colectomy is permanent. Note the protruding 'spout' produced by everting the ileum. **(f)** End colostomy in Hartmann's procedure sometimes becomes permanent.

TYPES OF STOMA

The way in which a stoma is fashioned depends on its purpose. The main types of stoma are described below and illustrated in Figure 20.16. Colonic stomas are designed with the bowel mucosa lying flush with the skin. Small bowel stomas are fashioned with a 'spout' of bowel protruding about 3 cm, to ensure that the irritant small bowel contents enter the ileostomy appliance directly rather than flowing on to the skin (see Fig. 20.15 above).

Caecostomy

A connection is established between the skin and the caecum and is held open with a large balloon catheter (see Fig. 20.16a). Its sole function is to decompress the bowel of gas; it is inappropriate for diversion of the faecal stream. Caecostomy is rarely used now because the stoma frequently becomes blocked with faeces and requires regular irrigation to maintain patency.

Loop stoma

This type of stoma is designed so that both the proximal and distal segments of bowel drain on to the skin surface (see Fig. 20.16b). This deflects proximal effluent to the skin surface and provides a 'blow-off' valve for the distal loop. Since the distal loop no longer has any functioning capacity, such stomas are often described as **defunctioning stomas**. They are used mainly as a temporary measure.

A loop of bowel (usually terminal ileum) is brought through a single skin aperture and held above the skin surface by a 'bridge' of plastic rod. An incision is then made in the side of the exteriorised loop to open both proximal and distal loops. The bridge is usually removed after about 1 week. When the stoma is closed, weeks or months later, the bowel is dissected from the skin, the bowel incision closed or a section of bowel resected, and the loop dropped back into the abdomen. The most common form of loop stoma is the **loop ileostomy**; occasionally a **loop transverse colostomy** is used. Both are usually sited below the waistline on the right. The former is smaller and easier to manage and therefore preferable.

A variant of the loop stoma is used if complete and prolonged defunctioning is required. The proximal colon is brought to the skin and opened as usual and the distal end is oversewn and sutured to the abdominal wall just under the skin next to the open proximal end. This allows complete defunctioning of the distal bowel but avoids the need for a laparotomy when closing the stoma as both ends are close together. This is an alternative to the older 'split stoma' operation in which proximal and distal ends were brought separately to the skin surface at different sites.

Double-ended stoma

This is a variant of the loop stoma and is used if complete and prolonged defunctioning is required. The 'bridge' is fashioned from a pedicle of abdominal wall skin, which remains in place until the stoma is closed.

Split stoma

This is the ultimate form of defunctioning stoma which is now rarely used, having been superseded by the loop stoma. The bowel ends are completely divided. Both proximal and distal ends are brought separately to the skin surface, the proximal one as an end stoma which passes stool into a stoma appliance; the distal defunctioned end produces a little mucus and is termed a **mucous fistula**.

Single end stoma

This type of stoma is most commonly used to 'resite the anus' on to the abdominal wall and is a permanent stoma. It may be employed as an ileostomy after pan-proctocolectomy or as a colostomy after removal of the rectum and anal sphincter (i.e. abdomino-perineal resection).

Hartmann's procedure

This technique is increasingly used after emergency resection of rectosigmoid lesions where primary anas-

tomosis is inadvisable because of obstruction, inflammation or faecal contamination. Hartmann's procedure may also be used in frail or debilitated patients. The lesion is resected, the proximal loop is made into an end colostomy and the distal remnant closed with sutures or staples (see Fig. 20.16f). The residual rectum is thus completely defunctioned but its secretions still pass through the anus. Several months later, when local inflammation has resolved, the bowel may be reconnected. The development of circular stapling instruments has simplified reconnection and is the main reason for the increasing use of Hartmann's operation. The colostomy is identical to the end colostomy employed after an abdomino-perineal resection. The colostomy is so well tolerated that some patients prefer to keep it permanently rather than undergo another major operation.

Double-barrelled colostomy

The term double-barrelled colostomy does not apply to any of those described above, but was applied to the stoma resulting from the old **Paul–Mikulicz operation**, now rarely used (see Fig. 20.16c). This operation enabled

Table 20.2 Complications of ileostomy and colostomy

Complication	Treatment
Early complications Mucosal sloughing or necrosis of the terminal bowel due to ischaemia	Reoperation and refashioning of the stoma
Obstruction of stoma due to oedema or faecal impaction	Exploration with a gloved finger and sometimes glycerine suppositories or softening enemas
Persistent leakage between skin and appliance causing skin erosion and patient distress, often due to inappropriate location of stoma (e.g. over skin crease)	May respond to stoma nursing care or require a resiting operation
Late complications Prolapse of bowel	Refashioning of stoma
Parastomal hernia due to abdominal wall weakness	Resiting of stoma
Parastomal fistula	Refashioning of stoma
Retraction of 'spout' ileostomy	Reoperation and refashioning of a new ileostomy
Stenosis of stomal orifice	Refashioning of stoma
Perforation after colonic irrigation	Emergency operation
Psychological and psychosexual dysfunction	May require counselling or measures to reverse stoma

safe resection of proximal sigmoid or descending colon where an anastomosis would have been unsafe and there was sufficient bowel length for both ends to be brought to the skin. At the first operation, the lesion and nearby colon were mobilised so it could be brought completely outside the abdominal wall (exteriorisation). The two limbs of the loop were sutured together for about 10 cm deep to the abdominal wall to resemble a double-barrelled shotgun and the exteriorised bowel was cut off flush with the skin leaving a double stoma. Later, the spur between the two stomas was crushed using an enterotome and the colostomy gradually closed spontaneously. The operation had the advantage that a major laparotomy was not required to 'reverse' the procedure and close the stoma, unlike a Hartmann's operation. In most cases, however, the distal bowel was too short to reach the skin.

IRRIGATION TECHNIQUE FOR MANAGING A COLOSTOMY

An ileostomy tends to work continuously during the day whereas a colostomy is intermittent. Some patients with a colostomy prefer to dispense with a stoma bag by using a technique of colonic irrigation. Once every few days the patient passes a litre or more of water into the colostomy via a special spout; then the water is allowed to drain out, with the aim of emptying the entire colon. Once this has been done the stoma is covered with a dry dressing and a stoma bag is not needed until the next irrigation.

COMPLICATIONS OF COLOSTOMY AND ILEOSTOMY

These are summarised in Table 20.2.

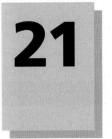

21 Chronic inflammatory disorders of the bowel

INTRODUCTION

The term **inflammatory bowel disease** is usually used to describe two chronic remittent bowel disorders, **ulcerative colitis** and **Crohn's disease**, which are described in the bulk of this chapter. These disorders share many pathophysiological and clinical features. Both conditions usually present with chronic diarrhoea, but recurrent bouts of abdominal pain are peculiar to Crohn's disease. Medical and surgical gastroenterologists working as a team help to obtain the best outcomes. Most patients can be managed on an outpatient basis but acute exacerbations or complications often necessitate hospital admission. Surgery is usually indicated when medical management has failed or when complications such as fulminant colitis, obstruction, haemorrhage or perforation occur.

Ulcerative colitis and Crohn's disease are relatively common in developed countries but they must be distinguished from **parasitic infestations** which also cause chronic inflammation of the large bowel. Infestations such as **amoebiasis** and **giardiasis** are common in developing countries and may be contracted by overseas travellers; they are described briefly at the end of the chapter. **Ischaemic colitis** is included here but **antibiotic-associated colitis** is covered in Chapter 47.

EPIDEMIOLOGY AND AETIOLOGY OF INFLAMMATORY BOWEL DISEASE

The aetiology of the inflammatory bowel diseases remains obscure despite extensive epidemiological, clinical and laboratory research. Ulcerative colitis and Crohn's disease are considered to be separate entities but a clear distinction cannot be made in 10–15% of cases; this is termed **indeterminate colitis**. The diseases may share some aetiological factors or even represent different facets of the same disease.

Despite problems of reliable diagnosis, epidemiological studies indicate that ulcerative colitis and Crohn's disease are relatively common in the developed communities of Western Europe, North America, Australasia and South Africa. The incidence appears to be much lower in Southern and Eastern Europe and Japan. The diseases are rare in most of Africa, Asia and South America. In the West, the incidence of Crohn's disease appears to have increased over the past 50 years, while ulcerative colitis has remained static or has even declined.

Most cases of inflammatory bowel disease develop in the late teens and twenties with little difference between males and females. Social class seems to be irrelevant as does urban versus rural living. In the USA, white people are three times more susceptible to ulcerative colitis than black people and five times more susceptible to Crohn's disease.

A wide variety of dietary factors, infective agents and immune responses have been proposed for the aetiology of inflammatory bowel diseases but none has been clearly implicated. There is a familial incidence, with 6–8% of patients with ulcerative colitis and about 20% of those with Crohn's disease having first-degree relatives with the same condition. There is a high concordance of Crohn's disease in monozygous twins, though this is not so for ulcerative colitis. One conclusion is that both conditions have a polygenetic hereditary predisposition, with the more complete genotype tending to Crohn's disease and the less complete to ulcerative colitis. A genetic link between the two diseases is supported by the association of both conditions with a range of non-gastrointestinal disorders of which the most common is **ankylosing spondylitis**. Pericholangitis, in contrast, occurs commonly in ulcerative colitis and occasionally progresses to **sclerosing cholangitis**, but is rare in Crohn's disease.

Infection is believed to play a part in initiating some cases of both ulcerative colitis and Crohn's disease as many cases follow an acute attack of gastroenteritis. One strain of *Escherichia coli* has been implicated in causing an acute colitis very similar to ulcerative colitis, and it seems likely that other organisms, as yet unidentified, may be found responsible for initiating these acute inflammatory disorders.

ULCERATIVE COLITIS

Ulcerative colitis is an inflammatory disorder of the mucosa and submucosa of the large bowel. It is characterised by recurrent acute exacerbations and intervening periods of quiescence or chronic low-grade activity. The severity of symptoms corresponds to the level of disease activity. Systemic features affect a small proportion of patients, and these include anaemia, inflammation of joints (**arthropathy**) and inflammation of the uveal tract of the eye (**uveitis and iritis**). The disease always involves the rectum but often extends proximally in continuity to involve a variable length of colon. In nearly 20% of cases (but only those with pancolitis), the distal end of the ileum is secondarily affected; this is described as **backwash ileitis**.

PATHOPHYSIOLOGY OF ULCERATIVE COLITIS

Initially, the colonic mucosa becomes acutely inflamed. Neutrophils accumulate in the lamina propria and within the tubular colonic glands to form small, highly characteristic **crypt abscesses**. This is followed by sloughing of the overlying mucosa to produce small superficial ulcers. If the inflammatory process persists, the ulcers coalesce into extensive areas of irregular ulceration. Residual islands of intact but oedematous mucosa project into the bowel lumen; these inflammatory lesions are called **pseudopolyps** (see Fig. 21.1). The inflammation is confined to the mucosa and submucosa, only extending into the muscular wall and peritoneal surface in **fulminating colitis**.

Acute inflammatory episodes range from several days' to several months' duration. After subsiding, they recur months or even years later. During quiescent periods, the acute inflammation resolves and the mucosa regenerates. The lamina propria, however, remains swollen by a chronic inflammatory infiltrate of lymphocytes and plasma cells. The colonic glands show a marked reduction in the number of mucin-secreting goblet cells, histologically termed '**goblet cell depletion**'.

After the disease has been present for some time, **dysplastic changes** appear in the epithelium. After prolonged or repeated episodes of inflammation, the epithelium becomes even more dysplastic, and may develop **adenocarcinoma**. In young patients with total colitis for 10 years, the risk of developing carcinoma is about 5–7%. A diagnosis of cancer may be delayed if symptoms are mistaken for a relapse of colitis and not investigated. Cancers in these patients are often particularly aggressive. In longstanding colitis, the mucosa and submucosa undergo fibrosis, resulting in loss of haustration and a shortened colon, the so-called **lead pipe colon** (see Fig. 21.2c, p. 294). This has a characteristic radiological appearance.

CLINICAL FEATURES OF ULCERATIVE COLITIS

Acute inflammatory attacks are marked by loose blood-stained stools streaked with mucus. Diarrhoea may be severe, with the patient suffering up to 20 loose stools per day, often preceded by cramping abdominal pain. In many patients, the urge to defaecate is so precipitate that incontinence ensues unless a lavatory is immediately available. Fear of incontinence keeps many patients at home and may profoundly limit social life and employment. This, rather than the frequency of defaecation, is the worst handicap in ulcerative colitis.

Any attack of ulcerative colitis may be **fulminant**, and the patient may become prostrated by dehydration, severe

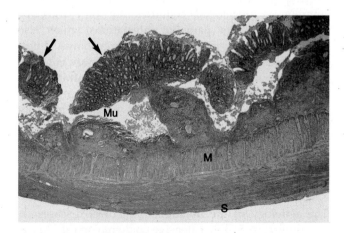

Fig. 21.1 Ulcerative colitis—histopathology
Erosion and undermining of the mucosa **Mu** by the inflammatory process has produced typical pseudopolyps (arrowed). Inflammation spares the muscle wall **M** and serosa **S**. Mucosal glands show reactive and regenerative changes.

electrolyte disturbance and blood loss. Occasionally, the colon dilates considerably and eventually patchy necrosis occurs. The patient is systemically ill with high fever, marked tachycardia and dehydration. This process, known as **toxic megacolon**, culminates in perforation and fatal peritonitis unless emergency colectomy is performed.

Ulcerative colitis is a systemic disorder sometimes accompanied by one or more non-gastrointestinal manifestations, summarised in Box 21.1. During active phases of the disease, the erythrocyte sedimentation rate (ESR) is elevated and moderate anaemia is common. The anaemia is normochromic and normocytic, described as 'anaemia of chronic disease'. A similar non-specific anaemia is found in other, chronic inflammatory disorders like rheumatoid disease. Both ulcerative colitis and Crohn's disease can cause an arthropathy of large joints similar to ankylosing spondylitis or rheumatoid arthritis; this occurs in up to 20% of patients. Serum tests for rheumatoid factor are negative, making this a **seronegative arthropathy**. Joint involvement can occur without active colitis and may even present before the colitis.

CLINICAL EXAMINATION AND INVESTIGATION OF SUSPECTED ULCERATIVE COLITIS

The typical patient referred for investigation of suspected ulcerative colitis is a young adult who gives a history of

---

SUMMARY

Box 21.1 Systemic manifestations of ulcerative colitis

Weight loss
● Frequent during exacerbations

Anaemia
● Typically chronic and non-specific (normochromic, normocytic)

Arthropathy
● Sacroileitis/ankylosing spondylitis or rheumatoid-like arthritis, especially of large joints (approximately 20% of cases)

Uveitis and iritis
● Painful red eye or eyes (approximately 10%)

Skin lesions
● Erythema nodosum, i.e. tender red nodules on the shins (uncommon), pyoderma gangrenosum, i.e. purulent skin ulcers (rare)

Sclerosing cholangitis
● Progressive fibrosis of intrahepatic biliary system leading to cirrhosis, progressive liver failure, jaundice and eventually death (rare)

---

several weeks of frequent loose stools, later streaked with blood and mucus. The attack often starts with an attack of gastroenteritis or traveller's diarrhoea which fails to settle. Careful questioning often elicits a story of similar previous attacks. There is sometimes a history of associated symptoms like arthropathy or uveitis.

General examination often reveals anaemia but abdominal examination is usually unremarkable. Rectal examination, followed by proctoscopy and sigmoidoscopy, is mandatory to palpate, inspect and, if necessary, biopsy the rectal mucosa. Other diseases of the rectum and anus such as carcinoma and benign solitary ulcer must be excluded. Ulcerative colitis always involves the rectum and extends proximally for a variable distance. Thus, diseased bowel is always accessible to sigmoidoscopic diagnosis. The diseased mucosa ranges in appearance from mildly hyperaemic and easily traumatised, to more severe involvement with extensive patchy ulceration. Biopsies should be taken from representative areas. Typically, blood-streaked loose faeces leak down into the lumen during examination.

At least three separate fresh stool samples should be microscoped and cultured to exclude bacterial or parasitic causes of diarrhoea as these conditions may closely simulate ulcerative colitis.

Contrast radiology

If the clinical picture and histological findings are consistent with inflammatory bowel disease, the extent and degree of colonic involvement can be assessed by barium enema examination. Radiological appearances are illustrated in Figure 21.2.

Colonoscopy

Colonoscopy, using flexible instruments up to 180 cm long, enables direct inspection of the entire colonic mucosa and the taking of multiple biopsies (see Fig. 21.3). It is a useful adjunct (or alternative) to radiological examination and permits excision or biopsy of polyps or other suspicious lesions (e.g. inflammatory pseudopolyps) to exclude malignancy. Furthermore, colonoscopy is used for periodic surveillance for dysplastic change in patients with longstanding total colitis, known to have an increased risk of developing carcinoma.

PROCTITIS

In ulcerative colitis, the mucosal abnormality usually extends beyond the reach of the sigmoidoscope. Some patients with colitic symptoms, however, have inflammation confined to the lower rectum. The mucosa often has a granular appearance and the condition is described as **proctitis** or **granular proctitis**. Its cause is unknown

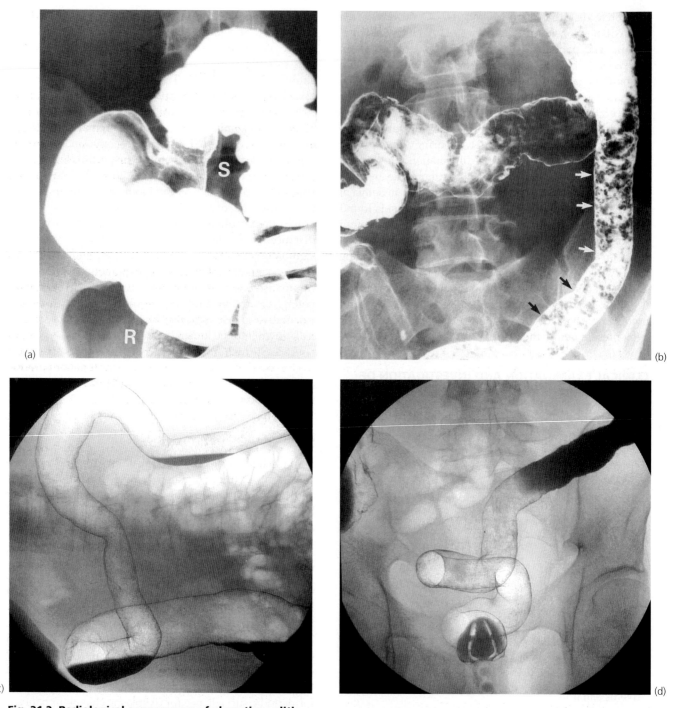

Fig. 21.2 Radiological appearances of ulcerative colitis

(a) This 35-year-old woman presented with a 3-month history of blood-streaked diarrhoea and passing mucus per rectum. Sigmoidoscopy showed marked superficial ulceration, and histology of biopsies confirmed ulcerative colitis. This barium enema shows extensive ulceration of the rectum **R** and lower sigmoid colon **S**, although this is a subtle sign. It is shown here only by fuzziness of the bowel wall caused by barium filling the mucosal ulcer craters. The rest of the colon was normal. Ulcerative colitis always affects the rectum and a variable amount of colon proximal to it, and always in continuity. **(b)** Severe and longstanding ulcerative colitis in a man of 50. The whole colon is affected (pancolitis) with loss of the normal haustral pattern. There is extensive pseudopolyp formation, particularly in the descending and sigmoid colon, manifest by multiple small filling defects (arrowed). Prolonged severe ulceration stimulates mitotic activity and is probably responsible for dysplastic changes and eventual malignant change in longstanding severe ulcerative colitis. **(c)** and **(d)** 'End-stage' or 'burnt-out' ulcerative colitis in a 49-year-old office worker. He had suffered episodic, but not incapacitating, diarrhoea for 34 years, but presented on this occasion because of urgency and incontinence. Sigmoidoscopy showed only moderate rectal ulceration. This barium enema shows a typical smooth, shortened 'lead pipe' colon, with complete loss of haustration. Note that **(c)** is orientated in the lateral decubitus position. He failed to respond to medical treatment and underwent proctocolectomy and ileostomy.

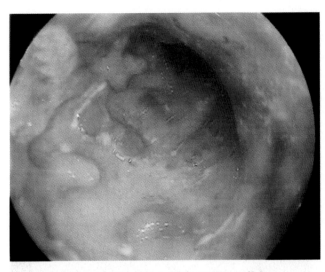

Fig. 21.3 Colonoscopic view of ulcerative colitis
This colon is quiescent, with no evidence of current ulceration but inflammatory polyps are seen as memorials to past severe inflammation and ulceration.

and its course self-limiting, though it tends to recur at times of stress, often at protracted intervals. Proctitis usually responds to short courses of local corticosteroid therapy but can occasionally progress into a distal or even a total colitis. Colonoscopy (or barium enema) is required if lesions higher up the colon such as carcinoma or Crohn's disease cannot be excluded on clinical grounds.

FULMINANT ULCERATIVE COLITIS

Fulminant attacks of ulcerative colitis sometimes occur, with extremely frequent watery, blood-stained stools and systemic illness. An attack may progress to toxic dilatation and eventual perforation. Urgent colectomy may be judged necessary to treat fulminant colitis which is resistant to medical therapy or toxic megacolon. Fulminant bloody diarrhoea with prostration may also occur in infective colitis, e.g. *Salmonella* colitis, cholera or amoebiasis, and these diagnoses should be excluded by microbiological examination of the stool.

Whatever the cause, patients with acute colitis require urgent hospital admission and resuscitation including fluid, electrolyte and blood replacement. Sigmoidoscopy and biopsy are performed to establish the diagnosis. Plain abdominal radiography is performed to monitor for dilatation which might indicate toxic megacolon (defined as colonic diameter greater than 6 cm). In the absence of megacolon, plain radiography may demonstrate other features of acute ulcerative colitis as shown in Figure 21.4. An urgent barium enema may be performed without bowel preparation ('**instant enema**') if the diagnosis is in doubt and there is no evidence of toxic dilatation on plain film. Colonoscopy is rarely

indicated in fulminant cases as it carries a risk of perforation.

MANAGEMENT OF ULCERATIVE COLITIS

The management of ulcerative colitis varies from patient to patient and from episode to episode. The choice of treatment depends on the severity of individual attacks, the amount of colon involved, the extent of chronic symptoms and the risk of long-term complications. The treatment options for ulcerative colitis are summarised in Box 21.2.

Corticosteroids

Mild to moderate attacks can usually be controlled with locally active rectal steroid preparations once or twice daily. These may be in the form of prednisolone enemas or hydrocortisone foam. Foam is more easily retained and appears just as effective as fluid enemas. Short courses of high-dose oral corticoids are used for more severe exacerbations (e.g. prednisolone 60 mg daily for 2 weeks, phased out over the next month). Intravenous administration is advisable in seriously ill patients. There is no evidence that 'bowel rest' (i.e. nil by mouth) and total parenteral nutrition (TPN) are of any value in ulcerative colitis. Immunosuppressive drugs, especially **azathioprine**, are occasionally tried in patients who fail to respond to corticosteroids.

SUMMARY

Box 21.2 Main treatment measures for ulcerative colitis

Local corticosteroid preparations (e.g. prednisolone suppositories and enemas, hydrocortisone foam)
● Employed in all cases of active disease

Systemic corticosteroids
● Suppress moderate or severe exacerbations (oral or intravenous administration according to severity of disease)

Oral (or sometimes rectal) aminosalicylate preparations, e.g. sulphasalazine, mesalazine or olsalazine
● Long-term maintenance therapy to minimise relapse

Oral antidiarrhoeal drugs, e.g. codeine phosphate, loperamide

Surgical removal of the colon
— emergency operation: incipient or actual perforation, serious haemorrhage, failure of fulminant colitis to improve on medical treatment
— elective operation: failure of medical treatment, risk of malignancy

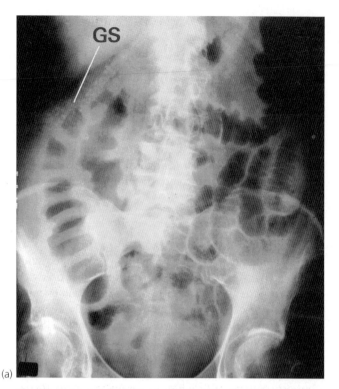

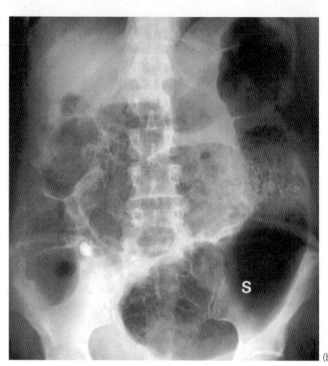

(a)

(b)

Fig. 21.4 Acute ulcerative colitis and toxic megacolon
(a) This 44-year-old woman presented with fulminant ulcerative colitis. She was prostrated by frequent diarrhoea and consequent electrolyte abnormalities. This plain supine radiograph shows acute right-sided colitis. The caecum, ascending colon and proximal transverse colon are affected. In this area, there is absence of the normal 'convex outward' pattern and there are thick folds crossing the bowel lumen. This appearance is caused by oedema of the bowel wall; note the incidental finding of gallstones **GS**. **(b)** This patient presented in a similar way but became toxic while in hospital undergoing intensive medical treatment. There was an increasing tachycardia, fever and abdominal tenderness. Serial plain abdominal radiographs showed an increasing diameter of the left colon. This film shows the sigmoid colon **S** dilated to 10 cm and in imminent danger of perforation. This is known as toxic dilatation of the colon; it occurs most commonly in ulcerative colitis and usually affects the transverse colon.

Aminosalicylate preparations

Oral 5 aminosalicylic acid (5-ASA) preparations have long been employed as maintenance therapy in mild to moderate ulcerative colitis to prevent relapse; they substantially reduce the severity and frequency of attacks. A range of 5-ASA preparations is now available including the original drug, sulphasalazine, which is a combination of a sulphonamide and aminosalicylic acid that dissociates in the large bowel to release the therapeutic agent 5-ASA. Other drugs in this group include mesalazine and olsalazine. The drugs are usually well tolerated but may cause lupoid skin rashes or rarely, serious blood dyscrasias.

Other supportive measures

Anti-diarrhoeal agents such as codeine phosphate or loperamide and bulking agents like methylcellulose may help to reduce stool frequency.

Patients with moderately severe chronic disease frequently become anaemic and lose weight, in part because of persistent loss of protein in the stool. These problems may be helped by medical treatment, a diet high in calories and protein, and oral iron supplements.

Surgery for ulcerative colitis

Surgery is required only in about 20% of patients with ulcerative colitis. Colectomy may be needed in the following:

- Fulminant cases which fail to respond to intensive medical treatment
- Acute cases which progress to toxic megacolon, perforation or haemorrhage
- Patients with chronic disabling symptoms of intractable diarrhoea with urgency, recurring anaemia and failure to maintain adequate weight and nutrition
- Children with failure to thrive and retardation of growth (both are exacerbated by corticosteroid therapy)
- Patients with longstanding persistent total colitis, to prevent malignant change particularly if colitis started in childhood. Biopsy evidence of dysplasia strengthens the case for surgical treatment

As a general principle, surgery for ulcerative colitis requires removal of the entire large bowel and is curative. There are two surgical options:

- **Proctocolectomy** which leaves the patient with a permanent ileostomy after the anal sphincters have been removed. This is psychologically distressing, especially for a young person
- **Sphincter-preserving operations** which avoid a permanent ileostomy. In these operations, the rectal stump remaining after total colectomy is excised and a neo-rectum or **ileo-anal pouch** is fashioned from

two or more loops of terminal ileum. This was originally described by Parks. The outlet of the reservoir is brought down through the pelvis and anastomosed to the upper anal canal. Many patients have excellent continence and can evacuate the bowels in the normal way. In a sick patient, or one on high-dose corticosteroids, a total colectomy and ileostomy is often undertaken initially. The patient can then recover from the acute illness and stop steroid treatment before a second operation for completion proctectomy and ileo-anal pouch formation

CROHN'S DISEASE

Crohn's disease is a chronic relapsing inflammatory disorder of the gastrointestinal tract which predominantly affects younger people. About 60% of patients are under 25 years at the time of initial diagnosis, and on average, symptoms will by then have been present intermittently for 5 years. It potentially affects any part of the tract from mouth to anus. The small bowel alone is affected in 50% of patients, the large bowel alone in 20% and both together in 30%. In contrast to ulcerative colitis, the inflammation involves the whole thickness of the bowel wall (**transmural inflammation**). The disease often affects one or more discrete segments of the bowel with intervening parts of the bowel being completely spared (discontinuous disease). The affected areas are known as 'skip lesions' (see Fig. 21.9, p. 303).

The terminal ileum is affected most commonly and in up to half of all cases, the disease is confined to the terminal ileum. When Dr Crohn first described the condition in 1932, he thought it only affected the terminal ileum, hence the original name 'terminal ileitis'. Later, it became clear that other segments of the bowel could also be affected. The name was thus changed to **regional enteritis**, a term still widely employed in the USA. As mentioned above, the large bowel is affected in at least 30% of cases, either alone or in association with disease elsewhere in the gastrointestinal tract. Crohn's disease may also affect the perianal region, whether or not the large bowel is involved. Occasionally, the disease involves the stomach, duodenum, oesophagus or mouth. With each exacerbation, previously affected or new areas may become involved. The disease tends to run a protracted and unpredictable course.

PATHOPHYSIOLOGY AND CLINICAL CONSEQUENCES OF CROHN'S DISEASE

The essential pathological feature of Crohn's disease is chronic inflammation of one or more discrete segments

of bowel with the inflammation extending diffusely through the entire thickness of the bowel wall. The wall becomes markedly thickened by inflammatory oedema, especially in the submucosa. The epithelium remains largely intact but is criss-crossed by deep **fissured ulcers**. These ulcers, and the intervening areas of dome-shaped mucosa and submucosa, give a typical 'cobblestone' surface appearance.

Granulomas containing multinucleate giant cells (see Fig. 21.5) are usually scattered throughout the inflamed bowel wall as well as in local lymph nodes. Although granulomas are diagnostic of Crohn's disease, they are not always found. Longstanding inflammation leads to progressive **fibrosis** of the thickened bowel wall, which encroaches on the lumen, producing **elongated strictures**.

Effects of mucosal inflammation

Mucosal inflammation causes diarrhoea which, if the colon is involved, may be streaked with mucus and blood. Luminal narrowing results in partial obstruction which causes grumbling, colicky abdominal pain. There may also be acute episodes of more severe pain and vomiting which precipitate hospital admission. Pain is a prominent feature in Crohn's disease in contrast to ulcerative colitis.

If the small bowel is inflamed, diarrhoea occurs and digestive and absorptive functions may be adversely affected. Extensive disease results in general malabsorption causing protein-calorie malnutrition, iron and folate deficiency, and anaemia. In children, Crohn's disease may cause marked growth retardation. Ileal inflammation disrupts bile salt reabsorption. Excess bile salts in the faeces cause colonic irritation (and more diarrhoea) while diminished recirculation of bile salts may result in gallstone formation. Involvement of the terminal ileum may also reduce vitamin B_{12} absorption but serious deficiency usually occurs only after surgical resection.

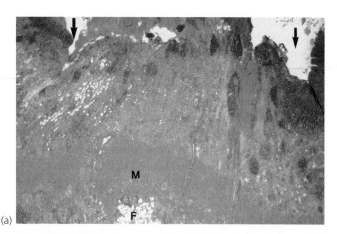

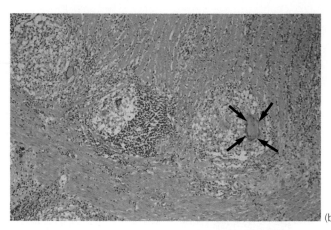

(a)

(b)

Fig. 21.5 Crohn's disease affecting the colon—histopathology
(a) Inflammation has produced fissure ulcers (arrowed) which extend into the muscle wall **M**. Lymphoid aggregates are also present and the inflammatory process extends into serosal fat **F**. **(b)** High-power view showing well-formed granulomas with typical giant cells (arrowed), enabling a confident diagnosis of Crohn's disease to be made.

Effects of transmural inflammation

Crohn's disease causes additional problems if serosal inflammation extends to adjacent structures. If inflamed bowel impinges on the parietal peritoneum, pain becomes localised and more severe, and signs of local peritonitis develop. Indeed, Crohn's disease of the terminal ileum may mimic acute appendicitis. At laparotomy, the terminal ileum is seen to be inflamed and the bowel wall abnormally thick to palpation. In this case, the terminal ileum should not be excised; a firm diagnosis of Crohn's disease can be made if other 'skip lesions' are found in the small bowel, if typical histological changes are found in excised mesenteric lymph nodes or if small bowel barium studies performed later show characteristic lesions. *Yersinia ileitis* (see Ch. 19, p. 273) has a similar clinical presentation but the disease is acute, completely reversible and confined to the terminal ileum.

Fulminant colonic Crohn's disease occasionally causes toxic dilatation which is clinically identical to ulcerative colitis, but this presentation is rare.

Serosal inflammation may cause a segment of diseased bowel to adhere to nearby abdominal structures. Several complications may occur if these become matted together by the inflammatory process:

- **Adhesions**. These tough, fibrotic post-inflammatory adhesions are rarely symptomatic, but constitute a formidable obstacle if operation is needed later
- **Perforation**. Free perforation is rare but a contained perforation may occur which causes localised pericolic or pelvic abscess formation
- **Fistulae**. These may develop between diseased bowel and other hollow viscera causing unusual clinical phenomena. For example, a gastrocolic fistula may result in faecal vomiting; an ileorectal fistula may aggravate diarrhoea. Entero-vesical fistulae cause

severe urinary tract infections and pneumaturia (passage of 'soda-water' urine), and fistulae between bowel and uterus or vagina lead to vaginal passage of faeces. Entero-cutaneous fistulae between bowel and skin occasionally develop as a complication of bowel resection for Crohn's disease

Perianal inflammation

Perianal inflammation is common in Crohn's disease. Symptoms include recurrent perianal abscesses, characteristic blueish, boggy 'piles' (see Fig. 21.6) and antero-lateral anal fissures. The last two are quite distinct from ordinary haemorrhoids and posterior anal fissures. Multiple fistulae commonly develop between rectum and perianal skin. These are sometimes so numerous as to cause a 'pepper-pot' or 'watering-can' perineum (see Fig. 21.7). Paradoxically, this is more often associated with small bowel disease than colorectal disease.

Systemic features

Like ulcerative colitis, Crohn's disease is a systemic disorder and has a similar range of non-gastrointestinal manifestations (see Box 21.1, p. 293). It is common for patients to feel generally ill during an acute attack, in contrast to ulcerative colitis. Specific systemic features affecting skin, joints or the eye are relatively uncommon and not necessarily related to intestinal disease activity.

SYMPTOMS AND SIGNS IN CROHN'S DISEASE

Symptoms of Crohn's disease can be similar to those of ulcerative colitis, particularly when the large bowel is involved (see Table 21.1, p. 302). Diarrhoea is usually less distressing and less likely to contain blood. Other

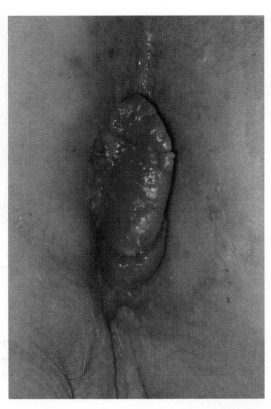

Fig. 21.6 Crohn's 'piles'
This appearance is typical of Crohn's 'piles'. They are pale and
oedematous in contrast to ordinary haemorrhoids.

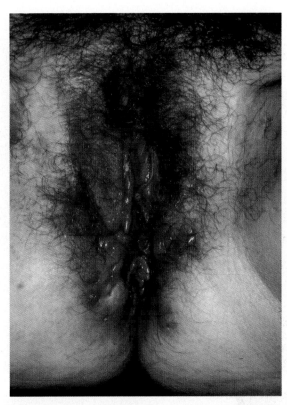

Fig. 21.7 Multiple anal fistulae in Crohn's disease
This 30-year-old woman had several 'skip lesions' of Crohn's disease in
her small bowel and was troubled by recurrent perianal sepsis. This
photograph shows a typical 'pepper-pot perineum', with several
fistulous openings (arrowed) seen around the circumference of the
anus. Anal skin tags are also visible.

characteristic symptoms of Crohn's disease include cramp-
like abdominal pain, weight loss and general malaise.

Physical examination may reveal generalised wasting
and anaemia and sometimes other features like arthropathy. On abdominal examination, there may be areas
of tenderness, an inflammatory mass or the scars of previous surgery. The perianal skin should be examined for
fissures, fistulae, Crohn's 'piles' or stenotic scarring from
previous disease. Diseased rectal mucosa, with its typical
firm surface nodularity, may be felt on digital examination.
Sigmoidoscopic examination is usually normal but there
may be mucosal oedema if the rectum is involved. In
more severe cases, the typical 'cobblestone' appearance
with fissured ulceration may be seen. Biopsies may be
positive even when the mucosa is apparently normal.

APPROACH TO INVESTIGATION OF SUSPECTED CROHN'S DISEASE

Investigation of suspected Crohn's disease is similar to
that for ulcerative colitis in respect of the large bowel,
but follows a different pattern when there is suspected
small bowel disease.

Isotope scanning using radioactive indium-labelled
white blood cells is useful as an initial assessment of the
extent of disease and indicates which parts of the bowel
to examine radiologically. Abnormalities on barium
enema may be difficult or impossible to distinguish from
ulcerative colitis. The definitive diagnosis in these patients
may depend on histological examination of a surgical
specimen or a clinical course characteristic of Crohn's
disease.

Barium 'follow-through' is the traditional method of
examining the small bowel but is being supplanted by
'small bowel enema'; the latter, despite its name, is
performed via the oral route, and involves the controlled
instillation of barium into the duodenum through a
nasogastric tube. Typical radiological appearances of
Crohn's disease include narrowing of the lumen due to
mural oedema and fibrosis, nodularity and cobblestoning
of the mucosal surface, deep fissured ulceration extending
into the muscular wall, spiky 'rose thorn' ulcers and
possibly evidence of fistula formation. Radiological
changes in small and large bowel are shown in Figure
21.8. Colonoscopy may enable a histological diagnosis to
be obtained in colonic disease.

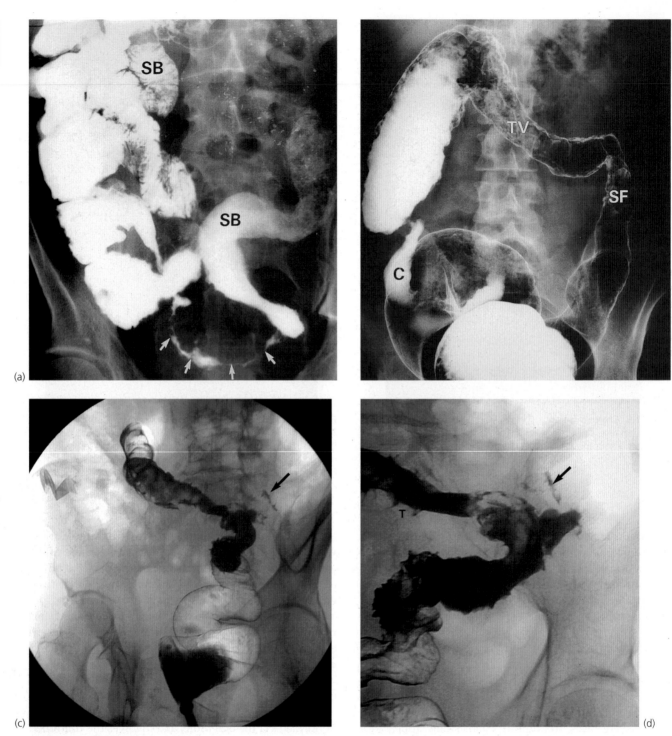

Fig. 21.8 Radiological appearances in Crohn's disease

(a) This man of 51 had recurrent attacks of colicky abdominal pain, with diarrhoea and loss of weight. This barium follow-through examination shows one of the characteristic radiological appearances of Crohn's disease. The terminal ileum is extremely narrowed by inflammation of the whole wall thickness (arrowed); this is known as the 'string sign of Kantor' and causes the symptoms and signs of partial obstruction. This film also shows dilatation of small bowel **SB** proximal to the stricture. **(b)** This man of 48 presented with 8 months of diarrhoea and feeling generally unwell. The barium enema shows Crohn's disease of the caecum **C**, transverse colon **TV** and splenic flexure **SF**. The descending colon and sigmoid are normal. Here, the features of Crohn's disease are discontinuous skip lesions with normal bowel between, a ragged luminal outline due to ulceration, and loss of haustration. **(c)** Double contrast barium enema in a 28-year-old woman who complained of 8 months' history of recurrent abdominal pains and diarrhoea. She had not lost weight. This film shows a 'ragged' segment in the sigmoid colon with narrowing and 'rose thorn' ulcers **T**, better seen in the close up view in **(d)**. In both views, contrast is visible outside the colon (arrowed). In fact, this is in small bowel because of a fistula between colon and small bowel.

MANAGEMENT OF CROHN'S DISEASE

Drug therapy is the mainstay of treatment for Crohn's disease but surgery is usually required in patients with chronic obstructive symptoms. Medical treatment employs a similar range of drugs to that used for ulcerative colitis, including oral prednisolone and aminosalicylate preparations (5-ASA); sometimes the antimetabolite azathioprine is used as a steroid-sparing agent in extensive small bowel granulomatous disease. High-dose oral corticosteroids (30–60 mg daily for 2–3 weeks) are used to induce remission in acute attacks of Crohn's disease. New-generation steroids such as budesonide are destroyed in the first pass through the liver and in principle, deliver topical anti-inflammatory effects to the small bowel without the adverse systemic effects. Such treatment is useful in mild to moderate Crohn's, as are the 5-ASA preparations, e.g. sulphasalazine. Any of these drug treatments can be effective for acute attacks but maintenance therapy conveys no additional benefits.

Topical steroid enemas and foams are of some benefit in acute distal colonic disease but have little value in perianal disease. In the latter case, secondary bacterial infection is probably responsible for much of the pain and purulent discharge. Treatment with oral metronidazole for 1–2 months often helps to alleviate symptoms.

Anti-diarrhoeal drugs and bulk-forming agents may help to control fluid stools and urgency. Supportive treatment is often required for complications such as anaemia and malnutrition.

Dietary modification has become an established treatment for the long-term management of Crohn's disease to prevent acute exacerbations without risking the side effects of drug treatment and reducing the need for surgery. There is some evidence that intolerance to certain foods plays a part in provoking acute attacks, and acute attacks can often be settled by restricting intake to elemental diets. Later, certain food groups can be reintroduced one at a time to determine whether any particular group exacerbates the inflammatory process. Some patients can be maintained on a limited diet for years without recourse to medication or surgery. However, in a disease with relapses and remissions like Crohn's disease, proof of benefit can be hard to obtain.

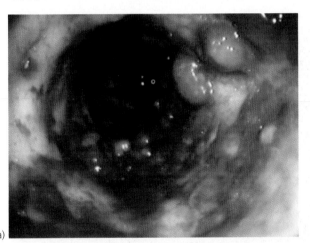

(a)

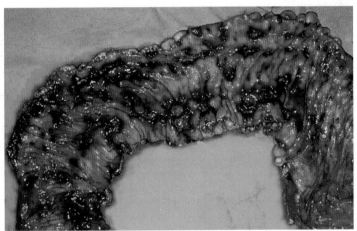

(b)

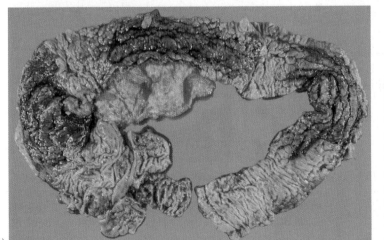

(c)

Fig. 21.9 Appearances of Crohn's colitis
(a) This is a typical colonoscopic view of florid Crohn's colitis. Note the nodular appearance producing a 'cobblestone' surface with linear ulcers between the nodule, seen more clearly in **(b)**. **(b)** Specimen of Crohn's colon from another patient with similar symptoms. Here 'aphthous type' ulcers are clearly visible. **(c)** This subtotal colectomy specimen was removed from a man of 54 with a long history of weight loss, diarrhoea and abdominal pain. There are three 'skip lesions' typical of Crohn's disease, in the ascending colon, the transverse colon and the hepatic flexure showing thickening of the wall, cobblestone mucosal surface and narrowing of the lumen.

Table 21.1 Comparative features of ulcerative colitis and Crohn's disease

	Ulcerative colitis	Crohn's disease
Pathology		
Inflammation	Recurrent acute inflammation with intervening quiescent phases	Chronic relapsing inflammation
General distribution	Continuous involvement of affected part of colon	Skip lesions in any part of gastrointestinal tract
Rectal involvement	Always	About 25%
Ileal involvement	Backwash ileitis only	Involved in 80% of cases; exclusive to ileum in 50% of cases
Depth of wall involved	Mucosa only	Transmural, including serosa
Mucosal changes	Widespread irregular superficial ulceration with or without pseudopolyps	Fissured ulceration causing 'cobblestone' appearance
Granuloma formation	Absent	Characteristic but not always present
Mesenteric adenopathy	Reactive hyperplasia only	Lymph nodes often enlarged; granulomas may be present
Fibrosis of wall	Minimal	Marked
Main clinical features		
Diarrhoea	Severe during acute attacks, often causing incontinence	Less prominent
Rectal bleeding	Very common	Less common
Abdominal pain	Mild cramping 'pre-defaecation' pain with diarrhoeal attacks	Dominant feature—persistent or grumbling pain with severe acute attacks
Abdominal mass	No	Relatively common
General debility	Unusual	Characteristic
Complications		
Strictures	Rare	Common and often multiple
Fistulae	Rare	Common
Anal and perianal lesions	Uncommon	Common
Massive haemorrhage	Occurs in fulminant disease	Rare
Intestinal obstruction	Rare	Incomplete obstruction is common
Perforation	Complication of toxic megacolon	Free perforation rare but perforation causing local abscess formation or internal fistula common
Toxic megacolon	May occur in fulminant attacks	Rare
Malignant change	High risk with severe/longstanding disease	Low risk
Management		
Local steroids	All active disease	Less effective
Systemic steroids	Severe exacerbations	Severe exacerbations
Aminosalicylates (5-ASA)	Long-term maintenance	Less effective
Immunosuppressives	Occasionally in intractable cases—'steroid sparing'	Rarely effective
Surgery	Uncommon—usually in longstanding disease to prevent malignancy or in fulminant colitis	Commonly required

THE ROLE OF SURGERY IN CROHN'S DISEASE

Surgery plays a larger part in Crohn's disease than ulcerative colitis but no matter how much bowel is removed or subjected to stricturoplasty, it does not influence subsequent recurrence elsewhere.

The main indications for surgery may be summarised as follows:

● Acute exacerbations unresponsive to steroids
● Acute complications, e.g. abscess, perforation, major haemorrhage
● Persistent local ileal disease
● Intolerable long-term obstructive and other symptoms, e.g. abdominal pain, perianal disease, general ill-health
● Entero-cutaneous fistulae and symptomatic internal fistulae

The choice of operation depends on the site and extent of disease. The former belief that all disease must be resected has been abandoned. Surgery for multiple small bowel strictures now involves multiple **stricturoplasties**, a technique of enlarging the lumen of diseased bowel without losing potential absorptive length. If the disease is limited, resection of the diseased segment with a small margin of normal tissue may be performed, followed by end-to-end anastomosis. About 50% of patients with terminal ileal disease develop further lesions elsewhere after initial resection. If ileal Crohn's disease is found incidentally at appendicectomy, the affected segment is best left alone. For large bowel disease, the entire colon is generally removed (pan-proctocolectomy with ileostomy).

This is because there are usually several colonic 'skip lesions' and recurrence is likely. A blind rectal stump may be left in situ if unaffected by disease in order to reduce the extent of the operation. Pouch procedures are not recommended because of the risk of recurrent disease in the small bowel.

Recurrent disease often necessitates further surgery. Abscesses are usually treated by simple drainage with resection of the affected bowel at the same time or later. Fistulae between abdominal viscera are treated by removal of the diseased bowel. In contrast, entero-cutaneous fistulae, usually a complication of recent surgery, are a more formidable problem since they are often associated with complicating factors like intra-abdominal sepsis, gross fluid and electrolyte abnormalities, and a hyper-catabolic state. Patients with entero-cutaneous fistulae require intensive medical care and strategic surgical intervention before definitive treatment of the fistula is possible.

Intestinal bypass operations leaving inflamed segments of bowel in situ were popular at one time for Crohn's disease. The rationale was that diseased bowel would heal once 'rested'. The results and complications, including blind loop syndromes, were much worse than for resection and the technique has been abandoned in favour of resection or stricturoplasty.

A comparison of ulcerative colitis and Crohn's disease is shown in Table 21.1.

OTHER CHRONIC INFLAMMATIONS OF THE COLON

AMOEBIC COLITIS

Entamoeba histolytica is a protozoon parasite responsible for amoebic colitis. It is an endemic bowel commensal in many developing countries but is also found in a few people in developed countries. Most of those infected have no symptoms but they are all carriers. Less than 5% of those infected suffer amoebic colitis. In these, the organism invades the large bowel mucosa, causing chronic relapsing symptoms similar to ulcerative colitis or Crohn's disease. Encysted parasites are shed by carriers in their faeces and infection is readily transmitted to new individuals via contaminated hands or uncooked food.

The incidence of amoebiasis is likely to increase in the West as tourism expands into endemic areas. If sufferers are mistakenly treated with systemic steroids for inflammatory bowel disease, the result may be fatal.

PATHOLOGY OF AMOEBIC COLITIS

Initial penetration of bowel mucosa by the parasite causes small surface erosions. Lateral spread from the depths of the crypts produces **flask-shaped mucosal ulcers**. These are multiple and discrete, and are characteristic of amoebic colitis. Amoebae can often be seen near the edge of ulcers on standard histological preparations, but can best be demonstrated when stained magenta by the periodic acid-Schiff method. The mucosa between the ulcers is remarkably normal. Large granulomatous colonic lesions also occur. These are known as **amoebomas**.

Occasionally, rampant invasion causes widespread mucosal sloughing and muscle wall involvement. This progresses to local perforation and a pericolic abscess or toxic megacolon leading to massive perforation and generalised peritonitis.

In any case of amoebic colitis, amoebae passing to the liver in the portal veins may occasionally produce **hepatic abscesses**. These are usually solitary and are filled with reddish-brown necrotic material, said to resemble anchovy sauce.

CLINICAL FEATURES OF AMOEBIC COLITIS

The disease usually affects the proximal colon, causing colicky abdominal pain, erratic bowel habit with episodes of blood-stained loose stools, and right iliac fossa tenderness. If the distal colon is involved, the patient suffers chronic watery diarrhoea with blood and mucus. When the entire colon is involved there is generalised abdominal tenderness as well as systemic features, e.g. pyrexia and progressive weight loss. A large **amoeboma** may be palpable and must be differentiated from carcinoma or diverticular disease.

If the patient develops an amoebic liver abscess, systemic features become more marked, with general ill-health and a swinging pyrexia with sweating attacks. There is pain in the liver area and an enlarged tender liver on palpation. The abscess may rupture spontaneously into the peritoneal cavity (causing peritonitis) or through the diaphragm into the chest. Secondary lung abscesses may then rupture into the bronchi and the patient coughs up 'anchovy sauce' sputum.

DIAGNOSIS OF AMOEBIASIS

In developed countries, amoebic colitis should always be considered in the differential diagnosis of ulcerative colitis or Crohn's colitis.

Amoebic colitis can be diagnosed on histology of biopsy specimens. Alternatively, parasites containing ingested red cells can be sought in fresh stool specimens or scrapings from bowel lesions; this is diagnostic of invasive amoebiasis. Contrast radiology does not differentiate amoebic colitis from other forms of colitis.

Liver abscesses cause serological tests for amoebiasis to become positive. The lesions are readily demonstrated by hepatic ultrasound and the diagnosis is confirmed by needle aspiration.

TREATMENT OF AMOEBIASIS

Metronidazole is the drug treatment of choice, given orally (400 mg three times daily) or parenterally if the disease is severe. When small liver abscesses are present, the dose is doubled and this may eliminate them without need for surgery. Emergency surgery is occasionally necessary in fulminating amoebic colitis or less urgently for large liver abscesses.

GIARDIASIS

Giardiasis is caused by the flagellate protozoal parasite *Giardia lamblia* and is an infection of small bowel. It is included here for convenience. Giardiasis is endemic in many developing countries as well as in Russia and other Eastern European countries. The organism thrives when sanitation is poor and water supplies are contaminated. Sporadic outbreaks of giardiasis sometimes occur in developed countries but it is most often seen in young travellers returning from long holidays abroad. In Australia, native animals are a reservoir for *Giardia*, resulting in contamination of water courses, leading to human infections after 'bush' camping holidays. In a typical attack, explosive foul-smelling diarrhoea continues for several days or a few weeks, eventually settling spontaneously. Less commonly, the disease may take a protracted course, with chronic diarrhoea, pain and abdominal distension. There may also be anorexia, nausea and weight loss.

Diagnosis is made on stool microscopy; at least three samples from different days should be examined to ensure that the parasite is not missed. The disease responds rapidly to oral **metronidazole** although other antiparasitic drugs may be preferred.

ISCHAEMIC COLITIS

Ischaemic colitis is a condition of the elderly which usually presents with rectal bleeding. The history is characteristic; there is a bout of cramp-like abdominal pain lasting a few hours, followed by an attack of rectal bleeding. Usually the bleeding is dark red, often without faeces, and occurs one to three times over about 12 hours. The episode then ceases spontaneously. The differential diagnosis includes acute bleeding from diverticular disease. The cause is transient ischaemia of a segment of large bowel, the splenic flexure being most vulnerable. Further attacks occasionally occur but most patients have no further trouble. Investigation by barium enema in the acute stage may reveal colonic oedema in the affected segment (see Fig. 21.10). A rare late complication is fibrotic stricturing of the area originally affected by ischaemia.

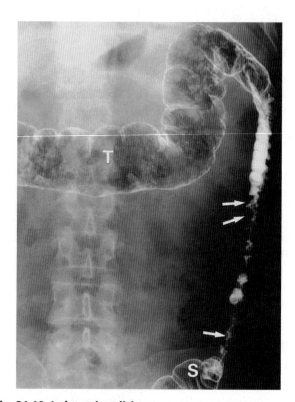

Fig. 21.10 Ischaemic colitis
This 72-year-old man presented with a bout of severe abdominal pain 48 hours before this barium enema was performed. Soon after the pain, there was a single episode of fresh rectal bleeding. This film shows typical (though extensive) changes of acute ischaemic colitis, which characteristically involved the proximal descending colon. The transverse colon **T** and sigmoid colon **S** are normal. Note the extremely narrowed lumen of the ischaemic segment and the characteristic thumb-printing (arrowed) caused by mucosal oedema.

22 | Disorders of large bowel dynamics

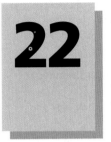

INTRODUCTION

Irritable bowel syndrome, **chronic constipation** and **diverticular disease** all arise from disordered peristaltic function and are largely attributable to a modern highly refined diet. These conditions could be regarded as endemic in developed societies. They make considerable demands on the time of family practitioners, physicians and surgeons, yet they are largely preventable. A hundred years ago, they were largely unknown in the West (apart from the obsession with constipation), as they still are in many rural communities in developing countries.

Apart from symptoms needing treatment, the main surgical importance of these conditions is that they must be distinguished from large bowel cancer.

The large bowel conditions mentioned above have several symptoms in common:

● Intermittent attacks of abdominal pain
● Erratic bowel habit
● Abdominal bloating and passage of excessive flatus

Sigmoid volvulus is an acute condition resulting from massive chronic dilatation of the sigmoid colon and consequent twisting of the sigmoid loop on a narrow mesentery. In Western countries, it is seen mainly in the elderly and patients with learning difficulties or mental illness. In developing countries, it is common in areas of very high fibre intake.

MODERN DIET AND DISEASE

EPIDEMIOLOGICAL OBSERVATIONS

Little scientific attention was paid to diet-related disease until the 1970s although Gaylord Hauser had written on the subject in the 1930s. In the 1970s, the ideas of Surgeon Captain T. L. Cleeve, a Royal Navy physician, and later the remarkable epidemiological observations of Denis Burkitt, a long-time missionary surgeon in Africa, began to be published. Now the subject of diet is not only respectable in surgical circles but has made enormous contributions to the understanding and management of many common diseases. Diseases such as irritable bowel syndrome, diverticular disease, appendicitis and colorectal cancer, which are common in Western society, are largely unknown in the developing world and this difference is almost certainly related to diet. Thus, it follows that a dietary history is important in evaluating patients with these conditions, and dietary change is often a fundamental part of their management.

Over millions of years as 'hunter-gatherers', humans subsisted on a staple diet of vegetables and fruits, grains, legumes and nuts, supplemented by small quantities of meat and fish. The human gastrointestinal and metabolic systems are thus perfectly adapted to that diet. During the brief period of the last 100 years, the average Western diet has changed dramatically, largely due to affluence, fashion, convenience and food processing. Since the 1980s there have been similar trends in the more prosperous parts of developing countries, particularly in the cities. The modern diet compared with the hunter-gatherer diet contains many more calories. These are largely in the form of refined carbohydrates and fats, especially saturated animal fats. Equally important, the modern diet contains far less unabsorbable fibre residue.

MECHANISMS OF DISEASE CAUSED BY MODERN DIET

While the increase in calories and nutrients has brought many benefits, just as many problems have arisen. The modern diet has had an adverse effect on both bowel function and metabolism, particularly of lipids, and this has led to a multiplicity of disorders. The ways in which modern diet may induce disease and dysfunction are outlined in Box 22.1. In relation to diseases of the bowel, the most important factors are faecal volume and consistency and gastrointestinal transit time. The average Western adult passes between 80 and 120 g of firm stool each day with a transit time of about 3 days. Transit time can be as long as 2 weeks in the elderly. In contrast, rural dwellers in the developing world, with a diet similar to that of the hunter-gatherer, pass between 300 and 800 g of much softer stool each day with an average transit time of less than a day and a half.

INCREASING DIETARY FIBRE CONTENT

An essential part of managing many bowel conditions and preventing others is a substantial increase in daily dietary fibre intake. Box 22.2 lists the readily available foods with a high fibre content which can be eaten regularly with little effort or extra expense. Increasing the fibre content of the normal diet almost inevitably leads to reduced consumption of refined carbohydrates and saturated animal fats and lower total energy intake. Patients should be advised to introduce dietary fibre gradually as a sudden increase is likely to cause abdominal discomfort and distension and increased production of flatus. Bulking agents (**ispaghula husk** preparations) can be taken in the early stages to achieve a rapid result while avoiding these unpleasant side effects.

IRRITABLE BOWEL SYNDROME

Irritable bowel syndrome (IBS) has only been accepted in recent years as a pathological entity although the symptom complex has been described in the past under other names such as '**spastic colon**'. The condition is very common, particularly in young and middle-aged women.

CLINICAL FEATURES OF IRRITABLE BOWEL SYNDROME

The patient typically complains of episodic 'cramping' abdominal pain occurring at any time of day and lasting from about 15 minutes to several hours. The pain is un-related to meals or other provoking factors. It may occur anywhere in the abdomen but tends to occur peripherally, i.e. in either iliac fossa or the epigastrium, and usually recurs in the same general area in any one patient.

Symptoms occur daily for weeks at a time and then resolve for weeks or months, only to return later. The patient may recognise that symptoms are worse at times of stress and are absent during weekends and holidays. The pain may provoke an urge to open the bowels and

---

KEY POINTS

Box 22.1 Mechanisms by which refined diet may cause disease

Slowed gastrointestinal transit time
- Increases duration of contact between stool and bowel mucosa; this increases duration of contact of carcinogens, predisposing to colorectal cancer

Increased intra-abdominal pressure due to straining at stool
- Obstructs venous return making haemorrhoids and varicose veins more likely
- Predisposes to hiatus hernia, inguinal hernia and rectal prolapse

Reduced bulk and more solid consistency of faeces
- Make peristalsis less effective and constipation more likely
- Increase intraluminal pressure predisposing to diverticular disease
- Hard stool increases friction, causing anal fissure and perhaps haemorrhoids
- Small stool bulk increases concentration of carcinogens
- May contribute to pathogenesis of appendicitis by obstructing appendiceal orifice

Decreased loss of bile salts in the faeces
- Increased bile salt pool predisposes to gallstone formation
- Increased bile salts in lumen may result in formation of carcinogens

Changes in bacterial flora of the bowel
- May result in formation of carcinogens
- May be implicated in appendicitis

Increased refined carbohydrate intake
- Predisposes to diabetes
- Contributes to excess calorie intake causing obesity

Increased dietary fat intake, particularly saturated animal fats
- Predisposes to atherosclerosis
- Predisposes to gallstone formation
- Contributes to excess calorie intake and obesity

Increased absorption of dietary fat because of reduced binding by fibre
- Increases fat absorption and blood lipid levels

Obesity
- Weakens abdominal wall muscles predisposing to hiatus hernia, abdominal wall hernias and vaginal prolapse
- Predisposes to thromboembolism
- Contributes to musculoskeletal and joint disorders

Box 22.2 Foods with a high fibre content

- Whole-grain and bran-enriched breakfast cereals, e.g. muesli, All-Bran, Weetabix (not cornflakes, puffed rice, etc.)
- Wholemeal bread (not white or 'brown')
- Other wholewheat products, e.g. wholewheat pasta, wholemeal pastry, digestive biscuits
- Other whole grains, e.g. brown rice, cracked wheat
- Pulses of any kind, e.g. haricot beans (including canned baked beans), kidney beans, chick peas, other dried beans and lentils
- Potatoes (skins should be left on)
- Unpeeled fruit and vegetables (actually low in fibre compared with grains and pulses)

evacuation may bring some relief from the pain. An erratic bowel habit is a characteristic feature of irritable bowel syndrome. Passage of loose stools alternates with constipation, with small hard stools described as looking like rabbit pellets. Patients may also complain of abdominal distension and excess flatus.

PATHOPHYSIOLOGY AND AETIOLOGY OF IRRITABLE BOWEL SYNDROME

The pathophysiology of irritable bowel syndrome is poorly understood but a low-fibre diet seems to play a major part. Colonic motility studies in these patients show abnormal rises in intraluminal pressure and disordered peristalsis resulting in segmenting, non-propulsive contractions. The small volume of faeces (because of little residual fibre) thus becomes excessively dehydrated and fragmented. Food intolerance (wrongly called food allergy) has been found to play a part in a proportion of patients with irritable bowel syndrome. The three common culprits are dairy products, gluten and wheat, and exclusion of these items can produce dramatic improvements. Some patients with irritable bowel syndrome appear to be hypersensitive to gut distension and their symptoms may be exacerbated by a high-fibre diet. These patients in particular may benefit from a low-fibre diet with the addition of methylcellulose fibre substitutes which do not ferment, e.g. Celevac. Thus the patient avoids constipation without the usual fermentation associated with a high-fibre diet.

Air swallowing (**aerophagia**) may also cause similar symptoms of bloating and discomfort and can be treated by physiotherapy. Psychological factors are probably important in some cases; these patients tend to be tense and introspective. Perhaps the condition represents an imbalance in intestinal hormonal and autonomic control systems, both centrally and locally mediated.

MANAGEMENT OF IRRITABLE BOWEL SYNDROME

There is no specific test for irritable bowel syndrome. Diagnosis is made on the basis of a typical history after excluding other disorders and often after a trial of treatment. In the young patient, where carcinoma is unlikely, abdominal and rectal examination (probably including sigmoidoscopy) is all that is required. These will be normal except perhaps for mild tenderness in the area of pain. In a patient over the age of 50, the diagnosis of irritable bowel syndrome is unlikely and carcinoma and diverticular disease must be excluded by sigmoidoscopy and barium enema or colonoscopy before it can be accepted.

Treatment involves reassurance, adjusting the diet to include adequate fibre, and prescribing bulking agents and antispasmodic drugs such as mebeverine. Codeine phosphate is useful as an analgesic for occasional use. This combination of treatment given early in an attack produces rapid relief of symptoms and confirms the diagnosis. There is probably little benefit in giving continuous treatment. For selected patients, relaxation therapy may be useful.

CONSTIPATION

CLINICAL FEATURES OF CONSTIPATION

Whether or not they regard it as a problem, many patients suffer from chronic constipation. Constipation is difficult to define but the essence is an inability to evacuate the bowels with sufficient frequency, ease, completeness or satisfaction. Perception of the norm varies greatly; some patients insist that daily evacuation is essential whilst others tolerate a bowel movement only once a week.

Constipation is often considered in two groups. The first is **slow transit constipation** where there appears to be a general failure of colonic propulsion. The other group includes patients with evacuation difficulties who are labelled as having an **evacuation disorder**. These patients often complain of incomplete rectal evacuation and the sensation of obstructed defaecation. They are particularly difficult to treat as the pathophysiology of the condition is not understood.

From a medical viewpoint, evacuation less than twice a week is abnormal. In the uncomplaining elderly, defaecation may occur much less frequently, causing vague discomfort and anorexia, and predisposing to urinary retention, incontinence and urinary tract infection. Severe constipation may lead to faecal impaction and complete bowel obstruction necessitating admission to hospital. Faecal fluid may intermittently escape past the impacted faecal mass and cause soiling, overflow incontinence or apparent (**'spurious'**) **diarrhoea**.

Abdominal pain may be the presenting symptom of constipation. The pain may be sufficiently severe to result in emergency hospital admission with suspected appendicitis (usually children) or intestinal obstruction (usually the elderly). As many as 25% of patients in these age groups admitted with abdominal pain are diagnosed as suffering from constipation. There is no fever, tachycardia or vomiting, and signs of peritoneal inflammation are absent. There may, however, be mild abdominal tenderness. The faecally loaded left side of the colon often forms a palpable column which may indent on palpation and have a putty-like consistency. Rectal examination usually reveals a palpable mass of faeces, although in the elderly the faeces may be impacted higher up. Thus, an empty rectum does not exclude constipation.

PATHOPHYSIOLOGY OF CHRONIC CONSTIPATION

For surgeons, chronic constipation is mainly a problem of children and the elderly. Patients present both as emergencies and in the outpatient clinic. For general practitioners and gastroenterologists, constipation is more a problem of young women. In most cases, the cause is a combination of low-fibre diet, poor fluid intake, obesity, inactivity and persistent failure to respond promptly to the urge to defaecate. Long-term use of **purgative drugs** such as senna derivatives may have an adverse effect on peristalsis. Some drugs, particularly **codeine** and **opiates**, slow large bowel motility, whilst other drugs such as **aluminium hydroxide mixtures** and **iron preparations** solidify the stool. Constipation is a characteristic feature of **hypothyroidism** and is also seen in **hypo-** and **hypercalcaemia**.

MANAGEMENT OF CONSTIPATION

Diagnosis of constipation in children can usually be made on the history and clinical examination; successful treatment confirms the diagnosis. If chronic severe constipation persists in infants despite treatment, the diagnosis of **ultra-short segment Hirschsprung's disease** (see Ch. 44) should be considered. In the elderly, carcinoma or the complications of diverticular disease should be excluded by sigmoidoscopy and barium enema once the constipation has been treated.

In severe constipation, immediate treatment involves the following local measures, in increasing order of desperation!

- Lubricant glycerine suppositories
- Stimulant suppositories (e.g. bisacodyl)
- Small phosphate enemas (disposable or 'mini' enemas)
- Stool-softening arachis oil enemas
- Large-volume soap and water enemas ('high, hot and a helluva lot')—rarely used these days

- Manual disimpaction (may require general anaesthesia)
- Oral sodium picosulphate or mannitol (1 L 10% mannitol with an equal quantity of other fluid)

Many patients take a high-fibre diet but do not drink enough, failing to recognise that both are necessary for the effect of fibre to be produced. Many women fail to benefit from a high-fibre diet. In these patients, increasing their fibre even more does not improve matters. If the condition is not severe, then eating more figs, apricots, prunes etc. may solve the problem. Otherwise, a low dose of a stimulant laxative taken from time to time should help.

If there is any suspicion of bowel obstruction, oral laxatives of any kind are contraindicated.

Managing chronic constipation involves treating the acute problem as above (and see Box 22.3), followed by long-term prophylactic measures. Most patients should be encouraged to increase dietary fibre and fluid intake and to heed the urge to defaecate but to avoid straining. Bulking agents may be appropriate in the medium term. In chronic laxative abuse, the laxative may have to be continued.

SIGMOID VOLVULUS

PATHOPHYSIOLOGY OF SIGMOID VOLVULUS

Patients with longstanding chronic constipation tend to develop a capacious, elongated and relatively atonic colon, especially in the sigmoid region. This is sometimes described as **acquired** or **idiopathic megacolon**.

Occasionally, a huge sigmoid loop, heavy with faeces and distended with gas, becomes twisted on its mesen-

---

KEY POINTS

Box 22.3 Oral laxative agents

- Stimulant/irritant laxatives, e.g. danthron, bisacodyl, senna derivatives
- Faecal softeners and lubricants, e.g. dioctyl, liquid paraffin
- Osmotic laxatives, e.g. lactulose, mixtures of magnesium hydroxide or magnesium sulphate
- Proprietary preparations, e.g. Milpar (liquid paraffin and magnesium hydroxide emulsion), Ex-Lax (phenolphthalein)
- Strong laxatives for single-dose use for bowel preparation or very stubborn constipation, e.g. sodium picosulphate (stimulant), mannitol solution (osmotic)

Note: bulking agents do not have a laxative effect in the short term

teric pedicle to produce a closed-loop obstruction (see Fig. 22.1). If this sigmoid volvulus is not corrected, venous infarction ensues, followed by perforation and catastrophic faecal peritonitis. This full picture is uncommon but when it occurs, there is often a history of several episodes of transient obstruction which probably represents incomplete volvulus. Some episodes of abdominal pain diagnosed as constipation may in fact be sigmoid volvulus, resolving spontaneously as constipation is treated. Volvulus of the caecum, small bowel or stomach, however, is unrelated to constipation.

CLINICAL FEATURES OF SIGMOID VOLVULUS

In developed countries, sigmoid volvulus is rarely seen except in the elderly, those with severe learning difficulties and long-stay patients in mental institutions; in contrast, it is very common in parts of the world where diet is extremely high in fibre. The patient is mildly unwell with abdominal distension and a variable degree of abdominal pain. There is also absolute constipation (of both faeces and flatus) for at least 24 hours. On digital examination, the rectum is empty but capacious. The abdomen is visibly distended and tympanitic but rarely tender. This is true even if the colon has reached the stage of venous infarction. Once perforation occurs, the full picture of faecal peritonitis will be evident.

MANAGEMENT OF SIGMOID VOLVULUS

Plain abdominal X-ray usually shows a single grossly dilated sigmoid loop, often reaching the xiphisternum (see Fig. 22.2). An erect film may reveal a characteristic 'inverted U' or 'coffee-bean sign' of bowel gas in the upper abdomen, with fluid levels at the same height in the two bowel limbs in the lower abdomen; an abdominal lateral decubitus X-ray may reveal two parallel fluid levels running the full length of the abdomen.

If sigmoid volvulus is diagnosed, a sigmoidoscope is gently passed as far as possible into the rectum and a flatus tube inserted through it. The end of the **flatus tube** is then gently manipulated through the twisted bowel into the obstructed loop. If this is successful, there is a gush of liquid faeces and flatus, relieving the obstruction. The flatus tube can be left in situ for 24 hours to maintain decompression, discourage retwisting and allow recovery of the vascular supply of the bowel wall. Despite this, volvulus is likely to recur later.

If plain X-ray and sigmoidoscopy do not confirm volvulus but large bowel obstruction is still suspected, a **limited barium enema** is performed, without bowel preparation. This differentiates volvulus from other causes of obstruction such as carcinoma and diverticular disease, or pseudo-obstruction. In volvulus, pressure from the barium enema may cause the bowel to untwist, releasing a torrent of faeces and flatus.

If a volvulus cannot be released, operation is performed urgently. In most cases, the bowel is still viable but sigmoid colectomy is often required to prevent recurrence. The usual procedure is to bring the two divided ends of bowel out on to the abdominal wall to form a **double-barrelled colostomy** (see Ch. 000), rather than risk a primary anastomosis in dilated and unprepared colon. For recurrent volvulus, **sigmoid colectomy** or suturing the bowel to the abdominal wall to prevent twisting may be performed electively.

DIVERTICULAR DISEASE

Diverticular disease is a common condition of uncertain aetiology. There is evidence that it can be caused or at least aggravated by a chronic lack of dietary fibre but there is probably also a genetic element. It occurs in at least one-third of the population of developed countries over the age of 60. Females are affected more often than males. (Note that the singular noun is *diverticulum* and the plural *diverticula*, not *diverticulae*; the adjectival form is *diverticular*.)

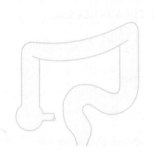

Normal colon

(a)

Megacolon of chronic constipation/laxative abuse

(b)

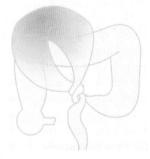

Sigmoid volvulus

(c)

Fig. 22.1 Mechanism of sigmoid volvulus
(a) Normal colon. (b) Megacolon of chronic constipation/laxative abuse—a large, floppy transverse colon and huge sigmoid loop.
(c) Sigmoid volvulus showing a grossly distended fluid-filled sigmoid colon twisted about its narrow neck, producing a 'closed-loop' obstruction.

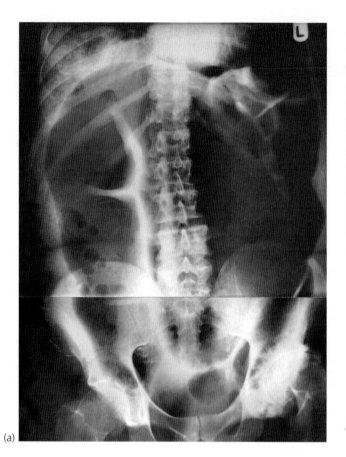

(a)

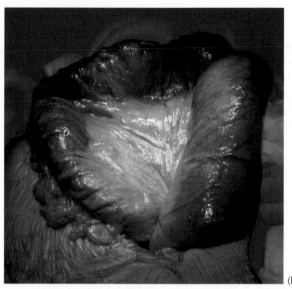

(b)

Fig. 22.2 Sigmoid volvulus
This 35-year-old man with Down's syndrome presented with a massively swollen abdomen and total constipation. **(a)** The clinical and radiographic diagnosis was sigmoid volvulus but the volvulus could not be relieved by gentle passage of a flatus tube. At operation, **(b)** the hugely distended sigmoid emerged from the laparotomy wound. The loop had twisted three times around its narrow base and the colon was of doubtful viability. This sigmoid colon was resected without untwisting the volvulus.

PATHOPHYSIOLOGY OF DIVERTICULAR DISEASE

In diverticular disease, the colonic muscle wall is thicker than normal, not because of hypertrophy but because of an excess of elastic tissue between the muscle fibres. This abnormal distribution of elastin is the most marked pathological abnormality and may be related to the pathogenesis of the disease. The functional sphincter at the rectosigmoid junction probably fails to relax, leaving a high pressure in the proximal bowel. In addition, **hypersegmentation** is the probable mechanism for the formation of diverticula. In this, two segments of colon close to each other contract at the same time, sending a peristaltic wave towards each other. This causes very high luminal pressure in short segments of the colon which results in pockets of mucosa herniating through weak points in the bowel wall. These potential defects occur where mucosal blood vessels penetrate the wall from outside, between the longitudinal muscle bands (**taenia coli**). The sigmoid colon is the segment most commonly affected by diverticular disease and the condition extends for a variable distance proximally. Right-sided diverticular disease is more common in Japanese, Chinese and Polynesian races and is particularly common in Hawaii. In the West, isolated diverticula

sometimes occur alone in the caecum but these are probably congenital rather than acquired.

The presence of uncomplicated diverticula is probably unimportant; this asymptomatic condition was formerly described as '**diverticulosis**'. An individual diverticulum may, however, become inflamed as a result of obstruction of the narrow outlet. This results in the formation of a **diverticular abscess**. The abscess effectively lies outside the bowel wall and leads to other complications described below. The microscopic anatomy is demonstrated in Figure 22.3.

COMPLICATIONS OF DIVERTICULAR DISEASE

Diverticular inflammation may lead to a variety of complications:

- Spreading pericolic inflammation
- Pericolic abscess
- Intraperitoneal perforation
- Acute rectal haemorrhage
- Fistula formation into other abdominal or pelvic viscera
- Bowel-to-bowel adhesions
- Fibrous strictures of bowel

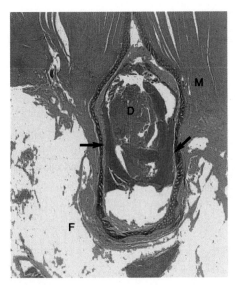

Fig. 22.3 Diverticular disease—histopathology
Low-power view of muscle wall **M** showing a diverticulum lined by mucosa (arrowed) and extending into fat **F**. Faecal material is present within the diverticulum **(D)**.

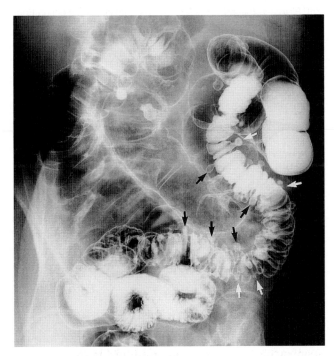

Fig. 22.4 Diverticular disease
Barium enema showing the typical appearance of multiple diverticula (arrowed) in the sigmoid and descending colon in a 77-year-old woman. A few diverticula are also present in the transverse colon.

CLINICAL PRESENTATIONS OF DIVERTICULAR DISEASE AND THEIR MANAGEMENT

The pathological consequences of diverticular inflammation are collectively described as **diverticulitis** and are summarised in Figure 22.5. Most patients with diverticula are asymptomatic, and diverticula are a common incidental finding when the colon is investigated by barium enema or colonoscopy. The typical appearances are shown in Figures 22.4 and 22.5.

Chronic grumbling diverticular pain (see Fig. 22.5b)

This is probably the most common manifestation of diverticular disease, and is usually managed in family practice. Peridiverticular inflammation is chronic, low-grade and recurrent. Local irritation provokes bowel wall spasm causing chronic pain and erratic bowel habit. There is chronic constipation with small pellet-like faeces and episodic diarrhoea. On clinical examination, there is little abnormal to find except perhaps mild left iliac fossa tenderness and faecal loading. Barium enema is often performed to confirm the diagnosis and exclude malignancy.

In most patients, symptoms can be relieved by taking a high-fibre diet and bulking agents. In the past, however, before the importance of dietary fibre was realised, many patients with severe chronic symptoms were subjected to colectomy, with all its attendant complications.

Acute diverticulitis (i.e. spreading pericolic inflammation—see Fig. 22.5c)

This represents local extension of the inflammation described above. The local inflammation involves the pericolic tissues and parietal peritoneum. Typically, the patient complains of continuous left iliac fossa pain and is systemically ill with a pyrexia and tachycardia, often requiring admission to hospital. Abdominal findings range from mild left iliac fossa tenderness to obvious local peritonitis.

Antibiotic treatment is directed against the usual faecal organisms. In severe cases, a combination of intravenous antibiotics such as a cephalosporin and metronidazole is used, and the bowel 'rested' by stopping oral intake and giving intravenous fluids. Less severe cases can be managed at home with oral antibiotics, e.g. metronidazole alone or with amoxycillin or a cephalosporin.

Pericolic abscess (see Fig. 22.5d)

Pericolic abscess represents a further extension of the pathological process just described. The clinical presentation is similar at first but fails to resolve with antibiotics. The patient suffers persistent pain and tenderness, a swinging pyrexia and incomplete obstruction due to spasm of the bowel wall muscle. Sometimes a pericolic abscess presents as sepsis or 'pyrexia of unknown origin'. The pericolic abscess may drain spontaneously into the bowel producing an attack of purulent diarrhoea; the

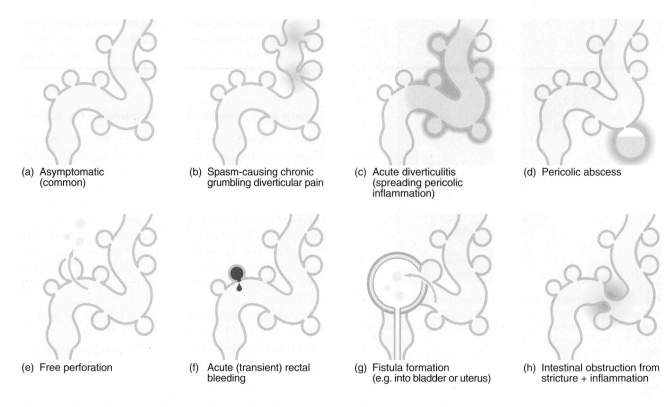

(a) Asymptomatic (common)

(b) Spasm-causing chronic grumbling diverticular pain

(c) Acute diverticulitis (spreading pericolic inflammation)

(d) Pericolic abscess

(e) Free perforation

(f) Acute (transient) rectal bleeding

(g) Fistula formation (e.g. into bladder or uterus)

(h) Intestinal obstruction from stricture + inflammation

Fig. 22.5 Clinical presentations of diverticular disease

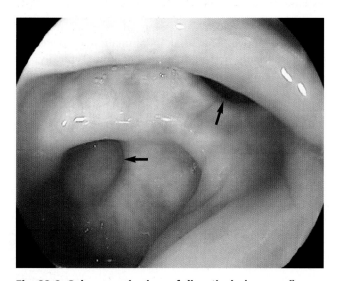

Fig. 22.6 Colonoscopic view of diverticula (arrowed)

condition then resolves. Diagnosis of a pericolic abscess can often be made by ultrasonography. A barium enema may show leakage of contrast into the abscess cavity (see Fig. 22.7).

Antibiotic therapy, as for acute diverticulitis, is the first line of treatment. Ideally, this contains the abscess, allowing it to drain spontaneously into the bowel. If antibiotic treatment fails, operation is required. This is a major procedure involving diversion of the faecal stream via a colostomy, and exploration and drainage of the abscess. In addition, the affected segment of bowel must be removed (Hartmann's operation—see Ch. 20, p. 289). This is best done at the first operation if the inflammation is not too extensive and the surgeon is sufficiently experienced. If not, resection is performed electively several months later when inflammation has subsided. The colostomy is closed at the same time or later. Perforated carcinoma can present in a similar way and the diagnosis should be excluded if resection is to be delayed.

Diverticular perforation (see Fig. 22.5e)

A small, asymptomatic diverticular abscess may rupture spontaneously, i.e. perforate, resulting in the escape of gas or bowel contents into the peritoneal cavity. The patient presents with an acute abdomen, the severity of clinical signs depending on the size of the perforation and degree of peritoneal contamination. The perforation may be anything from a pinhole size, allowing only bowel gas and a little fluid to escape, to a hole up to 1 cm in diameter causing generalised faecal peritonitis and septicaemia. With small perforations, the symptoms and signs may be little more than those of acute diverticulitis; diagnosis is confirmed by the presence of free gas under the diaphragm on an erect chest X-ray.

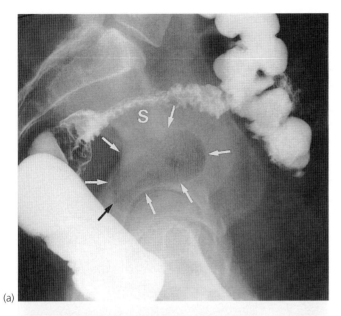

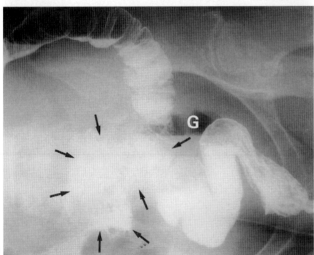

Fig. 22.7 Pericolic abscess due to perforated diverticular disease

Barium enema films from a 49-year-old woman who presented with abdominal pain and tenderness, a mass in the left iliac fossa and a swinging pyrexia. She was treated with antibiotics but the pyrexia failed to settle. **(a)** Right lateral view of the recto-sigmoid region showing marked narrowing of the distal sigmoid **S** due to spasm and inflammatory oedema. The radiolucent area antero-inferiorly (outline arrowed) represents a bubble of gas in a large pelvic abscess. **(b)** Lateral decubitus film (left side upwards) of the same patient taken later during the same examination. This shows barium which has leaked into the abscess cavity (outline arrowed). Note also a fluid level with a gas bubble **G** above it, within the abscess. At laparotomy, a large pericolic and pelvic abscess was found to be walled off. This was drained surgically, the sigmoid colon excised and the end of the descending colon brought out as a terminal colostomy in the left iliac fossa. The rectal stump was oversewn; 3 months later, the bowel was reconnected.

Treatment usually involves immediate parenteral antibiotics to prevent septicaemia, followed by laparotomy to perform peritoneal toilet, diversion of the faecal stream and resection of the diseased bowel (Hartmann's operation), as previously described.

Acute rectal haemorrhage (see Fig. 22.5f)

Diverticular disease may present with an episode of acute rectal bleeding, probably resulting from erosion of a bowel wall artery by a small diverticular abscess. Blood loss is variable but the bleeding almost always stops spontaneously. The patient typically complains of having passed a mass of fairly fresh blood instead of the expected stool and is admitted to hospital urgently. The main differential diagnosis is **ischaemic colitis** but other causes of rectal bleeding such as carcinoma and haemorrhoids must be considered.

Management is rarely surgical. After any necessary resuscitation, the patient is kept under observation for several days, after which it is safe to perform a barium enema.

Fistula formation into other abdominal or pelvic structures (see Fig. 22.5g)

Fistula formation occurs when an inflamed diverticulum lies in close proximity to another hollow viscus. An inflammatory adhesion develops between them and the diverticulum then ruptures into the other viscus, leaving a persistent channel between the two. A fistula between the large bowel and a loop of small bowel (see Fig. 22.8) causes diarrhoea. A vesico-colic fistula causes **pneumaturia** and severe urinary tract infection. A fistula into the vagina after a previous hysterectomy causes a purulent vaginal discharge. Diverticular disease is the most common cause of these kinds of fistula but they may also be caused by Crohn's disease or sometimes colorectal cancers.

Surprisingly, fistulae rarely show up on barium enema examination. Diagnosis is made on the history, at operation or at cystoscopic examination in the case of bladder fistula. Surgical treatment involves excision and histological examination of the affected segment of bowel.

Intestinal obstruction (see Fig. 22.5h)

Diverticular disease occasionally presents with complete large bowel obstruction due to a combination of acute inflammatory thickening, muscle hypertrophy and spasm. **Incomplete obstruction** is much more common and presents as severe constipation. Chronic diverticular inflammation sometimes causes isolated fibrous strictures, particularly in the sigmoid colon, which cause intermittent bouts of constipation. When seen on barium enema (see Fig. 22.9) these strictures must be distinguished from malignancy or Crohn's disease. This may require colonoscopy.

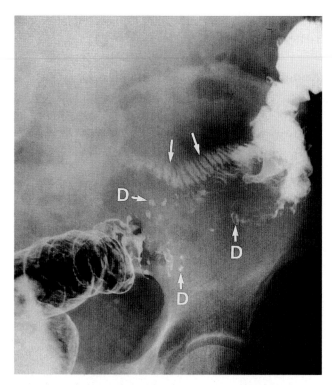

Fig. 22.8 Diverticular fistula into the distal ileum
Barium enema of a 61-year-old man with a recently erratic bowel habit, who presented with pain and tenderness in the left iliac fossa. The X-ray shows the sigmoid colon, although part of it is poorly filled with barium which is only seen in the diverticula **D**. There is a loop of small bowel which contains contrast (arrowed), indicating the presence of a colo-ileal fistula caused by peridiverticulitis.

When acute diverticular inflammation involves the pericolic tissues, small bowel may become entangled in the process. Thus, adynamic small bowel obstruction may be the presenting feature.

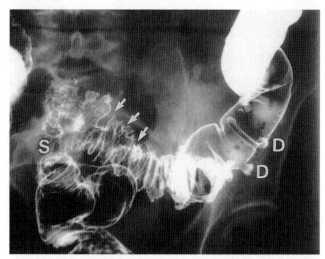

Fig. 22.9 Diverticular stricture in the sigmoid colon
This 64-year-old man suffered several attacks of diverticulitis which settled with antibiotics. This frontal view of a barium enema shows diverticula **D** in the upper sigmoid colon and circular muscle hypertrophy in the distal sigmoid colon (arrowed) typical of diverticular disease. There is a stricture **S** near the recto-sigmoid junction. This stricture does not show the typical 'shouldering' of a carcinoma, although carcinoma could not be excluded on barium enema. Colonoscopy confirmed that it was benign. This patient later had a severe attack of diverticulitis which required surgery and a Hartmann's operation was performed.

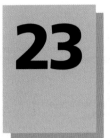

23 Anal and perianal disorders

INTRODUCTION

Anal and perianal disorders make up about 20% of general surgical outpatient referrals. Although trivial in pathological terms, these conditions are extremely distressing and embarrassing. Patients often tolerate symptoms for a long time before seeking medical advice. The common anal symptoms are summarised in Box 23.1 and their interpretation is discussed in Chapter 11.

Disorders of the anus and perianal area are illustrated in Figure 23.1. Haemorrhoids and other common benign anal conditions must be distinguished from carcinoma of the rectum and the rare carcinoma of the anus, particularly in older patients. Most anal and perianal conditions can be treated on an outpatient basis, although abscesses, and haemorrhoids that have become strangulated or thrombosed may present as surgical emergencies.

ANATOMY OF THE ANAL CANAL

The anal canal is approximately 4 cm long and is surrounded by the anal sphincter mechanism (see Fig. 23.2). There are four areas of differing epithelium lining the anal canal. At the anal verge, there is stratified squamous epithelium with associated skin appendages—sweat glands, hair follicles and sebaceous glands. The appendages are then absent up to the level of the anal valves at the **dentate (pectinate) line**. From here, the epithelium becomes cuboidal for a variable distance and this is called the **anal transition zone** (ATZ). Towards the upper part of the anal canal this gives way to rectal mucosa proper. On proctoscopic inspection, the rectal mucosa is pink but in the anal canal where it overlies the submucosal venous plexus, it is a darker reddish-blue.

The mucosa of the upper part of the anal canal is thrown into 6–10 longitudinal folds, the **columns of Morgagni**, each containing a terminal branch of the superior rectal artery and vein. The folds are most prominent in the left lateral, right posterior and right anterior sectors where the vessels form prominent **anal cushions**. These are important in maintaining continence and may enlarge to form haemorrhoids, complex collections of arterioles, arteries, venules, venous saccules and connective tissue. The anal columns are not readily visible on proctoscopy but the transition between glandular rectal mucosa and anal skin is clearly visible. The lymphatics of the upper part of the anal canal drain to the pelvic and abdominal lymph node chain, whereas the lower part of the anal canal drains to the inguinal lymph nodes. All of the anal canal below the rectal mucosa is exquisitely sensitive, for example, to injection. In contrast, the rectal mucosa is relatively insensitive.

The anal sphincter mechanism has three constituents, the **internal sphincter**, the **external sphincter** and **puborectalis**. The internal sphincter represents a downward but thickened continuation of the rectal wall musculature. The encircling external sphincter and the puborectalis sling (which is part of levator ani) arise from the pelvic floor. Continence is maintained principally

KEY POINTS

Box 23.1 Common anal symptoms

- Anal bleeding
- Anal itching and discomfort
- Pain on defaecation
- Perianal itching and irritation
- 'Something coming down'
- Perianal discharge

Haemorrhoids

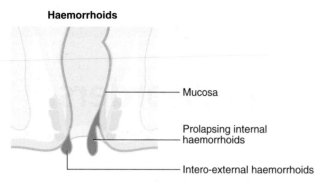

— Mucosa

— Prolapsing internal
   haemorrhoids

— Intero-external haemorrhoids

**Thrombosed external
haemorrhoid**

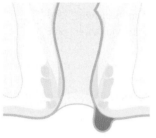

Anal fistula

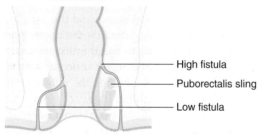

— High fistula
— Puborectalis sling
— Low fistula

Rectal prolapse

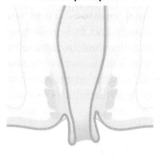

Prolapsing low rectal polyp

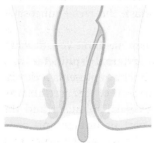

Anal fissure

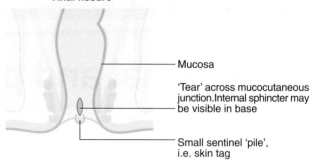

— Mucosa

'Tear' across mucocutaneous
junction. Internal sphincter may
be visible in base

— Small sentinel 'pile',
   i.e. skin tag

Abscess

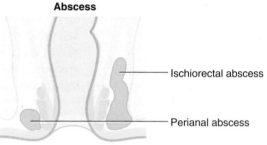

— Ischiorectal abscess

— Perianal abscess

Perianal warts

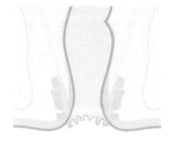

Anal carcinoma

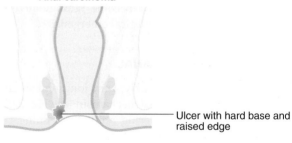

— Ulcer with hard base and
   raised edge

Low rectal carcinoma

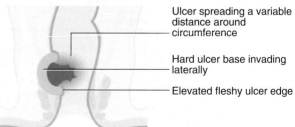

Ulcer spreading a variable
distance around
circumference

Hard ulcer base invading
laterally

Elevated fleshy ulcer edge

Fig. 23.1 Anal and perianal disorders

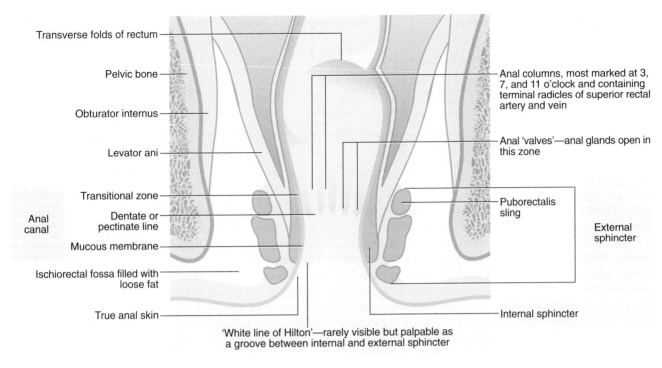

Transverse folds of rectum

Pelvic bone

Obturator internus

Levator ani

Transitional zone

Anal canal — Dentate or pectinate line

Mucous membrane

Ischiorectal fossa filled with loose fat

True anal skin

Anal columns, most marked at 3, 7, and 11 o'clock and containing terminal radicles of superior rectal artery and vein

Anal 'valves'—anal glands open in this zone

Puborectalis sling

External sphincter

Internal sphincter

'White line of Hilton'—rarely visible but palpable as a groove between internal and external sphincter

Fig. 23.2 Anatomy of the anal canal

by the pressure generated by the anal sphincters squeezing on the three anal cushions causing them to occlude the lumen between them. Continence is assisted by the fact that the rectum proximally forms a compliant reservoir to store stool. The angle maintained by the action of puborectalis is no longer thought to be important as regards continence.

HAEMORRHOIDS

Haemorrhoids (piles) are extremely common, affecting nearly half of the population at some stage in their lives. Men tend to suffer more often and for longer periods, whereas women are particularly susceptible in late pregnancy and the puerperium.

PATHOGENESIS OF HAEMORRHOIDS

It is likely that heredity plays an important part in predisposing individuals to haemorrhoids. This predisposition is brought to light by pregnancy, constipation or diarrhoea. Lack of fibre in the modern Western diet is probably also a factor in predisposed patients. Haemorrhoids are probably initiated by straining to pass small hard stools. Straining raises intra-abdominal pressure which obstructs venous return and the venous plexuses become engorged. The bulging mucosa is then dragged distally by the hard stool. Furthermore, persistent straining at stool causes the pelvic floor to sag downwards, extruding the anal mucosa and causing a minor degree

of prolapse. In pregnancy-related haemorrhoids, venous engorgement and mucosal prolapse are probably the main mechanisms. Progesterones mediate venous dilatation, and the fetus obstructs pelvic venous return.

Anatomically, haemorrhoids are enlarged, engorged anal cushions and these may bleed, prolapse or result in minor mucus or faecal leakage, particularly when passing flatus. Bleeding from the arterial component of the anal cushion results in the characteristic bright red rectal bleeding. The venous component only causes a problem if it becomes thrombosed to form a **thrombosed external venous saccule** (sometimes wrongly labelled a perianal haematoma). Haemorrhoids are usually located in the three, seven and eleven o'clock positions when viewed with the patient in the supine lithotomy position. These correspond to the anatomical positions of the anal cushions.

CLASSIFICATION OF HAEMORRHOIDS

Haemorrhoids (piles) are classified into first, second and third degrees according to the extent to which they prolapse through the anal canal. **First degree piles** never prolapse; **second degree piles** prolapse during defaecation and then return spontaneously into the anal canal; **third degree piles** remain outside the anal margin unless replaced digitally (see Fig. 23.3). Most haemorrhoids can be described as 'internal' because they are covered by glandular mucosa. Large neglected haemorrhoids may extend beneath the stratified squamous epithelium so that their lower part becomes covered by

317

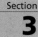

First degree   Second degree   Third degree

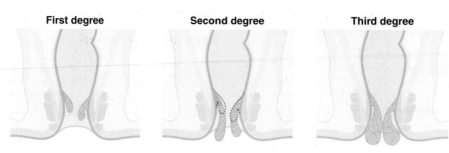

Fig. 23.3 Classification of haemorrhoids

skin. These are correctly described as **'intero-external' haemorrhoids**, or more commonly 'external piles'.

Any haemorrhoids may bleed from stool trauma during defaecation. Large haemorrhoids may thrombose if they prolapse and their venous return is obstructed by sphincter tone. Such piles then become solid and cannot be effectively replaced within the anal canal. In extreme cases, the haemorrhoid undergoes venous infarction (strangulation) and ulceration. The local pain and irritation caused by haemorrhoids results in increased anal sphincter tone and spasm, thus aggravating the problems of defaecation and prolapse. Longstanding haemorrhoids eventually atrophy, probably by thrombosis and fibrosis, leaving small **skin tags** at the anal margin.

SYMPTOMS AND SIGNS OF HAEMORRHOIDS

Haemorrhoids often produce symptoms intermittently. Attacks last from a few days to a few weeks, often with complete freedom from trouble between times. Episodes of constipation are often a precipitating factor.

The symptoms of haemorrhoids are:

- Perianal irritation and itching (pruritus ani)
- Aching discomfort and pain exacerbated by defaecation
- Haemorrhoidal prolapse
- Rectal bleeding (fresh blood, on the paper or separate from stool)

Most patients reaching the surgeon have already tried various anaesthetic and sedative creams and suppositories, self-administered or prescribed by the general practitioner. Reasons for referral are persistent symptoms and the need to exclude malignancy as a cause of bleeding.

With imperfect closure of the anal cushions, leakage of mucus together with low-grade secondary infection by faecal bacteria or *Candida* cause both skin maceration and perianal irritation. Scratching exacerbates the problem.

On examination, external piles or skin tags may be visible in the anal area. Digital examination is essential to exclude carcinoma and provides a useful measure of anal tone. Haemorrhoids, however, are not palpable unless they are large since they empty with pressure from the examining finger. **Proctoscopy** is necessary to demonstrate internal piles, which are seen bulging into the lumen as the proctoscope is withdrawn. **Sigmoidoscopy** is important in patients over 40 years, if there is a history of bleeding or any symptoms suspicious of malignancy; occasionally a rectal polyp will be diagnosed in this way.

ACUTE PRESENTATIONS OF HAEMORRHOIDS

Thrombosed or strangulated haemorrhoids present with acute pain and many patients are admitted to hospital as an emergency. These complications are common in the late stages of pregnancy and soon after delivery. The diagnosis of **thrombosed haemorrhoids** is usually obvious on inspection—an oedematous, congested purplish mass is seen at the anal margin. Tight spasm of the anal sphincter makes digital rectal examination extremely painful. **Strangulated haemorrhoids** are even more painful than thrombosed haemorrhoids, and the strangulated mass may become necrotic or even ulcerated. Symptomatic relief is given by bed rest and applying ice packs and topical local anaesthetic gel over a few days; this may be the only treatment that can safely be offered in late pregnancy. Acute haemorrhoidectomy under antibiotic cover provides definitive management for both thrombosed and strangulated haemorrhoids but carries a higher risk of complications.

CONSERVATIVE MANAGEMENT AND PREVENTION OF HAEMORRHOIDS

The most important means of preventing and treating haemorrhoids is avoiding constipation and ensuring a bulky stool. This is often best achieved by taking a diet high in fibre. This change in diet may be supplemented initially with an ispaghula husk bulking agent. The patient should be advised to heed the call to evacuate as when this occurs there appears to be a reflex release of lubricating mucus which may be absent later. In addition, the patient should be strongly encouraged to avoid straining and to spend minimal time in defaecating. Many sufferers regularly spend a long time on the lavatory reading. This ritual easily leads to unnecessary straining at the end of defaecation, and a mild haemorrhoidal or mucosal prolapse can be interpreted as incomplete evacuation of faeces, prompting further straining. Prolonged straining occasionally leads to the formation of a 'solitary ulcer' on the posterior wall of the proximal anal canal, which may be clinically indistinguishable from a malignant ulcer. In many patients with symptomatic haemorrhoids, these simple measures are enough to relieve the symptoms.

Pruritus ani can be greatly helped if the perineum is washed and dried after defaecation and kept dry by applying talcum powder. Washing the perianal area with soap aggravates the symptoms, so it is better to apply aqueous cream and then wash it off with plain water. With prolapsing third degree haemorrhoids, symptoms can often be relieved by the patient replacing the haemorrhoids digitally after defaecation. Many creams, suppositories and other topical preparations are available with or without prescription, and are very widely used. Many contain local anaesthetic agents and steroids. They are useful to help a patient recover from an episode of haemorrhoidal symptoms but do nothing to treat the underlying condition and may cause local allergic reactions. Overuse causes maceration of the perianal skin and predisposes to secondary infection.

SURGICAL TREATMENTS FOR HAEMORRHOIDS

Injection of sclerosants

First degree haemorrhoids which do not regress with dietary change and avoidance of straining, and most second degree haemorrhoids are best treated by sclerosant injection. An irritant solution is injected submucosally around the pedicles of the three major haemorrhoids. This provokes a fibrotic reaction, effectively obliterating the haemorrhoidal vessels and causing atrophy of the haemorrhoids.

The procedure can be performed on an outpatient basis and does not require any anaesthetic. The haemorrhoids are first assessed by external inspection, with the patient both at rest and 'straining down'. A proctoscope is then inserted to its full length so that the distal end of the proctoscope lies beyond the external sphincter and projects into the lower rectum (see Fig. 23.4). The instrument is then slowly withdrawn and the haemorrhoids are seen to bulge into the lumen. The proctoscope is reinserted as before and 3–5 ml of 5% phenol in oil is injected just beneath the mucosa. Usually three injections are given, near the sites at which each vessel enters or leaves the haemorrhoidal plexuses, i.e. at positions three, seven and eleven o'clock as viewed with the patient in the lithotomy position i.e. supine. A specially designed aspirating syringe and a shouldered needle are intended to help avoid injecting directly into a vein or injecting too

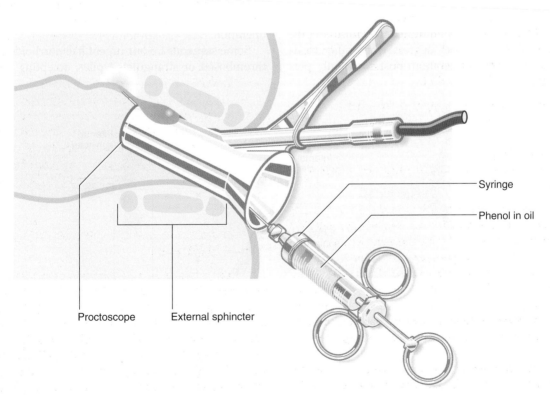

Syringe

Phenol in oil

Proctoscope   External sphincter

Fig. 23.4 Technique of injecting haemorrhoids

deeply, although aspiration is not routinely employed in practice. Injection must be placed superficially and is painless provided the needle is placed correctly into the neck of the haemorrhoid above the anal canal; direct injection into the haemorrhoid itself is extremely painful. Injection may be repeated on 2–3 occasions at intervals of 4–6 weeks.

Banding

An alternative to injection is the application of **Barron's bands** to obliterate the haemorrhoidal vessels (see Fig. 23.5). Contrary to popular belief, the bands are not placed around the stalk of prolapsing haemorrhoids; this would be unbearably painful because of the somatic innervation of anal skin. Instead, a cone of mucosa just above the haemorrhoidal neck is picked up in special forceps and drawn into the banding instrument. The bands are then released around the base of the cone, constricting the haemorrhoidal vessels. The result is that the haemorrhoid gradually shrinks.

Lord's stretch

This technique, which was in vogue in the 1980s, involved manual dilatation of the anal sphincter under general anaesthesia. This procedure is not recommended because of the high risk of causing permanent incontinence for flatus and sometimes for stool, especially in the elderly.

Haemorrhoidectomy

Haemorrhoidal excision is indicated for third degree haemorrhoids and for lesser degrees when other treatments have failed. The operation most commonly per-

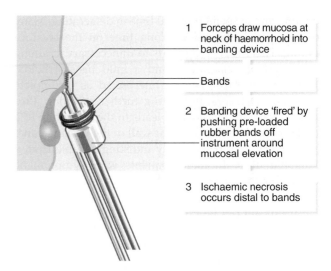

1 Forceps draw mucosa at neck of haemorrhoid into banding device

Bands

2 Banding device 'fired' by pushing pre-loaded rubber bands off instrument around mucosal elevation

3 Ischaemic necrosis occurs distal to bands

Fig. 23.5 Barron's banding technique for haemorrhoids
Note that the haemorrhoid itself is not banded.

formed is the one described by **Milligan and Morgan** and shown in Figure 23.6, in which the haemorrhoidal masses are excised together with overlying mucosa and some skin. This leaves skin and mucosal defects which heal by secondary intention and wound contraction. A skin bridge **must** be preserved between each wound to prevent the serious late complication of anal stenosis.

Before operation, stool softeners such as bulking agents and gentle laxatives should be given to avoid constipation afterwards. The painful early postoperative period can be greatly eased by caudal analgesia given at operation.

Some surgeons favour urgent haemorrhoidectomy for thrombosed or strangulated piles, accepting the higher

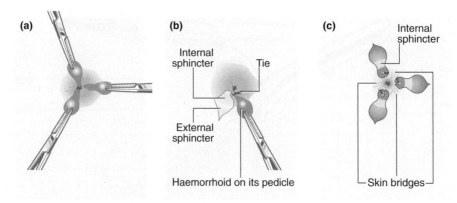

Fig. 23.6 Technique of Milligan–Morgan haemorrhoidectomy
(a) Identification of the main haemorrhoids; the external part of each is clamped with a haemostat and retracted outwards. **(b)** Scissors are used to incise the skin around the external haemorrhoid, any excess skin being excised at the same time. The haemorrhoid is then raised on its pedicle by dissection from the external sphincter and the internal sphincter. The pedicle is transfixed and ligated at its base with an absorbable suture. The skin is not closed. **(c)** The same process is repeated for the other primary haemorrhoids, ensuring that skin bridges are preserved between each raw area. The completed haemorrhoidectomy has a 'cloverleaf' appearance. After haemostasis is ensured, wounds are dressed with paraffin gauze (tulle gras) and a surgical pad applied, held in place by a perineal 'T' bandage.

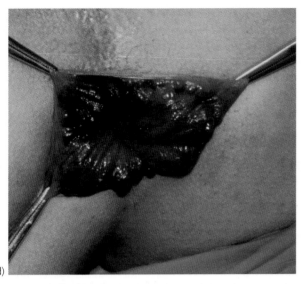 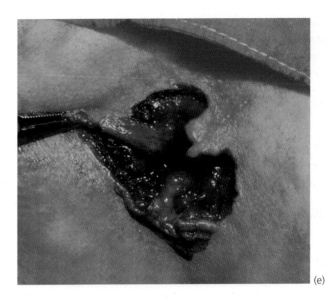

(d)   (e)

Fig. 23.6 Continued
(d) Intero-external haemorrhoids prolapsed and held with artery forceps. **(e)** 'Clover-like' appearance after haemorrhoidectomy. It is vital that skin bridges are retained between the areas of resection or anal stenosis will occur as healing proceeds ('If it looks like a dahlia, it's a failure').

risk of complications in exchange for a more rapid return to normal life. Prophylactic antibiotics should be given because of the risk of infection in necrotic tissue. Hospital stay and recovery period are generally shorter with urgent haemorrhoidectomy than with any conservative approach.

THROMBOSED EXTERNAL HAEMORRHOIDS

A thrombosed external haemorrhoid or pile is an acutely painful anal condition (Fig. 23.7). The onset is sudden and there is persistent pain over 1–2 weeks which is worse on defaecation. A thrombosed external haemorrhoid is sometimes called a perianal haematoma but this is inaccurate for it is not a haematoma but a thrombosis of perianal venous saccules. The condition often occurs

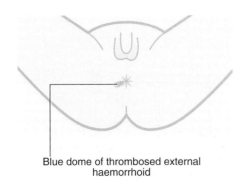

Blue dome of thrombosed external
haemorrhoid

Fig. 23.7 Thrombosed external haemarrhoid

in patients with haemorrhoids but can be seen in isolation. On examination, a blue-black hemispherical bulge is seen in the skin near the anal margin; haemorrhoids may or may not be present.

Most thrombosed external haemorrhoids subside over a few days and patients need only oral analgesia. Most topical anaesthetic creams are not absorbed by the skin and are useless. If pain is intolerable, the thrombosis may be incised and drained under anaesthesia.

ANAL FISSURE

An anal fissure is a longitudinal tear in the mucosa and skin of the anal canal caused by passing a large, constipated stool. The tear is nearly always in the midline of the posterior anal margin. The fissure causes acute pain during defaecation and sphincter spasm, both of which persist for up to an hour. The result is fear of defaecation and this aggravates the constipation. There is often a small amount of fresh bleeding at defaecation. This history alone is diagnostic of an anal fissure. On inspection, the fissure is concealed by the anal spasm but a small skin tag (sentinel pile) may be seen at the superficial end of the fissure (see Fig. 23.8). Rectal examination is extremely painful and rarely possible.

Patients sometimes manage to tolerate the pain of an acute fissure by using local anaesthetic creams and then present after a long period with a chronic anal fissure prevented from healing by anal sphincter spasm and repeated tearing open of the healing fissure during passage of stools.

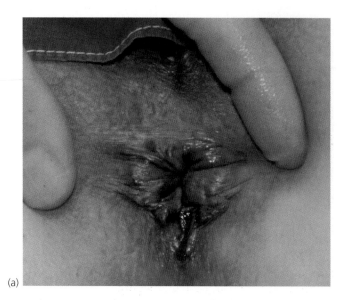

(a)

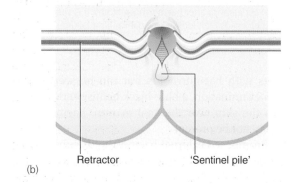

(b)   Retractor   'Sentinel pile'

Fig. 23.8 Anal fissure
(a) Chronic anal fissure with a 'sentinel pile'. Simple fissures are typically posteriorly located, as in this patient. **(b)** Explanatory diagram.

MANAGEMENT OF ANAL FISSURE

Anal fissure can be managed conservatively or operatively. Modern conservative treatment involves the use of topical glyceryl trinitrate (GTN) ointment 0.2%, applied three times a day for a month. Patients need to be warned that it may cause headaches. This treatment can cure up to 60% of anal fissures. For the rest, the GTN concentration can be increased to 0.3 or 0.5% for a further month if tolerated.

Surgery in the form of **lateral submucous (internal) sphincterotomy** brings more immediate relief, but there is a 10–15% incidence of incontinence of flatus following this procedure. Surgeons tend to be reluctant to offer sphincterotomy to women because their sphincters are shorter and less robust, and because occult sphincter injury from childbirth may already have occurred. However, if a prolonged course of GTN fails to work and the patient is suitably informed of the risks, an internal anal sphincterotomy may be performed. **Anal stretch** used to be performed for fissure, but the frequency of

incontinence is unacceptable; the procedure is dangerous because it dilates the external sphincter unnecessarily and produces global damage to the internal sphincter which is exceptionally difficult to correct later. Dietary advice regarding fibre intake should be given to help prevent recurrence.

ANORECTAL ABSCESSES

PATHOPHYSIOLOGY AND CLINICAL FEATURES OF ANORECTAL ABSCESSES

Abscesses in the anorectal area are common surgical emergencies. They present with constant and often severe perineal pain and local tenderness.

Anorectal abscesses begin as acute purulent infections of **anal glands**. These lie between the internal and external sphincters and drain into tiny pits, the anal crypts, near the dentate line. The ducts are very narrow and duct obstruction may be the factor that initiates the infection. Rarely, an abscess remains confined between the sphincters and an **intersphincteric abscess** results. The only symptom may be chronic anal pain and there is little to find on clinical examination to explain it. The only clue may be localised tenderness on rectal examination.

From the intersphincteric plane, infection tends to spread in one or more of three directions (see Fig. 23.9):

● **Downwards** between the sphincters towards the anal verge, forming a **perianal abscess**. This is the most common presentation and accounts for 80% of anorectal abscesses. The patient presents with a painful, tender, red swelling close to the anal verge
● **Outwards** through the external sphincter into the loose fibro-fatty tissue of the ischiorectal fossa, forming an **ischiorectal abscess**. There is little barrier to spread of infection in this space and a neglected or inadequately treated abscess may become enormous. Ischiorectal abscesses make up about 15% of anorectal abscesses. The patient presents with systemic signs of infection and perineal pain. There is tenderness over

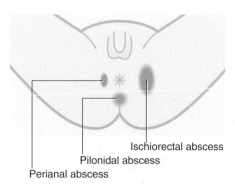

Ischiorectal abscess
Pilonidal abscess
Perianal abscess

Fig. 23.9 Abscesses in the anorectal region

the ischiorectal fossa lateral to the anus but there may be no visible redness or swelling; rectal palpation reveals a tender mass lateral to the rectum

● **Upwards** between the sphincters to form a **supralevator abscess**, involving the pararectal tissues above the pelvic floor. These make up less than 5% of anorectal abscesses and present with systemic signs of infection, rectal pain and difficulty in micturition. On rectal examination, a tender mass is palpable near the tip of the finger

TREATMENT OF ANORECTAL ABSCESSES

If perianal infection is seen very early, oral antibiotic treatment may abort it. The use of antibiotics in this way by general practitioners, coupled with early referral, has reduced the number and severity of cases reaching the surgeon. However, once an abscess is diagnosed, **surgical drainage** is needed; antibiotics are only indicated when there is spreading infection. Drainage is performed under regional or general anaesthesia. Careful **examination under anaesthesia** is performed first to establish the extent of the abscess. An intersphincteric abscess is drained by an internal sphincterotomy; perianal and ischiorectal abscesses are drained via the perianal skin, ensuring all loculations are broken down. Large ischiorectal abscesses require packing or placement of a drain to keep the neck of the cavity open whilst granulation tissue gradually fills the space from its depths. Further examinations under anaesthesia after a few days are often planned to ensure complete drainage and to inspect for fistulae. Supralevator abscesses are often more complicated and require complex staged surgical procedures including drainage by incising the rectal wall from an anal approach.

Incising a perianal abscess results in complete resolution in about 50% of cases; the other half develop an **anal fistula** (see below). The fistula is usually undetectable at the time of drainage but is recognised by a persistent discharge through the area of the skin incision continuing for several weeks afterwards.

Differential diagnosis of abscesses in the perianal area includes:

● **Crohn's disease**—may cause multiple abscesses and complex fistulae (see Ch. 21) and must be excluded
● **Hidradenitis suppurativa**—originates in perianal apocrine glands; it is easily distinguished from perianal abscesses by careful inspection
● **Pilonidal abscess**—occurs in the skin of the natal cleft (see Fig. 23.9 and page 538) but may mimic a genuine perianal abscess if near the anal margin; careful examination shows the presence of embedded hairs but no communication with the anal canal. Treatment is also by incision and drainage but further

procedures may be required to treat the associated pilonidal sinus (see Ch. 40, p. 538)
● **Tuberculous abscess and fistula**—very rare

ANAL FISTULA

Anal fistulae usually develop as a complication of perianal, ischiorectal or supralevator abscesses. A fistula consists of a chronically infected tract extending from an internal opening at the level of the dentate line, and passing through the site of the previous abscess to an external opening on the perianal skin near the old drainage scar. The communication between abscess cavity and bowel is established by spontaneous drainage into the bowel either before surgical drainage or after incomplete surgical drainage. Thus any abscess in the anal region should be drained early and thoroughly.

The patient typically complains of intermittent discharge of mucus, often faecally stained, in the perianal region. On examination, a small papilla of granulation tissue is seen on the skin within 2–3 cm of the anal margin (see Fig. 23.10 and 11.1). This clinical picture is diagnostic of an anal fistula; unfortunately, this apparently trivial skin lesion may be dismissed as a pustule or an incompletely healed perianal abscess.

Most anal fistulae are simple and relatively superficial, with the internal opening located in a crypt at the level of the dentate line (well below puborectalis), most often in the posterior midline. These are known as **low anal fistulae**. For successful treatment, it is crucial to locate the internal opening. **Goodsall's rule** helps to predict

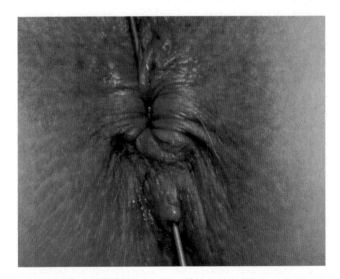

Fig. 23.10 Anal fistula
A probe has been passed from the skin surface through a low anal fistula to emerge in the anal canal at the level of the dentate line. Treatment consisted simply of cutting down onto the probe, thus laying open the fistula along its length. The wound was left to heal by secondary intention.

whether a fistula is likely to have a short direct tract to the anal canal (if the external opening is in front of an imaginary transverse line across the anus) or likely to have a curved course towards an internal opening in the posterior midline (if the external opening is behind the transverse line). Horseshoe fistulae confound this rule with an anterior external opening and a posterior midline internal opening.

Assessment and treatment require general or regional anaesthesia. Examination under anaesthetic (EUA) is performed first. A malleable probe is gently manipulated through the fistula to try to demonstrate the internal orifice. If this is not found, hydrogen peroxide can be gently injected into the external opening. This has replaced methylene blue as the best way of finding the internal opening.

Provided the fistula is entirely below the puborectalis muscle (which is palpable at operation), treatment is by laying open the tract by cutting down on to the probe with a scalpel, transsecting the anal margin and opening the whole length of the fistula. This is known as **fistulotomy** and involves dividing some of the internal sphincter and often part of the external sphincter. The wound heals gradually by secondary intention. There is no loss of faecal continence, but flatus may be less well controlled.

If the internal opening lies above puborectalis, surgical treatment is difficult and highly specialised because of the need to retain the functional integrity of the sphincters (including puborectalis) to preserve continence. Where complex fistulae are suspected, the anatomy can be very well defined preoperatively by magnetc resonance imaging (MRI). If the fistula involves more than half the length of the external anal sphincter complex, surgical division of the fistula track would cause incontinence. In these cases, slow division of the muscle using a non-absorbable suture threaded through the fistula can avoid this problem; this is known as **seton**.

Anal fistulae sometimes occur as a manifestation of **Crohn's disease**. Such fistulae tend to be multiple and in the most extreme cases form a 'pepper-pot' perineum (see Fig. 21.6, p. 299).

PILONIDAL SINUS AND ABSCESS

These conditions arise from the skin of the natal cleft rather than the anus and are covered in Chapter 40 (p. 538).

ANAL WARTS (CONDYLOMA ACCUMINATA)

Warts in the perianal region (see Fig. 23.11) have the same pathology and viral aetiology (human papilloma virus) as warts elsewhere but are usually transmitted by sexual activity. Referral to a genitomedical unit may be appropriate if other sexually transmitted diseases are suspected.

In small numbers, anal warts can be treated by topical applications of **podophyllin**. When large numbers are present, surgical excision under general anaesthetic is the only practical option. This involves meticulous excision of each individual wart by electrocautery. The normal skin between the warts is carefully preserved to avoid delayed healing or the disastrous complication of anal stenosis.

RECTAL PROLAPSE

Rectal prolapse is mainly seen in young children and the elderly. In children, it is usually a relatively minor and self-correcting problem. In the elderly, it is a chronic problem with no easy surgical solution (see Fig. 23.12). In pathophysiological terms, a rectal prolapse is a hernia of the rectum through the pelvic floor. In effect, the mucosa and muscle wall intussuscept through the anal canal. In the early stages, the prolapse occurs only with defaecation and retracts spontaneously. At a later stage, the rectum may prolapse when the patient merely stands up. The patient is thus reluctant to leave home and often becomes socially isolated.

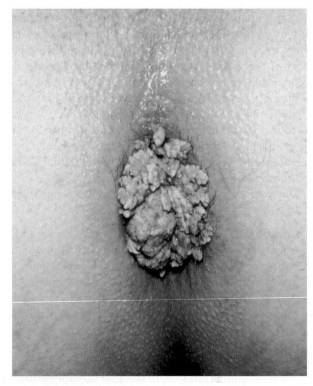

Fig. 23.11 Anal warts (condyloma accuminata)

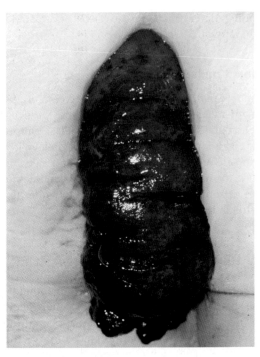

Fig. 23.12 Rectal prolapse
This complete rectal prolapse was in an 80-year-old woman. It emerged spontaneously whenever she stood, causing considerable discomfort and inconvenience, to say the least!

In childhood, rectal prolapse usually occurs around the age of 2 years. It tends to occur during toilet training and causes parental anxiety. Parents should be reassured that the prolapse will return spontaneously after defaecation; gentle manipulation using water-soluble lubricant jelly may be required. These children should be given a high-fibre diet and taught not to strain during defaecation. More sophisticated treatment is rarely required.

In the elderly, rectal prolapse is either remarkably well tolerated or else concealed. The patient becomes accustomed to reducing the prolapse manually after defaecation and rarely complains about it. A high-fibre diet makes little difference to the problem since the anatomical defect will never recover spontaneously. If the prolapse occurs on standing or if incontinence develops, the patient is likely to require surgical treatment. Incontinence is not directly due to the prolapse but to dilatation of the internal anal sphincter by the prolapse.

MANAGEMENT OF RECTAL PROLAPSE

There are four operations commonly employed to treat rectal prolapse, two via an abdominal route and two via a perineal route. The abdominal operations include **suture fixation rectopexy**, where the rectum is mobilised and the mesorectum sutured to the sacral promontory and the presacral fascia, and **resection rectopexy**, where the rectum is mobilised and sutured in the same way, but

a sigmoid colectomy is also performed to try to prevent the constipation that often accompanies simple suture fixation. Older procedures using mesh slings or plastic foam wrappers to hitch the rectum in place are rarely used nowadays.

The popular perineal procedures include **Delorme's operation** (most common in the UK). In the USA the preferred perineal procedure is (Altemeirer's procedure). Both of these involve a perineal excision of the rectum and sigmoid colon and a colo-anal anastomosis. There is a continuing debate about which of these procedures is best with regard to functional outcome including avoiding constipation.

In the very unfit, a subcutaneous circumanal silicone rubber ring may be inserted (a modification of the old Thiersch wire procedure). This is a minor procedure but is apt to fail because the ring is too tight (causing constipation) or too loose (allowing recurrent prolapse).

ANAL AND PERIANAL NEOPLASMS

Anatomically, the anal canal is the terminal part of the large intestine; it begins at the upper surface of the anorectal ring (a palpable ring surrounding the anal canal at the upper surface of the pelvic floor) and ends at the puckered pigmented hair-bearing true skin surrounding the anus.

NEOPLASMS OF THE ANAL MARGIN

Pre-invasive carcinoma

Paget's disease of the anal margin is histologically similar to Paget's disease of the breast; it is not invariably accompanied by invasive carcinoma, although it can transform into adenocarcinoma. Paget's disease causes severe pruritus, and scaly plaque-like lesions are visible. Treatment is by wide excision. **Bowen's disease** is squamous carcinoma in situ occurring in the elderly. It presents as a brownish plaque or diffuse fleshy nodular area. About 10% of these lesions become invasive. Treatment is by wide excision.

Squamous cell and basal cell carcinoma

Carcinoma of the anal margin is a cutaneous tumour presenting as an elevated ulcer with rolled everted edges. These lesions of the anal margin occur most frequently in men and are usually well differentiated. They often present late with inguinal lymph node metastases. Treatment is by wide local excision, preserving the anal sphincters. Basal cell carcinoma in this site behaves similarly to basal cell carcinoma elsewhere; local excision is the treatment of choice.

NEOPLASMS OF THE ANAL CANAL

Squamous carcinoma of the anal canal

Squamous carcinoma of the anal canal arises from the anal transitional zone and has several different histological forms (e.g. basaloid, mucin-producing) which behave in a similar manner. The disease is uncommon and forms less than 5% of anorectal malignancies. It is mainly a disease of elderly females. The symptoms—fresh rectal bleeding, anal pain, discomfort and discharge—are similar to those of haemorrhoids and other common benign anal conditions; the patient may ignore them or the doctor may miss the diagnosis at first. Anal canal carcinoma metastasises to superior rectal as well as to inguinal lymph nodes, reflecting the mixed drainage of the anal canal. By the time of presentation, 50% already have superior rectal node metastases and 30% inguinal node metastases.

On palpation, squamous carcinoma feels hard and woody due to invasion of perianal tissues. This is in contrast to the other perianal conditions described above. Diagnosis is confirmed by proctoscopic biopsy.

Until the 1980s, the standard treatment was surgical **abdomino-perineal resection** of rectum and anus with a permanent end colostomy in the left iliac fossa. The cure rate was less than 50%. Improved results have been claimed for a non-surgical approach, employing a combination of radiotherapy and chemotherapy. The indications for surgical, oncological or combined treatment are not yet clear. Inguinal lymph node metastases developing later may be excised or treated with radiotherapy.

Malignant melanoma

The anal canal is the third most common site for malignant melanomas after the skin and the eye. They cause non-specific anal symptoms of discomfort and bleeding, and diagnosis may thus be delayed. These tumours are usually non-pigmented and need biopsy evidence to make a firm diagnosis. Melanomas in this site are extremely malignant with a cure rate of about 10% with abdomino-perineal proctectomy.

LOW RECTAL POLYPS AND CANCER

Rectal adenomas may sometimes develop a long pedicle and be dragged down into the anal canal. They may be mistaken for haemorrhoids if they appear at the anal verge. This emphasises the importance of proper investigation of patients with persistent haemorrhoid-like symptoms by palpation, proctoscopy and sigmoidoscopy. Treatment of low polyps is by excision with a diathermy snare and histological examination to check for malignancy.

Adenocarcinomas arising low in the rectum sometimes present with anal bleeding and discharge. Again, these symptoms should be properly investigated rather than dismissed as haemorrhoids.

24 Thoracic surgery

INTRODUCTION

Although most respiratory disease is managed by non-surgical methods, non-cardiac thoracic surgery includes diagnosis and management of a range of benign and malignant respiratory diseases including chest trauma, oesophageal reflux and tumours (also managed by some upper gastrointestinal surgeons), and various mediastinal disorders. This chapter deals with surgical respiratory problems and mediastinal disorders. The principles of oesophageal surgery are covered in Chapter 15 and chest trauma in Chapter 10.

INVESTIGATIVE TECHNIQUES

IMAGING

Computerised tomography (CT) of the chest offers high-resolution images of the entire lung fields in cross-section and provides quantitative information about tissue density in all parts of the chest; most pathological lesions can thus be diagnosed with a fair degree of confidence. In particular, the progress of apparently benign intrapulmonary masses can be followed accurately with serial CT scans, thus avoiding unnecessary surgical resection.

For staging bronchogenic carcinoma, CT scanning is invaluable. Positron emission tomography (PET) is being evaluated for its potential to provide improved diagnostic accuracy for intrathoracic malignancy.

LUNG FUNCTION TESTS

Formal lung function tests are mandatory before chest surgery and serve two main purposes:

- Measurement of airflow into and out of the alveoli, i.e. FEV_1, FVC, peak air flow, total lung capacity, alveolar ventilation

- Measurement of gas diffusion across the alveolar–capillary interface, i.e. tests of involving rates of diffusion of carbon monoxide

Lung function tests provide a detailed portrait of the pathophysiology of the particular chest disease and can be used to demonstrate changes over time or as a result of treatment. When surgery is contemplated, lung function tests are employed to assess ventilatory capacity to withstand chest wall incision or lung resection.

BRONCHOSCOPY

Bronchoscopy gives direct access for biopsy of lesions within the airways and, with **transbronchial biopsy**, provides access to lesions in the lung parenchyma. In many centres, diagnostic bronchoscopy is performed mainly by chest physicians using flexible instruments, with more difficult and potentially complicated cases passing to thoracic surgeons. Flexible bronchoscopy is performed under similar conditions to gastroscopy, using topical local anaesthesia and sometimes intravenous sedation.

Rigid bronchoscopy

Direct visual access to the large airways first became possible with the rigid bronchoscope. Its limitations include the need for general anaesthesia, the technical difficulty in achieving a thorough, reliable and satisfactory examination, and limited access to airways beyond lobar level. Rigid bronchoscopy remains a useful tool for certain therapeutic manoeuvres, e.g. removing inhaled foreign bodies and aspirating inspissated mucus responsible for postoperative lung or lobar collapse; the latter, however, may now best be done with a flexible bronchoscope.

Despite the popularity of rigid bronchoscopy in some centres, its use is certain to decline for most applications in the face of competition from flexible bronchoscopy.

Flexible bronchoscopy

There has been steady progress in the development of flexible bronchoscopes employing fibre optics and microchip cameras. Endoscopes have become narrower (yet with larger biopsy channels), more manoeuvrable and capable of producing better-quality colour images and instruments can be introduced using local anaesthesia or via an in situ endotracheal tube. Access can easily be achieved to the level of individual lung segments and adequate-sized biopsies obtained of masses lying within the airway or in the adjoining lung parenchyma, the latter by transbronchial needle biopsy under X-ray guidance.

PLEURAL ASPIRATION AND PERCUTANEOUS BIOPSY

In the case of pleural effusion, pleural aspiration may be performed for cytological examination using a standard wide-bore needle and syringe. Blind pleural biopsy can be performed at the same time using an **Abram's needle**. Many deeper intrathoracic masses are amenable to percutaneous biopsy under X-ray or CT guidance.

MEDIASTINOSCOPY

The mediastinoscope is used to biopsy paratracheal and sometimes subcarinal lymph nodes. The instrument is a rigid tube incorporating fibreoptic light guides; it is inserted via a skin incision above the suprasternal notch and passed caudally along the plane of the pretracheal fascia (see Fig. 24.1). The route passes close to the superior vena cava on the right, the innominate artery, the arch of the aorta and the left atrium anteriorly, the descending aorta on the left and the recurrent laryngeal nerves posterolaterally on each side. All these structures are at risk of damage and, although rare, this must be explained to the patient (and recorded as such) as part of obtaining informed consent. Mediastinoscopy gives access to the entire middle and posterior mediastinum except for the subaortic fossa (the area below the arch of the aorta which often contains lymph nodes). Access to this area is obtained by anterior mediastinotomy.

ANTERIOR MEDIASTINOTOMY

Anterior mediastinotomy (see Fig. 24.2), a form of minithoracotomy, may be used to obtain tissue from lesions in the anterior mediastinum, e.g. thymic tumour. The approach may be made to the left or right of the sternum, either intercostally or by resection of a costal cartilage. Left anterior mediastinotomy affords good access for diagnostic biopsy of masses in the subaortic fossa.

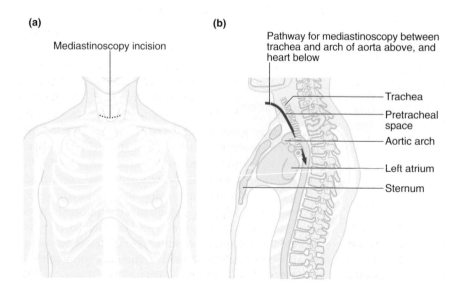

(a)

Mediastinoscopy incision

(b)

Pathway for mediastinoscopy between trachea and arch of aorta above, and heart below

- Trachea
- Pretracheal space
- Aortic arch
- Left atrium
- Sternum

Fig. 24.1 Mediastinoscopy
(a) For investigation of the posterior mediastinum. **(b)** Sagittal section.

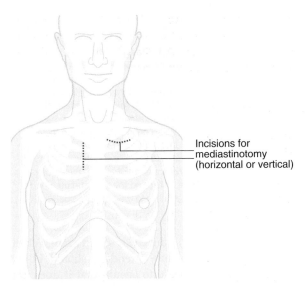

Incisions for
mediastinotomy
(horizontal or vertical)

Fig. 24.2 Mediastinotomy

THORACOTOMY

Thoracotomy, described on p. 335, gives full access for biopsy of paratracheal, subcarinal and hilar lymph node groups, the great vessels, oesophagus, lung and pericardium and is used when less invasive procedures are inappropriate or have failed. Immediate examination of frozen sections of specimens taken during surgery is often helpful in determining the extent of surgery required and the completeness of resection achieved.

THERAPEUTIC PROCEDURES

PROBLEMS AFFECTING THE PLEURAL SPACE

Between the chest wall and the lung is a potential space, the pleural cavity, lined by mesothelium. Pleura lining the chest wall is known as **parietal pleura** and that covering the lung as **visceral pleura**. The pleural space normally contains a minute amount of serous fluid which lubricates the movement of the opposed shiny pleural surfaces and causes them to adhere by surface tension. This, and the negative pressure that would result if the surfaces were separated, keep the lungs expanded. Disease or injury may result in accumulation within the pleural cavity of air (**pneumothorax**), fluid (**pleural effusion**), pus (**empyema**) or blood (**haemothorax**), causing potentially serious (or even fatal) disturbances of respiratory and, in some cases, cardiovascular function. Pus in the pleural cavity, as in any other location, must be drained before infection can be controlled.

The basic principles of pleural drainage are illustrated by the management of pneumothorax. The management of pleural effusion, empyema and haemothorax involves variations of the technique to accommodate the particular pathologies of such fluid collections.

PNEUMOTHORAX

Spontaneous pneumothorax usually results from rupture of a bulla on the pleural surface of the lung. This is a congenital air-filled cavity which communicates with the bronchial tree. Rupture causes air to escape into the pleural space and the lung to collapse. **Traumatic pneumothorax** usually results from blunt chest injury, often as a result of rib fractures penetrating the visceral pleura. Sharp chest injury, e.g. stab wounds, may also be responsible. Different types of pneumothorax are illustrated in Figure 24.3.

A pneumothorax requires treatment under the following circumstances:

● When the lung volume is compromised by more than about 25% as calculated on a PA chest X-ray
● If the pneumothorax is increasing in size
● When a small pneumothorax is having a disproportionate effect on lung function because of pre-existing lung disease
● Where there is a tension pneumothorax

Sometimes the site of air leakage acts as a one-way valve, creating a **tension pneumothorax**. The valve effect allows air to escape into the pleural space but not to return to the airway, causing collapse of the lung on the affected side. Rising intrapleural tension pushes the mediastinum towards the opposite side, compressing and compromising the contralateral lung and obstructing systemic venous return. The physiological upset is extreme and poses an immediate threat to life so the condition must be treated urgently.

Treatment of pneumothorax

Aspiration

An uncomplicated pneumothorax in an otherwise fit patient can often be treated by aspiration. A 20 ml syringe

329

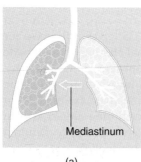
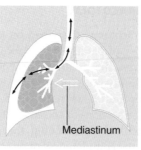
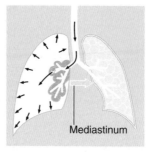
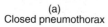

(a)
Closed pneumothorax

(b)
Open pneumothorax

(c)
Tension pneumothorax

Fig. 24.3 Classification of pneumothorax
(a) In closed pneumothorax the pleural defect closes spontaneously, leaving a fixed amount of air in the pleural space. **(b)** In open pneumothorax there is free passage of air via an open defect in the visceral pleura. **(c)** In tension pneumothorax the pleural defect acts as a flap valve allowing progressive entry of air into the pleural space, collapsing the lung and pushing the mediastinum to the opposite side.

is connected to a three-way tap and a needle. The needle is inserted into the pneumothorax via an intercostal approach and 20 ml of air aspirated. The tap is turned to exclude the needle and the air evacuated from the syringe. This is repeated until no more air can be withdrawn. Progress is monitored by chest X-ray. The process can be repeated, but formal tube drainage may become necessary if the pneumothorax continues to recur.

In the case of tension pneumothorax, rapid emergency relief can be obtained by plunging a large needle into the pleural space via an intercostal space. However, a formal apical chest drain must be inserted soon afterwards.

Intercostal tube drainage
The technique of intercostal chest drainage is described in Box 24.1 and Figure 24.4; see also Figure 24.5. For treatment of a pneumothorax, a single apical drain is used which may be of small size, e.g. 16F gauge.

Intercostal tube drains must be connected to an apparatus which prevents lung collapse due to air refluxing into the chest as a result of negative intrapleural pressure. The usual mechanism is to connect a tube from the drain into a water bottle such that the end of the tube is below the water level so as to form an underwater seal. The bottle is placed below the level of the patient so that gravity creates a small vacuum. As the patient breathes, excess air and fluid in the pleural space are gradually expelled into the bottle and air bubbles out of the exhaust tube. If there is an air leak from the lung via a breach in the visceral pleura, this is manifest by continued bubbling in the bottle and failure of the lung to expand. Suction should then be applied to the outlet of the underwater seal for a few days; this usually enables the lung to expand and adhere to the chest wall, thereby remaining inflated and blocking the site of the air leak.

Patients with intercostal drains must be transported with care to prevent reflux of fluid into the chest. At one time it was recommended that chest tubes should be clamped when patients were to be moved but this advice is now rarely given. If drainage tubes are clamped, the drain fails to function and lung collapse can occur. When a patient is transported, one attendant should be in charge of the drainage bottle to ensure that it does not tip over and that it always remains below the level of the patient.

Intercostal drains are removed when their purpose is complete. In all cases the lung must be fully expanded. For pneumothorax, cessation of bubbling in the bottle for 24 hours is an indication for removal; for fluid drainage, the duration varies according to the underlying problem.

Treatment of persistent or recurrent pneumothorax
More extensive surgical intervention may be required for persistent or recurrent pneumothorax. Approaches

---

KEY POINTS

Box 24.1 Technique of intercostal tube drainage of chest

- Make a 2 cm incision near the upper border of the rib and parallel to it
- Bluntly dissect the intercostal muscles down to the parietal pleura with artery forceps. Stay near the upper border of the rib to avoid intercostal vessels
- Palpate the lung with a gloved index finger to free adhesions and ensure free entry for the drain
- Remove the trocar from a large-bore chest drain tube (at least 28F gauge). Grasp the distal end with artery forceps and guide the drain into the chest in an apical or a basal direction according to purpose. *Never* insert a chest drain with the trocar in position as this is highly dangerous
- Attach the drain to an underwater seal and suture the drain to the chest wall. Snug the skin around the drain with a purse string suture. Apply an airtight dressing around the tube and tape the tube to the chest wall. Sit the patient up to 45°
- Take a chest X-ray to confirm the position of the tube

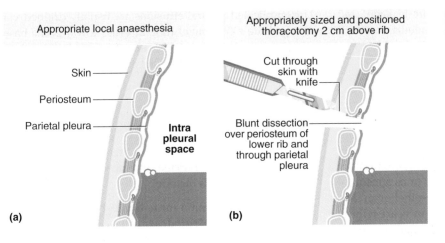

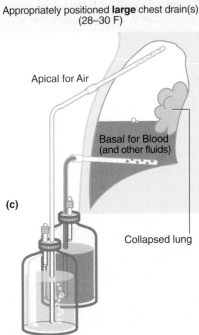

Fig. 24.4 Technique of intercostal tube drainage of chest
(a) Three structures with somatic sensory innervation. **(b)** After thoracotomy a finger should pass easily into the intrapleural space. **(c)** Chest drains should always be attached to an underwater seal. Note: A small diameter can be employed for pneumothorax alone.

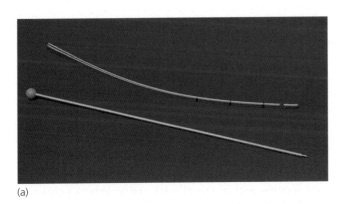

(a)

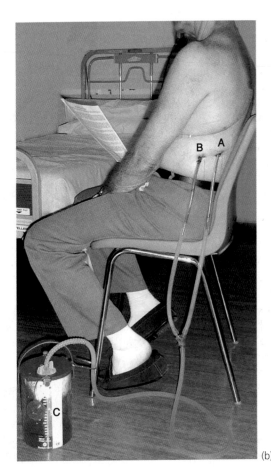

Fig. 24.5 Chest drain
(a) 30 F gauge tube (10 mm) with stylet removed (and thrown away!). Note the radiopaque line and the side holes near the tip. **(b)** Post thoracotomy and lobar resection of lung for cancer. This patient has two chest drains in situ, and **A**pical drain for Air and a **B**asal drain for Blood. Both are connected to an underwater seal, **C**, to prevent inflow of air that would cause a pneumothorax.

(b)

331

include stapling of bullae to prevent air leakage, and pleurectomy, which causes the visceral pleura to attach permanently to the bare chest wall (see Fig. 24.6).

EXCESS PLEURAL FLUID

There is normally a very small amount of fluid lying between visceral and parietal pleura. This may substantially increase in response to lung disorders secondarily affecting the pleura (e.g. infection, inflammation, primary lung cancers, metastatic cancer of breast) or as a result of primary pleural disorders such as mesothelioma. The fluid may be a watery transudate (e.g. in heart failure) or an exudate of variable viscosity (e.g. due to pleural infection). Indications for draining a pleural effusion include:

- **Diagnostic**
  — empyema
  — suspected malignancy
  — traumatic haemothorax
- **Therapeutic**
  — removing the compressive effects of a large pleural fluid collection on the lung
  — draining pus from an empyema
  — arresting haemorrhage from damaged intercostal vessels causing haemothorax

Uncomplicated pleural effusions are usually drained via a large-bore (30F guage) tube inserted towards the base of the pleural cavity in the most practical dependant position. If the fluid collections are loculated, more than one drain may be required.

Malignant effusions

Malignant effusions (e.g. from breast cancer) usually recur after simple drainage and need to be treated in other ways. Methods include:

- Stimulating **adhesion formation** between visceral and parietal pleura (**pleurodesis**). This can be achieved by aspirating the fluid, injecting an irritant such as tetracycline and maintaining tube drainage until permanent adhesions have developed. An alternative is to perform **pleural abrasion**. Via a small thoracotomy, the parietal pleura is widely abraded using a surgical swab. Again, chest drainage allows adhesions to form between the two layers of pleura with permanent prevention of effusion. This and the following technique both obliterate the pleural space
- **Parietal pleurectomy**. This open thoracotomy operation involves the stripping of the parietal pleura which results in diffuse adhesion of the lung surface to the chest wall (see Fig. 24.6)
- **Pleuro-peritoneal shunting** using a tubular device connecting the two cavities. This is implanted beneath the skin and incorporates a one-way valve. The pleural fluid is then reabsorbed via the abdominal peritoneum. This may be the treatment of choice in patients with a short life expectancy

EMPYEMA

When pleural fluid becomes infected, pus accumulates in a loculus within the pleural cavity; this is known as an **empyema**. In the early stages, an empyema can be treated by dependent intercostal tube drainage with irrigation if necessary; early loculi may respond to treatment with urokinase. In chronic cases, a thick fibrous wall or **cortex** gradually forms around the pus-filled space. Treatment options then include prolonged closed tube drainage or open tube drainage involving removal of a segment of rib, and surgical 'decortication' of the entire abscess wall (see Fig. 24.7). This releases the tethered chest wall and diaphragm and allows the lung to re-expand.

HAEMOTHORAX

Following chest trauma, blood may accumulate in the pleural space. This is usually drained via two large

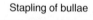

Stapling of bullae

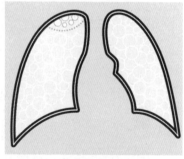

Pleurectomy

Visceral pleura ———

Removal of the parietal pleura of upper half of affected pleural space ———

Parietal pleura ———

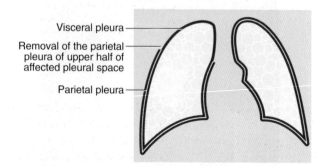

Fig. 24.6 Surgical approaches for treatment of persistent pneumothorax

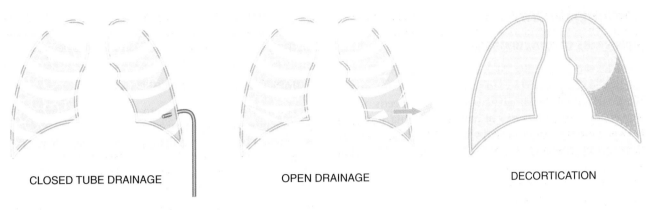

CLOSED TUBE DRAINAGE   OPEN DRAINAGE   DECORTICATION

Fig. 24.7 Treatment of empyema thoracis
(a) Closed tube drainage. **(b)** Open drainage—a segment of rib is removed and a red rubber tube inserted. **(c)** Decortication—the 'abscess' wall of the empyema is removed.

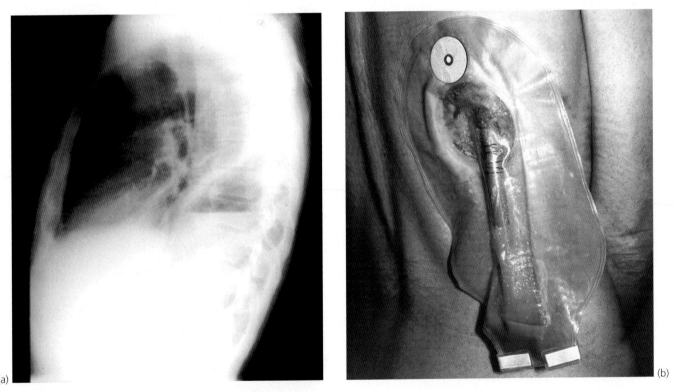

(a)   (b)

Fig. 24.8 Empyema thoracis
This 51-year-old man underwent a thoraco-abdominal oesophagogastrectomy for proximal gastric cancer. He suffered a small intrathoracic anastomotic leak and developed an intrapleural empyema, shown by the fluid level in **(a)**. **(b)** Drainage of empyema. A section of rib overlying the cavity is resected and a large red rubber tube inserted to give dependent drainage into a bag. The drain is gradually shortened as the cavity closes. This patient was alive and well 15 years later.

drains, one apically and one basally located. A similar strategy is employed after open chest surgery. However, recently clotted blood will not drain successfully and thoracotomy may be required. Later, clot liquefies and may be removed by drainage. Removing blood allows the lung to expand against the chest wall and helps to arrest continuing haemorrhage from intercostal vessels. Persistent or increasing drainage of blood indicates continuing intrathoracic bleeding which often necessitates surgical intervention. Continued bleeding is usually from the systemic circulation (e.g. intercostal or great vessels) rather than from the lung parenchyma.

TRACHEOSTOMY

PRINCIPLES OF TRACHEOSTOMY

A tracheostomy (see Fig. 24.9) is an artificial opening into the trachea and is performed to provide a secure airway when the pharyngeal airway or larynx needs to be bypassed. With time, an epithelialised fistula develops between the skin and trachea which allows tracheostomy tubes to be changed and the airways cleaned without difficulty.

Indications for tracheostomy include:

- Permanent functional obstruction of the upper airway, e.g. carcinoma of larynx
- Temporary or potential upper airway obstruction, e.g. facial fractures, major head and neck operations
- Patients requiring long-term ventilatory support; prolonged endotracheal intubation is likely to cause permanent laryngeal damage and prevent swallowing and speech. Tracheostomy also provides continuous access to the lower airways for bronchial toilet

Tracheostomy should be a planned procedure performed in the operating room under general anaesthesia. It is not an emergency procedure for patients with upper airway obstruction. For these patients endotracheal intubation or cricothyroidotomy (see Fig. 24.10) should be used.

COMPLICATIONS OF TRACHEOSTOMY

- **Haemorrhage** caused by erosion of the innominate (brachiocephalic) artery
- **Tracheo-oesophageal fistula**, particularly where a nasogastric tube is in place
- **Displacement of the tracheostomy tube** may occur before the 'fistula' is established, making it difficult to reintubate the trachea
- **Tracheal stenosis**, usually the result of prolonged use of a high-pressure cuff

THORACOTOMY

POSTEROLATERAL THORACOTOMY

Posterolateral thoracotomy is the standard approach for lung and oesophageal resections as well as for surgery of the descending aorta. The incision is sited below the

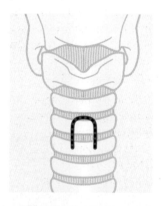
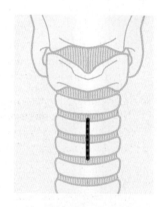
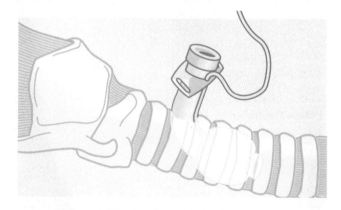

(a)   Bjork flap tracheostomy   Vertical incision in trachea   Tracheostomy tube in situ

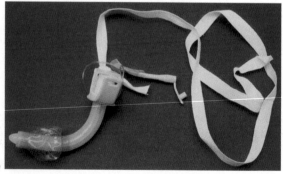
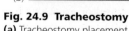
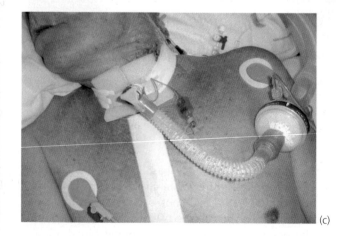

(b)   (c)

Fig. 24.9 Tracheostomy

(a) Tracheostomy placement.. (b) Disposable tracheostomy tube. Note distal balloon which is inflated via the small tube to provide a snug fit inside the trachea. (c) Patient being ventilated via an elective tracheostomy after cardiac surgery.

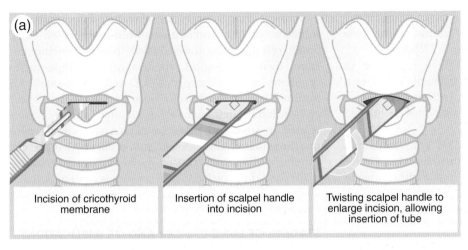
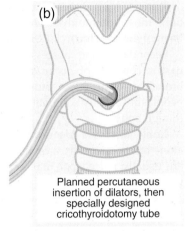

(a) Incision of cricothyroid membrane | Insertion of scalpel handle into incision | Twisting scalpel handle to enlarge incision, allowing insertion of tube

(b) Planned percutaneous insertion of dilators, then specially designed cricothyroidotomy tube

Fig. 24.10 Cricothyroidotomy
(a) In a dire emergency, this life-saving procedure can be rapidly employed to gain time. **(b)** Modern mini-cricothyroidotomy can be performed percutaneously by making a small incision through the cricothyroid membrane and progressively dilating it with graded dilators before insertion of a specially constructed small-diameter tube, e.g. Minitrach or Quicktrach. These are used in accident victims and often in intensive care units.

inferior angle of the scapula, latissimus dorsi is divided and the chest is entered through the bed of the (unresected) fifth or sixth rib. If necessary, the incision can be extended into the abdomen (thoraco-abdominal incision) so that the operative field extends above and below the diaphragm, e.g. for oesophago-gastrectomy or thoraco-abdominal aortic aneurysm.

LATERAL THORACOTOMY

Lateral thoracotomy involves an incision extending between anterior and posterior axillary lines. It is used for limited access, most often for surgical treatment of pneumothorax.

ANTERIOR THORACOTOMY

This is used for diagnostic biopsy (p. 329). It is less likely to cause post-thoracotomy neuralgia than other thoracotomy approaches.

THORACOSCOPY

This is the thoracic equivalent of laparoscopy or 'keyhole' surgery and is sometimes known as **video-assisted thoracotomy**. Rigid instruments for viewing and operating are inserted through small incisions in the chest wall and the image is displayed on a monitor so that the whole team can view the procedure.

As with laparoscopic surgery, these techniques are evolving and being evaluated and the indications and contraindications are gradually emerging. For some applications, such as thoraco-dorsal sympathectomy and pleural biopsy, thoracoscopy is the treatment of choice, whilst for others, e.g. lobar resection, hiatus hernia repair, further appraisal is needed.

Disadvantages of thoracoscopic techniques include:

● Thoracoscopic operations often take much longer than equivalent open procedures (e.g. pleurodesis, pleurectomy, stapling of apical bullae)
● The completeness of thoracoscopic excision of malignant lesions is difficult to evaluate
● Post-thoracotomy neuralgia may also complicate thoracoscopy incisions

MEDIAN STERNOTOMY

Median sternotomy or 'sternal split' gives wide access to the heart and the entire anterior mediastinum including the great vessels. It is the standard incision for coronary artery bypass surgery as well as for excision of thymic lesions and retrosternal parathyroid tumours and, occasionally, resection of a goitre with massive retrosternal extension.

SPECIFIC THORACIC DISORDERS

LUNG ABSCESS

Lung abscesses have become much less common with effective antibiotic treatment of pulmonary infections.

Onset of symptoms may be insidious with clinical features including a swinging pyrexia, foul-smelling sputum and the finding of a cavitating shadow on chest X-ray.

Primary lung abscess may follow bacterial lung infection, most commonly with *Staphylococcus aureus*, beta haemolytic streptococci, *Pseudomonas or Klebsiella*.

Secondary lung abscess may follow aspiration of gastric contents or occur in lung segments distal to a bronchial obstruction caused by a centrally placed neoplasm (usually squamous cell carcinoma) or inhaled foreign body.

Lung abscesses are usually treated with antibiotics alone but occasionally a cavity requires drainage. Drains are usually placed percutaneously under ultrasound or CT guidance.

CANCER OF THE LUNG

Lung cancers arise as primary bronchogenic tumours or as metastatic deposits from cancers elsewhere in the body. Of the primary tumours, only 20% will not have metastasised by the time of presentation. Lymph nodes in the hilar area are usually involved first, followed by other mediastinal nodes. Bone and brain are common sites of distant metastatic spread and may be responsible for initial presentation.

Primary lung cancers are classified into **small cell tumours** (10–15%) and **non-small cell tumours** (85–90%). Small cell tumours (often called 'oat-cell carcinomas' from their histological appearance) are thought to originate from pulmonary APUD cells. Non-small cell tumours are derived from bronchopulmonary tissues and include squamous cell carcinoma (almost always related to smoking), adenocarcinoma and large cell or undifferentiated carcinomas, and broncho-alveolar cell tumours. Many lung cancers grow rapidly and assessment should not be delayed if surgery is contemplated.

STAGING OF LUNG CANCER AND ITS IMPLICATIONS

TNM staging of lung cancer is fundamental to planning appropriate treatment. The staging system follows the general TNM pattern described on page 100 and is shown in Figure 24.11.

In staging bronchogenic carcinoma, CT scanning is invaluable. Intravenous injections of contrast improve its reliability by enabling blood vessels to be discriminated reliably from lymph nodes. The likelihood of enlarged lymph nodes being malignant increases with size, from

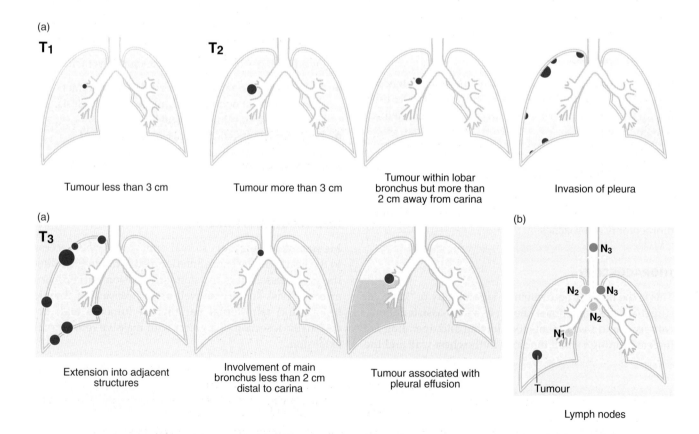

(a)

T_1 T_2

Tumour less than 3 cm   Tumour more than 3 cm   Tumour within lobar bronchus but more than 2 cm away from carina   Invasion of pleura

(a)

T_3

Extension into adjacent structures   Involvement of main bronchus less than 2 cm distal to carina   Tumour associated with pleural effusion

(b)

N_3

N_2 N_3

N_2

N_1

Tumour

Lymph nodes

Fig. 24.11 Tumour staging using the TNM classification
(a) Tumour size and extent. **(b)** Lymph node involvement.

7% for nodes less than 1 cm in diameter to 40% for nodes 1–2 cm in diameter and 66% for nodes larger than 2 cm.

The role of surgery in the management of lung cancer varies according to the type of tumour, the known responsiveness of the tumour type to other therapies (i.e. radiotherapy and chemotherapy), the general state of respiratory function and the age and fitness of the patient for major surgery. As a general principle, surgery is reserved for patients who are potentially curable. Surgery usually involves removing one or more affected lung lobes (**lobectomy**) or the whole lung (**pneumonectomy**), sometimes with resection of involved chest wall.

For carcinoma in nodal stage N_0 (no nodal involvement) or N_1 (metastasis to ipsilateral hilar or peribronchial nodes only) with no known distant metastases (M_0), excising the primary tumour and local nodes by lobectomy or pneumonectomy (with or without chest wall resection) gives a 5-year survival of about 50%. N_2 disease is diagnosed when there are metastases to ipsilateral mediastinal or subcarinal lymph nodes or both. When diagnosed preoperatively (e.g. by mediastinoscopy and biopsy), complete resection is possible in less than 10% of patients and 5-year survival following resection is only 2%.

N_3 disease is defined by metastases in contralateral mediastinal lymph nodes, scalene or supraclavicular lymph nodes. If N_2 or N_3 disease (or M_1 disease with distant metastases) is confirmed during initial staging, the results of surgery are so poor that it is rarely offered and other methods of palliation need to be considered. If preoperative staging of mediastinal lymph nodes is negative but N_2 disease is discovered at thoracotomy (occult N_2 disease), 50% of patients can undergo a histologically complete resection and this subgroup would expect a 5-year survival of 30%.

For disease too advanced for useful surgery, radiotherapy can increase life expectancy and provide effective palliation for troublesome complications such as lobar collapse, haemoptysis, superior vena caval obstruction or symptomatic metastases in brain or bone. Radiotherapy has also proved useful for managing symptomatic tumour recurrence after surgery. The role of adjuvant chemotherapy in treating lung cancer is currently under scrutiny.

SURGICAL TREATMENT OF LUNG CANCER

Surgical treatment of lung cancer involves wide resection of the primary cancer with sampling of loco-regional (mediastinal) lymph nodes to establish accurate TNM staging. Accurate pathological staging of the surgical specimen influences the decision to employ adjuvant chemotherapy or radiotherapy.

The standard surgical approach is via a postero-lateral thoracotomy. For lobectomy, one or more lobes are excised. Both lungs have three 'surgical' lobes; the right has upper, middle and lower lobes, the left has upper, lingular and lower lobes. For pneumonectomy, the entire lung is removed.

The empty thoracic space left by resection is soon taken up by hyperinflation of the remaining lung tissue, mediastinal shift and elevation of the hemidiaphragm.

Apart from treatment of malignant disease, indications for lung resection include:

● **Trauma**—major sharp injury to a lobe or lung, or cases of blunt trauma where a bronchus has been ruptured
● **Infection**—consequences of infection including bleeding due to bronchiectasis or secondary fungal infection of a persistent, antibiotically 'sterilised' abscess cavity
● **Benign tumours**—if curative excision via bronchotomy is impracticable
● **Lung transplantation**—transplantation of a single lung is sometimes performed for non-malignant disease when there is minimal respiratory reserve and one lung is significantly more affected than the other. Bilateral lung transplantation is performed in patients with lung diseases involving infection, e.g. cystic fibrosis or bronchiectasis. Heart–lung transplantation is offered when both lungs are irreparably damaged by cardiovascular disease, e.g. severe pulmonary hypertension (see Ch. 4)

DISORDERS OF THE MEDIASTINUM

Disorders of the mediastinum of surgical importance are summarised in Figure 24.12.

ANTERIOR MEDIASTINUM

Retrosternal thyroid

Rarely, the thyroid gland is ectopically located in the anterior mediastinum where it may become enlarged by any of the processes discussed in Chapter 42. Alternatively, an inferior extension of a normally located thyroid gland may spread retrosternally into the anterior mediastinum as a result of similar pathological changes. The adverse effects of retrosternal thyroid enlargement are usually related to progressive displacement of the trachea. Sudden enlargement of restrosternal thyroid tissue caused by haemorrhage can threaten the airway. Most retrosternal thyroids can be removed through a standard thyroidectomy collar incision and only rarely is a median sternotomy required.

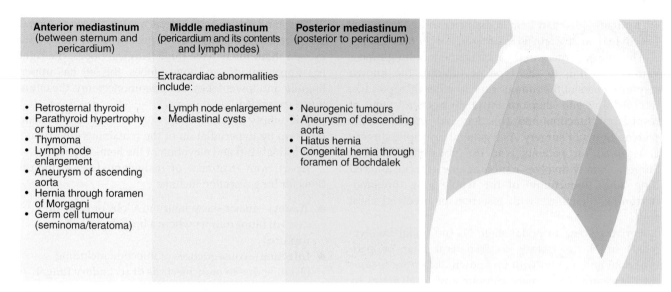

Anterior mediastinum (between sternum and pericardium)	**Middle mediastinum** (pericardium and its contents and lymph nodes)	**Posterior mediastinum** (posterior to pericardium)
	Extracardiac abnormalities include:	
• Retrosternal thyroid • Parathyroid hypertrophy or tumour • Thymoma • Lymph node enlargement • Aneurysm of ascending aorta • Hernia through foramen of Morgagni • Germ cell tumour (seminoma/teratoma)	• Lymph node enlargement • Mediastinal cysts	• Neurogenic tumours • Aneurysm of descending aorta • Hiatus hernia • Congenital hernia through foramen of Bochdalek

Fig. 24.12 Disorders of the mediastinum

Thymus

The thymus causes few pathological problems with the exception of the rare thymic tumour (**thymoma**) which may be benign or malignant. Distinguishing between the two is difficult on histological grounds and diagnosis has to be based on morphological characteristics, such as the presence of a capsule. For malignant thymomas, surgical excision is the only treatment and achieves a 5-year survival rate of about 65%.

Myasthenia gravis is an unusual clinical condition associated with certain thymic tumours or thymic hyperplasia. After thymectomy, the paroxysmal fatigue of myasthenia is usually improved and the need for anticholinesterase therapy reduced. However, the symptoms are rarely completely eliminated.

Parathyroid

Benign and malignant parathyroid tumours usually occur in the neck but may occasionally occur anywhere between the retrothyroid area and the arch of the aorta. If retrosternal lesions are suspected, exploration of the anterior mediastinum accompanied by thymectomy permits the abnormal parathyroid tissue to be removed.

MIDDLE MEDIASTINUM

This contains the pericardium and hila of both lungs. Disorders requiring surgical intervention include:

● **Lymph node enlargement**—bronchogenic malignancy or lymphoma are the most common causes. Tumour type may be defined by biopsy and the extent by CT scanning

● **Aneurysms**—those of the ascending aorta or the arch of the aorta are usually degenerative but may also appear as a late complication of aortic trauma or dissection. Syphilitic aneurysm is now rare
● **Developmental cysts**—these include pericardial, bronchogenic, enterogenous and cysts of uncertain origin. Mediastinal cysts occasionally become infected and even more rarely undergo malignant change
● **Germ cell tumours**—primary or secondary teratoma or seminoma occasionally occur. These tumours are diagnosed by histology or raised serum markers and can usually be treated successfully with chemotherapy

POSTERIOR MEDIASTINUM

The posterior mediastinum lies behind the pericardium. Surgery may be required for the following conditions:

● **Aneurysms of the descending aorta**
● **Benign tumours of neurological origin**—these may be bilobed and extend into the spinal canal
● **Diaphragmatic hernia**—hiatus hernia is common but is not always associated with gastric reflux. Most sliding hernias can now be treated with acid-reducing drugs, weight loss and other simple advice (see Ch. 15). The more unusual **para-oesophageal** or **rolling hiatus hernia** may lead to gastric infarction and many believe its presence is an indication for surgery. Congenital herniation into the posterior mediastinum (**hernia of Bochdalek**) is very rare. Discussion continues as to whether hiatus hernias requiring surgery should be approached from above or below the diaphragm

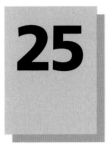

25 Diagnosis of problems in the groin and scrotum

INTRODUCTION

This chapter describes the clinical presentation and diagnosis of lumps and swellings in the groin and scrotum. The specific conditions causing these problems along with their management are covered in the following two chapters.

Groin lumps and swellings account for about 10% of general surgical outpatient referrals. In both sexes, the commonest lumps in the groin are **hernias**, either inguinal or femoral. Both are caused by abdominal contents protruding through defects in the abdominal wall. In the male, the testis descends into the scrotum via the inguinal canal, and this area remains potentially weak throughout life; inguinal hernias are therefore more common in males. If large, an **inguinal hernia** may present as a scrotal lump rather than a groin lump. In the female, the uterine round ligament pursues a course similar to the spermatic cord in the male; this explains the occasional occurrence of inguinal hernias in females. The femoral canal, below the inguinal ligament, is another potential weakness in the abdominal wall and may give rise to a **femoral hernia**.

Enlarged lymph nodes due to infection or malignancy also cause groin lumps or swellings. Less common are vascular abnormalities such as a **saphena varix** or a **femoral artery aneurysm**. Very rarely nowadays, a **psoas abscess** may track beneath the inguinal ligament to present in the groin. This used to be a complication of tuberculous disease of the spine but is now more commonly a result of colon-related sepsis.

The embryology and anatomy of the groin, testis and perineum provide a good starting point for understanding many surgical problems in this area and are explained in Figures 25.1–25.5.

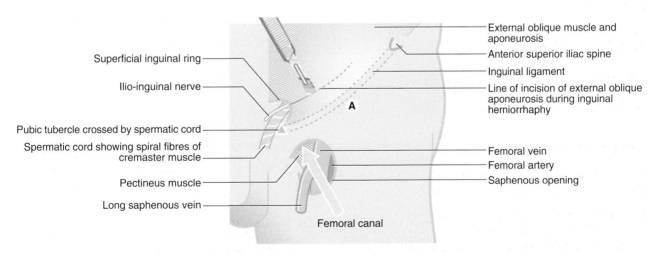

Fig. 25.1 Structure of the inguinal and femoral canals
A is the surface marking of the femoral pulse, midway between the pubic symphysis and the anterior superior iliac spine; the deep ring lies 2.5 cm above it.

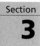

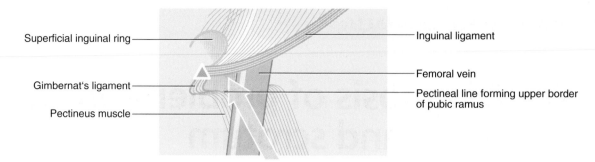

Superficial inguinal ring —⎯ Inguinal ligament

Gimbernat's ligament —⎯ Femoral vein

Pectineus muscle —⎯ Pectineal line forming upper border of pubic ramus

Fig. 25.2 Structure of the femoral canal
The abdominal opening seen from below.

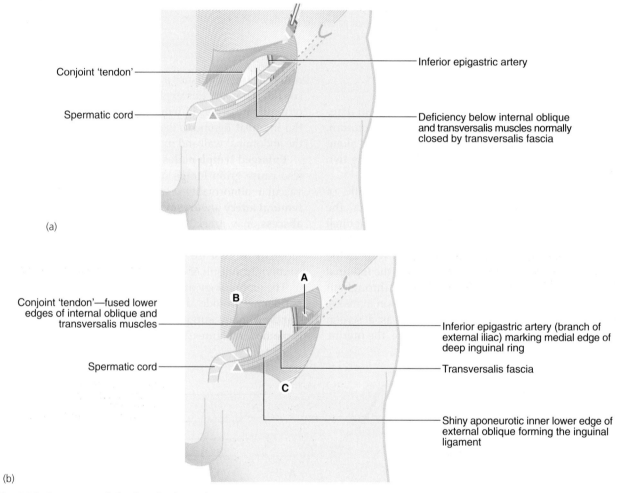

Conjoint 'tendon' —⎯ Inferior epigastric artery

Spermatic cord —⎯ Deficiency below internal oblique and transversalis muscles normally closed by transversalis fascia

(a)

Conjoint 'tendon'—fused lower edges of internal oblique and transversalis muscles —⎯ Inferior epigastric artery (branch of external iliac) marking medial edge of deep inguinal ring

Spermatic cord —⎯ Transversalis fascia

A
B
C

⎯ Shiny aponeurotic inner lower edge of external oblique forming the inguinal ligament

(b)

Fig. 25.3 Structure of the inguinal canal
(a) Inguinal canal displayed by opening the anterior wall (external oblique aponeurosis). **(b)** Inguinal canal with the spermatic cord removed. **A** is the proximal end of the spermatic cord where it leaves the deep inguinal ring. **B** and **C** are the upper and lower edges of the incised external oblique reflected to show the inguinal canal.

Testicular tumours are usually of germ cell origin; they are relatively uncommon but important not least because curative treatment is now available for most of them. The lymphatic drainage of the testis (to the intra-abdominal nodes) is different from that of the scrotal skin (towards the inguinal nodes) and is determined by the embryology of testicular descent.

When pain in the groin or scrotum is the main presenting symptom, the usual cause is a newly developed inguinal hernia, a strangulated inguinal or femoral

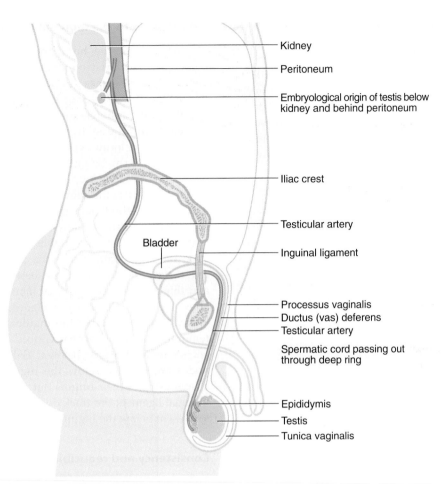

Kidney

Peritoneum

Embryological origin of testis below
kidney and behind peritoneum

Iliac crest

Testicular artery

Bladder

Inguinal ligament

Processus vaginalis
Ductus (vas) deferens
Testicular artery

Spermatic cord passing out
through deep ring

Epididymis
Testis
Tunica vaginalis

Fig. 25.4 Embryological descent of the testis
The testicular artery marks the line of descent of the testis towards the scrotum. In the embryo, the arterial supply is direct from the aorta, and
this persists even when the testis has reached the scrotum.

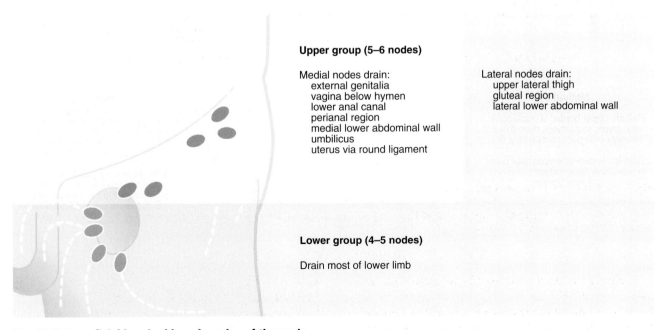

Upper group (5–6 nodes)

Medial nodes drain:
external genitalia
vagina below hymen
lower anal canal
perianal region
medial lower abdominal wall
umbilicus
uterus via round ligament

Lateral nodes drain:
upper lateral thigh
gluteal region
lateral lower abdominal wall

Lower group (4–5 nodes)

Drain most of lower limb

Fig. 25.5 Superficial inguinal lymph nodes of the groin
The lower group lie around the termination of the long saphenous vein. Both upper and lower groups drain to the external iliac nodes.

hernia, an acute infection of the scrotal contents or testicular torsion. All but the first of these are acute surgical emergencies.

Disorders of the penis (other than problems with the foreskin) are uncommon in adults; the most serious is carcinoma. In children, penile disorders are either developmental or minor inflammatory conditions; these are discussed in Chapter 45. Disorders of the female genitalia are usually seen by gynaecologists and are not covered here.

LUMPS IN THE GROIN

Lumps in the groin or scrotum may or may not be painful. The groin and scrotum must both be examined when either is swollen to discover the anatomical origin of the swelling. The patient must be examined both lying and standing to avoid missing an inguinal hernia which reduces spontaneously or a varicocoele which empties when the patient is supine.

CLINICAL EXAMINATION

Lumps in the groin are examined in the same way as lumps elsewhere but there are two special points to note as follows:

- The relationship of the groin lump to the inguinal ligament
- The consistency and reducibility of the lump

Relationship to the inguinal ligament

The position of the lump in relation to the inguinal ligament should first be identified. The ligament is not visible but stretches between two palpable bony prominences: the **anterior superior iliac spine** laterally and the **pubic tubercle** medially (see Fig. 25.1). Usually, the iliac spine is easy to find but the pubic tubercle can be difficult to locate, especially in obese patients. The pubic tubercle can be found by palpating outwards from the midline along the upper border of the pubic symphysis (care is needed as the spermatic cord can be tender). This is a better method than invaginating the scrotum with the index finger from below (see Fig. 25.6).

The pubic tubercle is higher than might be imagined from the skin contour, and the inguinal ligament does not correspond to the crease between lower abdomen and thigh. Rather, the inguinal ligament is 2 cm or more above the crease. As shown in Figure 25.7, inguinal hernias always originate above the inguinal ligament, whereas femoral hernias, saphena varices and femoral artery aneurysms always arise below it. Enlarged inguinal lymph nodes are usually below the inguinal ligament. Psoas abscesses have their origins out of reach well above the inguinal ligament but track down within the psoas sheath to present below the inguinal ligament.

Consistency and reducibility

The consistency and reducibility of a groin lump can be useful diagnostic features. Hernias are usually soft but

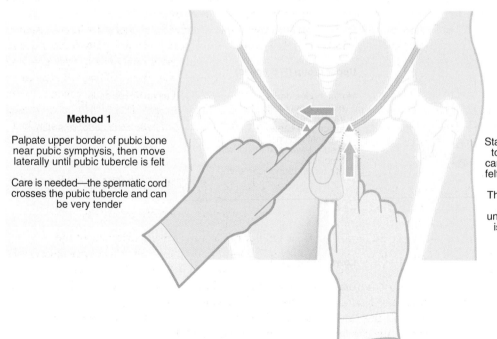

Method 1

Palpate upper border of pubic bone near pubic symphysis, then move laterally until pubic tubercle is felt

Care is needed—the spermatic cord crosses the pubic tubercle and can be very tender

Method 2

Starting low in the scrotum anterior to testis, invaginate scrotal skin carefully until the pubic tubercle is felt on upper border of pubic bone

This gives very good palpation of the tubercle but can be uncomfortable for the patient and is therefore not recommended

Fig. 25.6 Digital palpation of the pubic tubercle

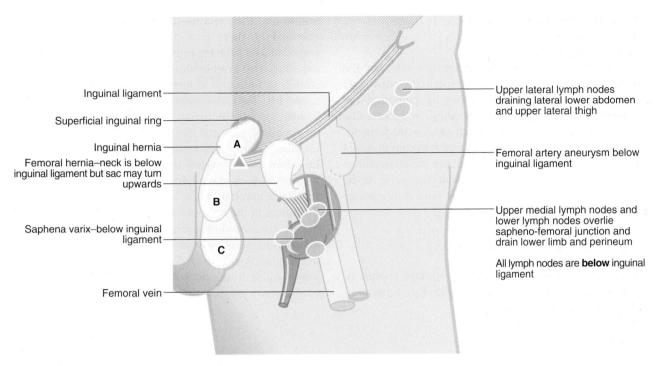

Inguinal ligament

Superficial inguinal ring

Inguinal hernia

Femoral hernia–neck is below inguinal ligament but sac may turn upwards

Saphena varix–below inguinal ligament

Femoral vein

Upper lateral lymph nodes draining lateral lower abdomen and upper lateral thigh

Femoral artery aneurysm below inguinal ligament

Upper medial lymph nodes and lower lymph nodes overlie sapheno-femoral junction and drain lower limb and perineum

All lymph nodes are **below** inguinal ligament

Fig. 25.7 Significance of the relationship of groin lumps to the inguinal ligament
A, **B** and **C** are stages in the enlargement of an indirect inguinal hernia. Note that the neck is above the inguinal ligament. A direct inguinal hernia enlarges forwards in position **A**.

the most reliable diagnostic sign is whether the lump reduces spontaneously when the patient lies flat or reduces with gentle manipulation. Most inguinal hernias are at least partly reducible, although longstanding hernias gradually become irreducible because of adhesions within the sac. These are said to be **incarcerated**. Another characteristic of an inguinal hernia is a palpable **expansile impulse** when the patient coughs. If bowel is present within (and the hernia is not strangulated), auscultation will reveal bowel sounds. In contrast, femoral hernias are usually irreducible and have no cough impulse since the femoral canal is so narrow. Bowel sounds are not heard unless the hernial orifice is so large as to admit a large and reducible mass of bowel. This is rare, however.

Distinguishing between direct and indirect inguinal hernias may be clinically difficult and is of little practical importance. Despite this, it is a useful exercise in eliciting clinical signs and frequently comes up in student examinations! The patient's age is perhaps the most useful indicator of the type of inguinal hernia, with indirect hernias most common under the age of 50 and direct hernias more common after that age. By definition, an **indirect inguinal hernia** is one in which the hernial sac leaves the abdomen via the deep (internal) inguinal ring to enter the inguinal canal. Thus, if the hernia can be completely reduced, finger pressure over the deep ring (2.5 cm above the femoral pulse – see on Fig. 25.1) will

prevent it reappearing on coughing. In contrast, a **direct inguinal hernia** leaves the abdomen through a weakness in the posterior wall of the inguinal canal, i.e. medial to the deep ring, and so cannot be controlled by digital pressure over the deep ring.

Enlarged inguinal lymph nodes vary in consistency, number and size depending on the pathological cause; they are not reducible. A **saphena varix** is very soft and completely disappears on palpation, refilling when pressure is released. **Femoral artery aneurysms**, however, are firm and pulsatile. These vascular conditions must be diagnosed correctly as injudicious operation could be catastrophic!

SCROTAL LUMPS AND SWELLINGS

A lump or swelling in the scrotum may be:

- A solid or cystic mass arising from one of the components of the scrotal contents or spermatic cord. These anatomical structures include testis, epididymis, epididymal appendage, vas deferens and pampiniform venous plexus
- A collection of fluid in the tunica or processus vaginalis (**hydrocoele**)
- An inguinal hernia extending along the embryological path of testicular descent

343

CLINICAL EXAMINATION

The origin of a scrotal lump

The first clinical objective is to determine whether the swelling arises in the groin, in the spermatic cord itself or in the scrotum. This is achieved by palpating the spermatic cord at the neck of the scrotum. In the case of a hernia, the spermatic cord is much greater in diameter than normal and the hernia can be shown to communicate with the abdominal cavity. Spermatic cord swellings (varicocoele or cyst) are usually easy to recognise. If the lump is purely scrotal, the spermatic cord is normal in diameter.

Testicular and epididymal lumps

When the abnormality is scrotal, an attempt should be made to palpate the testis and epididymis separately,

and to find their relationship to the lump. If the testis is enlarged or there is a lump within it, this must be regarded as a primary tumour until proven otherwise by expert clinical examination, surgical exploration or ultrasound scanning; if doubt remains, excision biopsy is necessary. Testicular swellings due to lymphoma, leukaemia or granulomatous infections (e.g. tuberculosis or syphilitic gumma) tend to be softer, but this is an unreliable sign. Any testicular pathology may cause a little fluid to accumulate in the tunica vaginalis resulting in a small **secondary hydrocoele**. This rarely interferes with testicular palpation.

Lumps in the epididymis (cysts, chronic epididymitis or rarely, tuberculous granulomas) are discrete from, but attached to, an otherwise normal testis. Tiny focal lumps in the epididymis are rarely clinically important. Infective lesions cause diffuse thickening of the epididymis, whereas epididymal cysts are almost always located at the upper

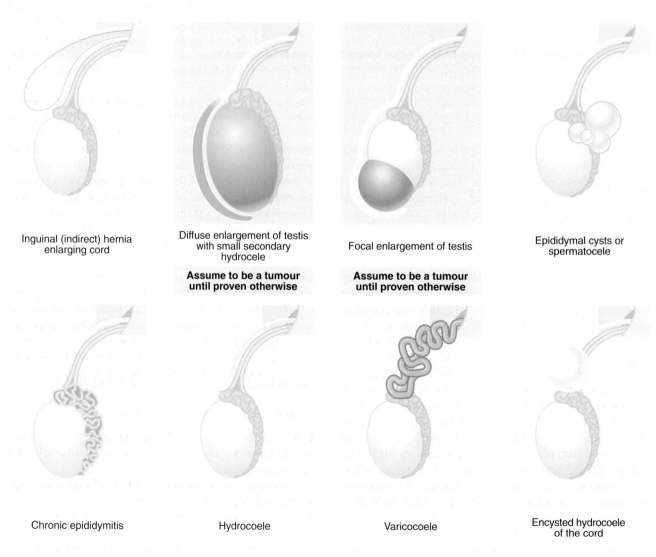

Inguinal (indirect) hernia enlarging cord

Diffuse enlargement of testis with small secondary hydrocele

Assume to be a tumour until proven otherwise

Focal enlargement of testis

Assume to be a tumour until proven otherwise

Epididymal cysts or spermatocele

Chronic epididymitis

Hydrocoele

Varicocoele

Encysted hydrocoele of the cord

Fig. 25.8 Causes of a lump or swelling in the scrotum

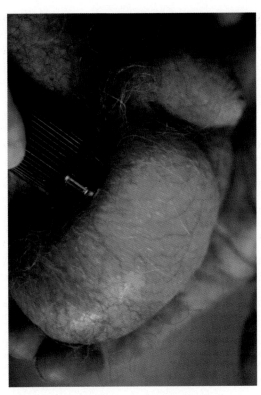

Fig. 25.9 Transillumination of a scrotal cyst
This 30-year-old man complained of a swelling in the right scrotum. On clinical examination, there is a 3 cm soft rounded swelling at the upper pole of the epididymis. A confident diagnosis of epididymal cyst can thus be made.

pole. Epididymal cysts are filled with clear fluid and therefore transilluminate. **Transillumination** (Fig. 25.9) is demonstrated by shining a strong beam of light from a (torch or fibreoptic cable) through the scrotum in a partly darkened room. If the lesion is fluid-filled, it will glow (except in the case of blood). About 10% of cysts in the epididymis, and most of those in the cord, are filled with an opalescent fluid containing spermatozoa. These **spermatocoeles** also sometimes transilluminate brilliantly.

Other scrotal lumps and swellings

Slow accumulation of fluid within the tunica vaginalis produces a **primary hydrocoele** surrounding the testis. Primary hydrocoeles are common in the elderly. They are often ignored by the patient until they become very large (300 ml or more) because they do not cause pain. The testis is not palpable separately from the swelling but occasionally, the hydrocoele is lax enough to allow the testis to be palpated through it; more often the hydrocoele is too tense for this. Diagnosis is confirmed if the swelling transilluminates.

In young boys, the tunica vaginalis may sometimes remain in continuity with the peritoneal cavity via a

patent processus vaginalis. This is so narrow that herniation does not occur but it allows peritoneal fluid to accumulate by gravity during the day. This causes a scrotal swelling which may disappear overnight, and is known as a **communicating hydrocoele**.

Abnormalities of the spermatic cord are usually varicocoeles or cysts. **Varicocoeles** are common, often asymptomatic, and represent dilatation of the venous network making up the pampiniform plexus. They feel like a 'bag of worms' on palpation and disappear in the supine position. **Cysts of the cord** are usually small, spherical and transilluminable. They represent either an **encysted hydrocoele** arising from a remnant of the processus vaginalis or a **spermatocoele**.

GROIN AND SCROTAL PAIN

ACUTE PAIN

Several common conditions can present with acute pain in the groin or scrotum. These are listed in Box 25.1 with their typical signs and symptoms. A **strangulated hernia** will usually be readily diagnosed by finding an irreducible hernia which is tender and often red, although strangulated femoral hernias may be grape-sized and unimpressive. Strangulated hernias, particularly femoral hernias, sometimes present with abdominal pain or signs of obstruction but without localised pain. This emphasises the importance of examining the hernial orifices in every patient with an acute abdomen.

Testicular torsion must always be excluded clinically if there is acute scrotal pain since the testis can be saved if operation is performed promptly; an exploratory operation is mandatory if torsion of the testis cannot be confidently excluded. Torsion occurs mainly in adolescents but occasionally in young adults. The main differential diagnosis at all ages is acute bacterial **epididymitis. Torsion of an epididymal appendage** (hydatid of Morgagni) produces symptoms similar to testicular torsion in children but less severe; surgical exploration is usually still required to exclude it. A **traumatic haematocoele** is also associated with acute pain but the trauma or surgery which preceded it will point to the likely diagnosis.

CHRONIC PAIN

Chronic pain in the groin or scrotum which occurs without any clues in the history and without swelling is difficult to diagnose and treat.

Groin pain may be caused by **inflamed inguinal lymph nodes** secondary to infection in their field of drainage. **Strained muscle attachments** to the bony pelvis sometimes cause groin pain; this particularly affects the hip adductor attachments near the pubic tubercle; and is usually associated with extreme physical activity. Groin

Table 25.1 Summary of disorders of the groin and scrotum and their clinical features

Disorder	Anatomical/developmental basis	Clinical features
1. GROIN LUMPS AND SWELLINGS		
a. Inguinal hernia		
Direct	Simple bulging of abdominal contents due to inadequate support given by weak posterior wall of inguinal canal	Discomfort; lump disappears on lying down; risk of incarceration if large; low risk of strangulation
Indirect	Passage of abdominal contents, often including bowel, through inguinal canal towards scrotum or labium majus	Potential for incarceration and strangulation; much more common in men
b. Femoral hernia	Passage of abdominal contents, often including bowel into femoral canal	Rarely has a cough impulse; rarely reducible; very likely to become strangulated
c. Inguinal lymphadenopathy	Inguinal nodes drain lower limb, abdominal wall below umbilicus, anal canal, scrotal skin, penis (but not testes, which drain to para-aortic and para-iliac nodes)	Enlarged nodes indicate infection, lymphoma or secondaries in drainage area
d. Saphena varix	Dilatation of long saphenous vein superficial to deep fascia before it enters the femoral vein	Can be mistaken for femoral hernia but empties on pressure and disappears on lying down, unlike femoral hernia; other varicose veins present in the leg
e. Femoral artery aneurysm	Dilatation of common femoral artery just below inguinal ligament	Found in patients over 65 years, mostly male; classic clinical sign is expansile pulsation; could be mistaken for femoral hernia
f. Psoas abscess	Classically, a tuberculous abscess of lumbar vertebra tracking down inside sheath of psoas muscle; occasionally a pyogenic abscess originating within the abdomen presents via the same route	TB presents as swelling or 'cold abscess' below inguinal ligament; rare nowadays but may be confused with lymph nodes; pyogenic abscess typically 'hot'; rarely may be due to abscess from renal stones
2. TESTICULAR DISORDERS		
a. Incompletely descended testis (for children, see Ch. 45)	Failure of complete descent from retroperitoneal site into scrotum; testis may be arrested at any point of descent or in an ectopic site	Mainly a problem of infancy and childhood requiring orchidopexy; possible cause of lump in groin; predisposition to malignancy; fertility may be impaired
b. Torsion of testis	Rotation of testis in scrotum; twisting of the spermatic cord result in venous obstruction which may culminate in infarction; recurrent incomplete torsion may occur	Complete torsion causes severe acute scrotal pain (and sometimes abdominal pain); partial torsion may cause episodic pain
c. Inflammation of epididymis or testis	'Epididymo-orchitis' is a term often used incorrectly for acute epididymitis. Usually caused by common urinary tract pathogens	Acute epididymitis is painful; must be distinguished from testicular torsion; usually associated with UTI
	Acute orchitis is often viral (mumps)	Testicular pain and swelling
	Chronic orchitis may be caused by tuberculosis or syphilitic gumma	Usually presents as painless testicular enlargement
d. Testicular tumours	Derived from germ cells of testis; metastasise via lymphatics to para-iliac and para-aortic nodes or via bloodstream, commonly to lung	Present as painless swelling of testis usually with small secondary hydrocoele
3. DISORDERS OF OTHER SCROTAL CONTENTS		
a. Hydrocoele	Abnormal collection of fluid in space around testis; in children may still be in communication with peritoneal cavity (communicating hydrocoele)	Presents as a painless scrotal swelling which transilluminates; testis may be difficult to palpate within it until fluid is drained
b. Haematocoele	Collection of blood around testis; usually early result of trauma or surgery	Presents like a hydrocoele after trauma but does not transilluminate
c. Varicocoele	Dilatation of pampiniform venous plexus of spermatic cord	Presents as a scrotal swelling separate from testis and epididymis; feels like a 'bag of worms'; disappears on lying down, thus patient must be examined standing
d. Epididymal cyst and spermatocoele	Cyst derived from epididymal tissue	Epididymal cyst presents as a scrotal swelling which transilluminates; separate from the testis, often multiloculated; spermatocoele is unilocular, in cord or epididymis and may be transilluminable
e. Torsion of hydatid of Morgagni	Torsion of epididymal appendage	Occurs in children; may present late as a small hydrocoele; in the acute phase, presents as scrotal pain and oedema and may simulate testicular torsion

SUMMARY

Box 25.1 Common causes of acute pain in the groin and scrotum

Strangulated inguinal or femoral hernia
● Painful, irre...... tender groin lump
● Som........... as intestinal obstruction or

......ilateral scrotal pain with or
......alised abdominal pain
......testis is high in the scrotum and
......r, and the cord is thickened; later
......ften obscured by oedema
......stis may lie horizontally (bell-clapper

......didymal appendage (hydatid of

......s in children
......t of unilateral scrotal pain; the testis
......lly. There is a tenderness only at its
......and minimal overlying oedema

......mitis
......Moderate or severe scrotal pain and tenderness with marked redness and oedema
● Often preceded by symptoms of urinary tract infection; urine usually contains white cells, nitrites and organisms

Haematocoele following trauma or scrotal surgery (e.g. vasectomy)
● History may be diagnostic although torsion is sometimes precipitated by trauma

pain may also be **referred** from a diseased hip joint. An early **inguinal hernia** sometimes causes groin pain before the hernia becomes clinically detectable.

Chronic scrotal pain is most often due to **inflammation**. It can often be traced back to a vasectomy, although the cause is often obscure and the treatment ineffective. Patients present weeks or months after the operation, complaining of localised tenderness at the operation site or a general ache in one side of the scrotum. If there is a small tender lump due to a stitch granuloma, this is usually cured by excision.

Pain is also a feature of chronic bacterial **epididymitis**, which usually follows an acute episode.

Recurrent, incomplete **testicular torsion** may cause transient episodes of severe pain in the inguino-scrotal region or poorly defined lower abdominal pain. In these cases, the anatomical relationship of the testis to the tunica vaginalis is often abnormal so the testes lie horizontally rather than vertically when the patient is standing. These 'bell-clapper' testes are susceptible to torsion.

The important disorders of the groin and genitalia are summarised in Table 25.1, together with their anatomical and clinical significance.

THE MISSING OR ECTOPIC TESTIS

Scrotal examination may reveal the absence of one testis or both testes. The problem is very common in children but is sometimes discovered incidentally in adults. The testis is very rarely truly absent but lies somewhere along the normal path of testicular descent, usually in the inguinal canal but occasionally within the abdomen. **Incompletely descended testes** (often called undescended testes) are usually small and atrophic and, being histologically dystrophic, are predisposed to malignant change; indeed an inguinal mass may sometimes be a testicular tumour in an incompletely descended testis. Previous **orchidectomy** should of course be excluded. This is often performed bilaterally for treating metastatic prostatic cancer or unilaterally for torsion associated with a necrotic testis or during surgery for recurrent inguinal hernia.

Occasionally, an adult testis may become displaced upwards towards the inguinal canal following trauma or surgery; this is known as a **trapped testis**. The testis is normal in size but is fixed in position by adhesions. If trauma was the cause and there were other major injuries, the scrotal injury may have been overlooked.

Trauma, including operative trauma during operations for hernia or incompletely descended testis, may damage the blood supply and cause **testicular atrophy**. The resulting testis is abnormally small and soft. When both testes are small, the cause is usually hypoplasia, androgen insufficiency or hormonal therapy for prostatic carcinoma.

26 Hernias and other groin lumps

INTRODUCTION

This chapter covers the individual entities which make up the common surgical lumps in the groin area. These include inguinal and femoral hernias, enlarged inguinal lymph nodes, saphena varix and femoral artery aneurysm. Diagnosis of these lesions is covered in Chapter 25.

INGUINAL HERNIA

Inguinal hernia is one of the most common complaints in general surgical outpatient departments. In a typical district general hospital, inguinal hernias account for about 7% of surgical outpatient consultations and about 12% of operating theatre time.

As shown in Figure 26.1, inguinal hernias in males are by far the most common groin hernia. Femoral hernias are uncommon in males—97.5% inguinal versus 2.5% femoral. Even in females, inguinal hernias occur twice as often as femoral hernias yet femoral hernias are twice as common in females as in males. Inguinal hernias are eight times more common in males because of the potential abdominal wall weakness caused by testicular descent.

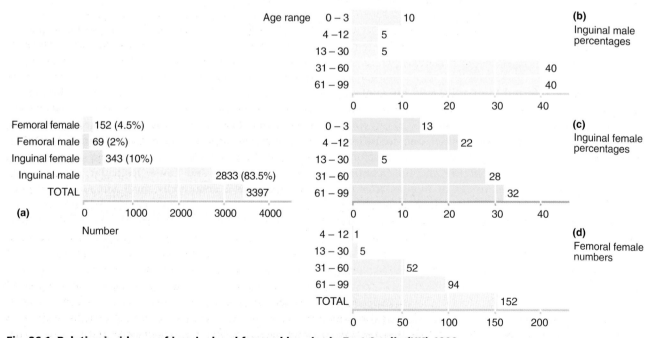

Fig. 26.1 Relative incidence of inguinal and femoral hernias in East Anglia (UK) 1990
(a) Number of hernias by type and sex. Percentage of all hernias is shown in brackets. **(b)** Incidence of inguinal hernias in males. **(c)** Incidence of inguinal hernias in females. **(d)** Incidence of femoral hernias in females.

Inguinal hernias occur at any age. In childhood they are always of developmental origin and are particularly common in premature infants. In males, hernias are most common before the age of 5 and after middle age. A smaller peak occurs in the late teens and early twenties. Hernias in these young men probably result from a congenital predisposition, exacerbated by work or sport. Inguinal hernias should be repaired early to reduce the risk of strangulation and the need for emergency operation.

ANATOMICAL CONSIDERATIONS

Details of the surgical anatomy of the inguinal and femoral canals are shown in Figure 26.2. In this diagram, the external oblique aponeurosis (or fascia) which forms the anterior wall of the inguinal canal is shown opened as it would be after the first stage of a hernia repair operation.

In the diagram, the external oblique aponeurosis has been split obliquely from the external ring along the line of its fibres for about 5 cm laterally and the cut edges reflected upwards and downwards to expose the inguinal canal. Note that the internal oblique and transversus abdominis muscles are deficient above the medial half of the inguinal ligament. Their inferior borders fuse in this area to form the conjoint tendon. This 'tendon', which is usually just the fused lower edge of the muscles, forms a shallow arch stretching from the lateral half of the inguinal ligament to the pubic crest. The D-shaped defect in the muscular abdominal wall leaves the transversalis fascia as the only restraint to herniation of the abdominal contents. It is normally particularly strong in this area.

The spermatic cord passes through the transversalis fascia in the most lateral part of the muscular defect. The inferior epigastric artery passes upwards immediately medial to it. Thus, the deep (internal) ring is bounded by inguinal ligament below, conjoint tendon above and laterally, and the inferior epigastric artery medially. The posterior wall of the inguinal canal consists of transversalis fascia and the medial insertion of the conjoint tendon.

MECHANISMS OF INGUINAL HERNIA FORMATION

Inguinal herniation may be direct or indirect. A **direct hernia** protrudes directly through the transversalis fascia and enters the inguinal canal through its posterior wall. An **indirect hernia** leaves the abdomen via the deep inguinal ring to follow an oblique course along the inguinal canal through the abdominal wall (see Fig. 26.3). In either case, the herniated abdominal contents are contained within a sac of peritoneum. The hernia may consist merely of peritoneum and its associated extra-peritoneal fat, but the sac usually contains omentum or

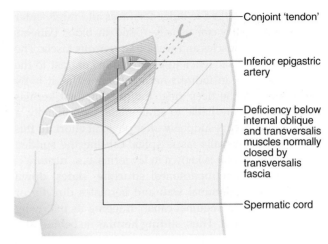

Fig. 26.2 Relations of the deep inguinal ring

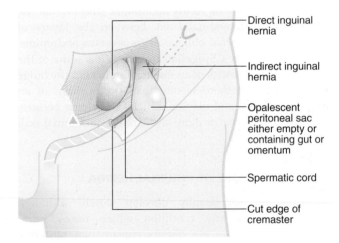

Fig. 26.3 Direct and indirect inguinal hernias
A direct inguinal hernia bulges medial to the inferior epigastric artery and is not attached to the spermatic cord. An indirect inguinal hernia leaves the deep inguinal ring lateral to the artery and *within* the cremaster.

small bowel. Less commonly, the sac contains large bowel or appendix, or rarely bladder. Occasionally, the contents of the sac are diseased, e.g. large bowel carcinoma, an inflamed appendix (appendicitis) or peritoneal tumour secondaries, and this may be the reason for the emergency operation at which the condition is discovered.

Distinguishing clinically between direct and indirect hernias is often difficult and is unimportant except at operation. It should be noted that an indirect and a direct hernia can occur together on the same side.

In an indirect hernia, the peritoneal sac may represent a patent or reopened processus vaginalis. It may extend as far as the tunica vaginalis surrounding the testis. It is easy to accept that indirect hernias have a congenital origin in children or in young muscular men, but this is less convincing in flabby older men.

Direct hernias tend to bulge forwards and rarely enter the scrotum. They are usually found in older patients with deficient muscles and weak transversalis fascia. The neck of a direct sac tends to be broad, in contrast to the narrow neck of an indirect hernia, confined as it is by the borders of the deep ring. Indirect inguinal hernias are therefore more liable to strangulate. Occasionally, a direct hernia occurs suddenly after physical effort. In this case, the transversalis fascia splits, causing the sudden appearance of what is known in lay terms as a 'rupture'.

Sometimes a retroperitoneal structure 'slides' down the posterior abdominal wall and herniates directly or indirectly into the inguinal canal, dragging its overlying peritoneum with it. Thus, **sliding hernias** lie behind and outside the peritoneal sac (see Fig. 26.4). Diagnosis can only be made at operation.

Rarely, herniation occurs through a fascial defect at the lateral border of rectus abdominis. The hernial sac comes to lie interstitially, i.e. between the layers of internal and external oblique or transversus abdominis. This is known as a **Spigelian hernia**. It has some of the clinical characteristics of an inguinal hernia but the bulge lies higher and more medial than the position of an inguinal hernia, and may be difficult to palpate because it is covered by one or more layers of the abdominal wall (see Fig. 26.5).

NATURAL HISTORY OF INGUINAL HERNIA

Inguinal hernias usually develop slowly, although exacerbated by any condition which raises intra-abdominal pressure, e.g. obesity, constipation, straining at micturition or chronic coughing; continued heavy lifting probably has a similar effect. In adults, a single episode of increased intra-abdominal pressure, e.g. an extreme bout of heavy lifting, may 'rupture' the abdominal wall, resulting in the sudden appearance of a direct hernia. In infants, a period of severe coughing may precipitate an acute indirect hernia which may become irreducible.

Initially in adults, the peritoneal sac and its contents are completely reducible into the abdominal cavity. This usually occurs spontaneously when the patient lies down, but larger hernias may need manipulating by the patient if they are to be reduced. In general, the longer a hernia remains and the larger it becomes, the more difficult it is to reduce. This increases the likelihood of fibrous adhesions developing within the sac which prevent complete reduction. A chronically irreducible hernia which is not strangulated is described as **incarcerated**. However, the term is often used inaccurately when a clinician is uncertain whether an acutely irreducible hernia is strangulated. It is safer to assume such a hernia is strangulated until proved otherwise.

Hernial strangulation

Inguinal hernias may become irreducible or strangulated at any time; those with a narrow neck that are difficult to reduce or that cause pain are at special risk. Strangulation occurs if the hernial contents become constricted by the neck of the sac or by twisting. Obstruction of venous return then leads to swelling and later to arterial obstruction. If strangulation is not relieved by manual or operative reduction, **infarction** follows. The strangulated inguinal hernia first becomes irreducible and then tender and later red. Symptoms and signs of bowel obstruction develop over the next few hours, followed by peritonitis if the bowel perforates (Fig. 26.6).

MANAGEMENT OF INGUINAL HERNIAS

Inguinal hernias in adults should ideally be repaired by **herniorrhaphy**. Performing elective repair soon after

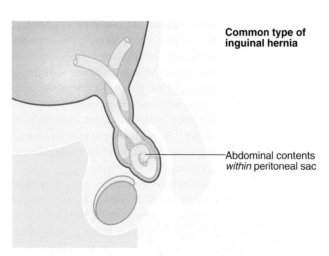

Common type of inguinal hernia

Abdominal contents *within* peritoneal sac

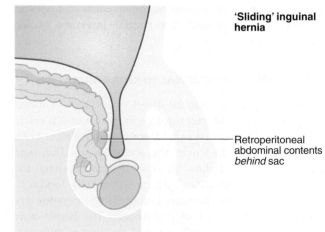

'Sliding' inguinal hernia

Retroperitoneal abdominal contents *behind* sac

Fig. 26.4 Common and sliding inguinal hernias

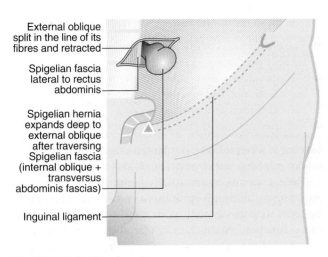

External oblique split in the line of its fibres and retracted

Spigelian fascia lateral to rectus abdominis

Spigelian hernia expands deep to external oblique after traversing Spigelian fascia (internal oblique + transversus abdominis fascias)

Inguinal ligament

Fig. 26.5 Spigelian hernia

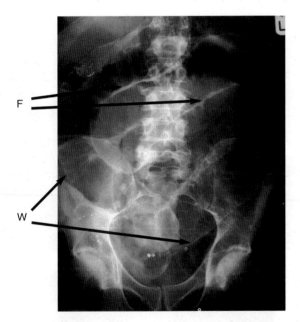

Fig. 26.6 Wrigler's sign
This 40-year-old man presented with symptoms and signs of distal small bowel obstruction due to a strangulated inguinal hernia. At first, the abdomen, though distended and tympanitic, was not tender. However, during resuscitation, the abdomen became tender. This X-ray shows a clear outline of the outside of parts of the small bowel **W**, representing Wrigler's sign. A false Wrigler's sign is seen in other parts **F** and this is where two loops of thickened small bowel lie in contact.

diagnosis reduces the risk of strangulation and minimises stretching of the abdominal wall musculature. The latter probably lowers the rate of recurrence. If age or infirmity makes an operation hazardous, a **truss** may be the only treatment but it is markedly inferior to herniorrhaphy.

With time, an enlarging hernia may become irreducible. Urgent operation is not essential provided there are no problems with the hernia. Some patients give a history of episodes in which the hernia becomes temporarily

irreducible. These episodes may be accompanied by local pain and tenderness or even symptoms of bowel obstruction (vomiting, colicky abdominal pain, distension and absolute constipation). These warning episodes should be taken as an indication for operation very soon. More severe and prolonged symptoms usually precipitate emergency admission to hospital, in which case strangulation must be assumed to have occurred (the term strangulation prompts rapid action!) and operation should be performed urgently.

Very large 'wheelbarrow' hernias are invariably of long standing and are found in elderly men (see Fig. 26.7). They only present when size becomes a handicap, if bowel strangulates within the hernia or if the anatomical distortion interferes with micturition. Bowel adhesions may make operation difficult and postoperative wound infections are common. Despite this, surgery for strangulation cannot be avoided. If the hernia is not strangulated, a bag truss (see p. 353) may be the most appropriate treatment.

Inguinal herniorrhaphy and herniotomy

Until recently, the standard open techniques of herniorrhaphy were all based on Bassini's 19th century extraperitoneal approach. Many variations have been described but all remove or reduce the peritoneal sac and employ non-absorbable sutures to repair the abdominal wall. Success with these methods of herniorrhaphy is

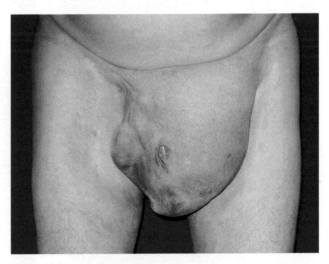

Fig. 26.7 Inguino-scrotal hernia
This man of 76 lived alone and only presented to a doctor when he had increasing difficulty with controlling the direction of his micturition. His penis had disappeared altogether as the hernia had enlarged. The right testis is visible in the scrotum but the left side of the scrotum is filled with a large hernia. At operation, the abdominal wall defect was surprisingly small and was easily repaired by a standard method.

undoubtedly operator-dependent and, in competent hands, any standard technique gives good results and low recurrence rates. The lowest reported recurrence rates, close to zero, were from the Shouldice hernia clinic in Canada using the Shouldice variation of a Bassini repair.

In recent years, the Lichtenstein technique has over-shadowed the various Bassini techniques and has widely become the preferred standard operation. This operation is similar to the Bassini up to the point of repair. Then it employs a **no tension** technique, using a patch of non-absorbable open-weave mesh to repair and reinforce the defect rather than suturing muscle and fascial layers together under tension. Figure 26.8 shows the principles of the Bassini and Lichtenstein types of inguinal hernia repair.

The mesh technique has several distinct advantages:

● The technique is easily learned and junior doctors can reliably produce good results
● Postoperative pain is substantially reduced allowing increased mobility and early return to normal activities such as work and driving
● Recurrence rates appear to be exceptionally low

Having a foreign body implanted ought to increase the risk of infection but in practice, this is exceptionally rare.

Hernia operations are usually performed under general anaesthesia, although epidural or spinal anaesthesia may be used in patients with poor cardiovascular or respiratory function. Many hernia operations are performed under local anaesthesia, particularly in specialised clinics.

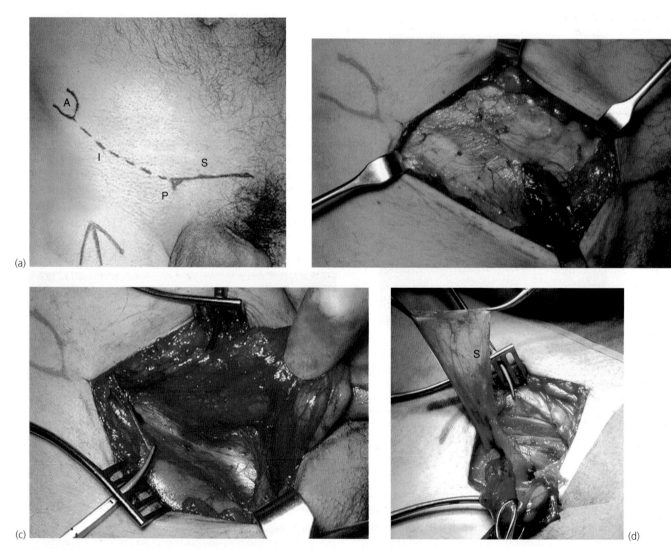

(a)

(b)

(c)

(d)

Fig. 26.8 Technique of Lichtenstein hernia repair

(a) Skin markings demonstrating the upper border of the public arch **S**, the anterior superior iliac spine **A**, the pubic tubercle **P** and the inguinal ligament **I**. Note the side of operation has been marked with an arrow on the thigh. **(b)** The dissection down to the external oblique aponeurosis. The external (superficial) ring is arrowed. **(c)** External oblique aponeurosis opened, demonstrating the shiny inguinal ligament, which is its inturned lower edge. **(d)** The indirect hernia sac **S** dissected out from the spermatic cord and held upwards before ligation and excision. The inferior epigastric artery and vein lie at the medial border of the deep inguinal ring.

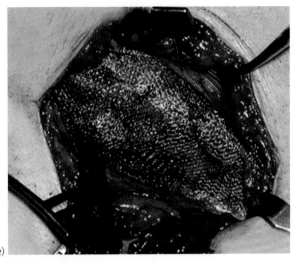
(e)

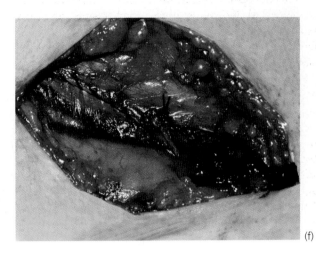
(f)

Fig. 26.8 Continued
(e) Polypropylene mesh is cut to shape before insertion and sutured in place along the inguinal ligament and tacked to the surface of the internal oblique with 'starry sky' sutures. **(f)** External oblique closed to recreate the inguinal canal before skin closure.

In infants, the patent processus vaginalis is merely ligated and excised (**herniotomy**); formal repair of the abdominal wall defect is usually unnecessary. If the defect is enormous, a single stitch should be used on the medial side to narrow the deep ring.

Complications of herniorrhaphy are unusual but scrotal haematoma or wound infection occasionally occurs soon after operation. Late complications include chronic groin pain due to inadvertent trapping of the ilio-inguinal nerve in the repair and to testicular atrophy caused by inadvertent damage to the testicular artery, usually with diathermy. The latter is a particular problem with recurrent hernias.

To minimise complications in obstructed and strangulated hernias, the first step is to ensure that the patient is fully resuscitated; more patients die of fluid and electrolyte problems than of delaying an operation for a few hours. The hernia is approached via a standard groin incision.

Laparoscopic inguinal hernia repair

Laparoscopic repair of inguinal hernias by transperitoneal or retroperitoneal routes is possible but has not shown any convincing advantages over open techniques for primary hernia repair. The technique is probably most useful for hernias which have recurred several times or for bilateral repair, and is described in Chapter 6.

Recurrent inguinal hernia

Even when a recognised operative technique is competently performed, hernias recur in about 0.5–10% of cases over a lifetime. The rate is greatly increased when inadequate attention has been given to operative principles. Apart from technical failure, recurrence is probably due to inherently poor musculature, chronic cough, urinary obstruction, constipation or resumption of heavy work too soon after repair. Operations for recurrent hernia are often more difficult and have a higher potential for complications than a primary repair. A laparoscopic approach has the advantage that it allows the repair to be placed in virgin territory.

Postoperative care and return to normal activities

Most inguinal hernias are now repaired on a day case basis although some patients stay in hospital for 24–48 hours to allow early recovery under controlled conditions.

During the first postoperative week, patients should avoid activities likely to strain the repair, such as heavy lifting or driving a car. Over the next 2 or 3 weeks, they should gradually return to normal activity, including usual sexual activity. Return to work depends on the physical nature of the job and whether activities cause pain, but usually varies from 2–6 weeks.

Trusses (see Fig. 26.9)

A truss may be used to control certain types of hernia when surgery is either inappropriate or unacceptable to the patient. A pressure truss can be safely used if the hernia is easily reducible and can be kept reduced and free of symptoms. Pressure trusses made of padded webbing have superseded various spring contraptions. For very large hernias which cannot be reduced, a 'bag truss' can be used to support the hernia.

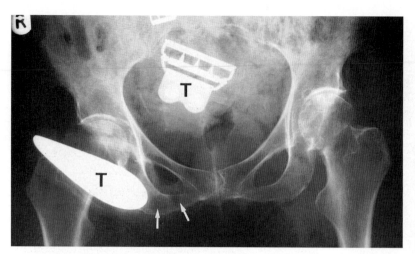

Fig. 26.9 Truss with unreduced inguinal hernia
X-ray of the pelvis in an 82-year-old woman following a fall causing a fractured neck of the left femur. She happened to be wearing a truss **T** for a longstanding, large right inguinal hernia. This was not kept reduced by the truss as indicated by the presence of bowel gas (arrowed) in the inguinal area.

FEMORAL HERNIA

Femoral hernias are formed by a protrusion of peritoneum into the potential space of the femoral canal. The sac may contain abdominal viscera (usually small bowel) or omentum. In males, inguinal hernia is 40 times more common than femoral hernia, but in females, inguinal hernia is only twice as common. Increased intra-abdominal pressure and other factors related to pregnancy may be important in females since the incidence of femoral hernia is higher in parous than nulliparous women. In both sexes, femoral hernia is assumed to be acquired; no evidence of a congenital sac has ever been found. Thus, femoral hernias, unlike inguinal hernias, are rare but not unknown in children.

CLINICAL FEATURES OF FEMORAL HERNIA

A femoral hernia is usually small, appearing as a grape-sized lump immediately below the inguinal ligament and just lateral to its medial attachment to the pubic tubercle. The anatomy of the femoral canal is shown in Figure 25.2, p. 340. If a femoral hernia becomes large, it tends to be deflected upwards and may seem to arise above the inguinal ligament. This explains the importance of careful examination to determine the origin of a hernial neck.

Since the femoral canal is narrow, a cough impulse can rarely be detected, and the hernia is usually irreducible. Thus, small femoral hernias may be difficult to distinguish from other lumps arising in the femoral canal such as a lipoma or enlarged Cloquet's lymph node. However, a hernia is deeply fixed whereas the others tend to be more mobile.

Strangulated femoral hernia

In contrast to strangulated inguinal hernia, there are usually no localising symptoms and signs in strangulated femoral hernia, and the classic presenting features are those of distal small bowel obstruction. The diagnosis of strangulated femoral hernia is easily missed unless the femoral region is carefully examined for a lump, which is usually small, the size of a large grape, and often unimpressive.

In nearly 30% of strangulated femoral hernias, only part of the bowel circumference is trapped in the hernial sac. Although the bowel lumen remains patent and the patient continues to pass flatus, peristalsis is sufficiently disrupted for other signs of obstruction to occur, notably vomiting. This is known as **Richter's hernia** (see Fig. 26.10). Resuscitation and urgent operation are required.

MANAGEMENT OF FEMORAL HERNIA

The abdominal orifice of the femoral canal is small and indistensible. Consequently, abdominal contents finding their way into the canal strangulate much more readily than they do in inguinal hernias. Thus, all femoral hernias, even if asymptomatic, should be repaired without delay. Use of a truss is dangerous.

Elective repair is performed by emptying and excising the peritoneal sac (see Fig. 26.11). The femoral canal is then closed with non-absorbable sutures between pectineus fascia and inguinal ligament. The canal can be exposed by several different methods. The most common are the **femoral** or low approach, the **Lotheissen** or high approach via the posterior wall of the inguinal canal, and the **McEvedy** or pararectus extraperitoneal approach.

ENLARGED INGUINAL LYMPH NODES

The lymph nodes of the inguinal region are clustered into the three anatomical groups shown in Figure 25.5, p. 341. These drain the lower abdominal wall and lower back, perineum (including vulva and vagina), anal canal,

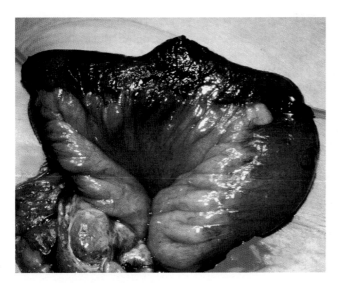

Fig. 26.10 Richter's hernia
This 71-year-old woman presented with symptoms and signs of incomplete small bowel obstruction; these included vomiting, abdominal distension and colicky abdominal pain, but she continued to pass flatus. She had a grape-sized femoral hernia which was not tender. At operation, part of the wall of the ileum was trapped in the hernia. The photograph shows bruising around the area trapped in the hernia. Luckily, the bowel was viable and did not need resection. The hernia was repaired before closure.

penis and scrotal skin and the whole lower limb. The testes, derived from the retroperitoneal area, drain to the upper para-aortic nodes within the abdomen rather than the inguinal nodes.

Inguinal lymph nodes may become secondarily enlarged as a result of local disease in their field of drainage.

Examples include infections of the foot, skin diseases, sexually transmitted infection or tumours. Inguinal lymph node enlargement may also be part of a generalised lymphadenopathy in lymphoma or a systemic infection such as glandular fever or AIDS. Multiple small hard ('shotty') nodes are commonly found, especially in men, and are accepted as normal. These nodes probably result from minor infections of the lower limb, and are easily palpable in males because they have less subcutaneous fat.

CLINICAL FEATURES OF ENLARGED INGUINAL LYMPH NODES

Enlarged inguinal lymph nodes present with pain or a lump in the groin but are often discovered incidentally. When they are small, it can be difficult to determine clinically whether nodes are abnormal. Enlarged lymph nodes are recognised by their anatomical position and by excluding hernias or vascular abnormalities. Enlarged nodes are usually mobile but become fixed to the surrounding tissues when infiltrated by tumour. If doubt exists as to whether the nodes are enlarged, ultrasound scanning will usually give a definitive answer, and can be used to guide percutaneous needle biopsy. If enlarged and fixed inguinal lymph nodes are confirmed, the history may need to be reviewed for clues as to the origin. A history of systemic manifestations of lymphoma or acquired immunodeficiency syndrome (AIDS) should be sought. These include malaise, periodic fevers and weight loss. There may be a history of a 'mole' or 'wart' having been removed, even many years before. If this was a malignant melanoma or squamous carcinoma,

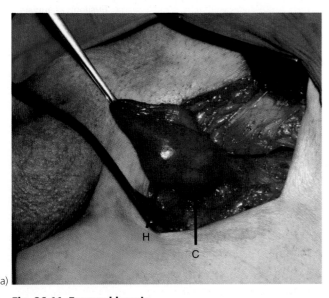

(a)

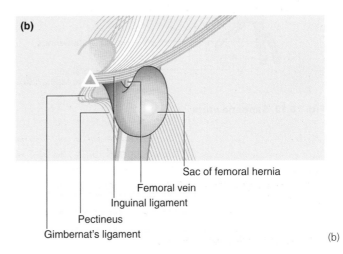

(b)

Sac of femoral hernia
Femoral vein
Inguinal ligament
Pectineus
Gimbernat's ligament

(b)

Fig. 26.11 Femoral hernia
(a) An average-sized femoral hernia **H** at operation. The patient's genitalia are to the left of the photograph. The line of the inguinal ligament is marked with an interrupted line and the opening of the femoral canal is seen at **C**. **(b)** The four margins of the femoral canal.

it could now have metastasised. Other symptoms of tumours that could metastasise to inguinal lymph nodes should be sought. For example, anal pain or bleeding might indicate an anal carcinoma.

The examination should include palpating lymph nodes in the neck and axillae, and palpating the liver and spleen. The skin of the whole drainage field should be examined closely, paying particular attention to the back, perineum and feet, including between the toes and beneath the toenails. The examination may reveal infection, squamous cell carcinoma or malignant melanoma. Rectal examination is mandatory to exclude anal carcinoma. A blood test for human immunodeficiency virus (HIV) may be indicated.

If enlarged lymph nodes cannot be explained by simple local factors or a systemic illness, nodes should be sampled for histological examination by fine needle aspiration or needle core biopsy, or should be surgically removed. If only a single node is enlarged, histology often shows non-specific reactive changes. The patient usually recovers fully and a diagnosis is never made.

SAPHENA VARIX

A saphena varix is a dilatation of the long saphenous vein in the groin, just proximal to its junction with the femoral vein (see Fig. 26.12). The varix is caused by valvular incompetence at this point; there are usually varicose veins elsewhere in the long saphenous system.

The varix can reach the size of a golf ball or even larger. On examination, the swelling is soft and diffuse. The diagnostic feature is that it empties with minimal pressure and refills on release ('the sign of emptying'). A cough impulse is invariably present. If these physical signs are not sought and the patient is only examined standing, the varix can be mistaken for a solid mass.

Treatment is high saphenous ligation, as for saphenofemoral reflux associated with varicose veins (see Ch. 34).

FEMORAL ARTERY ANEURYSM

Femoral aneurysms are uncommon as a cause of a lump in the groin. They may occur as part of generalised aneurysmal disease of the abdominal aorta, iliac and lower limb arterial system but can also occur in isolation. Diagnosis is made on clinical examination; the lump lies below the midpoint of the inguinal ligament (see Fig. 26.13) and has a characteristic expansile pulsation. Distinguishing an aneurysm from a femoral hernia is clearly vitally important. The management of aneurysms is discussed in Chapter 35.

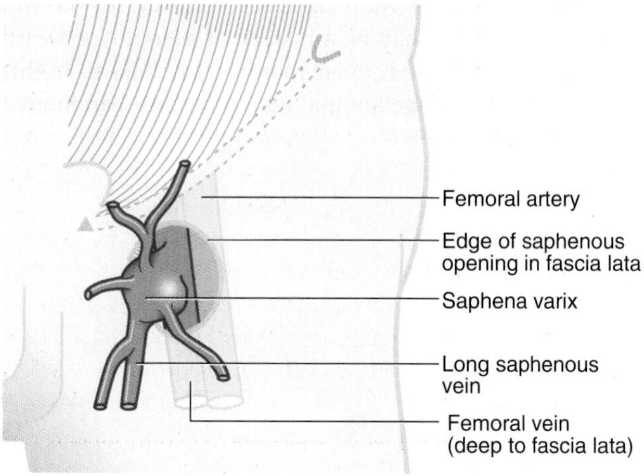

Femoral artery

Edge of saphenous opening in fascia lata

Saphena varix

Long saphenous vein

Femoral vein (deep to fascia lata)

Fig. 26.12 Saphena varix

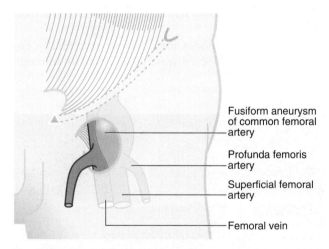

Fusiform aneurysm of common femoral artery

Profunda femoris artery

Superficial femoral artery

Femoral vein

Fig. 26.13 Femoral artery aneurysm

27 Disorders of the male genitalia

DISORDERS OF THE SCROTAL CONTENTS

INTRODUCTION

Abnormalities of the scrotal contents include disorders of normal scrotal contents, i.e. the testis and its coverings and the spermatic cord as well as inguino-scrotal hernias (see Chapter 26). Distinguishing between them is usually a matter of simple clinical examination. The diagnosis which must not be missed is the testicular tumour. Other problems include inflammation, hydrocoeles and cysts, maldescent, torsion and testicular trauma, as well as varicocoele. Male sterilisation is also covered in this chapter.

INFLAMMATION OF THE EPIDIDYMIS AND TESTIS

EPIDIDYMITIS

The most common inflammatory disorder of the scrotal contents is bacterial epididymitis. This is usually secondary to a urethral infection conducted via the vas deferens. The primary infection is either a urinary tract infection with coliforms (50–65 age group) or a sexually transmitted infection with *Chlamydia* or *Neisseria gonorrhoeae* (common in the 15–30 age group). Epididymitis is often incorrectly referred to as orchitis or epididymo-orchitis. The testis is rarely infected, although the surrounding inflammation may cause testicular tenderness. The differential diagnosis includes sperm leakage following vasectomy causing a **sperm granuloma**, and **vasitis nodosa**. Epididymitis is painful and usually begins acutely. It may present as a surgical emergency and be indistinguishable clinically from testicular torsion. On examination of a patient with acute epididymitis, the affected side of the scrotum and its contents are swollen, oedematous and tender, and the scrotal skin is red and warm. It may be difficult to palpate the testis and epididymis separately once the infection has become established. Epididymitis must never be diagnosed in a boy under 15 in the absence of urinary symptoms, or a proven urinary infection or urethritis. Such an 'acute scrotum' must be explored to exclude torsion (see p. 366).

Treatment of acute epididymitis is with bed rest for pain relief and at least 1 month of an appropriate broad-spectrum antibiotic. The infecting organism is often not identified but attempts should be made to pin it down using urine cultures, blood cultures or culture of urethral discharge after prostatic massage. Ciprofloxacin is often favoured on a 'best-guess' basis and is continued if culture confirms sensitivity of the organisms.

Persistent or chronic epididymitis may cause the patient to present with chronic scrotal tenderness. This usually follows an initial acute episode. Chronic epididymitis may also result from inadequate antibiotic therapy of an acute episode.

Tuberculous epididymitis

Tuberculosis may involve the epididymis via bloodstream spread from a pulmonary focus. A tuberculous urinary tract infection may spread to the epididymis and epididymal swelling may be the presenting complaint.

357

Typically, the whole length of the epididymis is thickened, non-tender and 'cold'. In contrast to bacterial epididymitis, the epididymis can be readily distinguished from the testis on palpation. If untreated, the testis may also become involved.

Diagnosis requires the analysis of serial early morning urine specimens (EMUs) for mycobacteria or, more reliably, histological examination of percutaneous needle biopsies. If tuberculosis is confirmed, a search must be made for pulmonary and urinary tract disease (see Ch. 32).

ORCHITIS

Primary bacterial orchitis is rare and may result from pyogenic infection in the genital tract or elsewhere in the body. **Tertiary gummatous syphilis** may involve the testis, producing diffuse non-tender enlargement; this is now extremely rare. There is usually a history of primary and secondary lesions. Sometimes a gumma is found unexpectedly during investigation of a suspected testicular tumour.

Viral orchitis is most often caused by **mumps**. In postpubertal males, bilateral mumps orchitis produces infertility in 50% of cases; elevated follicle-stimulating hormone (FSH) blood levels following orchitis usually indicate the patient is infertile. Mumps orchitis manifests 4–6 days after the onset of parotitis with extreme testicular tenderness and an inflammatory hydrocoele. Treatment is directed at symptomatic relief. Other viruses affecting the testis include Coxsackie, human immunodeficiency virus (HIV), Epstein–Barr, varicella, and in earlier times, smallpox.

HYDROCOELE

PRIMARY HYDROCOELE

A hydrocoele is an excessive collection of fluid within the tunica vaginalis, the serous space surrounding the testis. Like the peritoneal cavity, the tunica vaginalis contains a small amount of serous fluid which is normally produced and reabsorbed at the same rate.

In infants and children, a hydrocoele is usually an expression of a patent processus vaginalis (PPV). Provided there is no hernia present, hydrocoeles below the age of 1 year usually resolve spontaneously. For older children ligation of the PPV is required.

Primary hydrocoeles may develop in adulthood, particularly in the elderly, by slow accumulation of serous fluid, presumably caused by impaired reabsorption. These hydrocoeles can reach a huge size, containing several hundred millilitres of fluid. The lesions are otherwise asymptomatic. The swelling is soft and non-tender on examination and the testis cannot usually be palpated. The presence of fluid is demonstrated by transillumination.

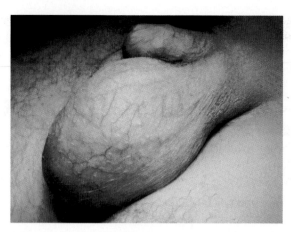

Fig. 27.1 Testicular hydrocoele
This man of 67 had a painless swelling of the left side of the scrotum for several years that was slowly enlarging. On examination, the swelling was confined to the scrotum and did not involve widening of the cord at the neck of the scrotum which might indicate a hernia. The testis was not palpable separately from the testis and the swelling transilluminated, confirming the diagnosis.

Note that a secondary hydrocoele may develop in response to tumour or inflammation of the testis. In most cases, the hydrocoele is small and the testis can easily be palpated to reveal the primary abnormality.

Management

If a testicular tumour is a possibility, hydrocoeles must not be aspirated as malignant cells can be disseminated via the scrotal skin to its lymphatic field. If tumour cannot be excluded clinically, ultrasonography is indicated. Provided there is no suspicion of tumour, the hydrocoele can be **tapped**, i.e. aspirated with a needle and syringe. Clear straw-coloured fluid and a palpably normal testis confirm the diagnosis; otherwise surgical exploration of the testis is needed.

After aspiration of a primary hydrocoele, fluid reaccumulates over the following months and periodic aspiration, sclerotherapy or operation is needed. For younger patients, operation is usually preferred, whereas the elderly or unfit can have aspirations repeated whenever the hydrocoele becomes uncomfortably large. Sclerotherapy is an alternative; after aspiration, 6% aqueous phenol (10–20 ml) together with 1% lignocaine for analgesia can be injected and this often inhibits reaccumulation. Several treatments may be necessary.

HYDROCOELE OF THE CORD

Rarely, a hydrocoele develops in a remnant of the processus vaginalis somewhere along the course of the spermatic cord. This hydrocoele also transilluminates, and is known as an **encysted hydrocoele of the cord** (see

Fig. 27.2). In females, a multicystic **hydrocoele of the canal of Nuck** sometimes presents as a swelling in the groin. It probably results from cystic degeneration of the round ligament.

FOURNIER'S SCROTAL GANGRENE

Occasionally, elderly men develop an acute unilateral infection within the tunica vaginalis which rapidly extends outwards to cause spreading gangrene of the scrotal skin (see Fig. 27.3). It is a form of **necrotising**

fasciitis and does not involve the testes. There is often an associated septicaemia. The underlying causes are varied and include pre-existing primary hydrocoele, genito-urinary trauma, either accidental or iatrogenic, perirectal abscess and urethral stricture. Predisposing factors include diabetes mellitus, corticosteroids, chemotherapy and alcohol abuse. The infecting organism is principally an anaerobe but there is often synergistic aerobic infection. Treatment is urgent and includes intravenous antibiotics and surgical excision of all the necrotic tissue, with the wound being left open to heal by secondary intention.

EPIDIDYMAL CYST AND SPERMATOCOELE

Multiple cysts may develop in the upper pole of the epididymis and present as a painless scrotal swelling (see Fig. 27.4). One cyst is usually larger than the others. Epididymal cysts affect a slightly younger age group than hydrocoeles. The testis can be palpated separately from the cysts, which lie near the upper pole of the testis. Epididymal cysts transilluminate.

Less common is the **spermatocoele**, a single cyst containing spermatozoa. Spermatocoeles usually occur in the head of the epididymis and may present like a third testis. They are clinically similar to epididymal cysts but may or may not transilluminate. Occasionally they occur in the spermatic cord. They probably arise from the **rete testis** (a plexus of spaces upon which the seminiferous tubules converge) and the 10–20 small ductuli efferentes connecting the rete testis to the epididymis; thus surgical excision may cause obstruction to the passage of sperm. If a patient wishes to remain fertile and the cysts are bilateral, excision may be contraindicated.

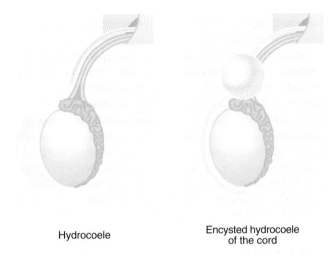

Hydrocoele

Encysted hydrocoele of the cord

Fig. 27.2 Hydrocoele and encysted hydrocoele of the cord

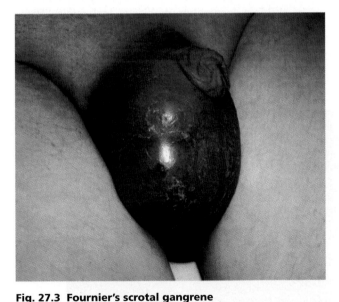

Fig. 27.3 Fournier's scrotal gangrene
This 81-year-old man presented with scrotal pain and a rapidly rising temperature. The right side of the scrotum was red and oedematous on admission to hospital; within 2 hours, the black necrotic areas seen at the lower pole appeared and rapidly extended. He was treated with intravenous antibiotics and wide surgical excision to remove all necrotic tissue. The patient had a pre-existing hydrocoele.

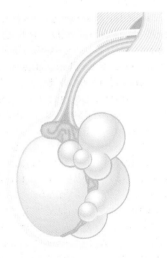

Fig. 27.4 Epididymal cysts

VARICOCOELE

A varicocoele (see Fig. 27.5) represents dilatation and tortuosity of the veins of the pampiniform plexus of the spermatic vein in the spermatic cord. The cause is unknown, but since the condition is much more common on the left (90%), it may result from the different venous drainage on the two sides. On the left, the testicular vein drains into the high-pressure renal vein, whereas the right testicular vein drains directly into the inferior vena cava.

Varicocoele is common, affecting as many as 10% of young adult males. It is usually asymptomatic but is often discovered during general physical examination for infertility. Varicocoele increases scrotal temperature which may inhibit normal sperm function and eventually cause testicular atrophy. In the supine position, the distended veins collapse and are impalpable. Varicocoele can only be diagnosed if the patient is examined while standing, when the varicocoele feels like 'a bag of worms'.

Rarely, a varicocoele may be caused by obstruction of the left renal vein by an invading renal adenocarcinoma. Such varicocoeles do not collapse when the patient lies supine. If the history of varicocoele is short, particularly in the elderly, or if it is on the right side, then ultrasound investigation for renal adenocarcinoma may be appropriate.

In adults, surgical treatment of varicocoele is only indicated for the relief of pain or the treatment of low sperm count (oligospermia). In the child or adolescent, treatment is advised to preserve spermatogenesis. The treatment can be laparoscopic, clipping the veins posterior to the sigmoid colon, or open surgical ligation can be performed at or above the groin level. Embolisation of testicular veins can be performed percutaneously via the femoral vein; this may become the treatment of choice in the future.

TESTICULAR TUMOURS

Testicular tumours are the most common solid tumours in males between the ages of 25 and 35 years. In males of all ages, they comprise about 1% of all malignancies. About 1 new case occurs in 20 000 males per annum and half have metastases by the time of presentation. Undescended testes are at least 30 times more likely to become malignant, although the individual risk is still low. Such tumours are usually seminomas.

More than 90% of primary testicular tumours are derived from germ cells; the rest include gonadal, stromal, mesenchymal and ductal tumours. Germ cell tumours are categorised as either **seminomas**, derived from spermatocytes, or **non-seminomatous germ cell tumours** (NSGCTs). **Teratomas**, derived from multipotent germ cells, make up the majority of the NSGCT group with the rest mainly undifferentiated embryonal cell carcinomas, choriocarcinomas or tumours of mixed cell type. Non-germ cell **Leydig cell tumours** derived from the gonadal stroma often present with excess hormone secretion rather than a testicular lump, which causes precocious puberty in a child and testicular feminisation in an adult.

The testes may also be involved in more widespread malignancy: lymphoma, chronic lymphocytic leukaemia or, in children, acute lymphoblastic leukaemia. These rarely present as lumps in the testis but the surgeon may be asked to perform a testicular biopsy as part of the monitoring process.

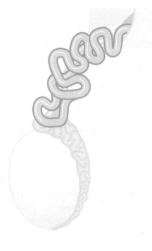

(a)

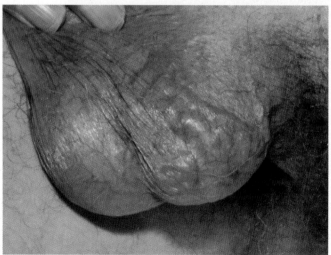

(b)

Fig. 27.5 Varicocoele

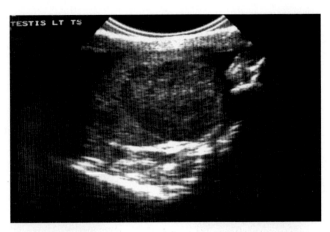

Fig. 27.6 Seminoma
This ultrasound scan was performed on a 23-year-old man with a short history of an enlarged testis. There was no clinical sign of a hydrocoele. The scan shows a solid mass involving the whole testis with no evidence of fluid. The scan is fairly homogeneous, suggesting seminoma. Teratomas tend to be more variegated but a definitive diagnosis requires surgical exploration.

PATHOLOGY OF TESTICULAR TUMOURS

Seminomas

Seminomas—derived from spermatocytes—make up more than half of the malignant testicular tumours. Their peak incidence is at 35 years and they occur mainly between the ages of 20 and 45 years. The cut surface of seminomas is typically pale, creamy-white and **homogeneous**. Histologically, the tumour cells are uniform and tightly packed. A distinct but rare form of seminoma, the **spermatocytic seminoma**, occurs between the ages of 50 and 70 years and almost never metastasises.

Teratomas

Teratomas are slightly less common than seminomas and their peak incidence is a decade earlier. Since they are derived from multipotent cells, teratomas may contain tissue from all three germ cell layers: ectoderm, mesoderm and endoderm. Teratomas exhibit a wide range of differentiation. Differentiated and intermediate tumours contain a collection of tissues resembling mature adult tissues: in particular, squamous epithelium (ectodermal), cartilage and smooth muscle (mesodermal), and respiratory epithelium (endodermal). Consequently, the cut surface of teratomas often appears **variegated**, with cystic areas and areas of necrosis and haemorrhage; this is easily distinguished from seminoma with the naked eye.

Undifferentiated germ cell tumours are regarded as variants of teratoma and are generally known as non-seminomatous germ cell tumours. In some of these tumours, described as **embryonal carcinomas** in the USA, no organoid elements are evident. Another variant

contains tissues with malignant syncytiotrophoblastic and cytotrophoblastic features. These are known as **trophoblastic teratomas** or **choriocarcinoma**. Some germ cell tumours contain mixed cell types with areas of poorly differentiated teratoma and areas of seminoma, but one or the other tumour type usually predominates. These mixed tumours behave as teratomas and should be treated as such.

Box 27.1 shows the current classification of primary malignant testicular tumours used in the UK. Other classifications are used in other countries. All classifications are frequently updated as new information emerges.

CLINICAL FEATURES OF TESTICULAR TUMOURS

A malignant testicular tumour usually presents as a painless, progressively enlarging testicular lump. If the capsule becomes involved, a **secondary hydrocoele** may develop but this is usually small and does not hinder palpation of the lump.

Both seminoma and teratoma spread via lymphatics to para-aortic nodes at the level of L1/2. Spread is then proximally along the lymphatic chain and thoracic duct to the supraclavicular nodes and systemic circulation. Lung secondaries are particularly common in teratomas. Poorly differentiated testicular tumours metastasise early and may present as enlarged abdominal or cervical lymph nodes or with symptoms of lung metastases. The primary testicular lesion may be very small or even impalpable.

A solid testicular lump must be assumed to be a tumour until proven otherwise. The history is rarely helpful but may include an episode of trauma which merely drew attention to the lump. On examination, the testis is either diffusely enlarged or contains a discrete lump

---

KEY POINTS

Box 27.1 Classification of malignant testicular tumours*

- Seminoma
- Differentiated teratoma (TD)
- Malignant teratoma intermediate (MTI)
- Malignant teratoma undifferentiated (MTU)—also known as embryonal tumour
- Subvariant: Malignant teratoma trophoblastic (MTT) also known as choriocarcinoma
- Yolk sac tumour

* Testicular Tumour Panel and Registry of the Pathological Society of Great Britain and Ireland. Unlike the WHO classification, this groups all non-seminomatous tumours under the heading of teratoma

which is firm and non-tender. A small hydrocoele may be present. Systemic examination may reveal evidence of metastases. Malignant cervical nodes will be palpable but enlarged para-aortic nodes can rarely be palpated unless they are huge. Inguinal nodes are not involved unless the tumour has spread to the scrotal skin. This is rare except when biopsy or orchidectomy has been performed through a scrotal incision, which is bad surgical practice if malignancy is suspected.

INVESTIGATION AND TREATMENT OF TESTICULAR TUMOURS

The outlook for treated testicular tumours, even with metastases, is often good. Cure rates have improved dramatically over the past 25 years with the use of CT scanning and tumour markers for staging and monitoring the disease and with the evolution of scientifically based treatment protocols. Investigation and treatment usually take place in parallel. The aims are to confirm the diagnosis, to detect any metastases and to stage the disease, and to treat according to the stage.

The first investigation is ultrasonography of the scrotal contents. If this confirms a solid testicular mass, direct surgical examination will be required, as described on page 365. Preliminary staging investigations are usually performed beforehand, including chest X-ray to look for hilar node involvement and lung secondaries (see Fig. 27.7), and blood levels of tumour markers. Tumour markers are useful for tracking residual or recurrent tumour metastases as blood levels correlate closely with tumour bulk. A preoperative measurement is important as it may become negative later; serial postoperative measurements help monitor disease progress and the impact of therapy.

Tumour markers

Human chorionic gonadotrophin (βHCG) is secreted by syncytiotrophoblastic cells and levels may rise in any tumour type, particularly poorly differentiated germ cell tumours. **Alpha-fetoprotein** (AFP) is produced by yolk sac elements. About 75% of patients with metastatic teratoma have elevated AFP levels but this marker is not expressed in seminoma. **Lactic dehydrogenase** (LDH) is elevated in more than half of all patients with metastatic seminoma. Tumour markers are repeated at intervals during follow-up and are invaluable for predicting the appearance of new metastases.

Surgical exploration

Orchidectomy is the only appropriate treatment for the primary tumour and is usually performed as part of the

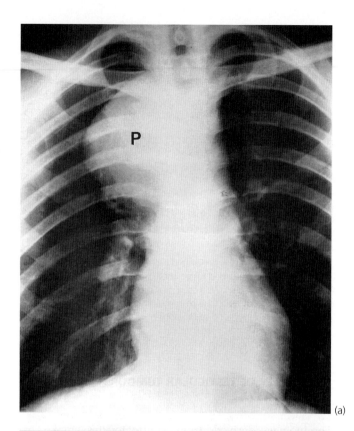

(a)

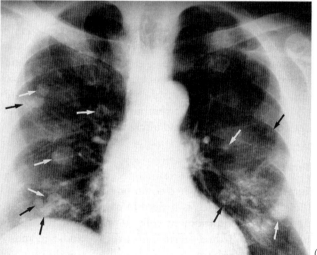

(b)

Fig. 27.7 Metastatic testicular tumours
(a) This 24-year-old man presented with a small testicular lump. An orchidectomy was performed and the cut surface of the tumour was cystic and haemorrhagic. Histology confirmed the expected diagnosis of testicular teratoma. This chest X-ray shows a large mediastinal mass which represents a grossly enlarged paratracheal lymph node **P**. Para-aortic node involvement occurs in teratoma but not seminoma. This patient's disease was defined as stage III because the disease was not extralymphatic. **(b)** Multiple bilateral pulmonary metastases (arrowed) in a 27-year-old man with a testicular swelling. The cut surface of the orchidectomy specimen was homogeneous and histology confirmed seminoma. Pulmonary metastases occur in both teratoma and seminoma, and in either case indicate stage IV disease.

diagnostic process. The surgical approach involves an exploratory operation performed via an inguinal incision to avoid involving the scrotal skin. The spermatic cord is temporarily clamped to preclude venous spread of tumour cells and the testis is brought out for visual examination and palpation. If the testis is obviously malignant, orchidectomy is then performed, dividing the cord at the internal inguinal ring. If there is any diagnostic doubt, a testicular biopsy is taken and examined immediately by frozen section. The other testis is usually unaffected and can be preserved. Further treatment is planned according to tumour type and stage.

Imaging for staging

If malignancy is confirmed, computed tomography is performed to establish the sites and degree of involvement of abdominal, thoracic and pelvic lymph nodes. CT may demonstrate pulmonary metastases not shown on chest X-ray. A standard method of staging testicular tumours is shown in Figure 27.8 and Box 27.2 opposite.

Management of seminoma

For stage I seminoma, i.e. disease confined to the testis, many oncologists recommend no further initial treatment. Seminoma is, however, very radiosensitive and many advise para-aortic radiotherapy as there is a 30% relapse rate with orchidectomy alone. For stages IIa and b (i.e. abdominal lymphadenopathy up to 5 cm diameter), radical radiotherapy to the ipsilateral para-aortic and iliac nodes gives a cure rate of about 95%. Oligospermia of the contralateral testis may occur even if the latter is lead-shielded but this is usually transient. There is also a vogue for single-dose chemotherapy with **carboplatin** for all stages, avoiding radiotherapy altogether. For more advanced disease, chemotherapy is nearly always indicated.

Management of teratomas and other non-seminomatous germ cell tumours

Up to 25% of patients with stage I disease would relapse within a year of orchidectomy without further treatment. Radiotherapy has no curative role in these types of tumour. Further treatment for stage I disease has three options:

● Immediate chemotherapy
● Retroperitoneal lymph node dissection
● Surveillance and treatment if metastases occur

In the USA, lymph node dissection is often employed and provides a good cure rate but risks ejaculatory failure from autonomic nerve damage. In the UK, meticulous surveillance is the preferred option. Chemotherapy for relapse is virtually always successful and thus 75% of patients are spared additional treatment.

Chemotherapy is indicated for all patients with known metastatic disease, including those in whom the only evidence of metastatic disease is elevated tumour markers. Results of chemotherapy for metastatic disease were transformed in the 1970s by the use of **cis-platinum**. The Einhorn regimen from Indiana combined this with **vinblastine** and **bleomycin** and gave even better cure rates of 70%. Later, **etoposide** replaced vinblastine (bleomycin, etoposide, cis-platin—'BEP') with improved overall cure rates of 85%. Three-quarters of patients with teratomas and other non-seminomatous germ cell tumours have low-volume disease, and in these cure can be expected in 95%.

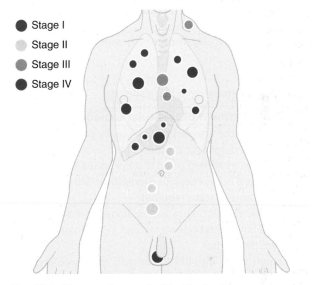

● Stage I
○ Stage II
● Stage III
● Stage IV

Fig. 27.8 Stages of spread of testicular tumours

KEY POINTS

Box 27.2 Stages of spread of testicular tumours

Stage I
● Tumour confined to testis

Stage II
● Retroperitoneal lymph node involvement
— IIa nodes < 2 cm
— IIb nodes 2–5 cm
— IIc nodes > 5 cm

Stage III
● Metastasis above the diaphragm confined to lymph nodes

Stage IV
● Extralymphatic metastases (usually lungs and liver)

Long-term surveillance

After chemotherapy, surgical debulking ('salvage') of residual lymph node masses is occasionally indicated. In the long term, tumour markers and sequential CT scans are used to monitor the success of treatment. Recurrent disease can often be successfully treated by radiotherapy, chemotherapy or surgery.

Fertility

Many patients with testicular tumours are subfertile at presentation and chemotherapy with BEP has unpredictably adverse effects on fertility. Patients need to be counselled carefully and, if appropriate and required, semen should be collected and stored before treatment so that artificial insemination or in vitro fertilisation may be performed later. However, the success rate is poor.

Treatment of testicular tumours is summarised in Box 27.3.

KEY POINTS

Box 27.3 Treatment of testicular tumours

1. Removal of the affected testis—usually performed as part of the diagnostic process
2. No further treatment given if stage I disease (i.e. no metastases) but meticulous surveillance with tumour markers and CT scans required
3. Radiotherapy—local irradiation alone for moderate abdominal lymph node metastases in seminoma (stages IIa and IIb)
4. Chemotherapy with BEP (bleomycin, etoposide and cis-platinum)—for all cases of metastatic teratoma, and metastatic seminoma beyond stage IIb
5. Debulking surgery for lymph nodes treated by chemotherapy—sometimes necessary

---

MALDESCENT OF THE TESTIS

The testis may fail to descend normally from the posterior abdominal wall into the scrotum where it should lie at birth in the full-term infant. If the testis is not in the scrotum, it usually lies at some point along its normal path of descent, most commonly in the inguinal canal. Alternatively, it may be found in an **ectopic** position, most often in the superficial inguinal pouch just above the external inguinal ring.

Maldescended testes are often structurally abnormal, and this may be responsible for the failure of normal descent. The maldescended testis is known to be at increased risk of malignancy, which may also be due to

developmental abnormalities. Unless the testis is successfully relocated in the scrotum before the age of 10, the risk of malignancy persists despite operation.

In developed countries, the condition is usually identified at screening during early childhood and surgically corrected (orchidopexy) at a young age (see Ch. 45); the ideal age is probably around 2 years. Delaying treatment until puberty is disastrous for spermatogenesis.

A few cases of absent testis are missed in childhood, however, and present in adulthood with:

- An 'absent' testis—confirmed if a vas is found at groin exploration. Laparoscopy appears to be the best investigation to search further if no vas is found
- A groin lump which is the testis or a testicular tumour
- Groin pain due to acute or recurrent torsion

TORSION OF THE TESTIS OR EPIDIDYMAL APPENDAGE

TESTICULAR TORSION (see Fig. 27.9)

In infants, the newly descended testis and its investing tunica vaginalis are mobile within the scrotum and may undergo **extravaginal torsion**. This presents as a hard, swollen testis. Later, the testis becomes suspended in the scrotum in a near vertical position, anchored by the spermatic cord and by attachments to the posterior wall

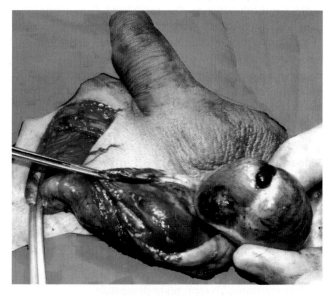

Fig. 27.9 Torsion of the testis
This 15-year-old boy experienced sudden severe lower abdominal pain extending to the scrotum during a football match. A provisional diagnosis of torsion was made and the scrotum explored within 2 hours of the onset of pain. At operation, the testis was twisted 2½ times around on its cord (arrowed) and was near infarction. On untwisting however, it soon regained normal colour. Both testes were fixed to prevent future torsion.

of the scrotum. This prevents rotation of the testis. Minor anatomical variations can produce a narrow-based pedicle with a horizontal ('bell-clapper') testicular lie, which allows the testis to become twisted about its axis within the tunica vaginalis (**intravaginal torsion**). When this occurs, the veins in the pampiniform plexus are compressed, causing venous congestion. After a few hours, venous infarction will occur unless the torsion is corrected. Trauma during sport may sometimes initiate the process of torsion. Torsion of the testis is a surgical emergency requiring prompt diagnosis and urgent surgical treatment if the testis is to be saved.

Testicular torsion presents with a sudden onset of severe testicular pain often accompanied by poorly localised central abdominal pain and sometimes vomiting. The abdominal pain occurs because the testis retains its embryological nerve supply within the abdomen. In the early stages of torsion, the affected testis is tender, slightly swollen and drawn up into the neck of the scrotum where the cord may be palpably thickened. With these features, the diagnosis is seldom in doubt. At a later stage, the overlying scrotal skin tends to become red and oedematous, making accurate palpation difficult. At this point, torsion may be difficult to distinguish clinically from acute epididymitis and the scrotum must be explored surgically.

TORSION OF THE EPIDIDYMAL APPENDAGE (HYDATID OF MORGAGNI)

A small embryological remnant at the upper pole of the testis is known as the hydatid of Morgagni (see Fig. 27.10). This may undergo torsion and produce symptoms similar to those of testicular torsion, out of proportion to the size of the infarcted tissue. Infarction of

the hydatid is of no consequence except that it must be distinguished from testicular torsion.

MANAGEMENT OF SUSPECTED TESTICULAR TORSION

Differentiating between acute epididymitis and torsion can be difficult; if a firm diagnosis cannot be reached, surgical exploration is mandatory. Investigations are of little value: both radionuclide studies and Doppler ultrasound examination may be employed to show testicular blood flow but results can be misleading. If torsion is seen at an early stage, it is sometimes possible to untwist the testis without operation. The testis is gently rotated outwards, if necessary using local anaesthetic infiltration in the cord. Successful reduction relieves the emergency, but the testis should be surgically secured as soon as practicable to prevent recurrence.

In most cases, urgent operation is imperative as delay leads to testicular necrosis after about 8 hours. A scrotal incision is made and the testis is examined and untwisted. If the testis is black and fails to recover its colour, it is necrotic and should be removed to prevent it inducing a sympathetic contralateral orchiopathy. If some colour is restored, biopsy can be performed to check for viability; otherwise the testis is best left, although it may later atrophy. The untwisted testis is then sutured to the tunica vaginalis or placed into a dartos pouch to prevent recurrence. Both testes should be secured since predisposition to torsion is usually bilateral.

TRAUMA TO THE TESTIS

The testes may be injured during contact sports or fights. The dense fibrous capsule which invests the testis (tunica

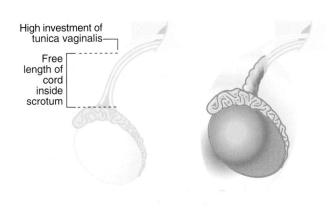

High investment of tunica vaginalis

Free length of cord inside scrotum

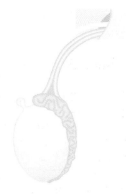

Pedunculated hyatid of Morganii

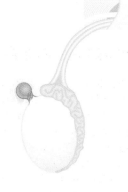

Torsion of hyatid of Morganii

(a)

(b)

Fig. 27.10 Torsion of the testis and Hydatid of Morgagni

albuginea) may remain intact or split but the testis is extremely painful in either case. If the tunica remains intact, a **testicular haematoma** results; if it splits, the testicular parenchyma bursts and bleeds into the tunica vaginalis cavity, resulting in a **haematocoele**.

If pain is severe and persistent, the scrotum can be explored surgically. Pain from a testicular haematoma can be relieved by incising the tunica albuginea. Evacuating a haematocoele, however, may be impossible because blood tends to infiltrate the tissues. If the haematocoele can be evacuated, a rupture of the tunica albuginea is best repaired.

MALE STERILISATION

Male sterilisation by vasectomy is a simple, effective method of birth control. It can be performed under local anaesthesia at little cost and requires no special equipment. The essential prerequisite is that the couple involved should have already completed their family, since reversal is technically difficult and unreliable. A technique of vasectomy is illustrated in Figure 27.11.

Most techniques involve removal of a section of the vas (ductus) deferens and ligation or cauterisation of the cut ends. For medico-legal reasons, the nature of the excised portion is often confirmed histologically. Spermatozoa remain in the proximal duct system for several months after vasectomy. Thus, the operation cannot be considered a success until at least two successive sperm counts performed about 1 month apart after 20–25 ejaculations are negative. Despite correct operative technique and negative sperm counts, there is a late failure rate of about 1 case in every 500. Failure due to spontaneous reconnection of the vas should be proved by a positive sperm count; note the problems of determining paternity in the case of unexpected pregnancy!

Early complications of vasectomy include postoperative scrotal haematoma (operator error) and wound infection. Later, failure of sterilisation may become apparent or a **sperm granuloma** may present as a tender scrotal swelling near the cut end of the vas. Further excision is usually required. Chronic debilitating pain can occur in the testis and the patient must be warned of this possibility at the time of consent. The patient must also be warned of the possibility of spontaneous reversal.

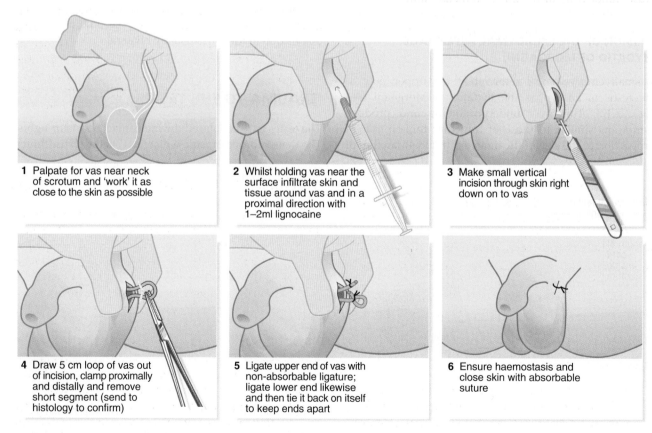

1 Palpate for vas near neck of scrotum and 'work' it as close to the skin as possible

2 Whilst holding vas near the surface infiltrate skin and tissue around vas and in a proximal direction with 1–2ml lignocaine

3 Make small vertical incision through skin right down on to vas

4 Draw 5 cm loop of vas out of incision, clamp proximally and distally and remove short segment (send to histology to confirm)

5 Ligate upper end of vas with non-absorbable ligature; ligate lower end likewise and then tie it back on itself to keep ends apart

6 Ensure haemostasis and close skin with absorbable suture

Fig. 27.11 Technique of vasectomy
Note that each side is dealt with separately.

DISORDERS OF THE PENIS

Problems with the foreskin (prepuce) are common and form the majority of surgical disorders of the penis. They include **balano-posthitis** (inflammation of the glans and foreskin), **phimosis** (stricture of the preputial meatus), **paraphimosis** (acute constriction of the glans by a tight retracted foreskin) and **balanitis xerotica obliterans** (idiopathic sclerosis of the foreskin).

Carcinoma of the penis is uncommon but obviously important. **Peyronie's disease** (idiopathic fibrosis of the corpora cavernosa) is now a frequent presentation in urological outpatient clinics (below). Exclusion of cancer is usually the first requirement.

FORESKIN PROBLEMS IN ADULTS

PHIMOSIS

The most common foreskin problem in adults arises when the foreskin will not retract fully and causes pain on intercourse. This is called phimosis and is usually caused by fibrosis of the foreskin. This fibrosis may be due to chronic or recurrent low-grade *Candida* infection. Phimosis is aggravated by attempts at retraction which cause minor tears of the inner epithelial lining inducing further fibrosis. Phimosis may be accompanied by stenosis of the urethral meatus, also due to recurrent inflammation and fibrosis. Treatment involves circumcision.

BALANO-POSTHITIS (BALANITIS)

The term balano-posthitis refers to overt inflammation of the glans penis and foreskin (Greek: *balanos* gland, *posthe* foreskin); it is the correct term to use in preference to the short form balanitis, which, has, however, passed into common usage. The condition occurs most commonly in children. Inflammation is most often caused by Candida or faecal bacteria but this problem rarely reaches the surgeon.

Balanitis xerotica obliterans is a fibrotic condition of the foreskin of unknown aetiology and analogous to lichen sclerosis of the vulva in females. It produces a thickened, stenosed, often depigmented foreskin which is often adherent to the glans. Circumcision solves the problem but the process can involve the urethral meatus causing meatal stenosis, sometimes requiring meatotomy or meatoplasty at the same time.

PARAPHIMOSIS

If a phimotic foreskin is forcibly retracted, the tight meatal band may lodge in the coronal sulcus making reduction impossible. This is known as paraphimosis. Progressive oedema of the glans penis and foreskin then exacerbates the difficulty of reduction. It may occur at any age, but is particularly common in elderly men in whom the foreskin is not correctly pulled forwards after retraction for catheterisation or washing the glans (female nurses and junior doctors are the main culprits). Paraphimosis also occurs in children and adolescents experimenting with foreskin retraction. In most cases, the foreskin can be reduced by firm manual compression of the glans and foreskin. Local anaesthetic jelly is applied first for lubrication and pain relief. Sometimes, it may be necessary to incise the tight ring under local or general anaesthesia to effect reduction. Preputioplasty, in which the band is incised longitudinally and the skin sutured transversely, can often be performed at the same time to solve the problem in the long term. If not, circumcision or preputioplasty is usually performed at a later date when the oedema and inflammation have resolved.

CIRCUMCISION

Circumcision for phimosis, paraphimosis and recurrent balanitis in children has largely gone out of favour. Most cases will respond to local treatments or to preputioplasty. Misguided circumcision may predispose to ammoniacal nappy rash and meatal stenosis.

Circumcision should be reserved for unresolved phimosis, recurrent balanitis and sclerosis from balanitis xerotica obliterans. The surgical technique is shown in Figure 27.12. During the operation, the urethral meatus should be checked for stenosis. If present, a meatotomy may be required. An occasional early postoperative complication is haemorrhage which usually requires surgical re-exploration. Postoperative bleeding can best be prevented by meticulous haemostasis at operation.

PEYRONIE'S DISEASE

This disease of unknown aetiology occurs in young to middle-aged adults. Some cases are thought to result from penile trauma during sexual activity and some cases are associated with Dupuytren's contracture. Slowly progressive asymmetrical fibrotic plaques develop in the fascia surrounding the corpora cavernosa of the penis. The corpus spongiosum including the glans is spared. The plaques may become calcified and visible on X-ray. The condition causes the penis to bend towards the affected side on erection, making intercourse difficult and painful. There may be spontaneous partial resolution with time.

Severe cases require surgery. **Nesbitt's operation** involves creating pleats in the corpus on the contralateral side. Another approach involves excision of the plaques which are replaced by a patch of tunica vaginalis. Either procedure may restore symmetrical erection. Penile pros-

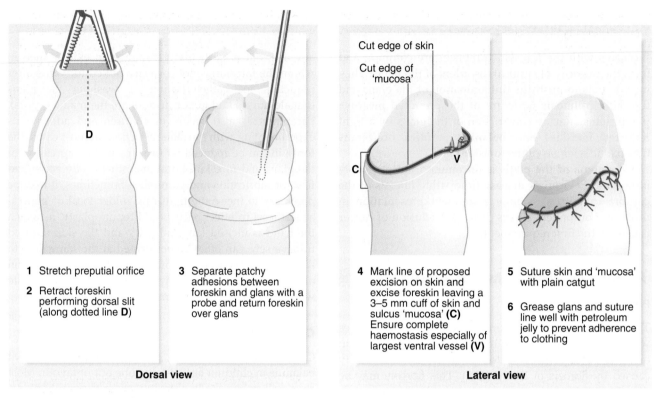

1 Stretch preputial orifice

2 Retract foreskin performing dorsal slit (along dotted line **D**)

3 Separate patchy adhesions between foreskin and glans with a probe and return foreskin over glans

Dorsal view

4 Mark line of proposed excision on skin and excise foreskin leaving a 3–5 mm cuff of skin and sulcus 'mucosa' **(C)** Ensure complete haemostasis especially of largest ventral vessel **(V)**

5 Suture skin and 'mucosa' with plain catgut

6 Grease glans and suture line well with petroleum jelly to prevent adherence to clothing

Lateral view

Fig. 27.12 Technique of circumcision

thetic implants may be required if erection is inadequate for satisfactory sexual intercourse. 'Medical treatments', i.e. steroid injections or radiation, are of no benefit.

CARCINOMA OF THE PENIS

Carcinoma of the penis is rare in developed countries and almost unknown in circumcised males. Poor hygiene and accumulation of smegma are suspected aetiological factors but there is growing evidence of a viral aetiology linked to that of carcinoma of the uterine cervix in females (human papilloma virus).

Histologically, the tumours are squamous cell carcinomas, usually well differentiated, which arise from the inner surface of the foreskin or the glans penis in the region of the coronal sulcus. The tumour invades locally and tends to invade the distal urethra (Fig. 27.13a).

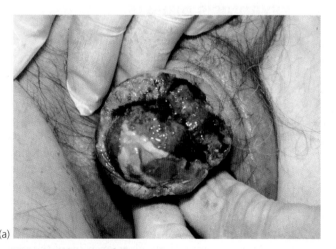

(a)

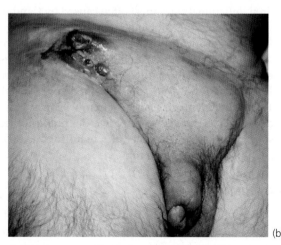

(b)

Fig. 27.13 Carcinoma of the penis
(a) An obvious carcinoma of the penis, revealed when the foreskin is retracted. **(b)** Unfortunately, this patient already had extensive spread to the inguinal lymph nodes.

Metastatic spread is to the inguinal lymph nodes (see Fig. 27.13b). **Erythroplasia of Queyrat** is the term given to severe dysplasia and carcinoma in situ of the glans and may represent a precursor of invasive carcinoma.

Most cases of carcinoma of the penis are found in the elderly. The disease is usually well advanced before an irregular lump, bleeding or discharge is noticed. In un-circumcised males, the lesion may be hidden by the foreskin. Figure 27.14 illustrates staging of the disease.

Surgical excision usually requires at least partial amputation of the penis, and block dissection of the inguinal lymph nodes if they are involved. Radiotherapy can be used in stage I disease if the urethra is not involved and for palliation in stage IV disease.

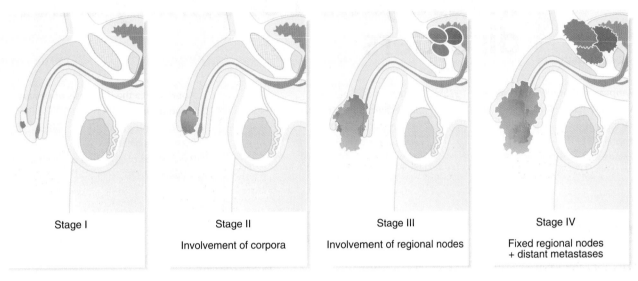

	Stage I	Stage II	Stage III	Stage IV

Stage I

Stage II
Involvement of corpora

Stage III
Involvement of regional nodes

Stage IV
Fixed regional nodes
+ distant metastases

Fig. 27.14 Stages in the spread of carcinoma of the penis

28 Symptoms, signs and investigation of urinary tract disorders

INTRODUCTION

Urinary tract disorders are common and comprise a significant part of the workload of family practitioners, general physicians, paediatricians and surgeons. In recent decades, the specialty of urology has become well established. Despite this, the general surgeon still deals with many urological problems, especially in smaller hospitals, where they make up about 25% of the general surgical workload.

Disorders of the prostate account for at least half the workload in urological surgery. The main conditions are benign prostatic hypertrophy, which affects about 10% of ageing males in Western countries, and prostatic carcinoma, which is now the second most common cancer in men. The remaining surgical disorders of the kidney and urinary tract can be divided into five broad groups: tumours, stone disease (**urolithiasis**), infections, congenital abnormalities and finally, local and systemic disorders which secondarily involve the urinary tract.

This chapter deals with the symptoms, signs, approach to investigation and diagnosis of urinary tract disease. The various disease entities are then discussed in the following five chapters.

SYMPTOMS OF URINARY TRACT DISEASE

The common symptoms of urinary tract disease fall into eight categories:

- Abdominal pain
- Passage of blood in the urine (**haematuria**)
- Pain associated with micturition (**dysuria**)
- Disorders of micturition such as frequency or hesitancy
- Retention of urine (acute or chronic)
- Urinary incontinence
- Passage of bowel gas in the urine (**pneumaturia**)
- Passage of blood in the semen (**haemospermia**)

The pattern of symptoms usually suggests the diagnosis and guides appropriate investigations. This section explains how the various symptoms relate to the underlying causes.

URINARY SYMPTOMS CAUSED BY DISEASE OF THE URINARY TRACT

Outflow of urine from the kidney may sometimes become impeded by obstruction of the urinary tract, and this may interfere with renal function. If there is chronic obstruction to bladder outflow or bilateral upper tract obstruction, the patient may develop renal failure, often without any localising symptoms.

Benign prostatic hypertrophy is the most common prostatic disorder, and usually presents with symptoms of bladder outflow obstruction (i.e. disorders of micturition or urinary retention or both) and sometimes with haematuria. Prostatic obstruction predisposes to bladder infections or stones, and the patient may present with these.

Carcinoma of the prostate is undoubtedly becoming more common. It may present with bladder outflow obstruction similar to benign prostatic disease or it may be discovered at an asymptomatic stage at a medical check-up, either by digital rectal examination or blood test (prostate specific antigen, PSA). Many cases are first diagnosed by the symptoms of metastases, such as bone pain.

Chronic prostatitis may be bacterial or abacterial (properly called **prostadynia**) and usually presents with chronic perineal ache and often aching testes. In the acute form, bacterial prostatitis may present as a systemic illness (or even Gram-negative septicaemia) with urinary symptoms and an exquisitely tender prostate. Occasionally, a prostatic abscess develops.

The important urinary tract tumours, stone diseases and infections are briefly outlined in Table 28.1. Any of these disorders may present with haematuria. Some of the conditions cause urinary obstruction and abdominal pain. The severity and character of the pain are determined by the site and degree of obstruction and, perhaps most importantly, the rapidity of onset. Disorders which cause urinary stasis also predispose to urinary tract infection.

Table 28.1 Pathophysiology and clinical features of urinary tract tumours, stones and infections

Disease	Pathophysiology	Clinical features
TUMOURS		
Renal cell carcinoma (also known as renal adenocarcinoma and formerly as 'hypernephroma')	Occurs in adults. Derived from renal tubular cells	Presents either incidentally (e.g. on CT scan) or with symptoms of haematuria, a mass or constitutional signs such as pyrexia or polycythaemia or is asymptomatic
Nephroblastoma (Wilms' tumour); see Chapter 45	Developmental origin; usually diagnosed before age 5	Presents as an abnormal mass with or without pain and haematuria
Transitional cell carcinoma	May arise in transitional epithelium anywhere from pelvicalyceal system to urethra, but most commonly in bladder	Usually presents with haematuria. Predisposes to urinary tract infections. May cause ureteric obstruction
Squamous cell carcinoma (very uncommon)	Arises in metaplastic squamous epithelium. Secondary to chronic stone or schistosomal irritation, especially in bladder. Also arises *de novo* in squamous epithelium of distal urethra (very rare)	As for transitional cell carcinoma
Adenocarcinoma of bladder (very rare)	Arises from columnar epithelium of urachal remnant	As for transitional cell carcinoma
STONE DISEASE		
Stones may develop in pelvicalyceal system or bladder. Pelvicalyceal stones can pass into the ureter	Stones in situ may cause irritation of urinary tract epithelium	Present as pain or haematuria or recurrent infection
	Chronic—renal stones may cause chronic pelviureteric or ureteric obstruction either directly or by causing fibrotic strictures	Present with chronic pain (due to back pressure) or recurrent infection
	Acute—renal stones may cause ureteric obstruction as they pass down the tract	Present as acute colicky pain often with renal tenderness (renal or ureteric colic). Infection may supervene, destroying the kidney if untreated
INFECTIONS		
'Common' infections due to bowel organisms	Infection develops either via bloodstream (haematogenous) or lower urinary tract (ascending). Any urinary tract abnormality or stasis predisposes to infection	Typically present with dysuria and frequency with or without haematuria
Tuberculosis (uncommon)	Kidney involvement via bloodstream from pulmonary or other primary disease. May spread via urine to ureters and bladder	May present as haematuria, persistent sterile pyuria, or as an incidental finding in pulmonary tuberculosis
Urinary schistosomiasis (bilharzia—very common in some developing countries; probably the world's most common cause of haematuria)	Induces chronic inflammation and fibrosis in bladder wall leading to gross bladder distortion, stones and squamous cell carcinoma	Presents with haematuria and various symptoms of infection and bladder fibrosis
Urethritis	Caused by gonococcus or *Chlamydia*. Sexually transmitted	Presents with urethral discharge and dysuria

Many different congenital abnormalities may involve the kidneys, ureters, bladder, urethra and genitalia, either alone or in combination. Most of the serious abnormalities are recognised at birth or in early childhood. The exceptions are polycystic disease and medullary sponge kidney, which usually present in adulthood. Less serious congenital abnormalities such as duplex systems may predispose to urinary tract infections because of abnormal flow dynamics. These abnormalities may be discovered at any age during the investigation of recurrent urinary tract infections. Congenital disorders which present mainly in adulthood are discussed in Chapter 33 and those presenting mainly in childhood in Chapter 45.

URINARY SYMPTOMS CAUSED BY NON-URINARY DISEASE

The urinary tract sometimes becomes secondarily involved in local inflammatory conditions such as Crohn's disease or diverticular disease. Fistulae may form, resulting in the passage of flatus or faeces in the urine or both (pneumaturia and faecuria). Retroperitoneal fibrosis, diverticulitis, tumours of the prostate, cervix or colon, and sometimes aortic or iliac aneurysms may secondarily involve the ureters and cause upper urinary tract obstruction.

ABDOMINAL PAIN

Most urinary tract diseases cause symptoms which are obviously referable to the urinary tract. When urinary symptoms are associated with abdominal pain, the cause is usually found to arise in the urinary tract. Urinary tract disorders may, however, cause abdominal pain without urinary symptoms; the diagnosis is then not so obvious and other characteristic clinical features must be sought.

PAIN ARISING FROM THE KIDNEYS AND UPPER TRACT

Renal inflammation or stretching of the renal capsule causes pain in the renal angle, the posterior space between the lowest rib and the iliac crest. This area may also be tender to palpation or percussion.

Renal stones, tumours or polycystic disease may cause dull and persistent loin pain even without obstruction.

In acute infections such as pyelonephritis or bladder infection, the pain is severe and is usually associated with systemic features and urinary tract symptoms.

Acute obstruction and distension of the pelvicalyceal system produce excruciating loin pain which often radiates to the hypochondrium or groin (see Fig. 28.1). If the ureter is obstructed, the pain is colicky (due to ureteric peristalsis) and often radiates down to the iliac fossa and groin. When obstruction is low in the ureter, the pain may radiate to the genitalia. This pain is known as **renal** or **ureteric colic**.

PAIN ARISING FROM THE BLADDER

Pain originating in the bladder (e.g. in cystitis) is felt in the suprapubic area. Pain may be referred to the penis or vulva if the bladder trigone is involved. In adults, clear-cut urinary symptoms such as dysuria and frequency are usually also present, but children may have no localising symptoms or complain only of pain, making the diagnosis less obvious. Dysuria is usually the predominant symptom of urethral disorders, but pain arising in the male urethra (e.g. in sexually transmitted infections) is usually referred to the tip of the penis. Finally, the pain of prostatic inflammation (prostatitis) is usually felt deep in the perineum. The prostate is tender on rectal examination in the acute but not the chronic form.

PAIN SIMULATING URINARY TRACT DISEASE

Pain from other abdominal pathology may sometimes mimic pain arising from the urinary tract. Acute appendicitis may present with suprapubic pain and biliary tract pain may be referred to the right thoraco-lumbar region, while posterior duodenal ulcers and pancreatic disease may cause pain in the central lumbar region. An expanding or leaking abdominal aortic aneurysm may sometimes mimic the pain of urinary tract disease, particularly if a ureter is compressed. Diseases of the thoraco-lumbar spine, such as metastatic cancer, tuberculosis, spondylosis and disc lesions, may also simulate upper urinary tract disorders. Suspected renal colic with a local rash is usually due to shingles (herpes zoster); the rash may not appear for several days after the onset of pain; perineal zoster may cause retention of urine. In

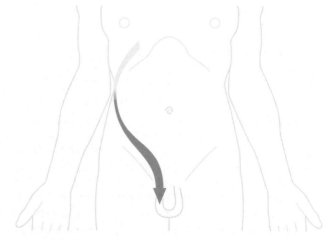

Fig. 28.1 Renal pain and its referral

women, pain arising from the ovaries or genital tract (e.g. pelvic inflammatory disease) may be confused with bladder pain.

HAEMATURIA

Patients may notice blood or even clots in the urine (**frank haematuria**) and this needs to be distinguished from urethral bleeding. More often, blood is discovered on 'dipstick' testing or microscopy of a midstream urine specimen (**microscopic haematuria**). Haematuria is often episodic rather than persistent, whatever the cause. 'Dipstick' testing for haematuria is extremely sensitive and yields many false positive results. Thus a positive dipstick result should be confirmed by urine microscopy, and if confirmed, freshly voided urine should be examined for malignant cells by exfoliative cytology.

CAUSES OF HAEMATURIA (see Fig. 28.2)

Tumours are a common cause of frank and microscopic haematuria and must be suspected, even if another possible cause is found. Haematuria from tumours is typically painless. However, carcinoma in situ, a dysplastic condition with a high likelihood of progression to frank carcinoma, usually presents with irritative voiding, dysuria and haematuria. Irritation from infection or stones may also cause bleeding, but this is usually accompanied by pain or dysuria. If the urethra is obstructed by prostatic enlargement, straining at micturition may cause bleeding from dilated veins at the bladder neck.

Trauma to a normal kidney may cause frank haematuria if considerable force has been applied, but microscopic haematuria is common after minor trauma in contact sports and rarely indicates a significant injury. Enlarged kidneys are more susceptible to trauma, whatever the primary pathology. In hydronephrosis or polycystic kidneys, minor blunt trauma may cause gross haematuria.

Sometimes urine becomes red with haemoglobin rather than blood. In young people this may be induced by vigorous exercise such as jogging (**exercise haemoglobinuria and haematuria**). These patients are believed to have defective red cell membranes which makes them more vulnerable to trauma. Exercise haemoglobinuria is self-limiting and requires no treatment.

Haematuria also occurs in renal parenchymal inflammations such as glomerulonephritis or arteritis. Renal haematuria may also be caused by microemboli settling in the kidneys, as in atrial fibrillation or infective endocarditis. Any urinary tract disorder with a potential for haematuria is more likely to be revealed when a patient is on anticoagulant therapy or develops a bleeding diathesis.

DIAGNOSTIC FEATURES OF HAEMATURIA

Gross bleeding results in the passage of clots. The stage of micturition at which blood appears is sometimes diagnostically useful. Blood from the kidneys, ureters or bladder wall will completely mix with the urine, and be present throughout the urinary stream. Urethral bleeding may leak out independently of micturition, or be seen only at the beginning or end of the urinary stream. Blood arising from the bladder neck or posterior urethra may sometimes present as terminal haematuria.

Haematuria on dipstick testing should be confirmed by urine microscopy, which can also check for infection by culture and sensitivity. Microscopic haematuria may represent a significant lesion anywhere in the urinary tract and must be taken seriously. However, in 5–10% of cases of isolated episodes of microscopic haematuria, a cause is never found.

DYSURIA

Dysuria describes pain or discomfort on micturition, often accompanied by difficulty in voiding. The pain is often described as 'burning' or 'scalding'. Any irritation of the urethra may cause dysuria. The most common cause is urinary tract infection, but urethral instrumentation, or the presence of a catheter, also commonly causes dysuria.

DISORDERS OF MICTURITION

The normal bladder has a capacity of 350–500 ml. When this is reached, the detrusor muscle undergoes reflex contraction, initiating the desire to void. Micturition is normally initiated by conscious sphincter relaxation; a voluntary detrusor contraction then empties the bladder completely.

FREQUENCY OF MICTURITION

This is defined as the frequent passage of small quantities of urine, but with a normal daily urine volume. If severe, frequency may sometimes result in incontinence.

There are five main causes of frequent micturition:

- **Bladder irritation**—infection is the most common cause of urinary frequency and is usually accompanied by dysuria. The patient feels an almost constant need to pass urine regardless of the amount of urine in the bladder
- **Incomplete emptying of the bladder**—this is most commonly caused by bladder outlet obstruction as in prostatic hypertrophy, but it may also be caused by neurological disorders such as multiple sclerosis or

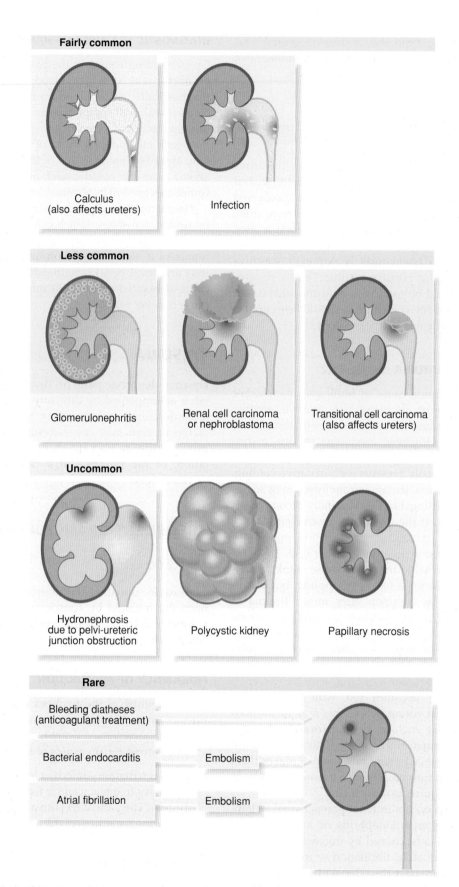

Fairly common

Calculus
(also affects ureters)

Infection

Less common

Glomerulonephritis

Renal cell carcinoma
or nephroblastoma

Transitional cell carcinoma
(also affects ureters)

Uncommon

Hydronephrosis
due to pelvi-ureteric
junction obstruction

Polycystic kidney

Papillary necrosis

Rare

Bleeding diatheses
(anticoagulant treatment)

Bacterial endocarditis

Embolism

Atrial fibrillation

Embolism

Fig. 28.2 Renal causes of haematuria

spinal trauma. Voiding is incomplete so the bladder soon reaches full capacity again. The increased volume of residual urine in the bladder after micturition predisposes to infection

- **Detrusor instability (the unstable bladder)**—in this condition, the voiding reflex is activated before the bladder is properly filled. Small volumes of urine are thus passed more frequently. This may be a secondary effect of obstruction to bladder outflow
- **Small or indistensible bladder**—this is a rare cause of frequency and may be due to surgical resection, inflammatory fibrosis such as tuberculosis, schistosomiasis, idiopathic interstitial fibrosis or following radiotherapy
- **Psychosomatic frequency**—this characteristically occurs during the daytime and not at night

Frequency must be distinguished from **polyuria**, in which the amount of urine produced is excessive and normal voiding volumes are passed at more frequent intervals. Polyuria is usually accompanied by polydipsia (excessive drinking). Excess urine production is not a surgical problem; it most commonly results from diabetes mellitus, less commonly from renal failure and occasionally from diabetes insipidus.

NOCTURIA

Nocturia describes the need to pass urine at night. The patient may wake with the urge to void hourly, if not more frequently. Nocturia usually accompanies frequency or polyuria. Patients with cardiac failure may experience nocturia as peripheral oedema is returned to the general circulation in the supine position and renal perfusion is thereby increased. Elderly patients, in particular, elaborate more urine at night due to enhanced renal blood flow when recumbent. Thus they may pass more urine at night than in the daytime. Some class II calcium channel antagonists are sometimes associated with nocturnal polyuria.

URGENCY

Urgency is the sudden desire to void, which, if ignored, may result in incontinence. Urgency results from irritation of the bladder neck as in cystitis, or from the abnormal entry of urine into the proximal urethra as in prostatic enlargement. If the bladder is overfilled as a result of outlet obstruction, spasms of abnormally high detrusor pressure can cause urgency or even incontinence. Other urinary symptoms are usually present.

HESITANCY

Difficulty in initiating micturition, known as hesitancy, usually occurs in males. In extreme cases, the patient may have to stand for several minutes before urinary flow begins. The usual cause is prostatic obstruction, which prevents entry of sufficient urine into the proximal urethra to initiate sphincter relaxation. Hesitancy may occur in young males because the bladder neck will not relax. The symptom is common, and often intermittent and situational, e.g. in a urinal when other men are nearby; the problem is not organic but rather psychosomatic.

POOR URINARY STREAM

Urinary stream is often reduced when there is urethral narrowing. The most common cause is prostatic enlargement or bladder neck hypertrophy, which may limit the urine flow to a dribble despite straining. A poor stream may be caused by a urethral stricture, in which case other urinary symptoms may be minimal or absent.

POST-MICTURITION DRIBBLING

With this symptom, urine flow does not cease completely at the end of micturition. Dribbling may simply involve the leakage of a few drops of urine or be so severe as to amount to incontinence. Post-micturition dribbling may result from abnormal sphincter function, but is usually due to incomplete emptying of the urethra by a weakened bulbospongiosus muscle. This symptom is not indicative of prostatic obstruction. When occurring in isolation in women, it may denote weakness of the pelvic floor. Urine trapped below a healthy sphincter and above a urethral stricture dribbles out after bladder emptying but more commonly presents with terminal dribbling.

'PROSTATISM'

This term is often applied to the symptoms of hesitancy, poor stream, terminal dribbling and incomplete bladder emptying with frequency, nocturia, urgency and urge incontinence. Any of these may occur in prostatic obstruction, but the term should be used with care because it implies a diagnosis, and may prejudice proper evaluation of symptoms. This symptom complex is now sometimes termed **lower urinary tract symptoms (LUTS)**.

RETENTION OF URINE

Urinary retention means the inability to void when the bladder is full. It occurs when the sphincter is unable to relax or when there is proximal urethral obstruction. Both factors may occur together.

ACUTE RETENTION

In its simplest form, acute urinary retention can occur in normal individuals, usually males, particularly postoperatively. At this time, fluid overload, drugs, pain, the supine posture, anxiety or embarrassment are responsible. Similar factors may precipitate an episode of acute retention in individuals with asymptomatic prostatic enlargement. Occasionally acute retention is caused by an obstructing blood clot (**clot retention**) or stone.

In the female, acute retention can occur after abdominal surgery, perhaps as a side effect of anaesthetic or analgesic drugs. It may also occur in pregnancy if the enlarging uterus becomes jammed in the pelvis at about 14 weeks' gestation. An ovarian cyst or uterine fibroid of similar dimensions may also cause obstruction of this type. Otherwise, multiple sclerosis should be suspected.

CHRONIC RETENTION

Chronic retention may occur with abnormalities of structure or function of the bladder muscle or sphincter mechanism. Less commonly, it is caused by persistent urethral obstruction. In chronic retention, voiding of urine is often incomplete. The problem progresses until the residual volume approaches maximum bladder capacity. Voiding then usually occurs by 'overflow' and the bladder tends to become abnormally distended. When obstruction is prolonged and severe, the bladder muscle hypertrophies, bladder diverticula may develop, and back pressure on the kidneys may cause uraemia and renal failure. At any stage, complete cessation of flow, i.e. **acute-on-chronic retention**, may be precipitated by over-filling (often alcohol-induced), urinary tract infection or severe constipation. The most common cause of chronic retention is bladder outflow obstruction caused by a thickened bladder neck or prostatic enlargement. It may also be caused by lower spinal neurological problems, e.g. central protrusion of lumbar intervertebral discs damaging the S2, 3, 4 innervation of the detrusor.

URINARY INCONTINENCE

Involuntary passage of urine is a distressing and socially debilitating symptom. It may occur in a variety of disorders with a structural or functional abnormality of the bladder or sphincter mechanism. The normal bladder has a capacity of approximately 350–500 ml. During filling, the detrusor muscle relaxes so that the intra-vesical pressure does not rise until bladder capacity is approached. Once the bladder is filled, voiding occurs by detrusor contraction and sphincter relaxation. Both are mediated via a spinal reflex at the level of S2, 3, 4. Super-imposed on this system is an inhibitory mechanism under cortical (conscious) control, which delays voiding if it is socially inappropriate. Conscious control, including nocturnal control, develops during early childhood. Nocturnal incontinence is known as **enuresis**.

The pathophysiology of incontinence can be divided into three categories based on disorders of structure and function which are described below and summed up in Box 28.1. Some disease processes may produce incontinence by more than one mechanism.

LOSS OF CORTICAL CONTROL

Loss of inhibitory control over reflex voiding may occur in disease of the cortex, such as senile atrophy (dementia), or in disease of the spinal cord above the sacral reflex level, such as multiple sclerosis. Traumatic paraplegia is a common cause of complete loss of cortical control. The resulting incontinence may be described as the **supra-sacral neurogenic bladder**. The bladder fills to normal capacity and then empties spontaneously, and more or less completely, leaving little residual urine.

DISORDERS OF SACRAL REFLEX CONTROL OF DETRUSOR AND SPHINCTER FUNCTION

If the sacral reflex arc is damaged on its afferent or efferent sides, reflex contraction of the detrusor and relaxation of the sphincter are lost. This may occur in low spinal trauma or nearby disease, such as myelomeningocoele, diabetic neuropathy or invasive pelvic tumours. The bladder consequently becomes grossly distended and urine passively overflows causing constant dribbling incontinence. This can be alleviated considerably by regular manual emptying of the bladder, achieved by applying abdominal pressure or more effectively by

---

SUMMARY

Box 28.1 Causes of incontinence

Loss of cortical control
- Cortical disease
- Spinal cord disease, i.e. supra-sacral neurogenic bladder

Abnormalities of the sacral reflex mechanism
- Sacral neurogenic bladder
- Detrusor instability
- Infection producing bladder hyperactivity
- Hypotonic bladder

Detrusor or sphincter abnormalities
- Stress incontinence
- Post-prostatectomy
- Tumor invasion
- Urethral trauma
- Contracted bladder
- Rare congenital abnormalities

intermittent self-catheterisation (ISC). This form of incontinence may be described as a **sacral neurogenic bladder**. The large residual volume of urine strongly predisposes to infection, which must be prevented.

In some patients, typically middle-aged women, the reflex control of detrusor activity becomes hypersensitive so that the voiding reflex is initiated when the bladder volume is well below full capacity. The cause is unknown. This hypersensitivity results in small volumes of urine being passed frequently, and often so precipitously as to produce **urge incontinence**. The condition is known as **irritable bladder syndrome** or **detrusor instability**, a minor but distressing form of incontinence.

Bladder infection produces excessive sensory irritation and activation of the voiding reflex. In young children and the elderly, this may be responsible for incontinence without the usual symptoms of infection.

Persistent bladder outflow obstruction—prostatic enlargement—causes progressive stretching of the bladder and in some way damages the voiding reflex. The result is a hugely distended, flaccid, **hypotonic bladder**. Dribbling overflow incontinence may persist even when the obstruction has been removed.

STRUCTURAL ABNORMALITIES OF THE BLADDER OR SPHINCTER

Many disorders may directly interfere with normal detrusor or sphincter function. In some cases, an additional contributory factor is damage to the afferent or efferent components of the neurogenic reflex mechanism.

The most common condition in this category is **stress incontinence**, in which the sphincter is weak. Any sudden increase of pressure on the bladder (while coughing, sneezing or laughing, for example) causes small quantities of urine to leak out. Stress incontinence is usually seen in parous women and results from pelvic floor damage during childbirth. There is often a degree of uterine prolapse and cystocoele.

Prostatectomy (transurethral or open) may damage the sphincter, as may locally invasive tumours or pelvic fractures which involve the proximal urethra. Tuberculosis, radiotherapy and **interstitial cystitis** in its severest form may cause severe bladder contraction and frequency to the point of incontinence.

Incontinence is a feature of several rare congenital abnormalities such as epispadias or ectopic ureter opening below the sphincter mechanism. These should be excluded in a child who fails to develop continence.

PNEUMATURIA

Pneumaturia is the passage of gas mixed with urine. It is caused by perforation of gut into the urinary tract, or rarely, vice versa, resulting in fistula formation. The commonest causes are diverticular disease and Crohn's disease, although it sometimes occurs in carcinoma of the colon or bladder (see Fig. 28.3). Gross urinary tract infection is inevitable. The patient typically complains of symptoms of urinary infection (dysuria and frequency) and may also describe bubbles or even faeces in the urine.

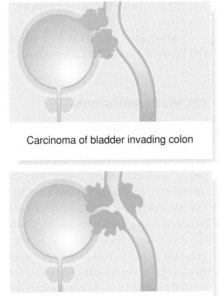

Carcinoma of bladder invading colon

Colonic carcinoma invading bladder

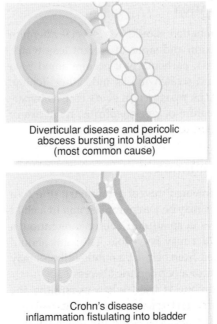

Diverticular disease and pericolic abscess bursting into bladder (most common cause)

Crohn's disease inflammation fistulating into bladder

Fig. 28.3 Causes of vesicocolic fistulae

HAEMOSPERMIA

Haemospermia describes the presence of blood in semen. It is usually innocent but can be caused by prostatitis or a stone in an ejaculatory duct. In the older male patient it is a rare presenting symptom of prostatic carcinoma.

APPROACH TO DIAGNOSIS OF URINARY SYMPTOMS

SPECIAL POINTS IN THE HISTORY

A detailed history of the urinary tract symptoms should be taken, together with a general history to elucidate any systemic causes or contributing factors, e.g. diabetes or multiple sclerosis. A full history of medication, past and present, should be recorded.

In patients with haematuria, the occupational history may be important. Exposure to aniline dyes and other industrial chemicals that were once widely used in the rubber and cable industries greatly increased the risk of transitional cell carcinoma of the urinary tract. Tobacco smoking has been calculated to cause 50% of bladder cancers.

Haematuria can also be caused by infestation with *Schistosoma*, which is endemic in parts of the Middle East and Africa and is transmitted by water snails. A history of residence or travel in affected regions should therefore be sought. Similarly, tuberculosis is common in developing countries and can easily be overlooked in immigrants.

PHYSICAL EXAMINATION

GENERAL EXAMINATION

A full general examination should pay special attention to a sallow complexion and signs of weight loss which may indicate uraemia, particularly if accompanied by a uriniferous smell and scratch marks indicating itching. Blood pressure must be measured in every case as hypertension may be a feature of pyelonephritis, renal artery stenosis, polycystic kidneys or glomerulonephritis.

ABDOMINAL EXAMINATION

Abdominal inspection may reveal asymmetry due to a huge renal mass; this may be a nephroblastoma in a child or polycystic kidneys in an adult. In chronic retention, a large, lopsided bladder may be visible. The loins should be carefully inspected from behind; a subtle fullness may indicate a renal mass or a perinephric abscess.

A bimanual technique is used when examining the abdomen for urinary tract disease. One hand palpates the subcostal region anteriorly while the other hand is placed in the renal angle to push the kidney forward on to the palpating hand. The kidneys are impalpable unless they are enlarged or displaced, except in a very thin patient. A renal mass will usually move with respiration and, because it is retroperitoneal with gut anteriorly, should also have an overlying area of resonance to percussion. The main causes of an enlarged kidney are hydronephrosis, polycystic disease, renal cell carcinoma and, in children, nephroblastoma (Wilms' tumour). Loin tenderness is uncommon in non-acute renal disorders except in chronic perinephric abscess. Tenderness is usually found in acute conditions, such as pyelonephritis or acute obstruction. Renal tenderness can be distinguished from vertebral tenderness by gently tapping the spinous processes. This will cause pain if the tenderness is vertebral.

The lower abdomen is palpated for the bladder. A distended bladder is felt as a soft mass arising from the pelvis, sometimes asymmetrically. It is dull to percussion and pressure on it may induce an urge to void; bladder distension is easily confirmed on ultrasound examination. A suprapubic mass in the male usually indicates urinary retention, but occasionally it is a colonic carcinoma, a huge bladder tumour or stone. In the female, ovarian masses, pregnancy or uterine fibroids are more common causes of a suprapubic mass than urinary retention.

Auscultation along the 12th rib posteriorly may reveal the bruit of renal artery stenosis.

RECTAL EXAMINATION

Rectal examination should be performed in both sexes. In females, a vaginal examination may also be indicated. In the male, the prostate is palpated per rectum for size, shape and consistency (see Fig. 28.4). The prostate is about 3 cm in diameter and weighs 10–15 g. When moderately enlarged, it is approximately the size of a golf ball and weighs about 30–40 g; when greatly enlarged, the prostate may weigh as much as 800 g. When the prostate gland is this large, its upper edge may be out of reach of the examining finger. Note that most prostatectomy operations leave a capsular remnant so that the prostate is still palpable and may be of firmer consistency on palpation. Note that it is impossible to make an accurate assessment of the volume of the prostate digitally (see Fig. 28.5).

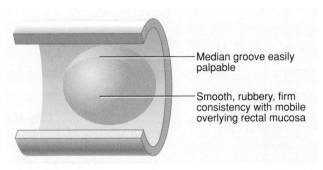

Median groove easily palpable

Smooth, rubbery, firm consistency with mobile overlying rectal mucosa

(a) Benign prostate

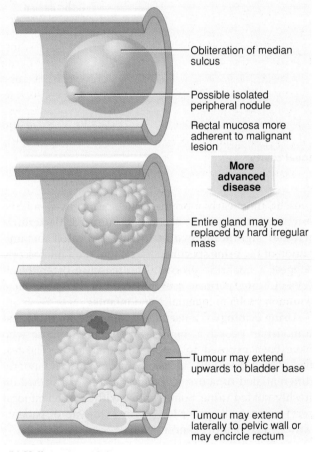

Obliteration of median sulcus

Possible isolated peripheral nodule

Rectal mucosa more adherent to malignant lesion

More advanced disease

Entire gland may be replaced by hard irregular mass

Tumour may extend upwards to bladder base

Tumour may extend laterally to pelvic wall or may encircle rectum

(b) Malignant prostate

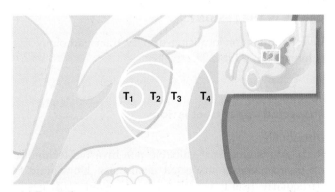

T_1 T_2 T_3 T_4

(c) Prostatic cancer

The severity of prostatic obstructive symptoms depends on the extent of encroachment upon the urethra and not the prostatic diameter. In some cases, an enlarged median lobe lying posteriorly above the bladder outlet may act as a flap valve, intermittently obstructing urine outflow.

On palpation, the normal prostate has a smooth surface and a firm consistency, and is divided into two lateral lobes by a midline groove. In prostatic hyperplasia, enlargement is usually symmetrical, and the midline groove is maintained. Consistency remains normal. In contrast, a prostate infiltrated with carcinoma is irregular and asymmetrical. There are often hard nodules, and the median groove may be lost. In advanced cases, the tumour may be felt invading laterally into the pelvis or forward around the rectum. Digital examination may distinguish benign from malignant prostatic enlargement in gross cases, but if carcinoma is suspected, **transrectal needle biopsy** is performed blindly (i.e. by palpation) or preferably under ultrasound guidance. Note, however, there is a 2% risk of systemic sepsis and the procedure needs to be covered with a single dose of a prophylactic antibiotic, e.g. gentamicin. Prostatic tenderness is uncommon and may indicate prostatitis.

INVESTIGATION OF SUSPECTED URINARY TRACT DISEASE

In common conditions like prostatic hyperplasia or urinary tract infection, the diagnosis is usually evident from the history and examination. Investigation is limited to confirming and refining the diagnosis before treatment is initiated. Symptoms such as haematuria, however, suggest several diagnostic possibilities and other diagnoses must be excluded.

A simple approach to investigation of urinary tract disease is to consider the following questions:

● Are any blood tests likely to be helpful in diagnosis?
● What urine tests are indicated?
● Where is the lesion?

ARE ANY BLOOD TESTS LIKELY TO BE HELPFUL IN DIAGNOSIS?

The blood tests that can be useful in diagnosing urinary tract disease are summarised in Box 28.2.

When prostate cancer is suspected, **prostate specific antigen (PSA)** levels should be estimated and fractionated into **free PSA**, **total PSA** and their **ratio**. The

Fig. 28.4 Palpation characteristics of the prostate
(a) Benign prostate. (b) Malignant prostate. (c) Prostatic cancer: TNM tumour grades on palpation. Note that palpation is more accurate when performed under general anaesthesia.

379

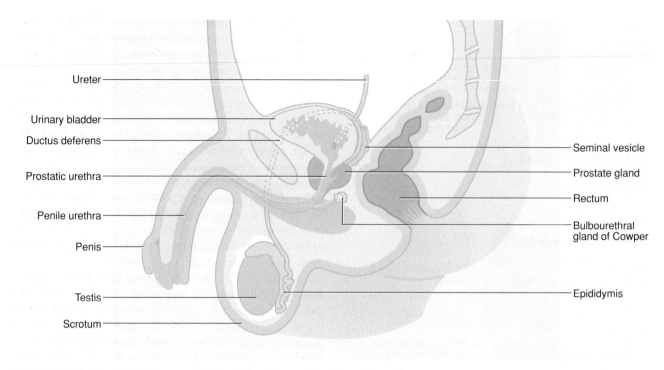

Ureter

Urinary bladder

Ductus deferens

Prostatic urethra

Penile urethra

Penis

Testis

Scrotum

Seminal vesicle

Prostate gland

Rectum

Bulbourethral
gland of Cowper

Epididymis

Fig. 28.5 Relationship of the prostate to the rectum and peritoneal cavity

free PSA is more likely to be raised in carcinoma and is a reliable indicator if the level is markedly elevated. In biopsy-proven prostatic cancer, persistently raised PSA levels above 20 are likely to indicate metastatic disease. However, the level may be normal in the presence of a small-volume cancer.

Total PSA rises with age and in benign hyperplasia tends to rise in proportion to prostate mass. Acute retention, urinary tract infection, any urethral instrumentation or biopsy of the prostate causes elevation of the PSA for up to 6 weeks; standard digital rectal examination does not affect PSA level.

WHAT URINE TESTS ARE INDICATED?

Any urinary symptoms should prompt collection of a clean **midstream urine specimen (MSU)** for microscopy and bacteriology. Microscopy will show the presence or absence of significant numbers of red blood cells (**microscopic haematuria**), white cells (**pyuria**) and bacteria (**bacteriuria**) (see Fig. 28.6). However, the cells can lyse if the specimen is kept overnight at room temperature.

Bacteriuria of more than 5×10^5 per cubic millimetre is considered to indicate significant infection. The urine is cultured to identify the organisms, and the organisms tested for antibiotic sensitivity. Culture-negative urine (**sterile pyuria**) is characteristic of urinary tract tuberculosis, urinary stone, bladder tumour, prostatitis or (most commonly) a partly treated urinary tract infection. If present, three early morning urine specimens should be examined for acid-fast bacilli and cultured. **Bacteriuria without significant pyuria** usually indicates contamination of the urine specimen. **Casts** found on microscopy suggest a nephritic process. The presence of epithelial cells indicates perineal contamination of the specimen, a common problem in females and infants.

Urine cytology is a useful screening test for urothelial tumours in people at high risk, particularly those who have been exposed to industrial carcinogens. The test has a high positivity in carcinoma in situ and poorly differentiated tumours. Cytology must be performed on freshly voided urine. Some centres with an efficient local service use cytology for long-term follow-up of patients with treated bladder cancer.

WHERE IS THE LESION?

Investigations for localising urinary tract pathology are summarised in Table 28.2, p. 383.

Suspected upper tract lesions

Ultrasound
Renal ultrasound is a valuable non-invasive technique for investigating a suspected renal mass. Ultrasound is particularly useful in differentiating solid from cystic lesions, and for demonstrating dilatation of the renal

Box 28.2 Blood tests useful in diagnosing urinary tract disease

Full blood count
- Hypochromic microcytic anaemia: chronic iron deficiency anaemia due to haematuria (rare)
- Normochromic normocytic anaemia: chronic renal failure (lack of erythropoietin), chronic inflammatory disorders, e.g. tuberculosis
- Polycythaemia: renal adenocarcinoma
- Leucocytosis: infection

Erythrocyte sedimentation rate (ESR)
- Raised in chronic and acute infections, renal adenocarcinoma and retroperitoneal fibrosis

Urea, electrolytes and ceatinine
- Impaired renal function in bilateral obstructive uropathy or chronic renal failure associated with hypertension, diabetes etc.

Prostate specific antigen
- Raised in metastatic carcinoma of prostate (see text). A normal level does not exclude prostatic carcinoma. Moderate elevations occur in benign disease, especially with acute retention of urine, urinary tract infection and following urethral instrumentation or prostatic biopsy

Alkaline phosphatase (bone isoenzyme)
- Raised in multiple bony metastases from any type of tumour

Calcium, phosphate, uric acid and parathyroid hormone levels
- Useful investigations in stone disease

pelvis. If bladder pathology is suspected, the bladder can easily be examined at the same time. The bladder is particularly well seen if it is distended with urine; patients should be advised to take copious fluids before the investigation is performed. Ultrasound can demonstrate stones in the kidney or bladder even if they are radiolucent (urate), but can rarely demonstrate a stone in the ureter.

Intravenous urography

Intravenous urography (IVU) is the traditional radiographic technique for demonstrating the urinary tract, although it provides poor assessment of function. Comparative renal function is best investigated by radionuclide scanning. An IVU involves intravenous injection of an aqueous solution of iodinated benzoic acid which is rapidly filtered by the glomeruli and excreted. This radiopaque solution opacifies the urinary system, dem-

onstrating the renal parenchyma, the renal pelvis and the ureteric anatomy. The cortical concentration of contrast (**nephrogram**) gives an indication of the shape, thickness and bilateral symmetry of the renal cortex.

Cysts and tumours of the kidneys are usually revealed by the distortion of normal anatomy they cause, although they are often indistinguishable from each other by this investigation. Tumours opacify with contrast to a variable extent and sometimes show a characteristic 'vascular blush'.

If the collecting system (renal pelvis, calyces and ureter) is dilated, this is usually easily seen, and the level of an obstruction can often be demonstrated. When obstruction is almost complete, films may have to be taken at long intervals since back pressure delays cortical excretion.

Congenital abnormalities of the pelvicalyceal system, such as duplex systems, are often found incidentally. Transitional cell tumours may show as filling defects in collecting systems or bladder. If an abnormality is seen in the kidney or renal pelvis, **tomography** can be performed during the same examination to reveal more structural detail. If renal excretion is poor, as in chronic renal failure or gross obstruction, IVU examination may be improved by using a high-dose infusion of contrast. However, this is a dangerous technique in diabetic nephropathy as it may precipitate acute renal failure.

The imaging investigation of choice in the initial assessment of urological symptoms is ultrasound though an IVU is a better option in stone disease or when greater detail of the ureters is required.

CT scanning

In urology, CT scanning is usually performed after injection of intravenous contrast. This helps distinguish renal malignancies from hamartoma or other benign diseases. It can also distinguish the rare angiomyolipoma of the kidney. Modern spiral CT machines give more rapid image capture and better definition. In renal cell carcinoma, CT can demonstrate direct spread of tumour thrombus along the renal vein and into the inferior vena cava so that surgery can be better planned. Enlarged lymph nodes may be diagnosed and biopsied percutaneously and the liver examined for metastases. CT may demonstrate malignancy so advanced that it is inoperable, saving the patient a fruitless operation. In bladder or prostatic cancer, it can demonstrate whether the disease is organ-confined, aiding in staging. Increasingly spiral CT is indicated for the investigation of stone disease, particularly ureteric colic.

Special contrast investigations

Ascending ureterography is especially useful for defining ureteric tumours. Its use has considerably reduced as radiological experience and technology have advanced.

(a)

Date of onset: 2/52
Antibiotics Current / Intended: nil
Clinical details:

Intermittent haematuria
No pain

Signed:

PATIENT STATUS	
Please tick box	
NHS	
PP	
OSV	
CAT 2	
Consultant/GP	

Surname:
Hospital No.:
Forenames:
Date of Birth: 2 Oct 1940
Ward/Address:

USE BALLPEN FIRMLY

MICROSCOPY		T. Vaginalis		1 AMP/AMOX	2 CEPHALEXIN	3 C/SULPHONAMIDE	4 NITROFURANTOIN	5 NALIDIXIC ACID	6 COTRIM/TRIMETH	7 TETRACYCLINE	8 CERYTHROMYCIN	9 PENICILLIN	10 FLUCLOX	11 FUCIDIN	12 NEOMYCIN	13 CMETRONIDAZOLE	14 GENTAMICN	15 CEFOTAXIME		
Pus cells	0	Gr. Pos. Cocci	Gr. Pos. Rods																	
Red Cells	>25	Gr. Neg. Rods	Gr. Neg. Cocci																	
Epithelial Cells		Yeasts	Vincents																	
Casts		1. no growth																		
Crystals		2.																		
		3.																		
Glucose	G%																			
Protein	trace mg%																			

S – Sensitive R – Resistant
M – Intermediate
Phoned:

Specimen Request: MSU Micro C & S
Date taken: / Received: / Lab. No.: / Reported:

BACT.

(b)

Date of onset: 4 days
Antibiotics Current / Intended: nil
Clinical details:

burning dysuria
frequency

Signed:

PATIENT STATUS	
Please tick box	
NHS	
PP	
OSV	
CAT 2	
Consultant/GP	

Surname:
Hospital No.:
Forenames:
Date of Birth: 18.6.28
Ward/Address:

USE BALLPEN FIRMLY

MICROSCOPY		T. Vaginalis		1 AMP/AMOX	2 CEPHALEXIN	3 C/SULPHONAMIDE	4 NITROFURANTOIN	5 NALIDIXIC ACID	6 COTRIM/TRIMETH	7 TETRACYCLINE	8 CERYTHROMYCIN	9 PENICILLIN	10 FLUCLOX	11 FUCIDIN	12 NEOMYCIN	13 CMETRONIDAZOLE	14 GENTAMICN	15 CEFOTAXIME		
Pus cells	>50	Gr. Pos. Cocci	Gr. Pos. Rods																	
Red Cells	>100	Gr. Neg. Rods	Gr. Neg. Cocci																	
Epithelial Cells	±	Yeasts	Vincents																	
Casts	−	1. >10⁵ orgs/ml Enterococci		S		R	S		R											
Crystals	−	2.																		
Bacteria ++		3.																		
Glucose	− G%																			
Protein	++ mg%																			

S – Sensitive R – Resistant
M – Intermediate
Phoned:

Specimen Request: MSU C & S
Date taken: / Received: / Lab. No.: / Reported:

BACT.

(c)

Date of onset: 3/12
Antibiotics Current / Intended: none
Clinical details:

Pain (L) loin
Evening fevers
Frequency

Signed:

PATIENT STATUS	
Please tick box	
NHS	
PP	
OSV	
CAT 2	
Consultant/GP	

Surname:
Hospital No.:
Forenames:
Date of Birth: 12/4/50
Ward/Address:

USE BALLPEN FIRMLY

MICROSCOPY		T. Vaginalis		1 AMP/AMOX	2 CEPHALEXIN	3 C/SULPHONAMIDE	4 NITROFURANTOIN	5 NALIDIXIC ACID	6 COTRIM/TRIMETH	7 TETRACYCLINE	8 CERYTHROMYCIN	9 PENICILLIN	10 FLUCLOX	11 FUCIDIN	12 NEOMYCIN	13 CMETRONIDAZOLE	14 GENTAMICN	15 CEFOTAXIME		
Pus cells	>25	Gr. Pos. Cocci	Gr. Pos. Rods																	
Red Cells	0	Gr. Neg. Rods	Gr. Neg. Cocci																	
Epithelial Cells	0	Yeasts	Vincents																	
Casts		1. no growth																		
Crystals		2.																		
		3.																		
Glucose	G%																			
Protein	trace mg%																			

S – Sensitive R – Resistant
M – Intermediate
Phoned:

Specimen Request: MSU Micro C & S
Date taken: / Received: / Lab. No.: / Reported:

BACT.

Fig. 28.6 Typical MSU reports
(a) Haematuria. **(b)** MSU indicative of urinary tract infection. **(c)** MSU showing 'sterile pyuria' (possible tuberculosis).

Table 28.2 Summary of investigations for localising urinary tract pathology

Investigation	Indications	Findings
Plain erect abdominal X-ray ('KUB' film)	Follow-up of radiopaque stones	Renal calcification; stones in kidney, ureter and bladder
	(Incidental finding)	Abnormal renal size, shape and position
Ultrasound scanning	Renal masses	Differentiates solid from cystic renal lesions
	Suspected upper tract obstruction	Shows dilatation of renal pelvis or ureters
	Symptoms of bladder outflow obstruction	Estimates bladder volume after micturition; bladder wall thickness; complications of upper tract obstruction
	Rectal ultrasound probe for assessing prostatic symptoms or enlargement	Useful for detecting foci of carcinoma and guidance of biopsy needles
	Chronic renal disease and chronic urinary obstruction	Thickness of renal cortex
	General investigation of urinary symptoms	Morphology of upper tracts and bladder
	Investigation of urethral strictures	Definition of stricture and periurethral fibrosis
Intravenous urography (with or without tomography)	Haematuria	If tumour present, may show non-functioning part of cortex and/or distorted anatomy
	Suspected urinary tract stone	Back pressure effects of obstruction on upper tract; position of stone
CT scanning (plus intravenous contrast)	Renal mass suspicious of tumour	Abnormal mass and blood supply typical of renal tumour
	Palpable loin mass; differentiation of a pelvic mass from a prostatic or bladder tumour	Size, nature of lesions and extent of invasion
	Loin pain	Definition of cause particularly in calculous disease
Special contrast examinations of upper tract, e.g. retrograde or percutaneous (antegrade) ureterography	Obstruction of upper urinary tract not shown by other means	Site and perhaps nature of obstruction
Micturating cystography	Recurrent urinary tract infections or 'failure to thrive' in children	Severity of vesicoureteric reflux
Radionuclide renal scans	Definition of renal blood flow, function or morphology. Diagnosis or follow-up of upper tract obstruction	Renal morphology, excretory function (total and differential), presence and sites of obstruction
	Vesicoureteric reflex	Indirect evidence of vesicoureteric reflux and less intrusive
Radionuclide bone scans	Bone pain in prostatic carcinoma	Bony metastases
Cystourethroscopy (with or without biopsy or bladder resection)	Haematuria	Urothelial tumours of urethra or bladder
	Investigation of bladder neck obstruction and treatment, e.g. transurethral resection of bladder neck or prostate	Visual inspection of bladder neck and prostate
	Treatment of bladder stones	Litholapaxy (stone crushing)
Ureteroscopy	Lower ureteric problems, particularly stones	Direct visualisation of lower ureter and guidance for instrumentation to destroy or retrieve stones
Urine flow rate	Measurement of urinary flow in bladder outlet obstruction. Poor flow indicates obstruction or poorly functioning detrusor	Assessment before and after prostatectomy or bladder neck incision
Cystometrography (usually video)	Investigation of incontinence	Nature of incontinence
	Sometimes used in assessment of bladder outflow obstruction and results of treatment	To confirm bladder outflow obstruction in equivocal outflow obstruction
		To differentiate between primary and secondary detrusor instability in irritative voiding
Renal arteriography	Occasional use in renal tumours	Demonstrating abnormal tumour blood supply (rarely used nowadays)
		Therapeutic embolisation for bleeding or pain in inoperable tumours

Radionuclide scanning

Radionuclide scanning techniques can be used to assess differential renal function. They are particularly useful in monitoring kidney function after relief of obstruction. They can demonstrate renal scars and are a non-invasive method of demonstrating vesicoureteric reflux in children.

Suspected lower tract lesions

Radiography and ultrasound

Ultrasound examination has largely replaced IVU as the standard investigation for lower tract disease. Modern high-resolution ultrasound equipment can demonstrate tumours, cysts and other abnormalities of bladder and prostate shape and volume, but can seldom define lesions smaller than 5 mm. Ultrasonography can also define the size, shape and position of stones. In addition, it can be employed to estimate the volume of residual urine where there is any degree of bladder outlet obstruction. **Transrectal ultrasound** using colour duplex can be used to give high-resolution images of the prostate (to reveal size and nodularity) and the bladder neck (for hypertrophy). Carcinomas of the prostate are classically hypoechoic and have a typical blood flow pattern. Ultrasound can be used for accurate guidance of transrectal biopsy of abnormal areas, especially impalpable lesions in the transitional zone of the gland.

Cystourethroscopy

Cystourethroscopy (cystoscopy), using rigid or flexible instruments, is an important diagnostic and therapeutic tool for disease of the urethra, prostate and bladder. Flexible cystoscopy can usually be performed under local anaesthesia on an outpatient basis.

A similar but longer rigid instrument, the **ureteroscope**, can now be used for retrieving stones from the ureter and a flexible device allows passage to the kidney and treatment of calyceal stones by laser lithotripsy.

When a bladder tumour or urethral pathology is suspected, cystoscopy is the investigation of choice. Flexible cystoscopy allows the same 'instant' availability as outpatient flexible sigmoidoscopy. It allows direct visual examination, but if biopsy and immediate treatment are required, cystoscopy is usually performed under general or regional anaesthesia which also permits deep bimanual palpation.

Other investigations

If clinical examination suggests local spread of a bladder or prostatic tumour, **CT or MRI scanning** may be used to assess the extent of invasion. In carcinoma of the prostate, **radionuclide scanning** is the most accurate non-invasive method for diagnosing bony metastases.

Urethrography is the best investigation for assessing suspected urethral rupture in perineal injuries and pelvic fractures and may be combined with a **suprapubic contrast cystogram**. It is also used for urethral stricture examination. For suspected urethral obstruction, **contrast urethrography** or urethral ultrasound can be used to localise the site of obstruction or stricture. If a colovesical fistula is suspected, **barium enema** may demonstrate the colonic lesion responsible (but rarely the fistula itself).

Urine flow rate provides a quick assessment of degree of obstruction and can be used after treatment to assess change. It is easily measured and can be simultaneously plotted on a graph. The patient simply passes urine into a funnel leading to the machine, although it should be noted that urine volumes voided below 250 ml can be misleading. When incontinence and bladder instability are being investigate, **cystometrography** is usually performed as a video-cystogram combined with urodynamic measurements to assess the relationship between bladder pressure and volume. It is particularly useful in the case of high-pressure bladders with outlet obstruction and in diagnosing urge and stress incontinence in women.

29 Disorders of the prostate

Benign hyperplasia and carcinoma are the most common prostatic disorders and have an increasing importance in an ageing population. Inflammation and infection of the prostate (**prostatitis**), is a less common condition occurring in a younger age group and rather poorly defined clinically.

ANATOMY

The normal prostate gland is small, about 3 cm in length and diameter and weighing about 10–15 g. The gland is situated immediately below the bladder neck so that the first 3 cm of the urethra lies within the gland (see Fig. 28.5, p. 380). Thus, the walls of the proximal urethra are composed of glandular tissue and this part is known as the **prostatic urethra**. The urethra then penetrates the muscles of the pelvic floor that incorporates the distal sphincteric mechanism. Prostatic hyperplasia or carcinoma may cause local effects of urethral obstruction, and carcinoma may invade and disrupt the sphincter mechanism.

The posterior aspect of the gland is palpable rectally (see Fig. 28.4, p. 379) and a **median groove** can usually be identified. This groove is described as dividing the gland into two lateral lobes. The median groove tends to be obliterated in advanced prostatic carcinoma but is usually exaggerated in benign hypertrophy.

When the prostatic urethra is examined cystoscopically, an important landmark is the **veru montanum** (urethral crest), an elongated mound on the posterior wall. The size and prominence of the veru may vary considerably. At its midpoint is a small depression that may be visible into which the two **ejaculatory ducts** open. The posterior part of the gland above the ejaculatory ducts is known as the **median lobe**. If this becomes hypertrophied it may

form a pedunculated mass in the floor of the bladder (often described as the surgical 'middle lobe'); this may occasionally act as a flap valve and obstruct the bladder outlet.

As seen in Figure 29.1, the bulk of the normal prostate consists of up to 50 peripheral **glandular lobules**. These converge into about 20 separate ducts that open into the prostatic urethra lateral to the veru montanum. In addition to this glandular tissue proper, there is a zone of small paraurethral glands immediately adjacent to the urethra, the **transition zone**.

From middle age onwards, the transition zone tends to enlarge to cause **benign prostatic hyperplasia**. At the same time, the peripheral glandular tissue becomes compressed to form a fibrous outer 'surgical capsule'. In contrast, carcinoma of the prostate arises most often in the peripheral glandular tissue, tending to spread outwards into adjacent structures more often than obstructing the centrally located urethra. Cancer occasionally arises in the glands of the remnants of the peripheral zone even after prostatectomy.

The normal prostate gland is surrounded by a filmy true capsule of little surgical significance; outside this is a rich venous plexus which, in turn, is invested by a dense fascial sheath. During open or endoscopic prostatectomy, it is important not to disturb this venous plexus as it is a common source of haemorrhage during and after the operation. There are direct venous connections between the prostatic plexus and the vertebral extradural venous plexus which provide an easy route for blood-borne dissemination of prostatic cancer. Posteriorly, the prostatic fascial sheath is fused with the dense **fascia of Denonvilliers**. This provides something of a barrier against direct spread of cancer from the prostate to the rectum and vice versa.

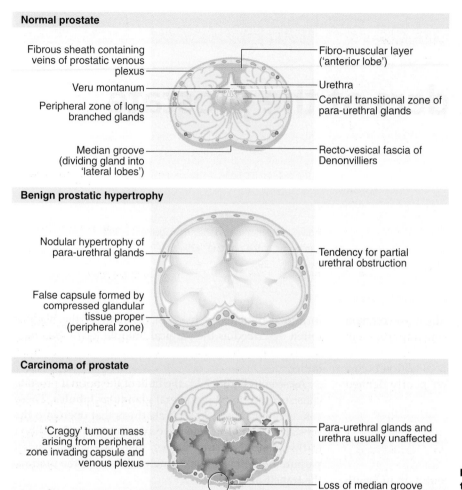

Normal prostate

Fibrous sheath containing veins of prostatic venous plexus

Veru montanum

Peripheral zone of long branched glands

Median groove (dividing gland into 'lateral lobes')

Fibro-muscular layer ('anterior lobe')

Urethra

Central transitional zone of para-urethral glands

Recto-vesical fascia of Denonvilliers

Benign prostatic hypertrophy

Nodular hypertrophy of para-urethral glands

False capsule formed by compressed glandular tissue proper (peripheral zone)

Tendency for partial urethral obstruction

Carcinoma of prostate

'Craggy' tumour mass arising from peripheral zone invading capsule and venous plexus

Para-urethral glands and urethra usually unaffected

Loss of median groove

Fig. 29.1 Horizontal sections through normal, hypertrophic and malignant prostate glands

BENIGN PROSTATIC HYPERPLASIA

Benign prostatic hyperplasia (BPH) affects half of all men aged 50 and the proportion increases with advancing age such that BPH is ubiquitous at 70 years. Approximately half of those affected have either no symptoms or mild symptoms acceptable to the patient and his family. In about 50% of men over 60, however, hyperplasia produces sufficient symptoms for treatment to be considered.

PATHOPHYSIOLOGY OF BENIGN PROSTATIC HYPERPLASIA

In pathological terms, the paraurethral transition zone glands undergo **nodular hyperplasia**. This causes progressive symmetrical enlargement of the gland up to several times its normal size. Patients occasionally present with a gland of 150 g but most are less than 50 g. The largest glands (of up to 800 g) may be fibrosarcomatous. The prostatic glandular tissue proper is compressed peripherally to form a false or surgical capsule. Occasionally,

the process is predominantly fibrotic, resulting in a small dense gland. Similar symptoms and signs of bladder outflow obstruction may be caused by the apparently independent disorder of bladder neck hypertrophy and fibrosis. Bladder outflow obstruction can be caused entirely by enlargement of the prostatic gland, by bladder neck obstruction or by a combination of the two.

The size of the prostate is best assessed by ultrasound and cannot be estimated reliably by digital examination. Moreover there is little relationship between prostatic volume and symptoms, and the presence of a large prostate without symptoms is no indication for treatment. Urine flow is determined by detrusor contractility and by the length and calibre of the prostatic urethra, not by the prostatic bulk. Prostatic urethroscopy provides further anatomical detail but no functional information.

CLINICAL FEATURES OF BENIGN PROSTATIC HYPERPLASIA

The symptoms of bladder outlet obstruction are summarised in Box 29.1. Symptoms usually develop gradually

Box 29.1 Symptoms of bladder outlet obstruction

These may be formally assessed using the International Prostate Symptom Score (I-PSS) for the purposes of comparing the efficacies of treatment

- **Hesitancy, worse with a full bladder or at night**
- **Poor stream, made worse by a full bladder or by straining**
- **Incomplete bladder emptying**
- **Frequency**
- **Urgency**
- **Nocturia**
- **Intermittent flow and terminal dribbling**
- **Post-micturition dribbling**
- **Double micturition ('pis-à-deux')**

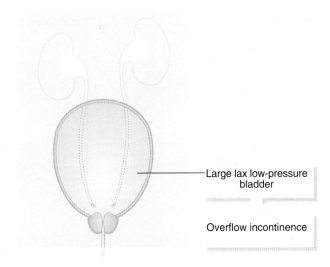

Large lax low-pressure bladder

Overflow incontinence

Fig. 29.2 Atonic bladder due to outlet obstruction

until eventually they interfere with daytime activity and sleep. Acute retention of urine may occur suddenly at any time and is commonly precipitated by bladder overfilling after excessive fluid intake. It is also a hazard of many general surgical, orthopaedic or ophthalmic operations on older men and also of pelvic or perineal operations after adolescence. In some patients, the severity of prostatic symptoms fluctuates from month to month (and even perhaps with the season!), making it difficult to decide whether an operation is necessary.

COMPLICATIONS OF BLADDER OUTLET OBSTRUCTION

Prostatic obstruction can progressively interfere with the patient's ability to empty his bladder but only 20–30% of patients have progressive symptoms and 50% remain unchanged over a 5-year period. In the progressive cases, the volume of **residual urine** gradually increases over weeks and months (i.e. chronic retention) and the intravesical pressure rises. The threshold for the voiding reflex is therefore reached more quickly and calls to void become more frequent. The stagnant residual urine is prone to infection and infection exacerbates the symptoms. In chronic retention, the bladder becomes vastly distended and atonic, leading to **overflow incontinence** (see Fig. 29.2). In other cases, the detrusor muscle undergoes hypertrophy in an attempt to overcome the outflow obstruction. The normally smooth bladder lining then becomes trabeculated. Eventually, muscle fibre bundles are replaced by non-contractile fibrous tissue; this may explain why some patients fail to improve after the prostatic obstruction is relieved. With a further rise in pressure, the depression between the muscle bands deepen (sacculation) and eventually form **bladder diverticula**. Urinary stasis in the diverticula predisposes to stone formation (see Fig. 29.3).

A small proportion of patients with bladder outlet obstruction experience little in the way of local symptoms. In these, rising intravesical pressure can be transmitted back into the ureters and kidneys causing hydronephrosis and **progressive renal parenchymal damage**. The patients often present with severe systemic illness or symptoms such as anorexia, apparently of non-renal origin. The renal failure may be accompanied by anaemia, dehydration, acidosis and infection. Bladder outflow obstruction in these patients is easily overlooked unless the bladder is examined for distension.

MANAGEMENT OF BENIGN PROSTATIC HYPERPLASIA

The principles of management of bladder outlet obstruction believed to be due to benign prostatic hyperplasia are outlined in Box 29.2, p. 389.

Diagnosis

A detailed history is first taken to assess the nature of the symptoms and how much they interfere with the patient's life. This, together with the patient's general condition, are the principal factors determining the need for treatment. The abdomen is examined for bladder size and the prostate palpated rectally. These clinical examinations, however, will reveal only gross abnormalities.

The next step is to investigate the effects of outlet obstruction on the bladder by estimating the volume of residual urine using ultrasound examination. This is reliable, quick, non-invasive, safe and cheap. At the same time, the upper tracts are insonated for distension which indicates back pressure transmitted from the bladder. When urinary symptoms are severe but residual volume is insignificant, the alternative diagnosis of an **irritable bladder** should be investigated. Measuring urinary flow

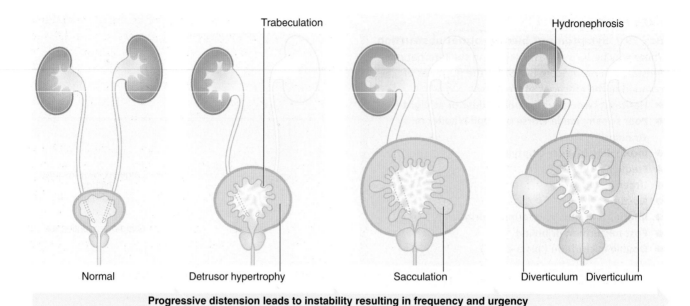

Progressive distension leads to instability resulting in frequency and urgency

Fig. 29.3 Back-pressure effects of bladder neck obstruction

during micturition is simple and is recommended but does not always give the answer; cystometrography is more complex and involves measuring the filling and emptying pressures of the bladder but it may be invaluable if doubt remains about the nature of the problem.

Renal function is assessed by estimating serum urea, creatinine and electrolytes. If these are abnormal, further metabolic investigations may be necessary and renal tract ultrasound is mandatory.

A midstream specimen of urine should be examined by microscopy and culture as urinary infection alone may be responsible for the presenting symptoms or may have precipitated an episode of urinary retention. In addition, if surgery is intended, it is important that infection is eradicated because of the risk of peri-operative septicaemia and secondary haemorrhage.

If the prostate feels nodular, carcinoma should be suspected, particularly if the **prostate specific antigen** (PSA) is elevated. Transrectal ultrasound scanning of the prostate and needle biopsy of suspicious areas should be performed even if operation is planned because a pre-operative diagnosis of carcinoma is likely to alter the plan of management. Marked elevation of serum PSA level is diagnostic of prostatic cancer but a mildly elevated PSA may be due to benign disease or infection. A normal result does not, however, exclude cancer.

Relief of chronic retention and obstructive effects on the kidney

In chronic retention associated with a large volume of residual urine (750 ml or more), abnormal renal function

or upper tract dilatation on renal tract ultrasound, the patient is usually catheterised for a period to drain the bladder. This allows detrusor tone to recover over the course of a few days. Drainage also allows any reversible component of renal failure to correct itself; it may take 3 weeks of catheter drainage to improve the biochemical renal function tests after which spontaneous improvement is unlikely. Fluid and electrolyte balance is monitored and restored if necessary by infusing intravenous fluid. In patients with chronic outflow obstruction and obstructive renal failure, catheterisation may produce a massive diuresis and this should be anticipated and treated appropriately. Such patients may need blood transfusion, intravenous antibiotics and other preparatory measures before surgery can be contemplated.

Cystoscopy

Despite the above investigations, the anatomical nature of the bladder outlet obstruction can be accurately assessed only by direct cystoscopic examination. At the same time, the bladder can be examined for other problems such as trabeculation, diverticula, tumours and stones. In patients with complications from bladder outlet obstruction or severe symptoms not responding to medical treatment, transurethral resection (TUR) of the obstruction is performed under the same anaesthetic (see 'TURP' below). In elderly or unfit patients, placement of a urethral stent may be considered. However, these devices are prone to problems of displacement, haemorrhage, local irritation and blockage. Only very occasionally are patients too unfit for some form of intervention. It is now rarely necessary to leave a patient with a long-term

SUMMARY

Box 29.2 Management of chronic bladder outflow obstruction

- Assess the symptoms and the likely need for treatment from the history, particularly how much the symptoms bother the patient
- Estimate the severity of bladder outlet obstruction by ultrasound and by measuring urine flow rate or cystometrography
- Investigate any disturbance of upper tract function and structure with renal function tests, ultrasound (and perhaps intravenous urogram)
- Exclude urinary tract infection by urine microscopy and culture
- Exclude prostatic carcinoma clinically, biochemically (prostate specific antigen) and by transrectal diagnostic ultrasound; if necessary, perform guided needle biopsy of abnormal areas
- Treat renal failure and other systemic problems
- Consider whether catheter drainage of the bladder is desirable
- Cystoscope the patient to rule out other pathology and to define the anatomical problem
- Discuss with the patient what can be offered and at what risk, i.e. drug treatment, transurethral resection of prostate (TURP), other local treatments under evaluation (such as laser vaporisation or microwave heating), urethral stenting or, as a last resort, long-term catheterisation
- Implement appropriate non-surgical treatments

If operation becomes necessary, diagnose the cause and extent of obstruction by cystoscopy, then either:

- Resect benign prostatic hyperplasia, divide bladder neck hypertrophy transurethrally, or obtain biopsy material by TURP if carcinoma seems likely and prior confirmation has been negative

   or

- Consider any other operative measures such as open prostatectomy or excision of diverticula where appropriate

catheter; in this event a suprapubic catheter is far preferable to a urethral catheter because of the much lower risk of infection and much greater patient comfort.

Drug treatments

Finasteride blocks the enzyme 5-alpha reductase from converting testosterone to dihydro-testosterone and thus reduces the size of hyperplastic prostate glands. A satisfactory response occurs in 60% of men and a 6-month trial of treatment is required; if successful, symptoms may improve to the extent that surgery can be delayed or avoided. Some herbal remedies such as Saw-Palmetto contain naturally occurring 5-alpha reductase substances. The place of finasteride and similar drugs in managing prostatic hyperplasia is still being defined but they can reduce the rates of surgical intervention and acute retention.

Alpha-adrenergic A_1 receptors are present in the bladder neck and prostate. If bladder neck hypertrophy or a prostate less than 50 g is responsible for the symptoms, selective alpha-adrenergic blocking drugs may enable the prostatic urethra to open more readily, relieving symptoms. Newer drugs, e.g. tamsulosin, terazosin or alfuzosin, have fewer side effects than earlier drugs such as prazosin.

Transurethral resection of prostate (TURP)

Transurethral prostatectomy reduces postoperative mortality and morbidity compared with open retropubic prostatectomy and requires a shorter hospital stay. Whilst TURP remains the gold standard for prostatic surgery, various other physical treatments have given varying degrees of success. Cryo-prostatectomy (freezing the gland) and cold punch prostatectomy are obsolete procedures. Modern alternatives include microwave thermotherapy, transurethral needle ablation (TUNA), transurethral laser incision of the prostate (TULIP) and laser ablation. Laser techniques can be valuable in special circumstances such as a patient on warfarin and have shown promising results approaching those of TURP. However, to date, evaluation is incomplete and follow-up relatively short.

The aim of prostatectomy is to remove the bulk of the prostate and leave the compressed but normal peripheral tissue. This protects the subcapsular venous plexus which might otherwise bleed catastrophically. A series of 'chips' or strips of tissue are excised with the resectoscope using a cutting diathermy wire loop; the chips drift into the bladder out of the way. A transparent isotonic irrigation solution is used during the process and this washes away blood and debris to allow continuous visibility. Sterile **glycine solution** is most often used for irrigation instead of water. Some fluid is inevitably absorbed and major plasma electrolyte changes can occur, producing the **TUR syndrome**; however, unlike water, glycine solution does not cause haemolysis but if absorbed in large volumes may cause dilutional hyponatraemia and hyperammonaemia. Various isotonic sugar solutions can now be safely used as alternatives. The enlarged gland is progressively sliced away as shown in Figure 29.4, taking great care to preserve the sphincter mechanism immediately distal to the veru montanum. The prostatic chips are always examined histologically and may reveal unsuspected carcinoma.

(a) Transurethral resectoscope

Handle

Flexible fibre optic light guide from light source

Cutting loop

Cutting loop wire in guide
Fibre optic light guide
Telescope for viewing
Space for flow of irrigation fluid
Insulated sheath

Eyepiece or videochip camera

Inlet for irrigation fluid

Cable for diathermy current to cutting loop

(b) Technique of transurethral resection

Cystoscopic view of normal prostate and bladder neck

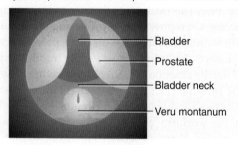

Bladder

Prostate

Bladder neck

Veru montanum

Transverse section to show position of 'scope and bladder neck in normal prostate

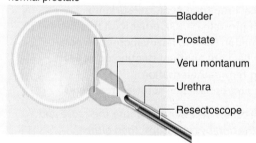

Bladder

Prostate

Veru montanum

Urethra

Resectoscope

Cystoscopic view of enlarged prostate

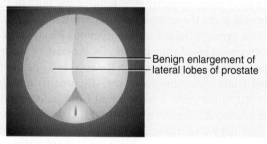

Benign enlargement of lateral lobes of prostate

Transverse section in benign enlargement of prostate

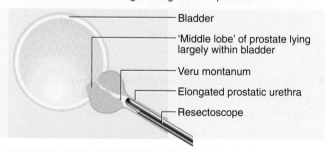

Bladder

'Middle lobe' of prostate lying largely within bladder

Veru montanum

Elongated prostatic urethra

Resectoscope

Transurethral resection of prostate

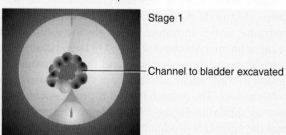

Stage 1

Channel to bladder excavated

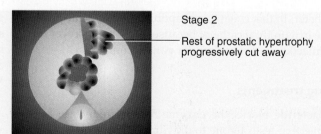

Stage 2

Rest of prostatic hypertrophy progressively cut away

Fig. 29.4 Transurethral prostatectomy

(a) Transurethral resectoscope. 'Divots' or chips are cut by squeezing the handle towards the eyepiece while turning the diathermy current on. This 'cheese-wires' the cutting loop through tissue. **(b)** Technique of transurethral resection.

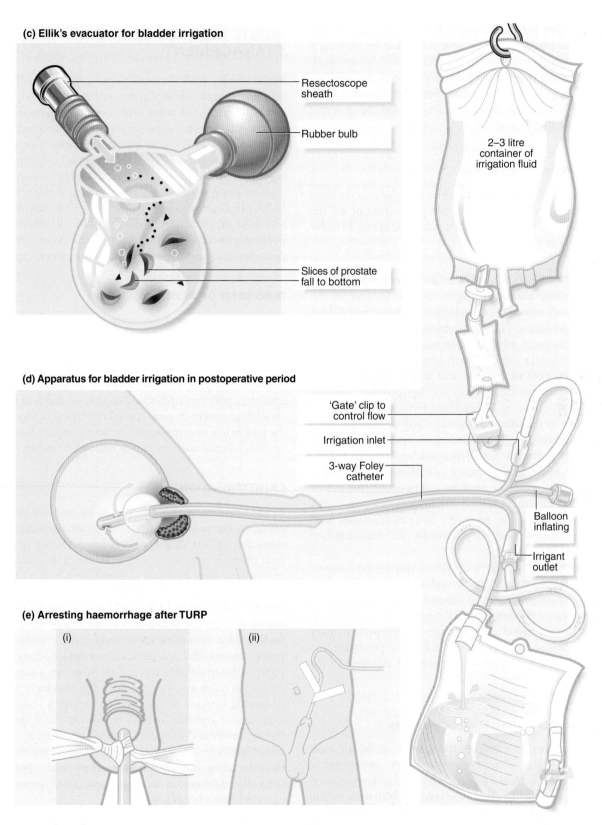

(c) Ellik's evacuator for bladder irrigation

Resectoscope sheath

Rubber bulb

Slices of prostate fall to bottom

2–3 litre container of irrigation fluid

(d) Apparatus for bladder irrigation in postoperative period

'Gate' clip to control flow

Irrigation inlet

3-way Foley catheter

Balloon inflating

Irrigant outlet

(e) Arresting haemorrhage after TURP

(i)

(ii)

Fig. 29.4 Continued
(c) Elik's evacuator for bladder irrigation. The instrument is completely filled with irrigation fluid and then attached to the resectoscope sheath which is left in the bladder after withdrawal of the main instrument. Squeezing the bulb flushes fluid alternately in and out of the bladder, bringing the cut prostatic slices with it which then settle to the bottom of the glass container. **(d)** Apparatus for bladder irrigation in the postoperative period. The rate of fluid flow is adjusted to be fast enough to prevent clotting within the bladder. In practice the effluent should be pink rather than red. **(e)** Arresting haemorrhage after TURP. Excessive bleeding after transurethral resection can often be controlled by inserting a special large balloon catheter and exerting traction on the catheter for 20 minutes (but not more). Tension is maintained by (i) tying a swab around the catheter, or (ii) attaching the catheter to the anterior abdominal wall with adhesive tape.

391

When obstruction is caused by bladder neck hypertrophy, the bladder neck muscle is divided by making a longitudinal incision in the bladder neck (bladder neck incision, BNI) using a diathermy point via the resectoscope. The prostate is not usually resected. This is equally effective where the obstruction is caused by a small prostate (< 30 g).

Retropubic prostatectomy

Open prostatectomy is used when the gland is so large that transurethral resection is not practicable or on the odd occasion where there are accompanying bladder diverticula or huge stones.

Complications of TURP and open prostatectomy

Prostatectomy usually disrupts the mechanism at the bladder neck which prevents semen entering the bladder during ejaculation. Thus, patients usually fail to ejaculate through the penis after prostatectomy (**retrograde ejaculation**), although the sensation of orgasm is unaffected. This affects 60% of patients and it is essential that the patient is informed and accepts this possible complication preoperatively. Maintaining fertility is not usually important in this older age group, but should the need arise, urine can be filtered to recover sperm for artificial insemination. Erectile impotence follows TURP in 5–15%, a similar rate to other major operations in the pelvis perineal area; patients must be informed of this before consent is obtained. Urethral strictures develop in 1–10% of cases, reflecting the relatively large instruments used and the employment of potentially harmful urethral catheters.

Minor haematuria can be expected during the first few weeks after prostatectomy. Secondary haemorrhage (due to infection or unsuspected cancer) can be more profuse and may cause **clot retention**, i.e. retention of urine caused by obstructing blood clot. Recovery of complete urinary continence is sometimes delayed following prostatectomy but there is only occasional permanent damage to the sphincter mechanism.

Long-term catheterisation or stenting

Operation greatly improves the quality of life in most patients. Even in patients over 80 years, perioperative morbidity and mortality are acceptably low. Nevertheless, a small proportion of severely debilitated, immobile or demented patients are better managed by long-term suprapubic or urethral catheterisation, changed regularly by the family practitioner or in the hospital department (see catheter management, below). An alternative is in situ urethral stenting, although this currently has a high rate of failure and other complications.

ACUTE URINARY RETENTION AND ITS MANAGEMENT

Acute urinary retention may occur in patients with long-standing symptoms of bladder outlet obstruction; indeed in the majority of men with chronic retention, acute retention is the first presentation. It is often precipitated by overfilling of the bladder, faecal loading or urinary tract infection but infarction of the gland substance may play a role in some cases. Acute retention is a common cause of emergency surgical admission. It is also a frequent early complication after any operation, especially in males, and may occur at any age even without bladder neck hypertrophy or prostatic enlargement. Management of postoperative acute retention is described in Chapter 47.

DIAGNOSIS OF ACUTE RETENTION

In a patient with no urine output, acute retention must be distinguished from anuria. However, the diagnosis is usually not difficult—the patient in retention is acutely distressed with abdominal or perineal pain and an easily palpable bladder. A brief history of previous similar episodes, previous urological surgery or accidental injury should be sought in case special treatment is required. If the problem is uncomplicated, a more complete history can be delayed until after the pain is relieved by catheterisation.

CATHETERISATION

Acute retention is usually treated by urethral or suprapubic catheterisation. Suprapubic catheterisation is no more demanding of the trained junior doctor or patient than urethral catheterisation. In either case, strict aseptic precautions must be taken to avoid introducing infection. Certain factors should discourage an attempt at urethral catheterisation. These include a history of previous difficult catheterisation, prostatectomy or urethral stricture or the finding of a non-retractile foreskin; for a patient with pelvic trauma and a suspected urethral fracture suprapubic catheterisation is mandatory. Inserting a suprapubic catheter is quick and safe provided the bladder is palpably distended tumour. If the problem appears complex, an experienced opinion should be sought early on before risking urethral damage by unwise attempts at urethral catheterisation. A surgeon with urological training may elect to carry out cystourethroscopy and appropriate surgical treatment as a single scheduled procedure if catheterisation is not urgent.

EVALUATING THE UNDERLYING CAUSE AND ANY PRECIPITATING FACTORS

A catheter is usually left in situ for a day or two after relieving the acute retention until the patient has been fully assessed. At this point, the decision is whether to attempt a **trial without catheter** (i.e. test whether the patient can void urine satisfactorily when the catheter is removed, or clamped off in the case of a suprapubic catheter) or whether to proceed directly with surgical or other treatment. Any urinary tract infection must be vigorously treated before a trial without catheter or an operation.

Common indications for cystourethroscopy and prostatectomy or bladder neck resection are:

- A huge volume of retained urine released by catheterisation—indicates chronic retention
- Raised levels of plasma urea and creatinine which improve after catheterisation—indicates chronic obstructive uropathy
- Previous episodes of acute retention
- Bladder outflow obstruction caused by carcinoma of prostate
- Failure of 'trial without catheter'
- Presence of vesical (bladder) calculi
- Acute retention in combination with a history of prostatism—sufficient in itself to warrant surgery

'TRIAL WITHOUT CATHETER'

If appropriate, the catheter should be removed either around midnight or very early in the morning so that if the trial is unsuccessful, a catheter can be replaced before the patient's and the surgeon's bedtime. Success is judged if the patient can pass reasonable volumes of urine with each voiding, i.e. more than about 100 ml. Even if passing good volumes, the patient must be examined at intervals to ensure that the bladder is not distending with retained urine which would indicate chronic retention with over-flow. Unsuccessful trial without catheter is an indication for cystourethroscopy and probable surgical treatment on the next available operating list. Approximately 50% will pass urine successfully, yet of these, 50% will have a further period of retention within 1 week and 68% within 1 year. Men with low flow rates, large residual volumes and palpably large prostates are more likely to develop further retention.

INDWELLING CATHETERS AND THEIR MANAGEMENT

The majority of patients with permanent catheters are elderly men with bladder outflow obstruction in whom surgery either is contraindicated or has failed. Indications for permanent catheterisation include:

- Patient unfit for prostatectomy
- Incontinent, elderly patient who is severely debilitated, demented or immobile

- Incontinence due to external sphincter damage caused by previous prostatectomy or invading carcinoma
- 'Sacral neurogenic bladder', e.g. in multiple sclerosis

Improvements in urological care, anaesthesia and peri-operative care have meant that many more patients can tolerate prostatectomy safely and are no longer condemned to long-term catheterisation.

For the rare patient who needs long-term catheter-isation, either the **urethral** or the **suprapubic** route may be used. An indwelling suprapubic catheter (inserted directly through the abdominal wall) may have fewer complications.

For either type, the major problems are **recurrent catheter blockage** and **infection**. Catheters readily be-come blocked by epithelial debris or by gradual accretion of calculus. Modern silicone or silicone-coated 'long-term' catheters are better in this respect but must still be changed regularly (every 10–12 weeks) to avoid this. In most cases, they can be changed at home by the general practitioner or community nurse using full sterile pre-cautions and intravenous antibiotic cover to prevent septicaemia. Once infection becomes established in the presence of a catheter, it is difficult to eradicate. However, low-grade infection is almost constantly present in elderly patients and cause little discomfort; antibiotics should be prescribed only if local symptoms become troublesome, if systemic signs of infection develop or when the catheter is changed.

CATHETERS IN PARAPLEGIC PATIENTS

In paraplegic patients, ureteric reflux predisposes to recurrent upper urinary tract infections. Established

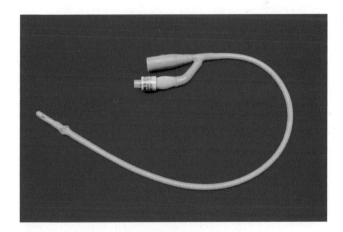

Fig. 29.5 Foley urinary catheter
The most commonly used self-retaining catheter. The main tube is made of latex, silicone coated latex, silicone rubber or plastic. After passing the catheter into the bladder, the distal balloon is inflated with water or saline according to its capacity, usually between 5 ml and 20 ml, and a drainage bag attached to the distal end of the catheter.

infections lead to progressive renal failure and death at an early age. For these patients, special care must be taken to avoid introducing infection, and urine specimens should be regularly microscoped and cultured and any infections treated promptly. Intermittent catheterisation rather than an indwelling catheter may be a better form of management, provided it is performed correctly; in many cases, patients successfully perform intermittent self-catheterisation themselves.

CARCINOMA OF THE PROSTATE

PATHOPHYSIOLOGY OF PROSTATIC CARCINOMA

Carcinoma of the prostate is common after the age of 65 years and is becoming increasingly common in the two decades before 65. The rising incidence is partly, but not entirely, explained by an enormous increase in early cases discovered on screening, particularly in the USA; it may also be related to high meat and fat consumption. East Asians living on a predominantly vegetarian diet have the lowest incidence of prostate cancer.

Carcinoma usually arises in the peripheral prostatic glands rather than in the paraurethral tissue and thus is often slow to become symptomatic. For the same reason, malignant change may occur in the **pseudocapsule** of compressed peripheral glandular tissue which remains after prostatectomy for benign hyperplasia. Prostatic cancers are nearly all adenocarcinomas with variable degrees of differentiation reflected in the aggressiveness of local and metastatic spread. The exception is carcinoma of the prostatic ducts which is urothelial and behaves like bladder cancer.

Most adenocarcinomas are well differentiated and contained within the capsule, slowly invading adjacent prostatic tissue and sometimes involving the bladder neck or sphincter mechanism. In many cases, the prostate is already enlarged by benign hyperplasia. Prostatic cancer metastasises to pelvic lymph nodes and via the bloodstream to bone (for which it has a particular affinity) and other organs. Tumour cell drain via the subcapsular venous plexus directly into the spinal venous system and this may explain the frequent occurrence of bone metastasis in the pelvis and spinal column. The average survival time after diagnosis of metastases is about 2 years.

In the UK 60% of tumours present with either locally advanced or metastatic disease and are therefore incurable. The converse is true in the USA where approximately 70% are organ-confined and potentially curable. This is believed to be the result of the Food and Drug Administration (FDA) recommendation that men over 50 years undergo annual digital rectal examination and PSA estimation.

Most prostatic cancers secrete a glycoprotein, **prostate specific antigen** (PSA), which is detectable in the blood

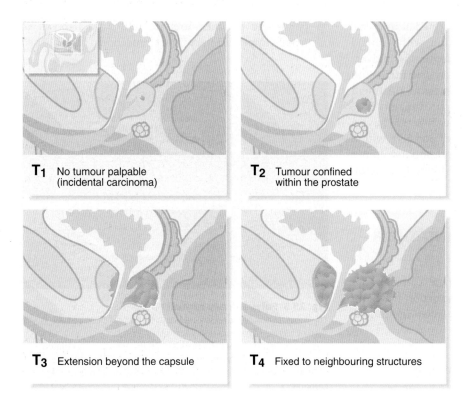

T₁ No tumour palpable
(incidental carcinoma)

T₂ Tumour confined
within the prostate

T₃ Extension beyond the capsule

T₄ Fixed to neighbouring structures

Fig. 29.6 TNM staging system for prostatic cancer

even when the tumour remains confined within the gland. More advanced tumours appear to produce greater amounts and hence detectable blood levels of PSA. Other prostatic conditions (e.g. hyperplasia, prostatitis) may cause elevation of PSA but levels over 10–15 nanograms/ml are likely to be caused by cancer, provided urinary infection can be eliminated as a cause.

Most tumours depend on the presence of male sex hormones for their growth and are rendered quiescent, at least for a time, by surgical or chemical castration. Localised tumours may be so slow-growing as to be effectively dormant but an unknown proportion of these will later metastasise. The main prognostic indicators are the presenting PSA level, the PSA velocity (i.e. the rate at which it rises) and the histological grading. These factors have complicated the debate about the value of screening for prostatic cancer and the appropriateness of radical 'curative' surgery for localised asymptomatic disease. Prostate cancer screening has not yet been recommended in the UK and Australia although there is growing evidence that it may be worthwhile.

Many patients have asymptomatic, localised or dormant disease diagnosed incidentally at TURP for presumed benign disease. At autopsy, one-third of men over 50 and 90% of men over 90 dying of other causes have microscopic cancer in the prostate and it must be assumed that this is true for the population at large. The natural history of such occult cancers is unknown and it seems that many do not progress to become clinically relevant. Some elderly patients with occult metastatic disease suffer troublesome non-specific symptoms, e.g. malaise and fatigue, which may be dismissed at first if prostatic cancer is not considered in the differential diagnosis. Even after characteristic local symptoms appear, the disease often pursues a prolonged course and many patients over 70 years die with their prostate cancer rather than from it. On the other hand, 50% of patients aged less than 70 years with moderately or poorly differentiated cancers will eventually die from the disease and a greater proportion will develop significant morbidity. Patients who suffer other life-threatening co-morbid conditions should be offered a 'watchful waiting' policy unless their metastases are symptomatic. A carcinoma of low histological grade comprising less than 5% of prostatic volume

can be safely left untreated and followed up with PSA monitoring. An untreated intracapsular lesion (T_1, T_2) takes about 7 years to progress to extracapsular spread.

Symptoms and signs of prostatic cancer depend on the degree of local and systemic spread. Clinical staging is most commonly based on the TNM system (see Fig. 29.6). See also Table 29.1 for the incidence of positive pelvic lymph nodes. The palpation characteristics of the malignant prostate are illustrated in Figure 28.4 (p. 379).

SYMPTOMS AND SIGNS OF PROSTATIC CANCER

Patients with stage T_1 or T_2 tumours may be asymptomatic; they may be discovered incidentally or on routine check-up, or present with lower urinary tract symptoms identical to those of benign hyperplasia. Provided the PSA is below 20, systemic disease is unlikely. Those with T_3 and T_4 tumours may present similarly and many develop other local symptoms from advancement of the primary, e.g. encirclement of the rectum or occlusion of ureters, and present with renal failure. Patients with nodal disease (N+) may have symptoms from local compression (swollen legs) and impaired lymphatic drainage (penile and genital oedema) T_3 and T_4 lesions have frequently already metastasised at presentation (M^+) and may present with symptoms of metastases such as bone pain, pathological fractures or spinal cord compression. Some patients present with pathological fractures of spine or neck of femur. Thus older men presenting to a doctor with backache should always have a rectal examination and PSA assay. In more advanced cases, non-specific symptoms of malaise, fatigue, weight loss and anaemia may develop and escape recognition for many months. Respiratory problems from pulmonary carcinomatous lymphangitis are an occasional presentation.

Rectal examination will usually reveal the primary diagnosis. On rectal palpation, a T_1 tumour appears normal or smoothly enlarged by benign hyperplasia; stage T_2 presents typically with a nodular, asymmetrical surface, and staged T_3 with a large, hard, irregular gland with evidence of extension beyond the capsule or into the seminal vesicles. A tumour fixed to bone or adjacent pelvic organs is stage T_4. Once cancer spreads more widely outside the prostatic capsule, characteristic symptoms and signs develop and the prognosis becomes substantially worse. Local spread may involve the rectum (causing change in bowel habit) or the bladder neck and ureters (causing incontinence, impotence or rarely obstructive renal failure). At this late stage, the tumour is obvious on rectal palpation. In very advanced cases where cancer has invaded laterally to involved the pelvic walls or encircle the rectum, the pelvis may appear 'frozen' solid with tumour. Some patients develop major deep venous thrombosis affecting the lower limb.

Table 29.1 Incidence of positive pelvic lymph nodes according to T category

T category	%
T_1 (focal)	2
T_2 (diffuse)	20
T_3	25
T_4	50
T_5	85

Modes of presentation of carcinoma of the prostate are summarised in Box 29.3.

APPROACH TO INVESTIGATION OF SUSPECTED PROSTATIC CARCINOMA

Obstruction of the bladder outlet by the prostate is usually caused by benign disease but may be caused by carcinoma. Unless the prostate feels malignant or there are obvious bony metastases, it may be impossible to distinguish between them clinically. Rectal ultrasonography is used to image the prostate irrespective of the findings on palpation and to guide transrectal needle biopsy if necessary. Serum PSA should be measured but results must be interpreted with caution, taking into account the rising levels with advancing age which are accepted as normal. Elevated PSA may indicate metastatic disease or aggressive localised disease but a normal result does not exclude disease confined to the gland and

is found in 25% of cases. False positive results sometimes occur in benign prostatic hyperplasia or inflammation (prostatitis). If carcinoma can be excluded, any obstruction may be treated in the usual way by TURP and the chips examined histologically. At prostatectomy, carcinoma is suspected if the gland lacks the usual clear plane of cleavage.

If a patient has skeletal pain, X-rays and radionucleotide bone scans are indicated. On X-ray, prostatic bony metastases are typically **sclerotic** or osteoblastic (i.e. dense, appearing white on X-rays) rather than **lytic** (as in most other bony secondaries), giving the characteristic patchy 'cotton-wool' appearance shown in Figure 29.7. Some lesions, however, are radiolucent. An isotope bone scan can reveal metastases when a plain X-ray is normal.

MANAGEMENT OF PROSTATIC CARCINOMA

Screening

Prevention of the disease would be ideal but this is impossible while the cause remains unknown. Screening is being evaluated for detection of early curable disease. Ideally, management would avoid treating cancers unlikely to advance, would ablate cancers confined to the gland (stages T_1 or T_2; N_0, M_0) but which are expected to advance, and would provide long-term palliation for locally advanced tumours (stage T_3; N_0, M_0) and metastatic disease (stages T_{1-4}; N^+ and/or M^+). Uncertainty will remain, however, until it becomes possible to identify accurately those local cancers which will advance to become clinically important, and those early cancers which have already metastasised and progressed beyond cure. In the USA the growing trend towards aggressive treatment of all operable cancers (by total prostatectomy) may be leading to a perception of falling mortality despite increased prevalence. If confirmed in the longer term, this suggests that surgical intervention may be genuinely curative.

> **SUMMARY**
>
> **Box 29.3 Modes of presentation of carcinoma of the prostate**
>
> - Asymptomatic—screening by rectal examination and PSA
> - Asymptomatic—incidental finding of nodular prostate on rectal examination
> - Symptoms of bladder outflow obstruction—tumour suspected by finding nodular prostate on rectal examination or a suspiciously raised serum PSA or found on histology after TURP
> - Symptoms of spread to surrounding pelvic tissues, e.g. change in bowel habit, loss of continence, recent impotence, ureteric obstruction
> - Symptoms of bony metastases, e.g. bone pain, malaise, anaemia, pathological fractures

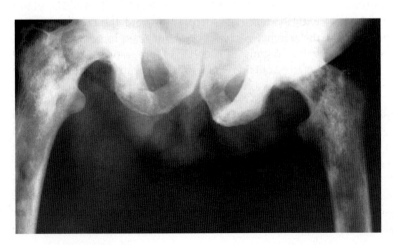

Fig. 29.7 Osteosclerotic bony metastases from prostatic carcinoma

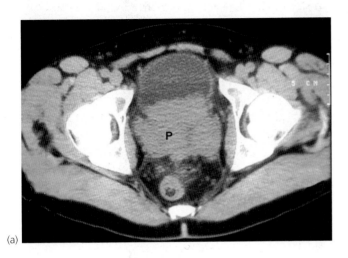

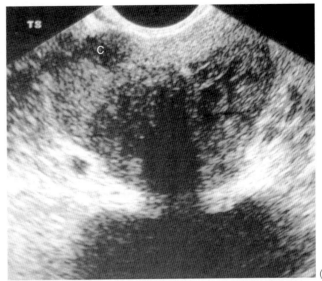

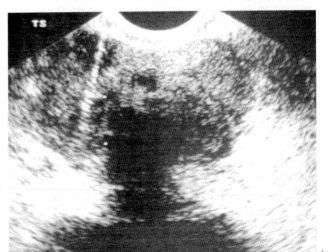

Fig. 29.8 Carcinoma of the prostate

(a) CT scan showing a large carcinoma of the prostate **P** invading extensively into the bladder anteriorly and posteriorly towards the rectum. This was a late and aggressive form of the disease and the patient lived less than 1 year. **(b)** and **(c)** Ultrasound guided biopsy. **(b)** Transrectal ultrasound scan of prostate showing a small cancer **C** within the peripheral zone and an acoustic shadow beyond it. The larger central zone is enlarged by benign hypertrophy. **(c)** After transrectal biopsy. The white line represents bubbles of air left after successful needle biospy of the tumour.

Early-stage disease (stages T_1 or T_2; N_0, M_0)

Total prostatectomy or radical radiotherapy is potentially curative for organ-confined disease, i.e. disease confined to the prostate, 'true' stage T_1 and T_2, and there is enthusiasm for such radical local treatment at specialist centres. If external beam radiation therapy is chosen, it is delivered so as to provide a high local tumour dose without adversely affecting the rectum. A fall in PSA level to 1.0 or less within 12 months of treatment is an indication of success without which relapse can be expected. There is a revival in the use of radioactive iodine seed implants (brachytherapy) as an alternative to external beam therapy; the seeds can be placed accurately under ultrasound control and provide the necessary high but localised dosage.

The effectiveness and side effects of these treatments must be compared with the standard alternative of 'watchful waiting', i.e. no treatment until disease advances locally or metastases appear. Neither radical treatment has yet been shown to be clearly superior in terms of survival, and the risk of unacceptable complications such as incontinence or impotence after radical surgery is high (although better results are claimed for 'nerve-sparing' radical prostatectomy). For these reasons, much more research needs to be done before radical methods can be adopted as standard treatment. At present, centres performing radical treatment consider patients individually, searching carefully for metastases and taking account of patient preference, age, sexual activity and preparedness to risk complications; inevitably, more patients prove unsuitable for radical treatment than undergo it.

Thus, the question remains open as to whether radical treatment of early prostatic cancer can be justified in the light of uncertainty about indications, cure rate, cost-effectiveness and quality of life. Only if early radical treatment is beneficial is it likely that screening for prostatic cancer will prove practicable.

Locally advanced disease (stages T_3 or T_4, N_0, M_0)

For patients presenting with bladder outlet symptoms, standard transurethral resection may relieve urinary symptoms; TURP may, however, risk permanent incontinence if the tumour has invaded the sphincter mechanism or the nerves controlling it. Further treatment then depends on local practice and patient preference. Locally advanced primary disease (stage T_3) is usually treated by **neoadjuvant** (before the principal therapy) or adjuvant radiotherapy with or without hormone therapy.

Metastatic disease (stage N^+ and/or M^+)

Many patients still present with metastatic disease. In these, the aim of treatment is to control symptoms and to retard the progression of disease. For patients presenting with bladder outlet symptoms, standard transurethral resection or 'channel TUR' usually restores urinary flow. Further treatment depends on local practice and patient preference.

Most prostatic cancers are androgen-dependent, at least initially, and hormonal manipulation is the mainstay of treatment of advanced disease. Local radiotherapy is frequently effective for treating painful metastases. Pathological fractures in the sclerotic metastates of prostatic cancer are much less common than in lytic metastases. This is fortunate since the dense bone is more difficult to cut and drill than normal bone if internal fixation is needed. Total prostatectomy or radical radiotherapy is a potentially curative treatment for organ-confined disease, i.e. disease confined to the prostrate, 'true' stage T_1 and T_2, and there is enthusiasm for such radical local treatment at specialist centres. However, for T_1 disease, 'watchful waiting' may be the best option, i.e. no local treatment until the disease advances locally or metastases appear. Some clinicians are using finasteride for T_1 patients in the hope that it will reduce tumour proliferation and spread.

If external beam radiation therapy is chosen, it is planned to be delivered in such a way that it provides a high local tumour dose without adversely affecting the rectum. As a measure of success, the PSA must fall to a low point of 1.0 or less by 12 months after treatment or relapse can be expected. There is a revival of radioactive iodine seed implants (brachytherapy) as an alternative to external beam therapy; the seeds can be placed accurately under ultrasound control and provide the necessary high but localised dosage. Currently, this treatment is a more expensive option. However, the effectiveness and side effects of these treatments must be compared with the

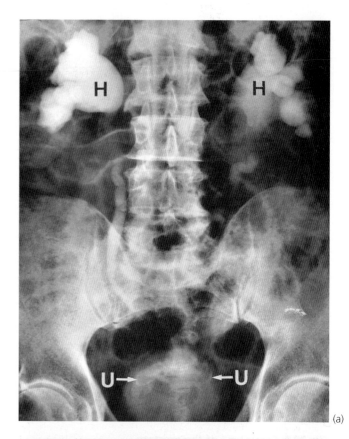

(a)

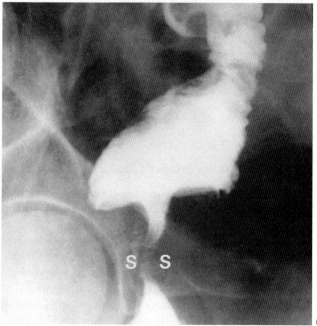

(b)

Fig. 29.9 Local effects of advanced prostatic carcinoma
(a) Intravenous urogram from an elderly man with advanced prostatic carcinoma. He presented with renal failure due to retroperitoneal spread of tumour which had caused bilateral distal ureteric obstruction. Note the gross bilateral hydronephrosis **H**; the distal ureters can be seen to narrow at **U**; this is better shown on the original film. **(b)** Barium enema from a 76-year-old man with known prostatic carcinoma who developed a change in bowel habit. The tumour has compressed and invaded the rectal wall circumferentially causing a marked stricture **S**.

standard alternative of watchful waiting. Neither radical treatment has been shown to be clearly superior in terms of survival, and the risk of unacceptable complications. Spinal cord compression may be treated by local radiotherapy or laminectomy but the neurological prognosis is poor.

Hormonal therapy

There are now three main treatment options:

- **Removal of both testes by subcapsular orchidectomy**. This is a quick and simple scrotal operation and removes about 95% of the testosterone synthesised (the rest is from the adrenals), producing an immediate fall in plasma testosterone. The testicular capsules are left in situ and these fill with blood clot and preserve the scrotal contour. There are few side effects other than hot flushes and no serious long-term sequelae. Where there is intolerable pain from metastases, orchidectomy is the treatment of choice and many patients wake up from the operation free of pain.

  Stilboestrol is a synthetic oestrogen and in the early days was the standard treatment for symptomatic prostate cancer. Stilboestrol suppresses luteinising hormone releasing hormone (LHRH) secretion from the hypothalamus and may also be cytotoxic to prostatic cancer cells in its own right. Although effective, it was found to have a high rate of serious thromboembolic side effects and has now largely been abandoned in favour of other methods of achieving similar ends. However, it remains an alternative to orchidectomy, either as primary treatment or as a salvage treatment after other methods have failed. The dose must not exceed 3 mg a day and precautions must be taken to reduce the increased risk of thrombosis.

- **Monthly injections of depot LHRH agonists (LHRHa)**. LHRH or **gonadorelin** analogues such as goserelin are at least as effective as orchidectomy but are expensive and have to be given parenterally, at least initially. The drugs need to be administered at intervals ranging from 4 weeks to 12 weeks. Therapy causes initial stimulation of luteinising hormone (LH) release from the pituitary, which in turn causes increased testicular testosterone secretion for up to 2 weeks. This is followed by inhibition of LH release by competitively blocking the receptors, resulting in an 'anorchic' state. As with orchidectomy, hot flushes and sexual dysfunction are the major side effects. Many patients experience a 'flare' of symptoms in the first 2 weeks, aggravating bone pain or spinal cord compression. For this reason, the first dose is usually covered by anti-androgen therapy (e.g. cyproterone acetate or flutamide). There is probably no advantage in continuing combined gonadorelin and anti-

androgen therapy because the anti-androgen contributes to the hormone resistance of the tumour by blocking androgen receptors. In addition, anti-androgens are hepatotoxic.

- **Anti-androgen drugs such as cyproterone acetate or flutamide**. These block the binding of dihydro-testosterone to its receptor at cellular level and, in contrast to LHRH antagonists, block both testicular and adrenal testosterone. In patients with a small tumour load, this total androgen blockade probably improves survival as well as time to first recurrence. Flutamide may preserve the potential for sexual arousal for longer, though with occasional side effects of diarrhoea and gynaecomastia, and this may be the preferred treatment for younger patients with advanced disease. Cyproterone acetate can lead to depression and thromboembolic complications but is effective in suppressing hot flushes.

Almost inevitably, prostatic cancer eventually escapes its androgen dependency and becomes refractory to hormonal treatment. The mechanism is unknown but occurs at a mean of 2 years after commencing treatment in M+ and 5 years in N+ disease. When this occurs, secondary treatment with stilboestrol may be of value. Bone metastases can sometimes be palliated by intravenous radioactive strontium. Non-hormone chemotherapy has little to offer, and often only symptomatic and general palliative measures can be offered. The principles and techniques of palliative care are described in Chapter 7.

The management of prostatic carcinoma is summarised in Box 29.4.

PROSTATITIS

Bacterial prostatitis is an uncommon inflammatory disorder of the prostate usually caused by coliforms, *Chlamydia* or *Neisseria*. Mycoplasma may also have a role. It occurs in acute and chronic forms. Urinary tract infection or instrumentation may be predisposing factors. Prostatitis can present acutely or in a chronic form.

ACUTE PROSTATITIS

Acute prostatitis is characterised by perineal pain and fever. Prostatic swelling may also cause bladder outflow obstruction and urinary frequency. The prostate is exquisitely tender on rectal examination and prostatic massage is inadvisable as it may precipitate bacteraemia.

Initial treatment is with intravenous antibiotics such as gentamicin until the patient is apyrexial and then a

SUMMARY

Box 29.4 Management of prostatic carcinoma

Histological diagnosis

● By transrectal biopsy or after TURP for symptoms of bladder outlet obstruction

Staging

● If radical treatment is contemplated—rectal examination (often under general anaesthetic), PSA, transrectal ultrasound, CT scanning for local spread and lymph node involvement

Treatment by stage

● At any stage, transurethral resection ('channel TUR') for persistent bladder outlet obstruction
● Stage T_1—watch and wait with no active treatment (finasteride may be prophylactic)
● Stage T_2—a choice of 'watchful waiting' or radical local treatment, i.e. prostatectomy or radiotherapy
● Stage T_3—radiotherapy, often with neoadjuvant or adjuvant hormonal therapy
● Stage T_4
   — anti-androgen therapies (e.g. bilateral orchidectomy) plus radiotherapy for painful bony metastases or spinal cord compression

   or

   — drug treatment with gonadorelins

   or

   — drug treatment with anti-androgen drugs, e.g. cyproterone acetate, flutamide, biclutamide

quinolone antibiotic orally for 6 weeks. Infective prostatitis may be the first presentation of diabetes mellitus.

CHRONIC PROSTATITIS

Chronic prostatitis presents with chronic, low-grade perineal and suprapubic pain. Symptoms and signs are often vague and ill defined and the diagnosis is sometimes made on inadequate grounds. Around 5% of cases are due to chronic bacterial infection most commonly by coliforms, whereas in 95%, no infective cause can be defined. Other theories of causation have been proposed, such as autoimmunity and intraprostatic urinary reflux.

Treatment is with appropriate antibiotics according to culture and sensitivity of prostatic fluid obtained after prostatic massage. Anti-inflammatory drugs may be used in addition to or instead of antibiotics, particularly in the non-infective cases; alpha-adrenergic blockers may also be employed.

30 Tumours of the kidney and urinary tract

INTRODUCTION

Two types of cancer arise from the renal parenchyma: renal cell carcinomas and nephroblastomas. **Renal cell carcinomas** (also known as renal adenocarcinomas and by the old names of hypernephroma and Grawitz tumour) are confined to adults. **Nephroblastomas** (Wilms' tumours) are developmental in origin and present in infancy or early childhood. These are described in Chapter 45.

Tumours of the transitional cell epithelium lining the urinary tract (urothelium) are very common. They may arise anywhere in the tract, including the pelvicalyceal system of the kidney, the ureters, the bladder and occasionally the urethra. Pelvicalyceal tumours are uncommon generally but are common in some parts of the world, e.g. Balkan nephropathy. These **transitional cell carcinomas** occur exclusively in adults and are most common in the bladder. **Squamous cell carcinomas** sometimes occur in the urinary tract and probably arise from metaplastic squamous epithelium caused by chronic irritation from stones or schistosomiasis. Squamous cell carcinomas also occasionally arise in the squamous epithelium at the urethral meatus. Very rarely, an adenocarcinoma may develop in the bladder from glandular epithelial remnants of the embryological urachus or a sarcoma may develop from connective tissue elements.

RENAL CELL CARCINOMA

PATHOLOGY OF RENAL CELL CARCINOMA

Renal cell carcinoma accounts for about 3% of adult malignancies and is twice as common in males as in females. It rarely develops before puberty but may occur at any age thereafter, with the peak incidence between 50 and 70 years. Renal cell carcinoma, like prostate, breast and colon cancer, mainly occurs sporadically but there are rare familial forms, e.g. von Hippel–Lindau disease. There is no proven aetiological association with diet or smoking.

Renal cell carcinoma originates in the renal tubules. The tumour cells are characteristically large and polygonal with clear cytoplasm representing accumulation of glycogen and lipid. For this reason, these tumours are sometimes known pathologically as **clear cell carcinomas**. In other variants, the cells are granular and stain more intensely.

Renal cell carcinomas vary in their grade of malignancy. Small isolated tumours are often found at autopsy. Many pathologists regard tumours less than 2 cm in diameter as virtually benign as they rarely display local invasion or distant metastases. Bilateral tumours are present in about 5% of cases. Large tumours invade surrounding tissues and may metastasise to para-aortic lymph nodes. Advanced renal cell carcinoma characteristically extends into the lumen of the renal vein and into the inferior vena cava ('tumour thrombus'—see Fig. 30.1). Distant spread is typically to lung, liver and bone. Lung metastases are often typical discrete 'cannonball secondaries'. Isolated metastases occasionally develop in the brain, bone and elsewhere.

Occasional benign renal tumours also occur, e.g. oncocytoma, adenoma and angiomyolipoma (see Box 30.1).

STAGING OF RENAL CELL CARCINOMA

Stage I tumours are confined by the renal capsule; stage II tumours have penetrated the renal capsule but remain confined by Gerota's perinephric fascia; stage III tumours have renal vein involvement or nodal spread; stage IV have distant metastases.

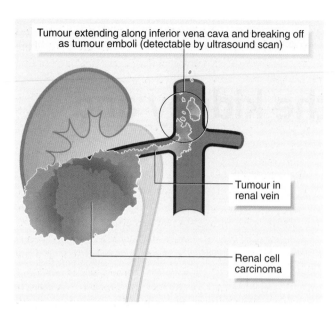

Tumour extending along inferior vena cava and breaking off as tumour emboli (detectable by ultrasound scan)

Tumour in renal vein

Renal cell carcinoma

Fig. 30.1 Venous spread of renal cell carcinoma

KEY POINTS

Box 30.1 Histological classification of adult renal tumours of the Union Internationale Contre le Cancer (UICC)

A. Malignant
1. Conventional clear cell carcinoma
2. Papillary or tubulo-papillary renal carcinoma
3. Chromophobe renal carcinoma
4. Collecting duct carcinoma

B. Benign
1. Oncocytoma
2. Papillary or tubular adenoma
3. Angiomyolipoma (may be neoplastic or hamartomatous)

CLINICAL FEATURES OF RENAL CELL CARCINOMA

The classic presentation of renal cell carcinoma is with the triad of **haematuria**, **a mass** and **flank pain**; however, all three occur in only about 15% of cases (see Fig. 30.2). One of these features is present in 40% of patients. Commonly, diagnosis is made incidentally by discovery of a tumour on ultrasonography or CT scanning. Renal cell carcinomas often reach a large size before discovery owing to their retroperitoneal position;

unfortunately, tumours larger than 8 cm have an 80% chance of having metastasised. About half the patients with renal cell carcinoma already have metastatic disease by the time of presentation.

Renal cell carcinoma can also present in a variety of unusual ways. Some tumours secrete excess **erythropoietin** which causes polycythaemia; **hypertension** may result from excess renin production. Similarly, ectopic production of a parathormone-like protein may cause **hypercalcaemia**. Renal cell carcinoma may cause pyrexia and should be considered in patients with a pyrexia of unknown origin. The erythrocyte sedimentation rate (ESR) is elevated in most cases. As with many other

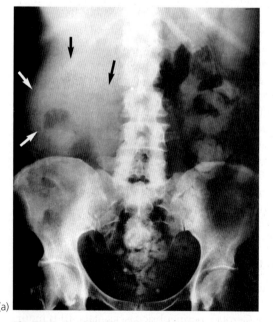

(a)

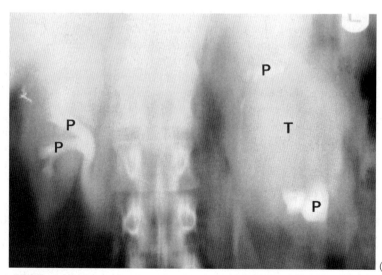

(b)

Fig. 30.2 Renal cell carcinoma: plain radiography and IVU
(a) This 50-year-old man presented with painless haematuria. The plain abdominal film shows a large soft-tissue mass in the right loin which obscures the psoas shadow (arrowed). **(b)** Tomogram taken during intravenous urography of a 58-year-old woman presenting with haematuria. The shape of the pelvicalyceal system **P** on the right is normal, but on the left it is grossly distorted by a tumour **T** in the middle of the kidney.

malignancies, metastases may be the presenting feature: for example, 'cannonball' secondaries discovered on a chest X-ray.

Common and uncommon presenting features of renal cell carcinoma are summarised in Box 30.2.

APPROACH TO INVESTIGATION OF SUSPECTED RENAL CELL CARCINOMA

When a renal cell carcinoma is suspected, ultrasonography is the first investigation and has superseded intravenous

---

SUMMARY

Box 30.2 Presenting features of renal cell carcinoma

Common presentations
- Frank haematuria
- Microscopic haematuria often discovered incidentally
- Loin pain
- Renal mass

Uncommon presentations
- Iron deficiency anaemia
- Polycythaemia
- Hypertension
- Hypercalcaemia due to parathormone-like protein production
- Pyrexia of unknown origin
- Elevated erythrocyte sedimentation rate
- Secondary lesions (e.g. 'cannonball' lesions on chest X-ray, pathological fractures)

---

urography. Ultrasound investigation reliably distinguishes simple benign cysts from solid masses that are most likely to be tumours. CT scanning with IV contrast can define renal vein and inferior vena caval spread (see Fig. 30.3a). CT scanning is also valuable for assessing invasion of perinephric tissues and for demonstrating regional lymph node or liver metastases. **Inferior vena cavography** is sometimes used if venous extension of tumour needs further delineation.

Arteriography is still occasionally employed in the case of solitary unilateral or bilateral tumours to assess the prospect of segmental resection. Renal tumours have a characteristic circulatory pattern distinct from normal kidney (see Fig. 30.3b). Arteriography is also employed if therapeutic embolisation is being considered to reduce the vascularity of a tumour a few days before surgery.

Full blood count is performed to look for anaemia or polycythaemia and a chest X-ray taken to look for pulmonary metastases (see Fig. 30.4). No other preoperative investigations are usually required.

MANAGEMENT OF RENAL CELL CARCINOMA

In most patients, the kidney involved by tumour is excised (**nephrectomy**). Most surgeons prefer an anterior transperitoneal approach. This allows clinical staging of the disease, permits control of the inferior vena cava and provides access to the renal artery and vein during extensive resections. A posterolateral thoraco-abdominal approach may be employed to allow early access to the inferior vena cava and renal arteries if the tumour is large. Wherever possible, the resection should be radical,

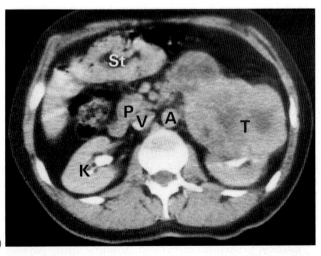

(a)

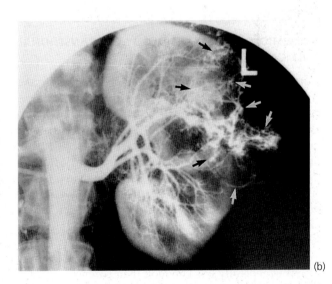

(b)

Fig. 30.3 Renal cell carcinoma: CT scan and arteriography
(a) CT scan showing a huge left renal tumour **T** in a 62-year-old man with left loin pain and a palpable mass; note the variable density of the tumour due to areas of necrosis and haemorrhage. Note also the normal right kidney **K**, aorta **A**, pancreas **P**, inferior vena cava **V** and stomach St. **(b)** Left renal arteriogram from a 68-year-old woman in whom a renal mass was demonstrated on intravenous urography. The arteriogram outlines the normal renal vessels and shows a large crescentic mass of abnormal vessels in the upper pole (outline arrowed) typical of renal cell carcinoma. Only part of the tumour vasculature is demonstrated, the rest having been destroyed by necrosis within the tumour.

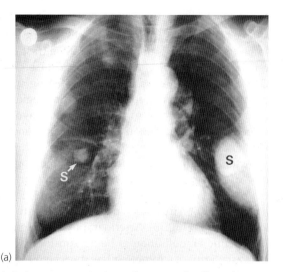

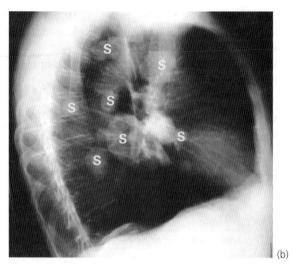

(a)

(b)

Fig. 30.4 Pulmonary metastases from renal cell carcinoma
(a) and **(b)** PA and lateral chest X-rays from the same patient as in Figure 30.3b, showing multiple 'cannonball' secondary lesions **S** of various sizes. These are typical of renal cell carcinoma.

with kidney, perinephric fat and lymph nodes taken *en bloc*. There is probably no role for radiotherapy, chemotherapy or hormonal therapy, although immunotherapy with interleukins or interferon may help, despite their toxicity.

Renal cell carcinoma is unusual in that surgical removal of isolated pulmonary or cerebral metastases occasionally results in cure. For palliation of multiple metastases, chemotherapy or immunotherapy is sometimes used but treatment is generally ineffective.

TRANSITIONAL CELL CARCINOMA

EPIDEMIOLOGY AND AETIOLOGY OF TRANSITIONAL CELL CARCINOMA

Tumours of urothelium are common. Histologically, they are nearly all transitional cell carcinomas (TCC); the rest are squamous cell carcinomas (7%) and adenocarcinomas (1%). Most arise primarily in the bladder but they also occur in the pelvicalyceal system and ureters and rarely in the urethra. Pan-urothelial transitional cell carcinoma occasionally develops in the renal pelvis, ureter, bladder and urethra but not necessarily simultaneously. Urothelial tumours are uncommon below the age of 50 and the incidence increases with age. Men are affected three times more often than women. TCC is at least four times more common than renal cell carcinoma; TCC of the renal pelvis is generally less common than parenchymal renal tumours. TCC occurs with a similar frequency to gastric cancer in men and about one-quarter the frequency of lung cancer.

Cigarette smoking is associated with a fourfold increase in incidence of urothelial tumours; this is probably mediated by urinary excretion of inhaled carcinogens. Urothelial cancers have been strongly associated with exposure to industrial carcinogens, once widely used in the rubber, cable, dye and printing industries. The likely carcinogens, benzidine, nigrosine and beta naphylamine, are now banned in most countries but history-taking should take account of possible exposure in earlier years. Hairdressers with prolonged exposure to various aniline dyes may also be at risk. Prolonged exposure causes a 20–60 times increase in risk of developing urothelial cancer. Tumours develop as long as 25 years after exposure and so a detailed occupational history should be taken in suspected cases. These carcinogens are excreted in the urine and the more prolonged presence of urine in the bladder compared with the rest of the tract probably explains why urothelial tumours most often arise in the bladder.

PATHOLOGY OF TRANSITIONAL CELL CARCINOMA

Well-differentiated TCC's histologically resemble normal transitional epithelium. Less well-differentiated tumours become increasingly unlike their tissue of origin so that the most anaplastic tumours can only be classified as urothelial because they are known to have arisen in the urinary tract. The degree of differentiation tends to be reflected in the tumour morphology as visualised at cystoscopy. Well-differentiated tumours form papillary frond-like lesions, whereas more aggressive tumours form plaque-like lesions which invade underlying muscle and surrounding tissues.

Most aetiological factors act on the whole urothelium, predisposing it to malignant transformation. Consequently, urothelial tumours are often **multifocal** and there may already be multiple tumours at the time of presentation. An affected individual is at high risk of developing further tumours despite complete eradication of an earlier tumour. When the primary tumour is in the pelvicalyceal system or ureter, there is a high risk of tumour developing later in the urothelium distal to the primary. About 30% of patients with upper tract urothelial tumours will ultimately develop bladder urothelial tumours. This was thought to result from 'seeding' of tumour cells shed from the proximal lesion but is more likely due in some way to the multicentric nature of the disease.

A sinister form of transitional cell carcinoma is **in situ carcinoma**. This presents with frequency and dysuria, aptly named 'malignant cystitis'. In the male these symptoms are often misdiagnosed as bacterial prostatitis. These lesions desquamate easily and have a high pick-up rate on urine cytology. Untreated, they infiltrate rapidly.

CLINICAL FEATURES OF TRANSITIONAL CELL CARCINOMA

TCC usually presents with painless haematuria (see Fig. 30.5). An upper tract lesion may cause ureteric colic (clot colic) and long stringy clots may be seen in the urine. If bleeding is gross, clots may cause ureteric obstruction. Rapid bleeding from a bladder tumour may cause **clot retention**, i.e. acute retention of urine due to clot obstruction. Bladder tumours arising near a ureteric orifice commonly obstruct one ureter causing hydronephrosis. Rarely, bilateral obstruction causes uraemia.

Bladder tumours also predispose to infection, and unexplained recurrent urinary tract infections need investigating to exclude TCC as a cause. Tumour invasion near the bladder neck may cause incontinence but this is usually preceded by haematuria or infection.

INVESTIGATION OF SUSPECTED TRANSITIONAL CELL CARCINOMA

Confirmed haematuria in the absence of infection must be investigated. A renal cell carcinoma which causes haematuria will usually be demonstrated by ultrasound. Intravenous urography outlines the upper tracts and a filling defect in the collecting system or ureter is suspicious of a urothelial tumour (see Fig. 30.6).

Ultrasound and IVU is followed by cystoscopy, the only reliable method for examining the lining of the bladder and urethra. If there is an upper tract tumour, cystoscopy may reveal blood emanating from one of the ureteric orifices. When bladder tumours are found, diagnosis and initial therapy go hand in hand. Where possible, lesions are completely excised down to muscle using a **transurethral resectoscope** (transurethral resection of bladder tumour, TURBT). The resected tissue is then sent for histological examination. This defines the degree of differentiation and the depth of tumour invasion into the bladder wall. Benign tumours do occur in the bladder—for example, 'inverted papilloma' or polyps with intestinal metaplasia; however, they are excessively rare. The term papilloma implies that a lesion is benign and its use should be avoided for labelling what is almost invariably a well-differentiated papillary transitional cell carcinoma.

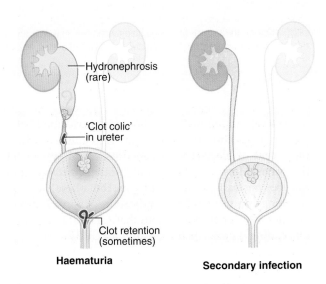
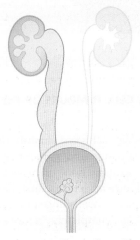
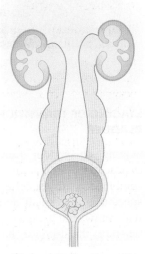

Haematuria **Secondary infection** **Unilateral obstruction with hydronephrosis** **Bilateral obstruction with uraemia (rare)**

— Hydronephrosis (rare)

— 'Clot colic' in ureter

— Clot retention (sometimes)

Fig. 30.5 Presenting features of urothelial tumours

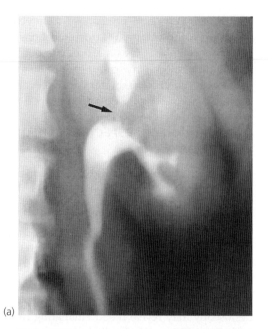

(a)

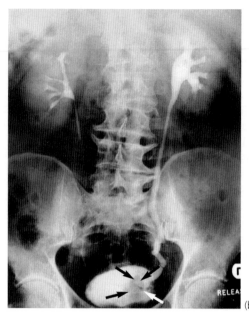

(b)

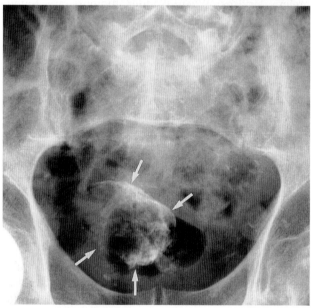

(c)

Fig. 30.6 Urothelial tumours at different sites
(a) This woman of 64 presented with persistent microscopic haematuria; a left renal tomogram during intravenous urography showed a stricture in the upper pelvicalyceal infundibulum (arrowed) caused by a urothelial tumour. **(b)** Intravenous urogram of a 67-year-old man complaining of loin pain and haematuria; on the left there is hydronephrosis and ureteric obstruction caused by a bladder tumour visible at the vesico-ureteric orifice (arrowed). **(c)** Plain X-ray of the pelvis in an 84-year-old man with recurrent urinary tract infections; note the calcified lesion in the bladder (arrowed), typical of calcification on the surface of a large bladder tumour. In a woman, this appearance would more likely be due to a calcified uterine fibroid.

STAGING OF TRANSITIONAL CELL TUMOURS OF THE BLADDER

Staging of bladder tumours is achieved mainly by cystoscopic examination and palpation under anaesthesia combined with histological examination of resected specimens. For small and superficial lesions, histology will show the extent of bladder wall invasion and whether the tumour has been completely removed. Apparently superficial lesions near a ureteric orifice should be treated as having invaded underlying muscle. For larger or deeper lesions, bimanual palpation of the bladder between a finger in the rectum and a hand on

the anterior abdominal wall should be performed before and after resection of the tumour. This gives an idea of the extent of bladder wall penetration and spread into the pelvis. However, the clinical 'bimanual examination' can be misleading, especially in the obese, and CT scanning is a more reliable indication of spread into the bladder wall or beyond. Note that CT scanning can be misleading if performed soon after a TURBT.

The Union Internationale Contre le Cancer TNM clinical system used in staging bladder tumours is illustrated in Figure 30.7 (the 'T' applies to the clinical stage of the tumour). In addition, some pathologists grade

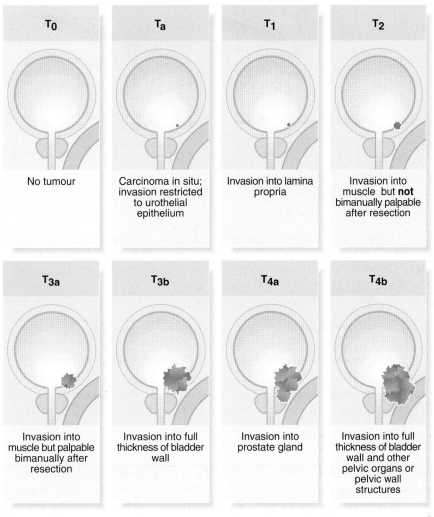

Fig. 30.7 System for staging bladder tumours
Note that ureteric involvement usually classifies a tumour as T_{3a} or T_{3b}.

bladder tumours according to P and G1 pathological criteria. **The 'P' system** (small p for the biopsy specimen and capital P for the whole specimen) classifies the extent of invasion on gross anatomical and histological grounds. **The 'G' system** grades the lesion according to the degree of differentiation (G1 = well differentiated, G2 = moderately differentiated and G3 = poorly differentiated or undifferentiated). Thus, as an example, a pathologist may report a biopsy as pT_2, G3. The pathological staging system is more precise than the clinical system alone.

MANAGEMENT OF TRANSITIONAL CELL CARCINOMA

Bladder tumours

Transitional cell tumours of the bladder display a range of morphological types ranging from small, discrete, often multiple, frond-like lesions through to extensive papilliferous or flat tumours. The first type is usually at a very early invasive stage and such lesions were formerly known as papillomas before their malignant potential was fully realised. Solitary T_1 or T_2 tumours without evidence of widespread carcinoma in situ have a 50% chance of not recurring after treatment. Four-quadrant biopsy of the rest of the bladder can help in formulating a treatment plan and prognosis. If papillary tumours coexist with carcinoma in situ, however, the long-term prognosis is ominous; these patients are usually treated by total cystectomy.

The initial management of bladder tumours is usually aimed at complete removal of tumour tissue by cystoscopic **transurethral resection**, even with large lesions. Further management then depends on the stage of tumour spread determined by examination under anaesthesia, CT scanning and histological staging.

As shown in Figure 30.8, bladder tumours classified as T_1 or T_2 can usually be completely resected. Single-

407

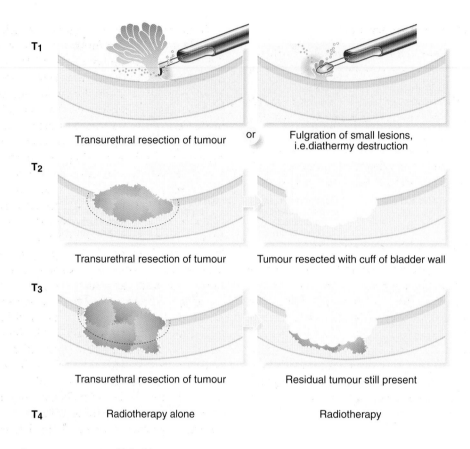

T_1

Transurethral resection of tumour   or   Fulgration of small lesions, i.e.diathermy destruction

T_2

Transurethral resection of tumour   Tumour resected with cuff of bladder wall

T_3

Transurethral resection of tumour   Residual tumour still present

T_4 Radiotherapy alone   Radiotherapy

Fig. 30.8 Cystoscopic management of bladder tumours

dose **intravesical chemotherapy** with mitomycin C or epirubicin has been shown to reduce the recurrence rate after the initial TURBT. T_1 lesions are notoriously re-current and if they recur repeatedly, a course of weekly intravesical chemotherapy or BCG (to stimulate local immunity) is the treatment of choice. For T_3 lesions, the preferred treatment in a fit patient is **total cystectomy**. The tumour can sometimes be downstaged before surgery by neoadjuvant systemic chemotherapy of the CMV or M:VAC types. Radiotherapy should be reserved for the unfit or older patient, or for relapse after initial cystectomy or initial systemic chemotherapy. There is no proven role for radiotherapy in superficial lesions.

When total cystectomy is necessary, some method of urinary diversion is required. The classic operation involves the isolation of a segment of ileum; both ureters are then anastomosed into one end of the ileal segment, creating an **ileal conduit**, whilst the other end is opened onto the abdominal wall as a urostomy. An earlier operation in which both ureters were diverted into the sigmoid colon has long been abandoned because of electrolyte disruption and a high risk of carcinoma at the uretero-colic anastomoses. Nowadays, most urinary diversions are into a continent pouch (a **neo-bladder**) constructed from a segment of ileum or large bowel and anastomosed to the urethra.

T_4 tumours are usually incurable; even total cystectomy rarely eliminates the entire lesion. Radiotherapy offers palliation and is valuable for controlling pain and haematuria.

Transitional cell tumours of the upper tract

TCCs of the pelvicalyceal system and ureter are un-common. Treatment usually requires excision of the whole upper tract on the affected side including kidney, ureter and a cuff of bladder wall surrounding the distal ureter. However, some small, isolated renal pelvic tumours can be dealt with endoscopically via a nephroscope passed into the pelvicalyceal system percutaneously.

Urethral tumours

Bladder tumours occasionally involve the urethra by direct spread. Very rarely a primary lesion occurs in the urethra; a pre-existing urethral stricture may be a predisposing factor. Management is by urethroscopic coagulation. Mitomycin C incorporated into urethral lignocaine gel can also be used. The surrounding penile vasculature allows early spread via the bloodstream and thus the ultimate prognosis is poor.

Unusual tumours of the urinary tract

The uncommon **squamous cell carcinoma** of the urinary tract is diagnosed and treated along similar lines to TCC. As previously mentioned, many develop as a complication of schistosomiasis. Distal urethral lesions are managed in the same way as penile carcinoma (see Ch. 27).

Adenocarcinoma is rare but can occur anywhere in the bladder, most often in a urachal remnant at the vault. Tumours of this type can often be removed by segmental resection of the bladder.

Follow-up and control of recurrent disease

Patients who have had potentially curative treatment for urothelial tumours (i.e. bladder stages T_1 to T_3 and all upper tract lesions) must be followed up for life. The goal is to detect recurrence of the original tumour and to diagnose new primary lesions at an early stage, bearing in mind the fact that the environmental factors that induced the initial lesion predispose the remaining urothelium to malignant change. It is not always easy to distinguish between small recurrences and new primaries; all of them tend to be labelled 'recurrences'.

Follow-up involves regular 'check' cystoscopies. Initially, these are performed at 3-month intervals and the interval is gradually extended to once a year if no further tumour is discovered. Flexible cystoscopy under local anaesthesia is employed for surveillance if there is a low risk of recurrence. This is quicker and more convenient than the former practice of repeated rigid cystoscopy under general anaesthesia but is not yet a suitable method of treating recurrences. After several years free of tumour, cystoscopy may be replaced by annual urine cytology. However, this is unreliable for patients with known well-differentiated papillary lesions. In these, dipstick testing for blood may be more useful. There is currently a vogue for using nuclear protein tumour markers which can pick up 50% of tumour recurrences; however, the reliability of the method needs to be improved before it can replace existing methods. Urine cytology may also be used for screening normal individuals with a high occupational risk.

Recurrent lesions are managed in the same way as the initial lesion, i.e. according to the stage of bladder wall invasion. The exception is when the initial treatment involved radiotherapy. For these patients, cure of recurrent cancer is improbable and palliative surgery ranging from TURBT to total cystectomy may be necessary to treat intractable problems such as severe haemorrhage.

31 Stone disease of the urinary tract

INTRODUCTION

Stone disease is second only to prostatic disease in the overall urological workload. Stones may occur in all parts of the urinary tract, including the pelvicalyceal system of the kidney, the ureter, the bladder and even sometimes the urethra. Stones most commonly provoke symptoms due to obstruction or by predisposing to urinary tract infections.

The pattern of stone disease has changed markedly over the last 150 years. Bladder stones were once extremely common, particularly in children, and were one of the few conditions successfully treated by surgery before the advent of anaesthesia and antisepsis. 'Cutting for stone', or **lithotomy** (lithos = stone), was often performed by itinerant surgeons. They used a perineal approach to the bladder, placing the patient in the manner still described as the **lithotomy position**. A **bladder sound** (i.e. a curved bougie) was placed via the urethra into the bladder to locate the stone. Meanwhile, fascinated onlookers held down the wretched patient for the surgeon's theatrical ministrations. The operation was often completed in seconds!

Nowadays, upper tract calculi are much more common than bladder calculi and the incidence is rising. The stones range from the uncommon **staghorn calculus** (7% of stones), which fills the pelvicalyceal system, to small stones developing in the pelvicalyceal system that may migrate and obstruct the ureter. Acute ureteric obstruction causes severe pain and presents as the surgical emergency known as **ureteric colic**. Most stone disease is, however, asymptomatic or else presents non-urgently to the outpatient clinic.

In developed countries stone disease in childhood is now rare. As shown in Figure 31.1, stone disease has a peak incidence in early adulthood and declines slowly thereafter. Males are affected two and a half times more often than females. Right and left upper tracts are equally affected. There is also a high incidence of recurrent stones.

PATHOPHYSIOLOGY OF STONE DISEASE

CHEMICAL COMPOSITION

Urinary calculi consist of crystalline compounds with a small proportion of matrix similar to ground substance. It is likely that most stones form around a nidus of organic material, e.g. necrotic renal papilla or infective debris. One stone constituent often predominates but sometimes there is a mixture. In other cases, the central

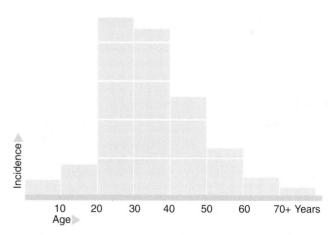

Fig. 31.1 Relative incidence of stone disease by age in developed countries

nucleus of the stone and the surrounding bulk of the stone are each composed of different materials. Thus, it is often difficult to reconcile the chemical classifications used in different analytical studies. Table 31.1 provides a simple chemical classification showing the relative frequency of the different types of stone as well as their important clinical characteristics and aetiology. Calcium is present in at least 90% of stones, either as oxalate or phosphate compounds or both.

MECHANISMS OF STONE FORMATION

Calcium-containing stones

In patients with stones containing calcium (the majority of cases) no specific is discovered. Some excrete excessive calcium (**idiopathic hypercalciuria**) without being hyper-calcaemic; in these, there may be increased intestinal absorption of calcium leading to increased urinary excretion. Experimental evidence suggests that some patients in this group are deficient in an as yet undefined urinary factor which prevents stone formation.

Idiopathic stone disease is probably caused not by a single factor but by interaction of several factors. The following examples illustrate some of these. Bladder stones composed of **urate** were once common in boys in England and are still common in some parts of Africa, Turkey and India. They are believed to be due to the combined effects of deficiency of protein, vitamin A and

trace elements, gastroenteritis and dehydration. All of these factors conspire to produce a small volume of concentrated acid urine which encourages uric acid to precipitate. Another factor is **prolonged immobilisation**, e.g. after multiple fractures or paraplegia, which causes generalised skeletal decalcification and increased calcium excretion. If there is also poor fluid throughput and incomplete bladder emptying, stone formation is likely. Inadequate fluid intake probably plays a part in the aetiology of many urinary tract stones.

Stones caused by excessive urinary excretion of a stone constituent

A minority of patients are found to have an underlying disorder responsible for excessive urinary excretion of the main constituent of the stone. Examples include **hyper-parathyroidism** (calcium), **hyperoxaluria** (oxalate), **gout** (uric acid), **cysteinuria** (cysteine stones) and **xanthinuria** (xanthine stones).

Other predisposing factors

A specific predisposing factor can be detected in a further minority of cases:

● **Chronic infection**. Infection, particularly with urea-splitting bacteria (e.g. *Proteus*), predisposes to magnesium-ammonium-phosphate stones

Table 31.1 Chemical composition, clinical features and aetiology of urinary tract stones

Chemical composition	%	Clinical features	Aetiology
Calcium oxalate	40	3 types of stone are described: — small smooth 'hemp-seed' stones — small irregular 'mulberry' stones — small spiculated 'jack' stones	Most cases are idiopathic; predisposing factors include urinary stasis, infection and foreign bodies. Some are due to metabolic disorders: — hyperparathyroidism — hyperoxaluria (rare inherited disorder)
Mixed calcium oxalate and phosphate stones	15	As above	Some are due to disorders associated with hypercalcaemia, e.g. sarcoidosis, multiple metastases, multiple myeloma, milk-alkali syndrome, overtreatment with vitamin D
Calcium and phosphate (hydroxyapatite)	15	as above	Some of these patients excrete abnormally large amounts of calcium (idiopathic hypercalciuria but without hypercalcaemia)
Magnesium ammonium phosphate	15	Typical of large 'staghorn' calculi of pelvicalyceal system and some bladder stones	Chronic infection with organisms capable of producing urease, typically *Proteus*. Urease splits urea, forming ammonia if the urine is alkaline
Uric acid	8	Stones tend to absorb yellow and brown pigments. Pure stones are radiolucent	Occur in primary gout and hyperuricaemia following chemotherapy for leukaemias or myeloproliferative disorders. Childhood urate bladder stones occur in some developing countries when urine pH is low
Cysteine or xanthine	2	Excess urinary excretion of cysteine or xanthine. Pure stones are radiolucent	Autosomal recessive inherited disorders

- **Urinary stasis**. There may be obvious or occult **urinary stasis** of the upper tract (e.g. **hydronephrosis** or rarely, **horseshoe kidney**) or the lower tract (e.g. **prostatic hypertrophy** or **neurogenic bladder**). Stasis becomes a particularly important predisposing factor when associated with recurrent or chronic infection
- **Foreign bodies**. Diseased tissue such as necrotic renal papillae (occurring in diabetes or analgesic nephropathy) may calcify. If a papilla sloughs into the renal pelvis, it can act as a nidus for calculus formation. Similarly, **foreign bodies** in the bladder act as foci for calcification. These may be inserted by the patient (e.g. ballpoint pen caps or hair clips) or be accidentally left behind after instrumentation or surgery (e.g. sutures, catheter fragments). **Schistosome ova** are responsible for bladder stones in some developing countries
- **Dietary causes**. These probably include overconsumption of dairy products. In areas with a high calcium content in the water, there is a slight increase in stone formation

Predisposing factors in stone formation are summarised in Box 31.1.

The clinical problem of urinary stones should not be confused with calcification of the renal parenchyma which is a feature of tuberculosis and medullary sponge kidney. These and similar diseases can usually be diagnosed on their characteristic X-ray appearance.

CLINICAL FEATURES OF STONE DISEASE

The nature of the adverse effects depends on the size, morphology and site of the stone(s). Many stones cause no symptoms but represent a potential problem. Other stones produce marked pathological effects which present with acute or chronic symptoms or are discovered incidentally on investigation of unrelated symptoms. The presentation of stones in the urinary tract is summarised in Box 31.2.

Urinary tract stones produce their injurious effects in three main ways:

- By obstructing urinary flow
- By predisposing to infection
- By causing local tissue irritation and damage

OBSTRUCTION OF URINARY FLOW

Pelvicalyceal obstruction

Obstruction of one or more renal calyces causes local urinary obstruction (**hydrocalyx**) and typically leads to chronic or recurrent loin pain. Similar pain may also

SUMMARY

Box 31.1 Predisposing factors in stone formation

- Idiopathic (most common)
- Stasis of urine, e.g. congenital abnormalities, chronic obstruction
- Chronic urinary infection (urea-splitting organisms, e.g. *Proteus*, cause alkaline urine and the development of magnesium-ammonium-phosphate stones, typically the 'staghorn' calculi of the renal pelvis—see Fig. 31.2)
- Excess urinary excretion of stone-forming substances, e.g. idiopathic hypercalciuria (calcium stones), hyperparathyroidism (calcium stones), hyperoxaluria (oxalate stones), gout (uric acid stones), cysteinuria (cysteine stones), xanthinuria (xanthine stones)
- Foreign bodies, e.g. fragments of catheter tubing, self-inserted artefacts, parasites (schistosome ova)
- Fragments of diseased tissue, e.g. renal papillary necrosis
- Multifactorial, e.g. prolonged immobility, children in the developing world

SUMMARY

Box 31.2 Presentation of stones in the urinary tract

- Incidental finding on X-ray
- Loin pain
- Ureteric colic
- Passage of small stones in the urine
- Cystitis
- Pyelonephritis
- Haematuria
- Impaired renal function

be caused by chronic, incomplete obstruction of the pelviureteric junction (PUJ) or ureter. The result is **hydronephrosis**, i.e. dilatation of the renal pelvis, both intrarenal and extrarenal. More severe obstruction may lead to progressive renal parenchymal damage and impaired renal function; if both kidneys are affected, the patient may develop renal failure.

Passage of stones into the ureter

If small renal stones pass into the ureter, there are several possible outcomes:

- Stones may pass to the bladder and exit via the urethra causing minor symptoms. The patient may intermittently pass 'gravel' or 'sand' (see Fig. 31.3) and experience dysuria and sometimes haematuria

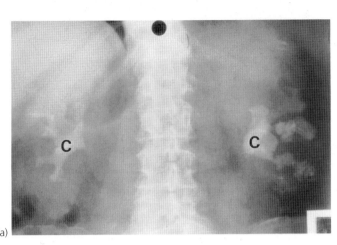
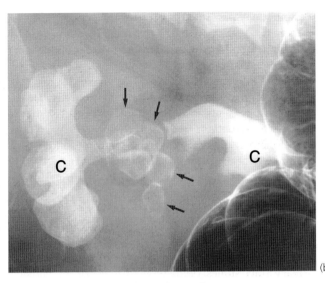

(a)

(b)

Fig. 31.2 Staghorn calculi
Plain abdominal X-rays showing staghorn calculi. **(a)** Asymptomatic bilateral 'staghorn' calculi **C**, found incidentally in a 61-year-old woman. **(b)** Huge 'staghorn' calculus C in upper middle parts of the right kidney; an incidental finding in a 69-year-old woman during barium enema examination; note also the multiple radiopaque faceted gallstones (arrowed), also asymptomatic!

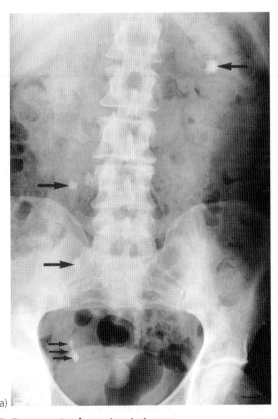
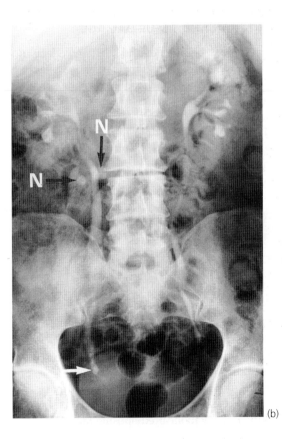

(a)

(b)

Fig. 31.3 Recurrent urinary tract stones
This man aged 40 had a 2-year history of passing small stones and 'gravel' in the urine. **(a)** Plain abdominal X-ray showing what appear to be several stones (arrowed) in the right ureter and in the upper pole of the left kidney. **(b)** Intravenous urogram (IVU) of the same patient showing partial obstruction at the lower end of the right ureter (arrowed); note that two of the radiopaque objects on the right side lie outside the area of contrast and thus probably represent calcified mesenteric lymph nodes **N** rather than ureteric stones; metabolic studies showed that this patient has idiopathic hypercalciuria.

413

- Stones may pass into the bladder and act as a nidus there for development of a larger bladder stone. Bladder stones occasionally cause bladder outlet obstruction and urinary retention
- A stone may impact in the ureter causing chronic partial obstruction and eventually hydroureter. This typically presents as loin pain but, surprisingly, may be asymptomatic
- A stone may impact in the ureter, causing sudden complete obstruction. The patient experiences extremely severe, unilateral colicky pain (**ureteric colic**) often with loin pain and tenderness due to renal distension

PREDISPOSITION TO INFECTION

Urinary tract stones predispose to infection by causing urinary stasis, by preventing proper 'flushing' of the tract and by providing niches in which bacteria multiply. Pelvicalyceal or ureteric stones may cause acute pyelonephritis and occasionally perinephric abscess. Bladder stones predispose to cystitis and ascending infections (see Fig. 31.4).

LOCAL IRRITATION AND TISSUE DAMAGE

Stones may present because of their irritant effects on local tissues. Simple inflammation may cause bleeding and thus present as **haematuria**. Chronic inflammation may lead to fibrosis; if this occurs at a narrow part of the tract, typically the PUJ or ureter, a **stricture** may form. Prolonged irritation of the bladder mucosa by stone may cause **squamous metaplasia** and eventually **squamous carcinoma**.

INVESTIGATION AND MANAGEMENT OF SUSPECTED URINARY TRACT STONES

APPROACH TO INVESTIGATION

When investigating a patient with urinary tract stones, the objectives are:

- To confirm a stone is present
- To locate the stone or stones
- To evaluate any deleterious effects of the stone(s) on renal function and urinary tract morphology
- To identify any structural disorders of the urinary tract acting as local predisposing factors
- To identify any metabolic predisposing factors

METHODS OF INVESTIGATION

In general, the above objectives will be met by performing the following investigations. For convenience, they are conducted concurrently:

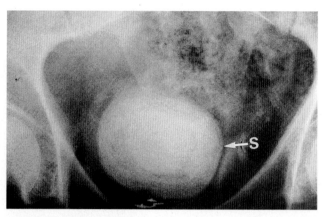

Fig. 31.4 Bladder stone
Plain X-ray showing massive bladder stone **S** in an 85-year-old man with benign prostatic hypertrophy and recurrent urinary tract infections; such stones are rare nowadays.

- Urine dipstick testing, microscopy, culture and sensitivity
- Tests of renal function, i.e. plasma urea, electrolytes and creatinine estimation
- Plain abdominal X-ray ('KUB'). Around 90% of stones are radiopaque because they contain calcium. Urate stones are radiolucent
- In acute cases, 'emergency' intravenous urogram (IVU). This consists of a pre-injection plain film of the abdomen and pelvis (KUB) and a further film 20 minutes after injection of radiopaque contrast and after micturition, with the patient prone (face down). Note: this is not the same as a full IVU with prior preparation. Figure 31.5 shows an IVU with the effects of stone obstruction. Urate stones show as filling defects on excretory films and look deceptively similar to a tumour
- Renal ultrasonography. This demonstrates hydronephrosis as well as the stones themselves
- Special contrast techniques. These are occasionally required, e.g. percutaneous (antegrade) pyelography or ascending (retrograde) ureterography
- Biochemical analysis of any recovered stones
- Tests for metabolic disorders (for recurrent stones), i.e. serum calcium, phosphate, oxalate, uric acid and alkaline phosphatase; 24-hour urinary excretion of calcium, uric acid and cysteine

INDICATIONS FOR STONE REMOVAL

The finding of a urinary tract stone is not an automatic indication for its removal or destruction. The exception is in airline or military pilots in whom ureteric colic could prove disastrous. The usual indications for stone removal are summarised in Box 31.3. Small stones in the pelvicalyceal system often remain unchanged and asymptomatic for many years and can safely be

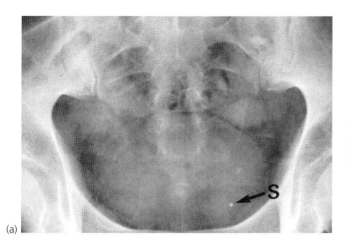

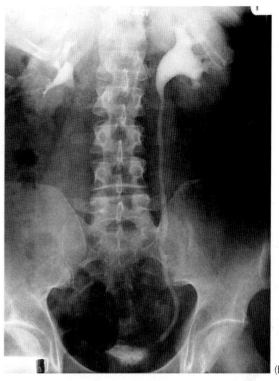

(a)

(b)

Fig. 31.5 Emergency IVU in ureteric colic
This 37-year-old man presented with left ureteric colic. **(a)** Part of the 'control' film showing a small radiopacity **S**, probably a stone, in the area of the left vesico-ureteric junction. **(b)** IVU taken 20 minutes after injection of contrast showing dilated left pelvicalyceal system and contrast-filled ureter down to the area of the stone. This confirms an obstruction at the vesico-ureteric junction.

KEY POINTS

Box 31.3 Indications for removal of urinary tract stones

- Obstruction of urinary flow
- Infection
- Persistent, recurrent or severe pain
- Stones likely to cause future obstruction or infection
- Small 'metabolic' stones likely to grow rapidly in size
- In patients where colic could be disastrous, e.g. airline or military pilots

---

monitored by annual radiography. Stones of 5 mm or less in diameter often pass right through the tract, although in doing so they may produce severe but short-lived symptoms of ureteric colic, haematuria or dysuria.

METHODS OF STONE REMOVAL

Stones can be removed by endoscopic methods, open surgery or a variety of percutaneous and less invasive techniques. The choice of technique depends on the size, nature and site of the stone, the availability of expertise and special equipment, and whether there is a need to correct congenital or acquired structural abnormalities.

Cystoscopic techniques

Cystoscopic methods (Fig. 31.6) are suitable for most bladder stones and for impacted stones in the lower

third of the ureter. Bladder stones can be broken into small fragments (**litholapaxy**) using a **lithotrite**, a modification of a cystoscope incorporating stone-crushing jaws. The fragments are then washed out by irrigation. Stones can also be fragmented by directly applied pulsed ultrasound, laser and other energy sources via a cystoscope.

A **Dormia basket** may be used to remove low ureteric stones less than 0.5 cm in diameter. This involves passing a special catheter into the ureter under cystoscopic vision and fluoroscopic radiographic guidance; the catheter used has a mechanism for capturing the stone. This does not always succeed, so the patient should be prepared for open surgery to follow immediately if endoscopic methods fail.

A **ureteroscope** can be used to examine the lower part of the ureter and assist with stone removal. The ureteric orifice is first dilated cystoscopically and then the slender rigid ureteroscope is passed (see Fig. 31.8a, p. 418). It can be used to help capture elusive stones with a Dormia basket or used to apply ultrasonic, electrohydraulic or lithoclast probes directly to the surface of a stone in order to destroy it. Flexible ureteroscopes are now becoming available and promise improved access.

Open surgical removal of renal or ureteric stones is rarely performed nowadays as renal stones can usually be removed by percutaneous methods or else fragmented by extracorporeal lithotripsy (see below). Ureteric stones can often be pushed back into the renal pelvis and destroyed or removed in the same minimally invasive way. Ureteric calculi impacted in the ureter can often

415

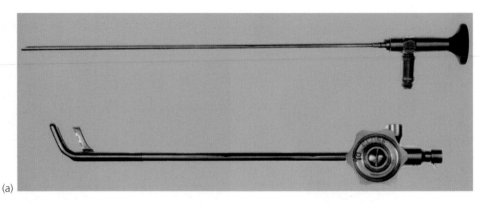

(a)

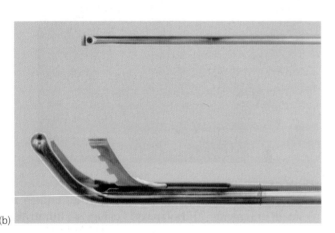

(b)

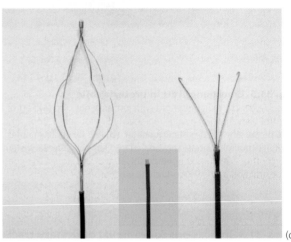

(c)

Fig. 31.6 Instruments for urinary stone removal
(a) Lithotrite. The telescope fits through the centre of the lithotrite, allowing a direct view as the stones are crushed between the jaws. Note: the jaws are closed before passing the instrument into the bladder via the urethra. **(b)** Close up of tip of lithotrite and telescope. **(c)** Dormia basket and grasping forceps. The Dormia basket (left) is advanced beyond the stone and then opened by advancing the centre wire from the proximal end. When open, the whole instrument is gradually withdrawn until the stone lodges within the wire basket. The centre wire is then withdrawn further until the stone is firmly held within the basket and the whole instrument withdrawn complete with stone. The trident grasper (right) operates in a similar way, grasping the stone as the wire is retracted.

be treated by lithotripsy, with or without prior stent placement. A **ureteric stent** is usually introduced after repeated instrumentation of the ureter to assist drainage or to prevent any stone displaced upwards from re-impacting in the ureter. If an impacted stone is causing complete ureteric obstruction leading to marked proximal dilatation, or if there is any suspicion of infection, a percutaneous nephrostomy should be inserted without delay (see Fig. 31.9, p. 419) to preserve renal function.

Open surgical methods

Before today's minimal access methods of removing or destroying urinary tract stones, open surgery was often required (see Fig. 31.7). For the pelvicalyceal system **pyelolithotomy** was performed; for the ureter, **uretero-lithotomy**; and for some bladder stones, **cystolithotomy**. 'Invasive' surgery is employed nowadays when the appropriate techniques are not available, are not indi-

cated or have failed. Open stone removal is also indicated at the same operation as elective correction of an anatomical abnormality which predisposes to stone formation. Examples are bladder diverticula, pelviureteric junction obstruction or ureteric stricture.

Percutaneous techniques

Direct percutaneous access to the renal pelvis can be obtained under local anaesthesia using radiological or ultrasound control. This allows a track to be created from the skin of the loin into the pelvicalyceal system (**nephrostomy**), through which progressively larger instruments can be passed. Small stones can be retrieved using a Dormia basket or a steerable grasping tool. Larger stones can be broken into fragments with electro-hydraulic or other probes, after which the fragments can be lifted out with special instruments (see Fig. 31.8b). Afterwards, the nephrostomy track closes spontaneously.

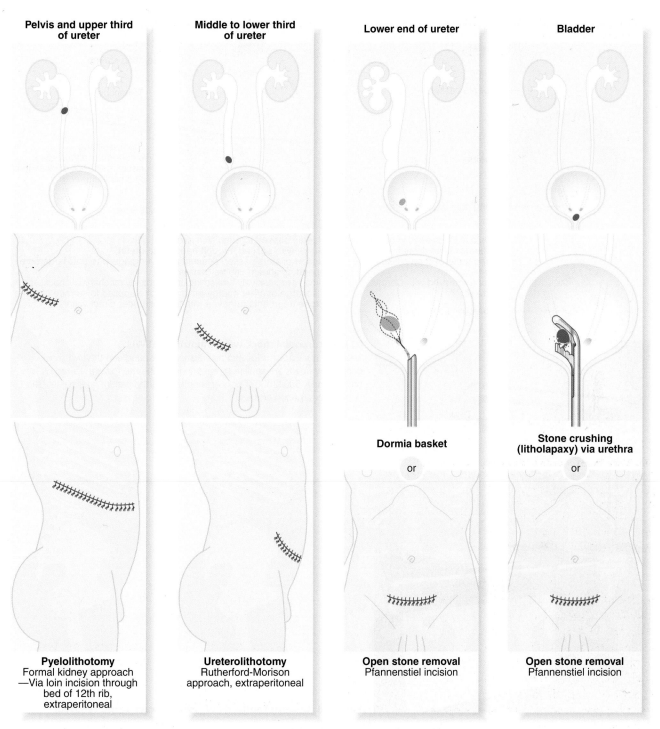

Pelvis and upper third of ureter

Pyelolithotomy
Formal kidney approach
—Via loin incision through
bed of 12th rib,
extraperitoneal

Middle to lower third of ureter

Ureterolithotomy
Rutherford-Morison
approach, extraperitoneal

Lower end of ureter

Dormia basket

or

Open stone removal
Pfannenstiel incision

Bladder

Stone crushing (litholapaxy) via urethra

or

Open stone removal
Pfannenstiel incision

Fig. 31.7 Conventional surgical and cytoscopic approaches for removal of urinary tract stones

Non-invasive stone removal technique

Extracorporeal shock wave lithotripsy (ESWL) is a non-invasive method of destroying stones using externally applied shock waves which pass into the patient to shatter the stone. The ultrasound beam is usually transmitted via water pads and focused on the stone by ultrasound or X-ray. The stone fragments are passed out in the urine and may cause ureteric colic or ureteric obstruction. For this reason, a ureteric stent is often placed before lithotripsy to prevent obstruction with stone fragments. The ureter dilates around the stent and stone debris is passed more easily after stent removal.

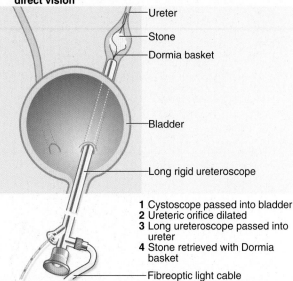

(a) Ureteroscopic retrieval of lower ureteric stones under direct vision

- Ureter
- Stone
- Dormia basket
- Bladder
- Long rigid ureteroscope
- Fibreoptic light cable

1 Cystoscope passed into bladder
2 Ureteric orifice dilated
3 Long ureteroscope passed into ureter
4 Stone retrieved with Dormia basket

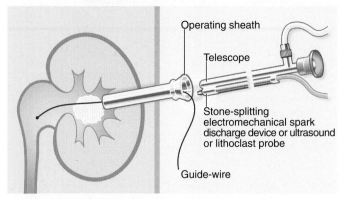

(b) Percutaneous stone splitting/retrieval

- Operating sheath
- Telescope
- Stone-splitting electromechanical spark discharge device or ultrasound or lithoclast probe
- Guide-wire

1 Needle passed through skin into renal pelvis
2 Guide-wire passed through needle into ureter
3 Hollow dilators passed sequentially over guide-wire until large bore operating sheath can be generated
4 Stone progressively broken into fragments by mechanical shock, spark discharge or other energy-emitting probe applied to surface of stone
5 Stone fragments removed with forceps under direct vision

(c) Extracorporeal shock-wave lithotripsy (ESWL)
The renal tract stone is located by biplanar ultrasound and the two shock-generating heads are applied to the skin in position to focus the shock waves on the stone. 500–2000 shocks are applied and the patient later passes 'sand' debris over a period of days.

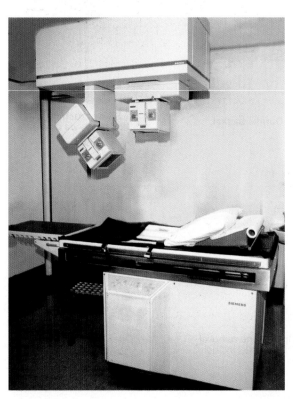

Fig. 31.8 Current methods of urinary tract stone removal

MANAGEMENT OF ACUTE URETERIC COLIC

Ureteric colic occurs when a stone causes sudden obstruction of a ureter. It presents typically with a sudden onset of severe unilateral pain radiating from one loin to the groin or tip of the penis. The pain is due to waves of ureteric peristalsis and episodes may last from several minutes to half an hour. At the peak of the pain, the patient writhes in agony. Indeed, the pain of ureteric colic can be so severe and incapacitating that military pilots known to have stones are grounded until the stones are removed. Most patients are seen urgently by their family practitioner or brought straight to the accident and emergency department. Non-steroidal anti-inflammatory drugs given as suppositories or injection have largely replaced intramuscular opiate analgesia to settle the pain. NSAIDs are more effective, longer-lasting and without risk of addiction or legal compromise. The drug of choice is diclofenac. Morphine should be avoided as it tends to provoke and prolong ureteric spasm and pain. The patient may have become pain-free by the time of first examination by the surgical staff, but the pain history is usually diagnostic. Occasionally, ureteric colic is not as severe but is more persistent, in which case it may mimic other acute abdominal conditions.

INVESTIGATION OF URETERIC COLIC

Ureteric colic almost always causes **microscopic haematuria**, and the first investigation is 'dipstick' testing of the urine for blood; if positive it should be confirmed on microscopic examination. A positive result reinforces the diagnosis. An IVU should then be performed urgently to confirm or refute the diagnosis (see Fig. 31.5, p. 415).

The characteristic radiological features of acute ureteric obstruction are:

● **Delay** of all phases of passage of contrast through the kidney and collecting system on the affected side; the more severe the obstruction, the longer the delay. If there appears to be no excretion, further films are taken every few hours for about 24 hours; usually contrast will eventually pass into the system, demonstrating the site of obstruction
● **Dilatation** of the collecting system above the point of obstruction

TREATMENT OF URETERIC COLIC

Most patients with ureteric colic initially require strong analgesics. These are usually non-steroidal anti-inflammatory drugs, e.g. diclofenac given by suppository or injection. Many patients settle on a single dose but two or three doses may be required. In most cases, the stone gradually passes down the ureter and into the bladder. Each stage of movement may be accompanied by an attack of colic. If a stone is retrieved, it should be chemically analysed. If there is complete obstruction of the ureter or infection above an obstructing stone, urgent intervention is usually required to prevent renal damage. Immediate treatment may involve placing a percutaneous nephrostomy tube to drain the renal pelvis (see Fig. 31.9), placing a stent beside the stone to allow urinary drainage or else removal of the stone endoscopically. After nephrostomy or stent placement, the stone sometimes passes spontaneously but more often requires further treatment later. In cases with persistent pain that do not need immediate intervention, plain abdominal X-rays will usually record changes in the position of the stone. If the stone is very large, it may have to be surgically removed. If the stone appears to be small enough to pass spontaneously, yet fails to progress,

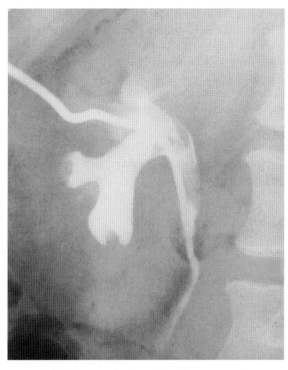

Fig. 31.9 Percutaneously placed nephrostomy drainage tube
A ureteric stone caused complete ureteric obstruction and the patient suffered continuing pain and developed a fever. Urgent drainage was required to prevent renal damage from a combination of obstruction and infection.

the patient can safely be allowed home if the criteria for urgent surgery mentioned above are not fulfilled. The IVU can be repeated after a week or two and a decision taken about the need for operation then.

LONG-TERM MANAGEMENT OF UROLOGICAL STONE DISEASE

MANAGEMENT OF METABOLIC ABNORMALITIES

Hyperparathyroidism is the only stone-forming metabolic abnormality that can be corrected by surgical treatment (parathyroidectomy). It is diagnosed by an elevated plasma calcium, lowered plasma phosphate and an elevated plasma parathormone level. Most patients are also hypercalciuric.

Dietary hypercalciuria should be treated by reducing the intake of milk, cheese, butter, bread and pastry. Local tap water and bottled water drunk by the patient should have its calcium level checked. **Idiopathic hypercalciuria** can be treated with thiazides. Allopurinol can be used in hyperuricaemia (see below) but may also prevent nidus formation in urine around which calcium crystals deposit during stone formation. Urate stones dissolve in alkaline urine and treatment may involve alkalinising the urine with sodium bicarbonate. Primary oxaluria is very rare; secondary oxaluria only occurs with huge intakes of tea, coffee, chocolate, strawberries and rhubarb.

The drug **allopurinol** may be given for hyper-uricaemia (gout) and is routinely given during chemotherapy for leukaemia. Allopurinol inhibits xanthine oxidase, an enzyme involved in synthesis of uric acid.

LONG-TERM FOLLOW-UP OF PATIENTS WITH URINARY TRACT STONES

For many patients, a symptomatic urinary tract stone manifests as an isolated episode with no apparent predisposing cause. Long-term follow-up for these patients is not usually required. Patients with stones that do not need removing or with recurrent stones require long-term follow-up with regular plain abdominal X-rays. Stones that enlarge during follow-up, that cause symptoms or obstruct need removing. Any patient with stone disease should probably be advised to increase fluid intake but apparently logically based diet changes are pointless or even harmful. Drinking excessive fluids during a bout of ureteric colic is misguided and likely to cause an increase in pain. For patients with recurrent stones or obsessive patients in search of help, a simple machine is available to measure relative urine concentrations at home to ensure adequate fluid intake. However, proof of benefit for any long-term therapy is difficult to obtain.

32 Urinary tract infections

INTRODUCTION

Urinary tract infections are a common problem in surgery. They may be responsible for abdominal pain or urinary tract symptoms that present to the clinician for diagnosis. More often, urinary tract infection is a secondary problem. It may occur after operation, particularly if a urinary catheter has been employed, or it may complicate surgical disorders of the urinary tract such as tumours or stones. Infections are usually caused by common bacteria of faecal origin.

Urinary tract infections may also be caused by special organisms, in particular *Mycobacterium tuberculosis*. Urinary tract infection with the tubercle bacillus in its early stages may produce the same symptoms and signs as ordinary bacterial infection. Tuberculosis is easily overlooked unless specifically sought.

On a world-wide basis, other organisms are more important causes of urinary tract infection, most notably the trematode *Schistosoma*. One manifestation of this causes severe bladder disease in developing countries.

Infections of the urethra are usually transmitted by sexual intercourse. Gonococci and *Chlamydia* are the organisms most commonly involved. A late result of gonorrhoea in males or its inappropriate treatment may be fibrous **urethral stricture**.

The most common cause of urethral stricture is trauma. This may follow prolonged catheterisation, instrumentation of the urethra or pelvic fractures with urethral involvement. Although most are not infective in origin, urethral strictures are covered in this chapter.

COMMON BACTERIAL INFECTIONS OF THE LOWER URINARY TRACT

PATHOPHYSIOLOGY OF LOWER URINARY TRACT INFECTIONS

The common infections of the urinary tract, i.e. those caused by faecal organisms, involve either the bladder or the upper tract (kidney, pelvicalyceal system and ureter) or both together.

The bladder is infected most often, with females being particularly susceptible; probably half of all females are affected at one time or another. Infection rate rises with pregnancy and with increasing age. In females, the infecting organisms probably enter via the urethra which is only 3 cm long. Organisms easily spread from the perineal skin, particularly during sexual intercourse.

Normally, the bladder is flushed clean by the frequent passage of newly produced urine, preventing the multiplication of bacteria in the urinary tract. Stasis of urine for any reason, such as incomplete bladder emptying, dehydration or immobility, interferes with this mechanism and predisposes to infection. Urethral instrumentation greatly predisposes to infection in either sex.

CLINICAL FEATURES OF LOWER URINARY TRACT INFECTIONS

Typical symptoms of bladder infection are **dysuria**, **frequency**, **urgency** and a sensation of **incomplete bladder emptying**. The term 'cystitis' is often used by patients to mean symptoms included on this list; however, infection is not always the cause of symptoms and to prevent confusion, the term is probably best avoided. Even when infection is present, symptoms may be trivial or absent, and this may make diagnosis difficult. Abdominal pain may be the only symptom; consequently, most patients with abdominal pain should have their urine tested as a matter of course.

In the elderly or the very young, there are often no localising symptoms, and the patient is just non-specifically unwell. Recurrent fever in a child can result from urine infection. In any ill patient in these age groups, the urine must be sent for examination before antibiotics are given. A sudden onset of enuresis or urinary incontinence in children or the elderly should also suggest bladder infection.

The different presentations of bladder infection are summarised in Box 32.1.

SUMMARY

Box 32.1 Presentations of bladder infection

- **Dysuria with frequency and urgency of micturition (very common)**
- **Lower abdominal pain (common—usually children or young adults)**
- **Unexpected development of incontinence (common in the elderly)**
- **Development of enuresis in a previously 'dry' child**
- **Non-specific ill-health in previously well infants or the elderly (including pyrexia of unknown origin and septicaemia)**

BACTERIOLOGICAL DIAGNOSIS OF LOWER URINARY TRACT INFECTIONS

Urinary tract infection is confirmed by examining a 'midstream' specimen of urine (MSU). If the specimen cannot be examined quickly, it should be refrigerated or it will become of no diagnostic value in a few hours (see Fig. 32.1). The specimen is centrifuged and the unstained sediment is then examined microscopically for white blood cells ('pus cells') and bacteria. The specimen is also cultured to identify the causative organism and determine antibiotic sensitivity. Bacterial contamination of urine specimens is common; a 'significant' infection is therefore defined as one in which pus cells are abundant and there are more than 100 000 (10^5) organisms per millilitre of urine. Enteric organisms are almost always responsible, the usual culprits being *Escherichia coli*, *Proteus* spp., *Enterococcus faecalis* and *Pseudomonas* (the last particularly in debilitated and catheterised patients).

Significant numbers of pus cells in the urine without bacterial growth most commonly result from patients taking antibiotics. If this is not the case, a stone, tumour, prostatitis or tuberculosis must be suspected and investigated. Infection often causes frank or occult haematuria; this only warrants further investigation if it persists after the infection is treated.

Some female patients experience typical symptoms of urinary infection but despite multiple laboratory examinations, no evidence of bacterial infection of urine is found. Non-specific urethral inflammation from the

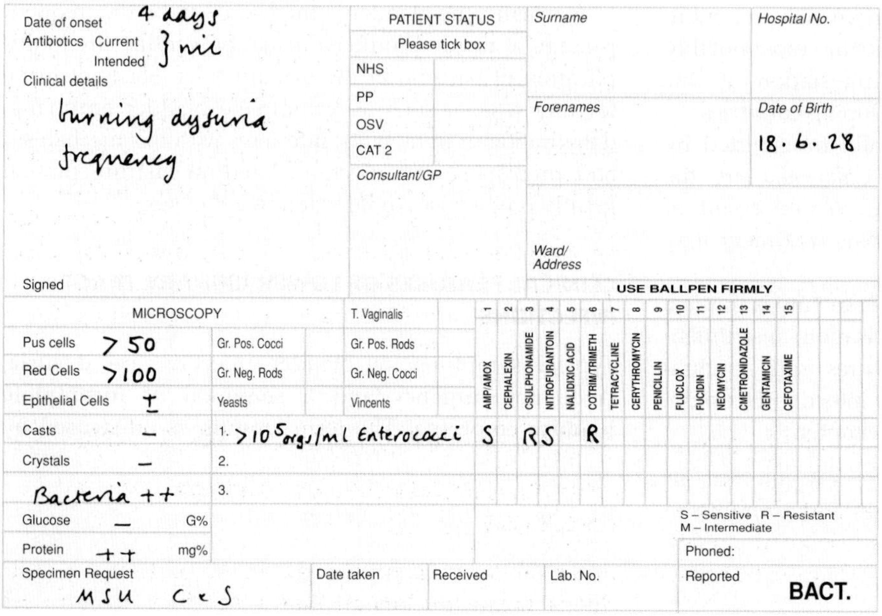
Date of onset 4 days
Antibiotics Current / Intended } nil
Clinical details
burning dysuria
frequency
Signed
PATIENT STATUS
Please tick box
NHS
PP
OSV
CAT 2
Consultant/GP
Surname
Hospital No.
Forenames
Date of Birth 18. 6. 28
Ward/ Address
USE BALLPEN FIRMLY
MICROSCOPY
Pus cells >50
Red Cells >100
Epithelial Cells +
Casts –
Crystals –
Bacteria ++
Glucose – G%
Protein ++ mg%
Gr. Pos. Cocci
Gr. Neg. Rods
Yeasts
T. Vaginalis
Gr. Pos. Rods
Gr. Neg. Cocci
Vincents
1. >10⁵ orgs/ml Enterococci
2.
3.
1 AMP/AMOX S
2 CEPHALEXIN
3 CSULPHONAMIDE R
4 NITROFURANTOIN S
5 NALIDIXIC ACID
6 COTRIM/TRIMETH R
7 TETRACYCLINE
8 CERYTHROMYCIN
9 PENICILLIN
10 FLUCLOX
11 FUCIDIN
12 NEOMYCIN
13 CMETRONIDAZOLE
14 GENTAMICIN
15 CEFOTAXIME
S – Sensitive R – Resistant M – Intermediate
Phoned:
Specimen Request MSU C & S
Date taken
Received
Lab. No.
Reported
BACT.

Fig. 32.1 Typical MSU report of urinary tract infection

trauma of intercourse may be responsible; this is probably the cause of 'honeymoon cystitis'.

MANAGEMENT OF BLADDER INFECTIONS

Antibiotic therapy is the principal treatment for bladder infection, initially chosen on a 'best-guess' basis. An MSU specimen should be collected for microscopy, culture and sensitivities (M, C & S) before therapy is commenced. If the initial antibiotic choice is inappropriate or unsuccessful, then the results of urine culture may suggest a more suitable alternative. An MSU should be repeated about 6 weeks after treatment, even if the infection appears to clear quickly. If there is doubt whether the infection has been eliminated, the MSU should be repeated several days after completion of the course of antibiotics.

Patients who have had urinary tract infections should be encouraged to increase their fluid intake. Indeed, this is often effective in dealing with early or mild symptoms and will probably cause many infections to resolve without drugs.

In **pregnancy**, the ureters and renal pelvis dilate under the effect of circulating progestogens and become more susceptible to infection. Where there is a risk of infection ascending from the bladder into the upper tracts, the urine should be tested routinely; evidence of significant bacterial growth must be treated actively with appropriate antibiotics, whether or not the patient is symptomatic. The antibiotic used must be known to be safe for use in pregnancy and non-teratogenic, e.g. a cephalosporin. Trimethoprim is also safe but may deplete folate. Standard texts such as the *British National Formulary* give specific information on prescribing in pregnancy and should be consulted.

RECURRENT BLADDER INFECTIONS

Patients who suffer recurrent infections tend to fall into three groups:

- The elderly, debilitated and infirm
- Young and middle-aged women
- Patients with unexpected urinary tract infections

Those in the first two groups can usually be managed without surgery.

The elderly, debilitated and infirm

These patients often have a multiplicity of simple predisposing factors such as constipation, incontinence, an indwelling catheter, poor fluid intake and diminished resistance. Correction of these problems and good nursing care (e.g. regular changes of indwelling catheter) may break the pattern.

Young and middle-aged women

Many of these patients can be helped by simple hygiene measures. These include 'wiping from front to back' after micturition or defecation, frequent and complete emptying of the bladder, increasing urine flow by raising fluid intake, and emptying the bladder soon after intercourse.

Patients with unexpected urinary tract infections

This group includes children or young men with a single episode of urinary infection, particularly if they fail to respond to simple measures, and anyone with recurrent urinary infections. These patients require investigation (e.g. ultrasonography, intravenous urography) and are often found to have a structural abnormality or pathological condition which encourages bacterial proliferation. Bladder stone or prostatic hypertrophy is commonly responsible. These predisposing conditions can often be corrected surgically. In the rest, however, no predisposing factor can be found.

As with isolated episodes of infection, recurrent infections are treated with antibiotics, but bacteriological investigation assumes a greater importance. Some patients lose their immunity against *E. coli* and need long-term, low-dose antibiotics to prevent recurrence.

The 'urethral syndrome'

This syndrome is only found in women and is characterised by episodic or persistent dysuria, frequency or urgency. Urinary symptoms occur without demonstrable infection or local anatomical abnormality such as uterine prolapse. The cause is not known, and the condition may be indistinguishable from recurrent urethral trauma due to sexual intercourse. Urethral dilatation under general anaesthesia may be successful in relieving symptoms, although the mechanism is obscure. If it fails, urethroscopy should be performed seeking a urethral diverticulum. Dysuria may also be a symptom associated with **atrophic vaginitis** in perimenopausal and postmenopausal women; this may be relieved by topical application of oestrogens to the vagina and introitus.

Some patients, particularly women and girls, experience persistent or recurrent low-grade symptoms, notably frequency and urgency. No cause is found, although some cases can be attributed to habit or to psychogenic or psychosexual factors.

UPPER URINARY TRACT INFECTIONS

PATHOPHYSIOLOGY OF UPPER URINARY TRACT INFECTIONS

Infections of the pelvicalyceal system and renal parenchyma (**acute pyelonephritis**) arise either by upward

423

extension of a lower tract infection or via the bloodstream (haematogenous).

Ascending infections occur most commonly when there is an abnormality causing ureteric reflux or stasis. Such conditions include ureteric obstruction, abnormal peristalsis (as in megaureter) and congenital incompetence of the cysto-ureteric antireflux mechanism. During pregnancy, the ureter becomes unusually dilated because of hormonal influences and this may contribute to the increased incidence of urinary infections during this time.

Haematogenous infection is often responsible when there is urinary stasis in the upper tract. Common causes are stones in the renal pelvis or obstruction of the pelviureteric junction (PUJ). In such cases, lower tract infection is a secondary phenomenon.

The factors initiating a renal infection are often unclear but pre-existing renal damage is a strong predisposing factor.

Pathological examination of an acutely infected kidney shows extensive neutrophilic infiltration of the renal parenchyma, often with small abscesses. Usually only one kidney is involved and the causative organisms are enteral, as in other urinary tract infections.

CLINICAL FEATURES OF UPPER URINARY TRACT INFECTIONS

The classic clinical features of acute pyelonephritis are unilateral loin pain and tenderness (see Box 32.2). The patient is generally unwell with systemic features of infection, i.e. pyrexia and tachycardia. The urine is usually cloudy, and microscopy and culture confirm the presence of pus cells and bacteria. There may also be typical symptoms of bladder infection. Often, the symptoms and signs are less specific and the patient presents with unilateral abdominal pain or discomfort. This may be mistaken for early acute appendicitis unless the urine is examined. Pyelonephritis may present without localising signs, especially in infants and the elderly, but patients are more unwell than in bladder infection and may even develop systemic signs of sepsis.

MANAGEMENT OF UPPER URINARY TRACT INFECTIONS

Diagnosis is made on the basis of clinical symptoms, signs and urine examination. Blood is also taken for culture when there are systemic signs of infection.

Treatment is with antibiotics, initially on a 'best-guess' basis, based on local microbiological advice. Dosage and route of administration depend on the severity of the illness; severe cases are treated with intravenous antibiotics.

Once the acute illness has been successfully treated, further investigation, usually ultrasonography and intravenous urography, may be indicated in the search for predisposing factors. In children, investigation should include a contrast micturating cystogram or equivalent

SUMMARY
Box 32.2 Presenting features of acute pyelonephritis
● **Unilateral loin pain and tenderness**
● **Less specific abdominal pain and discomfort**
● **Dysuria and cloudy, strong-smelling urine**
● **Haematuria**
● **Pyrexia and tachycardia**
● **Septicaemia (especially young children and the elderly)**

radionuclide scintigram to identify ureteric reflux (see Ch. 45).

COMPLICATIONS OF ACUTE PYELONEPHRITIS
(see Figs 32.2 and 32.3, p. 425)

Pyonephrosis

Severe infections may be complicated by obstruction of the pelviureteric outlet, resulting in the accumulation of pus in the renal pelvis (pyonephrosis). If untreated, this will destroy the renal parenchyma. Treatment involves surgical or percutaneous drainage followed by correction of the obstruction.

Perinephric abscess

If infection develops when a large 'staghorn' calculus is present, the accumulating pus may discharge through the renal capsule into the surrounding fat, resulting in a perinephric abscess (Fig. 32.3). This presents as a slowly expanding mass in the loin, often with only low-grade local and systemic symptoms. Urine investigation will reveal pyuria, whilst ultrasound and radiology will show a non-functioning renal mass containing fluid-filled areas. A large renal calculus may also be seen. A perinephric abscess sometimes develops as a result of haematogenous infection of a traumatic perinephric haematoma. The treatment of perinephric abscess is drainage, often followed later by nephrectomy of the end-stage kidney. The diagnosis should be considered in elderly patients with septicaemia from an unknown source. If a perinephric inflammatory mass partially resolves, it can result in **xanthomatous pyelonephritis**, a solid mass often suspected of malignancy and removed surgically.

GENITOURINARY TUBERCULOSIS

PATHOPHYSIOLOGY OF GENITOURINARY TUBERCULOSIS

About 4% of patients with tuberculosis have involvement of the genitourinary system. In developed countries,

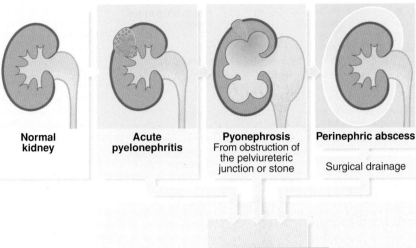

Normal
kidney

Acute
pyelonephritis

Pyonephrosis
From obstruction of
the pelviureteric
junction or stone

Perinephric abscess

Surgical drainage

Thinned cortex

Pitted external
surface

Reduced vertical
dimension
(shown on
intravenous
urogram)

End-stage kidney

**Fig. 32.2 Consequences of
untreated renal infection**

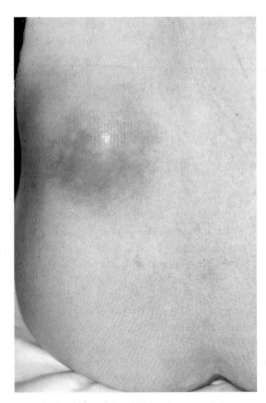

Fig. 32.3 Perinephric abscess
This woman of 55 presented with a 3-week history of left loin pain and
48 hours of rigors. The photograph shows a large abscess surrounding
the left kidney, pointing in the posterior loin. A plain abdominal film
showed a staghorn calculus in the kidney and isotope studies showed
no function in that kidney. The abscess was drained percutaneously
and she was treated with antibiotics. The kidney was later removed.

incidence is highest in debilitated elderly patients, often
with a history of treated tuberculosis. The other vulnerable group is immigrants from developing countries
where tuberculosis is endemic.

Mycobacteria reach the kidney or epididymis via the
bloodstream causing typical centrally caseating granulomatous lesions which may later calcify (see Fig. 32.4).
From the kidney, direct spread may occur to the ureter
(causing a fibrous stricture) or to the bladder. Tuberculosis of the bladder usually begins around a ureteric
opening and spreads more widely to cause patchy ulceration of the bladder wall and later fibrotic contraction.
Young adults are most commonly affected and there
is a seriously increased incidence among patients with
acquired immunodeficiency syndrome (AIDS). These and
other patients 'living rough' are poorly compliant with
treatment and provide a reservoir of infection for others.

CLINICAL FEATURES AND INVESTIGATION OF GENITOURINARY TUBERCULOSIS

Urinary tract tuberculosis is often asymptomatic and
is diagnosed during investigation of 'sterile pyuria'. If
there are symptoms, the usual ones are painless urinary
frequency, nocturia and sometimes haematuria. There
may also be systemic features such as weight loss and
night sweats, and respiratory symptoms if the lungs are
affected.

When urinary tuberculosis is suspected, at least three
early morning urine (EMU) specimens must be sent to

425

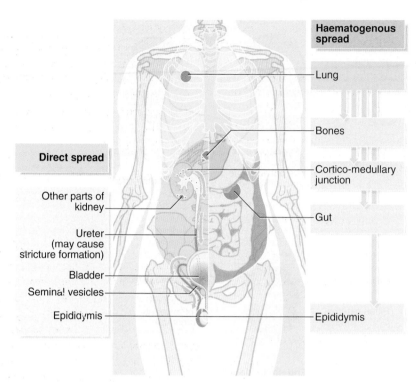

Haematogenous spread

Lung

Bones

Cortico-medullary junction

Gut

Epididymis

Direct spread

Other parts of kidney

Ureter (may cause stricture formation)

Bladder

Seminal vesicles

Epididymis

Fig. 32.4 Spread of tuberculosis to the genitourinary tract

the laboratory to be stained and cultured for tubercle bacilli (acid-fast bacilli, AFB). The entire volume of the first urine passed in the morning is collected and centrifuged to concentrate the small number of organisms. Culture usually takes 6–8 weeks but a negative result does not exclude urinary tuberculosis. Any acid-fast bacilli cultured need to be typed to exclude non-tuberculous varieties. If at cystoscopy there is a red patch around a ureteric orifice, this can be biopsied and examined histologically for caseating granulomas and stained for tuberculosis organisms, thus accelerating the diagnostic process. Blood is tested for anaemia, lymphocytosis and elevation of the erythrocyte sedimentation rate (ESR), and for biochemical indicators of renal function. A chest X-ray is taken to search for pulmonary disease. Renal calcification may be seen on plain abdominal X-ray (such as the control film of an intravenous urogram), while urography may show renal abnormalities or ureteric strictures.

MANAGEMENT OF GENITOURINARY TUBERCULOSIS

Chemotherapy is the mainstay of treatment, as for pulmonary tuberculosis, with the choice of agents made according to the local prevalence of particular strains of the organism and the results of culture and sensitivities. Surgery may be required later to treat ureteric strictures or a contracted bladder, or to excise damaged kidney tissue (partial or total nephrectomy). For ureteric tuberculosis, corticosteroids are usually given along with

antituberculous chemotherapy to reduce the risk of stricture formation. Plasma urea and creatinine should be monitored during the usual 6 months of therapy and signs of upper tract dilatation sought with periodic ultrasound examinations.

SCHISTOSOMIASIS

Schistosomiasis (bilharzia) is the most important parasitic disease of the urinary tract. It causes chronic inflammatory lesions in the bladder which lead to severe fibrotic damage. Schistosomiasis also predisposes to stone formation and squamous carcinoma.

Three schistosome species, *S. haematobium*, *S. mansoni* and *S. japonicum*, have a wide tropical distribution and are important human pathogens. The most destructive bladder disease, however, is caused by *S. haematobium*. This species is endemic to tropical and North Africa (particularly the Nile valley), and is also found in some Middle Eastern and southern European countries. More effective treatment with **praziquatel** has dramatically reduced the reservoir of infection and consequently the incidence of cases in Egypt, but treatment is relatively expensive and has made little impact in Sudan. Increasing world-wide travel makes it likely that the disease will be seen more frequently in travellers from Western countries.

The schistosome has a sophisticated life cycle which is dependent on poor sanitation. Humans (the main definitive host) are infected by working or bathing in contaminated water. The free-swimming adult forms (**cercaria**) penetrate the skin, usually of the feet, and pass through the venous circulation and lungs to the systemic arterial circulation, which disseminates them throughout the body. In the hepatic portal veins, male and female worms mate. The females, crammed with fertilised ova, then find their way via the mesenteric veins to the venous plexuses of the pelvic viscera, notably the bladder, where the ova are released. Aided by lytic enzymes, the ova then pass through the bladder wall into the urine and thence to the external environment.

On reaching water, the ova release mature ciliated forms (**miracidia**) which enter the intermediate host, a species of freshwater snail. The miracidia mature in the snail's liver before they are released as a new generation of adult cercarial worms. At this point, they are ready to enter human hosts, thus completing the life cycle.

CLINICAL PRESENTATIONS OF SCHISTOSOMIASIS

Initial skin penetration may cause mild local inflammation. Subsequently, the phase of haematogenous spread may cause general malaise, low-grade pyrexia and eosinophilia. About 2 months later, ova invading the bladder mucosa cause local inflammation, and manifest as frequency and haematuria at the end of micturition. The early symptoms may be trivial and may pass unnoticed in low-grade infestations.

The main bladder damage caused by schistosomiasis is due to an intense chronic inflammatory reaction to dead ova which have not passed out in the urine and are sequestered in the mucosa. Small granulomatous 'pseudotubercles' develop around each ovum and these later become fibrotic and calcified. Heavy or recurrent infestations result in a variety of destructive lesions including **ulcers**, **papillomata**, **cysts**, **giant granulomata** and **severe bladder contracture**. All predispose to secondary bacterial infection and formation of bladder stones. Squamous metaplasia is common and strongly predisposes to **carcinoma**, two-thirds squamous and one-third transitional cell.

The clinical features of schistosomiasis are summarised in Box 32.3.

MANAGEMENT OF SCHISTOSOMIASIS

Bladder or ureteric calcification is almost diagnostic of schistosomiasis. Diagnosis is confirmed either by microscopic examination of urine for ova (these are best found in the last few millilitres of a mid-morning specimen of urine) or more reliably by cystoscopic biopsy of bladder lesions.

Treatment is much simplified nowadays using the drug **praziquatel**. This is given in two doses on 1 day, 6 hours

---

SUMMARY

Box 32.3 Clinical features of schistosomiasis

- Skin rash at site of cercarial penetration
- Low-grade systemic illness with eosinophilia
- Urinary frequency and terminal haematuria
- Chronic inflammation of the bladder
- Bladder fibrosis and contracture
- Bladder stones
- Squamous cell carcinoma (two-thirds) or transitional cell carcinoma (one-third) of the bladder

apart, in a dose of 20 mg/kg body weight. **Metrifonate** is an alternative treatment if praziquatel is unavailable. Surgery is occasionally necessary later to correct or palliate residual deformities of the lower urinary tract.

About 5% of the world's population is affected by various forms of schistosomiasis and prevention must be the cornerstone of disease control. Improved sanitation and clean water supplies are essential. Ironically, the rapid expansion of water conservation and irrigation schemes has tended to spread the disease to previously unaffected populations. Effective treatment of affected individuals can substantially reduce the pool of infection and the number of new cases.

URETHRAL INFECTIONS AND STRICTURES

URETHRAL INFECTIONS

The only clinically significant infections of the urethra are sexually transmitted diseases. The most common are **gonorrhoea** and '**non-specific urethritis**', the latter usually caused by chlamydial infection. The acute condition usually presents with a urethral discharge and dysuria. The surgical importance of urethritis, particularly gonococcal urethritis, is that it may lead, months or years later, to a fibrous stricture in the posterior urethra. Fortunately, the condition is becoming uncommon as primary antibiotic therapy is more readily available and effective.

Serological tests for gonorrhoea are relatively unreliable, but serological tests for *Chlamydia* can demonstrate past infection. For current chlamydial infection, posterior urethral swabs examined on special slides are the only reliable test.

URETHRAL STRICTURES

Urethral strictures are now most commonly caused by inflammation resulting from **iatrogenic trauma**. Transurethral resection for prostatic surgery is the most common cause. Catheterisation with latex catheters in patients with poor tissue perfusion is another common cause, particularly catheterisation during cardiopulmonary bypass for cardiac surgery. These iatrogenic strictures involve the distal urethra or the meatus but strictures may also be a complication of traumatic instrumentation, in which case the membranous urethra is most vulnerable (see Fig. 32.5) A small proportion of strictures result from urethral tearing or rupture following displaced pelvic fractures. These usually require open surgical reconstruction.

The characteristic symptom of urethral stricture is a progressive diminution in urinary stream. If there is any associated chronic urinary retention, this may be accompanied by symptoms of bladder outlet obstruction, i.e. frequency and urgency. Diagnosis is made by direct inspection using a cystourethroscope.

Strictures may be short, elongated or multiple. An effective treatment involves stretching the scar tissue by repeated self-dilatation. This technique, performed once a week for 2 years, keeps the urethra open long enough for fibroblasts to remodel around it. An alternative with tight strictures is to cut the stricture longitudinally with a urethrotome under direct urethroscopic vision, and follow this by repeated dilatation. Recurrence after treatment is not only frequent, but almost to be expected; skilled urological follow-up is therefore desirable. More complicated strictures may require open surgical treatment: for example, excision of a short stricture and end-to-end anastomosis of the urethra. For some, inlays of bladder or oral mucosa may prove successful.

Urethral strictures may cause lifelong disability, and most can be avoided by extreme care of the urethra during catheterisation and urethral instrumentation. 'Routine' catheterisation appears to be an irresistible temptation to

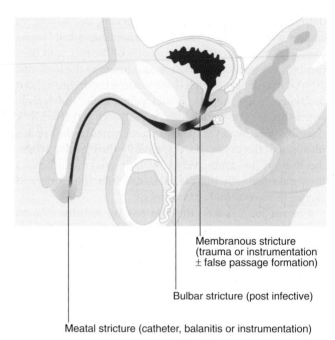

Membranous stricture (trauma or instrumentation ± false passage formation)

Bulbar stricture (post infective)

Meatal stricture (catheter, balanitis or instrumentation)

Fig. 32.5 Common sites of urethral strictures

all but urologists. As a general rule, the urethra should not be catheterised or interfered with unless absolutely essential. Sick patients should be catheterised only with a silicone urethral catheter or a suprapubic catheter to minimise local trauma. Any catheter or other urological instrument should be placed gently with minimal force or else under direct vision. If it proves difficult, an alternative means should be found or the procedure abandoned rather than risk urethral damage by forceful instrumentation.

33 Congenital disorders and diseases secondarily involving the urinary tract

CONGENITAL URINARY TRACT DISORDERS

INTRODUCTION

Serious congenital disorders of the kidneys and urinary tract nearly all present at birth or in early childhood and these are described in Chapter 45. The exception is **polycystic kidney** which may present in juveniles but more commonly presents in adulthood. There are also a number of lesser abnormalities of the upper tract which interfere with normal flow dynamics and predispose to infection, e.g. duplex systems or medullary sponge kidney. These are usually discovered during investigation of recurrent infections. Finally, asymptomatic abnormalities like unilateral renal agenesis, renal cysts or horseshoe kidney may be discovered incidentally during investigations (e.g. for hypertension) or surgery. With advancing age, a large proportion of the population develop benign renal cysts of varying size, usually of no clinical consequence.

A systematic summary of the important congenital disorders is presented in Table 33.1, with the conditions that present in adulthood signalled by an asterisk.

POLYCYSTIC KIDNEYS

The **adult polycystic kidney syndrome** is an **autosomal dominant disorder** characterised by multiple bilateral cysts of the renal parenchyma (see Fig. 33.1). The cysts slowly expand, compressing the renal parenchyma, and may lead to disruption of local control of blood pressure and eventually deteriorating renal function. Polycystic kidneys have three main variants: a juvenile form and

two adult forms. In one of the latter, the condition manifests in middle age with hypertension or progressive renal failure. In this form, the kidneys can be normal on ultrasound scanning in the first two decades of life. The second adult form is usually found incidentally in later life with almost normal renal function.

Thus, adult polycystic kidney may present with **hypertension** or progressive **chronic renal failure**. The enlarged cystic kidneys may cause loin pain or may be discovered

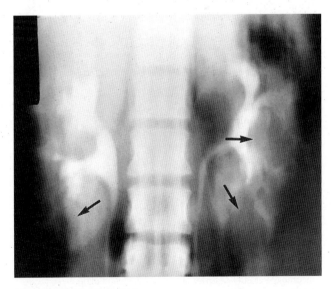

Fig. 33.1 Polycystic kidneys
IVU tomogram from a 52-year-old woman with hypertension and microscopic haematuria; both kidneys exhibit multiple lucent areas in the nephrogram representing cysts (arrowed), and the pelvicalyceal systems are slightly compressed.

Table 33.1 Congenital abnormalities of the urinary system

Nature of abnormality	Presentation
KIDNEY	
Bilateral agenesis (Potter's syndrome)	Oligohydramnios in pregnancy, stillborn infant with characteristic appearance of face and ears
Unilateral agenesis, aplasia or hypoplasia	Usually an incidental finding at any age. Often some abnormality on other side
Multicystic kidney Usually unilateral dysplasia of kidney with multiple cysts	Usually presents in the neonate as abdominal mass. Fatal if bilateral
Infantile polycystic disease Bilateral inherited disorder in which multiple small cysts replace renal parenchyma. Liver and pancreatic cysts often present also	Usually presents as gross abdominal distension in the neonate due to huge non-functioning kidneys. Invariably fatal
***Medullary sponge kidney** Cystic dilatation of collecting ducts of one or more medullary pyramids in one or both kidneys	May be found incidentally or during investigations for urinary infection. Cysts tend to become calcified and have characteristic X-ray appearance
***Adult polycystic kidney** Autosomal dominant disorder with multiple cysts throughout the parenchyma	Usually presents after age 30 with chronic renal failure, hypertension, haematuria or recurrent urinary tract infections
***Solitary cysts** Usually develop at one pole	Often incidental finding. May present with loin swelling or pain
***Horseshoe kidney** Fusion of lower poles of kidneys preventing normal developmental ascent	Often found incidentally but may cause hydronephrosis due to pelviureteric obstruction
***Ectopic kidneys and abnormalities of rotation** Due to failure of developmental ascent	Found incidentally or during investigation of complications such as pelviureteric obstruction
PELVICALYCEAL SYSTEM AND URETERS	
Pelvic hydronephrosis Dilatation of pelvicalyceal system due to congenital stenosis at pelviureteric junction	Usually presents in childhood or adolescence with loin pain or mass
Megaureter Abnormality of peristalsis of lower ureter resulting in gross proximal dilatation	Presents in young children as recurrent urinary tract infections
***Ureterocoele** Cystic dilatation of intravesical part of ureter due to stenosis of ureteric orifice	Incidental finding or may cause infection or symptoms of obstruction
Vesicoureteric reflux Unilateral or bilateral abnormality of ureteric insertion into bladder	Presents in children as recurrent pyelonephritis which can cause severe damage to developing kidney
***Duplex systems** Partial or complete duplication of a ureter	Often incidental finding or cause of recurrent infection
Ectopic ureter Ureter does not open into the bladder but into some other part of the genital tract, e.g. vagina	In females presents as dribbling incontinence and in males as recurrent urinary tract infections
BLADDER AND URETHRA	
Bladder hypoplasia Associated with some cases of hypospadias in boys or ectopic ureters in girls	Bladder distends once ureters or hypospadias is corrected
Urachal abnormalities i.e. Cyst, sinus, patent urachus; due to persistence of urachal remnants	Patent urachus usually presents in childhood with urine dribbling from umbilicus. Cysts and sinuses may present in adulthood. Adenocarcinoma sometimes develops in the urachal remnant
Bladder diverticulum Forms by herniation of mucosa through defect in muscular wall. In adults, usually due to bladder outlet obstruction; in children, due to congenital urethral valves	Usually presents as recurrent urinary tract infection
Bladder exstrophy Incomplete closure of lower abdominal wall in midline	Gross abnormality of genitourinary system obvious at birth
Urethral valves Usually occur in posterior urethra causing varying degrees of obstruction. More distal valves cause less obstruction	Severe cases present in the neonate with gross obstructive effects (palpable bladder after micturition), renal failure and infection. Milder cases present later with recurrent infection

Table 33.1 Continued

Nature of abnormality	Presentation
BLADDER AND URETHRA	
Epispadias	
Urethral meatus located in abnormal position somewhere on dorsum of penis. Often associated with major abnormality of penis	Obvious at birth with the urethra incomplete dorsally
Hypospadias	
Urethra opens in abnormal position on ventral aspect of penis due to defective urethral fold. The prepuce is 'hooded' and incomplete ventrally. Distal urethra is hypoplastic and shortened	Major cases obvious at birth. Minor cases have downward deviation of urinary stream. Sometimes a degree of **chordee** (downward bend of the penis)

*Conditions presenting in adulthood

incidentally on abdominal examination. These kidneys are particularly vulnerable to even minor trauma and **haematuria** is a common presentation.

Some of those affected with polycystic disease also have multiple cysts in the liver and sometimes in the pancreas. They present with massive abdominal swelling due to gross liver enlargement. There is no specific treatment for polycystic kidney disease and despite good conservative management, many patients will eventually require dialysis or renal transplantation. Surgical 'deroofing' of cysts, as may be appropriate in the management of solitary renal cysts (see below), is not appropriate here and often makes matters worse.

MEDULLARY SPONGE KIDNEY

This is caused by cyst-like dilatation (**ectasia**) of the collecting ducts of the renal medulla and may affect one or both kidneys. The cysts tend to become calcified, giving a characteristic radiographic appearance of streaky linear calcification in the renal papillae (see Fig. 33.2). On excretion pyelography, the tubular ectasia can be demonstrated as a 'flare' in the renal papilla. Marked degrees of medullary sponge kidney predispose to recurrent infection and stone formation because of intrarenal stasis of urine, but patients rarely present before adulthood. Minor degrees of change are often seen on intravenous urography (IVU) without symptoms.

DUPLEX SYSTEMS

The urinary collecting system may be duplicated to a greater or lesser extent. The duplication usually affects the renal end of the system and extends distally.

Complete duplex ureter is relatively common and may result in renal damage (see Fig. 33.3). The ureter draining the upper pole (upper moiety) of the kidney joins the bladder below the orifice of the lower pole ureter; this

ureter may have a defective antireflux mechanism at its junction with the bladder, thus predisposing to infection and renal parenchymal damage. In a child, the upper moiety may not show up on an excretion pyelogram (IVU) because an associated ectopic ureterocoele (region of abnormal ureteric dilatation) may have damaged the function of that part of the kidney. The diagnostic picture is of the calyces in the lower moiety looking like a 'drooping daffodil'. Lesser degrees of duplication are usually discovered by chance on IVU.

SOLITARY RENAL CYSTS

Isolated cysts of the renal parenchyma (see Fig. 33.4) are a common developmental abnormality and though rarely symptomatic, can be found in a large proportion

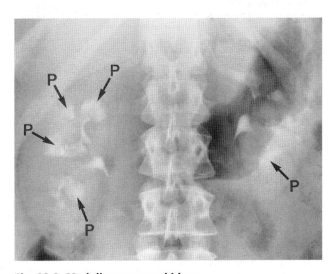

Fig. 33.2 Medullary sponge kidney
Bilateral medullary sponge kidney on an IVU from a 55-year-old woman with recurrent urinary tract infections; the renal papillae **P** have a typical 'flared' appearance and retain contrast because of the dilated collecting ducts. No radiopacity was visible on the control film although it can be seen in a considerable proportion of cases due to calcification in the ectatic ducts of the papillae.

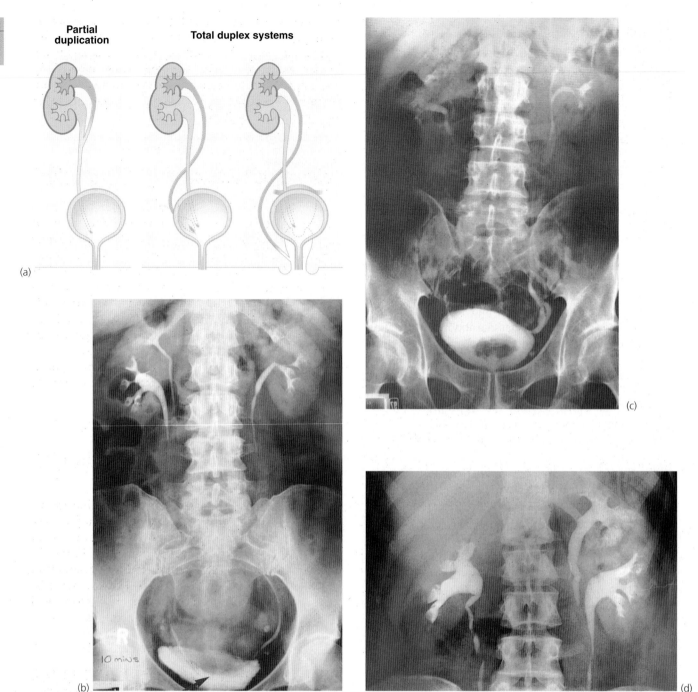

Partial duplication

Total duplex systems

(a)

(b)

(c)

(d)

Fig. 33.3 Duplex systems
(a) Partial and total duplication. In a total duplex system, the ureter from the upper renal moiety may open inferiorly in the bladder, or may open into the vagina (i.e. is ectopic). If vesicoureteric reflux occurs in the former case, it is via the **upper** ureteric orifice into the **lower** renal moiety. If a **ureterocoele** (dilated lower end of ureter) develops, it involves the lower ureteric orifice draining the upper moiety. An ectopic ureter causes continuous incontinence. **(b)** Duplication of the ureters on the right side; only one ureter can be seen passing as far as the bladder. The vesicoureteric junction is associated with a small, elongated ureterocoele (arrowed). **(c)** Complete left duplex system with both ureters visible all the way down to the bladder. **(d)** Partial duplication on the left side, the upper moiety of which exhibits the medullary sponge abnormality; this 25-year-old man presented with multiple ureteric stones, and the other abnormalities were incidental findings.

no value as the cysts rapidly refill. If intervention is required, cysts should be deroofed laparoscopically (in contrast to polycystic disease). Hydatid disease of the kidney should always be excluded before undertaking any surgical procedure on a 'renal cyst' to treat loin pain or ureteric obstruction, as inadvertent puncturing of cysts can lead to peritoneal spread.

HORSESHOE KIDNEY

This abnormality is caused by embryological fusion of the two developing kidneys at their lower poles. Normal renal ascent in the fetus is prevented by the inferior mesenteric artery so that the isthmus of the kidney comes to lie across the aorta at the level of the third or fourth lumbar vertebra. The condition is usually a chance finding on IVU investigation (where the diagnostic feature is of medially directed calyces—see Fig. 33.5), or at abdominal aortic surgery, when it may cause serious operative difficulties. Horseshoe kidney is sometimes associated with pelviureteric junction obstruction, which may lead to the diagnosis. Occasionally, a horseshoe kidney causes problems during pregnancy.

RENAL ECTOPIA AND OTHER RENAL ABNORMALITIES

A variety of other renal abnormalities (including ectopic kidneys (see Fig. 33.6, p. 435) rotational abnormalities, unilateral agenesis, aplasia or hyperplasia) may be found unexpectedly on investigation or at surgery. These abnormalities may confuse diagnosis and sometimes result in surgical mishap, e.g. excision of a pelvic kidney mistaken for an ovarian tumour. Note that transplanted kidneys are usually deliberately sited in the iliac fossa!

URACHAL ABNORMALITIES (see Fig. 33.7, p. 436)

During fetal development, the urogenital sinus communicates with the allantois via the urachus. Occasionally, this tract persists as a fistula between bladder and umbilicus. Sometimes the fistula does not open until adulthood. Similarly, a remnant may form a blind urachal sinus opening at the umbilicus or result in a urachal cyst in the midline of the lower abdomen. These structural abnormalities may then become infected. Very rarely, an adenocarcinoma develops in a urachal remnant in the bladder vault or in other urachal remnants.

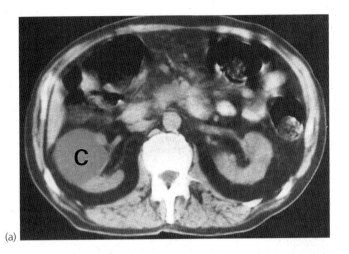
(a)

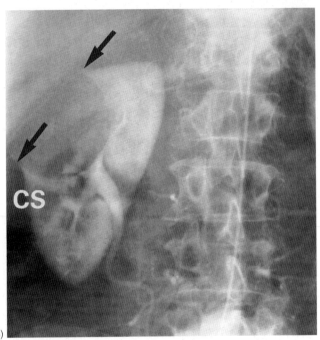
(b)

Fig. 33.4 Solitary renal cyst
(a) CT scan showing right renal cyst **C**. This was a chance finding in a woman of 45 under investigation for pancreatic pain. No treatment was necessary. **(b)** Another solitary renal cyst found by chance, this time on an aortogram. In this film, contrast has been injected into the aorta ('flush aortogram') rather than selectively; the typical animal-like 'claw sign' **CS** of a simple cyst (arrowed) is demonstrated.

of the population in later life, usually incidentally during renal ultrasound or IVU investigation. Their importance lies in distinguishing them from solid tumours and hydatid cysts, which is usually easily achieved with ultrasonography. Malignancy in association with a solitary cyst is very rare; if it does occur, it may show up as calcification in the cyst wall. Occasionally simple cysts cause pain or swelling. For these, aspiration alone is of

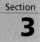
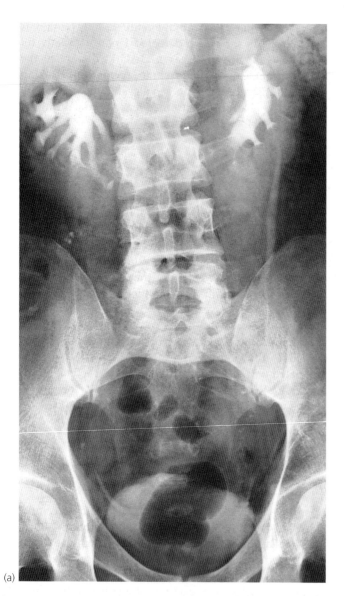

(a)

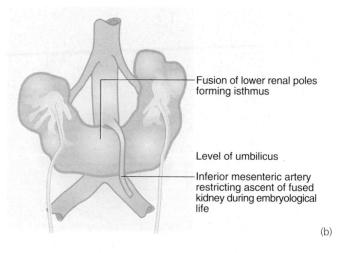

Fusion of lower renal poles forming isthmus

Level of umbilicus

Inferior mesenteric artery restricting ascent of fused kidney during embryological life

(b)

Fig. 33.5 Horseshoe kidney
Horseshoe kidney shown on IVU from a 51-year-old woman with recurrent urinary tract stones; the pelvicalyceal systems are oriented obliquely and converge inferiorly because the isthmus is stretched over the vertebral column. Each pelvis and ureter is more medially placed than normal and the whole renal mass lies much lower than would normal kidneys; the isthmus of a horseshoe kidney can rarely be demonstrated by IVU or ultrasound but can easily be imagined in this image.

DISEASES SECONDARILY INVOLVING THE URINARY TRACT

INTRODUCTION

A variety of abdominal disorders such as tumours, inflammatory bowel disease, aneurysms and retroperitoneal fibrosis may secondarily involve the urinary tract, as may iatrogenic (surgical) damage. These conditions affect the urinary tract by obstructing one or both ureters or occasionally by causing a fistula between bowel and urinary tract. Obstruction of one ureter alone may not be symptomatic although it may cause loin pain or predispose to infection; bilateral involvement usually presents with acute or chronic renal failure.

Of tumours outside the urinary tract, advanced **carcinoma of the uterine cervix** most commonly produces bilateral ureteric obstruction because of the close

anatomical relationship of the ureters to the cervix. This cancer may also ulcerate forwards into the bladder causing a **vesico-vaginal fistula**. This anatomical closeness makes the ureters vulnerable to trauma even at straightforward hysterectomy. Abdominal hysterectomy in particular can be associated with damage to the ureter causing stenosis and hydronephrosis or a uretero-vaginal fistula. An iatrogenic vesico-vaginal fistula can also occur. Carcinoma of the ascending or rectosigmoid colon may obstruct the right or left ureter respectively, although this is surprisingly rare. Most ureteric damage in relation to large bowel cancer results from colectomy operations.

Inflammatory disease which involves the bowel serosa may extend to involve nearby structures such as

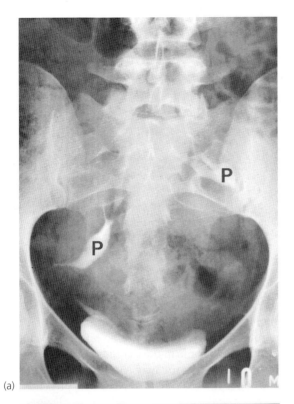

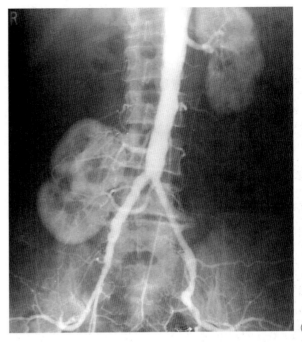

(a)

(b)

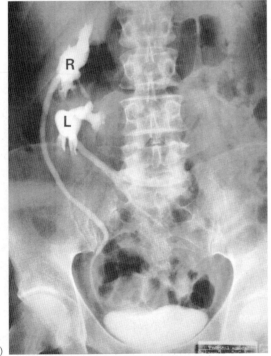

(c)

Fig. 33.6 Ectopic kidneys
(a) A 48-year-old woman with recurrent urinary tract infections; IVU shows abnormal pelvicalyceal systems **P** of bilateral pelvic kidneys.
(b) Right pelvic kidney discovered incidentally during arteriography for severe claudication. Its blood supply can be seen to arise from the distal aorta and iliac artery. She needed an aorto-femoral bypass but when faced with the technical difficulties, agreed to conservative management of her claudication. **(c)** Another middle-aged woman with recurrent urinary tract infections; the left kidney **L** is ectopically located on the apposite side and is fused to the right kidney **R** ('crossed renal ectopia').

the ureters and bladder, and this may lead to fistula formation. This is important in **Crohn's disease and diverticular disease**. A fistula between bowel and urinary tract presents as severe urinary infection, often with pneumaturia or faecuria.

An expanding abdominal mass may compress one or both ureters and cause symptoms from partial obstruction;

sometimes **aorto-iliac aneurysms** are responsible. An 'inflammatory' aneurysm near a ureter is likely to cause obstruction. This variant occurs in about 10% of aortic aneurysms. The cause is unknown but the effect is to produce retroperitoneal fibrosis across the anterior surface of the aneurysm. A much more common cause of ureteric dilatation is **pregnancy**, which tends to cause

435

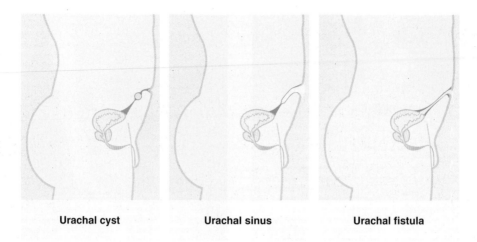

Urachal cyst   **Urachal sinus**   **Urachal fistula**

Fig. 33.7 Urachal abnormalities

bilateral megaureter due to the effects of progestogens. The main clinical significance of bilateral megaureter of pregnancy is that it predisposes to upper tract infection. Thus, significant bacteriuria in pregnancy, symptomatic or not, should be treated with antibiotics. Retention of urine can be caused by a pelvic mass such as a pregnancy of around 14 weeks or an ovarian lesion of similar size.

RETROPERITONEAL FIBROSIS

This relatively rare and obscure condition is characterised by progressive, intense fibrosis of the connective tissue lying posterior to the peritoneal cavity. About 50% of cases turn out to be caused by retroperitoneal spread of malignant disease. In the rest, the cause is unknown in many (i.e. idiopathic), but some drugs such as **methysergide** can induce the condition or it may be associated with an inflammatory aortic aneurysm. Retroperitoneal fibrosis sometimes causes hypertension via its effect on the kidneys.

Retroperitoneal fibrosis (RPF) compresses both ureters, causing bilateral hydronephrosis and eventually renal failure. Sometimes it is associated with inferior vena caval obstruction. Diagnosis is usually made on IVU, which shows bilateral hydronephrosis (see Fig. 33.8). The fibrotic process also draws the ureters closer together in the midline. The ESR is characteristically elevated.

Treatment usually involves a preliminary trial of high-dose steroids and insertion of **double-J stents** to maintain upper tract function whilst awaiting improvement. Surprisingly, ureters compressed by retroperitoneal fibrosis can usually be catheterised with ease. If medical treatment fails, the next step is usually dissection from the retroperitoneal tissue of the ureters (**ureterolysis**), which are then resited within the peritoneal cavity in an attempt to prevent recurrent obstruction. A biopsy of the retroperitoneal tissue should be taken to exclude malignancy and to confirm the diagnosis. If obstruction recurs, corticosteroid therapy may suppress the condition. Aortic grafting is indicated if an aneurysm is present.

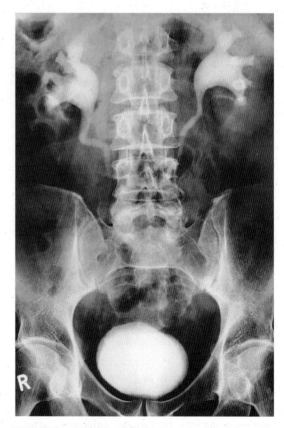

Fig. 33.8 Retroperitoneal fibrosis
This man of 62 presented with back pain. The IVU shows bilateral hydronephrosis due to ureteric compression; note how the ureters are tapered and characteristically drawn medially by the fibrotic process.

34 Vascular disorders of the lower limb—pathophysiology and clinical features

INTRODUCTION

The term 'vascular disease' is usually taken to mean disease of the arterial system, but it also includes diseases of veins and lymphatics. This chapter covers the presentation of vascular disorders of the lower limb, their clinical features and pathophysiology.

The active management of arterial disease only began in the 1950s and the sub-specialty of **peripheral vascular surgery** has evolved since then. Vascular surgery involves disorders of any arteries outside the heart and thoracic aorta as well as venous and lymphatic disorders and diabetic foot problems; it employs special techniques uncommon in general surgery. All clinicians should understand the principles of diagnosis and the scope and timing of treatment because complications of arterial diseases are seen across the whole field of medicine, e.g. acute ischaemia of a limb.

Arterial problems of the lower limb are covered in Chapter 35 and other arterial problems in Chapter 36.

Venous disorders are covered in Chapter 37 and encompass thromboembolic disease and its consequences, which are common, and **varicose veins**, which make up the largest single group of vascular problems.

Lower limb ulcers

Chronic lower limb ulcers are usually managed by general practitioners and community nurses with the more difficult cases referred to a dermatologist or surgeon. Many of these ulcers represent a complication of varicose veins or a late complication of deep venous thrombosis. The majority of the rest are caused by arterial insufficiency or diabetes and a few by vasculitis or ulcerating tumours. In developed countries, infection rarely plays a primary role. In intractable cases, persistent ulceration may be the result of a combination of factors, e.g. local trauma, diabetic neuropathy and obliterative atherosclerosis. Lower limb ulceration is covered later in this chapter.

PERIPHERAL ARTERIAL DISEASE

The bulk of arterial surgery is concerned with **lower limb ischaemia** and **carotid artery disease** (caused mainly by atherosclerotic obstruction) and degenerative **aneurysms**. Arterial trauma is an additional component, the volume of which depends on the local circumstances; for example, in wartime or civilian conflict, limbs are vulnerable to land mines and gunshot wounds and trauma to limbs is common in road traffic accidents.

LOWER LIMB ISCHAEMIA

Most lower limb ischaemia is **chronic** and ranges in severity from minimal to critical. The condition is often referred to as **chronic arterial insufficiency** or simply as **peripheral vascular disease** (PVD). **Acute lower limb ischaemia** occurs suddenly and often threatens the viability of the limb. The symptoms and signs of arterial insufficiency depend on the degree of ischaemia.

There are three main clinical presentations of lower limb ischaemia:

- **Intermittent claudication**—relatively mild ischaemia producing muscular pain only on exercise that is relieved by rest
- **Rest pain**—severe ischaemia presenting with pain in the affected foot, the pain becoming intolerable over a few days or weeks but without tissue loss. Many of these limbs are critically ischaemic

- **Critical ischaemia**—severe ischaemia with actual or potential tissue loss. Dry or wet gangrene or ulceration of part of the foot or leg may be present or likely to occur in the foreseeable future. By definition, the viability of the whole limb is threatened. The acutely ischaemic limb may be caused by embolism or acute thrombosis superimposed upon chronic atherosclerosis. In this situation, critical ischaemia may develop and progress very rapidly, with the leg becoming painful, cold and numb in a matter of hours. Emergency surgery or thrombolysis is required if the limb is to be saved.

OTHER CAUSES OF LOWER LIMB PAIN

Most arterial and venous disorders of the lower limbs can be recognised easily but in the acutely painful limb, differentiating between arterial insufficiency and deep venous thrombosis may require some clinical acumen; distinguishing the two is, however, highly important. Whatever the cause of the acutely painful limb, assessing the arterial element is an essential preliminary. In chronic cases, non-vascular causes of pain on walking such as **cauda equina compression** may be misdiagnosed as being arterial in origin.

ANEURYSMS

Aneurysms are an important degenerative disorder in older patients and most commonly affect the abdominal aorta, the ilio-femoral arteries and the popliteal arteries. Any aneurysm may rupture or leak and popliteal aneurysms in particular may thrombose or embolise and cause distal ischaemia. Although some aneurysms present acutely in one of these ways, the majority present as a painless pulsatile mass or are detected incidentally on ultrasound scanning, abdominal X-ray or CT. In addition, there is an increasing interest in population screening of older men for abdominal aortic aneurysms by ultrasonography. The way an aneurysm is managed depends on its site and its potential for serious complications.

VASCULAR INSUFFICIENCY OF THE LOWER LIMB

PATHOPHYSIOLOGY

Vascular disorders of the lower limb are caused mainly by atherosclerosis, arterial thromboembolism, aneurysms, complications of diabetes mellitus, and thromboembolic and varicose disorders of the venous system. In some patients, especially the elderly, several causes may interact. Accurate initial diagnosis of vascular disorders

depends largely on skilled clinical evaluation rather than special investigations. Symptoms and signs are best interpreted in the light of the underlying pathophysiological processes outlined in Table 34.1.

SYMPTOMS AND SIGNS IN THE LOWER LIMB

The principal symptoms and signs of lower limb vascular disease are pain, changes in skin texture, changes in skin colour and temperature, ulceration and swelling. The diagnostic importance of each of these is outlined in the following sections and summarised in Table 34.1.

PAIN

Most lower limb pain is due to trauma or musculoskeletal disorders rather than vascular disease. Where symptoms are caused by vascular disease, patients have minor pain and discomfort associated with varicose veins, have exercise-related pain, or have more severe pain caused by obliterative arterial disease or acute ischaemia.

INTERMITTENT CLAUDICATION

Chronic arterial insufficiency presents most commonly as muscular pain brought on by exercise which increases if walking continues. Symptoms usually predominate in one limb and the patient commonly **limps** with the pain, which accounts for the descriptive term 'intermittent claudication' (Latin *claudicare*: to limp). The patient is forced to stop walking, whereupon the pain subsides, usually within a minute or two. If exercise is then resumed, the pain recurs at about the same walking distance.

The pain of intermittent claudication is almost always in the calf whatever the level of the causative arterial obstruction. The pain may extend into the thigh or even buttock if walking is continued and this indicates arterial obstruction above the inguinal ligament. Absent foot pulses or foot pulses which become impalpable after exercise may be the only physical signs.

There is only one other condition which might reasonably be mistaken for arterial claudication after a thorough history has been taken; this is **cauda equina claudication**, caused by compression of the cauda equina within the spinal canal by central disc protrusion or spinal stenosis. In this condition, lower limb pain is also brought on by exercise but there are important differences; the claudication distance is very variable and is often absent on walking uphill or when cycling. The pain takes 30 minutes or so to subside and there is often a history of low back pain. On examination, there is usually evidence of a lower motor neurone lesion such as diminished or absent lower limb tendon reflexes. CT scanning of the

Table 34.1 Pathophysiology and clinical consequences of vascular diseases affecting the lower limb

Basic disease	Pathophysiological process	Clinical manifestations
OBLITERATIVE ATHEROSCLEROSIS AND ITS COMPLICATIONS		
Gradual luminal narrowing by atherosclerotic plaques, causing chronic ischaemia. May undergo sudden occlusion by superimposed thrombus. Affects aorta and large distributing vessels. More common in diabetics, particularly type II	Arterial supply adequate at rest but inadequate to supply metabolic demands of lower limb muscles (especially in calf) during exercise	**Intermittent claudication**–pain in lower limb muscles on walking, quickly relieved by rest. Popliteal and foot pulses not usually palpable. Femoral pulses present in 70%
	Arterial supply inadequate even at rest, resulting in ischaemia of all tissues, but just sufficient to sustain viability of the limb, although extreme peripheries may undergo patchy necrosis. Skin becomes atrophic, often with reactive dilatation of peripheral microvasculature causing redness. Healing severely impaired with risk of spreading infection if pressure or trauma (accidental or surgical) causes ulceration	**Severe ischaemia (critical ischaemia if viability threatened)**—pain in foot at rest (worse at night) relieved by hanging leg down. Symptoms develop over days or weeks. Skin of peripheries red/purple and dusky. Skin shiny and taut due to dependent oedema (patients often sleep with feet hanging down to gain relief). Foot becomes pale on elevation and red on dependency (Buerger's test). May be patchy dry or wet gangrene or ischaemic ulceration
	Acute severe ischaemia due to thrombotic obstruction of stenosed vessel. Leads to necrosis within 6–8 hours if untreated	**Acute-on-chronic ischaemia**—sudden onset of pain and pallor with gradual paralysis and numbness of leg. Later, skin becomes blue and blistered as necrosis supervenes. Symptoms and signs identical to acute embolic occlusion (see below)
Embolism arising from atherosclerotic lesions (obliterative or ulcerating)	Atherosclerotic debris or mural platelet thrombi (usually small) detach and pass to extreme peripheries. Showers of emboli may recur intermittently	Carotid atherosclerosis is a common cause of transient ischaemic attacks (TIAs). Aorto-ilio-femoral disease can cause lower limb embolism
ANEURYSMS		
Mainly affect aorta, illio-femoral and popliteal arteries. Aetiology uncertain—perhaps degeneration of elastin and/or collagen. Atherosclerosis may also be present	Progressive aneurysmal dilatation. May be self-limiting if hypertension and smoking controlled	**Asymptomatic**—discovered incidentally as pulsatile mass in abdomen, groin or popliteal fossa, on abdominal X-ray, CT or ultrasound scan, or on ultrasound screening. **Symptomatic**—abdominal or back pain with tender aneurysm. Needs urgent surgery
	Sudden rupture of aneurysm	**Sudden death**—acute, usually fatal, cardiovascular collapse. Often misdiagnosed as myocardial infarction
	Leakage of aneurysm into retroperitoneal tissues—usually leads to rupture within hours	**Leaking/ruptured aneurysm**—ill-defined back or abdominal pain often simulating ureteric colic or other abdominal emergency. Diagnostic if accompanied by transient collapse. Sometimes a history of recent similar episodes. Pulsatile abdominal mass palpable in 50%
	Sudden thrombotic occlusion of aneurysmal popliteal artery	Symptoms and signs of **acute severe leg ischaemia**; often pulsatile popliteal aneurysm on contralateral side
	Sudden distal ischaemia affecting lower limb due to embolism of thrombus from within aneurysm	If severe, as in thrombolic occlusion of popliteal artery above. If less severe, localised pain and reddish-blue areas of skin necrosis which do not blanch on pressure

Table 34.1 Continued

Basic disease	Pathophysiological process	Clinical manifestations
AORTIC DISSECTION		
	Blood passes out into a degenerated media and tracks distally and sometimes proximally; begins in thoracic aorta. Dissection may obstruct major aortic branches—mesenteric, renal and iliac arteries. May disrupt aortic valve or rupture into pericardium	Characteristically presents with shock and severe chest pain radiating to back. Renal artery involvement causes anuria. May present with acute bilateral lower limb ischaemia. Retrograde dissection to aortic valve causes acute left ventricular failure. Often fatal but some cases without aortic valve involvement recover with antihypertensive therapy; in others, thoracic aortic surgery may be successful
CARDIAC DISEASE CAUSING PERIPHERAL ARTERIAL SYMPTOMS		
Arterial thromboembolism secondary to myocardial infarction, mitral valve disease (especially rheumatic), atrial fibrillation, ventricular aneurysm (see also atherosclerosis above)	Embolism—usually large masses of mural thrombus become detached and impact at bifurcations of distributing arterial system causing acute critical ischaemia. May affect blood supply of upper or lower limb, brain or intestine	**Sudden onset** of symptoms and signs of **acute severe limb ischaemia**, stroke or mesenteric ischaemia. Often atrial fibrillation or recent history of myocardial infarction
Poor cardiac output, e.g. acute myocardial infarction, severe cardiac failure	Inadequate perfusion of all peripheral tissues, exacerbates pre-existing arterial insufficiency	**Progressive signs of severe ischaemia** with ulceration of legs, usually bilateral. Patient usually elderly with severe (often terminal) cardiac disease. Aortic thrombosis may be a terminal event
DIABETES MELLITUS—THE 'DIABETIC FOOT'		
May be 'pure' diabetic neuropathy but diabetes is often associated with accelerated atherosclerosis, and predisposition to infection	Pre-existing diabetic sensory neuropathy predisposes to traumatic injury and ulceration. Process exacerbated by abnormal intermediary metabolism and often complicated by pyogenic infection	Typical presentation of **neuropathic foot** is a deep, painless, infected ulcer with a characteristic 'punched out' appearance. Surrounding tissues well perfused (pink and warm). Peripheral pulses often palpable but there is generalised sensory impairment. Ulceration often recent, over a bony prominence and preceded by minor trauma. Infection may spread deeply and rapidly, causing limb-threatening necrosis and septicaemia
	Arterial supply may be compromised by atherosclerosis	Atherosclerosis may cause or complicate diabetic foot problems. Presentation similar to arterial disease in non-diabetic patients
VENOUS DISORDERS		
Deep venous thrombosis predisposed by pregnancy, oestrogen therapy, major surgery, trauma, obesity, abdominal or pelvic malignancy, immobility. May be complicated by **pulmonary embolism**	Spontaneous thrombosis in deep venous system of calf; may propagate proximally into illio-femoral veins. Obstructs venous return in short and long term. Spontaneous recanalisation may cause deep vein valvular incompetence, i.e. **chronic venous insufficiency**, and local venous hypertension. This obstructs capillary flow and inhibits metabolic exchange; leakage of red cells causes subcutaneous deposition of haemosiderin. Combined effects cause atrophy of skin and subcutaneous fat, fibrosis, poor healing and predisposition to ulceration	Classic acute presentation is **pain and swelling of calf and ankle** with calf tenderness. Dorsiflexion may cause pain (**Homan's sign**). Leg usually warm and normal colour but pulses may be impalpable due to oedema. If ilio-femoral veins involved, thigh also swollen. Late complication is **post-thrombotic limb** with chronic brawny oedema and narrow ankle due to lipo-dermatosclerosis. Skin atrophic, scaly and pigmented (**varicose/venous eczema**). Skin above medial malleolus most vulnerable to chronic ulceration after minor trauma

Table 34.1 Continued

Basic disease	Pathophysiological process	Clinical manifestations
Superficial venous thrombosis (i.e. thrombophlebitis). Usually occurs in tortuous dilated varicose veins; more common in pregnancy. Occasionally affects normal veins as **thrombophlebitis migrans** in patients with underlying malignancy elsewere	Spontaneous thrombosis in superficial veins; excites an inflammatory response in the vessel wall and surrounding tissues	**Rapid onset of acute, highly localised pain and tenderness**, associated with varicose veins. Overlying skin red and oedematous; underlying veins hard and nodular
Varicose veins—incompetent function of valves in veins connecting deep and superficial venous systems; often begins with sapheno-femoral valve. Basic abnormality may be in vessel wall	Blood is forced from deep venous system to superficial system through incompetent valves causing slowly progressive tortuous dilatation of superficial veins. Venous hypertension may cause chronic skin changes and sometimes ulceration. Dilated vessels are vulnerable to trauma and may bleed profusely	Slowly progressive development of prominent purple, dilated, tortuous superficial veins. Patient often complains of aching, especially after long period of standing. Patients may be upset by cosmetic appearance or, if there is a family history, fear of progression or ulceration. Pain relieved by elevation. Women more often affected than men; varicosities often first appear during pregnancy

spinal canal is diagnostic, demonstrating a narrow spinal canal or disc protrusions impacting on the cauda equina.

REST PAIN

With more severe arterial obstruction, ischaemic pain may occur when the patient rests in bed. Termed **rest pain** for obvious reasons, this usually occurs in the skin of the foot and is burning in character. It probably occurs at night because of several factors working together: loss of gravity assistance to arterial supply, physiological reduction in cardiac output at rest, and reactive dilatation of skin vessels to warmth. The pain is often relieved by hanging the leg over the side of the bed or even walking around.

In acute critical ischaemia, blood flow to the periphery is virtually absent and there may be no pain in the most severely affected area, presumably due to peripheral nerve ischaemia. Severe pain is usually present more proximally where the tissue is less ischaemic.

The pain of deep venous thrombosis is nearly always less severe than that of severe ischaemia. Physical examination will distinguish between the two conditions. In deep vein thrombosis, the limb is warm not cold, pulses are detectable (by palpation or Doppler flow meter) and there is no colour change (except in very severe cases). Swelling is often a feature of deep venous thrombosis but is not found in acute arterial ischaemia. It is vital to recognise acute arterial insufficiency as it rapidly progresses to irreversible necrosis. Beware of the trap in diabetic patients with neuropathy—severe ischaemia may be painless and disruption of small vessel control may mean the severely ischaemic foot is warm.

SKIN CHANGES

Changes in **skin texture, colour, pigmentation or temperature** (and the distribution of these changes) help to distinguish between the different types of lower limb vascular disorder. In the chronic disorder, the epidermis may be thin and atrophic because of deficient oxygenation and nutrition; this explains the use of the descriptive term **trophic changes**.

In arterial insufficiency, whatever the level of obstruction, the effects are most evident at the extreme periphery, i.e. the foot and toes. In contrast, the skin changes caused by chronic venous insufficiency are most severe around the medial side of the ankle above the malleolus, and are almost never seen on the foot. Furthermore, in venous disease, the cutaneous fat around the ankle may become thinned by atrophy and hardened by fibrosis (termed **lipo-dermatosclerosis** or, less accurately, **fat necrosis**). The leg above the ankle is oedematous. In extreme cases, there may be marked constriction at the ankle giving rise to a **champagne-bottle leg**.

CHANGES IN SKIN COLOUR AND TEMPERATURE

Colour change may suggest the underlying disease process, particularly if temperature change is also considered.

441

Many people, particularly the elderly, suffer from cold feet in cold weather. If both feet are pale when cold but have normal pulses, this is normal arteriolar constriction for temperature conservation.

THE ACUTELY COLD FOOT

The main pathological reason for a foot becoming acutely cold and white is a sudden complete arterial occlusion. This event is usually spontaneous but external precipitating events such as trauma or frostbite (see Fig. 34.1) will be evident from the history. Ischaemia is usually unilateral unless the abdominal aorta or both iliac arteries become obstructed. There are ischaemic changes in the foot extending a variable amount up the leg.

The cardinal clinical features of acute critical ischaemia are:

- **Pain**. This is variable in intensity and affects the distal part of the limb
- **Pallor** of the extremity. The ischaemic area is initially white but may be bluish though blanching on pressure with slow capillary refill. Later it becomes blue without blanching (fixed pigmentation) when necrosis occurs
- **Pulselessness** of the extremity. Foot pulses are absent and popliteal and femoral pulses may be lost, according to the level of occlusion
- **Paraesthesia** or **anaesthesia** of the periphery (i.e. altered or absent skin sensation). This only occurs if ischaemia is severe
- **Paralysis** of calf muscles. The patient is unable to flex or extend the toes or ankle. This only occurs if ischaemia is extreme. Pain may disappear at this stage

(As an aide-mémoire, the features of acute limb ischaemia are known as the five Ps: **P**ain, **P**allor, **P**ulselessness, **P**araesthesia and **P**aralysis. Not all of these are present all of the time; anaesthesia and paralysis are dire features.)

Once anaesthesia and paralysis occur, the viability of the limb is at immediate risk and urgent steps need to be taken to revascularise it. Even if these are successful, ischaemic changes may already be irreversible and there is a serious risk of muscle necrosis due to reperfusion injury. If the foot becomes dusky purple and fails to blanch on pressure, irreversible necrosis has occurred. These changes always involve the foot but may extend proximally (though rarely above the knee). The upper limit of the necrotic area is usually well demarcated from the proximal viable tissue. Blistering of the skin begins 24–48 hours after necrosis.

Colour change in venous thrombosis

Colour change is unusual in deep venous thrombosis but massive pelvic vein thrombosis may cause colour changes

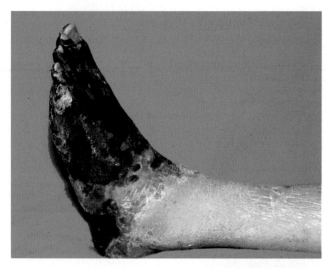

Fig. 34.1 Frost-bite
Ischaemic necrosis of the foot in an elderly man caused by sleeping outside in a very low temperature in winter. Below knee amputation was later performed.

sometimes mistaken for arterial occlusion. Such extensive thromboses are now unusual and occur mainly in high-risk patients. Massive thrombosis was once more common, especially during late pregnancy or the early puerperium. The condition was known as **white leg of pregnancy** or **phlegmasia alba dolens**. The whole of the lower limb is painful, pale and massively swollen. In contrast to the findings in arterial occlusion, the limb is warm and pulses are detectable despite the oedema. A rare but more serious variant is **blue leg** or **phlegmasia caerulea dolens** which represents incipient venous infarction.

THE CHRONICALLY COLD FOOT

In chronic arterial insufficiency with symptoms of severe claudication or rest pain, the onset of a dusky skin colour in the toes or foot suggests incipient tissue necrosis (**pre-gangrene**). If finger pressure is applied to the ischaemic skin, the rate of colour return gives an indication of skin perfusion. However, many elderly people with a slow refill time have cool, bluish feet with few symptoms and no skin breakdown. These patients rarely have arterial disease and this can easily be excluded by Doppler ankle pressure measurement.

Necrosis in chronic ischaemia may be patchy and localised if there is a developed collateral circulation. Such necrosis is usually confined to a toe or a limited part of the forefoot. The necrotic area slowly becomes hard, black and mummified (**dry gangrene**) and may eventually separate spontaneously from the viable tissue (see Fig. 34.2). However, there is always a danger that the necrotic area may become infected. The tissue then becomes boggy and ulcerated and the infection and

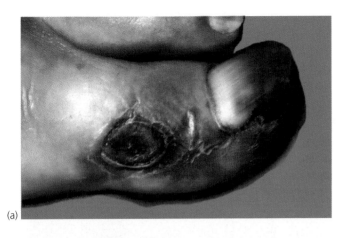
(a)

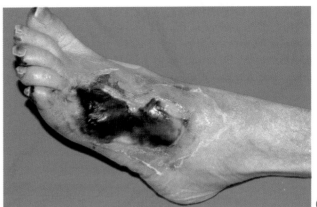
(b)

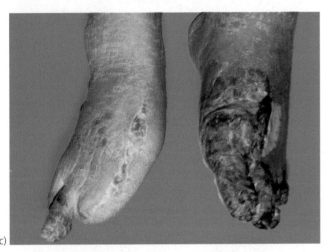
(c)

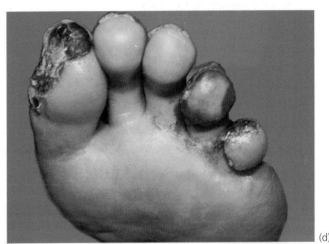
(d)

Fig. 34.2 Necrosis from severe ischaemia
(a) Acute ischaemic necrosis of big toe due to sudden, acute-on-chronic thrombosis of superficial femoral artery. **(b)** Acute ischaemic ulcer of dorsum of foot due to femoral artery embolism 24 hours before. **(c)** Left foot shows signs of severe chronic ischaemia with dry gangrene. Right foot has healed following successful femoro-popliteal bypass grafting and local amputation. **(d)** Chronic severe ischaemia with necrosis of toes as a result of obliterative aorto-iliac atherosclerosis.

gangrene spread proximally (**wet gangrene**). Wet gangrene requires urgent treatment, often with a combination of revascularisation and amputation.

Redness of the skin indicates that oxygenated blood is present in the capillaries. This implies there is no venous congestion or obstruction. With ischaemia, there is reactive dilatation of the microvasculature to hypoxia, a physiological attempt to extract the maximum oxygen from whatever blood is reaching the area. Thus severely ischaemic skin may feel cool, but paradoxically be red.

Buerger's test for severe ischaemia (see Fig. 34.3) involves high elevation of the leg for a minute or two. If the peripheral arterial pressure is inadequate to overcome the effects of gravity, the entire foot becomes white. When the leg is hung down, it gradually becomes bluish-red as blood flow returns. This test is easily misinterpreted—even in healthy people, the foot will blanch somewhat with elevation.

THE WARM FOOT

Inflammatory dilatation of the microcirculation also causes skin redness, but the skin is warm and slightly swollen because of enhanced blood flow. An example is low-grade bacterial **cellulitis** which may be seen in diabetes or chronic venous insufficiency, or may arise unexpectedly. Note that if infection develops in a severely ischaemic limb, the usual signs of inflammation may not develop and the extent of infection may be underestimated. If the blood supply is later restored surgically, signs of inflammation then develop.

ABNORMAL PIGMENTATION

In a **post-thrombotic limb**, valves in the deep veins have been disrupted by inflammation, organisation and recanalisation following deep venous thrombosis. The

443

valves thus become incompetent and allow **deep venous reflux**. This prevents the leg muscles from acting as a venous return pump and leads to chronic venous insufficiency. Standing erect causes venous stagnation, increased venous pressure in the leg (venous hyper-tension) and chronic leg swelling. Red cells extravasate into the tissues and form haemosiderin deposits which cause brown skin pigmentation. This, accompanied by dry, scaly, atrophic skin, is described as **varicose or venous eczema** (see Fig. 34.5).

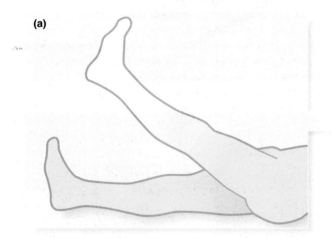

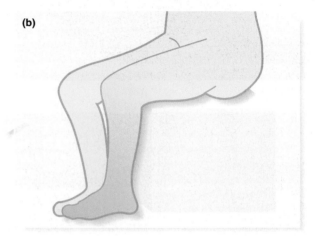

Fig. 34.3 Buerger's test in severe ischaemia of the lower limb

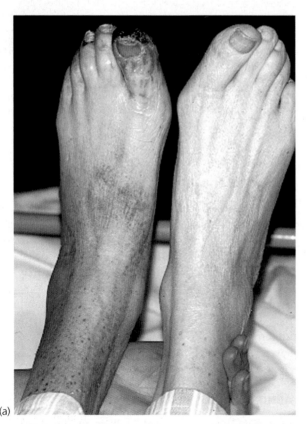

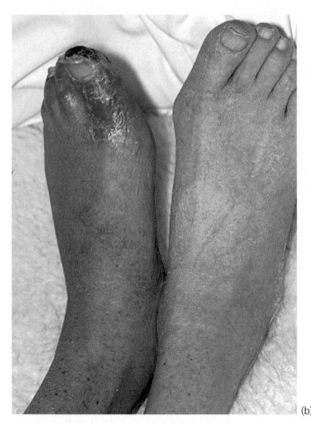

(a)   (b)

Fig. 34.4 This 78-year-old man had critical ischaemia of both legs. **(a)** Shows both feet elevated. The left big toe is seen to be necrotic distally. Both feet go pale but the right is dead white. **(b)** With dependency, both feet go blueish red, most marked this time on the right. Both feet would be Buerger's positive.

ULCERATION

Chronic ulceration of the lower limb is a common problem, particularly in the elderly. The causes are summarised in Box 34.1.

Effective treatment depends on clinical evaluation of the following factors, discussed in detail below:

● History of the origin and evolution of the ulcer
● The site of the ulcer
● The characteristics of the ulcer
● The nature of the surrounding tissues
● Relevant regional findings
● The patient's general condition

HISTORY OF THE ULCER

Details of the initial skin lesion and the circumstances in which it occurred may provide diagnostic clues. **Minor trauma** may be the initiating incident but failure to heal can usually be attributed to abnormal skin nutrition. The common causes include chronic venous insufficiency, arterial ischaemia and diabetic neuropathy. The ulcer often begins insidiously with minor breakdown in a patch of atrophic skin. In venous insufficiency, the skin often 'weeps' plasma.

In the elderly or in patients on long-term steroid therapy, minor trauma to the tibia may produce a V-shaped **flap laceration** (see Fig. 34.6). This invariably fails to heal because of poor blood supply both to the flap and the underlying tissue. Suturing a flap laceration increases tension and compounds the local ischaemia and must not be done; the result is even greater tissue loss and ulceration. The most effective management is often early excision of the flap and immediate split skin grafting.

In tropical countries, traumatic injuries and burns readily become infected. If they are not medically treated, these injuries develop into large chronic **tropical ulcers**. The infecting organisms are usually a mixture of spirochaetes and fusiform bacteria.

The duration of the ulcer, its healing, and subsequent recurrence or other changes give further clues to the diagnosis. Ischaemic ulcers present early because pain soon becomes intolerable and the ulcer refuses to heal (except in diabetics with coexisting ischaemia and neuropathy). In contrast, post-thrombotic and varicose ulcers are rarely painful and usually fluctuate between healing and breakdown. Rarely, squamous carcinoma develops in a longstanding ulcer and is recognised by proliferative change at the ulcer margin (see Fig. 34.7). These lesions are known as **Marjolin's ulcers** and were first described following burns which failed to heal. Primary skin malignancies on the leg may ulcerate, but these usually begin as a skin lump.

If a patient with a leg ulcer has claudication or rest pain, this suggests an ischaemic cause (see Fig. 34.8). Neuropathic or mixed diabetic ulcers tend to be painless

---

KEY POINTS

Box 34.1 Causes of chronic leg ulcers

● **Chronic venous insufficiency**
  — **Previous deep venous thrombosis (post-thrombotic limb)**
  — **Varicose veins (superficial venous insufficiency)**
  — **Congenital reflux—defective deep vein valves**
● **Chronic arterial insufficiency**
● **Diabetic neuropathy and other sensory neuropathies, e.g. leprosy**
● **Pressure sores**
● **Vasculitis, e.g. in rheumatoid disease and other collagen diseases**
● **Traumatic flap lacerations over the pretibial area**
● **Tropical ulcers involving bacteria or fungus infections**
● **Tuberculous ulcers**
● **Malignant tumours**

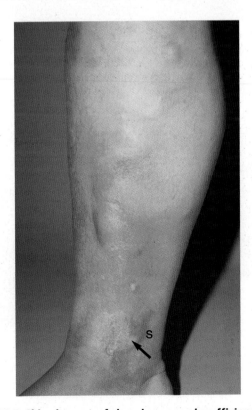

Fig. 34.5 Skin changes of chronic venous insufficiency
This 53-year-old woman suffered a deep vein thrombosis during her second pregnancy many years earlier. The leg is pigmented around the ankle and this tissue is woody on palpation (lipodermatosclerosis). The scar of a healed varicose ulcer **S** is seen above the medial malleolus (arrowed).

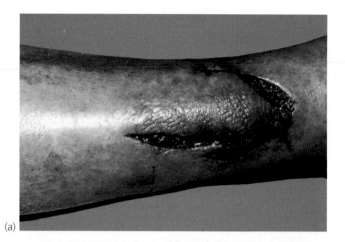

(a)

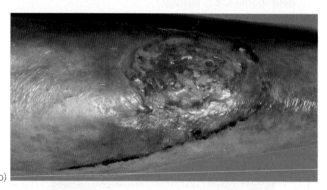

(b)

Fig. 34.6 Flap laceration
(a) This wound was caused by a fall in which the patient's shin was scraped on a stone step. It is tempting to suture such a wound but if this is done, the flap will invariably undergo necrosis as in **(b)**. Most of these types of wound require split skin grafting.

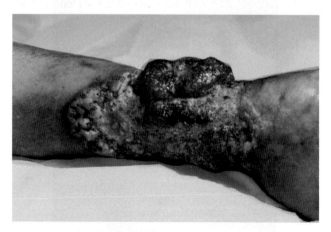

Fig. 34.7 Marjolins ulcer
Squamous carcinoma developing in a chronic venous ulcer. This very rare transformation followed 34 years of continuous venous ulceration. The leg was amputated below knee and the patient cured.

because of a sensory neuropathy (which may be the main predisposing cause). A history of previous deep venous thrombosis makes venous insufficiency the likely cause.

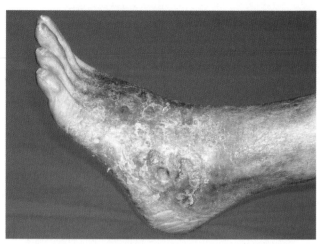

Fig. 34.8 Chronic ischaemic ulcers
This elderly man had intolerable pain in his foot, worse at night for 7 weeks. Note the foot is red and there are multiple ulcers over the lateral malleolus.

SITE OF THE ULCER

The site of the ulcer on the lower limb may point to its cause. Post-thrombotic and varicose ulcers arise typically just above the medial malleolus (the 'gaiter' area) and may extend circumferentially around the leg (see Fig. 34.9). They rarely occur in other sites. Diabetic (neuropathic) ulcers always occur on the foot either as perforating ulcers on the sole beneath the metatarsal heads or at other bony prominences; these include the toes, the ball of the great toe and the malleoli.

Ulcers due to arterial insufficiency may occur anywhere below the mid-calf, including the usual sites of venous or diabetic ulcers. **Pressure ulcers** occur mainly in debilitated, elderly or unconscious patients, especially at the back of the heel (see Fig. 47.9, p. 648). Even a few minutes in one position on a hard casualty trolley or operating theatre table may initiate skin necrosis in an already ischaemic limb. Pressure ulcers usually begin as a well-circumscribed patch of skin discoloration, which becomes necrotic and later ulcerates. The heels of vulnerable patients should be nursed carefully and regularly inspected to avoid this complication.

CHARACTERISTICS OF THE ULCER

Most ulcers are shallow, involving only the skin and subcutaneous fat. Diabetic ulcers, however, tend to penetrate deeply into the foot, where there is underlying necrotic and infected tissue. The base of any ulcer usually contains slough and fibrin but granulation tissue may be visible beneath. The slough should not be removed unless arterial insufficiency can be excluded, as

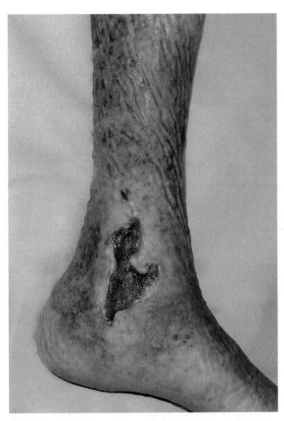

Fig. 34.9 Venous (varicose) ulcer
This longstanding ulcer is typical of venous ulceration by its site, the medial gaiter area of the ankle, its relative painlessness and the presence of venous eczema surrounding it. The visible corrugations in the skin above the ulcer are caused by four-layer bandaging.

NATURE OF THE SURROUNDING TISSUES

The characteristics of the surrounding tissues indicate the background on which the ulcer has formed. These characteristics include colour, texture and perfusion (shown by temperature, blanching response, venous filling and Buerger's test) as well as swelling and pigmentation.

REGIONAL FEATURES

Regional examination should search for diagnostic clues, e.g. peripheral pulses, inguinal lymphadenopathy (infection or malignancy), varicose veins or deep or superficial venous thrombosis.

GENERAL STATE OF THE PATIENT'S HEALTH

General history and examination may give useful diagnostic clues but are easily overlooked. Smoking is an important factor in atherosclerosis, and cardiac failure or arrhythmias may contribute to arterial insufficiency and cause chronic lower limb oedema. Paresis following a stroke makes a limb vulnerable to pressure ulcers. Maturity-onset diabetes may have developed insidiously, so the urine and blood sugar should always be tested. A diagnosis of diabetic neuropathy does not necessarily mean this is the cause of the ulceration as diabetics often have accelerated atherosclerosis and present with ischaemic ulcers or a mixed picture. Neuropathic complications and secondary infection are also common. A history of Raynaud's syndrome, rheumatoid disease, scleroderma or other collagen disorder may point to an arteritic cause.

this could aggravate ischaemia. If there is proliferating tissue in the ulcer, this should be biopsied.

The edge of most chronic lower limb ulcers slopes towards the base with no specific diagnostic features, although epithelial proliferation growing inwards from the edge suggests healing. Diabetic ulcers have a characteristic 'punched-out' edge with abrupt transition from normal skin to the necrotic crater. On the sole, diabetic ulcers have a hyperkeratinised edge in response to excess local pressure during walking caused by distortion of the foot. Malignant ulcers may have a raised margin.

SWELLING OF THE LOWER LIMB

Swelling of the lower limb (see Fig. 34.10 overleaf) may be bilateral or unilateral. The causes are summarised in Box 34.2. Systemic causes, and conditions listed under 'sluggish venous return' in the box cause bilateral swelling. The other causes tend to produce swelling of only one limb. Most causes of unilateral swelling are chronic and painless, except for acute deep venous thrombosis and cellulitis.

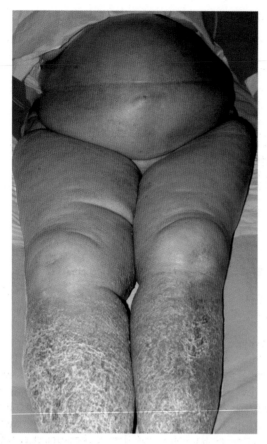

Fig. 34.10 Swollen limbs due to venous obstruction
Lower limb swelling due to pelvic compression caused by a massive
ovarian tumour. After excision of the tumour, the limbs gradually
returned to near normal over a period of 6 months.

KEY POINTS

Box 34.2 Causes of swelling of the lower limbs

Local causes

- 'Sluggish venous return', e.g. immobility, pregnancy, prolonged sitting in a chair, inefficient calf muscle pump (paralysis due to polio or hemiplegia)
- Acute obstruction of venous return, e.g. deep venous thrombosis
- Destruction of valves in deep venous system following previous deep venous thrombosis
- Congenital lymphatic aplasia or hypoplasia, e.g. Milroy's disease
- Cellulitis (usually streptococcal)
- Lymphatic obstruction by filariasis (in tropical Africa and Asia)

Regional causes

- Venous obstruction by pelvic mass, e.g. advanced pregnancy, ovarian cyst, pelvic malignancy
- Lymphatic obstruction by malignant involvement of inguinal or more proximal nodes, or after block dissection or radiotherapy
- Inferior venal caval obstruction

Systemic causes

- Congestive or right-sided cardiac failure
- Hypoalbuminaemia, e.g. malnutrition, nephrotic syndrome
- Fluid overload
- Side effects of drug therapy e.g. ACE inhibitors

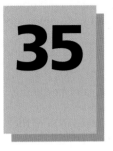

35 Principles of management of arterial insufficiency of the lower limb and the diabetic foot

INTRODUCTION

Chronic arterial insufficiency of the lower limb presents at any point along a scale of severity ranging from mild intermittent claudication brought on by severe exercise to gangrene of a large part of a limb. Between these two extremes are increasing severities of claudication, rest pain and trophic changes (including ulceration), or any combination of these.

Symptoms often develop suddenly, presumably signalling the acute event, or they may evolve over days or weeks or even arise so gradually as to be hardly noticed. Once present, symptoms and signs may remain stable or else progress; the latter is more likely if ischaemia is extreme and particularly if infection is present. In the advanced stages, the critically ischaemic limb is one which will undoubtedly be lost unless the blood supply is restored.

INTERMITTENT CLAUDICATION

SYMPTOMS OF INTERMITTENT CLAUDICATION

Intermittent claudication is the characteristic symptom of chronic lower limb ischaemia and the typical pain pattern is nearly always present. The patient experiences cramping pain in the lower limb muscles on walking and the pain is quickly relieved by rest. The calf is almost always involved first and is usually the only part involved. In some cases where there is more proximal arterial disease, the pain ascends into the thigh or even the buttock if walking continues. In nearly all cases, resting allows the pain to resolve within a minute or two, after which the patient can walk a similar distance before the pain recurs. An individual's **claudication distance** may range from 30 to several hundred metres; once established, the distance remains remarkably constant under similar conditions, e.g. on flat ground and at the same speed. Pain is worse on walking uphill and may be absent downhill.

The first symptoms appear unexpectedly and are often attributed to musculoskeletal causes. The patient usually only seeks medical advice when symptoms have persisted for several weeks or more. Two-thirds of patients are male and mostly aged 50–70 years; females are on average 10 years older. There is often a history of myocardial ischaemia in the form of angina or myocardial infarction or a history of coronary artery surgery or angioplasty. Nearly all are cigarette smokers or ex-smokers and most are hypertensive. In a few cases, claudication may be exacerbated by polycythaemia or by beta-adrenergic blocking drugs prescribed to control hypertension.

PHYSICAL SIGNS OF INTERMITTENT CLAUDICATION

Peripheral pulses are usually absent on the affected side but local examination is otherwise unremarkable. The dorsalis pedis, posterior tibial and popliteal pulses are almost invariably absent, and the femoral pulse is absent in about 30% of patients. Trophic skin changes are unusual except in patients towards the 'severe ischaemia' end of the scale. In these, there may be evidence of nail thickening and peripheral skin atrophy and Buerger's test may be positive (see p. 444); hair loss is probably of no significance. General systematic examination should seek other signs of atherosclerosis as summarised in Box 35.1; these may have an important bearing on management and prognosis.

449

NATURAL HISTORY OF INTERMITTENT CLAUDICATION

About one-third of patients experience spontaneous re-mission of all or most of their symptoms over a year or two without any treatment. It is well established that stopping cigarette smoking greatly improves the outcome. Another third remain stable in the long term with tolerable symptoms. The remaining third are either severely dis-abled by walking restriction or else progress to more severe ischaemic symptoms like rest pain. Indeed, about 10% of the total would progress to necrosis and ampu-tation if untreated.

Epidemiological studies show that patients with inter-mittent claudication have only half the life expectancy of unaffected people of the same age. Most die of other manifestations of atherosclerosis such as ischaemic heart disease and stroke.

SEVERE ISCHAEMIA

Severe lower limb ischaemia most commonly presents without a history of claudication but it may sometimes develop after a period of deteriorating claudication. In general, these patients are older and less physically active than typical claudicants. If untreated, a very small proportion improve and lose their pain, but the majority smoulder on with intolerable pain or progress to extensive necrosis. Once the deeper tissues of the foot become necrotic, local defences are overwhelmed and, infection spreads widely in the vulnerable ischaemic tissue. This results in wet gangrene and, ultimately, death from sepsis syndrome and multi-organ dysfunction. This sequence of events is rarely permitted to run its full course since

---

KEY POINTS

Box 35.1 General examination of the arteriopath

- Observe whether the patient can lie flat during examination (? orthopnoea)
- Inspect skin and mucous membranes for signs of polycythaemia, anaemia or cyanosis
- Examine for signs of cardiac failure—jugular venous pressure and lung bases
- Auscultate for cardiac murmurs
- Auscultate for arterial bruits in carotids, subclavians (in supraclavicular fossa), renals (in epigastrium or posteriorly in loins), mesenterics (in epigastrium) and femorals
- Measure blood pressure in both arms
- Palpate the abdomen for aortic aneurysm
- Inspect skin of legs (including pressure areas and between the toes) and toenails for ischaemic changes and signs of arterial embolism

---

rest pain is so severe and signs of systemic inflammatory response syndrome become so obvious that vascular re-construction or amputation becomes essential. Extremely elderly debilitated patients may be managed with opiate analgesia as for other terminally ill patients, since any form of surgery would probably be fatal.

The first manifestations of severe ischaemia develop in the foot and include:

- Intolerable rest pain initially at night, later becoming continuous
- Trophic skin changes—atrophic shiny red skin of the leg; ischaemic ulcers between the toes, in pressure areas of the foot or on the leg
- Patchy necrosis of the toes or skin of the foot
- Positive Buerger's test
- Failure of trivial injuries to heal
- Extreme vulnerability of ischaemic feet to pressure sores

CRITICAL ISCHAEMIA

Critical ischaemia occurs when arterial insufficiency is so severe as to threaten the viability of the foot or leg. This has been defined formally by a European consensus document as follows: persistently recurring rest pain requiring regular analgesia for more than 2 weeks, or ulceration or gangrene affecting the foot, plus an ankle systolic pressure of less than 50 mmHg (in diabetics, absent ankle pulses on palpation replace pressure measurement as calcification may render pressures artificially elevated).

In acute ischaemia, limb viability may be critically compromised from the outset but in chronic arterial insufficiency, critical ischaemia usually develops gradually over days or weeks. The underlying cause is blood flow restriction caused by progressive obliterative atherosclerosis exacerbated by secondary thrombosis.

INVESTIGATION OF CHRONIC LOWER LIMB ARTERIAL INSUFFICIENCY

The extent to which investigation is pursued in a patient presenting with symptoms of lower limb ischaemia depends on whether the clinical picture suggests inter-ventional treatment is likely to be necessary. As a minimum, most patients with claudication have resting ankle systolic pressures measured in the clinic and a full blood count to exclude polycythaemia or thrombocythaemia. Resting ankle systolic blood pressure can be measured using a **Doppler ultrasound blood flow detector**. Normal pressure is slightly above brachial systolic whilst patients with claudication usually range from 50 to 120 mmHg. Results are sometimes expressed as a ratio, the ankle/brachial index, with normal values from 0.8 to 1.2. Also in the clinic, it is simple to walk the patient along a corridor to measure claudication distance. Note, however, that Doppler

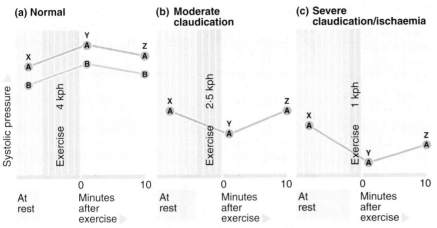

Fig. 35.1 Ankle pressure responses to exercise in intermittent claudication
X = systolic pressure at rest (A = ankle pressure; B = brachial pressure), Y represents pressure immediately after treadmill exercise (duration indicated by the breadth of the shaded zones) and Z = the pressure 10 min later. **(a)** Normal ankle pressure response to exercise. **(b)** Response in moderate claudication, i.e. reduced resting ankle pressure, reduced exercise tolerance, ankle pressure fall and recovery within 10 min. **(c)** Response in severe claudication or more severe ischaemia.

pressure measurements can be misleading. Considerable experience is needed in taking and interpreting the measurements and radical treatment should not be based solely on a random ankle pressure measurement.

THE VASCULAR LABORATORY

If available, more severe claudicants are often investigated in a vascular laboratory, which can provide useful objective information about blood flow under exercise conditions. Vascular laboratory assessment provides a useful baseline against which to measure improvement or deterioration (see below). Tests vary in type and complexity but the basic test is usually to measure the ankle systolic pressure before and after the patient has exercised on a treadmill (see Fig. 35.1). A fall in ankle pressure after exercise gives an indication of the severity of arterial disease and the recovery rate provides an indication of collateral compensation. In some hospitals, all claudicants are initially investigated in this way. This allows objective assessment of the disease and the response to conservative or operative treatment.

Other vascular laboratory tests include **duplex Doppler scanning** for arterial stenoses and occlusions. More experimental tests include plethysmographic measurement of blood flow and radionuclide scans for differential tissue blood flow.

ARTERIOGRAPHY

Arteriography should be reserved for patients thought to require intervention in the form of angioplasty or reconstructive surgery. It provides a map of the arterial system (see Fig. 35.2), showing sites and severity of vessel stenoses and occlusions, including the inflow (arteries feeding the area of concern) and the runoff (more distal arteries supplying the lower part of the limb). Arteriography is sometimes used wrongly by non-specialists to assess chronic arterial insufficiency. Arteriography does

not measure the rate of blood flow to the tissues nor the dynamic circulatory responses to exercise; it helps only with the mechanics of revascularisation.

A development in the field of angiography known as **digital subtraction angiography (DSA)** has now become standard. It involves electronic processing of the radiological image to 'subtract' non-contrast images including bone and gas to enhance the arteriographic profile. Much

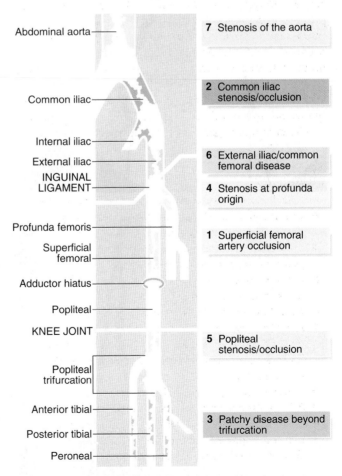

Fig. 35.2 Typical patterns of arterial disease

451

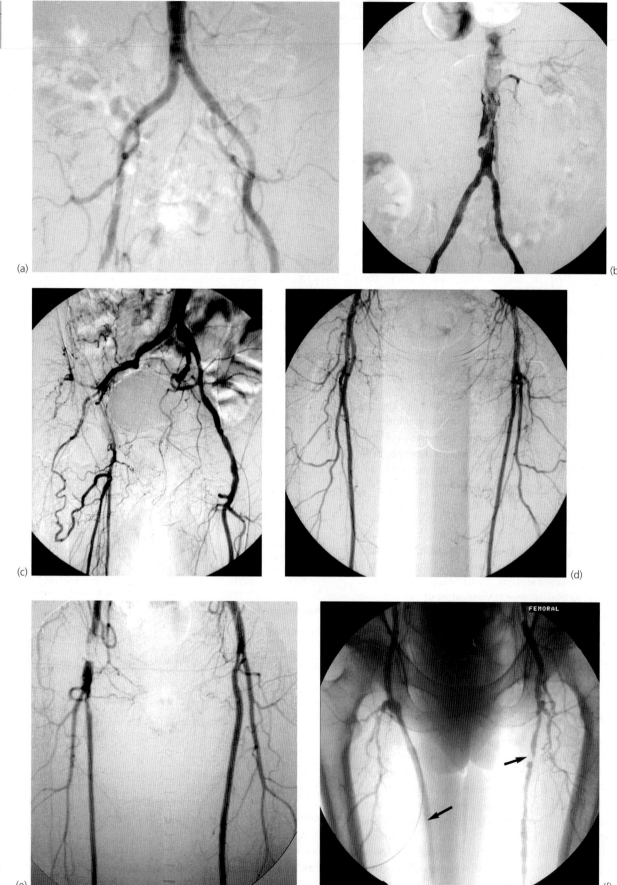

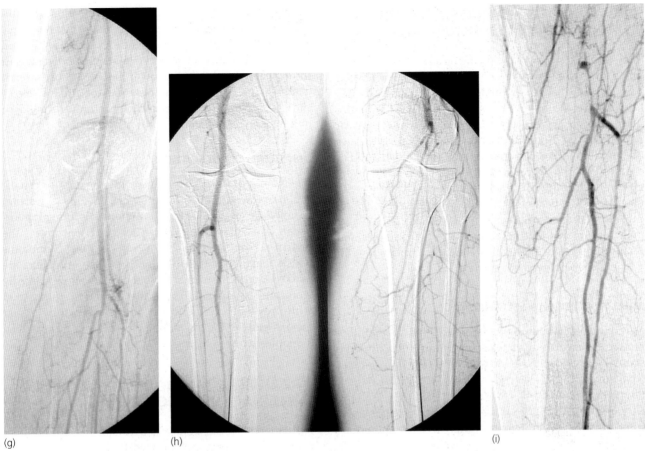

(g)　　　　　　　　　　(h)　　　　　　　　　　(i)

Fig. 35.3 Typical patterns of atherosclerosis affecting the lower limbs
(a) Normal aortoiliac segment. **(b)** 'Craggy' atherosclerosis of the distal aorta **(c)** Right external iliac occlusion. A large collateral is seen between the internal iliac and the common femoral. **(d)** Normal femoral segment. **(e)** Localised occlusion of right common femoral artery, easily treated by endarterectomy. **(f)** Atherosclerotic stenoses of left superficial femoral artery (SFA) (right arrow). This was successfully treated by angioplasty. Note the patent right fem-pop bypass (left arrow). **(g)** Normal infrageniculate (tibial) arteries. **(h)** Occlusion of the left popliteal artery (probably embolic) with no visible tibial arteries i.e. poor runoff. **(i)** Popliteal artery occlusion in another patient, with preserved tibial vessels being filled via collaterals.

smaller doses of contrast are required and contrast can be given intravenously (usually via a central venous line) or intra-arterially. This technique has several advantages over the older techniques. It is relatively non-invasive and safer than conventional arteriography because of reduced contrast load. It can also be used repeatedly for disease follow-up or for morphological screening of arteries where conventional arteriography might not be justified.

MAGNETIC RESONANCE ANGIOGRAPHY (MRA)

Magnetic resonance imaging (MRI) provides an alternative to non-invasive angiography. With MRI, there is a natural contrast between flowing blood within a vessel and the stationary soft tissues. This allows the characteristics of the vessel to be demonstrated without the need for intra-vascular contrast medium. Multiple contiguous images of slices of tissue can be put together to produce an MR angiogram by **volume acquisition**. Historically, data acquisition has been slow and the use of MRA has been restricted to relatively immobile areas of the body, i.e.

carotid arteries and the intracranial circulation. This limitation has now been overcome by the development of faster scanners and by enhancing the contrast between blood vessels and stationary tissue using special intra-venous contrast media. Successful angiography can now be performed in all regions of the body, apart from the coronary arteries, with scan times of no more than 30 seconds.

MRA is a quick outpatient procedure that requires no more preparation than an intravenous injection. It carries none of the risks of ionising radiation and is therefore ideally suited to repeated follow-up examinations. In situations where regular vascular surveillance is needed and cannot be performed by duplex ultrasound, MRA is a reliable though more expensive alternative. Over the next few years, contrast-enhanced MRA is likely to replace conventional diagnostic angiography in units with ready access to MR. Traditional angiography will be reserved for patients needing percutaneous intervention (angioplasty or stenting). Patients requiring open surgery will have this planned by virtually non-invasive imaging.

453

APPROACH TO MANAGEMENT OF CHRONIC LOWER LIMB ISCHAEMIA

The treatment options for chronic lower limb ischaemia range from conservative or 'expectant' treatment (e.g. advice about smoking, encouragement of walking exercise) to extensive reconstructive operations. These are summarised in Box 35.2. Severe and critical ischaemia are clear indications for revascularisation (or amputation) since the conditions are not tolerable in the long term. For claudication, the degree of handicap is assessed clinically by careful history-taking and perhaps by walking with the patient. The treatment depends on the degree of handicap, the patient's willingness to give up smoking, the potential for treating the pattern of atherosclerosis and finally the patient's overall preference. Further investigation is then planned accordingly.

MILD TO MODERATE CLAUDICATION

Most patients with mild or moderate claudication do not require revascularisation. The symptoms often improve spontaneously over 6–18 months, especially if the patient stops smoking, exercises regularly and loses excess weight. Simple advice to walk more slowly and use a walking stick will often greatly extend the claudication distance. Care of the feet and appropriate footwear should be strongly emphasised.

Numerous oral 'vasodilator' drugs are prescribed for claudication but none has withstood critical evaluation and they are not recommended.

SUMMARY

Box 35.2 Treatment options for chronic lower limb ischaemia

Mild to moderate claudication
- No active treatment except advice to stop smoking, exercise regularly, take statin, lose weight
- Balloon angioplasty

Disabling claudication
- Balloon angioplasty
- Reconstructive arterial surgery

Critical ischaemia
- Intravenous drug therapies such as prostacycline, vasodilators (e.g. naftidrofuryl oxalate)
- Lumbar sympathectomy (surgical or by phenol injection)
- Balloon angioplasty
- Reconstructive arterial surgery
- Amputation (below, through or above knee)
- Terminal pain relief

Investigation of this group of patients is usually unnecessary apart from baseline ankle pressure measurements and a full blood count to exclude polycythaemia and thrombocythaemia. In polycythaemia rubra vera, soft thrombi can develop in the lower limb and cause arterial insufficiency. Systemic manifestations of atherosclerosis such as hypertension, angina or arrhythmias should be investigated and treated if appropriate.

DISABLING CLAUDICATION

The main indications for further investigation of claudication are symptoms judged severe enough to warrant radiological or surgical intervention. Disabling claudication is usually an indication for treatment unless the patient is too unfit even for angiography. Symptoms which usually indicate the need for investigation are marked exercise restriction in younger patients or markedly worsening symptoms, especially if they are associated with proximal arterial obstruction (as shown by absent femoral pulses). Treatment is by percutaneous transluminal angioplasty or reconstructive surgery.

TREATMENT METHODS FOR CHRONIC ARTERIAL INSUFFICIENCY

All patients should be advised to stop smoking and if necessary to lose weight. Cigarette smoking is both a primary risk factor in the aetiology of atherosclerosis and a secondary risk factor in causing deterioration or graft occlusion after reconstruction. Symptoms of claudication are more likely to resolve without treatment if the patient ceases smoking. However, the overall success rate of persuading patients to give up smoking is depressingly low, probably less than 30%. Others in the household should also be encouraged to give up smoking to help motivate the patient.

PERCUTANEOUS TRANSLUMINAL ANGIOPLASTY (PTA)

In the 1950s, Dotter experimented with techniques for dilating local arterial stenoses with graded metal bougies. For technical reasons, the methods were not widely adopted. More recently, Gruntzig developed a dilatation technique in which a balloon, distensible to a fixed diameter and incorporated in the end of a catheter, is introduced percutaneously into the femoral artery (see Fig. 35.4). A guide-wire is first placed across the stenosis, then the balloon catheter manœuvred into position under arteriographic control. The balloon is finally inflated to a high pressure (5–15 atmospheres), crushing the atheroma into the arterial wall and relieving the obstruction. Success is particularly operator-dependent and is most effective for isolated short stenoses. With increasing experience, longer stenoses and occlusions in smaller vessels can be

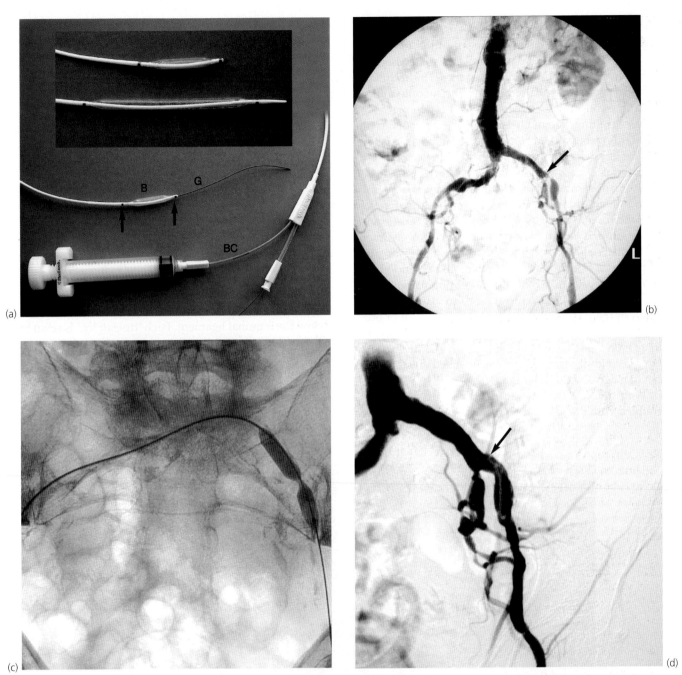

(a)

(b)

(c)

(d)

Fig. 35.4 Percutaneous transluminal angioplasty
(a) Balloon angioplasty equipment. This catheter is used for balloon dilatation of arterial stenosis. First, an artery some distance from the stenosis (usually the femoral) is punctured with a needle. A flexible guide-wire **G** is passed through the needle, along the artery and manipulated across the stenosis. The catheter is then threaded over the guide-wire until the distal balloon **B** (which can be inflated only to a pre-determined diameter) lies within the stenosis. The balloon is then inflated to high pressure using a special syringe attached to the balloon channel **BC**. Note the radio-opaque markers (arrowed) at each end of the balloon to allow it to be sited radiographically. **(b)** Arteriogram showing a tight stenosis at the distal end of the left common iliac artery. Catheter access proved impossible via the left femoral artery, so a guide wire was passed from the right femoral, over the bifurcation and across the stenosis. **(c)** An angioplasty balloon catheter was guided across the stenosis. As it was inflated the 'waist' caused by the arterial stenosis became clearly visible. With further inflation to 4 atmospheres pressure, the waist disappeared. **(d)** Appearance of the arteries post-angioplasty. This procedure was completed in under an hour on a day-case basis under local anaesthesia and proved durable over several years.

tackled successfully, avoiding the need for major surgery. Unfortunately, the method is less useful for distal calf arteries although results in this area continue to improve.

A similar technique is increasingly used for treating localised coronary artery stenoses as an alternative to coronary artery bypass surgery.

ARTERIAL RECONSTRUCTIVE SURGERY

Arterial reconstructive surgery began in the 1950s with the open removal of atheromatous plaques and associated thrombus from the aorta and iliac arteries. This technique, known as **thrombo-endarterectomy**, is technically difficult and time-consuming. It has largely been replaced by bypass grafting, although endarterectomy remains the standard operation for carotid artery stenosis (see below) and for isolated common femoral artery occlusions.

Arterial bypass grafting was first developed during the Korean war to treat arterial trauma using homografts from human cadavers. The initial results were excellent but within a few years, the grafts suffered from aneurysmal dilatation and rupture. This led to the use of synthetic graft materials for large arteries, and these are now available in a wide variety of shapes, sizes and cloths. Knitted polyester (Dacron) is the most popular and is the standard graft material for treating aorto-iliac obstruction. Many of these grafts are now sealed with gelatin or other proteins to minimise porosity. For smaller arteries, the long saphenous vein from the leg provides an excellent bypass conduit provided it is of suitable diameter and is not damaged by thrombosis.

With the availability and success of angioplasty, coupled with the recognition that conservative treatment may be as good as intervention for claudication, the volume of bypass grafting for arterial occlusive disease has fallen in most units. The majority of such surgery is now reserved for severely ischaemic limbs, either chronic or acute, and often when less invasive methods have proved unsuitable or unsuccessful. The most common bypass procedures are synthetic 'trouser' grafting for aorto-iliac (supra-inguinal) disease and femoro-popliteal bypass grafting, preferably using saphenous vein for infra-inguinal disease. However, a range of other bypass procedures and endarterectomy techniques sometimes have to be employed or used in addition to standard operations to cope with non-standard disease.

Aorto-iliac disease

The most common operation for aorto-iliac obstruction is the insertion of a trouser graft or 'Y' graft (see Fig. 35.5) between the aorta and the common femoral arteries just below the inguinal ligament. Each 'trouser leg' is sewn to a femoral artery, and the diseased vessels are left in situ posteriorly.

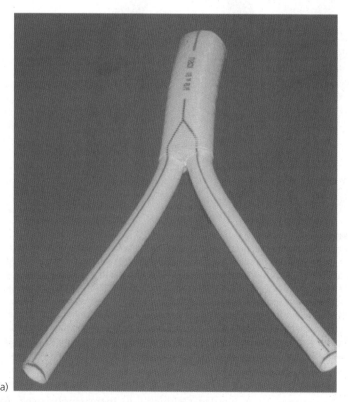

(b) Aorto-bifemoral bypass grafting

1 Proximal anastomosis—end of graft to side of aorta (occasionally aorta transsected and end-to-end anastomosis performed)

2 Distal anastomosis—end of graft to side of common femoral/profunda femoris junction, opening the profunda orifice to minimise future stenosis

(a)

(b)

Fig. 35.5 Trouser or 'Y' graft for aorto-iliac disease
A Dacron birfurcation graft **(a)** or prosthesis is used to bypass the aorto-iliac segment when it is occluded or stenosed, or to replace it when aorta and iliacs are aneurysmal. Note the guide-line down each limb which is to ensure they are not twisted during anastomosis.

Chapter 35

(a) Femoro-popliteal grafting

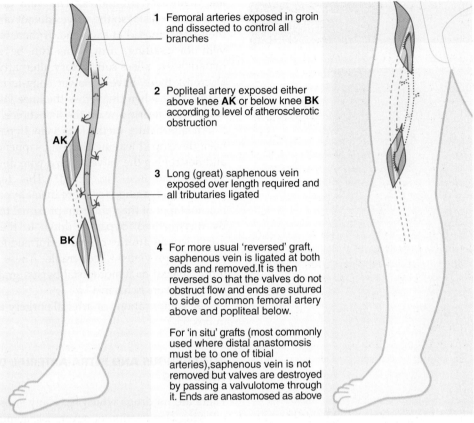

1 Femoral arteries exposed in groin and dissected to control all branches

2 Popliteal artery exposed either above knee **AK** or below knee **BK** according to level of atherosclerotic obstruction

3 Long (great) saphenous vein exposed over length required and all tributaries ligated

4 For more usual 'reversed' graft, saphenous vein is ligated at both ends and removed.It is then reversed so that the valves do not obstruct flow and ends are sutured to side of common femoral artery above and popliteal below.

For 'in situ' grafts (most commonly used where distal anastomosis must be to one of tibial arteries),saphenous vein is not removed but valves are destroyed by passing a valvulotome through it. Ends are anastomosed as above

(a)

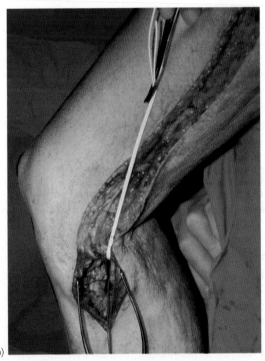

(b)

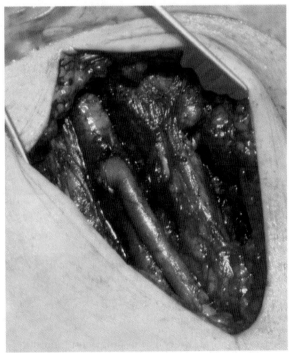

(c)

Fig. 35.6 Techniques of arterial bypass grafting
(a) Technique of femoro-popliteal grafting. **(b)** Long saphenous vein exposed in the thigh where it will be left in situ after destroying the valves with a valvulotome. The below knee popliteal artery is held in the white sling. **(c)** The vein graft anastomosed end-to-side to the common femoral artery in the groin.

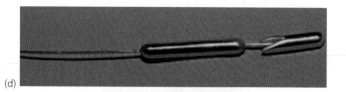

(d)

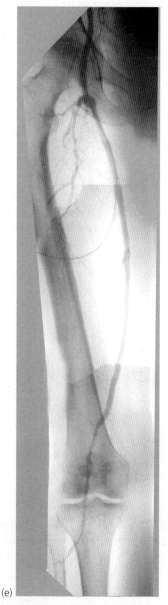

(e)

Fig. 35.6 Continued
(d) Head of Hall's valvulotome used to destroy valves for in-situ grafting. **(e)** Composite arteriogram showing patent fem-pop bypass.

Femoro-popliteal disease

The superficial femoral artery is the other common site of obstruction in the lower limb. This can be relieved by a bypass graft using the patient's long saphenous vein to link the common femoral artery and the popliteal artery; this is known as autogenous **femoro-popliteal bypass**

grafting (see Fig. 35.6). The usual technique is first to dissect out the long saphenous vein from groin to knee and ligate its tributaries. The vein graft is reversed proximal to distal so the valves do not obstruct flow, and then anastomosed at each end. If there is no suitable leg vein for grafting, arm veins can be used. Synthetic materials are a less satisfactory alternative (e.g. PTFE or Dacron); these have a lower long-term survival rate particularly when they cross the knee joint. A vein graft is therefore nearly always the first choice.

An alternative method of vein bypass grafting has been developed leaving the long saphenous vein in situ and destroying the valves with a wire device known as a **valvulotome** (see Fig. 35.6d). This technique has a particular advantage for more distal bypasses in that the natural taper of the vein from proximal to distal remains. By this method, bypasses down to the tibial or even dorsalis pedis arteries can be performed for distal disease that was previously inoperable. These are known as infrapopliteal or femorodistal bypass grafts and are only used for severe ischaemia.

The complications of arterial surgery are summarised in Box 35.3.

INTRAVENOUS AND INTRA-ARTERIAL DRUG THERAPIES

There are no drugs which have any substantial effect in relieving claudication or severe ischaemia, nor have any yet been discovered that can reverse atherosclerosis. The use of statins to lower blood cholesterol has not yet shown any proven benefit in peripheral arterial disease.

There has been extensive research into drug treatment for critically ischaemic limbs, aiming to improve peripheral perfusion or tissue viability where reconstruction is difficult or impossible. The goal is to allow time for the natural development of a collateral circulation. Intravenous

---

SUMMARY

Box 35.3 Complications of arterial surgery

- Complications of generalised arteriopathy: acute myocardial ischaemia, cerebrovascular accidents, renal failure, intestinal ischaemia—early or late
- Haemorrhage: arterial or venous—early
- Thrombosis of reconstructed vessels or graft leading to profound distal ischaemia (usually a technical fault)—early
- Embolism into limb vessels or renal vessels (particularly aneurysm surgery)—early
- Graft infection—late
- False aneurysm formation—late
- Progressive atherosclerotic lower limb ischaemia—late

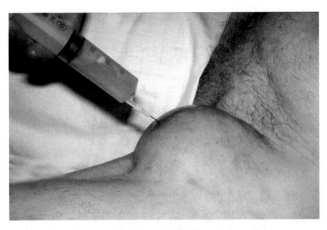

Fig. 35.7 Lymphocoele in groin following graft to femoral artery
Any operation in the region of the inguinal lymph nodes can interfere with lymphatic drainage and cause an accumulation of lymph known as a lymphocoele. In this case, the lymphocoele was aspirated periodically and finally stopped refilling about 4 months after the original operation. In fact, aspiration probably does not hasten the natural process of resolution.

prostaglandin analogues (e.g. Iloprost) and naftidrofuryl oxalate have shown some encouraging results but their serious side effects and the need for several days' intravenous infusion have limited their usefulness. Several research programmes are looking into stimulating new

vessel formation in unreconstructable limbs using locally applied intra-arterial growth factors but these are still some distance from everyday clinical practice.

SYMPATHECTOMY

Blood flow in the skin (but not muscle) is controlled by the sympathetic nervous system. Thus, even if the overall arterial supply is inadequate, rest pain in the skin may sometimes be relieved by sympathetic blockade. This can be performed by surgical excision of part of the lumbar sympathetic chain via an extraperitoneal approach or, less invasively and much more commonly, by translumbar injection of 6% aqueous phenol. This is known as **chemical sympathectomy** and is done under local anaesthesia and usually with radiographic control.

Unfortunately, only about 15% of patients with severe ischaemia obtain sufficient relief of symptoms to avoid a reconstructive operation or amputation and there appears to be no reliable way of selecting in advance those who will benefit. Sympathectomy is of no value in intermittent claudication as it does not influence muscle blood flow. It is most likely to succeed in early rest pain but is certain to fail where tissue loss (gangrene) has occurred. It may also be helpful in healing ulcers where moderate ischaemia is present in combination with some other factor such as chronic venous insufficiency.

ACUTE LOWER LIMB ISCHAEMIA

PATHOPHYSIOLOGY OF ACUTE LOWER LIMB ISCHAEMIA

The lower limb may become acutely ischaemic as a result of embolism or thrombosis. If a large embolus impacts in a major distributing artery, the distal blood supply is abruptly cut off. If the distal arteries are not atherosclerotic, an alternative collateral network will not have developed and the ischaemia is therefore all the more severe. Most large emboli originate in the heart, as a result of atrial fibrillation or mitral stenosis or both (left atrial thrombus), or of myocardial infarction (mural thrombus). Emboli usually impact at points where the arterial lumen narrows abruptly at branching points, in particular the aortic bifurcation (**saddle embolus**), the common femoral bifurcation and the popliteal trifurcation.

Sudden acute ischaemia may also develop if an essential distributing artery, already narrowed by atherosclerosis, becomes completely obstructed by secondary thrombosis of its lumen (acute-on-chronic occlusion). Another cause is thrombosis of a popliteal aneurysm or embolism from accumulated thrombus within an aortic or popliteal aneurysm. Occasionally, widespread thrombosis occurs in normal arteries causing acute ischaemia. This was

well recognised as a complication of the high-oestrogen contraceptive pill when it was in common use, but similar widespread thrombosis is sometimes seen as a complication of polycythaemia rubra vera, thrombocythaemia or leukaemias.

Acute thrombotic occlusion causes the most catastrophic results when it occurs in the popliteal artery (which has few useful collaterals), the external iliac/common femoral arterial trunk (the axial blood supply of the lower limb) or the profunda femoris (if the superficial femoral artery is already occluded).

CLINICAL FEATURES OF ACUTE LOWER LIMB ISCHAEMIA

Acute lower limb ischaemia presents clinically as a sudden onset of a painful, cold, white foot extending for a variable distance up the leg. After an hour or two of complete ischaemia, nerve ischaemia causes loss of sensation (although pain may be severe at the margin of the ischaemic area) and eventually muscle paralysis. Complete numbness indicates virtual cessation of blood flow (the five Ps—see p. 442).

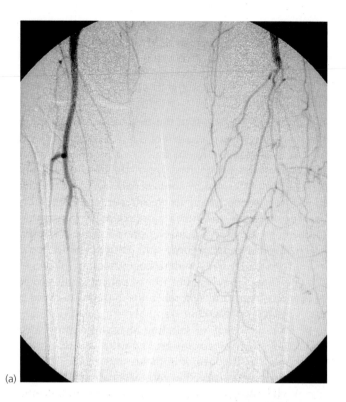

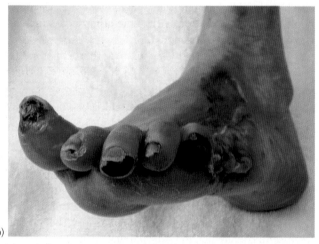

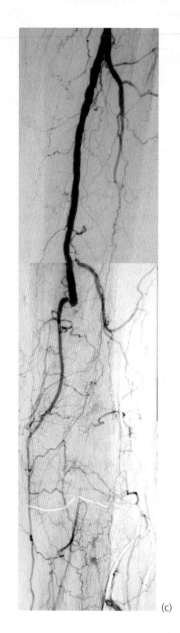

(a)

(b)

(c)

Fig. 35.8 Embolic occlusion of popliteal arteries
(a) Digital subtraction angiogram in a woman of 70 who presented with rest pain for 48 hours and necrosis of the dorsum of her foot and black toe tips for 24 hours. The right sided arteries are normal with no sign of atherosclerosis whilst the left popliteal is occluded with a sharp cut-off typical of embolism. The patient was in atrial fibrillation and the likely source of the embolus was the left atrium. She underwent a successful embolectomy, but because of the delay, a below-knee fasciotomy was performed to prevent compartment syndrome. **(b)** The foot ulcer 3 weeks after revascularisation. The ulcer gradually healed completely. **(c)** Arteriogram of another patient with chronic severe ischaemia of the foot. This strongly suggests embolism to be the cause. This patient has a moderate collateral supply consistent with the more chronic symptoms.

It is crucial that the diagnosis of acute complete arterial occlusion is recognised quickly because the resulting ischaemia is usually so profound that necrosis occurs within hours unless urgent treatment is undertaken. Unfortunately, because pain is often not a dominant feature, the urgency of the situation may not be appreciated by the patient, nursing staff or inexperienced doctors. Later,

necrosis becomes obvious as the affected area becomes mottled, dusky blue and discoloured. After about 24 hours, the skin becomes completely blue and blistered; tissue death is now irreversible.

The clinical features of acute severe lower limb ischaemia are listed in Box 35.4.

PRINCIPLES OF MANAGEMENT OF THE ACUTELY ISCHAEMIC LIMB

It is important to plan the general scheme of management of a patient with acute lower limb ischaemia at the outset. Time is likely to be limited before necrosis occurs and any delay or procrastination is likely to lead to excess morbidity or mortality. Cooperative vascular surgical and radiological expertise is usually required so that the full range of appropriate and timely treatment can be offered. As a first step, the patient should be anti-coagulated with a bolus dose of 10 000 U **intravenous**

KEY POINTS

Box 35.4 Clinical features of acute severe lower limb ischaemia

Symptoms and signs suggesting a predisposing cause for acute ischaemia (embolism or thrombosis)

- Recent chest pain or other evidence of myocardial infarction
- History of rheumatic heart disease
- History or finding of atrial fibrillation
- Previous arterial embolism
- History of intermittent claudication or other symptoms of peripheral arterial disease (thrombosis)
- Polycythaemia rubra vera (prone to intravascular thrombosis)
- Popliteal aneurysm in contralateral limb (possible thrombosis or embolism in affected limb)
- Aortic aneurysm (possible source of embolism)

Symptoms suggesting acute lower limb ischaemia

- Sudden onset of continuous pain, usually in one periphery
- Sudden and persistent coldness, usually in one periphery
- Sudden numbness or paraesthesia, usually in one periphery

Signs of acute lower limb ischaemia

- Unexpected coldness of the peripheral part of one or (less commonly) both legs
- Pallor or blueness of the periphery; in late cases, the fixed pigmentation of necrosis or skin blistering
- Poor peripheral capillary return after pressure blanching
- Strongly positive Buerger's test (pallor on elevation, slow return of redness on dependency)
- Progressive paralysis and foot drop (late sign)
- Absent lower limb pulses (particularly if known to have been present before)
- Ankle pulses undetectable by Doppler or very low ankle systolic pressure

---

heparin as soon as possible to prevent propagation of thrombus both proximal and distal to the occlusion. If the diagnosis is confirmed as embolism, then oral anticoagulation will usually be continued later.

The history may provide clues to the diagnosis. Evidence of mitral stenosis, an arrhythmia or recent myocardial infarction suggests embolism, whereas a history of claudication or a prothrombotic blood disorder points to thrombosis. Examining the affected limb does not help to distinguish embolism from thrombosis but the other limb provides evidence of the general condition of the peripheral arteries. If the other limb is well perfused with good peripheral pulses and normal ankle systolic pressure, then embolus is more likely. If a saddle embolus has lodged at the aortic bifurcation then both limbs may be ischaemic, although one side is usually affected more than the other. The popliteal fossa must always be palpated to exclude a thrombosed popliteal aneurysm.

Full blood count should be performed to exclude predisposing blood disorders and several units cross-matched if surgery is contemplated.

If clinical signs are strongly in favour of embolism, immediate surgical embolectomy may be undertaken, performing on-table **arteriography** if necessary. In most cases, the first intervention is not surgery but arterio-graphy which will demonstrate whether embolism or thrombosis is the diagnosis or whether there is an occluded popliteal aneurysm; it will also show which distal vessels are patent. Unfortunately, expediency is often the excuse for omitting arteriography but its omission places the patient at greater risk and removes the possibility of minimal access treatment with thrombolysis and angioplasty.

If acute-on-chronic thrombosis is the problem and the limb is likely to remain viable for 12 hours, **thrombolysis** may be undertaken, followed by angioplasty of any revealed underlying stenoses (see below). If the limb appears unlikely to remain viable that long, urgent re-constructive surgery should be performed if technically possible. Most patients needing arterial reconstruction for acute ischaemia require a **femoro-popliteal** or **femoro-tibial bypass** (see Fig. 35.6, p. 457).

Thrombolysis and angioplasty for acute thrombotic ischaemia

If arteriography reveals the cause of acute ischaemia to be thrombotic, the acute thrombus may be lysed using **streptokinase, urokinase** or **recombinant tissue plasmin-ogen activator** (rtPa). Systemic treatment with throm-bolytic agents is dangerous and not recommended, but direct instillation of one of these agents into the clot is often successful. This is usually performed via an arterial catheter manœuvred into place under radiological control from the other femoral artery. Dissolving the clot by this method usually takes 4–24 hours, which explains why it is unsuitable if the limb will not survive the duration of treatment. After successful lysis, the underlying stenosis can often be treated by transluminal angioplasty via the same femoral access puncture.

Embolectomy

Embolectomy is usually performed under local anaesthesia but the patient and theatre should be prepared for general anaesthesia in case it becomes necessary; full monitoring should be undertaken. The patient is usually already anticoagulated with intravenous heparin. A groin incision provides access to the arterial system. The

femoral artery bifurcation is exposed, all the vessels are temporarily clamped and an incision (**arteriotomy**) is made in the common femoral artery (see Fig. 35.9). This may reveal the obstructing clot. A **Fogarty balloon catheter** is then passed gently into each main vessel in turn, both proximally and distally. When catheter has been passed into the artery for 10 cm or so, the balloon is inflated gently and the catheter drawn back to sweep out any obstructing clot. This process is repeated at 10 cm intervals until the distal limit is reached. The operation is successful if clot is retrieved and blood flows back ('**back bleeding**') from each vessel as it is unclamped. If embolectomy is not possible, this usually indicates acute-on-chronic thrombosis. Immediate arteriography and treatment are required as delay carries a high rate of limb loss and death.

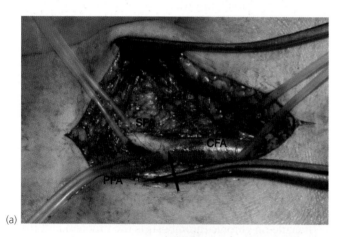

(a)

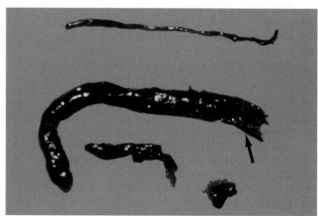

(c)

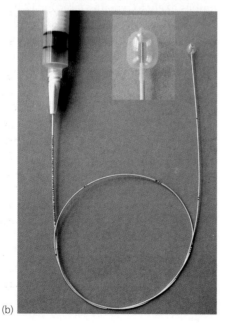

(b)

Fig. 35.9 Femoral artery embolectomy
(a) Surgical exposure of the femoral artery bifurcation, performed under local infiltration anaesthesia. The common femoral artery **CFA**, the profunda femoris **PFA** and the superficial femoral artery **SFA** are dissected cleanly and rubber slings placed around each artery. A transverse arteriotomy is made just proximal to the bifurcation (position arrowed). **(b)** A Fogarty balloon catheter is passed distally, the balloon is gently inflated and the catheter withdrawn to extract embolic and thrombotic material. This is performed in stages until the catheter can be passed to ankle level and back bleeding occurs. **(c)** Embolic material removed at operation from the superficial femoral artery and beyond using a Fogarty catheter. Note the paler embolic material (arrowed) and the darker thrombus propagated behind it.

THE DIABETIC FOOT

PATHOPHYSIOLOGY OF THE DIABETIC FOOT

Diabetic patients are particularly prone to serious ulceration and infection of the feet. The underlying disorder is believed to lie within the microcirculation (**microangiopathy**) but obliterative atherosclerosis also plays a part in some patients.

Several factors may contribute to diabetic foot problems:

- **Neuropathy.** Microangiopathy is believed to cause peripheral neuropathies which affect motor, sensory and autonomic nerves. The affected **motor nerves** supply the small muscles of the foot and the consequent unmodified traction of calf muscles produces distortion of the morphology and weight-bearing characteristics of the foot. **Sensory neuropathy** decreases pain sensation and hence awareness of injury from footwear and foreign bodies within shoes. Damaged **autonomic nerves** disrupt vascular control and cause loss of sweating. Neuropathic foot problems are painless and hence tend to be neglected by the patient
- **Arteriovenous communications.** These open beneath the skin, perhaps diverting nutrient flow away from it. Damaged tissue thus heals poorly and is vulnerable to infection, even if the injury or pressure damage is only minor
- **Arterioles.** These probably become narrowed and restrict capillary perfusion in a few cases
- **Impaired intermediary tissue metabolism** and a glucose-rich tissue environment. Both of these favour bacterial growth
- **Obliterative atherosclerosis.** Diabetics have an increased predisposition and are at greater risk of arterial insufficiency. Atherosclerotic disease follows the usual pattern (although often more distal) but tends to develop at a younger age

Most diabetic foot problems can be identified as being either primarily neuropathic or primarily atherosclerotic but some patients have elements of both. This makes diagnosis and management more difficult. Typically, the **neuropathic foot** is painless, red and warm with strong pulses, whereas the **atherosclerotic foot** is pale, painful, cold and pulseless. However, when both conditions occur together, the limb can be seriously ischaemic yet painless, warm and pink. If the foot is neuropathic and pulseless, only arteriography will demonstrate the arterial insufficiency.

Patients most at risk of neuropathic foot complications are elderly, poorly controlled, maturity-onset (type II) diabetics and younger patients with longstanding type I diabetes. Similarly, patients with diabetic renal or retinal complications appear to have an increased risk of foot problems. Recognising the **'at-risk' foot**, i.e. neuropathic foot, before trouble strikes is fundamental as virtually all neuropathic foot complications can be prevented with proper patient education and regular inspection and chiropody (podiatry) (see Box 35.5).

Management of atherosclerotic ischaemia is similar in diabetics and non-diabetics. For mixed disease, the arterial insufficiency should usually be treated first if there is to be any hope of healing.

CLINICAL PRESENTATIONS OF DIABETIC FOOT COMPLICATIONS

Foot complications of diabetic neuropathy present in four main ways (see Fig. 35.10):

- **Painless, deeply penetrating ulcers.** These usually develop beneath the first or fifth metatarsal head. The infecting organism is usually *Staphylococcus aureus*. The infection and necrosis tend to spread through the plantar spaces and along the tendon sheaths. Infection and local venous thrombosis appear to be the predominant factors in causing tissue destruction
- **Chronic ulceration** of pressure points and sites of minor injury. Skin perfusion is otherwise adequate

---

KEY POINTS

Box 35.5 The problem of the diabetic foot

- 'Diabetic gangrene is not heaven-sent but earth-born' (Joslin 1934)
- There is no such thing as 'mild' diabetes; all diabetics are potentially at risk
- Four out of five patients with diabetic foot problems have type II diabetes
- Foot problems are responsible for 47% of days spent in hospital by diabetics
- Diabetic foot problems are responsible for 12% of all hospital admissions in (internal) medicine
- In diabetics with new foot ulcers, 90% have peripheral neuropathy (compared with 20% in a diabetic control group), whereas only 14% have peripheral arterial disease compared with 10% in controls (Miami 1983–4)
- Patients with diabetic foot problems are incapacitated for an average of 16 weeks
- Diabetic foot problems are largely preventable
- Care and prevention of diabetic foot problems require specialist surveillance and management by a dedicated team; foot ulceration in diabetics represents a failure of medical management

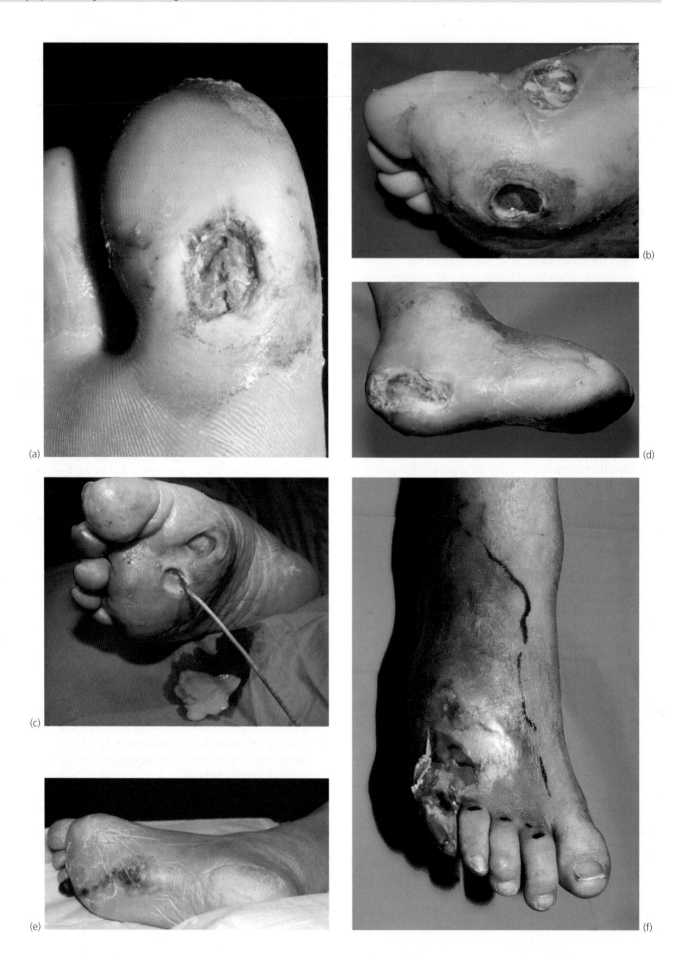

(a)

(b)

(c)

(d)

(e)

(f)

Fig. 35.10 Foot complications of diabetes (*facing page*)
(a) Penetrating ulcer of the great toe in a farmer of 35 with diabetic neuropathy and *hallux rigidus*. The ulcer was painless and contained necrotic slough. It healed after excision of the necrotic material and provision of special footwear to prevent undue pressure on the toe. **(b)** Chronic penetrating ulcers in a 60-year-old woman with maturity-onset diabetes. She had no evidence of major vessel disease but had signs of neuropathy. The deep ulcer beneath the head of the first metatarsal is characteristically surrounded with a thick keratin margin, and the ulcer on the medial side of the foot has an exposed tendon in its base. **(c)** Two penetrating ulcers in the sole of the foot. One ulcer is being probed and the probe passes right through the foot to the skin of the dorsum demonstrating extensive tissue destruction by infection. **(d)** This patient had already lost all his toes from neuropathic complications but presented later with this painful ulcer which proved to be due to arterial insufficiency. The ulcer healed after a successful superficial femoral angioplasty. **(e)** This patient has a combination of neuropathy and arterial insufficiency. This foot was painless despite spreading necrosis and a collection of pus in the sole of the foot. He underwent femoro-popliteal bypass and local excision of dead tissue and healing was eventually complete. **(f)** This man of 34 presented with a neglected infection in his foot. He had severe neuropathy but no arterial disease. The entire dorsum of his foot was necrotic and he had to undergo a primary below knee amputation. This complication would have been entirely avoidable had he sought and received treatment earlier.

- **Extensive spreading skin necrosis** originating in an ulcer and associated with superficial or deep infection. This develops very rapidly and spreads proximally, threatening both limb and life
- **Painless necrosis of individual toes.** These first turn blue then later become black and mummified, and may eventually be shed spontaneously. This usually occurs in mixed neuropathy and atherosclerosis and management hinges on whether local amputations will heal or whether arterial reconstruction is needed

MANAGEMENT OF NEUROPATHIC FOOT COMPLICATIONS

Control of infection

As a general rule, control of infection is the first priority in the management of diabetic foot problems. Minor foot lesions in the diabetic should always be taken seriously and treated early with **oral antibiotics** and frequent local cleansing and dressing.

If there is any sign of spreading infection or systemic involvement (i.e. pyrexia, tachycardia or loss of diabetic control), the patient should be admitted to hospital for more intensive treatment. This includes parenteral antibiotics, elevation, excision of any necrotic tissue and attention to blood glucose control.

Removal of necrotic tissue

Surgery may involve anything from simple **desloughing** of an ulcer to major amputation (see Fig. 35.11). If performed correctly, these surgical procedures result in complete and rapid healing. If good foot care is available, it is rare that amputation of more than single toes is required.

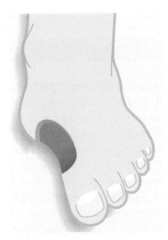

1 Excision of all necrotic tissue from ulcer, which is left to granulate

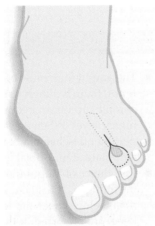

2 Digit amputation using racquet-shaped incision; toe is removed with both phalangeal bones and cartilage is nibbled from metatarsal (shaded)

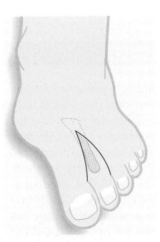

3 'Filleting' of digit and metatarsal if infection has spread more deeply. A 'cake-slice' is taken out of the foot and the wound left unsutured to heal by granulation

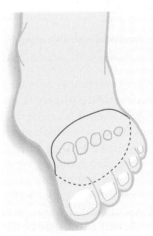

4 Transmetatarsal amputation for Symes amputation

(a)

Fig. 35.11 Operations on the diabetic foot
(a) Types of local amputation.

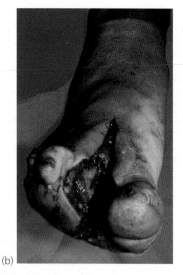

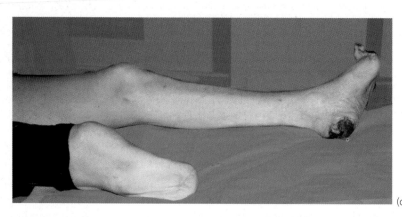

(b)   (c)

Fig. 35.11 Continued
(b) This is the same patient shown in Figure 35.10c. The second and third metatarsals have been excised, together with all the necrotic tissue in a 'cake slice' procedure. The wound was left open to heal by secondary intention, eventually giving a remarkably good functional result. **(c)** This elderly man suffered from a combination of neuropathy and obliterative atherosclerosis. He was blind as a result of diabetic complications. The right leg was eventually amputated below knee because of spreading infection, but the left was saved by angioplasty of stenosis in the iliac and superficial femoral arteries together with local surgery to remove necrotic tissue. Note the typical 'clawed foot' and distorted sole of motor neuropathy and that the great toe has already been amputated.

Prevention

All clinicians dealing with diabetics should place the highest priority on prevention. All diabetics should be screened for peripheral neuropathy and, for those at risk, detailed advice on self-care should be given and high-quality chiropody services provided. Careful attention should be given to footwear to correct abnormal pressure patterns. Special insoles or even special shoes may need to be made by an orthotist or surgical fitter. Careful follow-up and regular monitoring by a diabetic specialist nurse or clinic can successfully anticipate trouble.

AMPUTATION

Where practicable, strenuous efforts to preserve limbs by reconstructive surgery or interventional radiological techniques should be made, as the functional result and the success of rehabilitation are potentially far better than even the best major amputation. Mobility with artificial limbs is disappointing especially in the elderly or infirm. However, amputation cannot be avoided if revascularisation is technically impossible (particularly in diffuse distal arterial disease), if there is substantial tissue necrosis and a functionally useless foot, or deep spreading infection.

LEVEL OF AMPUTATION

Two principles guide the level of amputation (see Fig. 35.12):

● The amputation must be made through healthy tissue. If not, there is a high risk of wound breakdown and chronic ulceration, requiring further amputation at a higher level. When amputation is for (uncorrected) peripheral ischaemia, it is almost always necessary to amputate at mid-tibial level or above to ensure healing
● The choice of amputation level must take into account the fitting of a prosthetic limb. For this purpose, the mid-tibia (below-knee) and lower femoral levels (above-knee) are preferred. If the knee joint can be saved, the functional success of a prosthesis is much better. With improved prostheses, through-knee amputation is possible but healing rates are poor; most surgeons and prosthetists prefer above-knee to through-knee amputation, which has a better healing rate and easier prosthetics

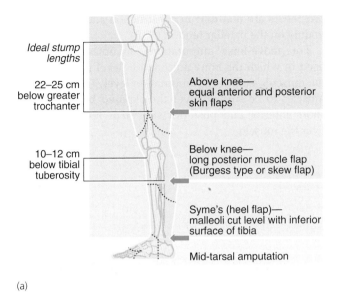

Ideal stump lengths

22–25 cm below greater trochanter

Above knee—
equal anterior and posterior
skin flaps

10–12 cm below tibial tuberosity

Below knee—
long posterior muscle flap
(Burgess type or skew flap)

Syme's (heel flap)—
malleoli cut level with inferior
surface of tibia

Mid-tarsal amputation

(a)

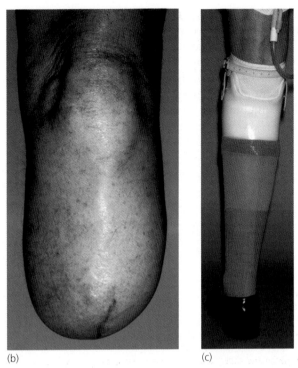

(b)   (c)

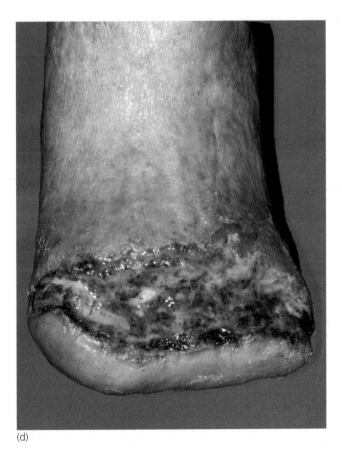

(d)

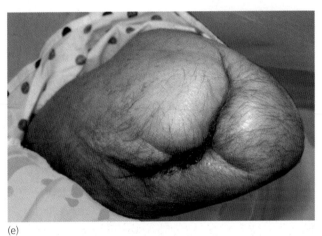

(e)

Fig. 35.12 Lower limb amputations
(a) Sites of election for lower limb amputations. **(b)** A well-healed below-knee stump at 6 weeks. The operation used a long posterior muscle flap and equal length 'skew' skin flaps. **(c)** The same patient fitted with a modular below knee prosthesis retained by a close fitting socket and a small strap above the knee. Note the urinary catheter. **(d)** Breakdown of below-knee stump because of inadequate arterial blood supply. **(e)** Above-knee stump in a diabetic patient. Unfortunately the original above-knee wound broke down and necrotic muscle had to be excised. The wound was left open and has nearly healed by secondary intention two months later **(e)**.

The traditional 'guillotine' amputation of the battlefield simply sliced off the limb, leaving the wound to heal by secondary intention. This reduced the risk of fatal gas gangrene or tetanus but the result for fitting limb prosthesis was poor.

There have been considerable developments in amputation techniques in recent decades in particular **myoplastic techniques**. For below-knee amputations, a long posterior flap of muscle and skin is now wrapped forward over the amputated bone and sutured in place.

467

This results in more reliable healing and a suitably shaped and cushioned stump. A more recent variation, the **'skew flap'** technique, uses a long posterior muscle flap but equal skin flaps. The healing rate is no better but the stump is better shaped for early prosthetic fitting. With these techniques and in experienced hands, about 70% of amputations for ischaemia will eventually heal, thus preserving the knee joint. Modern below-knee prostheses are **modular** in construction and bear weight mainly on the patellar tendon (PTB).

For above-knee amputations, myoplastic flaps are used in which the bony amputation level is proximal to the musculo-cutaneous amputation level. This allows the muscles to be sutured over the exposed bone end. The short anterior and posterior skin flaps are then closed over the muscle.

36 Aneurysms and other peripheral arterial disorders

ANEURYSMS

PATHOLOGY

In some patients with aneurysmal disease, all the major arteries are large in diameter (arteriomegaly) but an aneurysm is defined as a localised area of pathologically excessive arterial dilatation. Aneurysms of the abdominal aorta and the iliac, femoral and popliteal arteries are often labelled as complications of atherosclerosis but it is more likely that the primary disorder lies in degeneration of the elastin and/or collagen of the arterial wall. Atherosclerosis within aneurysms may be a less important secondary factor. Aneurysms are relatively uncommon; they are found mainly in males over 70 years of age and even less commonly in women an average of 10 years later. At least a quarter of these patients have more than one aneurysm.

Degenerative aneurysms are usually **fusiform** in shape, slowly expanding in diameter. As the aneurysm becomes larger, expansion accelerates and the risk of rupture increases. The majority of abdominal aortic aneurysms involve only the infrarenal aorta; some extend distally to involve one or both of the common iliac arteries and sometimes the internal iliac arteries (see Fig. 36.1). A few extend proximally to become **thoraco-abdominal aneurysms**.

CLINICAL PRESENTATION OF ANEURYSMS

Aorto-iliac aneurysms are often found incidentally as a pulsatile mass on abdominal examination, as calcification on plain abdominal X-ray, an obvious aneurysm on computed tomography (CT) or, most commonly, on ultrasound scanning for obstructive urinary symptoms (see Fig. 36.2). Occasionally the patient is the first to notice the abdominal pulsation. Despite this, nearly half of cases reaching the surgeon present because of symptoms of leakage into the retroperitoneal tissues. Elective surgery can have a mortality rate of less than 5%, whereas community and hospital mortality after rupture is in excess of 80%. There is a growing interest in ultrasound screening for aneurysms in elderly men in an attempt to detect and treat aneurysms before they rupture.

Pain is the most common symptom of a leaking aneurysm. The clinical picture ranges from an 'acute abdomen' to abdomino-lumbar pain of up to 1 week's duration. The diagnosis is usually suggested by finding a pulsatile abdominal mass. The patient often exhibits transient or more persistent **cardiovascular collapse** which should alert the clinician to the diagnosis.

Intraperitoneal rupture and often extraperitoneal rupture are rapidly fatal and are frequently the unrecognised cause of **sudden death** in the elderly. Cause of death is often wrongly attributed to 'myocardial infarction'.

Femoral and popliteal aneurysms are uncommon and usually present as a pulsatile mass. Femoral aneurysms occasionally rupture and popliteal aneurysms are liable to undergo thrombosis or cause embolism, in which case the patient presents with an **acutely ischaemic leg**. It is vital to exclude this diagnosis in a patient with an acutely ischaemic leg as successful treatment often requires thrombolysis in addition to surgery.

469

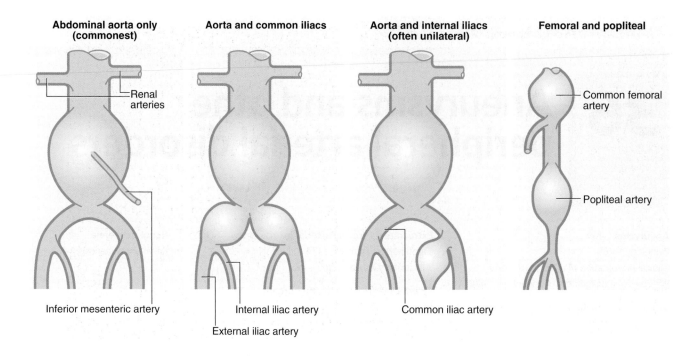

Fig. 36.1 Patterns of aneurysm formation
About 25% have more than one aneurysm either in continuity (common iliac, internal iliac) or not (femoral 10%; popliteal 20%). Abdominal aortic aneurysms rarely extend above the renal arteries.

PRINCIPLES OF MANAGEMENT OF ANEURYSMS

INDICATIONS FOR OPERATION (see Box 36.1)

A leaking or ruptured abdominal aortic aneurysm is a surgical emergency. Less than half the patients reach hospital alive, and only about half of these survive. The majority of patients die of shock before reaching the operating theatre or else of myocardial infarction or acute renal failure after operation.

On the other hand, the mortality after elective operation for aneurysm can be less than 5%. Thus, the decision to operate electively depends on the likelihood of leakage or rupture. If there are symptoms which can be attributed to the aneurysm, imminent rupture must be assumed and urgent operation performed. For asymptomatic aneurysms, the risk of rupture increases exponentially as the aneurysm dilates. Most vascular surgeons would consider operation for abdominal aortic aneurysms of 5 cm or more in diameter; 6 cm is generally considered to be critical since 40% of such aneurysms can be expected to rupture over the next 2 years. The indications for operation are summarised in Box 36.1.

INVESTIGATION OF ANEURYSM

If an aneurysm is obviously leaking, there is barely time to cross-match blood, let alone perform specific investigations on the way to theatre. For doubtful or non-acute cases, **ultrasound** or **CT scanning** is a rapid method of establishing the presence and size of an aneurysm. However, it should be emphasised that diagnosis of a leak or rupture must be made on clinical grounds; no test can reliably diagnose rupture until it is gross.

> **SUMMARY**
>
> **Box 36.1 Indications for operating on abdominal aortic aneurysms**
>
> **Leaking or ruptured aneurysms**
> ● If patient's state and general fitness permit
>
> **Symptomatic aneurysms**
> ● Aneurysms causing pain (particularly if tender), ureteric obstruction or embolism
>
> **Expanding aneurysms**
> ● Aneurysms which enlarge more than 0.5 cm in 1 year
>
> **Size**
> ● Most arterial surgeons now recommend operation on aneurysms of 5.5 cm diameter or greater, or any saccular aneurysm

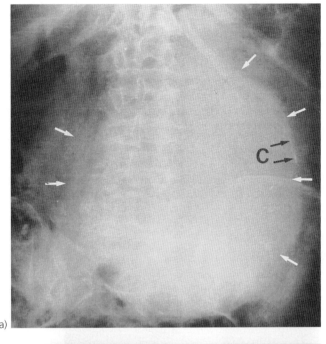

(a)

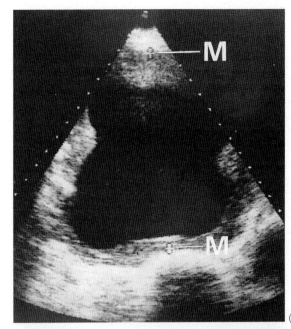

(b)

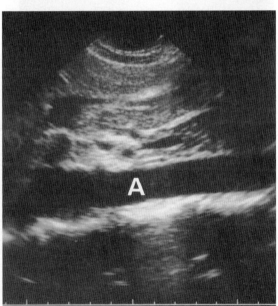

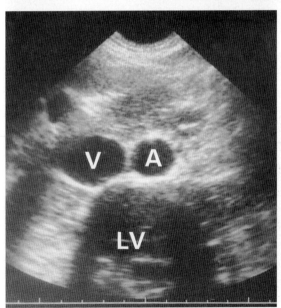

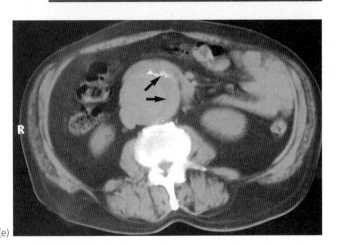

(e)

Fig. 36.2 Abdominal aortic aneurysm

This very obese 64-year-old man complained of continuous aching back pain for 2 weeks. **(a)** Plain abdominal X-ray showing huge abdominal aneurysm (outlined by arrows). Note calcification **C** along its left-hand aspect. **(b)** Abdominal ultrasound scan of the same patient. This shows the aneurysm is 11.5 cm in maximum antero-posterior diameter, as measured between the markers **M**, **M**. **(c)** and **(d)** Abdominal ultrasound scan in longitudinal and transverse sections showing size and position of a normal aorta **A**. The inferior vena cava **V** is also shown on the transverse scan (note that it is larger than the aorta). A lumbar vertebral body is labelled **LV**. **(e)** CT scan of a different patient with a 6 cm AAA. The thrombus lining the wall can clearly be seen (arrowed). Calcification is visible in the anterior wall where the third part of the duodenum is closely applied to it. Rarely, a primary aorto-duodenal fistula develops at this point.

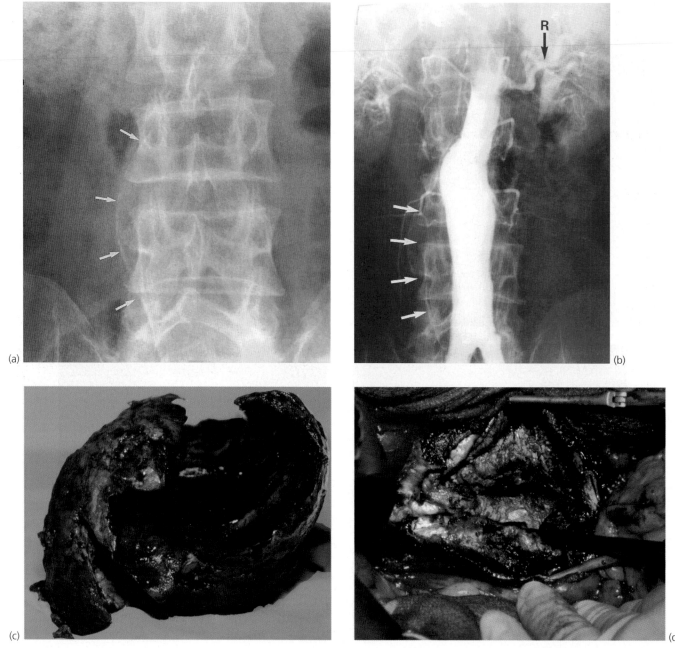

(a)

(b)

(c)

(d)

Fig. 36.3 A 70-year-old asymptomatic man in whom a pulsatile abdominal mass was an incidental finding. **(a)** Plain antero-posterior abdominal X-ray showing a mildly radiopaque mass in the midline with a line of calcification down its right-hand margin (arrowed). **(b)** Arteriogram from the same patient showing fusiform dilatation of the aorta beginning 2.5 cm below the origins of the renal arteries **R**. Note the calcification (arrowed) in the outer wall corresponding to that in (a); the space between this and the lumen of the aneurysm consists of old lamellated thrombus. **(c)** This cast of thrombus was removed from within the aortic aneurysm at operation; note the false lumen and concentric lamellae of thrombus progressively laid down as the aneurysm expanded over many months. **(d)** This shows the aneurysm sac opened at operation on a patient who had complained of chronic back pain. The posterior wall of the aorta is completely deficient in part and the anterior longitudinal ligament is visible in its base.

Ultrasonography is also used for periodic monitoring of asymptomatic aneurysms considered too small to warrant operation. Neither ultrasound nor CT scanning is completely reliable for showing the relationship of the aneurysm to the renal arteries and arteriography may be necessary for this. The 5% of cases where the aneurysm extends above the renal arteries require a thoraco-abdominal operative approach and the operation carries a greater risk. **Magnetic resonance angiography** which does not employ contrast material is developing rapidly.

It will probably supersede other investigations as further improvements in speed and convenience appear.

Arteriography is usually necessary if aneurysm patients requiring surgery also have evidence of lower limb ischaemia, in which case combined reconstruction may be required.

PRINCIPLES OF ANEURYSM SURGERY

The aneurysmal segment is surgically corrected by means of a graft. **Tube grafts** or **bifurcation grafts** of synthetic material (usually Dacron) are used for aorto-iliac and femoral aneurysms, while **autogenous saphenous vein** is preferred for popliteal aneurysms.

For abdominal aneurysms, the standard approach is a long midline abdominal incision. The aorta is usually reached via the peritoneal cavity or sometimes via an extraperitoneal approach. The patient is usually anti-coagulated with intravenous heparin to prevent distal thrombosis and the iliac arteries and the infrarenal aorta are clamped (see Fig. 36.5). The aneurysm is incised longitudinally and any clot within it removed. Bleeding lumbar arteries opening into the posterior aortic wall are oversewn.

The graft is sutured within the aneurysmal sac at each end and the sac is left in situ and later closed around the graft. This is known as an **inlay graft** and allows

separation of the graft from the intestine, reducing the risk of an aorto-intestinal fistula from the graft anastomoses. The graft is sutured proximally just above the

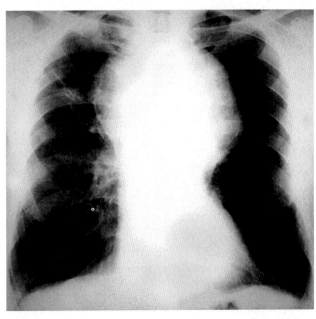

Fig. 36.4 Chest X-ray of thoracic aneurysm. This huge aneurysm of the aortic arch was discovered during workup prior to surgery for a large AAA. Unfortunately the thoracic aneurysm proved inoperable.

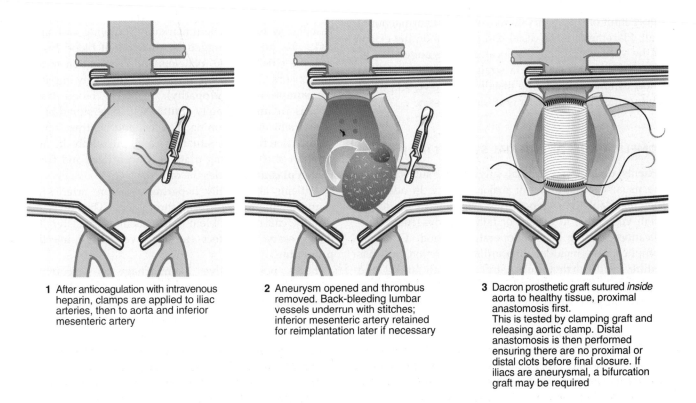

1 After anticoagulation with intravenous heparin, clamps are applied to iliac arteries, then to aorta and inferior mesenteric artery

2 Aneurysm opened and thrombus removed. Back-bleeding lumbar vessels underrun with stitches; inferior mesenteric artery retained for reimplantation later if necessary

3 Dacron prosthetic graft sutured *inside* aorta to healthy tissue, proximal anastomosis first.
This is tested by clamping graft and releasing aortic clamp. Distal anastomosis is then performed ensuring there are no proximal or distal clots before final closure. If iliacs are aneurysmal, a bifurcation graft may be required

Fig. 36.5 Technique of abdominal aortic aneurysm surgery

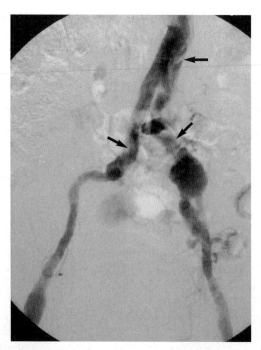

Fig. 36.6 Arteriography after aneurysm surgery
This arteriogram was performed for claudication 10 years after a
trouser or 'Y' graft for abdominal aortic aneurysm (arrowed). A new
aneurysm has appeared in the left common iliac artery and a small
aneurysm is also seen in the right common femoral. Neither was large
enough to require surgery but periodic follow up was continued using
ultrasound.

upper limit of the aneurysm to (relatively) normal aortic
wall. Placement of the distal end depends on the extent
of the aneurysm. It may be located in the aorta near its
bifurcation, in which case a straight tube graft is used
(most commonly), or more distally to iliac vessels when
a bifurcation graft ('trouser graft') is necessary.

COMPLICATIONS OF ARTERIAL SURGERY (see Box 35.3)

Patients undergoing arterial surgery are subject to all
the usual complications of major surgery. In addition,
they invariably have **generalised arteriopathy** rendering
them vulnerable to serious or fatal cardiovascular complications during the perioperative period. Common
complications include myocardial infarction, cardiac
failure, acute arrhythmias, strokes, renal failure and
intestinal ischaemia. Therefore, preparation for elective
arterial surgery must include meticulous preoperative
assessment and preparation. Any pre-existing medical
conditions like cardiac failure or hypertension should be
stabilised under expert advice.

For aortic and other major arterial operations, prolonged general anaesthesia, **aortic clamping** and heavy
operative blood loss place extra stress on a compromised
cardiovascular system. Thus patients require intensive

monitoring both during and after operation. This usually
means central venous and peripheral arterial catheterisation for accurate pressure measurements. For patients
with severe myocardial disease, a Swann–Ganz catheter
is often placed to monitor the pulmonary artery wedge
pressure (equivalent to left atrial pressure) as well as the
cardiac output. These and other high-risk patients should
be closely monitored in the early postoperative period
in an intensive care or high-dependency unit so that
complications can be recognised and treated early.

The local complications of arterial surgery include
haemorrhage, **embolism**, **thrombosis**, **graft infection** and
false aneurysm formation. The complications of arterial
surgery are summarised in Box 35.3 (p. 458) and discussed
in detail below.

Haemorrhage

During surgical access to the affected arteries, nearby
veins are vulnerable to tearing even when great care is
taken in dissection. For example, the iliac veins cross deep
to the iliac arteries and are often adherent to them. Venous
tears are often inaccessible and thus difficult to identify
and repair; they usually result in massive blood loss.

Making an arterial anastomosis is demanding under
the best conditions, but made even more difficult by
friable vessels and calcified atherosclerotic plaques. In
the high-pressure arterial system any defect is quickly
revealed and blood sprays everywhere! Fortunately the
vascular system can be remarkably forgiving and small
leaks are quickly plugged by platelets. If blood loss is
massive (10–25 units), platelets and coagulation factors
are consumed and haemostasis is progressively impaired
(**consumption coagulopathy**). Standard blood transfusions are unfortunately of little help since stored blood
is deficient in functioning platelets and clotting factors.
In this deteriorating situation (and preferably in anti-
cipation of it), infusing **platelet concentrates** and **fresh-
frozen plasma** provides the only answer.

Patients are usually heparinised before arteries are
clamped to prevent distal thrombosis. This does not
usually cause a problem with haemostasis later, but
if necessary the effect can be reversed by injecting
protamine.

Early postoperative haemorrhage is uncommon
provided adequate haemostasis is achieved before
completing the operation and closing the wound. When
bleeding does occur, it usually results from a pin-hole
leak at the anastomosis or a slipped ligature. Haemorrhage is manifest by generalised signs of hypovolaemia,
by progressive abdominal distension or, in the lower
limb, by swelling beneath the wound. Postoperative
haemorrhage will sometimes stop spontaneously following transfusion of blood and clotting factors, but if blood

loss continues or there is major haemorrhage, further operation is urgently required.

Embolism

In aneurysm surgery, embolism is usually caused by dislodging fresh or organised thrombus from the aneurysmal sac. It is largely preventable if the outflow vessels are clamped before the aneurysm is manipulated. Large emboli that lodge in femoral vessels can be retrieved with a Fogarty balloon catheter, but the more common fragmented distal embolism may cause infarction of digits or even the whole foot ('**trash foot**'). Infarction due to distal embolism is irreversible and usually necessitates amputation later.

Thrombosis

Thrombosis of the reconstructed vessels is a major problem in arterial surgery. It rapidly leads to profound distal ischaemia and results in loss of the limb unless urgently corrected.

Sluggish flow leads to thrombosis and may arise for a variety of technical reasons:

- Unrecognised stenosis proximal or distal to the reconstruction causing poor inflow or runoff
- Poor anastomotic technique with partial luminal obstruction
- Dissection of the layers of the distal vessel wall resulting in a flap of tunica intima and media which acts as a 'flap valve' occluding the lumen
- Twisting or kinking of a graft
- In situ thrombosis during arterial clamping

Thrombosis usually occurs in the first few hours after operation and becomes manifest by deterioration in the colour, temperature and pulses of the affected limb from the satisfactory state initially achieved at operation. Urgent reoperation is usually required.

Graft infection

Infection of a synthetic graft is uncommon but can be a devastating complication. It may occur in the early postoperative period or at any time months or years later. The infecting organisms are usually from the patient's own intestine. Infection is minimised by avoiding opening bowel, meticulous asepsis and haemostasis, and perioperative antibiotic cover. Antibiotics are normally given intravenously at anaesthetic induction and over the first 24 hours postoperatively. A cephalosporin (e.g. cefotaxime or cefuroxime), or a combination of gentamicin and flucloxacillin is suitable. In addition, gelatin-coated grafts can be soaked in an antistaphylococcal antibiotic e.g. rifampicin before placement.

Graft infection should be suspected if there is recurrent pyrexia and malaise or a persistently discharging wound sinus; occasionally, the wound breaks down, exposing the infected graft. Major graft infection has a bleak prognosis even when treated, the eventual outcome often being death from septicaemia or anastomotic breakdown with catastrophic bleeding. Standard treatment is to remove the infected graft and restore the distal circulation with an **extra-anatomic graft** (e.g. axillobifemoral), which bypasses the infected area.

False aneurysm formation

A false aneurysm is the result of a slow anastomotic leak confined by surrounding tissues. A slowly expanding blood-filled cavity results, which eventually ruptures or undergoes thrombosis. A false aneurysm usually presents as a palpable pulsatile mass. Occasionally a false aneurysm at an upper anastomosis with the abdominal aorta leaks into the overlying duodenum. This produces an **aorto-duodenal fistula** and presents with severe haematemesis. Aorto-duodenal fistulae may also result from graft infection. False aneurysms were formerly much more common because of the gradual breakdown of silk suture

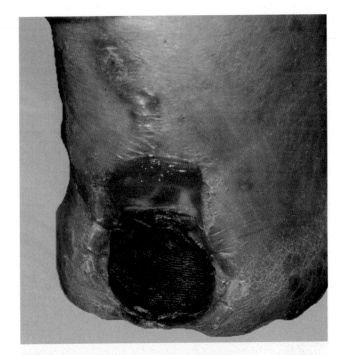

Fig. 36.7 Complication of arterial surgery
This patient was admitted to hospital with a ruptured aneurysm. He suffered arterial thrombosis of the lower limb during operation and a thrombectomy left him with an ischaemic foot. Poor attention to heel pressure relief during the early postoperative period led to this heel necrosis, which took several months to heal.

materials but suture durability has greatly improved with the introduction of polyester and polypropylene sutures.

LONG-TERM FOLLOW-UP AFTER ARTERIAL SURGERY

All patients with obliterative atherosclerotic disease are liable to progression of the disease and new ischaemic events. Thus, most patients are followed up long-term after surgery or angioplasty to monitor deterioration, to detect new disease and to enable timely intervention. Femoro-popliteal vein grafts can be examined at intervals using duplex Doppler scanning. Such **graft surveillance** can detect early graft stenoses, enabling them to be treated and the graft preserved. Aneurysm patients, on the other hand, can be discharged from follow-up 3 months after operation if there are no complications.

UPPER LIMB ISCHAEMIA

Ischaemia of the upper limb is rare. This is because atherosclerosis is very uncommon in the arteries supplying the upper limb. Furthermore, there is a rich collateral blood supply via the scapular anastomoses which can bypass occlusive disease of the subclavian artery. Upper limb ischaemia usually occurs when the subclavian artery is compressed at the thoracic outlet or when emboli obstruct the brachial or more distal arteries. Occasionally, vasospastic disorders like severe Raynaud's disease cause digital ischaemia.

THORACIC OUTLET COMPRESSION

The subclavian artery and vein and the brachial plexus pass through the narrow space between the first rib and the clavicle. If this space becomes narrow, neurological or arterial symptoms may appear; both of these are part of the **thoracic outlet syndrome**. The gap may be encroached upon by a healed fracture, by excess muscle development or some other unknown means. Upward pressure may also be exerted by a congenital **cervical rib** or fibrous band.

Symptoms of arterial compression include upper limb 'claudication' in people who habitually work with their arms above their heads, as the artery becomes further compressed in this position. In longstanding cases of subclavian artery compression, the artery beyond the stenosis often becomes dilated into an aneurysm (**post-stenotic dilatation**) which may collect thrombus. This may later embolise into the brachial artery causing acute ischaemia.

Neurological symptoms of thoracic outlet syndrome usually cause deficits in the T1 nerve root distribution.

Diagnosis of thoracic outlet syndromes is difficult and best performed in specialist centres with appropriate input from neurologists, surgeons, radiologists and physiotherapists. Operative intervention is becoming less common as conservative management improves. Occasionally the diagnosis is made by finding a lower blood pressure in the affected arm which varies with arm posture and obstruction can be confirmed by arteriography. Most cases are not, however, so straightforward.

Treatment is by excision of a cervical rib if present or else excision of the first rib. A subclavian aneurysm should be resected and replaced with a graft.

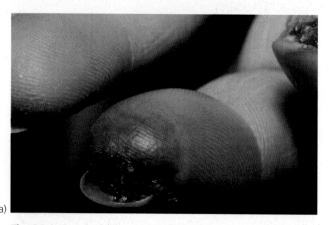

(a)

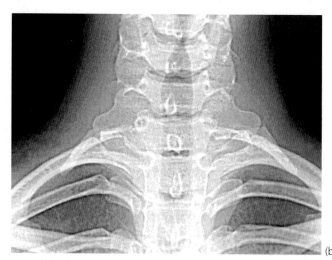

(b)

Fig. 36.8 Cervical rib causing subclavian artery compression.
(a) This 65-year-old butcher complained of a sudden onset of extreme pallor, coldness, weakness and paraesthesia in his right hand and forearm when handling meat in the cold room. **(b)** Plain X-ray of thoracic outlet showing bilateral cervical ribs.

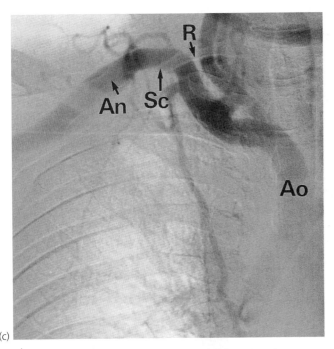

(c)

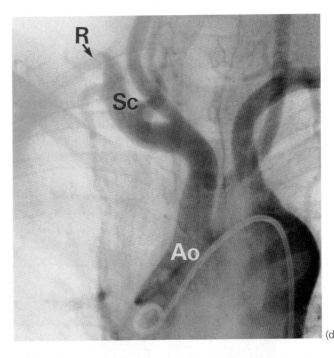

(d)

Fig. 36.8 Continued
(c) and **(d)** Show arch arteriography **(c)** With the shoulder adducted, there is normal blood flow through the subclavian artery **Sc**. Note the presence of a cervical rib R and dilatation of the subclavian artery just distal to it. This was a post-stenotic aneurysm **An** containing thrombus, which gave rise to distal embolism. The aorta is labelled **Ao**. **(d)** With the shoulder abducted and externally rotated ('the army saluting position'), subclavian blood flow is completely obstructed by the cervical rib; note the 'pigtail' arteriogram catheter in the aorta **Ao**.

EXTRACRANIAL CEREBRAL ARTERIAL INSUFFICIENCY

Extracranial atherosclerosis is common and is probably responsible for about one-third of all strokes. The common carotid bifurcation is the area most affected by atherosclerosis although obstructive disease may affect the distal internal carotid in the carotid siphon. The vertebral arteries are next most commonly affected. Less commonly, the orifices of the great vessels become obstructed where they leave the aortic arch.

CAROTID ARTERY STENOSIS

PATHOPHYSIOLOGY OF CAROTID ARTERY STENOSIS

Carotid artery atheroma often results in stenosis, with cerebral blood flow becoming critically impaired when luminal narrowing exceeds about 70% (Fig. 36.9). Rough atherosclerotic plaques without gross narrowing may also be the source of platelet emboli. Small emboli may cause transient ischaemic attacks (including transient blindness, known as **amaurosis fugax**), whereas large emboli or emboli into critical areas cause major strokes. Asymptomatic stenoses may be discovered on investi-

gation of carotid bruits or as part of the general investigation before major arterial surgery elsewhere in the body.

INVESTIGATION OF SUSPECTED EXTRACRANIAL VASCULAR DISEASE

A minority of patients suffering transient ischaemic attacks or stroke are found to have a **bruit** on auscultation of the carotid arteries. However, this finding does not indicate the degree of narrowing. Indeed, a significant stenosis may be silent, as of course is complete occlusion.

Patients with strokes, asymptomatic carotid bruits and transient ischaemic attacks should initially be investigated by non-invasive means. The preferred method is **duplex Doppler scanning**, an ultrasound technique which allows simultaneous imaging of the carotid arteries and measurement of blood flow velocity. The rise in velocity allows the degree of stenosis to be derived. If there is a high-grade stenosis (i.e. over 70%) in symptomatic disease, surgical intervention is the treatment of choice. With skilled duplex examination, many surgeons feel that

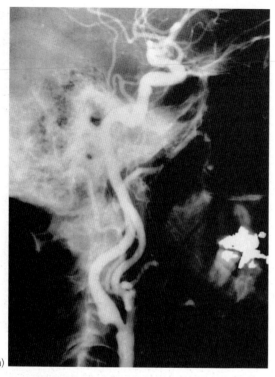

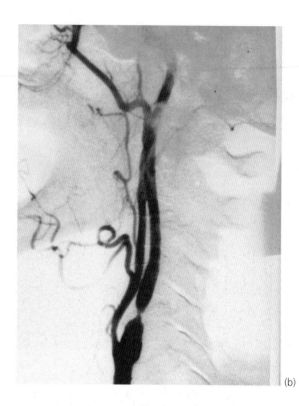

(a)

(b)

Fig. 36.9 Carotid artery disease

(a) This 71-year-old man suffered two transient episodes of left hemiparesis in one week ('TIAs'). Carotid angiography shows a localised 50% stenosis of the internal carotid artery just distal to the common carotid bifurcation; this degree of stenosis alone would not explain the symptoms. Note the typical post-stenotic dilatation immediately beyond the stenosis. The rest of the cerebral arterial system appears normal. At operation, an ulcerated atheromatous plaque was found, which was undoubtedly the source of emboli which caused the transient ischaemic attacks. Endarterectomy was performed and the patient has been entirely well since. Studies in the USA and Europe have shown surgery is definitely better than medical management in patients with a 70% or greater stenosis. **(b)** Subtraction film from a carotid angiogram in a different patient. This shows a 90% stenosis in the internal carotid artery which is haemodynamically significant, causing cerebral ischaemia on its own account.

carotid angiography is no longer necessary; this invasive technique carries a risk of stroke and is being replaced by duplex Doppler alone in uncomplicated cases.

TREATMENT OF EXTRACRANIAL ARTERIAL DISEASE

The role of surgery in managing extracranial vascular disease has become much clearer since publication of major randomised studies in the USA and Europe. The choice of treatment for symptomatic carotid artery stenosis is between **medical antiplatelet therapy** with aspirin 75–150 mg or clopidogrel 75 mg daily and **surgical endarterectomy**. Carotid endarterectomy enjoyed an enormous vogue in the 1970s and 1980s for treating transient ischaemic attacks, completed stroke and asymptomatic carotid stenosis, particularly in the USA. Scientific comparative studies have shown that in patients with carotid stenosis of greater than 70%, surgery reduces the annual stroke rate from about 6% in the medically treated group to about 1.5%. For lesser degrees of stenosis, surgery has not proved advantageous, although studies are continuing. Even in high-

grade stenosis, surgery does not reduce long-term mortality from carotid artery disease. The mortality rate of about 5% per annum over 5 years is comparable in medically and surgically treated patients, taking the operative mortality of 2–3% into account.

Currently about 2000 carotid endarterectomies are performed annually in the UK, but this is rising now the indications for surgical treatment of severe stenoses are clear. At present, seven males are treated for carotid artery stenosis for every three females.

The usual operation for carotid artery stenosis is **endarterectomy**. The carotid bifurcation is opened longitudinally after clamping the carotid arteries and anticoagulating the patient. A shunt is commonly used to maintain cerebral perfusion; this involves placing a tube in the common carotid below the stenosis and into the internal carotid above the stenosis, bypassing the operation site. The stenotic plaque is then removed and the carotid sutured directly or repaired with a vein patch sutured into the wall to maintain the diameter. Carotid surgery carries an appreciable risk of mortality or cerebral complications such as stroke which need to be taken into account when assessing individual departmental results and when comparing groups of patients treated medically and surgically.

SUBCLAVIAN STEAL SYNDROME

This unusual syndrome is caused by obstruction of the subclavian artery proximal to the origin of the vertebral artery. In consequence the subclavian is fed by retrograde flow from the vertebral artery via the carotids and circle of Willis. This situation remains tenable until there is excessive demand by the upper limb. At that point, blood becomes diverted ('stolen') from the cerebral circulation causing transient cerebral ischaemia. Figure 36.10 illustrates a classic example. Treatment is to bypass the obstruction with a graft.

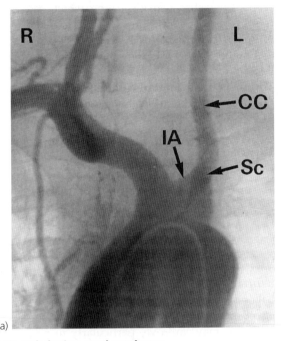

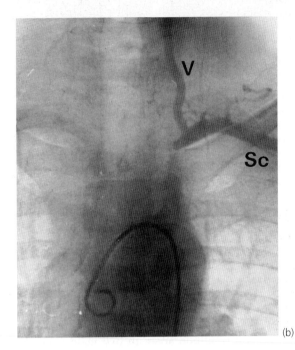

(a)

(b)

Fig. 36.10 Subclavian steal syndrome
Subtraction angiograms from a 55-year-old house-painter who complained of dizziness when painting walls and ceilings. **(a)** Aortic arch (with 'pigtail' arteriogram catheter visible) showing normal right innominate artery with its subclavian and common carotid branches. On the left, the arterial anatomy is anomalous, with the common carotid **CC** arising from an innominate artery **IA** rather than direct from the aorta. The left subclavian artery **Sc** appears to be occluded beyond a short stump. **(b)** X-ray exposure taken 4 seconds later; the aortic arch and its branches are now clear but contrast has appeared in the left vertebral artery **V**, flowing downwards from the circle of Willis. This has flowed onwards to fill the left subclavian artery **Sc** retrogradely. Thus there is complete obstruction of a segment of the left subclavian artery proximal to the origin of the vertebral artery, and the vertebral artery supplies the left upper limb at the expense of the cerebral circulation. The results in episodes of transient cerebral ischaemia at times of high vascular demand from the left upper limb.

ARTERIAL INSUFFICIENCY IN OTHER ORGANS

MESENTERIC ISCHAEMIA

Blood supply to portions of the bowel may be compromised in four main ways:

- **Strangulation.** This is a mechanical problem presenting as bowel obstruction. It is described in detail in Chapter 13. It may be the result of a **hernia** (see Ch. 26), **volvulus** (see Ch. 22) or **fibrous bands** resulting from previous surgery (see Ch. 47)
- **Acute thrombotic or embolic obstruction** (Fig. 36.11). This is analogous to acute thrombosis or embolism of the lower limb, as described in Chapter 35. The cause is usually superior mesenteric artery occlusion and the condition presents as an 'acute abdomen' (see Ch. 13)
- **Transient ischaemia.** This presents as inflammation of the bowel characterised by abdominal pain and rectal bleeding. The condition is known as **ischaemic colitis** and is discussed at the end of Chapter 21
- **Chronic mesenteric artery insufficiency.** This condition presents with gross weight loss and abdominal pain following eating; it is analogous to intermittent claudication due to arterial insufficiency in the lower limb and is described in the next section

479

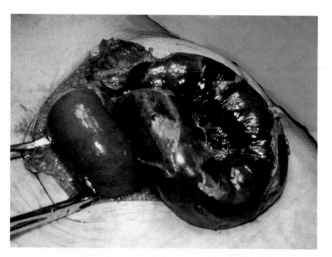

Fig. 36.11 This woman of 77 presented with moderate abdominal pain and circulatory collapse requiring vigorous resuscitation. She was in atrial fibrillation and was acidotic. Mesenteric embolism was suspected and was confirmed at operation. Unfortunately, as often happens, the entire mid-gut territory, between 20 cm along the jejunum to the mid-transverse colon was necrotic and no beneficial procedure was possible.

CHRONIC MESENTERIC ISCHAEMIA

The rare condition of chronic mesenteric ischaemia or '**gut claudication**' occurs when the visceral blood supply is restricted to a point where it is adequate at rest but inadequate during active digestion. This occurs when there is gross atherosclerotic narrowing of the three main mesenteric vessels (coeliac, superior mesenteric and inferior mesenteric arteries). These patients present with severe epigastric pain on eating which causes 'fear of food'. There is always gross weight loss and sometimes an epigastric bruit can be heard on auscultation.

Diagnosis is by arteriography with a lateral projection allowing the origins of the three main vessels to be seen. Treatment is by surgical reconstruction of the origins of one or more of the mesenteric arteries.

RENAL ISCHAEMIA

RENAL ARTERY STENOSIS

PATHOPHYSIOLOGY OF RENAL ARTERY STENOSIS

This uncommon condition arises in two main ways. In children and young adults, the cause is **fibromuscular hyperplasia**. In older patients, **atherosclerosis** is the usual cause. Renal artery stenosis may present with hypertension (ischaemia of one or both kidneys causes poor perfusion, thus activating the renin–angiotensin system) or functional renal impairment. It is sometimes discovered incidentally on urography as a non-functioning or poorly functioning kidney.

Fibromuscular hyperplasia responds well to balloon dilatation, which often results in the blood pressure returning to normal. Atherosclerosis may be treatable by balloon angioplasty or reconstructive surgery but the effect on hypertension is unpredictable; renal function, however, may improve, particularly in patients with a short history of hypertension or if the renal artery stenosis is bilateral.

It is important that renal artery stenosis is recognised in patients needing aortic reconstructive surgery, whether this is for occlusive or aneurysmal disease. This is because hypotension during the operation may initiate thrombotic occlusion of narrowed renal arteries. This causes postoperative renal failure. Renal artery stenosis should be treated before operation by balloon dilatation, or by reconstruction at the same time as the aortic operation.

37 | Venous disorders of the lower limb

VENOUS THROMBOSIS AND THE POST-THROMBOTIC LIMB

ANATOMY OF THE LOWER LIMB VENOUS SYSTEM

Blood is drained from the lower limb via two separate systems. The **deep venous system** drains the deep tissues of the foot and muscles of the lower leg and thigh. These deep veins lie within the mass of lower limb muscles, and include the large **soleal venous sinuses**. Muscle contraction during walking and other exercise provides an essential mechanism for pumping blood back towards the heart against gravity. Reverse flow is prevented by numerous valves in the system.

The skin and tissues superficial to the deep fascia drain mainly into the **superficial venous system** which comprises two main vessels, the **long (great) saphenous vein** and the **short (small) saphenous vein**. The long saphenous vein receives tributaries from the antero-medial aspect of the limb (and lower anterior abdominal wall), and penetrates the deep fascia in the groin to drain into the femoral vein. The short saphenous vein drains the posterior part of the leg and passes through the deep fascia of the calf to flow into the popliteal vein, part of the deep venous system. There are numerous other interconnecting superficial veins that will drain venous blood from the limb if refluxing long or short saphenous veins are removed. The superficial system has no muscular pump to aid venous return but valves normally guard against retrograde flow, particularly at the sapheno-femoral junction and the sapheno-popliteal junction. A number of **perforating veins** drain blood from the superficial system into the deep system; valves normally ensure one-way flow. Most of the perforators are on the medial part of the leg above the ankle but there is a fairly constant **'Hunterian perforator'** in the medial mid-thigh.

PRESENTATION AND CONSEQUENCES OF DEEP VENOUS THROMBOSIS

Deep venous thrombosis (DVT) in the lower limb most commonly occurs as a complication of a major operation, lower limb fractures, myocardial infarction or other severe illness. In the past, DVTs were commonplace after childbirth but early mobilisation has considerably reduced the incidence. About one-third of DVTs present with no apparent cause and these are usually managed by physicians. Many of these patients have a detectable **prothrombotic state**. The risk factors, clinical presentations and management of acute DVT and pulmonary embolism are discussed in Chapter 47.

Deep venous thrombosis in the lower limb is an acute local problem with the added risk of a potentially fatal pulmonary embolism; however, it may also lead to major long-term complications in the lower limb. The severity of post-thrombotic problems generally reflects the extent of the initial DVT. The affected extremity is known as a **post-thrombotic limb** or, less accurately, a **post-phlebitic limb**.

A high proportion of patients undergoing major operations who have risk factors for deep venous thrombosis can be shown (using sensitive radionuclide techniques) to develop asymptomatic thrombi in calf veins despite lack of clinical evidence of thrombosis. Such 'silent' thromboses may explain the occurrence of typical post-thrombotic changes in patients where there is no history of an acute thrombotic episode.

PATHOPHYSIOLOGY OF POST-THROMBOTIC PROBLEMS

Provided fatal pulmonary embolism has not occurred, deep venous thromboses gradually undergo organisation and recanalisation. In the process, valves in the deep veins can be damaged and become incompetent allowing reflux, thus leading to **chronic venous insufficiency**. The syndrome usually takes years to develop; the prolonged interval makes it easy to forget this important reason for trying to prevent deep venous thrombosis in hospital patients! In patients where the proximal veins have been completely occluded by thrombus, recanalisation may not occur at all or else is incomplete. This leaves venous outflow obstruction and the consequences are more marked and appear sooner.

In the normal adult limb, venous pressure at the ankle while standing is about 125 cm of water. This falls markedly during walking as a result of the calf pump. In contrast, in the post-thrombotic limb, where deep venous valves allow reflux or, worse still, veins are occluded, ankle venous pressure remains high during calf muscle activity. This leads to incompetence of valves in the perforating veins. Blood is forced into the superficial system, causing venous hypertension and disrupting the normal vascular dynamics of the skin and subcutaneous tissues. This may result in impaired skin vitality and healing ability.

The following factors probably contribute to the clinical outcome:

- Venous stagnation restricts arterial replenishment of capillary blood
- Arteriovenous shunts beneath the affected skin divert blood away from the dermal capillaries
- Venous hypertension causes dilatation of the local venules and capillary network, allowing plasma proteins to leak into the interstitial spaces. Fibrin polymerises forming **pericapillary cuffs** but these probably do not interfere with metabolic exchange between blood and tissues

Characteristic local signs of a gross post-thrombotic limb are listed in Box 37.1.

The post-thrombotic syndrome should also be suspected when a patient presents with lesser degrees of skin change. The majority, however, will prove to have only superficial venous insufficiency.

INVESTIGATION OF VENOUS INSUFFICIENCY

When a patient presents with ankle ulceration, a chronically swollen limb or typical skin change of venous insufficiency around the ankle, suspicion may be raised of chronic venous insufficiency due to superficial venous reflux or post-thrombotic changes or both. The diagnostic pathway develops in response to the following questions:

1. Is the condition venous in origin? This is suggested by a history of DVT, prolonged bed rest, lower limb fractures or a finding of varicose veins or a 'champagne-bottle' leg (Fig. 37.1). If the condition is not venous, another cause of ulceration and swelling should be sought
2. Is there superficial venous insufficiency (Fig. 37.2 later), deep venous insufficiency, or a combination of both?
3. How much of a contribution is made by superficial venous insufficiency? (This is likely to respond to surgery, unlike deep venous reflux)

When there are small areas of skin change or ulceration which correlate with the degree of superficial venous

---

KEY POINTS

Box 37.1 Signs of a gross post-thrombotic limb
- Chronic lower leg swelling with brawny oedema
- Varicose veins with incompetent perforating veins
- Inflammation and haemosiderin pigmentation in the area above the medial malleolus (the 'gaiter' area) and other parts of the lower half of the leg known as **varicose eczema**. This may be complicated by low-grade cellulitis
- Active or healed venous ulceration above the medial malleolus
- **Lipo-dermatosclerosis** around the ankle (replacement of soft subcutaneous fat with firm collagen). This causes the 'champagne-bottle leg' with oedema above and a narrow atrophic ankle below

---

incompetence, these can be treated surgically as uncomplicated varicose veins. If there are marked skin changes, the anatomy of the deep venous system and the competence of valves in the deep veins need investigation. **Venography** used to be the 'gold standard' but latterly, skilled assessment with **duplex colour-flow Doppler ultrasound** is proving more informative and less invasive than venography.

Ambulatory venous pressure can be measured at the ankle during repeated calf muscle contraction, using direct cannulation. As described earlier, high venous pressure during calf exercise is a feature of the post-thrombotic limb; however, it may also be caused by excessive pressure in the superficial venous system due to incompetence of the valve at the sapheno-femoral junction or other thigh perforators. If ambulatory venous pressure is high, the measurement is repeated with an above-knee tourniquet in place. Any fall in the ambulatory venous pressure is then attributable to superficial venous incompetence, which can be treated by surgery. Deep venous incompetence is not generally amenable to surgery, and treatment is necessarily conservative.

MANAGEMENT OF POST-THROMBOTIC PROBLEMS

The main post-thrombotic problems requiring active treatment are chronic ulcers and cellulitis.

Venous ulcers

Ulcers may develop spontaneously but are more commonly initiated by minor trauma which fails to heal, often complicated by secondary infection.

The majority of venous ulcers can be healed by simple non-operative methods, provided treatment is applied effectively and assiduously. Even if operative treatment is required, conservative measures should be used to prepare the limb. These include reducing swelling by

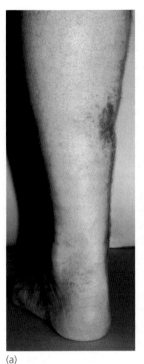
(a)

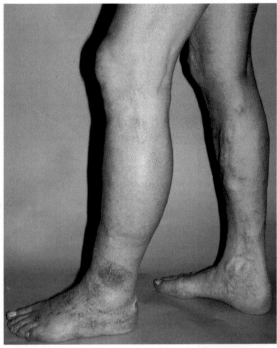
(b)

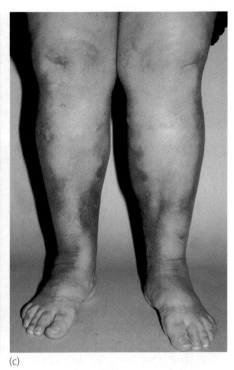
(c)

Fig. 37.1 Post-thrombotic limbs and venous eczema
(a) Healed venous ulcer showing local loss of subcutaneous fat and surrounding pigmentation. **(b)** Man of 66 with no history of DVT showing marked swelling of the left leg with pigmentation in the lateral gaiter area representing venous eczema. The right leg has moderate varicose veins; the blue discolouration around both ankles is an age change due to dilated venules and is of no clinical importance. On colour duplex ultrasound examination, there was evidence of deep venous thrombotic damage in the left leg. **(c)** Bilateral post-thrombotic limbs in a woman of 57 with gross venous eczema, fat atrophy, signs of healed venous ulceration and varicose veins.

bandaging, removing necrotic tissue from the ulcer base and controlling cellulitis. Support and compression of the skin and superficial tissues is the mainstay of treatment. This may be provided by elastic bandages or correctly sized graded compression stockings. In either case, the aim is for pressure to be greatest at the ankle (about 20 mmHg), reducing progressively up the limb. Great care must be taken to ensure that pressure does not cause ischaemia or abrasions over tendons or bony prominences. The main contraindication to the use of compression is severe chronic ischaemia, where pressure could further reduce arterial input. Most venous ulcers can be rapidly healed while keeping the patient ambulatory by competent multi-layer bandaging (the Charing Cross technique uses four layers), avoiding the need for hospital care except for complications or skin grafting.

Spreading cellulitis should be treated with systemic antibiotics. Infection confined to the ulcer is treated by excision of dead tissue if necessary and simple dressings such as saline soaks; use of antiseptics may retard granulation tissue and epithelialisation. Local applications of antibiotics have no place in the management of ulcers.

Surgical treatment may be indicated, particularly if there is superficial venous incompetence. Varicose veins should be ligated or removed. More controversial is surgical disruption or ligation of incompetent perforating

veins, even if performed by subfascial endoscopic surgery (SEPS). Intractable or large ulcers may require skin grafting once the ulcer base is clean.

Long-term care and prevention

The uncomplicated post-thrombotic limb is debilitating enough to the patient, who is often elderly, without the added complication of chronic venous ulceration.

As soon as the condition is recognised, the patient should be encouraged to use appropriate graduated compression stockings and to take great care to avoid even minor trauma to the limb, especially to the area above the medial malleolus.

For minor venous insufficiency, well-fitting class I **graduated compression elastic stockings** or tights provide adequate support but care should be taken that there is no proximal constricting band to impair venous return. In more severe venous insufficiency, class II or III graded compression stockings are extremely valuable and may reverse the tissue damage or at least arrest its progress. In addition, they provide protection from minor trauma. Ideally they should be worn at all times except in bed. The importance of correctly fitted stockings should be emphasised; ideally, they should be supplied by an experienced surgical fitter.

483

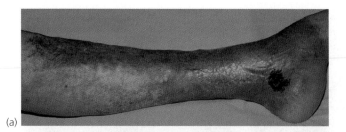

(a)

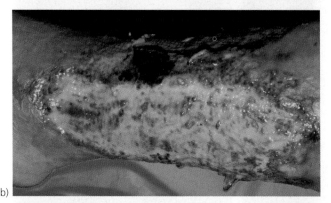

(b)

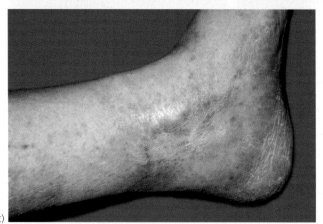

(c)

Fig. 37.2 Venous ulceration
(a) Post-thrombotic limb with marked venous pigmentation and a chronic ulcer which heals and breaks down periodically. **(b)** Chronic venous ulcer in a post-thrombotic limb. The ulcer is virtually circumferential and represents a serious management problem. **(c)** Chronic ulcer that healed several years before, following a Cockett's operation, an open procedure for subfascial ligation of perforators, the scar of which is visible. This operation can now be performed endoscopically in the SEPS procedure (see p. 483).

In many patients, effective elastic support will be required for life. Even so, subsequent episodes of cellulitis or ulceration are likely to occur.

AXILLARY VEIN THROMBOSIS

Axillary vein thrombosis is an uncommon condition representing the upper limb equivalent of DVT; it is usually managed by internal physicians, but may some-

times reach the surgeon. It usually presents with a sudden onset of swelling and aching pain in the whole arm. On examination, the hand, forearm and arm are swollen with a bluish tinge. Sensation is preserved. In most patients, no cause is found, but the condition can occur as a manifestation of visceral malignancy (**thrombophlebitis migrans**), or a blood disorder with raised viscosity, such as polycythaemia rubra vera. It is likely that most cases result from external compression of the subclavian vein between the first rib or a cervical rib and clavicle. The space may be congenitally reduced or excess physical activity such as weight lifting may cause local trauma. The usual treatment is anticoagulation to prevent propagation of thrombus and to encourage spontaneous clot lysis. Predisposing disorders should be sought. A few patients benefit from surgical excision of the first rib.

VARICOSE VEINS

Varicose veins are dilated, tortuous and prominent superficial veins in the lower limb (see Fig. 37.4). Varicose veins are very common, being present in about 20% of people aged 20 and increasing to 80% at 60 years. Nevertheless, only about 12% of those affected have symptoms or develop complications. Varicose veins are one of the most common reasons for surgical referral in developed countries, particularly when improved medical services are able to cope with the volume of more serious disease and where expectations for treatment are higher. The condition appears to be a product of an upright posture.

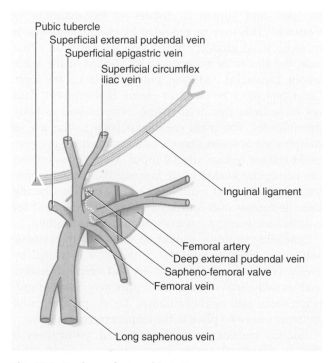

Fig. 37.3 Sapheno-femoral junction

PATHOPHYSIOLOGY OF VARICOSE VEINS

Abnormal communication between the deep and superficial venous systems appears to be the essential factor in the development of varicose veins. In most patients the process probably begins with failure of the valve at the sapheno-femoral junction. When this happens, an uninterrupted column of blood from the heart progressively dilates the veins down the leg (see Fig. 37.4a). Varicose veins usually develop slowly over 10–20 years, so that in most cases, surgical treatment is not urgent. The long saphenous system is involved in about 90% of cases and the short saphenous system in 25% (some have both systems involved).

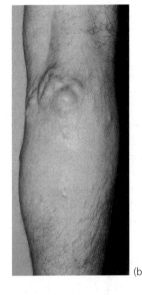

(a)   (b)

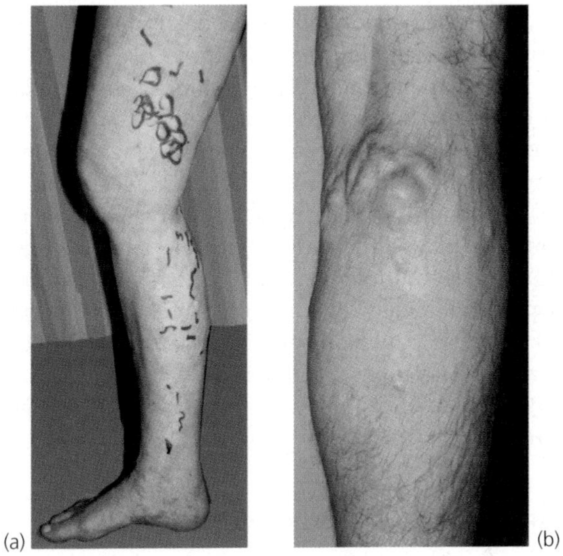

Fig. 37.4 Varicose veins
(a) Typical varicosities in the long saphenous territory evident both above and below knee and most prominent on the medial side of the limb. The black markings were made immediately prior to surgery by the operating surgeon. **(b)** Typical short saphenous varicosities, which do not extend above the knee. These veins could not be controlled with an above knee tourniquet and there was gross reflux evident on hand held Doppler examination, confirmed on colour duplex Doppler.

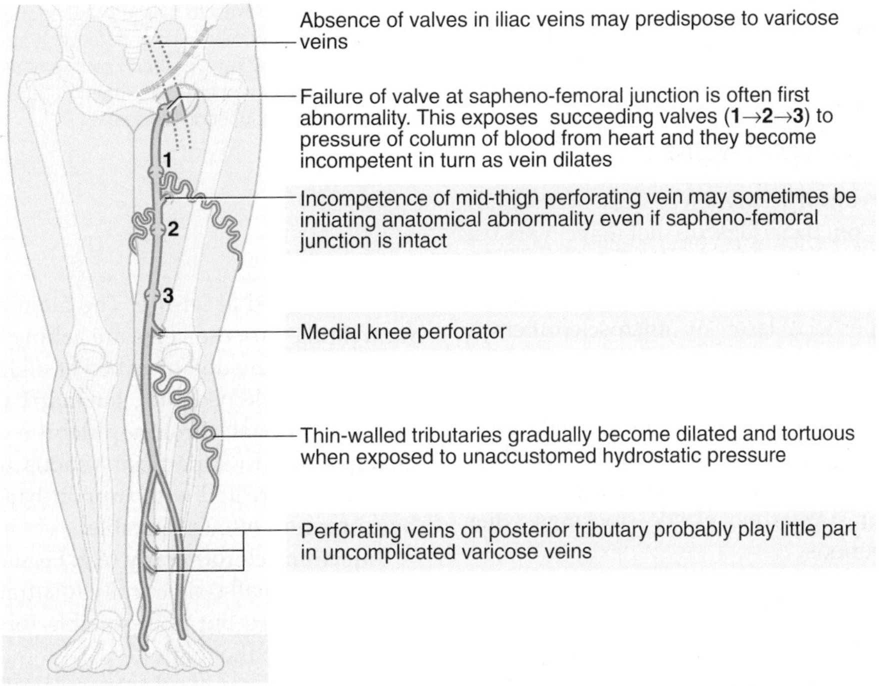

KEY POINTS

Box 37.2 Examination technique for varicose veins

● **Severity**—Examine the extent and severity of varicose veins with the patient standing. Many patients attend with unsightly 'spider veins' which are not varicose. Others attend for advice because they are worried their leg will break down with ulcers

● **Skin changes**—Examine the leg for swelling, ulcers and varicose eczema. Could this be a post-thrombotic limb?

● **Long or short saphenous**—Examine distribution of varicose veins. Are their varicosities above knee indicating probable sapheno-femoral incompetence? Could these be short saphenous system varicosities? i.e. postero-lateral calf feeding from popliteal fossa

---

Absence of valves in iliac veins may predispose to varicose veins

Failure of valve at sapheno-femoral junction is often first abnormality. This exposes succeeding valves (**1→2→3**) to pressure of column of blood from heart and they become incompetent in turn as vein dilates

Incompetence of mid-thigh perforating vein may sometimes be initiating anatomical abnormality even if sapheno-femoral junction is intact

Medial knee perforator

Thin-walled tributaries gradually become dilated and tortuous when exposed to unaccustomed hydrostatic pressure

Perforating veins on posterior tributary probably play little part in uncomplicated varicose veins

Fig. 37.5 Pathophysiology of varicose veins

Women are affected about six times more often than men, with the majority of varicose veins developing during or soon after the second or third pregnancy. An important factor is probably the high level of progesterone which causes changes in the structure of collagen (which may not later recover), as well as smooth muscle relaxation. Pressure on the pelvic veins by the enlarging uterus may contribute by restricting venous return.

In some patients, hereditary factors appear to play a part, especially in men, particularly those who develop varicose veins in their teens. Predisposing anatomical factors may include congenital lack of valves in the iliac veins or abnormal vein wall elasticity. Deep venous thrombosis plays little part in causing simple varicose veins. Rarely, multiple congenital arteriovenous fistulae (Klippel–Trynlawnay syndrome) cause gross varicose veins. In these patients, there is gigantism of the lower limb and often venous ulceration (see Ch. 40, p. 543).

A technique of examining varicose veins is shown in Figure 37.6.

SYMPTOMS AND SIGNS OF VARICOSE VEINS

The most common complaints related to varicose veins are:

- Aching legs, usually after standing all day
- Poor cosmetic appearance, especially in summer when the legs are exposed
- Fear of future leg ulcers ('like my mother had')
- Fear of varicosities progressing
- Worry about varicosities bleeding, particularly if traumatised
- Varicose eczema or ulcers
- Ankle oedema
- Recurrent superficial thrombophlebitis

MANAGEMENT OF VARICOSE VEINS

Many patients who consult a surgeon because of unsightly vascular markings on their legs do not have varicose veins. Instead, these are often 'spider veins' or dilated superficial venules. Cosmetic treatment includes covering cosmetics and superficial laser or microsclerotherapy using injected sclerosants. Many patients have long-standing varicose veins with no complications, and merely seek reassurance that they will not ulcerate in the future. Surgical treatment is not usually necessary for these patients but advice can be given to elevate the legs when sitting and to wear supporting elastic stockings when standing for long periods.

Indications for surgical treatment of varicose veins

Surgical treatment for varicose veins is to a large extent cosmetic or to prevent future complications, and operation

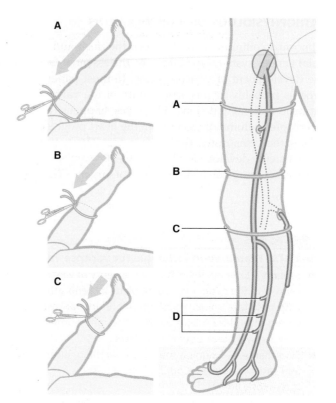

Fig. 37.6 Technique of examining varicose veins
Elevate limb and ensure veins are emptied by massaging distal to proximal. Apply tourniquet tightly around upper thigh **A** and stand patient up. Does tourniquet prevent veins filling and removing it cause rapid filling from above? If so, main communication is a sapheno-femoral junction. If veins fill rapidly despite tourniquet, repeat the test with tourniquet above knee **B**. If this controls filling, then main communication is mid-thigh perforator. If this tourniquet fails to control filling, repeat below knee **C**. If this controls filling, communication is likely to be short saphenous-popliteal incompetence or medial knee perforator incompetence. If no tourniquet controls filling, communication is probably by one or more distal perforating veins often post thrombotic **D**. Note that 90% of varicose veins involve the long saphenous system.

can be planned at leisure. The main medical indications for treating varicose veins are **aching legs** after standing, relieved by elevation or in bed at night (particularly with unilateral ankle oedema), **haemorrhage** from a varicose vein, **superficial thrombophlebitis** and **varicose skin changes** due to superficial venous insufficiency. All of these can be treated with support bandages or stockings, but surgery is often preferable.

Injection sclerotherapy (e.g. Fegan technique) is used for treating small cosmetically unattractive varicose veins below the knee but is unsuitable for major varicosities, particularly in the thigh.

The techniques of injection sclerotherapy and surgery for varicose veins are shown in Figure 37.7.

(a) Injection sclerotherapy for minor varicose veins (after Fegan)

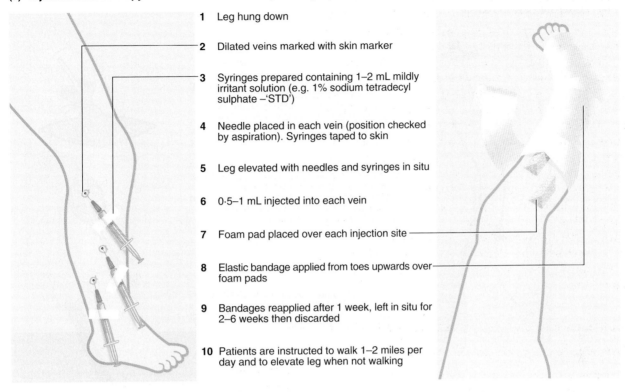

1 Leg hung down

2 Dilated veins marked with skin marker

3 Syringes prepared containing 1–2 mL mildly irritant solution (e.g. 1% sodium tetradecyl sulphate –'STD')

4 Needle placed in each vein (position checked by aspiration). Syringes taped to skin

5 Leg elevated with needles and syringes in situ

6 0·5–1 mL injected into each vein

7 Foam pad placed over each injection site

8 Elastic bandage applied from toes upwards over foam pads

9 Bandages reapplied after 1 week, left in situ for 2–6 weeks then discarded

10 Patients are instructed to walk 1–2 miles per day and to elevate leg when not walking

(b) Operations for varicose veins

(i) HIGH SAPHENOUS LIGATION

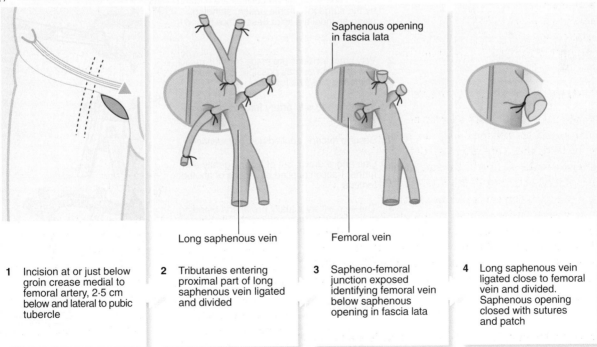

Saphenous opening in fascia lata

Long saphenous vein

Femoral vein

1 Incision at or just below groin crease medial to femoral artery, 2·5 cm below and lateral to pubic tubercle

2 Tributaries entering proximal part of long saphenous vein ligated and divided

3 Sapheno-femoral junction exposed identifying femoral vein below saphenous opening in fascia lata

4 Long saphenous vein ligated close to femoral vein and divided. Saphenous opening closed with sutures and patch

Fig. 37.7 Treatment of varicose veins

(b) **Operations for varicose veins**

(ii) LONG SAPHENOUS STRIP

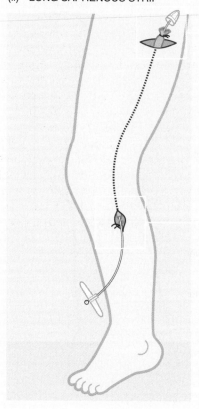

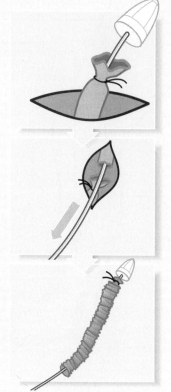

1 The stripper is a long flexible wire with a bullet-shaped knob on the 'business' end. The entry vein (proximal or distal, according to choice) is prepared as shown and the narrow end of the stripper passed down or up the long saphenous vein until it can be brought out to the surface

2 Stripping is usually downward. The vein is ligated to the wire at the bullet end and the narrow end is pulled smoothly and firmly, tearing off tributaries and any perforators on the way, emerging with the complete vein bunched up on the stripper

3 The wounds are closed and the limb firmly bandaged to minimise subcutaneous bleeding. Patients should be warned to expect postoperative bruising

(iii) AVULSION OF VARICOSITIES

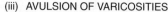

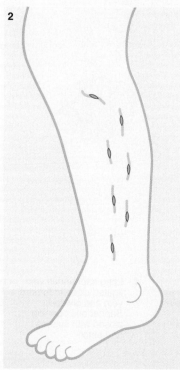

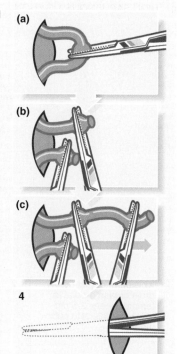

1 Before operation, all varicosities are marked by the surgeon with the patient standing, using an indelible spirit based fibre-tipped pen

2 Very small incisions are made over the marks and as much vein as possible is pulled out ('nick and pick') as follows:

(a) Vein grasped with artery forceps or special vein hook

(b) Second forceps applied and vein divided

(c) One end is drawn out of wound gently and further traction applied by means of another forceps

3 The vein will eventually break and bleeding is controlled by finger pressure. The process is repeated for the other end of vein

4 Forceps can be passed subcutaneously to retrieve nearby varices thus reducing the number of incisions required

5 Each wound is left open or closed neatly with 'steristrips', a fine suture or staple and non-adherent gauze applied to each one. The limb is bandaged firmly from toes proximally using an elastic bandage

Fig. 37.7 Surgical treatment of varicose veins (Continued)

Perioperative management of the patient having varicose vein surgery

Varicose veins must be **marked out** on the legs before operation. This should be done by the surgeon who will actually do the operation. An indelible marker must be used so that marks are not washed off by the patient or by skin preparation in the operating theatre. The patient must stand, often for some minutes, to allow the veins to fill, and marking should be performed in this position. Most surgeons mark all the prominent veins that are visible or palpable. Extra marks are often added for reas needing special surgical attention like suspected perforating veins.

Any patient with a history of venous thrombosis, whether deep or superficial, should be prescribed **low-dose subcutaneous heparin**. Patients with other risk factors for deep venous thrombosis, especially obese patients, should have the same prophylactic treatment. The first dose of heparin should be given 1 hour before operation.

Immediately after operation, non-adherent dressings are applied to all the incisions, and the whole leg is bandaged firmly with an elastic bandage. The patient should then be mobilised and encouraged to walk about. Twenty-four hours later, all dressings can be removed and the bandage exchanged for a graduated elastic stocking. On return home, patients should keep as active as possible, walking on a treadmill or outside the house for a few hundred metres or cycling a kilometre or two, several times a day for the first 2 weeks. When the patient is sitting, the legs should be elevated, and the patient should get up and walk around about every half-hour. All these measures are designed to discourage venous stagnation and venous thrombosis. Most patients can return to work after 1 week and can drive a car 24 hours after operation. The patient should be warned that the legs are likely to be bruised when the bandages are removed.

38 Cardiac surgery

This chapter is intended to give a flavour of the range and scope of work performed by cardiac surgeons and to provide an introduction to larger reference texts for those seeking greater detail. Heart and lung transplantation is discussed in Chapter 4.

INTRODUCTION

Surgery of the heart fascinated surgeons for many years. However, until the 1950s, only a very limited range of cardiac procedures was possible. These included **closed mitral valvotomy** for mitral stenosis and several ingenious methods of closing atrial septal defects in the beating heart. More extensive cardiac surgery became a reality when an effective mechanical device to circulate and oxygenate the blood during open heart surgery appeared in 1953. For the first time, a patient could be supported artificially with the heart and lungs bypassed whilst surgery took place in a motionless, blood-free field. Since then, the specialty of cardiac surgery has expanded and developed rapidly. Now very few cardiac operations are performed without bypass, and these are mostly palliative procedures for congenital heart disease. As a result of the availability of cardiopulmonary bypass, the early emphasis on uncomplicated surgery for congenital heart disease has shifted markedly towards more ambitious techniques for treating acquired heart disease. More recently, in keeping with the move towards minimal access in other areas, attempts are being made to perform coronary artery surgery via small incisions without bypass. However, further development is needed before this can become generally available.

For coronary artery surgery, a bloodless field is created by clamping the aorta at a point between the origins of the coronary arteries and the insertion point of the aortic cannula site through which the arterial blood returns from the bypass machine (see Fig. 38.1). Without coronary blood supply, however, the myocardium becomes anoxic and is at risk of infarction. Potential ischaemic damage is minimised by **cold cardioplegia** which reduces the metabolic demands of the heart as follows (see Table 38.1 below):

● The myocardium is cooled to between 4–12°C by infusing electrolyte solution at 4°C (see Table 38.1)
● The mechanical action of the heart is arrested by the high potassium content of the solution (16 mmol/L KCl)

Several actual and potential problems arise when blood is exposed to an extracorporeal circuit:

● The clotting cascade is activated, causing intravascular coagulation of blood. Preventing this by using heparin as an anticoagulant has been crucial in allowing cardiopulmonary bypass. High-dose heparin (300 IU/kg) is given systemically before the heart is cannulated. After the operation, the patient is weaned off cardiopulmonary bypass, the extracorporeal circuit removed and the heparin reversed with protamine sulphate

Table 38.1 Constituents of a typical infusate for cold cardioplegia (St Thomas's solution)

Constituent	Quantity
Sodium chloride	110.0 mmol/L
Potassium chloride	16.0 mmol/L
Magnesium chloride	16.0 mmol/L
Calcium chloride	1.2 mmol/L
Sodium bicarbonate	10.0 mmol/L
Procaine	16.0 mmol/L

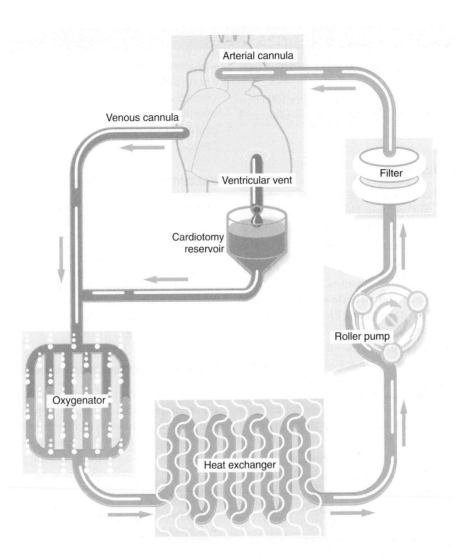

Fig. 38.1 The standard circuit for cardiopulmonary bypass

1. Systemic venous blood is siphoned into a reservoir by gravity
2. Collected blood is exposed to oxygen
3. Blood is passed through a heat exchanger allowing for body cooling or rewarming
4. Oxygenated and temperature-controlled blood is pumped under pressure into the systemic arterial circulation

Snares are placed around both superior and inferior vena cava to prevent air entering the right-sided cardiac chambers which would lock the gravity siphon. In this way any of the four cardiac chambers can be entered for surgical access.

- Clotting factors and platelets are consumed within the extracorporeal circuit (mainly within the oxygenator) leading to a bleeding diathesis. Blood products may be needed to reverse this
- The complement cascade and other factors involved in inflammation are activated to a variable extent

ASSESSING RISK IN CARDIAC SURGERY

Since the range of procedures in cardiac surgery is limited, the discipline is relatively easy to audit and nearly all cardiac units now undertake detailed audit. Comparison of results between units allows suitable standards to be developed and maintained. Apart from surgical and anaesthetic skill, there are many patient-related factors likely to affect the final outcome of, for example, aortic valve replacement. Several scoring systems have been devised to attempt to predict relative risk in such cases. None is completely reliable but the **Parsonnet scoring system** is perhaps the most widely used. Most systems predict the risk of perioperative death by totalling up a series of individual risk scores which take account of the surgical procedure and its urgency, and patient factors including pre-existing cardiac disease and general co-morbidity.

Section
3

CONGENITAL CARDIAC DISEASE

TYPES OF CONGENITAL HEART DISEASE

Congenital heart disease is found in about 2 per 1000 live births and falls into two main groups: those with and those without cyanosis.

CYANOTIC HEART DISEASE

Cyanotic heart disease occurs when there is mixing of systemic arterial and venous blood through a predominantly right-to-left cardiac shunt. The most common examples are:

● **Tetralogy of Fallot**—there is ventricular septal defect (VSD) with pulmonary artery stenosis, right ventricular hypertrophy and an aorta which overrides the ventricular septum, thus taking blood from both ventricles
● **Transposition of the great arteries**—the pulmonary artery arises from the left ventricle and the aorta from the right ventricle
● **Tricuspid atresia**—there is absence of a functional tricuspid valve
● **Truncus arteriosus**—pulmonary artery and aorta fail to develop separately
● **Total anomalous pulmonary venous drainage**—pulmonary venous blood drains into the right side of the heart
● **Eisenmenger's syndrome**—increased pulmonary blood flow due to a pre-existing left-to-right shunt (see next section) causes severe pulmonary hypertension resulting in spontaneous reversal of the shunt so that flow becomes right-to-left

ACYANOTIC HEART DISEASE

Acyanotic congenital heart disease may involve:

● A shunt from left to right sides of the heart (e.g. via an atrial or ventricular septal defect) or a ductus arteriosus which remains in its patent antenatal state (PDA)
● Failed or incomplete embryological development of parts of the heart or great vessels without shunting, e.g. coarctation of the aorta

MANAGEMENT OF CONGENITAL HEART DISEASE

Surgical management of congenital heart disease aims to palliate its effects or to correct the defect or defects mechanically, or else both in sequence.

Early in the history of cardiac surgery, palliation was often all that could be offered. Later, initial palliation was sometimes followed by a second-stage corrective operation carried out when the child was larger. Nowadays, corrective procedures are usually offered at the outset, as operations have become more customary, myocardial protection is more predictable and operative risks are lower.

PALLIATING CONGENITAL CARDIAC DISORDERS

When pulmonary blood flow is reduced (as in tricuspid atresia, tetralogy of Fallot or pulmonary artery stenosis), palliation aims to increase pulmonary flow by creating a shunt between the systemic arterial circulation and the pulmonary artery (see Fig. 38.2).

When pulmonary blood flow is too great (e.g. VSD or truncus arteriosus), the aim is to reduce the flow by artificially narrowing the main pulmonary artery using external banding.

CORRECTING CONGENITAL CARDIAC DISORDERS

Surgical correction of congenital heart disease is based on accurately identifying the lesion or lesions and performing procedures which restore the normal flow and functioning of the heart. Correction may be mechanically straightforward as in the following procedures:

● Closing a persisting ductus arteriosus (PDA)
● Resecting the narrowed segment of descending aorta in coarctation of the aorta
● Closing an atrial or ventricular septal defect

In other cases, correction may be complex: for example: total correction of Fallot's or of anomalous pulmonary venous drainage. Procedures such as these should only be performed in specialist paediatric cardiac surgical units.

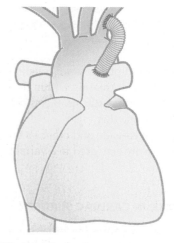

Fig. 38.2 Palliation of tetralogy of Fallot
Modified Blalock–Taussig shunt.

ACQUIRED HEART DISEASE

The different types of acquired heart disease are listed in Table 38.2.

CORONARY ARTERY DISEASE

PATHOPHYSIOLOGY

Coronary heart disease (ischaemic heart disease) is nearly always atherosclerotic in origin, with subintimal thickening due to deposition of cholesterol-containing lipid together with hyperplasia of smooth muscle cells in the media which migrate into the subintimal area. These changes all reduce the luminal diameter. As blood flow through a vessel is related to the fourth power of the radius (Poiseuille's Law), only small changes in cross-sectional area in small arteries are needed to cause a dramatic reduction in coronary artery blood flow. When coronary artery disease is being assessed on angiography, 50% reduction in cross-sectional area is regarded as significant.

Acute coronary ischaemia is usually brought on by thrombosis of already narrowed coronary arteries, in some cases precipitated by haemorrhage into atherosclerotic plaques.

The world-wide distribution of coronary atherosclerosis is patchy. It is predominantly a disease of developed

Table 38.2 Types of acquired heart disease

Type	Pathophysiology	Clinical presentation
Ischaemic heart disease	Usually caused by coronary atheroma and rarely by spasm, embolism or trauma	1. Reversible ischaemia presenting as angina 2. Painless or silent ischaemia discovered incidentally 3. Myocardial infarction
Valvular heart disease, affecting aortic, mitral, tricuspid or pulmonary valves	1. Congenital valve disorders (e.g. bicuspid aortic valve) predisposing the valve to later malfunction, degeneration or disease 2. Rheumatic valvular heart disease—mitral valve most common; also affects aortic valve (occasionally follows rheumatic fever, causing thickening and tethering of leaflets, shortening of mitral valve chordae and valve calcification) 3. Secondary involvement of valves caused by disruption of nearby structures: — aortic dissection involving the aortic valve — myocardial infarction involving the papillary muscles — myocardial ischaemia leading to scarring and contraction of the papillary muscles — autoimmune disorders, e.g. Libman–Sacks endocarditis — 'metabolic' defects, e.g. Marfan's syndrome 4. Infective endocarditis, usually on diseased valves	a. Disordered valve function — valve stenosis restricts blood flow — valvular incompetence causes reflux of blood b. Accumulation of 'vegetations' or thrombus which may embolise into the peripheral arterial tree c. Infection of vegetations or thrombus (bacterial endocarditis) — systemic symptoms (fever, anorexia, weight loss) — deteriorating valve function — infected systemic embolism to brain, kidneys etc.
Disease affecting the great arteries Aorta	1. Aortic dissection within the media resulting from atheroma or cystic medial necrosis 2. Aneurysm (connective tissue degeneration, syphilis, trauma, infection) 3. Traumatic transection	a. Acute severe chest pain b. Acute severe hypovolaemic shock with collapse or sudden death
Pulmonary artery	Peripheral deep venous thrombosis detaches and passes through the heart to impact in the pulmonary arteries	a. Acute occlusion by pulmonary embolism—may be silent, symptomatic or 'massive' and fatal b. Recurrent embolism may cause pulmonary hypertension
Pericardial disease	1. Pericardial constriction (scarring or tumour) 2. Pericardial effusion	Signs of constrictive pericarditis: systemic venous congestion with hepatomegaly and ascites; often atrial fibrillation Retrosternal pressure; muffled heart sounds; cardiac tamponade if acute and severe

countries, affecting both locally born people and certain immigrants with a genetic predisposition. Men are at greater risk than women, with 45% of men over 65 having some manifestation of the disease. Areas of particularly high incidence include Scotland and Finland. The rates in some countries, notably the USA, have been falling in recent years, perhaps as a result of reduced cigarette smoking and changes in other habits such as diet and exercise.

Risk factors for coronary atheroma (and atherosclerosis elsewhere) include unfavourable hereditary cholesterol and lipid profiles, cigarette smoking, diabetes, hypertension, obesity and a sedentary lifestyle (and perhaps a life of severe unrelieved stress).

The presentation of coronary heart disease is outlined in Table 38.3.

CONTROL OF PREDISPOSING FACTORS

The first step in treatment is usually to attempt to persuade the patient to modify risk factors known to contribute to disease progression. There are two motives here: firstly, if progression can be arrested, physiological development of collateral blood supply can proceed, and this means that intervention may become unnecessary. Secondly, the risk of occluding any form of arterial reconstruction is increased if risk factors, particularly

cigarette smoking, continue to act. Indeed, it has been shown that, on average, patients who continue to smoke after surgery gain no benefit from coronary artery bypass grafting. Smokers who fail to improve have thus suffered the risk and discomfort of surgery and at the same time squandered limited hospital resources. Nothing can yet be done about hereditary factors, but smoking, obesity and inactivity can be tackled. The benefits of modifying blood cholesterol levels are controversial, but it seems sensible at least to reduce the overall proportion of fat in the diet.

MANAGEMENT OF CORONARY ARTERY DISEASE

Coronary artery disease may be managed conservatively ('medical management') or by intervention, employing percutaneous techniques or surgical bypass grafting of coronary arteries. The anatomy of the coronary arteries is shown in Figure 38.3.

Percutaneous angioplasty techniques

A range of percutaneous minimal access techniques have been developed since the early 1980s to widen stenoses or recanalise occluded coronary arteries; these are usually performed by cardiologists. The mainstay of treatment is **percutaneous transluminal coronary (balloon) angio-**

Table 38.3 Presentation of coronary artery disease

Presentation	Secondary effects	Clinical effects
Ischaemic damage discovered incidentally in an asymptomatic patient	Potential risk of further MIs; developing complications of ischaemic heart disease; increased risk when performing an unrelated operation	Found incidentally, e.g. on ECG
A past history of myocardial infarction (MI)	Risk of further MIs; complications of ischaemic heart disease (IHD); risk during unrelated operation	History of typical pain (but note that 25% of MIs are painless)
Angina pectoris	Mortality/morbidity risks of unrelated operations increased	Typical pain brought on by exercise, anxiety or excitement
Complications of myocardial infarction	1. Rupture of part of the heart	Rupture of external wall of left ventricle Septal rupture causing a ventricular septal defect Papillary muscle rupture causing mitral or tricuspid regurgitation
	2. Fibrosis or scarring following myocardial infarction	Generalised fibrosis may cause cardiac failure through loss of contractile myocardium Localised fibrosis of an infarcted ventricular wall may cause a **ventricular aneurysm** Discrete fibrosis near a valve may cause tethering of a mitral leaflet resulting in mitral regurgitation Mural scars may disrupt the conducting system causing ventricular arrhythmias
	3. Mural thrombus may accumulate on a subendocardial infarct as an early response to injury	Thrombus may detach and cause systemic arterial embolism, e.g. to brain, lower limb or superior mesenteric artery; usually an early complication of myocardial infarction (1–6 weeks)

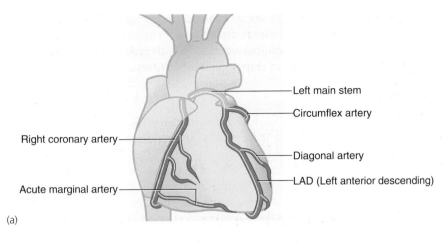

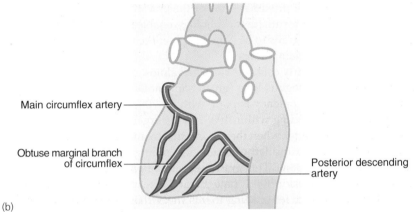

(a)

Fig 38.3 Anatomy of the coronary arteries
(a) Anterior view of coronary arteries.
(b) Posterior view of coronary arteries.
(c) Selective coronary angiography (A-P views as in (a)):
 (i) Normal right coronary artery
(ii) Normal left coronary artery.

Left main stem

Circumflex artery

Right coronary artery

Diagonal artery

Acute marginal artery

LAD (Left anterior descending)

Main circumflex artery

Obtuse marginal branch of circumflex

Posterior descending artery

(b)

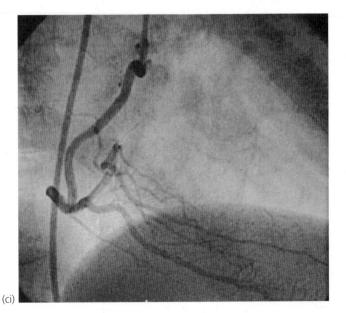

(ci)

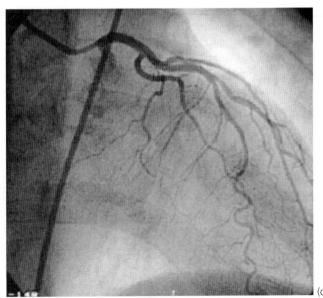

(cii)

plasty **(PTCA)**. Intra-coronary artery stents are being used in the ballooned segments in certain cases and a reduction in restenosis rate has been claimed. These stents are very expensive and their indications need to be more clearly defined by appropriately randomised trials.

When performed expertly, these techniques cause little disruption to the patient's life and recovery is rapid. However, set against this, there is a high early failure rate and a high medium-term restenosis rate (25% at 3 months). In addition, the patient and a surgical team have to be prepared to carry out an emergency operation on cardiopulmonary bypass at the time of angioplasty if things go wrong. This means tying up resources which are rarely required. Thus, the indications for percutaneous techniques currently depend as much on the availability of local expertise (and perhaps any local shortfall in surgical facilities for bypass surgery) as on strict medical indications. With improving medium-term results, the main indication for PTCA is for first-time intervention for relieving symptomatic single or double coronary artery stenoses.

Coronary artery bypass grafting (CABG)

Coronary artery bypass grafting is usually indicated in two categories of patient:

- Symptomatic patients with angina (including crescendo angina) who are not relieved by medical therapy or who are intolerant of it. This is by far the largest group
- Patients in categories believed to have a better prognosis after surgery than with medical therapy. Studies in the USA and Europe suggest improved survival after surgery is likely in patients with the following morphological characteristics:
  — Stenosis of the left main stem coronary artery (before it bifurcates into anterior descending and circumflex arteries)
  — Triple-vessel disease in conjunction with impaired left ventricular contractility (i.e. disease of the right coronary, the left anterior descending and the circumflex arterial systems)
  — Two-vessel disease which includes a proximal stenosis in the left anterior descending coronary artery

The results of CABG are encouraging, with between 85% and 90% of patients relieved of angina without the need for medication. A further 5% are substantially improved but require anti-anginal drug therapy.

Surgical technique
Coronary occlusive atherosclerosis is usually regarded as significant if there is a 50% reduction of cross-sectional area on angiography.

The aim of CABG is to bypass occlusive disease and provide a new source of inflow for the remaining patent coronary arteries using a saphenous vein graft as a conduit from the ascending aorta or by mobilising a nearby artery. Occlusive coronary artery disease is usually situated in the proximal third of the epicardial coronary arteries. This fortunate morphology enables the distal end of bypass grafts to be joined to patent recipient arteries beyond the main disease.

Early conduits consisted almost exclusively of reversed autologous long (great) saphenous vein. However, long-term patency is poor, with 50–70% of vein bypass grafts occluding within 10 years of surgery. Long-term patency is better when the left internal mammary artery is grafted on to the left anterior descending coronary artery (see Fig. 38.4). This graft seems to be particularly resistant to occlusion (90% patency at 10 years) and is the current choice for grafting to this site. Other nearby arteries have been used for CABG including the right gastro-epiploic artery and the inferior epigastric artery. Prosthetic materials give poor results for CABG but arterial grafts transplanted from other parts of the patient's body are becoming more popular, e.g. radial artery; long-term patency results are awaited. Thus, a combination of left internal mammary grafting to left anterior descending coronary artery and saphenous vein grafts to the other vessels remains the current surgical favourite.

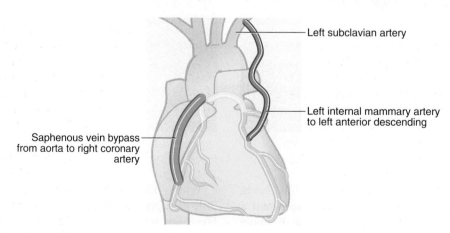

Fig. 38.4 Methods of coronary artery bypass grafting
Note that an explanted autogenous radial artery may be used as a bypass graft instead of saphenous vein.

Coronary artery surgery is performed under cardio-pulmonary bypass, usually with cold cardioplegia. In elective patients, the mortality risk is about 1%; in addition there is a 2% chance of stroke (especially after a previous stroke). Mortality rates for CABG are higher in patients with pre-existing heart failure as well as those requiring emergency operations. The rate also rises with increasing age.

In order to minimise the potentially damaging problems of cardiopulmonary bypass noted earlier, there is increasing interest in techniques of revascularising the ischaemic heart without bypass. However, operating conditions are more demanding and this may affect the accuracy of anastomoses and increase the occlusion rate of grafts and thus prejudice the success rate of the bypass procedure in abolishing ischaemia. These programmes are evolving and will no doubt become more widely employed as difficulties are ironed out.

Other types of surgery for ischaemic heart disease

In addition to CABG, other forms of surgery may be required for complications of myocardial infarction. These carry a higher risk than isolated CABG surgery. Types of surgery include:

- Excision of a left ventricular aneurysm—mortality about 5%
- Replacement or repair of a mitral valve leaking as a result of ischaemia—mortality about 15%
- Surgical identification and ablation of a ventricular arrhythmic focus—mortality about 15%
- Emergency repair of a post-myocardial infarction (MI) ventricular septal rupture—mortality about 30%
- Post-CABG heart failure necessitating ventricular support (intra-aortic balloon pump) or cardiac transplantation—mortality about 15% at 1 year

VALVULAR HEART DISEASE

In surgery for valvular heart disease, there has been a trend towards preserving the native valve where possible by repair. This has been particularly successful for myxomatous or degenerate regurgitation of the mitral valve. Mitral stenosis following rheumatic fever can also be successfully treated by valvotomy (separation of fused valve leaflets) provided surgery is performed before calcification has rendered the leaflets immobile.

The essence of conservative treatment for valve stenosis is to dilate the valve orifice mechanically. In the early days of cardiac surgery, Cutler and Levine (1925) introduced semi-closed, blind mitral valvotomy, performed via the left auricular appendage. With the heart still beating, the auricle was opened, a finger or one of a variety of mechanical devices inserted and the valve rapidly dilated. Symptomatic relief was usually satisfactory, but the valvotomy was often incomplete or else splits occurred in the leaflets rather than between them. The procedure often had to be repeated at intervals of a few years. Later, direct open valvotomy under cardiopulmonary bypass became popular. More precise and long-lasting results could be achieved by this method. More recently, there has been a return to closed valvotomy, with percutaneous trans-septal balloon dilatation of the stenosed valve. This can achieve satisfactory functional results with minimal upset to the patient.

Reconstructing the regurgitant mitral valve is becoming popular. Compared with valve replacement, this conservative technique has a lower perioperative risk and preserves left ventricular function. Thus, the overall functional result may be better than valve replacement. Repair techniques may also be employed for the diseased tricuspid or aortic valve. However, where regurgitant or stenosed valves are unsuitable for conservative treatment, valve replacement is the alternative.

VALVE PROSTHESES

There are two types of prosthesis for replacing heart valves: man-made or tissue grafts.

Many types of man-made mechanical valves have been tried, ranging from the original 'ball in cage' type, through tilting discs to bi-leaflet prostheses (see Fig. 38.5). The mechanical demands on replacement heart valves are extreme. They must cause minimal restriction to blood flow when open, yet prevent reflux when closed; they must be biocompatible, non-thrombogenic, resistant to infection and, most demanding of all, capable of opening and closing 70 times a minute for many years without mechanical failure. Modern mechanical valves are durable but thrombogenic and generally require lifelong anticoagulation. Anticoagulation carries its own risk with a mortality of about 2% over 5 years. Even with effective anticoagulation, there is a small risk of arterial embolism.

Replacement tissue valves may be either **homografts** (human) or **xenografts** (animal origin). Xenografts are almost exclusively harvested from pigs. In general, tissue valves are more resistant to thrombosis (anticoagulation is not necessary) but more prone to failure through degeneration as time goes by. Tissue valves can be expected to last between 8 and 12 years. Homograft (human) valves are believed to be resistant to early degeneration and are preferred for young patients to avoid exposure to the potential teratogenic effects of warfarin.

Infection of valve prostheses is devastating but fortunately rare. The risk is least for homograft valves. Prosthetic valve endocarditis carries a very high mortality and needs protracted treatment, often requiring the explanting (removal) of the infected prosthesis.

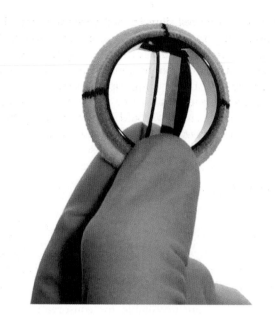

(a)

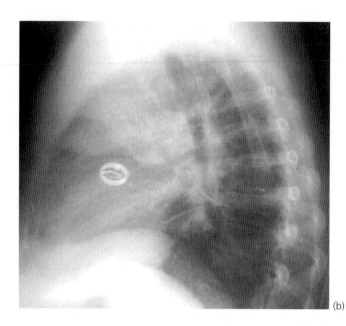

(b)

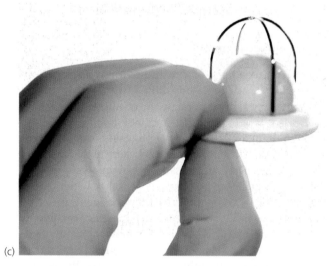

(c)

Fig. 38.5 Mechanical prosthetic valves
The two main types of artifical valve are shown here. **(a)** A tilting disc type valve (St Jude). Postoperative anticoagulation is often unnecessary with this type of valve. **(b)** A lateral chest X-ray showing a tillting disc mitral valve prosthesis in situ. **(c)** A ball and cage type of valve (Starr Edwards). These valves variously have metal or plastic balls. In most cases, lifetime anticoagulation is necessary.

INDICATIONS FOR VALVE SURGERY

The key to successful valvular heart surgery is to carry it out at the most appropriate moment in the natural history of the disease, when risks of surgery are least and potential benefits greatest, i.e. before irreversible ventricular dysfunction has occurred.

In aortic stenosis or regurgitation and mitral stenosis or regurgitation, indications include most patients with symptoms attributable to the valvular dysfunction. In addition, asymptomatic aortic stenosis should usually be treated if there is a pressure drop of 50 mmHg across the valve (this has a high risk of sudden death), and in aortic regurgitation when there is evidence of left ventricular dilatation.

AORTIC DISEASE

AORTIC DISSECTION

Aortic dissection is classified according to the part affected: the most widely used method is the Stanford system. Type A indicates that the ascending aorta is involved while type B describes the situation when any other part of the thoracic aorta is affected. An alternative classification method is De Bakey (see Fig. 38.6).

Without surgery, type A dissection carries an 80% mortality in the first month; with surgical management this falls to less than 20%. The operation involves resecting the ascending aorta and replacing it with a synthetic tube graft. If the dissection reaches the aortic valve, it is likely to be disrupted, causing acute severe regurgitation and perhaps occluding the coronary artery origins. In this case, the valve will need resuspending or replacing.

Uncomplicated type B dissections have a similar outcome (i.e. 20% mortality at 30 days after operation), whether managed surgically or medically (by control of hypertension). Surgery is required in type B dissection if there is aortic rupture, occlusion of vital branches, progressive dissection or subsequent aneurysm formation. Note that abdominal aortic aneurysms occur years later in up to 50% of patients with previous thoracic aortic dissection.

THORACIC ANEURYSMS

Aneurysmal dilatation of the thoracic aorta may occur in the ascending part, the arch or the descending part. There is a risk of rupture similar to that found in abdominal aortic aneurysms and surgical intervention is usually recommended when the aneurysm reaches a diameter of 6 cm. Replacing the descending aorta, particularly when there is thoraco-abdominal disease, threatens the main blood supply of the spinal cord (the artery of Adamkiewicz at about T10) so that paraplegia complicates 10–30% of these operations.

TRAUMA TO THE THORACIC AORTA

This may result from blunt or sharp injury. Blunt aortic trauma is usually associated with severe deceleration as occurs in head-on collisions in road traffic accidents. The common injury is partial or complete transection of the aorta at the junction between the relatively tethered arch and the relatively mobile descending aorta close to the ligamentum arteriosum. Complete transection is rapidly fatal; partial transection with an intact adventitia is liable to rupture and must be diagnosed to enable early treatment. Late aneurysm formation may also occur.

PULMONARY EMBOLISM

Emergency surgical removal of a massive pulmonary embolism has become increasingly rare with the introduction of effective thrombolytic agents. In pre-bypass days, an occasional Trendelenburg operation was performed, though rarely successfully. This involved a rapid

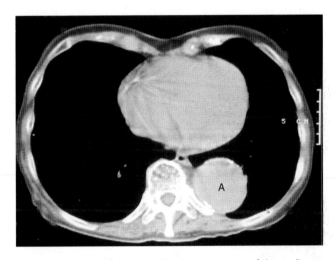

Fig. 38.7 CT scan of chest showing 5 cm aneurysm of descending thoracic aortic **A**.

Stanford type A (aortic valve may be involved)   Stanford type B

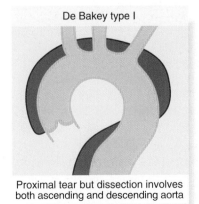

De Bakey type I

Proximal tear but dissection involves both ascending and descending aorta

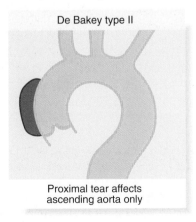

De Bakey type II

Proximal tear affects ascending aorta only

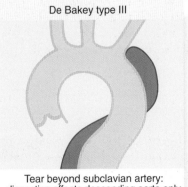

De Bakey type III

Tear beyond subclavian artery: dissection affects descending aorta only

Fig. 38.6 Thoracic aortic dissection

thoracotomy, opening of the pulmonary artery, removing the thrombus and rapid arterial closure. Nowadays, there are a few indications for a similar operation to be carried out under cardiopulmonary bypass—for example, after recent surgery or during pregnancy when thrombolytic therapy might carry unacceptable risks.

Surgical thrombectomy has recently found a place in managing chronic proximal obstruction of the pulmonary artery caused by recurrent embolism. This developing technique has avoided the need for heart and lung transplantation in a small number of patients.

PERICARDIAL DISEASE

Pericardial inflammation may result in constriction of the pericardium. World-wide, this occurs most commonly in tuberculosis. Constrictive pericarditis may also occur in certain autoimmune conditions such as rheumatoid arthritis or following pericardial trauma or mediastinal radiotherapy. Pericardial constriction impairs filling of the cardiac chambers and typically there is an equalisation of diastolic pressures in all four chambers of the heart. Clinical signs are of pulmonary and systemic venous congestion and a low cardiac output. Surgical treatment involves excision of the entire pericardium.

39 | Disorders of the breast

BREAST DISEASE IN GENERAL

INTRODUCTION

Patients with breast problems make up 15–20% of new referrals to general surgical outpatient clinics. Virtually every woman with a breast lump, breast pain or discharge from the nipple fears that she has cancer. The anxiety that results is made up of three components: the unknown course of the disease, the threat of mutilation and the fear of dying. Previously, this often prevented women from seeking early medical advice but in recent years public awareness and media publicity about self-examination and screening and the possible advantages of early treatment have encouraged earlier presentation.

Many patients have friends or relatives with breast cancer and their understanding of the disease will understandably be coloured by that experience. The possible effects of breast surgery on sexual attractiveness and femininity are often uppermost in a woman's mind, so consideration of this and other psychological aspects of breast disease should accompany every stage in the management process.

Despite their fears, fewer than 15% of patients presenting with breast problems to surgical outpatients departments in the UK have cancer. However, in Western societies about 1 woman in 10 will develop the disease and 1 in 18 will die from it. Early recognition of cancer offers the best hope of cure, so priority should be given to prompt diagnosis. In the UK, a government white paper insists that all breast referrals be seen within 2 weeks. Ideally, referrals should be seen in a 'one-stop' triple assessment clinic (clinical, imaging and cytology)

within 2–3 weeks for adequate counselling and, if appropriate, preparation for surgery.

EPIDEMIOLOGY OF BREAST DISEASE

The types of breast disease which are of surgical importance are described in Box 39.1.

BREAST CANCER

Breast cancer is predominantly a disease of Western civilisation and differences in incidence (the exceptionally low level in Japan, for example) are more likely due to environmental than racial differences. It used to be the most common cancer in women (having just been over-taken by lung cancer) and is the most common cause of death in women between the ages of 35 and 55. In the UK each year, about 24 000 new cases are diagnosed and over 13 000 women die of the condition. The incidence of breast cancer is rising but mortality has not risen, probably as a result of earlier detection and improved treatments. Breast cancer is not, however, a new disease; it was recognised by the ancient Egyptians and mastectomy was certainly performed in Roman times.

Breast cancer is extremely rare before the age of 25. It reaches a high incidence in the decade from 40 to 50 and continues to increase in frequency into old age. Breast cancer in the male accounts for less than 1% of new cases. Genetic factors are important in certain families with a

SUMMARY

Box 39.1 Types of breast disease of surgical importance

Malignant neoplasms
- Ductal or lobular *adenocarcinoma* by far the most common
- Rarely, a *sarcoma* or *metastasis* from elsewhere occurs in the breast

Benign tumour-like lesions
- This category comprises the common condition known as *fibroadenoma* and the less common conditions of *intraduct papilloma* and *lipoma*

Disordered physiological responses of breast tissue
- *Fibroadenosis* (also known as fibrocystic disease, benign mammary dysplasia and chronic mastitis) encompasses a variety of proliferative and other changes of the breast tissues
- All probably have an underlying hormonal aetiology and are regarded as *aberrations of normal development or involution (ANDI)*

Mammary duct ectasia
- Believed to be due to a chronic periductal inflammatory reaction to retained duct secretions

Infections
- *Cellulitis* and *breast abscess* are the main types of infection and usually occur during lactation
- Subareolar abscesses also occur in mammary duct ectasia

history of premenopausal breast cancer, particularly if several close relatives have been affected before the age of 50. The risk to female relatives is high and calls for genetic counselling and close surveillance. Genetic factors responsible have been identified as two genes (BRCA1 and 2) which also have a link to certain ovarian cancers. When a woman has a grandmother, mother or sister who has had breast cancer postmenopausally, the patient has only a modestly increased susceptibility.

Childless women or those having their first pregnancy over the age of 30 have double the breast cancer risk of women who have their first child before the age of 25. Nuns appear to be at extremely high risk. Protective factors include a short time between menarche and first pregnancy, early menopause and ovarian ablation below the age of 35. Breast feeding may be associated with a lower incidence of breast cancer. Although still controversial, present evidence suggests that prolonged use of the oral contraceptive pill has only a small adverse effect on risk and only if taken when the patient was young, seemingly delaying presentation. Hormone replacement therapy (HRT) probably plays little part in causing breast cancer but saves lives by substantially reducing the rate of myocardial ischaemia.

The only environmental factor known to promote the development of breast cancer is ionising radiation. Women exposed to large numbers of chest X-rays for monitoring tuberculosis (which occurred in the days before modern chemotherapy) have a moderately increased risk of breast cancer, and the women of Hiroshima and Nagasaki have a high risk of developing breast cancer even now.

NON-MALIGNANT BREAST DISEASE

Fibroadenosis and **fibroadenoma** account for most of the non-malignant breast disease which reaches the surgeon. Both occur almost exclusively in the reproductive years and they are probably both controlled by hormonal factors. Fibroadenoma is more common in young women, while fibroadenosis usually occurs in women between 35 and 45 (see Fig. 39.1).

Breast infections most commonly occur during pregnancy and lactation. Most are successfully treated early with antibiotics and do not reach the surgeon. If resolution is slow or incomplete or if an acute abscess develops (see Fig. 39.2), surgical intervention is required. Periareolar abscesses may occur in mammary duct ectasia but respond to antibiotic treatment and perhaps aspiration and should not be drained surgically.

Fat necrosis is rare and occurs in older age groups. The lump often appears long after the traumatic episode has been forgotten.

SYMPTOMS AND SIGNS OF BREAST DISEASE

The patient not only experiences the symptoms but is often the first to notice the physical signs. Both are

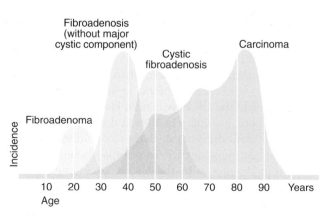

Fig. 39.1 Age incidence of common breast disorders

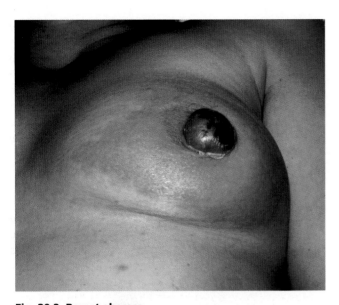

Fig. 39.2 Breast abscess
This woman of 40 presented with a neglected left breast abscess a few weeks after ceasing breast feeding. The abscess was drained at open operation but had destroyed much of the breast tissue. The organism was *Staph. aureus* as is commonly the case.

outlined in Table 39.1 along with their diagnostic importance.

SPECIAL POINTS IN HISTORY-TAKING

The duration of symptoms should be established, bearing in mind that a lump may have been present much longer than the woman is aware or will admit. Periodicity of pain or lumpiness in relation to the menstrual cycle suggests a hormone-related condition rather than malignant disease.

A history of previous breast problems such as cysts, abscess or trauma may provide a clue to the current diagnosis. Parity and age at first pregnancy might alter the statistical likelihood of a lesion being malignant.

Drug history should be recorded, including present or past use of hormone preparations. These include the contraceptive pill and hormone replacement therapy (HRT) for menopausal symptoms. A causal link between the use of these hormones and the development of breast cancer is unproven but cannot be discounted.

Table 39.1 Symptoms and signs of breast disease (see also Figs. 39.3, 4 and 5)

Symptom or sign	Clinical significance
1. Pain	
Varying with menstrual cycle	Suggests a physiological cause such as premenstrual syndrome or fibroadenosis. Both are responsive to treatment
Independent of menstrual cycle	Not helpful in diagnosis but may occur in carcinoma, fibroadenosis or infection
2. Lump in the breast	
Hard lump	The surface characteristics provide the most useful diagnostic information: a discrete mobile lump with a smooth surface is most likely to be a fibroadenoma if it is solid, or a fibroadenotic cyst if it is fluctuant. An ill-defined margin and any suggestion of tethering to superficial or deep structures strongly suggest carcinoma but are sometimes due to non-infective inflammation
Firm, poorly defined lump or lumpiness	This suggests fibroadenosis, especially if the outline is difficult to distinguish from normal breast tissue or if the breast is generally lumpy
Soft lump	Usually a lipoma or occasionally a lax cyst
3. Skin changes in the breast	
Skin dimpling	Sometimes a subtle sign but highly suggestive of carcinoma
Visible lump	Cyst, carcinoma or phylloides tumour. Cysts can appear with alarming speed
Peau d'orange (appearance of orange peel)	Over a lump, this is virtually pathognomonic of carcinoma. It is due to tumour invasion of dermal lymphatics causing dermal oedema. However, it may occur over an infective lesion
Redness	Usually infection, especially if skin is hot. Sometimes a feature of mammary duct ectasia
Ulceration	Neglected carcinoma in the elderly (often slow-growing)
4. Nipple disorders	
Recent inversion	Suggests a fibrosing underlying lesion such as carcinoma or mammary duct ectasia
'Eczema' (rash involving nipple or areola, or both)	If unilateral, this is the classic sign of Paget's disease of the nipple, a presentation of breast cancer
Nipple discharge	
Milky	Pregnancy or hyperprolactinaemia
Clear	Physiological
Green	Perimenopausal, duct ectasia, fibroadenotic cyst
Blood-stained	Possible carcinoma or intraduct papilloma

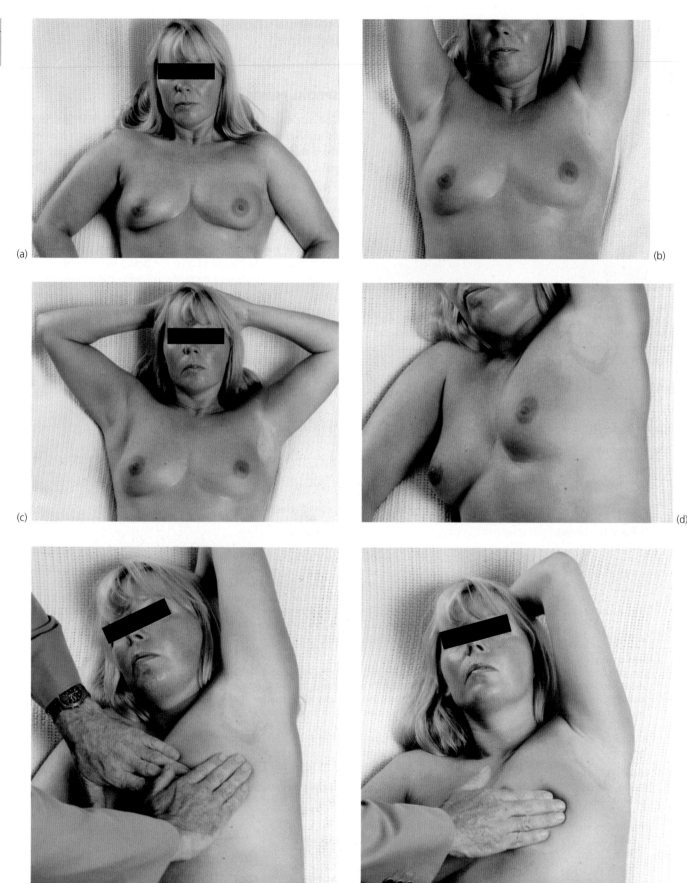

(a)

(b)

(c)

(d)

(e)

(f)

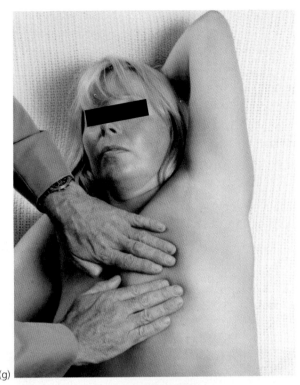

(g)

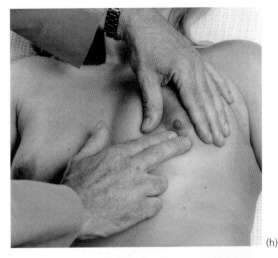

(h)

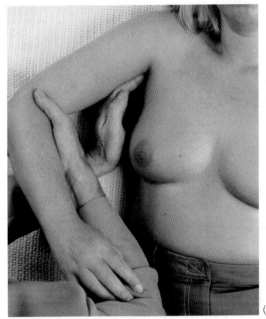

(j)

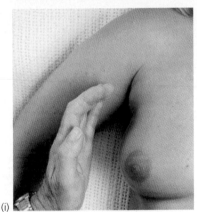

(i)

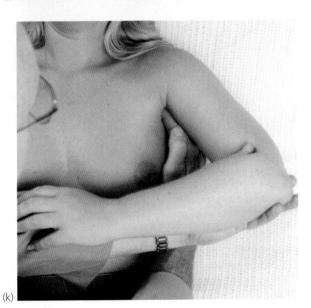

(k)

Fig. 39.3 Technique of breast examination

Inspection: the breasts should be inspected for asymmetry, skin tethering and dimpling, and changes in colour. This should be performed with the patient sitting comfortably, pressing hands on hips **(a)**, lifting arms in the air **(b)**, and pressing hands on top of the head **(c)**. *Palpation*: the patient should sit on an examination couch as shown in **(d)**, with the backrest at about 45° and rolled slightly to the contralateral side. The arm on the side to be examined should be elevated and the head rested on the pillow. The effect of these manoeuvres is to spread the breast over a greater area of the chest wall. With the smaller breast, the flat of the right hand is used to palpate the breast circumferentially by quadrants **(e)(g)**. The central part of the breast and the axillary tail must also be palpated. If there is a history of nipple discharge, the areola is pressed in different areas **(h)** to identify the duct from which it emanates and therefore the segment involved. Finally the **axillary lymph nodes** are palpated as shown in **(i)**, **(j)** and **(k)**. The left axilla is palpated with the right hand **(k)** and the right axilla is palpated with the left hand **(j)**. It is important to relax the axillary muscles by supporting the weight of the patient's arm as shown. The fingers of the examining hand are firmly held in a curve **(i)**, pressed high into the apex of the axilla against the chest wall and drawn downwards. The hand will then 'ride over' any enlarged axillary nodes.

505

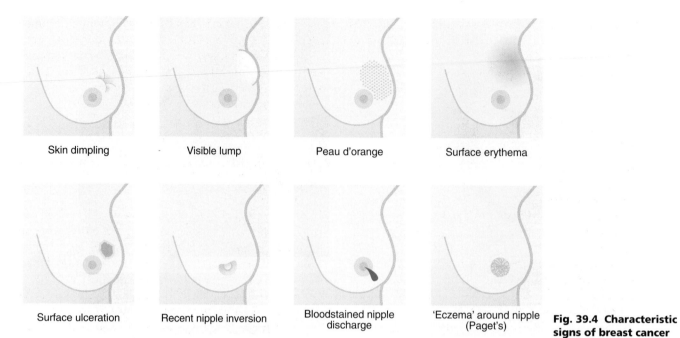

Skin dimpling

Visible lump

Peau d'orange

Surface erythema

Surface ulceration

Recent nipple inversion

Bloodstained nipple discharge

'Eczema' around nipple (Paget's)

Fig. 39.4 Characteristic signs of breast cancer

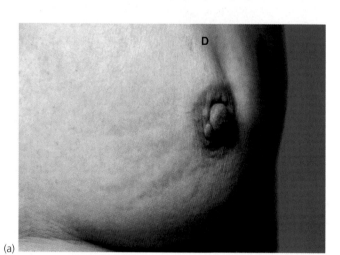

(a)

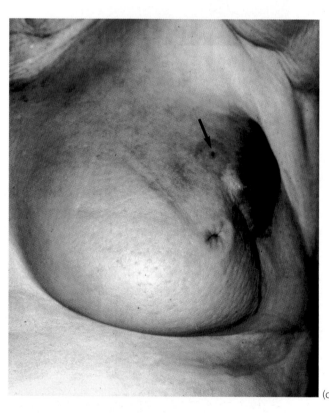

(c)

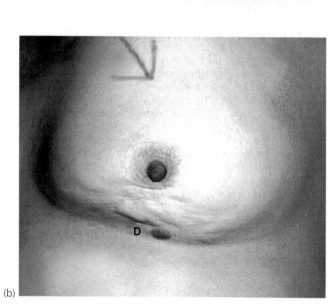

(b)

Fig. 39.5 Carcinoma of the breast

(a) and **(b)** Characteristic skin dimpling **D** over breast carcinomas. This may be a subtle sign and only be visible in tangential light. **(c)** Nipple retraction and widespread 'peau d'orange' resulting from a large central breast carcinoma. Peau d'orange is caused by a combination of cutaneous infiltration by tumour and skin oedema (and occasionally by infection). Locally advanced breast cancer may cause distortion of the breast. The colour change and ulceration are uncommonly seen and only occur in neglected cases. Note also the puncture wound of a core biopsy (arrowed). There was no obvious axillary node enlargement.

History-taking provides an opportunity for establishing a rapport with the patient, who usually fears cancer and its implications. A sympathetic approach and clear explanations lay the foundation for a trusting and co-operative relationship if malignancy is later diagnosed.

EXAMINATION OF THE BREASTS

The basic examination technique is shown in Fig. 39.3 and can be simplified for patient self-examination. Most women should be taught to examine their own breasts, although the value of self-examination remains unproven in detecting early breast cancer. During examination, the patient should be asked to identify any lump she has found herself so the surgeon can be sure of what she is worried about. Often no lump is found and it turns out she has palpated a part of a generalised breast lumpiness or the edge of the breast disc.

Breast examination involves six distinct manœuvres:

- Observation with the patient sitting up
- Observation with the patient raising and lowering her arms
- Examination of the nipples
- Systematic palpation of each breast
- Palpation of the axillae and supraclavicular fossae
- General examination for signs of distant metastases

The technique of palpating the breast may need to be modified according to the type of breast being examined. Palpation with the flat of one hand is usual, but it may be more appropriate to examine large pendulous breasts between two hands. The normal breast has a wide range of textures, ranging from soft, through nodular, to hard. This underlines the difficulties of clinical evaluation of a lump or lumpiness; what the patient or her doctor has felt may be physiological nodularity. Suspicious physical signs should be compared with the breast on the opposite side because physiological and other hormonally induced changes tend to be symmetrical. If a lump is found, the overlying skin must be examined for mobility and tethering. Fixation of the lump to the chest wall can be assessed by having the patient tense pectoralis major by pressing her hand on to her hip.

A history of nipple discharge can often be confirmed by applying pressure over the appropriate quadrant of the breast near the areola. The position of the duct on the summit of the nipple from where the discharge emerges can then be noted. Discharges that are not obviously blood-stained should be tested for blood using urinalysis dipsticks and should be smeared on slides and sent for cytology. Scrapings from suspected Paget's disease of the nipple can be sent for cytological analysis.

The experienced clinician can probably detect 85% of carcinomas bigger than 1 cm in diameter. None the less, a third of all carcinomas in asymptomatic women attending will be missed on clinical examination. Even among experts, there is at least a 25% error in detecting axillary node involvement by palpation. Because of the high rate of false negative examinations, clinical suspicion alone is enough to justify further investigations.

INVESTIGATION OF BREAST DISORDERS

There is no single test or combination of tests which can reliably detect all cancers. A definite lump on palpation should be sampled by **fine needle aspiration cytology (FNA)**; if the lump is indistinct on palpation but a suspicious area is revealed on imaging (ultrasound or mammography), a guided FNA or needle biopsy can be performed. FNA has now largely replaced open biopsy for diagnosis but a negative result does not exclude carcinoma. Core needle biopsies give the architecture of a cancer but may miss the relevant part of the breast. The multiple 'passes' of the FNA needle should confirm if a cancer is present. In the presence of a palpable lump, **mammography** gives up to 95% diagnostic accuracy on its own and this is increased by aspiration cytology or core (e.g. Trucut) biopsy. Unfortunately, the accuracy falls when mammography is used as a screening procedure for asymptomatic women without lumps. Mammography is also unreliable in women under 40 years because of dense breast tissue but may give useful information if a lump is palpable. The radiological features of carcinoma include a characteristic **fine calcification** (see Fig. 39.6) and puckering and distortion of breast tissue. These may be quite subtle signs, however, and the definitive interpretation should be left to an experienced radiologist. Two radiologists often 'double report' films for increased accuracy.

In the case of an apparently solid but discrete lump, **ultrasonography** can readily distinguish between a solid mass and a cyst and can often reveal characteristic changes of malignancy. However, a negative result does not exclude carcinoma.

If a cyst is suspected, aspiration should usually be attempted. Many clinicians prefer to arrange mammography and ultrasonography and aspirate under ultrasound control. The reason for this is that aspiration can distort the findings on imaging and reduce their discriminatory power. A simple cyst contains yellow or green fluid and the lump will disappear. The fluid is often sent for cytological analysis but this is not essential unless the aspirate is cellular or bloody. If the lump does not disappear or if the fluid is blood-stained, then a carcinoma should be suspected and the lump should be excised if cytology is unhelpful (see Fig. 39.20, p. 518). If

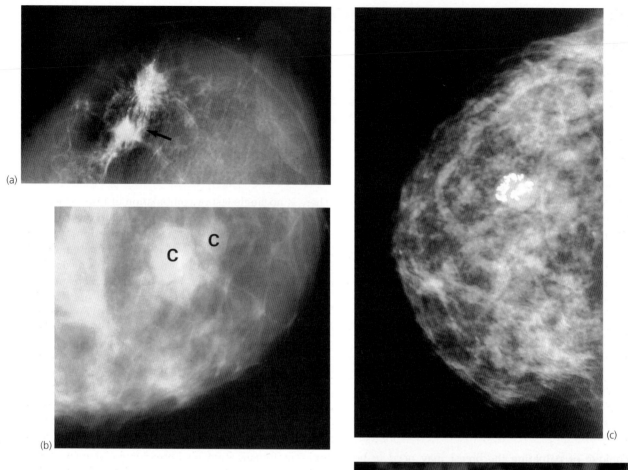

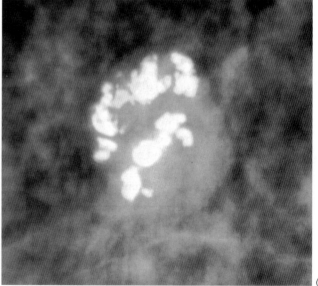

Fig. 39.6 Mammograms contrasting breast cancer fibroadenosis and fibroadenoma

(a) Two infiltrating spiculated (spiky) radiopaque masses are suggestive of malignancy but the nearby fine calcification (arrowed) clinches the diagnosis. Malignant micro-calcification is a subtle sign requiring careful examination of the films with magnification; it does not reproduce well in photographs. Coarser calcification is found in benign breast diseases. **(b)** This mammogram shows a fibroadenotic mass incorporating two well-circumscribed cysts **C**. **(c)** Shows the typical mammographic appearance of a fibroadenoma. **(d)** An enlarged view of the fibroadenoma, showing the much coarser calcification generally found in benign breast lesions.

mammography and ultrasound are reported as benign and the cyst refills within about 6 weeks, one more aspiration is performed. If it reappears again within a similar period, excision biopsy should be performed.

It is important to remember that no test can exclude carcinoma. If clinical suspicion remains, excision biopsy should be performed if appropriate, or the patient followed up and re-examined at intervals.

CANCER OF THE BREAST

PATHOLOGY

Virtually all cancers of the breast are adenocarcinomas; the exceptions are the occasional sarcoma or metastasis from elsewhere. Invasive carcinomas are predominantly **ductal carcinomas** (75%); 5–10% are described as **infiltrating lobular carcinomas** and may arise in the glands of the breast lobules; and 10–15% are part of a miscellaneous group, all of which have a better prognosis than the others. These include **tubular**, **colloid** and **ductal carcinoma in situ**. Most breast cancers show clear evidence of invasiveness at the time of presentation (see Fig. 39.7). In patients with breast carcinoma, other areas of the breast often contain atypical cells more than three layers thick, but still confined within the epithelial basement membrane of duct or lobule; this **'in situ' stage** probably precedes the development of infiltrating carcinoma. A histological diagnosis of intraduct or intralobular carcinoma in situ must be interpreted with caution because this may mean that an invasive carcinoma has been inadequately sampled. In situ carcinoma is common in screened patients and complete excision offers cure.

The distinction between ductal and lobular carcinoma is not merely of academic interest. Lobular carcinomas tend to arise multicentrically, so that bilateral tumours occur in a significant proportion of cases. Further, lobular carcinomas are more likely to bear oestrogen receptors and may be more responsive to anti-oestrogen therapy.

If **blood vessel or lymphatic invasion** is found in a histological specimen, this heralds a poor prognosis even if lymph nodes are negative.

Some patients with breast carcinoma (usually of ductal origin) present with reddening and thickening of the skin of the nipple and sometimes areola, often followed by fissuring and ulceration. This condition is most common in the elderly and is known as **Paget's disease of the nipple**. The epidermis of the nipple first and the areola later become infiltrated by neoplastic cells from the underlying carcinoma. These cells are believed to reach the surface by intra-epithelial spread along the mammary ducts (see Fig. 39.9).

NATURAL HISTORY OF BREAST CANCER

Before there is any clinical evidence of its presence, the breast tumour has usually reached at least 1 cm in diameter. Malignant cells may, however, have been proliferating during a long latent interval of about 8 years, and an in situ form may have been present for even longer. By invading locally, the tumour usually evokes a fibrous response in adjacent breast tissue which is largely responsible for the mass becoming palpable.

At some stage, tumour cells enter the lymphatics and spread to the regional lymph nodes of the axillary and sometimes internal mammary groups (see Fig. 39.10). Nodal metastasis is rare with tumours smaller than 0.5 cm diameter. In tumours of 1 cm diameter, axillary metastases are found in 25% and the incidence rises sequentially with tumour size up to 65% involvement with tumours larger than 5 cm. The nodes closest to the lesion are involved first, usually followed successively by other nodes in the chain, although 'skip metastases' can rarely occur. Recent research suggests that the sampling of a 'sentinel node' identified using a radio-isotope or injected dye may provide an accurate

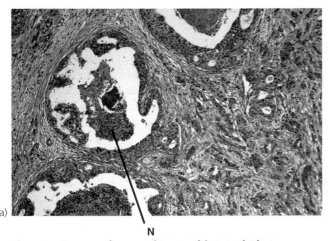

(a)

N

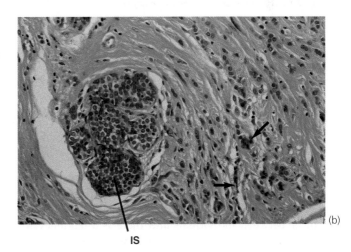

IS

(b)

Fig. 39.7 Breast adenocarcinoma—histopathology
(a) Ducts to the left of the picture contain highly atypical epithelium, with central necrosis **N**, a type of in-situ ductal carcinoma also known as *comedocarcinoma*. On the right of this micrograph is invasive ductal carcinoma composed of many small glandular structures diffusely invading breast tissue. **(b)** In situ **IS** and invasive (arrowed) lobular carcinoma. Malignant cells tend to be less atypical than in ductal carcinoma and do not form glands, but often invade in 'single-file'. Intracellular mucin is also characteristic of this variant of breast carcinoma.

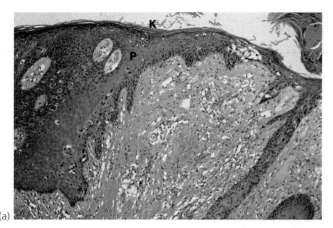

(a)

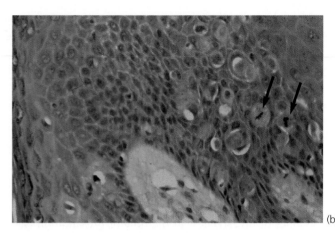

(b)

Fig. 39.8 Paget's disease of the nipple—histopathology
(a) Nipple epidermis containing numerous malignant Paget's cells **P** which have spread from an underlying in situ ductal carcinoma. The epidermis and keratin layer **K** show associated changes. **(b)** High-power view of Paget's cells showing intracellular mucin and mitotic activity (arrowed).

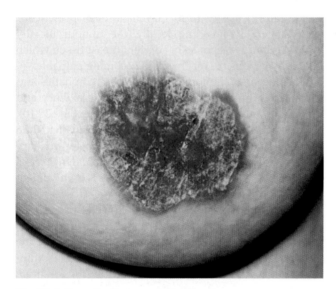

Fig. 39.9 Paget's disease of the nipple

indication of nodal involvement. Micrometastases are present in the nodes long before they are palpable; thus detecting nodal involvement requires histological proof. Later, tumour cells may breach the lymph node capsules to invade the surrounding tissues. In this way, the nodes become fixed and matted together. Systemic spread via the bloodstream may occur very early so that even a small localised lesion may have already metastasised widely. Nevertheless, systemic spread is more likely to have occurred once regional lymph nodes are involved.

There is great variation in the behaviour of breast cancer between individuals and there is a tendency for the disease to progress more slowly with advancing age. Indeed, 10% of untreated patients survive 10 years or more. In a minority of patients, usually the young, the disease follows a much more aggressive course. **Histological grade** is also a useful prognostic indicator: the

poorer the differentiation, the more likely is recurrence or early death. In some tumours, the cells possess oestrogen and other hormone receptors which can be demonstrated by immunological techniques. The clinical usefulness of this characteristic is not yet a subject of common agreement. Contrary to popular belief, pregnancy probably does not accelerate tumour growth when other factors such as youth are taken into account.

LIFE EXPECTANCY

Life expectancy for women with breast cancer (irrespective of the type of treatment) is shown in Figure 39.11, compared with unaffected women of equivalent ages. Metastasis can occur as late as 35 years after diagnosis but 60% of tumours that present with metastases will do so within the first 2 years. Two important facts emerge from this: firstly, women often survive many years after treatment for breast cancer but very few are completely cured of the disease.

That is, the majority of affected women will eventually die of breast cancer unless they die of some other disease in the meantime. Secondly, patients with a disease-free interval of 5 years after treatment clearly cannot be described as 'cured', as might be the case with other malignancies. Nevertheless, the survival after 5 and 10 years is improving.

SCREENING FOR BREAST CANCER

See Chapter 7, p. 101.

STAGING OF BREAST CANCER

The purpose of staging is to define the extent of tumour spread so that prognosis can be estimated and the most appropriate treatment planned. There are several systems

Regional lymphatic spread

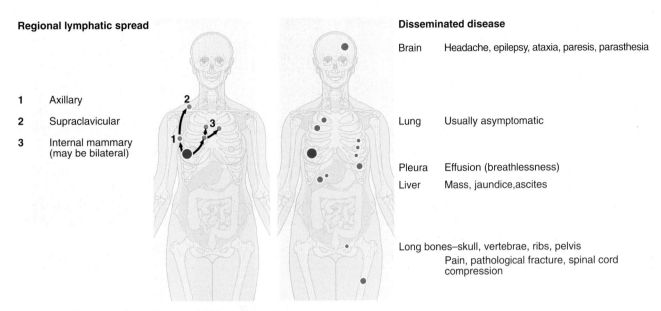

1　Axillary

2　Supraclavicular

3　Internal mammary
(may be bilateral)

Disseminated disease

Brain	Headache, epilepsy, ataxia, paresis, parasthesia
Lung	Usually asymptomatic
Pleura	Effusion (breathlessness)
Liver	Mass, jaundice, ascites
Long bones–skull, vertebrae, ribs, pelvis	
	Pain, pathological fracture, spinal cord compression

Fig. 39.10　Common sites of spread of breast carcinoma

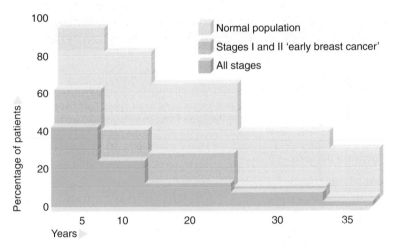

Fig. 39.11 caption area:

Normal population

Stages I and II 'early breast cancer'

All stages

Percentage of patients

Years ▶

Fig. 39.11　Life expectancy after diagnosis of breast cancer (after Brinkley and Haybittle)
Note that 5- and 10-year survival has improved in recent years with better diagnosis and treatment but it is too early to be sure that long-term survival will also improve.

of staging in common use; the simplest is based on clinical evidence of local and systemic spread. The more sophisticated use various additional methods such as grading of tumour histology, lymph node biopsy, chest X-ray or bone scans. Unfortunately, staging is still a crude tool since micrometastatic spread cannot be reliably detected by these methods. However, in the absence of detectable distant metastasis, axillary metastasis is the single most useful guide to expected survival.

The internationally accepted **TNM system** (see Fig. 39.13) uses clinical and investigation results to grade local **t**umour size and extent, regional spread to lymph **n**odes, and the presence or absence of **m**etastases. This allows more accurate recording of the extent of disease at any given time but it is still relatively imprecise. All breast cancer treatment trials now insist on recording pathological nodal status and histological tumour grade

to make comparison of responses to different treatments more scientific. Using the TNM system, breast cancer can be grouped into stages 0–IV and these stages are useful in planning treatment. An outline is given in Table 39.2.

PRINCIPLES OF MANAGEMENT OF BREAST CANCER

INTRODUCTION

The prognosis for patients with treated breast cancer has not changed substantially over the past 60 years despite extensive research into improved methods of treatment. However, disease-free intervals from treatment to first recurrence are gradually being extended. There are many variables in breast cancer—e.g. age of patient, aggressiveness of tumour, stage, response to therapy—and no

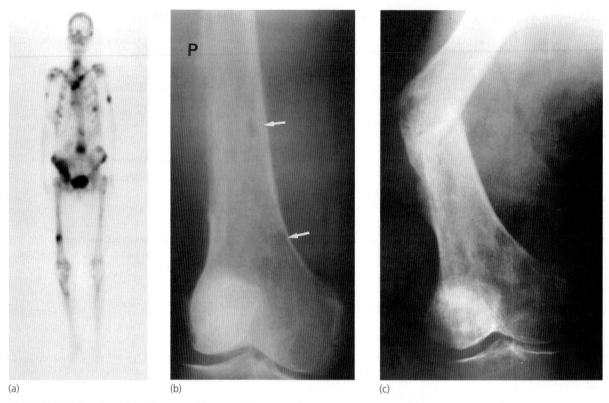

(a)   (b)   (c)

Fig. 39.12 Skeletal metastases from carcinoma of the breast
(a) Anterior view of radioisotope bone scan of a 48-year-old woman complaining of pain in the neck and right hip. She had had a mastectomy for carcinoma 8 years previously. The scan shows large metastatic deposits in the lower cervical and lumbar spine, right pelvis, right femur and left humerus as well as several smaller deposits in the ribs and elsewhere in the skeleton. **(b)** X-ray of the lower femur in a 79-year-old woman presenting with a fungating breast carcinoma and pain in the left knee. The X-ray shows radiolucencies (arrowed) in the distal femur and elevation of the periosteum **P** medially, indicating bony metastasis. Radiotherapy was arranged to alleviate the symptoms. **(c)** Some weeks later, despite treatment, the patient returned with this pathological fracture of the femur.

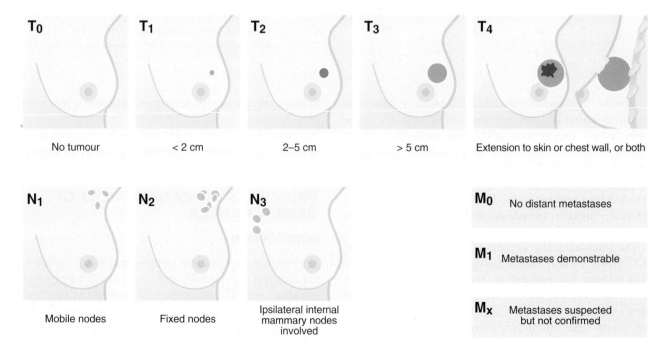

Fig. 39.13 TNM classification system for breast cancer

Table 39.2 Staging system for breast cancer using TNM classification

Stage	Description
0	Cancer in situ
I	T_1 without nodes or metastases
II	T_{1-2} + N_1 or T_3 + N_0
III	T_{1-4}, N_{2-3}
IV	Distant metastases (M_1)

single treatment is yet clearly superior for every patient. Clinicians generally agree on what is too little treatment or excess treatment, but opinions vary about the best treatments between these extremes (see Box 39.2). In practice, only small differences in disease-free interval or ultimate survival can be expected between currently accepted methods of treatment. This, and the long natural history of the disease, explains why specific details of management vary from one centre to another.

The standardisation of treatment is being encouraged with the help of government-backed 'evidence-based' guidelines. As factual information and reproducible results emerge from controlled trials, treatment methods will gradually evolve towards a series of consensus views which will be widely adopted. There is a strong trend towards patients with breast disease and especially cancer to be managed in specialist breast units. These can provide comprehensive and up-to-date care and monitoring but this may represent a counsel of perfection. Meanwhile, there are four universal principles of management which are summarised in Box 39.3. There is a reasonable prospect of long-term survival, if not cure, in **early breast cancer**

SUMMARY

Box 39.2 Major treatment options in breast cancer
- Excision biopsy alone (not recommended)
- Needle biopsy or aspiration cytology plus radiotherapy
- Wide local excision (lumpectomy) plus axillary node biopsy plus radiotherapy
- Simple mastectomy plus axillary node biopsy or clearance
- Modified (Patey) radical mastectomy
- Standard (Halsted) radical mastectomy (not recommended)
- Supra-radical (Urban) mastectomy (not recommended)

Note: The list starts with what is now generally regarded as inadequate treatment and progresses towards excessive treatment. Treatments near the centre of the list are the most commonly used. Axillary radiotherapy can be added to any type of mastectomy. Adjuvant chemotherapy or anti-oestrogen therapy can be combined with any treatment on the list.

but in **advanced breast cancer** palliation is the only realistic objective to improve the quality of life and only secondarily to extend life.

ESTABLISHING THE DIAGNOSIS

If there is clinical suspicion that a breast lump is malignant, the priority in most cases is to perform ultrasound scanning and mammography. This gives information about the lump in question but also surveys the rest of the breast tissue on both sides. The next priority is to obtain tissue for microscopic examination. This is best achieved by **fine needle aspiration cytology (FNA)** or **core needle biopsy**, if necessary guided by ultrasound or mammographic imaging. If this is negative or equivocal, a discrete lump should be completely excised with a wide margin of apparently normal breast tissue and the specimen examined histologically. This procedure, **excision biopsy**, can also form the first step in controlling local disease.

CONTROL OF DISEASE IN THE AFFECTED BREAST AND CHEST WALL

Removal of a discrete tumour mass along with a wide margin of normal tissue (**lumpectomy**) might be thought to effect a cure. Bitter experience, however, has shown that 40% of these tumours recur later within the same breast. Furthermore, distant metastatic spread may have already occurred or may occur later. Local recurrence takes place either because malignant cells had already penetrated beyond the margin of excision or because the remaining breast tissue is more susceptible to malignant change. The latter is particularly true for lobular carcinomas. Therefore, rational treatment must aim to eliminate tumour cells anywhere else in the affected breast. This can be achieved by surgical removal of the whole breast (**mastectomy**) or by radiotherapy.

Mastectomy

The traditional approach was to remove the entire breast once the diagnosis was confirmed. Patients were often prepared for possible mastectomy at the same operation

SUMMARY

Box 39.3 Principles of management of breast cancer
- Establish the diagnosis
- Control disease in the affected breast and chest wall
- Prevent and treat local and regional disease in early breast cancer
- Control advanced and disseminated disease

as excision biopsy, if a frozen section biopsy (performed while the patient remained on the operating table) showed cancer. However, this approach is no longer acceptable. Before such a mutilating operation, patients need the opportunity to discuss the diagnosis and the possible options for treatment; modest delays while this is accomplished do not adversely affect the outcome. Nowadays, most patients have a cytological or needle biopsy diagnosis before operation is planned and know what to expect as a result. There is a trend towards immediate reconstruction of the breast mastectomy (p. 517).

Breast-conserving surgery

There has been a gradual trend towards breast conservation in managing breast cancer, encouraged by improvements in radiotherapy and adjuvant treatment. In developed countries, only 25–30% of cancers are now treated by mastectomy. If technically possible (i.e. with non-central, single small tumours, particularly in the upper outer quadrant), wide local excision of the tumour mass is performed and the remaining breast tissue is irradiated. However, it is also important to obtain information on the axillary node status in addition, to guide therapy and provide prognostic information. The effectiveness of this conservative approach in preventing local recurrence is similar to that of mastectomy. Apart from its potential cosmetic and psychological advantages, wide local excision allows the option of later mastectomy if there is a local recurrence. Breast irradiation following local excision may form part of **radical radiotherapy**, designed to prevent local and regional recurrence.

Occasionally a patient presents with extensive local disease or widespread metastases. Surgery in these circumstances may be inappropriate and palliative measures such as radiotherapy may be used along with tamoxifen. Sometimes, such treatment 'downstages' the cancer, allowing subsequent mastectomy.

PREVENTION AND TREATMENT OF REGIONAL DISEASE IN EARLY BREAST CANCER

Even with a small primary tumour, micrometastatic disease may have already spread to local skin, chest wall or regional lymph nodes. Larger primary lesions may show local or regional secondary deposits at the time of initial presentation. Diagnosis in apparently early disease should include biopsy of axillary nodes, which is likely to determine whether adjuvant chemotherapy or hormonal therapy is used.

The options for managing axillary lymph nodes are:

- **An expectant policy** may be adopted. This involves treating regional metastases by surgery or

radiotherapy only if they become clinically apparent. This is rarely employed nowadays
- **Radical radiotherapy** may be given to all patients with breast cancer. This involves radiotherapy to the breast (if conserved) and the chest wall, as well as to lymph nodes in the axilla, and perhaps supraclavicular and internal mammary groups
- **Selective radiotherapy** may be given, based on the results of axillary node biopsy performed at the initial operation or at a second operation once cancer has been diagnosed. The nodes are subjected to radiotherapy only if they are histologically involved
- **Surgical removal of axillary lymph nodes** is employed in proven breast cancer as an alternative to radiotherapy by some surgeons, whether the nodes appear clinically involved or not. Prognosis is inversely related to the number of nodes involved. It is important diagnostically to remove 6–10 lymph nodes to avoid missing 'skip' metastases in higher nodes. Current practice is to perform a **level II dissection**, removing nodes up to the axillary vein and beneath pectoralis minor. In addition to the diagnostic benefits, some enthusiasts claim that complete surgical axillary node removal gives better shoulder mobility than radiotherapy. Complete axillary lymph node removal may be performed as an adjunct to breast-conserving surgery or as part of a simple mastectomy or a **modified radical mastectomy**. The latter preserves the pectoralis major muscle formerly removed in Halsted radical mastectomies. Radiotherapy should not be given to patients after radical lymph node clearance as this gives an unacceptable incidence of lymphoedema of the arm. Effective sentinel lymph node biopsy should help reduce the number of unnecessary complete axillary lymph node dissections.

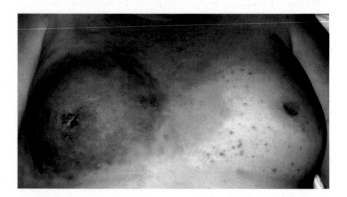

Fig. 39.14 Advanced breast cancer
This 60-year-old woman had been aware of a lump in her right breast for over a year before she could be persuaded to seek treatment. The whole breast is involved and malignancy has spread through the skin widely across the chest wall. The cancer was treated palliatively with tamoxifen and radiotherapy.

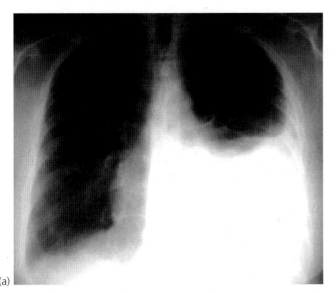

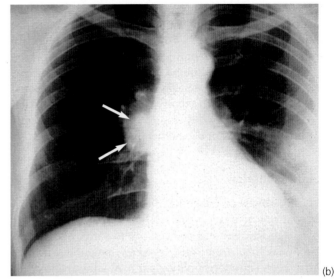

(a)　　　　　　　　　　　　　　　　　　　　　　　　　　　　　　　(b)

Fig. 39.15 Chest manifestations of metastatic breast carcinoma
(a) This 38-year-old woman had undergone a right mastectomy for ductal carcinoma 7 years before and presented with increasing shortness of breath. This chest X-ray shows a large left pleural effusion confirmed on cytology to be malignant. It was palliated by drainage and pleurodesis. **(b)** A different patient who had been treated 5 years before for lobular carcinoma of the breast. She presented with a chronic non-productive cough and was found to have a mass of lymph nodes at the right hilum (arrowed) and a right recurrent laryngeal nerve palsy due to invasion in the region of the carina.

Adjuvant chemotherapy

The unexpectedly low cure rate for apparently early breast cancer is due to occult metastatic spread. Surgery cannot adequately deal with metastases to mediastinal and supraclavicular nodes or elsewhere, but several pulses of systemic adjuvant chemotherapy have been shown to improve survival in certain groups of patients. This may be by destroying early metastases or malignant cells capable of metastasising or by the effects of chemotherapy causing ovarian ablation. Various combinations of cytotoxic drugs have been tested but the current consensus employs one of two main combinations, both of which contain **cyclophosphamide** and **5-fluorouracil**. In addition, the **CMF** regimen includes methotrexate and the **FAC** regimen includes adriamycin (doxorubicin). Adjuvant chemotherapy is currently employed for most premenopausal women shown to have high-grade tumours and axillary spread but without evident distant metastases. These regimens give an average 30% increase in survival in premenopausal women with more than four positive axillary lymph nodes on histology.

Systemic treatment with adjuvant chemotherapy is also sometimes used in some groups of node-negative patients and in some postmenopausal women but the benefits are not as clear-cut.

Adjuvant hormonal therapy

Tamoxifen, an oestrogen receptor blocker taken orally, is widely used as an adjuvant treatment. The drug has long proved beneficial for postmenopausal patients with breast cancer and, when taken for 2–5 years, conclusively prolongs the disease-free interval in this group (i.e. time to first local recurrence or metastasis). More recently, similar results have been demonstrated in premenopausal patients despite its disadvantage of causing symptoms of an early menopause. Oophorectomy gives survival equivalent to adjuvant chemotherapy and may prove to be an acceptable option. There is unconfirmed evidence that tamoxifen may safely reduce the risk of developing breast cancer if taken prophylactically.

CONTROL OF ADVANCED AND DISSEMINATED DISEASE

All the treatments so far described attempt to achieve a complete cure. In reality, about 65% of patients presenting with early breast cancer will eventually succumb to the disease despite the best treatments, though this may be as long as 35 years later. There is continued improvement, however, of 5- and 10-year survival rates. With current treatment modalities, the control of advanced and disseminated disease at any stage can only be palliative but worthwhile prolongation of life can often be achieved in addition to improving the quality of life.

Locally, tumour may spread within the breast, into the overlying skin or into the chest wall. **Pleural effusions** may appear and are usually the result of pulmonary metastases. Systemic spread commonly causes **osteolytic bone lesions** which are painful and may result in

515

pathological fracture (see Fig. 39.12, p. 512). Secondary deposits are common in the **liver** but less common in the **lungs** and **brain** (see p. 510); these metastases tend to become troublesome only at a terminal stage of the disease. **Lobular carcinoma** can metastasise to unusual sites such as skin (see Fig. 39.16) and bowel. Some metastatic sites, particularly bone, respond to local radiotherapy, while others may respond to systemic hormonal therapy or chemotherapy.

Local palliation

Locally advanced (stage III) disease in breast and axilla may appear to be inoperable at first sight. Current trends for stage III disease, however, are towards more interventional treatment using several modalities which have been shown to prolong survival substantially. For example, after diagnostic cytology or biopsy, three cycles of neoadjuvant (i.e. before surgery) chemotherapy will often convert the cancer into an operable prospect. Mastectomy and node biopsy are then performed, followed by radical radiotherapy and later by adjuvant chemotherapy or tamoxifen. In patients in whom this level of intervention is inappropriate, radiotherapy can be employed for palliation of advanced skin, breast, chest wall and lymph node disease or tumour recurrences, as well as for isolated bone metastases; all of these usually respond well. **Pleural effusions** can be aspirated or the pleural cavity obliterated by pleurectomy or instillation of tetracycline or various cytotoxic agents. Discrete lesions, for example in skin, can sometimes be removed surgically.

Hormonal manipulation

Hormonal palliative treatment of breast cancer is essentially empirical:

- **Tamoxifen** has been shown to extend survival in patients with metastases and is also worth giving in patients unfit for surgery. The drug has the side effect of causing menopausal symptoms in most women. Concern is now being expressed that long-term use may predispose to endometrial cancer. If tamoxifen fails, **megestrol** or other progestogens may prove beneficial. Specific aromatase inhibitors also show promise but are still being evaluated
- Surgical **oophorectomy** gives a good but temporary response in about a third of patients with intractable bone pain but it does bring about an immediate menopause with consequent side effects
- **Corticosteroids** may be used to suppress adrenal sex hormone production and may induce a sense of well-being
- **Adrenalectomy** and **hypophysectomy** are now seldom performed because of low response rate and

unpleasant side effects. Occasionally, the drug aminoglutethimide is used to perform a 'medical' adrenalectomy. Goserelin can also be employed as a luteinising hormone releasing hormone (LHRH) antagonist
- **Other agents**, e.g. the taxoids, are being evaluated

Systemic chemotherapy

Chemotherapy, using combinations of drugs, is sometimes employed for palliation of extensive metastatic disease and can give remissions in more than 70% of patients for up to 3 years. Gradual improvements in chemotherapeutic drugs and anti-nausea agents make this option worthwhile for certain patients, for example, young women or those with hepatic involvement.

LONG-TERM FOLLOW-UP

Women who have had one breast cancer have a 15% lifetime risk of developing a second tumour in the other

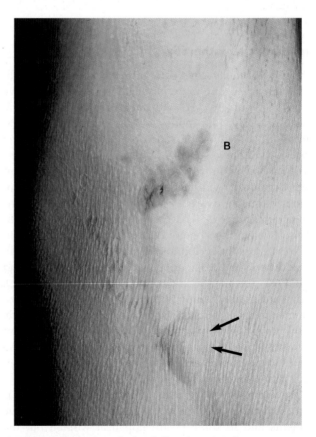

Fig. 39.16 Skin secondaries following simple mastectomy and radiotherapy
This patient presented with painless, slightly elevated nodules in the skin below the axilla 3 years after treatment for lobular carcinoma of the breast. In this photograph, the arm is elevated and one skin secondary can just be made out (arrowed); the site of excision biopsy of another is seen at **B**.

After mastectomy, it is important that lifelike prostheses are provided. Wherever possible, this should start with temporary prostheses in the immediate postoperative period. These may even be inserted before the patient leaves the operating theatre. Reconstructive surgery using myocutaneous flaps (transverse rectus abdominis (TRAM) or latissimus dorsi) and silicone implants (which cause continuing debate about safety) may be appropriate either at the initial operation or later in some patients. Self-help societies, like the British Mastectomy Association, can play a valuable part in helping the patient to return to normal life.

BREAST CANCER IN MALES

Up to 1% of all breast cancers occur in males. Presentation is often delayed because the diagnosis is not considered and it should be noted that unilateral breast enlargement in males deserves serious diagnostic effort. Management is similar to that in females. Chest wall and lymph node involvement may occur earlier because there is so little breast tissue and prognosis may be worse than for females.

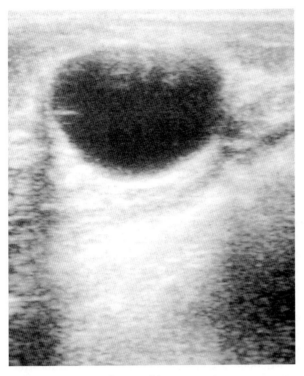

Fig. 39.17 Ultrasound scan of breast cyst
Showing the characteristic well defined dark area representing clear fluid, with a distinct acoustic shadow beyond it.

breast. The risk is higher if the original lesion was a lobular carcinoma. The breast tissue in these women may have an increased susceptibility to cancer, or breast cancer may arise at the same time in multiple foci. Thus women with breast cancer should be regularly followed up clinically and by mammography for many years after initial treatment. Patients should be instructed how to examine themselves and to return if they notice any new symptoms or signs.

PROSTHESES AND PREOPERATIVE PREPARATION FOR MASTECTOMY

The cosmetic effects of mastectomy are of great psychological importance to women and their families. Careful attention to this can alleviate distress and improve acceptance of disfigurement. Preoperative counselling by medical or specially trained nursing staff should prepare the patient for treatment.

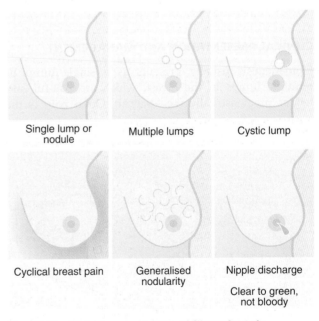

Single lump or nodule | Multiple lumps | Cystic lump

Cyclical breast pain | Generalised nodularity | Nipple discharge
Clear to green, not bloody

Fig. 39.18 Clinical presentation of fibroadenosis

BENIGN BREAST DISORDERS

The common benign breast disorders include fibroadenosis (including cystic disease), fibroadenoma, duct papilloma, fat necrosis, breast infections and mammary duct ectasia.

FIBROADENOSIS

PATHOLOGY

Fibroadenosis is a disorder of the breast in women of reproductive age, its peak incidence occurring between the ages of 35 and 45. It probably results from mildly disordered physiological responses to circulating hormones. Fibroadenosis is one of the 'aberrations of normal development or involution' (ANDI). In brief, the changes result from distortion and overgrowth of one or more of the various components of the breast, namely the **ducts**, the **lobules** and the supporting **fibrous tissue**. The fibrous tissue element becomes exaggerated, i.e. **fibrosis**, and the epithelial components undergo hyperplasia, i.e. **epitheliosis and adenosis**; hence the name fibroadenosis.

Although this book uses the general term of fibroadenosis, many other descriptive terms have also been applied, including benign change, mastitis, fibrocystic disease of the breast and cystic mammary dysplasia. Most of these terms are confusing, and some erroneously suggest that the condition is more than a simple proliferative disorder of breast tissue.

There is no evidence that fibroadenosis is a precursor of carcinoma. Fibroadenosis is common, however, and carcinoma will sometimes develop in a woman with fibroadenosis.

CLINICAL PRESENTATION AND MANAGEMENT

Fibroadenosis usually presents as a single lump or multiple lumps in the breast, which are painful and tender premenstrually (i.e. cyclical). Often pain is the presenting complaint rather than a lump. Lumpiness and tenderness are a cyclical feature of the normal breast; thus, diffuse fibroadenosis may just represent an extreme variation of the normal. Isolated lesions, however, may be difficult to distinguish clinically from carcinoma.

Breast cysts are a common form of fibroadenosis. The cysts are usually single, occasionally multiple, and they are most common in perimenopausal women. They sometimes develop with startling rapidity. On palpation, they can usually be recognised by their smooth rounded outline and characteristic tense fluctuation, similar to the texture of a table tennis ball. The diagnosis can be made by simple aspiration, preferably after mammography and ultrasonography. Carcinoma can be excluded if the criteria shown in Figure 39.20 are satisfied. The diagnosis of fibroadenosis thus depends on excluding cancer. This is done clinically, by ultrasound and/or mammography, aspiration cytology if appropriate or by excision biopsy if doubt remains. Note that cyst fluid only needs to be sent for cytological examination if cellular or bloody.

Once cancer has been excluded and the patient reassured, further treatment is often unnecessary. Isolated fibroadenotic lesions may have been surgically excised (and thus treated) in the process. When pain is severe and localised to a particular area, excision of the area may occasionally be justified, but if pain is more diffuse, oil of evening primrose or its purer form gammalinolenic acid may be tried. If the pain is severe and cyclical, drugs such as **danazol** and **bromocriptine** are sometimes used. Danazol inhibits pituitary gonadotrophin secretion but may have serious androgenic and other side effects which often limit its usefulness. Bromocriptine inhibits pituitary prolactin release and has fewer side effects.

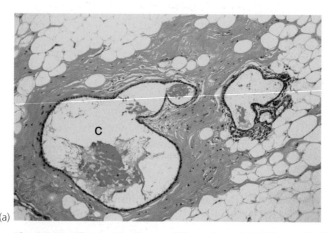

(a)

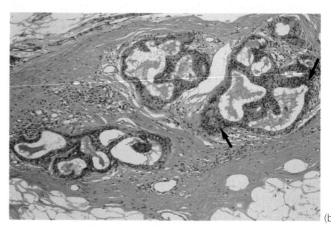

(b)

Fig. 39.19 Fibrocystic disease (fibroadenosis)—histopathology
Fibrocystic disease is known by a number of names, including fibroadenosis, reflecting the variety of changes seen. A number of these features are often present within a single lesion, or in different areas of the same or contralateral breast. The main components are: cyst formation, epitheliosis, fibrosis and proliferation of lobular acini, known as adenosis. Fibrosis may occur within areas of adenosis, splitting acini, known as sclerosing adenosis. **(a)** Dilated ducts form cysts **C** of various sizes, from microscopic to large palpable lesions measuring several centimetres. Often a cyst is lined by flattened ductal epithelium, however, this may also show secretory features, known as **apocrine metaplasia. (b)** Ducts show epithelial proliferation (arrowed), known as **epitheliosis**, which may give rise to single or multiple papillomas. The degree of hyperplasia within epitheliosis varies and may be associated with cytological atypia, which can indicate an increased risk of developing breast adenocarcinoma. At the extreme end of the spectrum, ductal proliferation may amount to ductal carcinoma in situ.

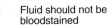

1   Fluid should not be bloodstained

2   Lump should disappear

3   Cyst should not recur

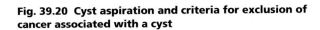

Fig. 39.20 Cyst aspiration and criteria for exclusion of cancer associated with a cyst

FIBROADENOMA

PATHOLOGY

Fibroadenoma commonly presents in younger women as a solitary breast lump. It is considered to be a benign neoplasm, but may represent a nodular form of fibroadenosis. The lesions are composed of epithelial and fibrous components; the epithelium forms glandular structures lined by mammary ductal cells and the connective tissue forms a loose cellular stroma (see Fig. 39.21). The lesions are well circumscribed by a condensed connective tissue capsule. As with fibroadenosis, there appears to be no association with breast cancer.

CLINICAL PRESENTATION AND MANAGEMENT OF FIBROADENOMA

Unlike fibroadenosis, fibroadenomas are usually found in women below the age of 30. The lesion usually presents as a discrete, non-tender, highly mobile lump. It may be found incidentally or during self-examination. Small lesions are sometimes described as **breast mice** since they slip away from beneath the palpating hand. Giant fibroadenoma-like lesions may occur in older women. These **phyllodes tumours** are usually benign but 25% are malignant and metastasise. Like fibroadenosis, the main clinical importance of fibroadenoma is to distinguish it from breast cancer. In patients under 25 years FNA can be relied upon; over 25, or if doubt remains, excision biopsy confirms the diagnosis and provides treatment.

DUCT PAPILLOMA

Duct papillomas are localised areas of epithelial proliferation within large mammary or lactiferous ducts (see Fig. 39.22). They are therefore benign hyperplastic lesions rather than neoplasms and are not premalignant, although they have been confused with in situ carcinoma.

Duct papillomas present with nipple bleeding or a blood-stained discharge. The differential diagnosis thus includes intraduct carcinoma and infiltrating carcinoma which must be excluded. The breast is carefully palpated for lumps and a mammogram is usually performed to search for frank carcinoma. Ductography may confirm the presence of a duct papilloma (Fig. 39.23). Duct papillomas are usually treated by surgical excision of the affected segment of breast (**microdochectomy**). The affected segment is identified during operation by passing a probe into the duct from where blood can be expressed.

TRAUMATIC FAT NECROSIS

Trauma to the breast, sometimes trivial or even unnoticed, may cause necrosis of adipose tissue. Initially, there is an acute inflammatory response but if necrotic fat remains,

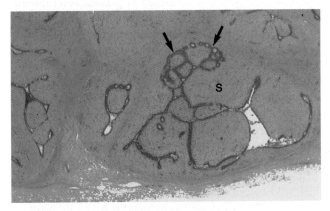

Fig. 39.21 Fibroadenoma—histopathology
This benign lesion shows proliferation of both glands (arrowed) and stroma **S**. In the variant illustrated, gland lumina are compressed by stroma. Fibroadenoma typically has a histologically well-defined edge.

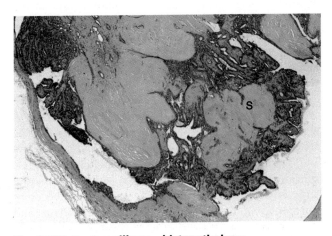

Fig. 39.22 Duct papilloma—histopathology
This is essentially a localised form of epitheliosis. Papilloma in a larger duct must be distinguished from papillary carcinoma, which lacks well-defined stromal cores **S**. Both lesions can present with blood-stained nipple discharge.

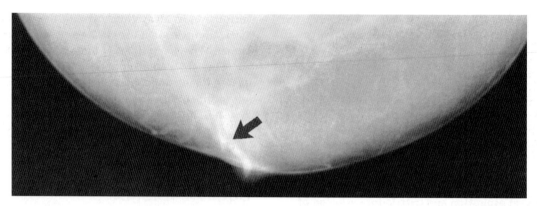

Fig. 39.23 Contrast mammogram (ductogram) outlining duct papilloma
This patient presented with bleeding from the nipple but no breast lump was palpable. The affected duct was injected with contrast material which outlines the duct system, revealing a small defect (arrowed) which represents a duct papilloma.

the inflammatory picture becomes more chronic. Plasma cells appear in large numbers and macrophages take up lipid material. A fibrotic response at the margins of the damaged area produces a hard, often irregular breast lump, which may cause skin dimpling if it is close to the surface. Thus the clinical picture may be indistinguishable from carcinoma. Traumatic fat necrosis is very rare and the diagnosis can only be made by excision biopsy.

INFECTIONS OF THE BREAST

Infections of the breast lobules present either as a **diffuse cellulitis** or as an **abscess** (Fig. 39.2). The latter is often the result of inadequately treated cellulitis. Less commonly, infections arise in the sebaceous (Montgomery's) glands of the areola, where they resemble common skin boils. Deep infections occur most commonly during late pregnancy and lactation. The organism is almost invariably *Staphylococcus aureus*. It gains access to the breast either through cracked nipple skin, through inverted nipples or via the bloodstream. Retention of breast secretions (engorgement) may be a predisposing factor. Abscesses can also occur in non-lactating patients with nipple inversion.

Diagnosis of an abscess is usually obvious, with local and systemic signs of acute inflammation. The patient is generally unwell with a tachycardia and fever. The affected segment of the breast is painful and tender, red and warm. If the infection is inadequately treated, a considerable amount of breast tissue is destroyed and a large amount of pus forms. The lesion then becomes fluctuant and eventually 'points' to the surface and discharges.

The early cellulitic phase is reversible if treated with appropriate antibiotics. Flucloxacillin is the antibiotic of choice on a 'best-guess' basis. If antibiotics are started too late or the wrong antibiotic is chosen, tissue damage and accumulation of polymorphs cause multiple loculi of pus to form which can only be effectively treated by surgical drainage. The need for surgical drainage has declined in recent years because of prompt and appropriate antibiotic treatment, sometimes aided by aspiration.

At operation, a skin incision is made over the most fluctuant area and the loculi are explored and broken down with a finger. If there is extensive damage, a drain may be inserted in the wound and if there is significant residual cellulitis, antibiotics should be prescribed after operation.

MAMMARY DUCT ECTASIA

Mammary duct ectasia means dilatation of the larger breast ducts. These usually contain green fluid and sometimes sterile pus. If an ectatic duct ruptures, a chronic inflammatory response develops in the surrounding breast tissue. Plasma cells are a characteristic feature of the histology, which is described as **plasma cell mastitis**. A few ducts may be involved or the whole duct system.

Mammary duct ectasia is most common in the decade around the menopause. Patients typically present with a green nipple discharge and tender lumpiness beneath or close to the areola and nipple inversion is a common accompanying feature. Occasionally mammary duct ectasia may produce abscess-like signs with localised reddening and tenderness in the breast but without overt signs of infection. The condition represents an inflammatory reaction to retained duct secretions with low-grade infection and usually settles with antibiotics. Infection associated with mammary duct ectasia should not be drained surgically as a ductal fistula will result.

Mammography sometimes shows typical diagnostic features (see Fig. 39.24). Management involves excluding

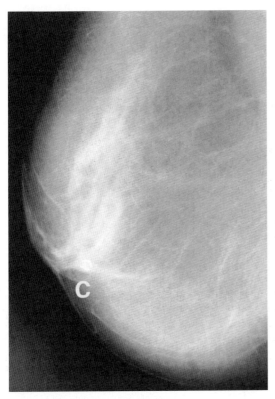

Fig. 39.24 Mammary duct ectasia
Radiopaque mass of dilated ducts with no features of malignancy.
Large duct calcification **C** is also seen. Note the skin indentation caused
by fibrosis. Clinically, this condition can be mistaken for carcinoma.

carcinoma and sometimes surgical excision of the affected tissue. If mammary duct ectasia is extensive or if sub-areolar pyogenic abscesses develop, sub-areolar excision of all the major ducts usually cures the condition (Hadfield's or Adair's operation).

Note that the term **plasma cell mastitis** describes a histopathological appearance rather than a clinical entity and is seen in different conditions such as fat necrosis or ruptured ectatic duct. These evoke an inflammatory response in which plasma cells predominate. Like any intense inflammatory response, this produces a firm irregular mass.

MALE BREAST DISORDERS

Any condition which occurs in the female breast can occur in the male. Only two conditions are clinically important: carcinoma (described earlier) and gynae-comastia. Any suspicious lumps should be removed. **Carcinoma** of the male breast is similar to that seen in women and is managed in the same way.

Gynaecomastia is benign hypertrophy of the breast disc and may have a hormonal basis. Clinically, one or both breasts become abnormally enlarged. Gynaecomastia may be present at birth in response to maternal oestrogens crossing the placenta; the condition resolves spontaneously over several weeks. Likewise, in pubertal males, the changing hormonal environment may cause temporary but distressing, commonly unilateral, breast enlargement which may require surgery. In older males, bilateral gynaecomastia may result from excess circulating oestrogens due to liver disease, certain testicular tumours or drugs such as cimetidine or spironolactone.

40 Disorders of the skin

INTRODUCTION

Only a small proportion of the enormous variety of skin disorders are surgically important. Unsightly lumps and possible malignant lesions fall into this category. **Ulcers** of the lower limb are common and usually of vascular or diabetic origin. Some venous ulcers are managed by dermatologists, but most of the remainder are managed by surgeons; these are discussed in Chapter 34. Ulceration also characterises many important, often malignant skin lesions.

Skin disorders comprise about 15% of new outpatient general surgical referrals. Many only require excision biopsy under local anaesthesia. A small proportion of skin lesions have a potentially sinister course, particularly malignant melanoma. These must be accurately diagnosed and treated. Suspected malignant skin lesions are often managed jointly by dermatologists or surgeons (including plastic surgeons) and radiotherapists. In general, the initial diagnostic referral should be made to the dermatologist, who sees many more skin conditions than the general surgeon. Some patients are referred after a skin lesion has been excised by a family practitioner and found to be malignant on histology.

Malignant melanomas comprise only 2% of all skin cancers in Northern Europe but, like basal cell and squamous cell carcinomas, their incidence closely correlates with sun exposure and fair skin. The incidence of all skin cancers is rising with the increase in foreign travel. Skin malignancies and their premalignant stages are much more common in sunny countries like Australia where they are reaching epidemic proportions.

Finally, the nails, which are specialised skin appendages, pose surgical problems in the form of infected **ingrowing toenails** and **onychogryphosis**. The rare subungual melanoma is an important diagnosis which should not be missed.

STRUCTURE OF NORMAL SKIN

The skin is made up of three main layers, the **epidermis**, the **dermis** and the **hypodermis**:

- The epidermis consists of four main layers—the basal layer, the prickle-cell layer, the granular layer and the keratin layer. Cell division normally occurs only in the basal layer
- The underlying dermis consists of dense, tough interlacing collagen fibres; their orientation determines the lines of tension in the skin known as **Langer's lines**. These are surgically important because incisions parallel to them heal with minimal scarring

- The deepest layer of the skin is the **hypodermis**, which consists of loose fibro-fatty tissue. The hypodermis contains the skin appendages—sweat glands, hair follicles and their associated sebaceous glands. The hypodermis is only loosely connected to the **superficial fascia**, which makes the skin mobile over the deeper structures. The exceptions are the palms of the hands, the soles of the feet and the scalp, where the skin is tightly bound to the fascial layer

A working classification of surgically important skin lesions based on site of origin is given in Figure 40.1.

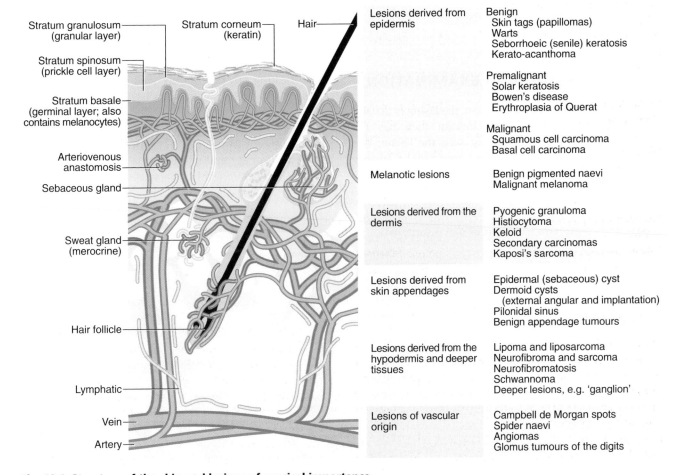

Fig. 40.1 Structure of the skin and lesions of surgical importance

SYMPTOMS AND SIGNS OF SKIN DISORDERS

The most common surgical skin complaint is a lump. This may be tender or painful, and it may have begun to bleed, discharge or ulcerate. The lesion may be pigmented or have changed colour. It may have appeared suddenly or enlarged rapidly, or there may have been some change in a longstanding lesion.

Any one of these symptoms may prompt the patient to seek medical advice, but the most frequent seem to be the ugliness or inconvenience of a lesion to the patient (e.g. getting in the way of a strap). Elderly patients may only come reluctantly and at the insistence of younger relatives. Some patients do not present until a lesion is huge, while others present with trivial lesions. Both types of patient may be worried by the thought of malignancy.

In practice (and in clinical exams) the diagnosis of skin lesions rarely follows the conventional pattern of history taking, physical examination and investigations. Rather, the lesion is thrust before the doctor's eyes and a 'spot' diagnosis or differential diagnosis is made. History and examination are then used to see whether they confirm the diagnosis or narrow the differential possibilities. Table 40.1 summarises the important clinical features of skin lesions and their diagnostic significance.

HISTORY TAKING AND EXAMINATION

As the patient describes the problem, the lesion is usually offered for examination. The clinician then has the questionable advantage of having seen the lesion; this may then guide the direction and emphasis of history taking. The patient should be questioned about other similar lesions or any regional lumps. Detailed inspection and palpation follow and by this time, a definite diagnosis or narrow differential diagnosis should have been established.

A **general history** must be taken at some point to establish whether there are any relevant systemic symptoms (e.g. weight loss suggesting malignant cachexia), concurrent disorders (e.g. diabetes predisposes to infection and may influence surgical management), any history of previous similar lesions, surgical treatment or trauma to the affected area. For example, a history of previous rodent ulcers (basal cell carcinoma) makes this diagnosis more likely another time. Previous surgery or trauma can cause implantation dermoids or a chronic inflammatory response to a foreign body.

Family history is occasionally valuable in rare genetic disorders such as neurofibromatosis. **Social history** should include occupational details as these may be relevant. For example, natal cleft pilonidal sinus is more common in truck drivers. Exposure to carcinogens such as lubricating oils persistently spilt on the same area of clothing may result in squamous carcinoma. Outdoor workers, especially those from the tropics, are predisposed to all types of skin cancer. Chronic ulcers may be contracted during **foreign travel**, e.g. tropical ulcers, Madura foot, tuberculous or atypical mycobacterial ulcers. Occasionally, patients deliberately injure themselves, producing mys-

---

Table 40.1 Symptoms and signs of skin disorders

Symptoms and signs	Diagnostic significance
1. Lump in or on the skin *Size, shape and surface features* Revealed by inspection — is the lesion smooth-surfaced, irregular, exophytic (i.e. projecting out of the surface)?	Epidermal lesions such as warts usually have a surface abnormality but deeper lesions are usually covered by normal epidermis. A *punctum* suggests the abnormality arises from an epidermal appendage e.g. epidermal (sebaceous) cyst
Depth within the skin Superficial and deep attachments. Which tissue is the swelling derived from?	Tends to reflect the layer from which lesion is derived (i.e. epidermis, dermis, hypodermis or deeper)
Character of the margin Discreteness, tethering to surrounding tissues, three-dimensional shape	A regular shaped, discrete lesion is most likely cystic or encapsulated (e.g. benign tumour). Deep tethering implies origin from deeper structures (e.g. ganglion). Immobility of overlying epidermis suggests a lesion derived from skin appendage (e.g. epidermal cyst)
Consistency Soft, firm, hard, 'indurated', rubbery	Soft lesions are usually lipomas or fluid-filled cysts. Most cysts are fluctuant unless filled by semi-solid material (e.g. epidermal cysts), or the cyst is tense (e.g. small ganglion). Malignant lesions tend to be hard and irregular ('indurated') with an ill-defined margin due to invasion of surrounding tissue. Bony-hard lesions are either mineralised (e.g. gouty tophi) or consist of bone (e.g. exostoses)
Pulsatility	Pulsatility is usually transmitted from an underlying artery which may simply be tortuous or it may be abnormal (e.g. aneurysm or arteriovenous fistula)
Emptying and refilling	Vascular lesions (e.g. venous malformations or haemangiomas) empty or blanch on pressure and then refill
Transilluminability	Lesions filled with clear fluid such as cysts 'light up' when transilluminated
Temperature	Excessive warmth implies acute inflammation e.g. pilonidal abscess

Table 40.1 Continued

Symptoms and signs	Diagnostic significance
2. Pain, tenderness and discomfort	These most often indicate acute inflammation. Pain also develops if a non-inflammatory lesion becomes inflamed or infected (e.g. inflamed epidermal cyst). Malignant lesions are usually painless
3. Ulceration (i.e. loss of epidermal integrity with the inflamed base formed by dermis or deeper tissues)	Tumours and kerato-acanthomas tend to ulcerate as a result of central necrosis. Surface breakdown also occurs in arterial or venous insufficiency (e.g. ischaemic leg ulcers), chronic infection (e.g. TB or tropical ulcers) or trauma
Character of the ulcer margin	In benign ulcers, the margin is only slightly raised by inflammatory oedema. The base lies below the level of normal skin. Malignant ulcers begin as a solid mass of proliferating epidermal cells, the centre of which eventually becomes necrotic. The margin is typically elevated 'rolled' and indurated by tumour growth and invasion
Behaviour of the ulcer	Malignant ulcers expand inexorably (though often slowly), but may go through cycles of breakdown and healing (often with bleeding)
4. COLOUR AND PIGMENTATION *Normal colour*	If a lesion is covered by normal coloured skin then the lesion must lie deeply in the skin (e.g. epidermal cyst) or deep to the skin (e.g. ganglion)
Red or purple	Redness implies increased arterial vascularity, which is most common in inflammatory conditions like furuncles. Vascular abnormalities which contain a high proportion of arterial blood such as Campbell de Morgan spots or strawberry naevi are also red, whereas venous disorders such as port-wine stain are darker. Vascular lesions blanch on pressure and must be distinguished from purpura which does not
Deeply pigmented	Benign naevi (moles) and their malignant counterpart, malignant melanomas, are nearly always pigmented. Other lesions such as warts, papillomas or seborrhoeic keratoses, may become pigmented secondarily. Hairy pigmented moles are almost never malignant. Rarely, malignant melanomas may be non-pigmented (amelanotic). Darkening of a pigmented lesion should be viewed with suspicion as it may indicated malignant change
5. Rapidly developing lesion	Kerato-acanthoma, warts and pyogenic granuloma may all develop rapidly and eventually regress spontaneously. When fully developed, these conditions may be difficult to distinguish from malignancy. Spontaneous regression marks the lesion as benign
6. Multiple, recurrent and spreading lesions	In certain rare syndromes, multiple similar lesions develop over a period. Examples include neurofibromatosis and recurrent lipomata in Dercum's disease. Heavy sun exposure predisposes a large area of skin to malignant change. Viral warts may appear in crops. Malignant melanoma may spread diffusely (superficial spreading melanoma), or produce satellite lesions via dermal lymphatics
7. Site of the lesion	Some skin lesions arise much more commonly in certain areas of the body. The reason may be anatomical (e.g. pilonidal sinus, external angular dermoid or multiple pilar cysts of the scalp) or because of exposure to sun (e.g. solar keratoses or basal cell carcinomas of hands and face)
8. Age when lesion noticed	Congenital vascular abnormalities such as strawberry naevus or port-wine stain may be present at birth. Benign pigmented naevi (moles) may be detectable at birth, but only begin to enlarge and darken after the age of two

terious chronic lesions; a **psychiatric history** is valuable here, though rarely forthcoming.

Drug history is rarely relevant to 'surgical' skin lesions, apart from agents applied topically. Silver nitrate stick, caustic agents and mechanical interference with wounds or lesions can distort the clinical picture.

The lesion is examined in detail, looking for the points described in Table 40.1. In addition, general clinical examination should search for other similar lesions, regional lymphadenopathy or a primary malignancy arising elsewhere and metastasising to skin. For example, if inguinal lymph nodes are enlarged, rectal and genital examination should be carried out to exclude concealed carcinoma. The lower limbs, including the soles of the feet, should also be examined, looking especially for malignant melanoma.

PRINCIPLES OF MANAGEMENT OF SKIN LESIONS

Many skin lesions can be diagnosed from the history and clinical examination, but wherever there is doubt, some form of biopsy is needed. This is particularly true if there is any risk of malignancy. Biopsy is usually performed as part of the treatment process. Incision and excision biopsy techniques are illustrated in Chapter 6 and Box 40.1 summarises the options in the surgical management of skin conditions.

KEY POINTS

Box 40.1 Principles of management of 'surgical' skin disorders

Simple excision or other physical methods, e.g. electrocautery, laser therapy or cryotherapy—for small, obviously innocent lesions

Excision biopsy—if there is any risk of malignancy or the clinical diagnosis is doubtful (only for small lesions)

Biopsy—for large lesions. Definitive therapy is then planned according to the histology

Wide local excision with or without skin grafting—for malignant melanomas and sometimes for other large malignant lesions

Radiotherapy—an alternative to excision for basal cell carcinoma and primary squamous cell lesions. Also sometimes used in squamous cell carcinoma if regional lymph nodes are involved

Lymph node clearance—if nodes are involved by malignant melanoma or squamous carcinoma

---

BENIGN LESIONS DERIVED FROM THE EPIDERMIS

SKIN TAGS (SQUAMOUS CELL PAPILLOMAS)

Skin tags are small benign polypoid lesions up to about 5 mm in diameter. They consist of a loose connective tissue core covered by normal, often excessively pigmented, keratinised epithelium. They are common in adults and may occur on any part of the body, particularly the trunk, neck, axillae and groins. In these locations, they may be irritated by clothing and bleed. Unsightly or inconvenient lesions may be easily removed by cautery or excision (under local anaesthesia), or by tying a fine thread around the stalk (also under local anaesthesia) which leads to ischaemic atrophy.

WARTS

Warts are small, virus-induced epidermal tumours. They are characterised pathologically by irregular thickening of the epidermis with grossly excessive keratinisation and exaggerated dermal papillae. The morphology of the lesion depends on its location on the skin.

The **common wart** (verruca vulgaris), a papilliferous lesion up to 1 cm in diameter, is most common on the fingers and back of the hands. In children, warts are often multiple, and commonly occur on the face. Facial lesions are often less keratotic with a smoother, more dome-like shape. They are often called **juvenile warts** (verruca plana juvenilis). Lesions on the sole of the foot, plantar warts (verruca plantaris), become extremely keratotic and flattened as a result of pressure. They may extend deeply into the foot, causing considerable pain. Warts may also occur on the genitalia, perineum and perianal area, usually spread by sexual contact. Genital warts sometimes grow to a large size; these are then known as **condylomata accuminata**.

Warts grow and regress spontaneously over several months, but they often require treatment to relieve pain, irritation or inconvenience. Many are treated for aesthetic reasons. Keratolytic applications (salicylic acid or podophyllin resin preparations) or cryosurgery (liquid nitrogen application) are often the first choice of treatment. If unsuccessful, electrocautery (with or without curettage) can be used.

SEBORRHOEIC KERATOSIS

Seborrhoeic keratoses (**seborrhoeic warts**) are extremely common skin lesions in elderly patients but occasionally appear in younger people (Fig. 40.2). The lesions are most often seen on the chest, face, neck and arms. There are often many lesions of different sizes with different intensities of pigmentation. They may be up to several centimetres in diameter. The lesions are slightly raised, sharply demarcated and plaque-like; they look and feel irregular and waxy. Sometimes they are so darkly pigmented that they cannot be distinguished clinically from superficial spreading malignant melanomas.

Histologically, a seborrhoeic keratosis is a localised proliferation of the basal layer of the epidermis. There is often hyperkeratosis in the surface crypts, resulting in round keratin nests. Seborrhoeic keratoses are sometimes called **basal cell papillomas** because of their origin, but they are not true neoplasms and are unrelated to basal cell carcinoma.

Treatment is only required for unsightly or easily traumatised lesions. As they are so superficial, they can be 'scraped off' with a curette or scalpel under local anaesthesia.

KERATOACANTHOMA

A keratoacanthoma is a nodular, usually single skin lesion, up to 2 cm in diameter (Fig. 40.3). It has an irregular central crater containing keratotic debris. As its name implies, the histological lesion consists of localised tumour-like epidermal proliferation, with a thick prickle cell layer (**acanthosis**) and marked keratinisation. Some epithelial cells are large and have atypical nuclei; the underlying dermis exhibits marked chronic inflammatory cell infiltration.

The importance of this benign lesion is that it can be difficult to distinguish clinically or even histologically from squamous carcinoma. Keratoacanthomas, however, tend to have a short lifecycle, appearing rapidly and

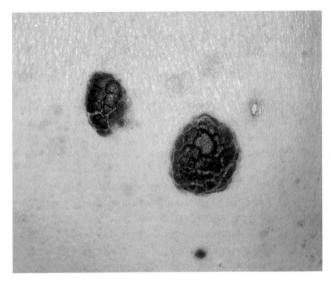

Fig. 40.2 Seborrhoeic keratoses

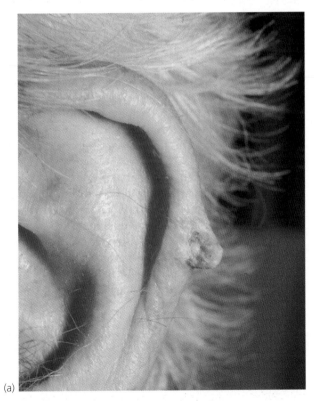

(a)

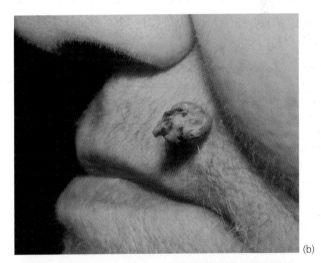

(b)

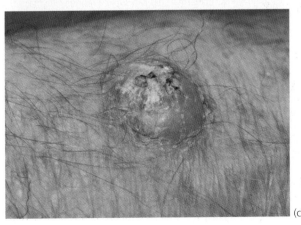

(c)

Fig. 40.3 Keratin horn and Keratoacanthoma
(a) Keratin horn on the pinna of an elderly man. If left, these can grow large. **(b)** This alarming looking lesion is a benign keratoacanthoma. The central keratin plug is characteristic. Resolution is spontaneous after a few weeks. **(c)** Similar lesion on the back of the hand. Squamous and basal cell carcinoma need to be excluded.

regressing spontaneously over 2–3 months, whereas squamous cell carcinomas continue to enlarge. Keratin horns may also look similar but rarely regress. The cause of keratoacanthoma is unknown but its behaviour suggests a viral origin.

Diagnosis and treatment is by local excision unless the lesion is obviously regressing. If there is still diagnostic doubt, the patient should be followed up as for squamous carcinoma.

PREMALIGNANT EPIDERMAL CONDITIONS

SOLAR (SENILE) KERATOSIS AND INTRA-EPIDERMAL CARCINOMA

PATHOLOGY AND CLINICAL FEATURES

Solar keratoses are flat, well demarcated, brown, scaly or crusty lesions with an erythematous base (Fig. 40.4). They bleed easily if traumatised or scratched. Solar keratoses are often multiple and are most common in middle-aged or elderly patients on sun-exposed parts of the body such as face, neck, arms and hands. The incidence is higher in farm workers, fishermen and other outdoor workers. Solar keratoses are especially common in fair-skinned people living in tropical or subtropical regions such as Australia or the southern USA.

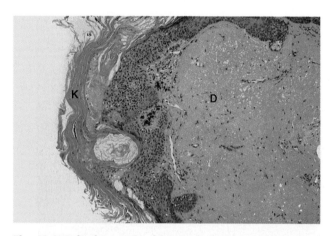

Fig. 40.4 Solar keratosis—histopathology
Occurring in sun-exposed areas, this lesion typically shows thickening of the keratin layer **K**. Epidermal cells can show a range of atypia, which may amount to squamous cell carcinoma in situ. The dermis **D** shows severe solar damage.

The characteristic histological features are marked thickening of the keratin layer (**hyperkeratosis**) and the prickle cell layer (**acanthosis**). Deep in the epidermis, there is a variable degree of dysplastic change and abnormal mitotic activity. These features suggest malignant transformation but most importantly, the basal layer remains intact.

The epidemiology and pathology of solar keratosis suggest that it is a premalignant condition which predisposes to squamous carcinoma. Any lesions in which the dysplastic changes extend from the basal layers to the surface are considered to be malignant. They are termed **carcinoma-in-situ** or **intra-epidermal carcinoma**. Clinically, these are more erythematous than the premalignant type and are sometimes described as **Bowen's disease**. Bowen's disease occurring on the glans penis is known as **erythroplasia of Queyrat**.

Management

Management of solar keratoses depends on the number, size and distribution of the lesions, the age of the patient, and whether or not the skin type predisposes to cancer. Isolated lesions are best excised. For multiple keratoses, excision biopsy of representative lesions should be performed initially to confirm the diagnosis. This is followed by excision biopsy, curettage or cryocautery of suspicious lesions. Patients should be advised repeatedly to minimise exposure to ultraviolet rays by wearing protective clothing and hats and applying total sunscreen creams. These patients should also be regularly examined for squamous cell carcinomas, basal cell carcinomas and melanomas, which are all more common in patients with marked sunshine exposure.

MALIGNANT EPIDERMAL LESIONS

SQUAMOUS CELL CARCINOMA

PATHOLOGY

Squamous cell carcinomas (Fig. 40.5) may occur anywhere on the skin or on stratified squamous epithelium of the mouth, tongue, oesophagus, anal canal, glans penis or uterine cervix. Squamous cell carcinoma also occurs in metaplastic squamous epithelium in the bronchus or bladder.

Squamous cell carcinoma usually occurs in older age groups, in areas of skin exposed repeatedly to ultraviolet light. Often, carcinoma develops from a pre-existing **solar (senile) keratosis**.

Much less commonly, squamous carcinoma develops

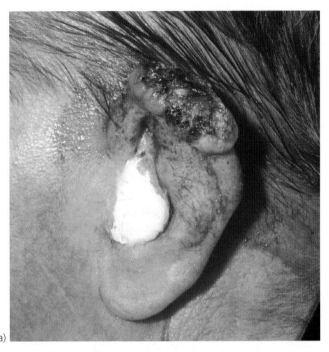
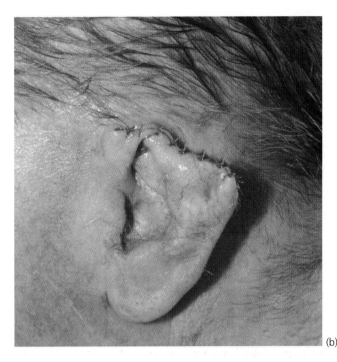

(a)
(b)

Fig. 40.5 Squamous carcinoma
(a) This 70-year-old farmer had worked in the fields exposed to the sun all his life. He presented with this obviously malignant lesion on the upper part of the pinna. It was confirmed on biopsy to be a well differentiated squamous cell carcinoma **(b)** after local resection.

in skin areas chronically exposed to **industrial carcinogens** such as ionising radiation, arsenic or chromium compounds, soot, tar, pitch or mineral oils. For example, carcinoma of the scrotum was common in chimney sweeps in the nineteenth century; the recognition of soot as the predisposing factor was a milestone in understanding carcinogenesis.

Chronic inflammation also predisposes to squamous carcinoma which may develop at the margins of osteomyelitic sinuses or longstanding ulcers. These are common in developing countries where burns are poorly treated. An ulcer in which carcinoma arises is known as a **Marjolin's ulcer**.

Histologically, squamous cell carcinomas of the skin are usually well differentiated, and the tumour cells resemble normal prickle cells. Keratin pearls and individual cell keratinisation are common features.

CLINICAL PRESENTATION

Squamous cell carcinoma usually presents as an enlarging painless ulcer with a rolled, indurated margin. Other lesions have an exophytic (outward growing, proliferative) cauliflower-like appearance with areas of ulceration, bleeding or serous exudation. Squamous cell carcinomas invade the dermis and deeper tissues such as bone or cartilage; further spread is usually to regional lymph nodes. Distant metastases are uncommon.

MANAGEMENT OF SQUAMOUS CELL CARCINOMAS

Management involves first confirming the diagnosis by biopsy. This is followed by local radiotherapy or sometimes by excision of the carcinoma with a margin of normal tissue. Infiltrated lymph nodes are treated with **radiotherapy** or sometimes **block dissection** (i.e. removing all the regional lymph nodes in a single block of tissue). In general, these tumours respond favourably to radiotherapy and recurrence is unusual. Patients are usually reviewed annually for about 5 years after successful treatment.

BASAL CELL CARCINOMA

PATHOLOGY AND CLINICAL FEATURES

Basal cell carcinomas are common, and nearly always result from exposure to excess ultraviolet sunlight. White-skinned people in tropical and sub-tropical regions have an extremely high incidence. Up to 50% of this group are affected at some time, often with multiple lesions. As with squamous cell carcinomas, basal cell carcinomas usually develop from middle age onwards, but their incidence is rising in younger 'sun-worshippers'. Males are affected at least twice as often as females, reflecting their greater occupational and recreational exposure to the sun.

529

Most basal cell carcinomas arise on the upper part of the face as shown in Figure 40.6, although any part of the skin can be involved. Most patients present early rather than late because the lesions are so visible.

Basal cell carcinomas begin as small pearly-white nodules with visible telangiectatic blood vessels. Early

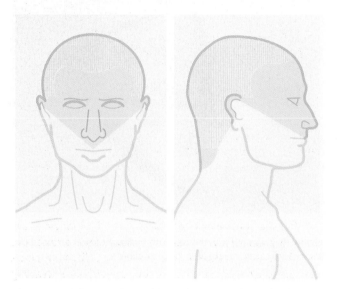

Fig. 40.6 Highest risk area for basal cell carcinomas shown in pink

lesions may ulcerate, bleed and then heal again, but as they grow larger they form irregular ulcers (**rodent ulcers**) with a pearly rolled margin. Although basal cell carcinomas almost never metastasise they are definitely malignant, invading underlying bone and cartilage. Neglected lesions on the scalp or neck may even invade the brain or spinal cord.

Histologically, the tumour cells have strongly basophilic nuclei and little cytoplasm. The cells at the periphery are arranged in a palisade pattern reminiscent of normal basal cells.

MANAGEMENT OF BASAL CELL CARCINOMAS

Small lesions are usually treated by radiotherapy, cryotherapy or curettage, although excision biopsy may be appropriate for isolated or suspicious lesions. Radiotherapy should be avoided on the nose or ear where cartilage is susceptible to radiotherapy and may undergo necrosis. Larger destructive lesions may require reconstructive plastic surgery and skin grafting.

MALIGNANT MELANOMA

This is discussed below under melanotic lesions.

MELANOTIC LESIONS

BENIGN NAEVI

The deeper layers of the epidermis contain scattered melanocytes which synthesise melanin. This pigment is then transferred to nearby epidermal cells where it is responsible for skin colour. The concentration of melanocytes in the skin is similar in all races but the degree of skin pigmentation depends on the amount of melanin produced. Although skin colour is mainly determined by genetic factors, it is enhanced by exposure to the ultraviolet rays of sunlight (tanning).

Melanocytes originate from the neural crest and migrate to the ectoderm during embryological development. Hamartomatous accumulations of melanocytes may appear in the epidermis or dermis or both to form raised, variably pigmented lesions known as **naevi** or **moles**.

Lesions range in diameter from about 3–30 mm. The surface may be smooth or irregular and may contain hairs. According to clinical and histological features, naevi can be subdivided into five types: **junctional, intradermal, compound, blue** and **juvenile naevi**. The first three are closely related pathologically. (See Fig. 40.8 for histopathology.)

JUNCTIONAL, INTRADERMAL AND COMPOUND NAEVI

Junctional and intradermal naevi

Junctional naevi develop at or before puberty by accumulation of small clumps of melanocytes deep in the epidermis. These appear as small papules, slightly raised above the surface, but deeply pigmented because the melanocytes are close to the skin surface. After puberty **intradermal naevi** predominate in these; the junctional naevus cells are thought to proliferate and migrate into the dermis to form a mass of cells, which present as raised papules. They are larger than junctional naevi and paler, as the melanin is masked by the thickness of overlying skin.

Some intradermal naevi continue to enlarge; pilosebaceous elements become exaggerated to produce fleshy, dome-shaped or polypoid skin nodules often with protruding hairs. These slightly pigmented naevi are probably the most common skin lumps occurring on the face and are particularly seen in the elderly and in women (see Fig. 40.7, the lateral lesion).

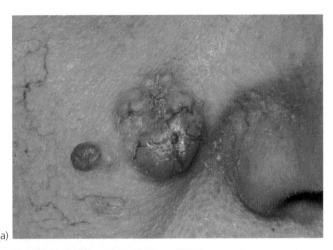 (a)

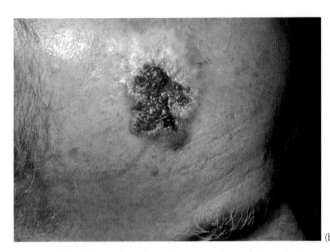 (b)

Fig. 40.7 Basal cell carcinoma (BCC)
(a) The larger nodular lesion on the cheek of this woman aged 77 is a typical BCC. Note the pearly appearance of the lesion which is beginning to ulcerate. In this position, treatment with radiotherapy avoids distortion of the nasolabial fold. The smaller lesion lateral to the BCC is a benign naevus. **(b)** Large BCC on the scalp of an elderly farm worker. Again, the typical pearly edge can be seen. After confirming the diagnosis on an incision biopsy of the edge, this was treated with radiotherapy.

Compound naevi

These uncommon lesions contain junctional and intradermal components and look like something between the two, i.e. slightly raised, moderately pigmented papules. Compound naevi are probably a late transition from junctional to intradermal naevi occurring in early adulthood (see juvenile naevi below). Compound naevi are believed to be susceptible to transformation into **aggressive malignant melanomas**.

BLUE NAEVI

Blue naevi are dark, blue-black, flat nodules formed by clumps of heavily pigmented melanocytes located deep in the dermis. The blue colour is an optical effect caused by the thick layer of overlying skin. Blue naevi occur at any age but are more common in the young; because of their dark colour they may be mistaken for malignant melanomas.

JUVENILE NAEVI

Juvenile naevi are most common in the young but may occur at any age. Histologically, they are compound naevi. The cells are large and pleomorphic which in adults would suggest malignancy. Despite this, the lesions are benign.

LENTIGO

Lentigenes (the plural of lentigo) are benign pigmented lesions which may need to be considered in the differential diagnosis of potentially malignant melanotic lesions. They are large, heavily pigmented plaques, which develop on the face and hands of the elderly. Melanocytes are more numerous, and melanin production is excessive but there is no accumulation of naevus cells. Lentigenes are benign but predispose to the superficial spreading variety of malignant melanoma.

MANAGEMENT OF PIGMENTED LESIONS

It is not particularly easy to distinguish clinically between the different types of benign naevi. Nor is it always easy to be sure that a pigmented lesion is not malignant. Excision biopsy is mandatory if there has been any recent change in a pigmented lesion or if there is any doubt about its nature. People are becoming increasingly aware that pigmented lesions can be malignant and so large numbers now seek medical advice. Fortunately, only a small proportion have malignant melanomas. If there is any suspicion of malignancy, specialist opinion should be sought. A dermatologist will usually be the first choice, but a surgeon will be involved if more than simple excision or biopsy is necessary.

In practice, if the patient or doctor is worried about a pigmented lesion, no matter how benign it looks, it is usually removed. Lesions subject to chronic irritation (e.g. at the waist, neck or palm) or in a site that is difficult to observe (e.g. sole of foot or genitalia) should certainly be removed. A fusiform incision removes the lesion together with a narrow margin of normal tissue (2–3 mm), enabling the skin edges to be readily opposed. All excised pigmented lesions should be examined histologically because a few benign-looking lesions will turn out to be malignant.

MALIGNANT MELANOMA

INTRODUCTION AND PATHOLOGY

Malignant melanoma (Fig. 40.9) arises by malignant transformation of melanocytes originating from the neural crest. Most malignant melanomas are poorly differentiated with numerous mitotic figures. The histological presence of melanin is diagnostic but **amelanotic** (non-pigmented) lesions need to be diagnosed by immuno-histochemical tests.

The tumour is the eighth most common malignancy and the world incidence is rising dramatically. The peak incidence is in the fourth decade. There has been an improvement in 5-year survival from about 40% in the 1940s to about 80% now. This may be due to greater public awareness, earlier detection and better treatment.

RISK FACTORS

The epidemiology of malignant melanoma is fascinating. About 80% occur in white-skinned people and the disease is extremely common in albinos of all races. Until recent times, malignant melanoma was quite rare in northern Europe but the incidence has risen dramatically over the last three decades. Overall, about 1 in 100 Americans will be affected at some time in their lives. The highest incidence in the world is in northern and western Australia and it is believed that ultraviolet radiation is the essential aetiological factor. Whilst a cumulative sun effect is the main factor for other skin malignancies, short periods of intense sun exposure causing blistering sunburn, for example on a 2-week holiday, appear to be more important for malignant melanoma. There is evidence that unaccustomed exposure to strong sunlight can suppress general immunological responses and, by implication, immunological tumour surveillance. This might explain malignant melanomas on parts of the skin not generally exposed to the sun, for example the soles of the feet.

Other risk factors include a family history of malignant melanoma, freckling of the upper back, red or blond hair, blue or green or grey eyes and the presence of solar (actinic) keratoses. Each of these factors increases risk by about 3.5 times.

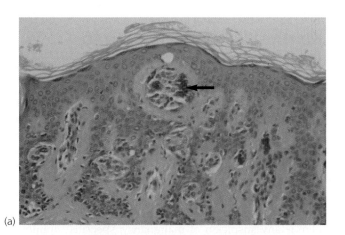
(a)

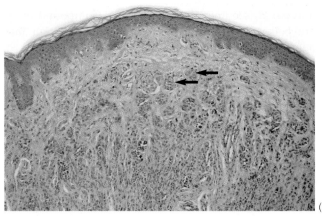
(b)

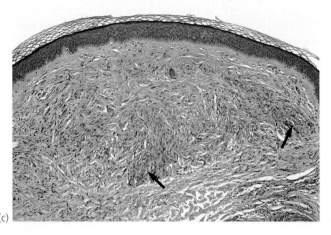
(c)

Fig. 40.8 Melanocytic naevi—histopathology
Increase numbers of melanocytes (naevus cells) may occur at various levels within the skin. **(a)** Nests of naevus cells (arrowed) at the dermo-epidermal junction, known as a **junctional naevus**.
(b) Intradermal naevus showing naevus cells (arrowed) within the upper and mid-dermis. A compound naevus is made up of both junctional and intradermal components. **(c)** Naevus cells having a spindle cell appearance (arrowed), rather than forming nests. This entity, known as **blue naevus**, may extend into deeper dermis. Sometimes a blue naevus component may be seen in association with the other types of naevi, a so-called **combined naevus**.

MELANOMA SUBTYPES

Melanomas may be classified as growing radially (**superficial spreading type**) or vertically (**nodular type**). About 80% are the superficial spreading type. These grow slowly and usually arise in pre-existing pigmented naevi. The lesions are flat with a variegated border and often have patches of regression. Nodular melanomas are more common in men and demonstrate an early vertical growth phase. They develop more rapidly and behave more aggressively than superficial spreading melanomas and tend to arise de novo in normal skin. Five per cent of nodular melanomas are **amelanotic**.

Lentigo maligna melanoma is uncommon and presents as large (> 3 cm) lesions on the face or neck of elderly women. These have a low metastatic potential but are locally invasive; they are distinct from **lentigo maligna**, a benign but precancerous melanosis.

Acral melanoma occurs on the palms or soles or under the nails. This is the only type that occurs in dark-skinned individuals and has a low incidence in white people. Most are larger than 3 cm at presentation and occur at a mean age of 60 years (see Fig. 40.25 below).

Mucosal melanoma occurs on any mucosal surface from mouth to anus, pharynx or paranasal sinuses or in the vagina. They tend to behave particularly aggressively. **Ocular melanoma** arises from uveal melanocytes and is the most common ocular malignancy. It is unique in metastasising to the liver, often years after treatment of the primary lesion.

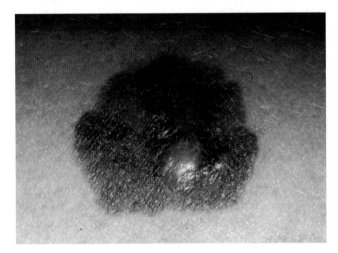

Fig. 40.9 Malignant melanoma.
Pigmented lesion of the forearm in a 33-year-old woman. A small black lesion had been present for many years before starting to spread to reach its present diameter of 2.5 cm. Histologically, this proved to be a mixed type of malignant melanoma with both 'superficial spreading' and nodular elements.

CLINICAL FEATURES OF MALIGNANT MELANOMA

Most malignant melanomas are black or dark brown, flat or nodular lesions which may bleed or ulcerate. If a pre-existing or new mole enlarges, darkens, bleeds, becomes inflamed, ulcerated or itchy, it should be regarded with great suspicion. Superficial spreading melanoma can

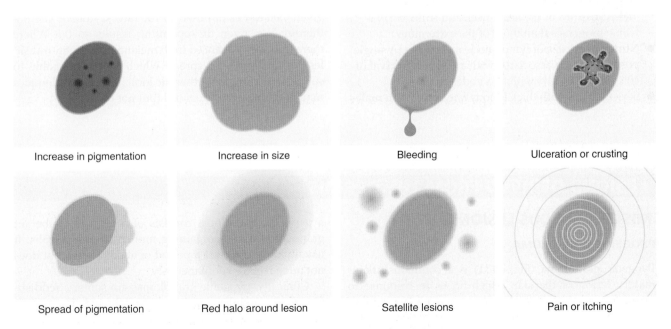

Increase in pigmentation Increase in size Bleeding Ulceration or crusting

Spread of pigmentation Red halo around lesion Satellite lesions Pain or itching

Fig. 40.10 Clinical features in a pigmented lesion suggestive of malignant melanoma

533

easily be mistaken for seborrhoeic keratosis. In general, spread to regional lymph nodes occurs early. Lateral spread in dermal lymphatics may produce **satellite lesions** around the primary nodule and 'in transit' lesions may appear along the course of the lymph node drainage.

Haematogenous spread occurs later, involving lung, liver, bone, brain and other tissues. The behaviour of malignant melanoma is unpredictable, although lesions arising before puberty or in the elderly tend to be less aggressive. Rarely, disseminated lesions undergo complete spontaneous regression, suggesting that immunological factors are involved. Melanomas that exhibit marked lymphocytic infiltration on histology have a better prognosis.

PROGNOSTIC FACTORS

Tumour thickness on histological examination (Breslow) is the most useful guide to prognosis and has proved more accurate than the level of invasion (Clark's levels). Tumour thickness correlates well with the likelihood of regional and distant metastases as shown in Table 40.2. Other factors affecting prognosis include:

- Pathological stage—nodal or distant involvement. If lymph node metastases are present, 10-year survival falls to about 30%, and if distant metastases are present, 2-year survival is only about 25%
- The presence of 'satellite lesions' around the primary or 'in transit' lesions between the primary and its lymph node field makes the prognosis worse
- The presence of ulceration of the primary lesion increases the risk of metastases and reduces survival
- Site of the primary—lesions of the scalp tend to recur locally. Lesions of the head, neck and trunk carry a worse prognosis than those of the extremities
- Number and size of lymph node metastases. A single positive node is associated with a 10-year survival of 40%, falling to 13% with two nodes or more
- Sex—females with thick lesions fare better than males

MANAGEMENT OF MALIGNANT MELANOMA

The first objective in managing a pigmented lesion is to establish whether it is malignant. Unless malignancy is clinically obvious, small lesions should be removed by excision biopsy and more extensive lesions sampled by incision biopsy. There have been two major changes in definitive management in recent years as a result of controlled trials. Firstly, it is no longer believed necessary to excise the lesion with a 5 cm margin all around and secondly, split skin grafting is no longer regarded as essential to achieve skin cover and provide early warning of local recurrence. For thin melanomas, less than 1 mm, a clear margin of 1 cm all around is sufficient. For thicker melanomas (1–4 mm) wider excision with 2 cm clearance is necessary to achieve optimum survival. For lesions thicker than 4 mm, a 3 cm clearance is believed desirable. In most cases, primary closure or local rotational flaps can safely achieve skin cover.

Debate continues about whether **elective lymph node dissection** improves survival for thicker lesions in the absence of involved nodes. Many specialised units carry out elective node dissection if practicable when the primary lesion is 1–4 mm thick, sometimes using lymphatic dye to locate 'sentinel' nodes, performing frozen section biopsy and proceeding to node dissection if positive. Other adverse prognostic factors also influence the decision to perform node excision (see earlier). Where regional lymph node involvement is clinically apparent, these nodes are excised.

Adjuvant radiotherapy is under trial and may reduce local recurrence rates and improve survival. Melanoma cells are sensitive to higher dose fractions than are normally given (600 rad as opposed to 180 rad). Cytotoxic chemotherapy has given disappointing results so far. Where there is locally advanced limb melanoma with 'in-transit' lesions and regional spread which is not amenable to surgical excision, hyperthermic local perfusion techniques may provide effective control (but not cure).

LESIONS DERIVED FROM THE DERMIS

MISCELLANEOUS LESIONS

PYOGENIC GRANULOMA

Pyogenic granuloma (Fig. 40.11) is a common inflammatory lesion of the skin which arises in response to minor penetrating foreign bodies such as splinters or thorns. Lesions are most common on the hands and feet but may also occur on the lips and gums. Pathologically,

a pyogenic granuloma consists of a mass of exuberant granulation tissue containing numerous polymorphs. It usually develops over a period of about 1 week but does not often regress spontaneously.

Clinically, pyogenic granulomas are solitary, reddish-blue fleshy nodules which may be polypoid. The surface may be ulcerated, in which case the lesion may be clinically indistinguishable from amelanotic malignant

Table 40.2 Risk of regional and distant metastasis in malignant melanoma according to Breslow thickless

Tumour thickness	Risk of regional metastases	Risk of distant metastases	10-year survival without nodal or distant metastases
Less than 1 mm	3–5%	3–5%	95%
1 to 4 mm	25–60%	10–20%	60–75%
More than 4 mm	> 60%	70%	45%

melanoma. Pyogenic granulomas should be excised and the base curetted or cauterised to prevent recurrence.

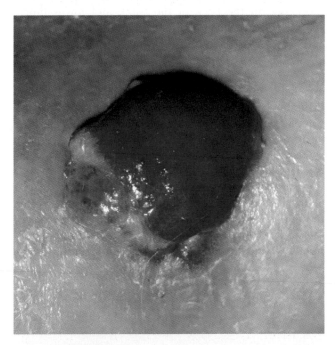

Fig. 40.11 Pyogenic granuloma
This man of 29 suffered a minor penetrating injury to his forearm from a piece of sharp metal. The wound did not heal as normal but produced this friable proliferative lesion. The appearance is typical of a pyogenic granuloma, composed largely of granulation tissue. It was removed by curettage under local anaesthesia and healing was uninterrupted.

KELOID SCARS

Keloids are formed by excessive deposition of collagen in the dermis during wound healing. The result is an elevated nodular lesion covered by normal epidermis. The chest and neck are particularly susceptible. The problem is much more common in black people.

Keloid formation may cause poor cosmetic results after injury, minor surgery, or even ear-piercing. Simply excising the lesion often makes scarring worse. Treatment is generally unsatisfactory; silicone gel under an occlusion dressing usually causes some regression. In extreme cases, excision of the scar followed by a low dose of local radiotherapy may suppress further keloid formation.

HISTIOCYTOMA

Histiocytomas, (also known as **dermatofibromas**), are common painless skin lesions occurring mainly on the limbs. They are firm nodules, usually about 5 mm in diameter and deep reddish-brown in colour. They are clinically important because they may be mistaken for malignant melanoma. Histologically, they contain numerous lipid-filled macrophages (**histiocytes**). One histological variant contains prominent vascular elements, and has given rise to the confusing term **sclerosing angioma**.

SECONDARY (METASTATIC) CARCINOMA

Metastatic tumour deposits may present as small hard painless nodules in the skin. They are usually located in the dermis and covered by normal epidermis. Visceral malignancy e.g. pancreatic or colon cancer may present with a metastasis at the umbilicus (Sister Joseph's nodule). There is usually a history of a treated malignancy elsewhere. Lobular breast carcinomas are the most common cause, but carcinomas of stomach, uterus, lungs, large bowel and kidneys can also metastasise to skin. Occasionally, biopsy of a mysterious skin lesion leads to the diagnosis.

Management of skin secondaries depends on the primary diagnosis but the prognosis is usually poor. Treatment is by local excision, radiotherapy or chemotherapy, depending on the severity of symptoms and the size, number and location of secondaries.

True skin metastases are a different entity from local spread of tumour or local implantation of cells during surgery, which are a particular feature of carcinoma of the breast. Laparoscopic surgery for malignancy has acquired a bad reputation, partly because of local recurrences at port sites.

KAPOSI'S SARCOMA

This once rare condition has leapt to prominence as one of the most frequent presentations of **acquired immune deficiency syndrome** (AIDS). The condition appears as multiple blueish-red to brown nodules or plaques, all of which are primary tumours (Fig. 40.12). They most commonly occur on the limbs. The tumours are characterised by proliferating dysplastic fibroblasts, accompanied by chronic inflammation, endothelial proliferation and

535

haemorrhage. Treatment of individual lesions is by excision biopsy.

FURUNCLE (BOIL) AND CARBUNCLE

A furuncle is a staphylococcal abscess which develops in a hair follicle in the dermis. Diabetes mellitus can be a predisposing factor. The lesion rapidly enlarges and eventually 'points' at the surface, spontaneously discharging pus. The centre often contains a core of necrotic tissue. Once the pus has discharged and the necrotic tissue has been shed, the lesion heals spontaneously; however, the necrotic core may need excision to speed the healing process. Drainage may be encouraged with poultices or dressings, such as magnesium sulphate paste, which are said to draw the pus to the surface by osmosis. Antibiotics should be avoided if pus is present, as they inhibit spontaneous drainage and may lead to the formation of a chronic abscess.

Furuncles are most common in young men with acne, especially on the back of the trunk and lower limbs. Axillary furuncles are common in middle-aged females, and tend to recur. Surgical drainage is necessary if a chronic abscess develops.

A furuncle may be the source of systemic sepsis, especially in uncontrolled diabetes. **Cavernous sinus thrombosis** is a rare but very serious (and often fatal) complication of a furuncle on the lateral aspect of the nose or infra-orbital area. This area drains into the cavernous sinus via the facial vein and inferior ophthalmic veins (see Fig. 40.17, p. 540).

A **carbuncle**, also staphylococcal in origin, is larger than a furuncle and consists of a honeycomb of abscesses, often draining (inadequately) via multiple sinuses. The back of the neck is the usual site (Fig. 40.13); here the skin is tightly bound by interlacing bundles of fibrous tissue.

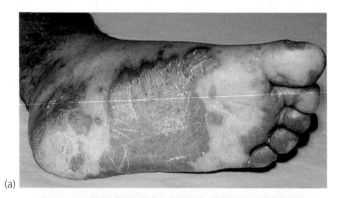

(a)

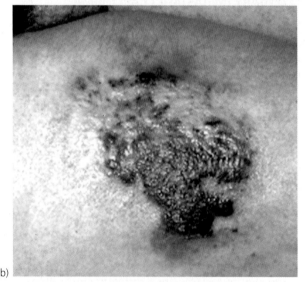

(b)

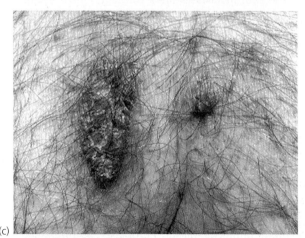

(c)

Fig. 40.12 Kaposi's sarcoma in various sites

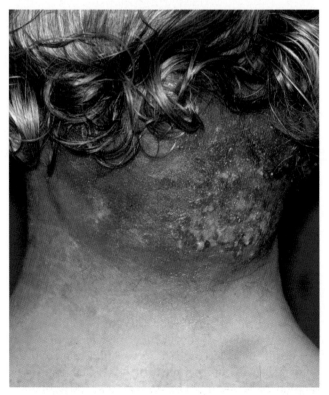

Fig. 40.13 Carbuncle on back of neck

Treatment is with anti-staphylococcal antibiotics such as flucloxacillin as early as possible. The aim is to minimise pus formation and necrosis that would lead to skin loss and delay healing. If pus has formed, thorough desloughing and drainage of the abscesses is required. Carbuncles are more common in diabetic patients, and may bring the diabetes to light.

CYSTS

Cysts are common skin lesions and by definition consist of an epithelium-lined cavity; this is filled with viscous or semi-solid epithelial degradation products. Most skin cysts probably arise from elements of hair follicles, possibly secondary to obstruction (**epidermal cysts** and **pilar cysts**). Occasionally, cysts also arise from develop-

mental epithelial remnants (**dermoid cysts**) or by traumatic implantation of epithelial fragments (**implantation dermoids**).

EPIDERMAL CYSTS

These are by far the most common skin cysts, and are often incorrectly described as '**sebaceous cysts**'. They are usually solitary and may be found anywhere on the body (except the palms or soles), most commonly on the scalp, trunk, face and neck. They range up to several centimetres in diameter. Epidermal cysts are smooth and rounded, and covered by normal epidermis in which a blocked duct (**punctum**) may be visible (Fig. 40.14b). On palpation, they have a doughy, fluctuant consistency and are usually not tender. They originate in the skin and are attached to it but are mobile over deeper tissues. Multiple

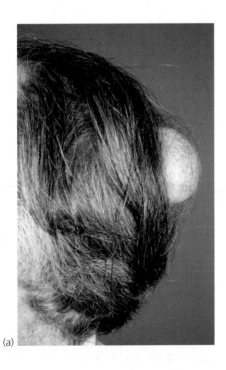

(a)

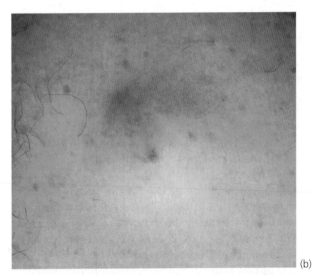

(b)

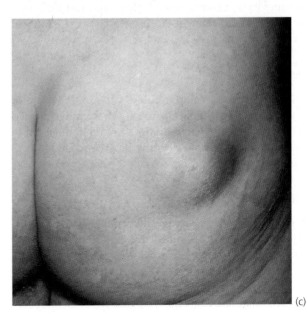

(c)

Fig. 40.14 Epidermal cysts
(a) This large epidermal (pilar) cyst of the scalp was clearly visible but several more were also palpable in the scalp hair of this 55-year-old man. **(b)** Non-inflamed epidermal cyst in the skin of the buttock. **(c)** Inflamed epidermal cyst of buttock.

small epidermal cysts sometimes develop on the scrotal skin or areola and cause considerable embarrassment.

Histologically, an epidermal cyst has a stratified squamous lining epithelium and is filled with keratin; this is consistent with its derivation from a hair follicle. The cyst contents are thick and waxy, and were originally thought to be sebaceous material. This gave rise to the erroneous name of sebaceous cyst.

Surgical removal (see Ch. 6, p. 93)

Epidermal cysts (Fig. 40.14) are mainly removed for cosmetic reasons, but sometimes because they interfere with clothing or combing the hair. An incision is made over the cyst beside the punctum, taking care not to puncture the cavity. The cyst is then enucleated by blunt dissection and delivered from the wound in its entirety. This ensures all the epithelium is removed and prevents recurrence.

Inflamed epidermal cysts

Trauma to epidermal cysts (often unnoticed), may cause some of the contents to escape into the surrounding tissues, exciting an intense foreign-body inflammatory response. The patient may complain of pain, swelling, redness and even spontaneous discharge of liquefied cyst contents; this looks like pus but is in fact sterile. These inflamed epidermal cysts are often described as 'infected' but this is rarely the case.

It is unwise to attempt removal of an acutely inflamed epidermal cyst because the tissue planes cannot be recognised and some of the epithelial lining is likely to be left. If pain is severe, liquefied cyst contents should just be drained as this provides rapid relief of symptoms. Culture of this material rarely yields any growth and so antibiotics are usually unhelpful. The residual cyst should be excised later in the usual way as it is almost certain to flare up repeatedly if left.

Pilar cysts

Some individuals develop multiple cysts on the scalp or less commonly on the face or neck. These range from a few millimetres to many centimetres in diameter, but grow very slowly. They can easily be excised under local anaesthesia.

DERMOID CYSTS

Dermoid cysts are pathologically similar to epidermal cysts in that they are lined by stratified squamous epithelium. As well as keratin, however, they contain hair, sebaceous glands and other ectodermal structures. Dermoids arise from cystic change in epithelial remnants left behind at lines of embryological fusion. They are usually found in the midline of the scalp, neck and lower jaw and at the outer angle of the eyebrow (**external angular dermoid**). Treatment is by excision.

IMPLANTATION DERMOIDS

These small keratin-filled cysts arise from epidermal fragments implanted in the dermis by minor penetrating injuries. Though not derived from epidermal appendages, they are pathologically similar to epidermal cysts, but may contain small foreign bodies. Implantation dermoids are most often seen on the fingers, often under the scar of a previous laceration.

PILONIDAL SINUS AND ABSCESS

As the name implies, pilonidal sinuses, cysts and abscesses contain 'a nest of hairs'. They are common in young adults, particularly hirsute men, and are found at the upper end of the natal cleft. Here, between the buttocks, there is often a congenital dimple or pit. Fragments of hair falling from the back or the head accumulate in this nidus. The hairs slowly work their way into the dermis, with the cuticular scales on the hairs acting like the barbs of an arrow. The process is encouraged by the massaging effect of sitting for long periods, for example when driving. Pilonidal sinus is thus common in truck and tractor drivers. They also occur between the fingers of hairdressers from implantation of their clients' hair (see below).

PILONIDAL ABSCESS

The mass of hairs and other skin debris in a pilonidal sinus excites a foreign-body inflammatory reaction, often merely resulting in a mildly or intermittently discharging sinus. If, however, the cavity becomes secondarily infected, an abscess develops and causes marked pain and swelling. Pilonidal abscesses are often multilocular. They sometimes drain spontaneously but rarely heal completely. Many require surgical drainage because of pain.

Pilonidal sinuses tend to run a long indolent course with chronic or intermittent purulent discharge via one or more sinuses to the skin surface. Periodic acute exacerbations may develop into abscesses which require urgent hospital admission for drainage.

TREATMENT OF PILONIDAL SINUS (Figs 40.15 and 14.16)

Definitive treatment aims to eliminate the nidus of hairs and associated cystic cavities, chronic abscesses and sinuses. At operation, obvious plugs of hair are first removed and then the sinus network is explored with probes, often aided by injecting blue dye into the sinuses. An elliptical wedge of tissue, incorporating the mass of sinuses, cysts

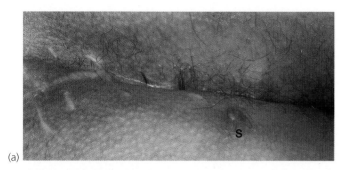

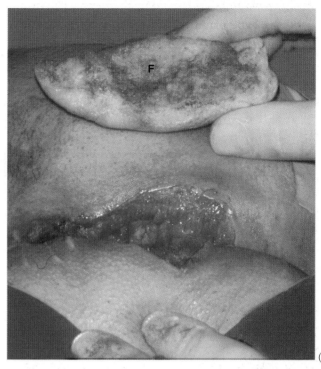

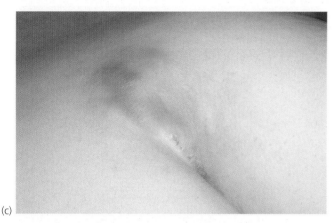

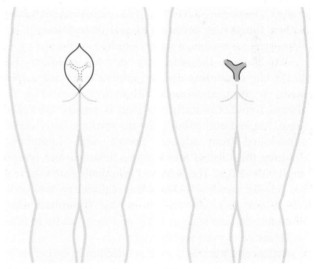

Fig. 40.15 Pilonidal sinus and abscess
(a) Recurrent pilonidal sinuses. The scar from a previous operation for this condition is visible. There are several tufts of hair emerging from sinuses in the midline and a typical sinus opening **S** to one side. **(b)** At operation, there was an extensive network of sinuses lined with granulation tissue and containing loose hairs. The entire network was excised and the wound 'saucerised' to prevent the cavity healing over. No attempt was made to close the defect as this is usually unsatisfactory because of breakdown or infection. A silicone foam **(F)** dressing was made by mixing the two components and pouring it into the wound. **(c)** Pilonidal abscess in a different patient of 24. This is a common presentation and usually requires formal surgical drainage and curettage of the sinuses.

and overlying skin is then excised. The incision may have to extend down to the sacral fascia. The resulting large defect bounded by healthy tissue is then packed and allowed to granulate from the base upwards. Healing takes several weeks but the patient can return home after a few days.

A less extensive surgical method known as **de-roofing**, shown in Figure 40.16, may be preferred. Another alternative treatment is **phenolisation**. In this, the sinus network is thoroughly curetted under general anaesthesia, and then filled with liquefied phenol for a minute or two. Phenol encourages fibrosis and may eliminate the cavity.

Despite surgery, pilonidal lesions commonly recur but this may be reduced by careful attention to hygiene. Daily baths and regular shaving of the area are recommended.

OCCUPATIONAL PILONIDAL SINUSES

Pilonidal sinuses occasionally develop in the web spaces between the fingers in hairdressers, caused by implanted hairs from customers. A similar condition occurs in farmers, with hairs implanted from farm animals.

(a) Radical excision of a wedge of tissue including all sinuses

(b) 'De-roofing' of sinuses and curettage of granulation tissue

Fig. 40.16 Surgical treatment for pilonidal sinus

SEBACEOUS HYPERPLASIA

Localised hyperplasia of sebaceous glands on the nose and in nearby skin creases is common in both men and women. Sebaceous glands are plentiful in this area. The condition probably reflects a mildly abnormal response to sex hormones.

Apart from their unsightly appearance, these small nodular lesions may on occasion be clinically indistinguishable from basal cell carcinomas; the diagnosis is made on histology after excision biopsy.

In **rhinophyma**, an extreme manifestation of sebaceous hyperplasia, the nose becomes enlarged and lumpy. It is mainly seen in older men, and is (unreliably) said to occur in heavy drinkers.

BENIGN APPENDAGE TUMOURS

A variety of benign tumours arise from skin appendages. The most common is the **cylindroma**, which is derived from sweat glands. Diagnosis is usually made unexpectedly on histological examination of an excised nondescript skin lump.

LESIONS IN THE HYPODERMIS AND DEEPER TISSUES

CELLULITIS

Cellulitis is a diffuse spreading infection of the subcutaneous tissues and deeper layers of the skin. It may be acute or chronic. Beta-haemolytic streptococci, usually Lancefield group A (*S. pyogenes*), are commonly responsible. These bacteria produce fibrinolysins and hyaluronidase which break down the protective intercellular barriers and promote spread of infection through the tissue planes. Although an intense neutrophil inflammatory response develops, pus rarely accumulates. Rather, the tissues become red and oedematous. If the skin surface is broken, a serous exudate is released.

Any part of the skin may develop cellulitis (Fig. 40.17), the organisms usually gaining entry via a traumatic or surgical wound, although a wound is not always found. Clinically, the skin is greatly thickened, tense, hot, red and painful; the margins are fairly clearly demarcated from adjacent normal skin. Lymphatics draining the affected area become inflamed and **lymphangitis** develops. The inflamed lymphatics are visible as red streaks passing towards the regional lymph nodes which are also swollen and tender (**lymphadenitis**). Systemic features such as fever and tachycardia indicate bacteraemia or even septicaemia.

Acute cellulitis was a serious infection in earlier times, not least as a complication of surgery. It is now readily treated with antibiotics.

CELLULITIS OF THE LOWER LIMB

Low-grade cellulitis may occur in the lower limb without evidence of any wound. This form of cellulitis is

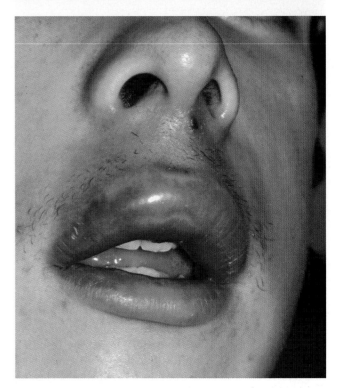

Fig. 40.17 Cellulitis of upper lip
This 18-year-old presented with 4 days of increasing swelling and pain affecting the upper lip following 'picking' of an acne spot. This infection lies in the 'danger triangle' involving the nose and upper lip where serious infection can be complicated by cavernous sinus thrombosis. This patient responded rapidly to intensive antibiotic therapy. The organism proved to be *Strep. pyogenes*.

usually found in older women, and presents as a localised, but not clearly demarcated, brawny inflammation of the leg, usually without regional lymph node involvement or systemic features of infection. Predisposing factors are lymphatic obstruction or oedema from any cause. These infections often recur and are difficult to document bacteriologically because there is no wound and no infected exudate. Nevertheless, they usually respond to antibiotics (such as tetracycline), rest, elevation of the limb and compression stockings when the inflammation has settled. Recurrence is common at intervals of months or years.

A similar low-grade cellulitis may occur in the upper limb or chest wall as a result of lymphatic obstruction following radiotherapy for breast cancer.

ERYSIPELAS

Erysipelas is an uncommon skin infection also caused by group A Streptococci. In this condition, the infection is more superficial, involving only the dermis. The spreading inflamed area is very well demarcated, with the margin raised above the normal skin.

LIPOMA AND LIPOSARCOMA

Lipomas are benign tumours of fat. They may occur anywhere that fat is normally present, most often in the hypodermis of the trunk and limbs and the aetiology is unknown, although mild trauma may be a factor. Typically, they present on the forearms (often multiple), in the supraclavicular fossa (Fig. 40.18), over the deltoid muscle or over the scapula. Lipomas can also be found within the peritoneal cavity, including the bowel submucosa, and within muscles or joints. They may also sometimes arise beneath the periosteum.

Pathologically, lipomas consist of a multilobular mass of fatty tissue with thin fibrous septa. A tenuous fibrous capsule usually defines the lesion clearly from the surrounding tissue. Lipoma cells are histologically indistinguishable from normal adipocytes. Lipomas vary in size from about 2–20 cm and are shaped like a flattened dome. The overlying skin is normal. Their consistency is soft and almost fluctuant. Lipomas are removed if they are inconvenient or unsightly. If the margin is poorly defined, recurrence is likely.

Liposarcoma is a rare malignant variant. It tends to occur in the retroperitoneal area and mediastinum rather than in the skin.

NEUROFIBROMA, NEUROFIBROMATOSIS AND SCHWANNOMA

Neurofibromas are benign tumours arising from the supporting fibroblasts of peripheral nerves. The tumour cells are loosely arranged in a gelatinous (myxomatous) intercellular material which often makes the lesion soft and pulpy to palpation. In the skin, neurofibromas may present as solitary sessile or pedunculated lesions in the vicinity of peripheral nerves. They are sometimes very tender to palpation.

The autosomal dominant inherited syndrome called **neurofibromatosis** (von Recklinghausen's disease) is characterised by multiple neurofibromas and café-au-lait spots; the latter are coffee-coloured skin patches. Sometimes, the neurofibromas are extremely numerous, and occasionally there is gross hypertrophy of subcutaneous tissues and skin folds. This extreme variation was immortalised by the famous 'elephant man' of Sir Frederick Treves. A small proportion of neurofibromas undergo malignant change into sarcomas.

Schwannomas are benign tumours arising from the Schwann cells supporting peripheral nerves. They present as firm, nodular lesions tethered to a nerve, and pressure on the tumour may cause pain in the area of distribution of the nerve. Treatment is by careful excision, attempting to preserve the affected nerve. This usually requires an operating microscope and microsurgical manipulation.

GANGLION

This extremely common and inappropriately-named condition is a cyst-like lesion derived from the lining of a synovial joint, tendon sheath or embryological remnants of synovial tissue. The 'cystic' space does not usually communicate with the associated joint or tendon sheath, and like synovial joint cavities, is not lined by epithelium.

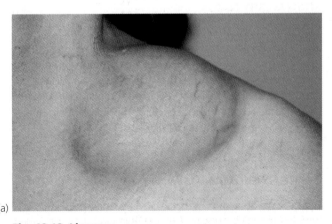
(a)

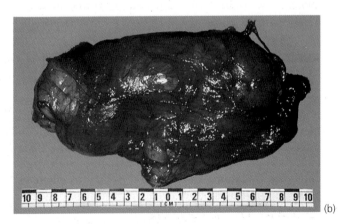
(b)

Fig. 40.18 Lipomas
(a) Large soft lipoma overlying the supra clavicular fossa in a 46-year-old woman. This is a common site for lipomas. It had been present for many years but had recently started to enlarge. **(b)** The surgical specimen. Note that it is larger than its clinical appearance would suggest.

It contains a colourless, gelatinous fluid. Ganglia present as superficial lumps, usually about 1–2 cm in diameter, though sometimes larger. They are most common on the dorsum of the forearm and hand (Fig. 40.19) and around the ankle. They are rarely painful but sometimes cause mechanical problems or interference with footwear. Ganglia are easily recognised by their smooth, hemispherical surface, and firm but slightly fluctuant 'cyst-like' consistency. The overlying skin is normal and mobile and the ganglion weakly transilluminable.

The age-old treatment for a ganglion was a sharp blow with a family bible, which dissipated the cyst contents into the tissues. Recurrence almost inevitably followed. Surgical excision is the accepted method of treatment now, but recurrence is still common.

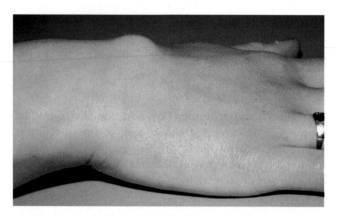

Fig. 40.19 Ganglion
This ganglion is in a common site, the dorsum of the hand.

LESIONS DERIVED FROM SKIN APPENDAGES

LESIONS OF VASCULAR ORIGIN

CAMPBELL DE MORGAN SPOTS

Campbell de Morgan spots are small, bright-red spots which appear on the trunk, usually in older patients. They represent highly localised capillary proliferation and have no clinical significance except for the titillation of bored examiners! Like other vascular lesions they blanch when compressed and then refill when pressure is removed.

SPIDER NAEVI

Spider naevi or telangiectases are small red lesions consisting of a central arteriole from which radiate dilated capillaries. This appearance explains their name. Isolated spider naevi may be found in normal individuals on the trunk, neck and face. Their numbers markedly increase in chronic liver disease, especially cirrhosis, and occasionally in pregnancy. Treatment is rarely required.

ANGIOMAS

Despite their name, angiomas are not true neoplasms but rather congenital hamartomas. They arise from localised excessive development of thin-walled blood vessels which may be of small diameter (**capillary haemangiomas**) or hugely dilated (**cavernous haemangiomas**). The histological appearance is often ambiguous, with most angiomas containing capillary and cavernous elements, as well as arteriovenous or even lymphatic components.

'PORT-WINE STAINS'

The most common haemangiomas are port-wine stains.

These can occur anywhere on the body, but especially the face, neck and scalp, and cause considerable cosmetic distress. They are present from birth and remain unchanged throughout life. Lesions are flat or slightly elevated and reddish-blue. They have an asymmetrical outline and range up to many centimetres in diameter. Trauma may cause bleeding or ulceration.

Surgical treatment, often urged by anguished patients, is rarely successful except for small lesions. Sclerosing agents can be injected to promote thrombosis, organisation and progressive devascularisation, but results are disappointing. Argon lasers tuned to the colour frequency of haemoglobin and other high energy light sources are an encouraging innovation and give promising results in some patients. Regrettably, the use of covering cosmetic preparations remains the best advice for most.

STRAWBERRY NAEVI

The strawberry naevus (Fig. 40.20) is a distinct type of angioma. These occur in early childhood as bright-red fleshy lesions and grow for a few years before involuting spontaneously. Although they disappear and leave no scar, parents often insist on excision for cosmetic reasons. In the long term, surgical excision is not good management as it leaves an unnecessary scar.

CYSTIC HYGROMA

Cystic hygroma is a lymphangioma that presents as a lump in the neck usually during childhood; it is described in more detail on p. 558. Characteristically, the lesion is highly transilluminable.

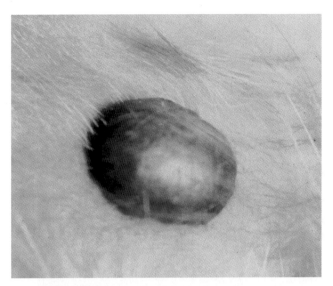

Fig. 40.20 Strawberry naevus
Strawberry naevus on the back of the neck in a 4-month-old infant.
This was present at birth and can be expected to grow with the child
for up to two years, then atrophy spontaneously, leaving no scar.

CONGENITAL SYNDROMES

Gross vascular malformations form part of a number of
rare congenital syndromes. These include **Sturge–Weber
syndrome** (angiomas of the face and intracranial contents)
and **Klippel–Trynawnay syndrome** (Fig. 40.21). The latter
syndrome usually affects one lower limb and the primary
abnormality is multiple arteriovenous fistulae. These lead
to hypertrophy of the limb (gigantism), gross varicose veins
with venous ulceration, and cutaneous capillary naevi.

GLOMUS TUMOUR

This is a benign tumour derived from the glomus body, a
small arteriovenous communication normally found in

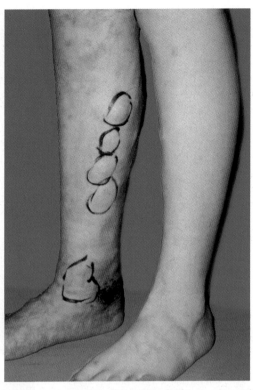

Fig. 40.21 Klippel–Trynawnay syndrome
Klippel–Trynawnay syndrome affecting the right leg in a male aged
19. The three characteristic features are gigantism due to multiple
congenital arterio-venous fistulae, gross varicose veins (outlined in
marking pen on the skin) and cutaneous capillary naevi. In addition,
this patient had a varicose ulcer, seen below the medial malleolus.

the peripheries. The glomus bodies are thought to play a
part in controlling local blood flow. Glomus tumours
occur singly, usually in the fingers and often beneath the
nail. They are tiny (1–3 mm) red flat lesions which are
exquisitely tender to the touch. Treatment is by surgical
excision.

DISORDERS OF THE NAILS

INGROWING TOENAIL

PATHOPHYSIOLOGY

Ingrowing toenail (Fig. 40.22) occurs when the distal
edge of the nail persistently cuts into the adjacent nail
fold. The problem almost exclusively affects the great toe
and usually affects teenagers and young adults. In effect
there is a laceration which cannot heal because of the
presence of a foreign body (the toenail). Superimposed
infection by a mixture of local bacterial and fungal flora
complicates the picture. The combination of acute inflam-

mation and attempts at tissue repair result in the formation of exuberant granulation tissue around the laceration
and surrounding inflammatory swelling. Swelling aggravates trauma caused by the nail edge.

Ingrowing toenail is mainly confined to teenagers and
young adults, particularly males. It probably results from
a combination of factors, including inadequate hygiene,
unsuitable footwear, cutting the nails too short at the
corners and the macerating effect of sweat on the skin.
High levels of circulating testosterone, as found in
adolescence may be an important aetiological factor.

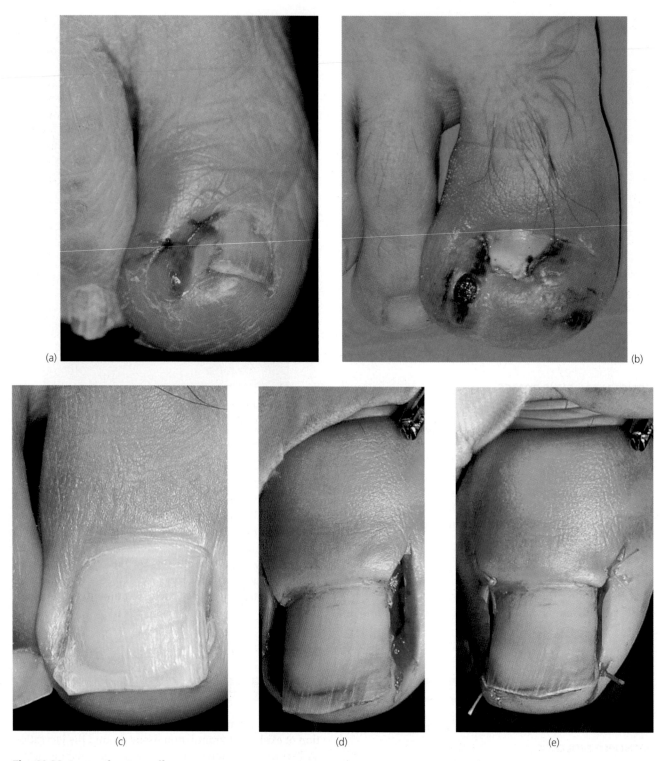

Fig. 40.22 Ingrowing toenail
(a) Infected ingrowing toenail on the lateral side of the toe. This patient had suffered recurrent attacks over many years which prevented him playing football. Note the swelling of the lateral side of the toe, the overgrowth of granulation tissue caused by chronic irritation and the purulent discharge. Surgical treatment was employed once the acute inflammation had settled with saline soaks and antibiotics. **(b)** Inflamed ingrowing toenail affecting medial and lateral sides. There is a great amount of hypertrophy, making suitable footwear hard to find. **(c)** Congenitally wide toenails. This man of 32 had suffered many bouts of inflammation over the years. **(d)** and **(e)** The same patient undergoing wedge resection and phenolisation of both sides of the nail. Note the use of a tourniquet.

MANAGEMENT

The main objective of treatment is to prevent persistent trauma by the nail edge. Surgical operations result in a week or more of discomfort and immobility, so conservative treatment should be tried first.

Conservative treatment

In all cases, simple conservative measures include regular bathing, frequent changes of socks (which should be made of cotton), avoiding tight or narrow shoes and avoiding trauma to the toe when inflamed, for example from kicking a football.

For an inflamed ingrowing toenail, foot soaks in warm saline should be carried out twice daily for at least 10 minutes. Surgical spirit applied twice daily may also help.

A useful further measure, once inflammation is settling, is to pack a small pledget of cotton wool beneath the corner of the nail to lift the nail out of the laceration. At the same time, the nail fold can be pushed away by packing a small elongated pledget between the nail fold and the nail edge. These tiny packs can be left in place for days but need to be increased in size as the corner of the nail rises away from its bed.

These conservative measures, all undertaken by the patient, are often successful in even severe cases but

Removal of nail alone

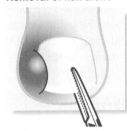

If badly infected and unresponsive to conservative treatment, 'first aid' is to remove the whole nail without disturbing the nail bed, under a local anaesthetic ring block
The nail can be lifted out by firmly grasping with artery forceps
Removal of the 'foreign body' allows inflammation to settle

Wedge resection/phenolisation for permanent narrowing of nail (If nail infected, give prophylactic antibiotics e.g. tetracycline)

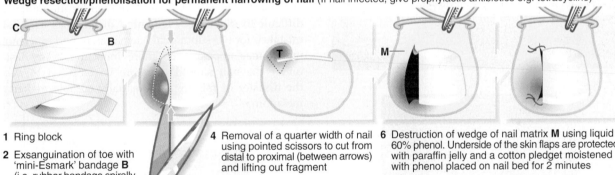

1 Ring block

2 Exsanguination of toe with 'mini-Esmark' bandage **B** (i.e. rubber bandage spirally applied)

3 Application of tourniquet **C** (e.g. thin rubber tube) around toe base before removing Esmark

4 Removal of a quarter width of nail using pointed scissors to cut from distal to proximal (between arrows) and lifting out fragment

5 Excision of a wedge of hypertrophic/inflamed tissue **T**

6 Destruction of wedge of nail matrix **M** using liquid 60% phenol. Underside of the skin flaps are protected with paraffin jelly and a cotton pledget moistened with phenol placed on nail bed for 2 minutes

7 Skin closure with absorbable sutures if necessary

8 Pressure dressing. Paraffin gauze and crepe bandage; then release torniquet

9 Redress at 24 hours

Zadik's operation for permanent abalation of nail and nail bed

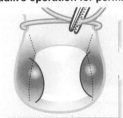 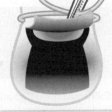 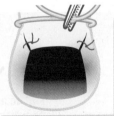

1 Nail and granulations removed and skin incised as shown (dotted lines)

2 Flap raised and germinal matrix treated by phenolisation as in 6 above

3 Flaps sutured back as shown

Fig. 40.23 Operations for ingrowing toenail

require perseverance. Systemic antibiotics should only be used if infection is spreading, and topical antibiotics are of little use.

Surgical treatment

Urgent surgical treatment involves avulsion of the whole nail, or one side of the nail. This immediately removes the 'foreign body' and permits rapid resolution. For recurrent ingrowing toenails, particularly if abnormal nail morphology is a contributory factor, part of the nail

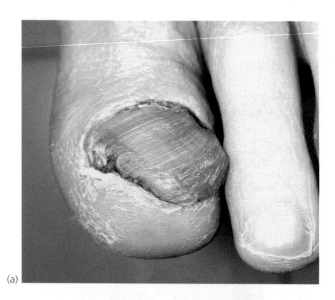

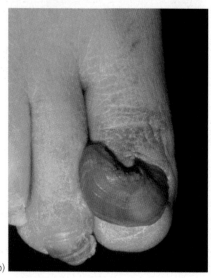

Fig. 40.24 Onychogryphosis
(a) Moderate degree of nail thickening and 'heaping up'. **(b)** More advanced and neglected case. Both of these were treated by chiropody, with careful and regular grinding down of the nails.

bed is best removed. The more popular procedures are illustrated in Figure 40.23. The operations are usually performed under local anaesthesia using a ring block and tourniquet. Local anaesthetic incorporating a vaso-constrictor such as adrenaline must *never* be used in the digits because of the risk of ischaemic necrosis.

ONYCHOGRYPHOSIS

Onychogryphosis ('ram's horn nail') (Fig. 40.24) is a gross abnormality of nail growth. It most commonly affects the great toenail, which becomes greatly thickened and distorted. Nail cutting with ordinary nail scissors then becomes impossible. Onychogryphosis is usually seen only in elderly patients, and probably results from previous trauma to the nail bed. This condition usually presents when it interferes with wearing shoes. A chiropodist (podiatrist) can treat onychogryphosis by using grinding instruments at regular intervals. Surgical removal of the nail and ablation of the bed is sometimes performed.

SUBUNGUAL MELANOMA

Malignant melanomas sometimes develop beneath finger- or toenails (Fig. 40.25). Because of their location, they are difficult to diagnose. Pigmented melanomas are easily mistaken for old subungual haematomas, and amelanotic melanomas appear even more innocuous. Any lesion under the nail should therefore be biopsied to avoid the disaster of missing a potentially curable malignant melanoma.

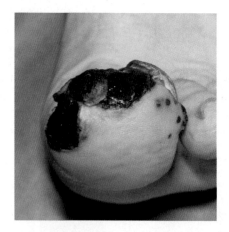

Fig. 40.25 Subungual malignant melanoma.
Aggressive malignant melanoma arising from beneath the nail of the first toe. Note the large main lesion and the satellite lesions nearby. This patient died of melanomatosis 1 year after this picture was taken.

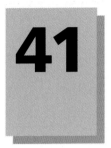

Lumps in the head and neck including salivary calculi

INTRODUCTION

The majority of head and neck disorders that reach the general surgeon are lumps of one sort or another. The main reasons for referral are either the need to exclude malignancy or for consideration of surgical treatment in the case of a metabolic disorder such as thyrotoxicosis or hyperparathyroidism. There is a large overlap with other specialities, particularly ENT, dental and oral surgery, plastic and reconstructive surgery and dermatology.

Swellings of the thyroid gland may be confused with other swellings in the front of the neck. Thus, a complete examination of the head and neck should include the thyroid area, as described in Chapter 43.

Although problems in the mouth are usually managed by dental or oral surgeons, patients will often seek advice from another clinician. For this reason, most doctors should understand the essentials of oral and dental disease and their management, particularly those working in an accident department.

HISTORY AND EXAMINATION IN THE HEAD AND NECK

The concentration of so many different tissues in and around the head and neck is responsible for the profusion of conditions causing lumps in this area. Box 41.1 provides a simple classification.

SPECIAL POINTS IN THE HISTORY AND EXAMINATION

As always, the history provides important clues to the diagnosis. Additional points such as the patient's age, the rate of growth of the lump and any associated symptoms such as pain, discharge or swelling related to eating may lead quickly to the diagnosis.

Most lumps in the head and neck are best examined with the patient sitting in a chair. This allows the examiner to palpate the lump from in front and behind. The

---

KEY POINTS

Box 41.1 Causes of a lump in the head or neck

1. **Thyroid disorders** (classified in Table 43.1)
2. **Lymph node enlargement:**
   — Lymphomas
   — Secondary tumour deposits
   — Local inflammatory lymphadenopathy from acute infections of the head and neck
   — Local inflammatory lymphadenopathy from chronic infections, e.g. tuberculosis
   — Inflammatory lymphadenopathy as part of a generalised lymphadenopathy, e.g. glandular fever or AIDS-related lymphadenopathy
3. **Congenital cysts**—thyroglossal, branchial and preauricular cysts, cystic hygroma and external angular dermoids
4. **Salivary gland disorders**—tumours, stones, rare autoimmune disorders such as Sjögren's syndrome
5. **Lumps in the skin**—any skin lesion may occur in the head and neck but the main problem is one of differential diagnosis, e.g. lipomas and epidermal cysts
6. **Rare tumours**—carotid body tumours, carcinoma of the maxillary sinus, tumours and cysts of the jaw
7. **Actinomycosis** (very rare)

examiner should establish the characteristics of the lump as summarised in Box 41.2. At the same time, he or she should try to visualise the relationship of the lump to overlying or underlying anatomical structures. For example, a lump in the cheek may lie in the skin, the superficial part of the parotid, the buccinator muscle, the oral mucosa or the parotid duct. In clinical examinations, it is often useful to try to describe the characteristics of the lesion as if to someone who cannot see the patient.

The whole of the scalp, the back of the neck and the skin behind and in the ears should be examined carefully. It is important to exclude primary tumours or infected lesions that may be producing lymph-node enlargement. The lymph nodes of the head and neck must also be palpated. A simple method is to think of them as lying in two planes, the horizontal and the vertical, as shown in Figure 41.1. The nodes in each plane can then be examined with two or three simple manoeuvres. For any lump in the lower half of the face or submandibular region, the oral cavity should be examined to exclude salivary gland lesions, oral malignancies or sources of infection such as a dental abscess. For any lump in the parotid region, the integrity of the facial nerve should be formally tested.

Examination of the oral cavity

For many doctors, asking the patient to open his mouth represents the entire oral examination. The following simple technique, illustrated in Figure 41.2a–d, will enable most significant lesions to be seen without any special instruments or lighting.

First, the patient should remove his or her dentures; the lips and their mucosal lining, and the lining of the cheeks and gums are then inspected. To do this, the lips are retracted by the examiner's gloved fingers or a wooden spatula and the mouth illuminated with a pen torch. At the same time, the teeth are inspected for gross decay and gingival inflammation. Painful inflammation is commonly related to a flap of gum over a partially erupted lower wisdom tooth.

If there is any suspicion of parotid disease, then the orifice of the parotid duct should be identified and palpated. This lies opposite the upper second molar tooth. The palate is examined easily if the patient tilts his head backwards. Finally, the tongue and floor of the

KEY POINTS

Box 41.2 Characteristics of a lump
- Site
- Size
- Shape
- Surface characteristics
- Fixation (superficial and deep)
- Anatomical origin
- Consistency
- Fluctuance
- Pulsatility
- Temperature
- Transilluminability
- Bruit
- Local lymphadenopathy

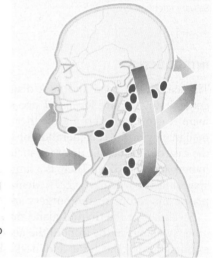

● 'Vertical' (internal jugular) nodes

● 'Horizontal' group of nodes

Fig. 41.1 Simple techniques for palpating head and neck lymph nodes

mouth are inspected for mucosal lesions. To assist the examination, the patient first protrudes, then elevates, the tongue inside the mouth.

Lumps in the floor of the mouth, submandibular area and cheeks should be palpated bimanually as shown in Figure 41.2f. Lumps in these areas are usually mobile and tend to move away from an examining finger.

DISORDERS OF THE SALIVARY GLANDS

There are three pairs of major salivary glands, the **parotid**, **submandibular** and **sublingual** glands. The parotid produces serous saliva, the submandibular produces a mixed sero-mucous saliva and the sublingual produces a mucous secretion. The parotid and submandibular glands each drain into the mouth via a single long duct, whereas the sublingual glands drain via many small ducts.

The surgical disorders of the major salivary glands are benign and malignant tumours, stones, bacterial infections and rare autoimmune disorders, all of which present as

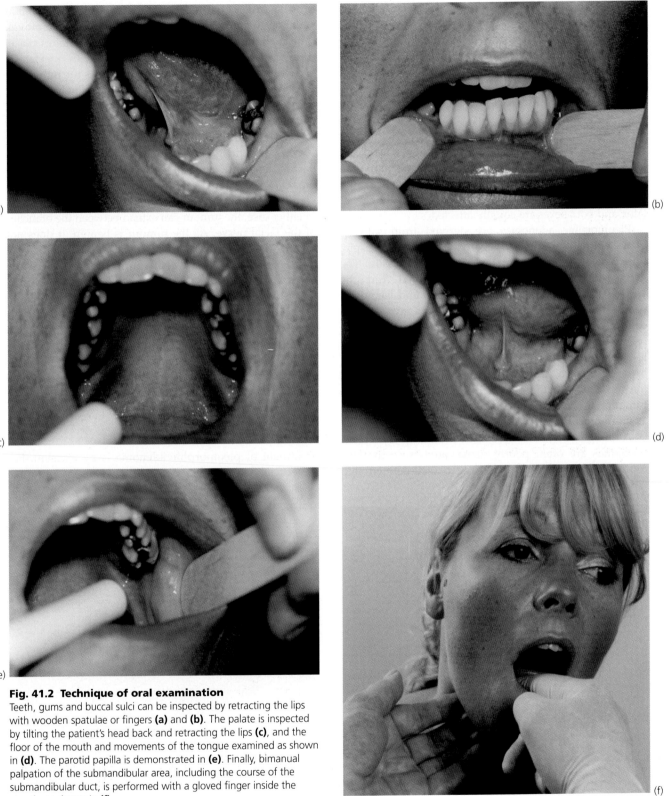

Fig. 41.2 Technique of oral examination
Teeth, gums and buccal sulci can be inspected by retracting the lips
with wooden spatulae or fingers **(a)** and **(b)**. The palate is inspected
by tilting the patient's head back and retracting the lips **(c)**, and the
floor of the mouth and movements of the tongue examined as shown
in **(d)**. The parotid papilla is demonstrated in **(e)**. Finally, bimanual
palpation of the submandibular area, including the course of the
submandibular duct, is performed with a gloved finger inside the
mouth, as shown in **(f)**.

salivary gland lumps. The oral mucosa also contains numerous small 'minor' salivary glands, any of which can undergo neoplastic change. Their main disorders are tumours and retention cysts.

SALIVARY GLAND TUMOURS

PLEOMORPHIC ADENOMA

Pleomorphic adenoma is by far the most common neoplasm of salivary gland neoplasms. It is also the most common cause of a lump in the parotid or submandibular gland. Most pleomorphic adenomas present in middle age or later, and both sexes are equally affected.

Pleomorphic adenomas are derived from salivary gland epithelium and are regarded as benign. Despite this, they show varying degrees of differentiation. The name **pleomorphic adenoma** was acquired from the varied histological appearance. Columns and islands of neoplastic epithelial cells are separated by a myxomatous connective tissue stroma which may contain areas resembling immature cartilage. This led early pathologists to believe that the tumour contained neoplastic tissue of both epithelial and connective tissue origin, thus generating the misleading name of **mixed salivary tumour**. Some tumours have no myxomatous tissue, and are described as **monomorphic** variants.

Although they do not metastasise, pleomorphic adenomas are often poorly demarcated from the surrounding tissue. There is usually a well-defined thin capsule, but the surface is usually nodular rather than smooth, an important point when attempting removal. True malignant transformation occasionally takes place, usually to squamous cell carcinoma, with metastasis occurring to cervical nodes and sometimes the lungs.

Clinically, the tumour presents as a very slowly growing, painless lump (see Fig. 41.3). Most are in the parotid, some in the submandibular gland, and a few in minor salivary glands.

Most parotid gland tumours occur in the superficial part of the gland, external to the plane of the facial nerve branches. Occasionally, they occur in the deep part of the gland in more intimate association with the facial nerve. In either case, the tumour can extend between the branches of the facial nerve. As the tumour is benign, it does not invade the nerve to cause a facial palsy. Facial nerve damage is, however, a risk during surgical excision, especially of deeper lesions. Patients should be warned of this possibility before operation.

If an older patient has a slowly growing solid parotid lump without a facial palsy, it is best to assume it is a pleomorphic adenoma. Definitive diagnosis can only be made histologically after excision.

Investigations may include ultrasonography and needle biopsy and CT scanning if malignancy is suspected.

Treatment

Treatment of pleomorphic adenoma is by excision. For superficial lesions, this is usually by the operation of

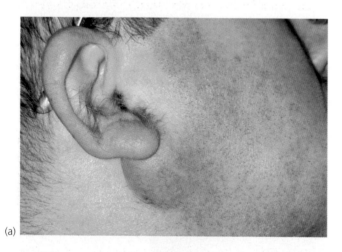

(a)

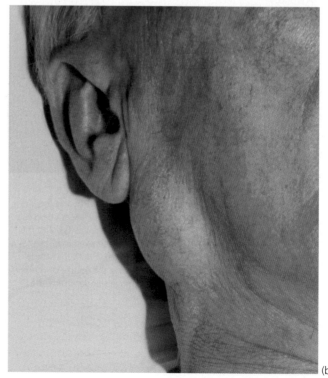

(b)

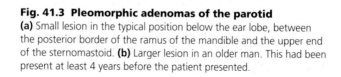

Fig. 41.3 Pleomorphic adenomas of the parotid
(a) Small lesion in the typical position below the ear lobe, between the posterior border of the ramus of the mandible and the upper end of the sternomastoid. **(b)** Larger lesion in an older man. This had been present at least 4 years before the patient presented.

superficial parotidectomy, which involves excising all glandular tissue superficial to the plane of the facial nerve. An alternative is meticulous enucleation, which has been shown to be as effective in curing the problem and to carry a lower rate of side effects. Recurrence is uncommon. For deeper lesions, an attempt should be made to excise the entire lesion, carefully identifying and preserving the branches of the facial nerve. Again, enucleation may be the safer option. If there is doubt about whether excision has been complete, postoperative radiotherapy may be advisable.

The main complication of parotidectomy is damage to branches of the facial nerve. Damage to the temporal or upper zygomatic branches may prevent complete closure of the eye, leading to corneal drying and damage. Division of the mandibular branch causes drooping of the angle of the mouth and embarrassing salivary dribbling. Similar damage may also complicate submandibular gland excision if the incision is incorrectly sited.

Salivary fistula is an occasional complication following parotid surgery, causing saliva to leak onto the face at meal times. The fistula usually resolves spontaneously after several weeks.

Frey's syndrome is a late complication of formal parotidectomy in 25% or more cases. It probably results from divided parasympathetic secretomotor fibres, originally innervating the gland, which then regenerate in the skin where they assume control of sweat gland activity. Facial sweating then occurs in response to salivatory stimuli, and is known as **gustatory sweating** and can be embarrassing.

ADENOLYMPHOMA (WARTHIN'S TUMOUR)

This unusual benign lesion constitutes less than 10% of salivary neoplasms, and occurs almost exclusively in the parotid glands. These tumours usually arise after middle age and there is a strong male predominance. They are sometimes occur bilaterally, either at the same time or at different times.

Histologically, the tumour is composed of large glandular acini. The epithelium, similar to large salivary ducts, is embedded in dense lymphoid tissue in which lymphoid follicles may be seen. The histogenesis is not understood, but the glandular part may be hamartomatous salivary duct tissue within a normal parotid lymph node. A strong association with cigarette smoking has been demonstrated.

Adenolymphomas are invariably benign. They present as a parotid lump, indistinguishable from pleomorphic adenoma. The diagnosis can sometimes be made by fine needle aspiration cytology, in which case simple enucleation can be performed to remove the tumour or it can be left alone. Adenolymphomas do not recur, but a satellite lesion may enlarge and present as another tumour.

MALIGNANT PRIMARY SALIVARY TUMOURS

Malignant tumours comprise only a small proportion of neoplasms of major salivary glands but form the major proportion of tumours of the minor (accessory) salivary glands scattered throughout the oral mucosa. With parotid lumps, facial nerve weakness is diagnostic of malignancy. The majority of malignant tumours are **adenocystic carcinomas** (also known as adenoid cystic carcinomas, and less accurately as cylindromas). The remainder include rare epithelial tumours such as **acinic cell carcinoma** and **squamous cell carcinoma**. In Australia, the most common parotid tumour is a malignant melanoma.

Adenocystic carcinomas have a characteristic cribriform (sieve-like) microscopic appearance due to numerous small spaces in the tightly-packed tumour cell mass. These tumours are highly invasive with early regional and systemic metastasis. Treatment involves wide mutilating surgery which usually destroys the facial nerve. Recurrence is unfortunately very common, and may occur as long as 5 years after apparently successful eradication. The tumours are unresponsive to radiotherapy and prognosis is almost uniformly poor.

SECONDARY TUMOURS IN SALIVARY GLANDS

The superficial part of the parotid gland contains lymph nodes which may become involved by secondary deposits from tumours of the face or scalp. In the same way, lymph node secondaries from the mouth may develop in the submandibular gland. The finding of a parotid or submandibular lump should therefore prompt a search for a primary tumour locally.

SALIVARY GLAND STONE DISEASE (SIALOLITHIASIS)

PATHOPHYSIOLOGY

The submandibular gland and duct are prone to formation of calcified stones (calculi), which obstruct salivary outflow and predispose to infection. Calculi may occur in the parotid duct but this is much less common. The aetiology of salivary calculi is not known, but the submandibular gland may be vulnerable because of its more viscid secretion and elongated duct.

Stones are not the only cause of salivary gland swelling and damage. For both the parotid and submandibular gland, trauma to the duct orifice may result in stenosis and salivary stasis.

Submandibular stones may be found anywhere along Wharton's duct (Fig. 41.4), including its course within the gland. Stones vary from several millimetres to a centimetre in diameter. Those in the distal part of the duct tend to have an elongated 'date stone' shape. (See Fig. 41.5.)

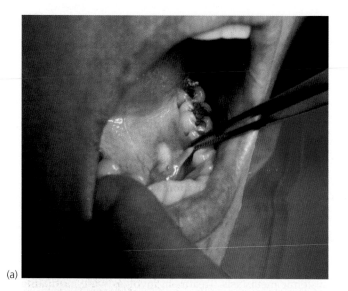

(a)

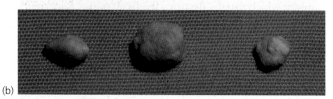

(b)

Fig. 41.4 Submandibular duct stone
(a) This photograph shows a stone visible in the anterior part of Wharton's duct; it was removed under local anaesthesia via a logitudinal incision in the duct. **(b)** Submandibular stones removed from a similar case.

CLINICAL FEATURES

Salivary calculi rarely cause complete obstruction but the patient usually experiences intermittent swelling or pain at meal times when salivary flow is high. The swelling subsides over the next hour. Acidic foods such as lemon juice stimulate rapid salivary flow, and can be used as a test in clinic. Pain is not a prominent feature; rather, patients describe a sensation of fullness. Salivary calculi occasionally present with acute or chronic bacterial infection (**sialadenitis**). Secondary infection in the obstructed system leads to rapidly worsening symptoms and even spreading cellulitis of the floor of the mouth (Ludwig's angina (Fig. 41.6)).

Most of the submandibular gland lies deep to the mandible and so there is little to see on external examination. Palpation of the submandibular area confirms that the gland is moderately enlarged and firm. On intraoral examination, the tip of a stone impacted at the orifice of Wharton's duct may be visible. Bimanual palpation is the only way to assess the size of the gland and will also confirm the presence of a stone in the duct. Palpation of the duct is performed from the back towards the front of the mouth to avoid displacing a mobile stone into the gland.

MANAGEMENT OF SALIVARY CALCULI

Plain X-rays (occlusal and lateral-oblique views) will demonstrate most calculi. Contrast radiography of the duct system (**sialography**) is sometimes indicated if the history suggests stone disease yet no stone is palpable or visible on plain X-ray. Sialography (Fig. 41.9 and 10)

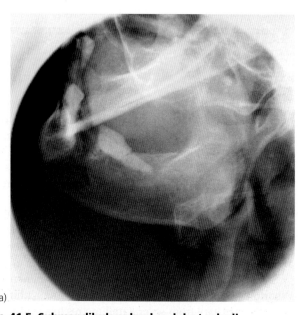

(a)

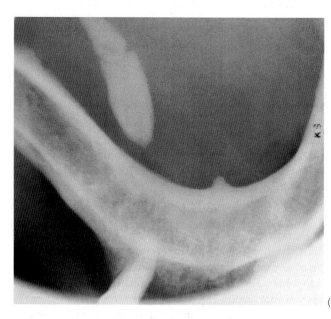

(b)

Fig. 41.5 Submandibular gland and duct calculi
(a) Lateral oblique plain X-ray, and **(b)** occlusal X-ray showing large 'date stone' calculus in the right submandibular duct. This was easily palpable bimanually in the floor of the mouth and removed via the oral route.

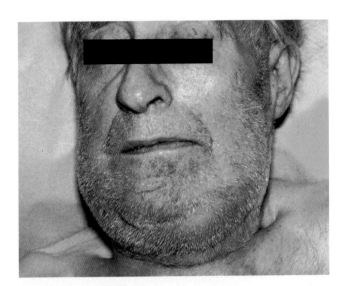

Fig. 41.6 Ludwig's angina
Spreading cellulitis of the submandibular region. This man of 70 had
large obstructing stones of the left submandibular duct and this had
led to infection in the duct and gland. This spread to the surrounding
tissues. He was beginning to develop respiratory embarrassment as a
result of laryngeal oedema but settled rapidly with antibiotics and
removal of the stones from within the mouth.

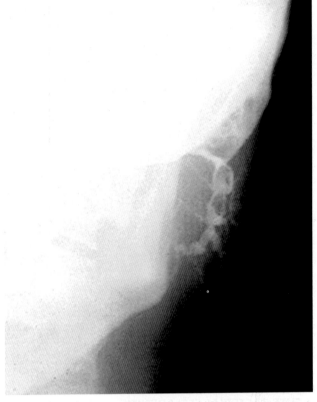

Fig. 41.7 Parotid sialography showing stones
This man of 58 complained of intermittent swelling in the region of
the left parotid gland, relieved on occasions by discharge of pus into
mouth. Contrast was injected into the orifice of the left parotid gland
to outline the duct structure. The main duct is dilated and contains
filling defects diagnosed as stones. This is an unusual finding as
stones are much more common in the submandibular gland.

requires cannulation of the salivary duct which may reveal
a stenosis of the duct orifice. Stenosis alone may produce
symptoms similar to obstruction by a salivary calculus.

Calculi in the anterior two-thirds of the duct in the
floor of the mouth are removed via an oral (Fig. 41.5)
approach. Immediately before operation, the continued
presence of the stone should be confirmed by palpation
or X-ray. At operation, if the stone is palpable, a longitudinal incision is then made in the duct over the stone
and the stone lifted out. If the stone is not palpable, the
duct is incised from the orifice backwards and the stone
can usually be removed with forceps. The incision is not
usually sutured but left open to improve salivary drainage.

Less commonly, calculi lie within the gland where
they are often multiple. The only way to remove the
obstruction is to excise the entire submandibular gland
through an incision below the mandible, carefully placed
to avoid damaging the mandibular branch of the facial
nerve (Fig. 41.10).

INFLAMMATORY DISORDERS OF THE SALIVARY GLANDS

The salivary glands are subject to infection both by viruses
(such as mumps) and bacteria. The glands may also be
affected by rare, apparently autoimmune phenomena
such as **Mikulicz's** and **Sjögren's syndromes**. Mumps is
rare outside childhood and young adulthood, is usually
bilateral, and resolves spontaneously. It is rarely a surgical
problem unless secondary bacterial infection supervenes.

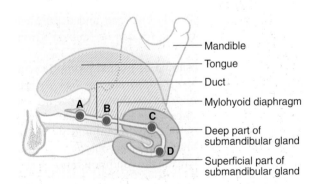

Note how the submandibular duct slopes downwards as it passes
posteriorly. Thus the more posterior stones are increasingly difficult
to remove from inside the mouth (**A→B**). **C** and **D** within the gland
can only be removed by removing the gland from the skin surface.
Note also how the gland is in two parts, superficial and deep, wrapped
around the posterior border of myohyoid

**Fig. 41.8 Submandibular gland and duct showing
common sites for stones**

553

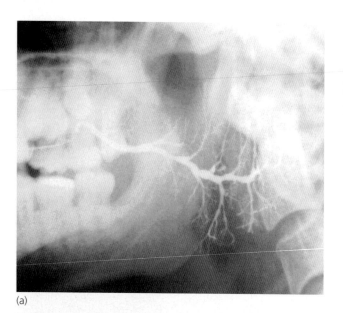

(a)

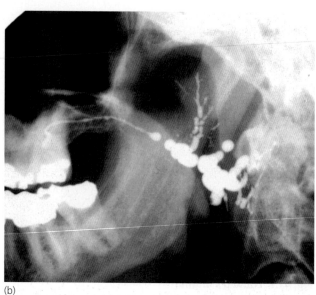

(b)

Fig. 41.9 Parotid sialography

(a) Normal sialogram showing regular duct diameter and branching. **(b)** Duct strictures and sialectasis. This 50-year-old man had recurrent bouts of parotid swelling complicated by infection. The sialogram shows several duct strictures with dilated ducts behind them. The dilatation is called sialectasis.

ACUTE BACTERIAL SIALADENITIS

This condition is now uncommon because of better mouth care in hospital; it almost always occurs in elderly or debilitated patients with poor oral hygiene but occasionally in children, in which case the underlying lesion is usually a suppurating lymph node within the parotid capsule. Dehydration and reduced salivary flow encourage ascending infection with oral flora, usually *Strep. viridans* or pneumococci.

The parotid gland is usually involved. The result is a painful, unilateral swelling accompanied by trismus, pyrexia and tachycardia. On examination, the parotid gland is tender and diffusely enlarged and a purulent discharge can be seen oozing (or can be 'milked') from the parotid duct orifice.

Bacterial sialadenitis should be treated promptly with parenteral antibiotics. If a parotid abscess has already formed, external surgical drainage should be performed. **Acute parotitis** was once common in postoperative surgical patients because of dehydration and poor oral hygiene. Intravenous fluids and close nursing attention to mouth care have now made the condition rare.

CHRONIC SIALADENITIS

Prolonged obstruction of a major salivary gland by a ductal calculus causes chronic inflammation of the gland. The glandular secretory elements progressively atrophy and are replaced by fibrous and adipose tissue. The duct system becomes dilated, fibrotic and infiltrated by chronic inflammatory cells. Chronic sialadenitis and salivary calculi usually involve the submandibular gland. The submandibular gland is swollen and there may be purulent discharge from the duct. The swelling is made worse by taking food.

Treatment is by removing the duct obstruction. In addition, antibiotics may be necessary. Glandular function may be irreversibly damaged if the process has been prolonged.

RECURRENT SIALADENITIS

This uncommon condition may occur at any age and usually affects the parotid gland. One gland or both glands are subject to recurrent attacks of painful swelling. This is caused by low-grade bacterial infection, although duct obstruction cannot usually be demonstrated. Recurrent attacks cause chronic swelling of the affected gland. Sialography shows dilatation of the duct system with terminal sacculation; this is described as **sialectasis**. The cause is most often a duct orificial stenosis, often caused by trauma from poorly fitting dentures or displaced teeth.

Immediate treatment includes antibiotics as indicated by culture of parotid duct discharge, as well as careful attention to oral hygiene. Ductoplasty to open the duct orifice is often successful. If sialography shows more remote duct stenoses, these can sometimes be dilated using balloons similar to angioplasty devices.

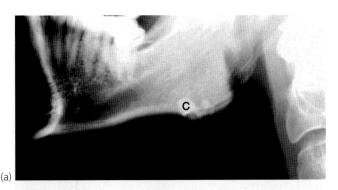

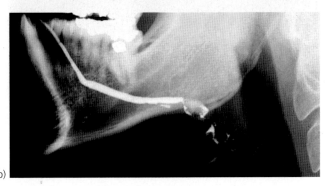

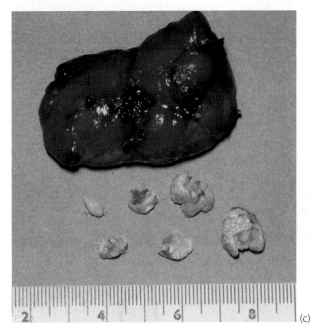

Fig. 41.10 Submandibular gland with stones
This 43-year-old man suffered chronic swelling and intermittent infection of the right submandibular gland: **(a)** Lateral plain X-ray showing calculi **C** within the gland. **(b)** Sialogram showing a normal Wharton's duct (note how rapidly it descends from the floor of the mouth). The stones within the gland are represented by filling defects in the contrast material. **(c)** The only means of dealing with the problem was excision of the gland via an extraoral (submandibular) approach. The gland contained six calculi.

AUTOIMMUNE SALIVARY GLAND DISORDERS

The salivary glands occasionally become involved in a chronic inflammatory process characterised by diffuse lymphoid infiltration and fibrosis. This is part of poorly understood autoimmune disorders which also involve lacrymal glands and mucous glands of the mouth and upper respiratory tract. The parotid and submandibular glands become diffusely and symmetrically enlarged, and salivary production is curtailed. The resulting dry mouth (**xerostomia**) not only causes distress and dysphagia, but predisposes to rampant dental caries. Diminished lacrymal secretion results in **kerato-conjunctivitis sicca**.

In isolation, the condition is known as **Mikulicz's syndrome**, but it may also occur in rheumatoid arthritis and other connective tissue disorders. In these cases, it is known as **Sjögren's syndrome**.

SALIVARY RETENTION CYSTS

Large retention cysts sometimes develop in the floor of the mouth. A cyst can reach several centimetres in diameter and is known as a **ranula** (frog mouth). The ranula typically appears as a blue-grey dome-like swelling beneath the tongue. It may burst spontaneously, discharging its contents and collapsing but it almost invariably recurs. The condition is painless but occupies space in the mouth and treatment is often requested for this reason. Excision is difficult because of the tenuous lining and because of the proximity to vital structures in the floor of the mouth; incomplete removal leads to recurrence. The usual treatment, therefore, is **marsupialisation**, i.e. de-roofing the cyst, so that it opens into the floor of the mouth (see Fig. 41.11).

LYMPH NODE DISORDERS OF THE HEAD AND NECK

Patients are often referred to a surgeon for biopsy of an enlarged lymph node in the cervical region. Often there are no other symptoms or signs. **Isolated lymph node enlargement** may be caused by local disease within its field of drainage. Examples include tonsillitis or dental infection, tonsillar tuberculosis or a malignant oro-

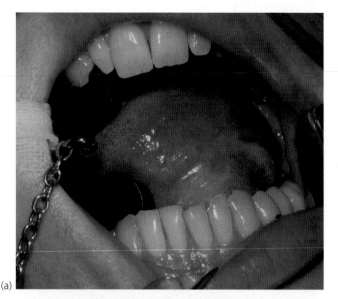
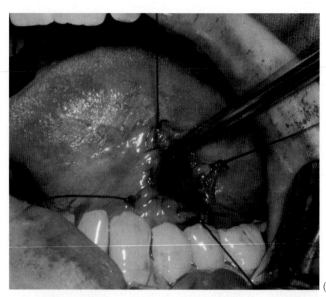

(a)   (b)

Fig. 41.11 Marsupialisation of a ranula
(a) Large salivary retention cyst in the floor of the mouth displacing the tongue towards the opposite side. **(b)** Operative photograph showing the 'de-roofed' cyst and the edges being sutured to the oral mucosa. The cavity rapidly 'filled in' from the base, obliterating the defect.

pharyngeal tumour. Nodes draining a bacterial infection may themselves suppurate, sometimes after the primary disorder has disappeared (see Fig. 41.12).

Alternatively, an enlarged cervical lymph node may be part of a **systemic lymphadenopathy** caused by glandular fever, lymphoma or HIV. Thus, any patient presenting with an enlarged lymph node requires careful general examination as well as examination of the head, neck and mouth. The latter often includes thorough endoscopy of the whole pharyngeal area, usually by a specialist ENT surgeon (otorhino-laryngologist). General examination should pay particular attention to axillary and inguinal lymph nodes, liver and spleen. A chest X-ray should be taken to look for enlarged thoracic lymph nodes. If cervical lymph node biopsy is necessary, improved histological techniques mean it can now be performed using a fine needle or core needle, usually under ultrasound control. If surgical removal of a gland is required, this should always be performed under general anaesthesia if practicable since the operation is often unexpectedly difficult. This is because lymph nodes are intimately related to so many vital structures and, furthermore, preoperative palpation tends to underestimate the size and extent of lymph node involvement.

CERVICAL TUBERCULOSIS

Tuberculosis involving the cervical glands (**scrofula**) was once common with the infection acquired by drinking milk from cattle infected with bovine tuberculosis. Cervical tuberculosis is now extremely rare in developed countries

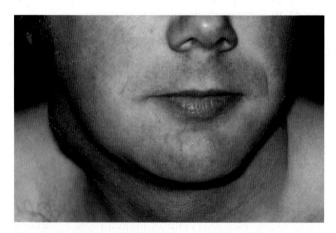

Fig. 41.12 Suppurating lymph node in the neck
This patient presented with a suppurating node in the neck which required external drainage. The primary site of sepsis was a dental abscess on a lower molar tooth.

but may be seen in recent immigrants from developing countries. The primary infection occurs in the tonsils but the condition presents with secondary involvement of the cervical nodes which become progressively enlarged and matted together. In advanced cases, liquefaction of the caseous material forms **cold abscesses**. If untreated, these eventually drain spontaneously onto the neck and leave disfiguring scars.

In the past, surgery was often required to drain and remove the affected glands. With modern chemotherapy this is now rarely necessary and surgery is mostly confined to excision biopsy for diagnosis.

LYMPHOMAS

An enlarged cervical lymph node is a common presentation of non-Hodgkin's lymphoma or Hodgkin's disease. The disease is often at an early stage and there may be no other symptoms or clinical signs. The diagnosis is then made by histological examination of a biopsy specimen.

SECONDARY (METASTATIC) TUMOURS

Cervical lymph node metastases may originate from primary malignant tumours in the head and neck, chest or abdomen. An enlarged lymph node may be the first indication of a tumour or a recurrence following treatment.

Tumours of the head and neck usually metastasise to nodes in the submandibular region and upper part of the anterior triangle. In contrast, tumours from the chest and abdomen usually metastasise to the lower part of the posterior triangle, particularly to **Virchow's node** (Fig. 41.13) which lies deeply in the angle between the sternocleidomastoid and the clavicle on the left side.

The following head and neck tumours commonly metastasise to cervical lymph nodes:

- Squamous carcinoma and melanoma of the skin of the neck, face, scalp and ear
- Squamous carcinoma of the mouth and tongue
- Squamous carcinoma of the nasopharynx,

oropharynx, larynx and paranasal sinuses; the primary tumour may be exceedingly small
- Adenocystic carcinoma of the major or accessory salivary glands
- Papillary (and occasionally medullary) carcinomas of the thyroid

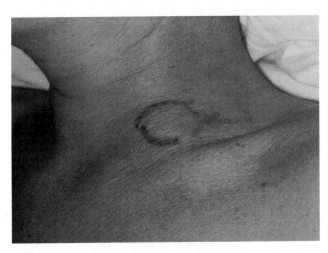

Fig. 41.13 Virchow's node
This 48-year-old woman noticed a painless lump in the left side of her neck. She had also lost a substantial amount of weight and had a poor appetite. Node biopsy revealed malignant adenocarcinoma cells and endoscopy showed an advanced carcinoma of stomach was the cause. Palpation of a malignant node in this site is known as Troisier's sign, after the French physician who diagnosed gastric cancer in himself.

MISCELLANEOUS CAUSES OF A LUMP IN THE NECK

CONGENITAL CYSTS AND SINUSES

A variety of cystic lesions of congenital origin occur in the head and neck and some of them may be associated with an external sinus opening. All are uncommon except in clinical 'short-case' examinations! They can be subdivided into thyroglossal cysts, branchial cysts, fusion-line dermoid cysts, preauricular cysts and sinuses, and cystic hygromas. All except for cystic hygroma are true epithelial cysts; cystic hygroma is a hamartomatous lymphatic malformation.

BRANCHIAL CYSTS, SINUSES AND FISTULAE

The precise embryological origin of these cysts is disputed but they probably arise from remnants of the second pharyngeal pouch or branchial cleft. Branchial cysts usually present in late adolescence or early adulthood but sometimes even later (Fig. 41.14). This late presentation is unusual for congenital lesions generally. The patient typically complains of a painless swelling in the side of the neck which may vary in size from time to time. Some

patients present with a painful red swelling due to inflammation of a previously unnoticed cyst.

The lump lies deep to the sternocleidomastoid, at the junction of its upper third and lower two-thirds. It protrudes forwards into the anterior triangle of the neck. The lump is soft and fluctuant on palpation. Provided it is not inflamed, the cyst usually transilluminates. Treatment is by percutaneous drainage or, if this is unsuccessful, by surgical excision. Inflamed cysts may require urgent drainage.

Branchial sinus and fistula presents as a discharging sinus near the lower end of the anterior border of the sternomastoid muscle. A **sinus** ends blindly on the lateral pharyngeal wall whereas a **fistula** communicates with the oropharynx near the tonsillar fossa. Surgical excision may be required.

FUSION-LINE DERMOID CYSTS

Dermoid cysts of congenital origin arise from epithelial remnants along lines of embryological fusion in the head and neck.

The most common are **external angular dermoids**, (Fig. 41.15), which are cystic swellings at the outer aspect of the supraorbital ridge. They are usually noticed soon after birth. On palpation these cysts are tense and firm and do not transilluminate because of their thick keratinous contents. They are deeply fixed and therefore immobile. External angular dermoids are usually removed surgically for cosmetic reasons during childhood.

Midline dermoid cysts are described as teratoid cysts because they contain a mixture of ectodermal, mesodermal and endodermal elements (e.g. nails and teeth, glands, blood vessels). As a rare phenomenon, dermoid cysts arise in the midline of the head or neck, usually during the first year of life. They should be removed surgically.

PREAURICULAR CYSTS AND SINUSES

Small cysts and sinuses may arise from developmental abnormalities of the first and second branchial arches (Fig. 41.15) which are involved in forming the external ear. The lesions become apparent in early childhood. They lie anterior to the tragus of the ear and present either as a small lump or a tiny discharging sinus which occasionally becomes infected. There may be an obvious associated abnormality of the auricle. Treatment is usually by surgical excision.

CYSTIC HYGROMAS

Cystic hygromas (Fig. 41.16) are not true cysts but lymphatic hamartomas which form multilocular cyst-like spaces. Cystic hygromas may be huge and disfiguring lesions present at birth. Smaller lesions may present in older children or adolescents as a painless lump in the neck just below the angle of the mandible. Cystic hygromas are soft and fluctuant and highly transilluminable.

Surgical excision may be difficult as these lesions often extend deeply into cervical and oro-facial tissues.

ACTINOMYCOSIS

Actinomycosis is a rare infection of the cervico-facial region. It is caused by *Actinomyces israeli*, an anaerobic Gram-positive bacterium with an unusual filamentous growth pattern similar to fungal mycelia. Actinomycosis is a chronic granulomatous infection which eventually forms multilocular abscesses which drain to the overlying skin via multiple sinuses. The pus exuding from the sinuses contains characteristic yellow clumps of organisms known as '**sulphur granules**'. The infection stimulates much fibrosis.

The organism is an oropharyngeal commensal but gains access to the tissues via carious teeth, tooth extraction sockets or traumatic wounds. Initially, there is a painful

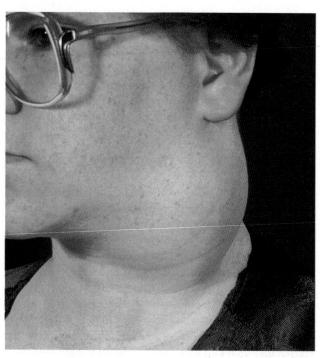

Fig. 41.14 Branchial cyst
This 30-year-old woman reported the sudden appearance of this large swelling in her neck associated with moderate pain over the previous week. The swelling was non-tender and fluctuant. Ultrasound confirmed it contained fluid. It was aspirated several times but failed to resolve and was eventually excised. It is not known why branchial cysts often come to attention so suddenly.

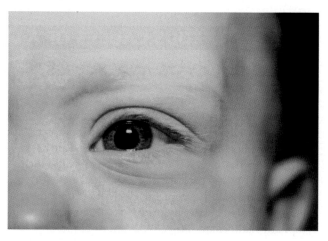

Fig. 41.15 External angular dermoid
This 4-month-old baby was noticed to have a swelling at the outer part of his left eyebrow. It was firm to palpation and was confidently diagnosed as a fusion line dermoid.

intraoral swelling. Inflammation then spreads slowly into the tissues, causing firm swelling of the cheek, mandible and submandibular region ('lumpy jaw'). The infection eventually erodes into the salivary glands, jaws and adjacent structures. Suppurative foci drain onto the surface of the face forming chronic discharging sinuses.

Actinomycosis is treated with a prolonged course (4–6 weeks) of high-dose penicillin. If necessary, the abscess network is surgically explored and drained.

Cervico-facial actinomycosis was once common and its decline in developed countries is probably the result of better oral hygiene and dental care. Actinomycosis also occurs in the ileo-caecal area, gaining access from an appendiceal perforation. Actinomycosis is now most often encountered in the pelvis as a complication of an intrauterine contraceptive device, although this remains rare.

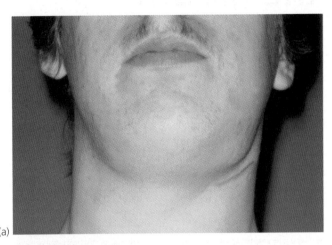

(a)

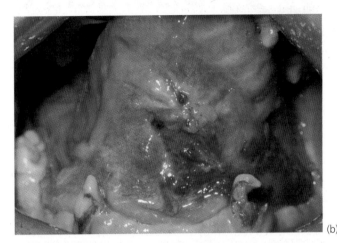

(b)

Fig. 41.16 Cystic hygroma
(a) This man of 23 had been born with a swelling under his left jaw which had not changed over recent years. The scar of a partial excision is visible. **(b)** Oral view of the same patient showing the haemangio-lymphangioma extends into the base of the tongue. It bleeds from time to time with minor trauma and this may have led him to neglect his teeth over the years.

42 Disorders of the mouth

DISORDERS OF THE ORAL CAVITY (EXCLUDING SALIVARY CALCULI)

The main disorders of the oral cavity are **dental caries** (decay) and its sequelae, inflammations of the gums and supporting bone (**periodontal disease**), tumours and premalignant conditions of the oral mucosa (leukoplakia and squamous carcinoma) and disorders of the accessory salivary glands such as retention cysts. Disorders of the main salivary glands are covered in Chapter 41. The main symptoms and signs of oral disease are summarised in Box 42.1.

advanced before it is visible, even with a dental mirror and probe, and may only be detectable on X-ray. In the meantime, the decay process is asymptomatic until close enough to the dental pulp to cause chemical inflammation and, eventually, bacterial invasion. The usual pathological process and corresponding symptoms are outlined in Figure 42.1.

DENTAL CARIES

PATHOPHYSIOLOGY AND CLINICAL FEATURES

Dental caries (dental decay) is one of the most common bacterial disorders in developed countries. The process begins when the protective enamel surface of the tooth is breached by the demineralising action of lactic acid. This is generated by commensal oral bacteria as a by-product of carbohydrate metabolism, particularly of refined sugar products. The most vulnerable sites for decay are the areas just below the contact points of adjacent tooth crowns and the deep pits and fissures on the biting (occlusal) surface of molars and premolars. These sites are inaccessible to the natural oral cleansing mechanisms and to tooth brushing.

Once the enamel is breached, proteolytic bacteria gain entry to the less densely calcified **dentine** beneath and cause its progressive destruction. The enamel remains intact until the supporting dentine is grossly undermined and the enamel fractures. Thus, dental caries may be well

---

KEY POINTS

Box 42.1 Symptoms and signs of oral disease and their main causes

Pain—dental caries and its sequelae, acute gingival inflammation such as pericoronitis and Vincent's infection (acute ulcerative gingivitis)

Bleeding—chronic gingival inflammation

Halitosis—dental caries and chronic periodontal disease

White lesions—epithelial dysplasia (leukoplakia), lichen planus and candidal infection

Oral ulceration—aphthous ulcers, squamous carcinoma, retained tooth roots, chronic tooth or denture trauma, and rare epidermal disorders (e.g. lichen planus or Behçet's syndrome)

Discharging sinuses—periapical tooth abscess ('gum boil')

Bony lumps in the jaws—fibrous dysplasia, tumours, cysts, ectopic teeth

Salivary glands and duct-related lumps—retention cysts, submandibular duct stones, tumours

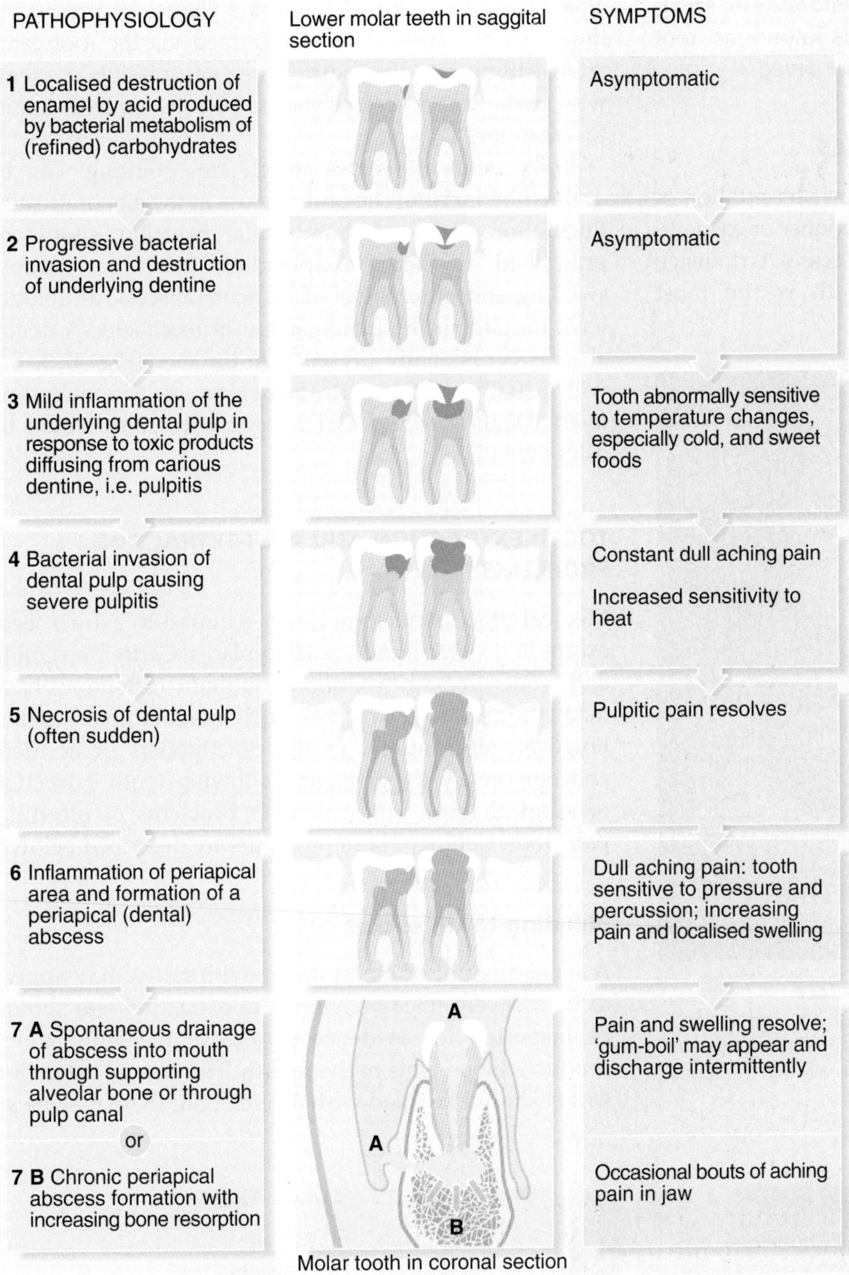

PATHOPHYSIOLOGY	Lower molar teeth in saggital section	SYMPTOMS
1 Localised destruction of enamel by acid produced by bacterial metabolism of (refined) carbohydrates		Asymptomatic
2 Progressive bacterial invasion and destruction of underlying dentine		Asymptomatic
3 Mild inflammation of the underlying dental pulp in response to toxic products diffusing from carious dentine, i.e. pulpitis		Tooth abnormally sensitive to temperature changes, especially cold, and sweet foods
4 Bacterial invasion of dental pulp causing severe pulpitis		Constant dull aching pain Increased sensitivity to heat
5 Necrosis of dental pulp (often sudden)		Pulpitic pain resolves
6 Inflammation of periapical area and formation of a periapical (dental) abscess		Dull aching pain: tooth sensitive to pressure and percussion; increasing pain and localised swelling
7 A Spontaneous drainage of abscess into mouth through supporting alveolar bone or through pulp canal or **7 B** Chronic periapical abscess formation with increasing bone resorption	A A A B Molar tooth in coronal section	Pain and swelling resolve; 'gum-boil' may appear and discharge intermittently Occasional bouts of aching pain in jaw

Fig. 42.1 Pathophysiology and symptoms of dental caries and its sequelae.

Once the pulp is exposed inflammation and bacterial invasion usually destroy the dental pulp and then spread to the periapical region where an **abscess** develops. This causes painful oral and facial swelling, and if untreated, eventually drains into the mouth or occasionally onto the face (Fig. 42.2). However, since the initiating cause remains, a chronic abscess will develop and flare up from time to time or continue with a persistent discharge.

The pain of dental caries is usually well localised and recognised as a 'toothache' by the patient. Dental pain may, however, be poorly localised and cause non-specific facial pain. Dental caries should always be considered

before rarer diagnoses are accepted. Overall, however, a surprising amount of dental caries, even with periapical infection, is asymptomatic.

MANAGEMENT OF DENTAL CARIES

Provided the dental pulp has not been invaded by infection (i.e. become 'exposed'), a dentist can usually remove the carious enamel and dentine and restore it (Fig. 42.3) with a lining of silver amalgam, synthetic resin or gold. This is usually placed over a sedative and insulating lining. Once bacteria have invaded the pulp, this necrotic tissue must be removed by **endodontic treatment**, and the pulp cavity filled; this is known as 'root filling'. In this way, the tooth can often be saved.

MANAGEMENT OF DENTAL ABSCESSES

A periapical abscess is the most common presentation of caries seen by the general medical practitioner or casualty officer. Primary treatment, as for other abscesses, is drainage of pus. Extracting the offending tooth is the most

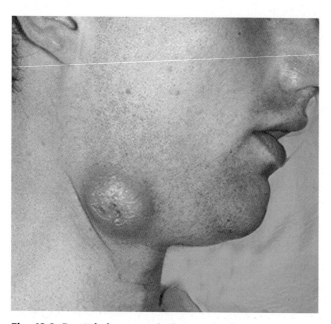

Fig. 42.2 Dental abscess pointing on the face
This young man presented to his doctor with an obvious abscess on the face; he was unaware that it arose from a tooth affected by dental caries. The abscess had to be drained externally and the tooth removed. The swelling then rapidly settled.

effective method, but if there is a chance of preserving the tooth, the abscess can be drained via the root canal after drilling into the tooth. Wherever possible, patients with periapical abscesses should be referred to a dentist for treatment.

Large acute abscesses which are 'pointing' can be drained by incising the oral mucosa at the site of greatest fluctuation. Oral or intramuscular penicillin should be prescribed if there is spreading infection. Without swelling and other signs of an acute abscess, antibiotics have no part in the management of toothache. A dental abscess occasionally presents on the face (Fig. 42.3) but will usually settle with extraction of the offending tooth. Dental abscesses are very rarely complicated by osteomyelitis.

TOOTH EXTRACTION AND POST-EXTRACTION PROBLEMS

Medical practitioners are rarely required to extract teeth except in geographically isolated places. Caries prevention and modern restorative and endodontic techniques have made the need for extraction much less common. Patients, however, often attend family practitioners or accident and emergency departments following tooth extraction or surgical tooth removal, with problems of bleeding, pain and swelling. These problems are described below.

Bleeding tooth socket

A small amount of blood mixed with saliva may appear to be a severe haemorrhage. The extraction site should be inspected for evidence of arterial bleeding, which produces blood clots in the mouth. The normal extraction socket should be filled with firm clot but there may be an

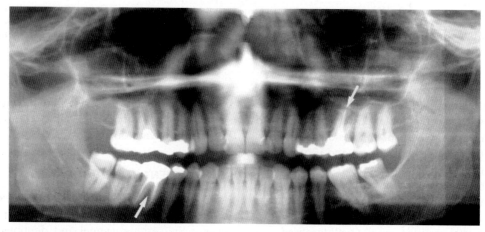

Fig. 42.3 Dental restorations and root fillings
This oral pantomograph (OPG) film shows silver amalgam restorations for caries in posterior teeth (shown as white radiopacities) and synthetic resin restorations in front teeth (shown as relative radiolucencies in the upper incisors). In addition, the upper left first molar and the lower right first molar (arrowed) have radiopaque root canal fillings, necessitated by dental caries invading the pulp.

ooze from the gingival margin. This is made worse if the anxious patient continually disturbs the clot by rinsing the mouth or 'exploring' the socket with the tongue. Aspirin as an analgesic may also promote bleeding by interfering with platelet activity.

Oozing or minor bleeding is easily controlled by the patient biting on a small dry pack such as a folded gauze swab. Pressure should be maintained for 10–15 minutes. More persistent bleeding is usually controlled by inserting several sutures through the gingival margins across the socket, partially closing the defect. This is illustrated in Figure 42.4. Afterwards, the patient should bite upon a small dry gauze pad. Suturing is performed under local anaesthesia, a small amount of which is infiltrated into the gingiva on each side of the socket. Absorbable polyglactin or catgut sutures are preferred as they do not leave irritating sharp ends. Absorbable sutures dissolve in 5–10 days.

If bleeding continues after these simple measures, the patient should be investigated for a coagulation or platelet abnormality.

Pain after tooth extraction

Forceps extraction or surgical tooth removal may lead to a great deal of pain soon afterwards. Removal of lower molar teeth may cause **trismus** (masseteric spasm) making jaw movements painful and restricted. If there is no sign of infection, treatment is with analgesia, not antibiotics. Pain appearing several days after extraction is usually due to a superficial osteitis of exposed bone within the socket caused by failure of the socket to fill with organised clot. This condition, known as **dry socket**, is intensely painful and requires dental treatment. Antibiotic therapy is not helpful.

Swelling after tooth extraction

Soft tissue swelling is not common after tooth extraction with the exception of surgically removed lower third

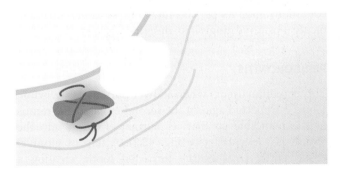

Fig. 42.4 Suture technique for bleeding tooth socket.
'Figure of eight' suture occludes bleeding gum edge on alveolar bone. Patient should bite for at least 10 minutes on a folded swab after suture to encourage clotting.

molars ('wisdom teeth'). Extraction of these teeth often causes marked swelling around the angle of the mandible, with trismus and pain. This swelling represents a normal inflammatory response and some interstitial haemorrhage rather than infection. The swelling subsides within a week or so postoperatively and again does not warrant antibiotic therapy.

INFLAMMATION OF THE PERIODONTAL TISSUES

GINGIVITIS AND PERIODONTITIS

Teeth are embedded in bony **alveolar ridges** in both upper and lower jaws. A thin layer of **cementum** (a bone-like material) on the root surface is joined to the bone of the socket by a tough collagenous tissue known as **periodontal membrane or ligament**. The oral mucosa is bound to the alveolar bone (the **gingiva** or gums) and normally forms a tight cuff around the tooth neck, protecting alveolar bone from bacteria and foreign material. A potential space between the gingival cuff and the enamel of the crown, known as the **gingival crevice** extends down to the cemento-enamel junction. At the free margin of the gingiva, the tough stratified oral epithelium becomes a thin vulnerable layer lining the gingival crevice.

If oral hygiene is inadequate, commensal bacteria colonise the gingival margin and form a white gelatinous **plaque** on the enamel (Fig. 42.5). If allowed to persist, plaque becomes adherent to the tooth surface and becomes mineralised. This is known as **calculus**, and cannot be removed by tooth brushing. Bacterial toxins then cause inflammation of the gingiva, known as **marginal gingivitis**. This appears as swelling and redness of the gums and slight bleeding during tooth brushing.

As seen in Figure 42.6, gingivitis causes eversion of the gingival margin. This encourages more bacterial plaque and calculus to form in the gingival crevice and also results in greater gingival trauma from food. These both lead to more extensive gingival inflammation.

If untreated, inflammation gradually extends to involve the deeper supporting tissues. This causes progressive resorption of alveolar bone and destruction of the periodontal membrane, known as **periodontitis**. By this stage, the gingiva is thickened and inflamed with a purulent discharge from the gums. This explains the old term 'pyorrhoea'. Despite this, the patient is remarkably pain free, although halitosis is obvious to others!

As periodontal inflammation progresses, more alveolar bone is destroyed and the gums recede. The root-surface becomes exposed to view, giving rise to the expression 'long in the tooth', once thought to be inevitable with advancing age. Teeth become increasingly mobile until they fall out or can be extracted with the fingers!

(a) Normal gingiva   **(b) Marginal gingivitis**

(c) Moderate gingivitis   **(d) Periodontitis**

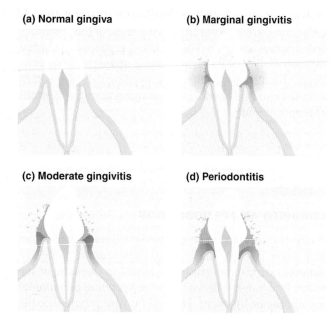

Fig. 42.5 Pathogenesis of periodontal disease
(a) Healthy pink gingiva forming tight cuff around base of crown.
(b) Plaque accumulates around gingival margins. Toxins are produced
by bacteria causing marginal inflammation; marginal gingiva becomes
red, slightly swollen and bleeds easily. **(c)** More severe gingival
inflammation: loss of tight protective cuff of gingiva allows
accumulation of bacterial plaque and calculus in gingival crevice.
(d) The inflammation involves the supporting alveolar bone which is
progressively resorbed so that adequate tooth support is eventually lost.

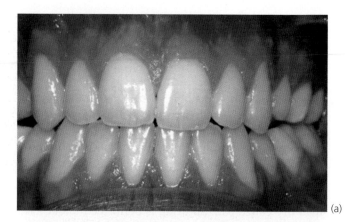

(a)

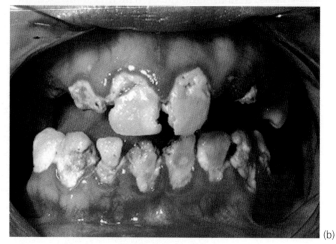

(b)

Fig. 42.6 Gingivitis and periodontitis
(a) Normal healthy gingivae. **(b)** Chronic gingivitis showing
accumulated plaque and calculus around the gingival margins. At this
stage, there has been no alveolar bone destruction and the
inflammatory process is potentially reversible. Many of these teeth
had to be extracted because of rampant caries.

An acute **periodontal abscess** may develop at some
point. On the whole, however, periodontal disease is an
insidious process commencing in early adulthood, but it
is almost entirely preventable. In adults, **periodontitis**
(not dental decay, as is commonly supposed) is responsible
for most lost teeth. The destruction of alveolar bone makes
it difficult to construct satisfactory dentures for many of
these patients, for lack of a retaining alveolar ridge.

Management of gingivitis and periodontitis

Gingivitis and periodontitis is almost entirely preventable
by thorough and regular tooth brushing and use of dental
floss, plus periodic dental scaling to remove inaccessible
plaque and calculus.

Initial dental scaling, and careful oral hygiene instruction
and supervision will cure gingivitis, which is a reversible
condition. During the early stages of improved oral hygiene,
bleeding will increase through brushing inflamed tissues.
This soon subsides unless further periodontal treatment
is needed.

Periodontitis also requires meticulous oral hygiene
once the teeth have been thoroughly cleaned of plaque
and calculus. Lost bone is never replaced, however, and
the gingival contour remains abnormal, making effective

oral hygiene difficult. Surgical recontouring of the gingiva
and underlying bone (**gingivoplasty**) may sometimes be
appropriate. It must be emphasised that antibiotics play no
part in the treatment of chronic gingivitis and periodontitis.
Antibiotics may, however, be useful for acute gingival
conditions such as pericoronitis and Vincent's infection
(acute ulcerative gingivitis), described below.

PERICORONITIS

This condition occurs when a lower third molar (wisdom
tooth) is impacted against the second molar or the ramus
of the mandible so that its normal eruption into the
mouth is prevented (see Fig. 42.7). A flap of gingival
tissue partly overlies the impacted tooth, creating a
space around the buried tooth crown. Food and bacterial
plaque collect here and lead to acute infection, which
may extend into surrounding tissues, and even into the
parapharyngeal area.

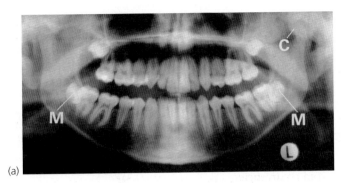

(a)

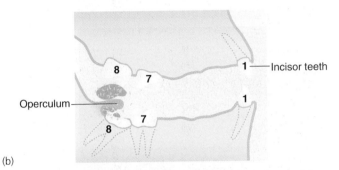

(b)

Fig. 42.7 Impacted lower third molars and pericoronitis
This OPG radiograph of a 16-year-old girl shows the whole lower jaw 'opened out'. Both lower third molars **M** are seen to be angled towards the second molars and impacted against them. The roots are not fully formed and there is little chance of these teeth erupting normally. These were an incidental finding, the X-rays having been taken to demonstrate a fracture of the neck of the left mandibular condyle **C**.

The patient complains of severe, poorly localised pain near the angle of the mandible. Pain is aggravated by closing the jaw because the opposing tooth bites on the swollen gingival flap. On examination, the pericoronal tissues of the affected tooth are red and swollen with a purulent discharge exuding from beneath the gingival flap. Oral examination may be difficult because of trismus. Externally, the submandibular lymph nodes are enlarged and tender.

Management of pericoronitis

Pericoronitis is a cellulitis with incipient abscess formation. It is caused by a mixture of organisms which are usually sensitive to penicillin. It is treated locally by irrigating beneath the flap with hydrogen peroxide and the patient is advised to rinse the mouth several times daily with warm salty water. Rapid relief can be obtained by removing the upper wisdom tooth which impinges on the flap over the lower wisdom tooth. Oral penicillin is required if the patient is systemically unwell. Once the acute infection is over, the lower wisdom tooth may need to be removed surgically, especially if attacks are recurrent.

ACUTE ULCERATIVE GINGIVITIS (VINCENT'S INFECTION)

This is an acute inflammatory condition with necrotising ulceration of the gingival margin. It is caused by a mixture of Gram-negative organisms, which are normal oral commensals. The most prominent bacteria are *Fusobacterium fusiformis*, *Borrelia vincenti* and *Bacteroides melaninogenicus*. Acute ulcerative gingivitis most commonly occurs in young adults who 'burn the candle at both ends' and become generally run down. Poor oral hygiene, pericoronitis and smoking may contribute. Acute ulcerative gingivitis is now uncommon, but was widespread among soldiers in the First World War when it gained the name 'trench mouth'.

There is an abrupt onset of gingival pain and bleeding, accompanied by a foul, often metallic taste and marked halitosis. Cervical lymph nodes are enlarged and tender, and there may be fever, malaise and anorexia. Oral examination reveals characteristic ragged, punched-out ulceration of the gingival margin, especially between the teeth (see Fig. 42.8). Ulceration elsewhere in the mouth is rare, except in severe cases where the pharyngeal mucosa becomes inflamed and ulcerated (**Vincent's angina**). Acute ulcerative gingivitis is easily distinguished from **herpetic gingivostomatitis**, the other acute ulcerative condition with systemic symptoms, as the former is confined to the gingival margin, whereas herpetic ulcers are scattered all over the oral mucosa.

Management of acute ulcerative gingivitis

Vincent's infection rapidly responds to metronidazole tablets, usually with full recovery of gingival morphology; penicillin is also effective. Tooth brushing is extremely painful during an attack and the mouth should be frequently rinsed with warm water or weak hydrogen

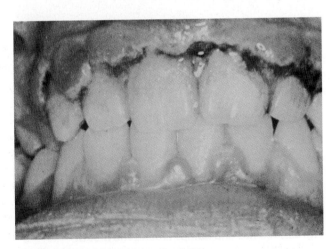

Fig. 42.8 Acute ulcerative gingivitis
This shows the typical appearance of acute ulcerative gingivitis (Vincent's infection); there is ulceration of the whole gingival margin with destruction of the interdental papillae, giving a ragged but almost straight gum margin compare this with Fig. 42.6(b).

peroxide to keep it clean. Afterwards, careful attention to oral hygiene will usually prevent recurrence.

EPULIS

An epulis is a benign, localised gingival swelling. Two types are recognised: fibrous epulis and giant cell epulis.

The **fibrous epulis** is simply a benign fibrous tissue tumour arising from the periodontal membrane or nearby periosteum. It forms a smooth, firm, slowly growing lump,

covered with normal gingiva. A fibrous epulis usually emerges between two teeth, which may be slightly pushed apart by pressure. Treatment is by local excision with curettage of the origin. Otherwise, the lesion may recur.

The **giant cell epulis** arises in a similar location but grows much faster. It forms an irregular red fleshy mass which ulcerates and bleeds. The lesion consists of numerous giant cells in a highly vascular stroma, which may invade local bone. Treatment involves extracting associated teeth and excising and curetting bone. This is the only way to avoid recurrence.

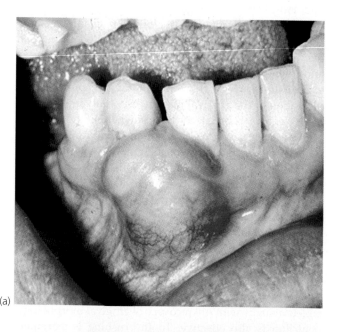
(a)

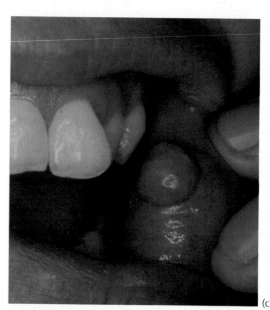
(c)

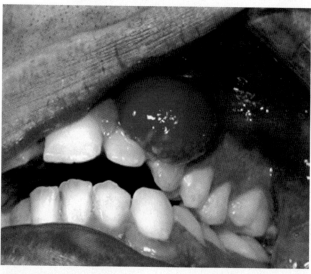
(b)

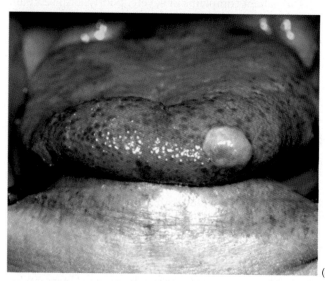
(d)

Fig. 42.9 Lumps and bumps around the mouth
(a) Fibrous epulis. This can be seen to be moving the nearby tooth out of alignment. **(b)** Giant cell epulis. Both of these are in typical interdental location. The fibrous epulis is the same colour as the gum, while the giant cell epulis is a deeper red. **(c)** Fibroepithelial polyp inside cheek. These lesions are common and are probably initiated by minor biting trauma to the cheek or lip. They are often inadvertently chewed upon and gradually become larger. Excision is usually straightforward. **(d)** Pyogenic granuloma of the tongue. These are probably initiated by injury and maintained by an excessive healing response. They can occur on the gum or anywhere else in the mouth.

Pyogenic granulomas may occur on the gums or oral mucosa of the lips. They have a similar appearance to pyogenic granulomas of the skin (see Ch. 40).

TUMOURS OF THE ORAL MUCOSA

PATHOPHYSIOLOGY AND AETIOLOGY

The whole oral cavity including the tongue is invested by stratified squamous epithelium. Squamous cell carcinomas of the mouth account for about 3% of all malignancies. Like their counterparts on the skin, squamous carcinomas in the mouth usually occur in older patients. Men are affected twice as often as women.

Smoking is the usual cause in developed countries. Pipe and cigar smokers appear to be at greatest risk. The tongue and lower lip are the common sites of oral cancer,

each accounting for about 25% of cases. Chronic irritation by ill-fitting dentures, jagged tooth restorations or alcohol abuse may contribute to the aetiology.

In India, Sri Lanka and Papua New Guinea and other countries the habit of chewing a small package of betel leaf, tobacco and lime causes a very high incidence of carcinoma of the buccal mucosa.

Leukoplakia is a premalignant dysplastic condition found in 50% of patients with oral carcinoma.

CLINICAL FEATURES OF ORAL CANCER

Oral cancer usually presents as a chronic indurated ulcer, which slowly enlarges and fails to heal (Fig. 42.10b and c). An early lesion may present as a non-ulcerated mucosal swelling. Lesions are usually painless, unless they become secondarily infected, although advanced

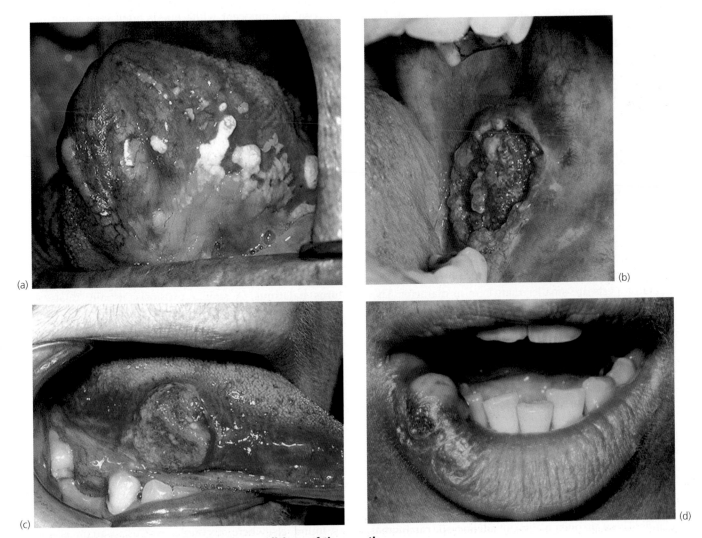

Fig. 42.10 Premalignant and malignant conditions of the mouth
(a) Leukoplakia under tongue. **(b)** Ulcerating squamous cell carcinoma (SCC) of the cheek. **(c)** Ulcerating SCC of the tongue. **(d)** Squamous cell carcinoma of the lip. This man of 60 had smoked a pipe most of his life. He tended to keep the pipe constantly in his mouth whilst he worked. He presented with a non-healing ulcer of the lip, proven to be a well differentiated SCC on biopsy. A wedge resection of the lip was performed and produced a cure.

lesions may cause pain as they invade deeply. Carcinoma of the tongue, for example, may cause pain referred to the ear or pharynx.

Oral squamous carcinomas are generally well differentiated. They invade locally but metastasise to submandibular and cervical lymph nodes only at a late stage. Spreading tumours of the posterior floor of mouth and tongue interfere with speech, mastication and swallowing. These are particularly distressing symptoms.

MANAGEMENT OF ORAL CANCER

A chronic oral ulcer which fails to heal after possible aggravating factors have been removed (such as ill-fitting dentures), should undergo incision biopsy to exclude cancer.

Oral cancers are excised with a margin of normal tissue. This may not be possible anatomically or cosmetically and often necessitates a major reconstructive surgical operation. Involved regional lymph nodes are removed by **block dissection**.

If excision is impractical, most of these tumours respond to radiotherapy. This may employ external beam treatment or radioactive implants. A disadvantage of radiotherapy, however, is that it damages salivary glands resulting in xerostomia (dry mouth). Apart from the discomfort, this predisposes to salivary gland infection.

Carcinoma of the lip has the best prognosis. The 5-year survival rate is over 60%, but for tumours of the tongue and floor of the mouth, this falls to only about 25%.

LEUKOPLAKIA

Leukoplakia means 'white plaque', and the term is used to describe white patches on the oral mucosa which cannot readily be scraped off (see Fig. 42.10a). This distinguishes them from candidal infections. White plaques may be caused by oral lichen planus or lupus erythematosus, but the main importance of leukoplakia is that it may represent epithelial dysplasia or even carcinoma-in-situ.

The cheeks and tongue are most often affected, although dysplastic patches may develop anywhere in the oral mucosa. An innocent white line is often seen along the inside of the cheek; this corresponds to the line of biting surfaces of the teeth and is caused by frictional hyperplasia.

Severe or extensive leukoplakia should be referred for specialist oral surgical opinion and biopsy. Areas of severe dysplasia require surgical removal, which may necessitate grafting.

MISCELLANEOUS DISORDERS CAUSING INTRAORAL SWELLING

RETENTION CYSTS OF THE ACCESSORY SALIVARY GLANDS

The oral mucosa contains numerous accessory mucous and serous salivary glands. Small retention cysts probably develop as a result of minor trauma to the duct. Most retention cysts are smaller than 1 cm in diameter. They commonly occur in the lower lip mucosa where they cause annoyance and are readily traumatised during speech or chewing. Retention cysts are blue-grey and are extremely soft to palpation. They often rupture spontaneously but usually reform. Small retention cysts can usually be completely enucleated under local anaesthesia; larger ones may need marsupialisation.

TUMOURS OF ACCESSORY SALIVARY GLANDS

Tumours occasionally arise in the accessory salivary glands. These are often malignant **adenocystic carcinomas**. They present as small, firm lumps in the oral mucosa or posterior palate, and are often noticed before invading deeply or metastasising. Treatment is by wide excision.

BONY EXOSTOSES

Local outgrowths of the jaw bones are common and may produce an intraoral lump. To the uninitiated doctor, this may be suspicious of neoplasia. The most common site is the centre of the hard palate, where it is known as a **torus palatinus**. A similar exostosis, usually bilateral, occurs inside the mandible, opposite the premolar teeth (**torus mandibularis**).

These lesions are extremely hard and covered by normal oral mucosa. Excision is rarely needed unless there are problems in wearing a removable denture.

CYSTS AND TUMOURS OF THE JAWS

Various cystic lesions and tumours arise in the jaws. Many are abnormalities of tooth-forming epithelium, either developmental or acquired. Most are rare and can usually be diagnosed radiologically. The jaws are occasionally the site of benign or malignant bone tumours, as found elsewhere. Examples are osteosarcomas and osteoclastomas.

Growth disorders of bone such as fibrous dysplasia and Paget's disease of bone may also affect the jaw.

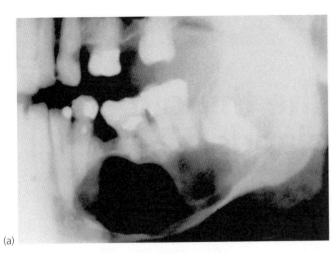

(a)

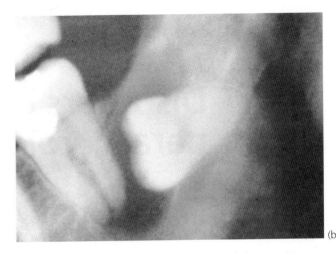

(b)

Fig. 42.11 Dental cyst and dentigerous cyst
(a) Large dental cyst in the mandible. This arose from tooth-forming epithelial remnants in the apical area of the lower left second premolar tooth which was extracted several months beforehand due to chronic periapical infection. **(b)** Dentigerous cyst associated with the crown of an unerupted lower third molar. These cysts originate from epithelial remnants of the tooth bud.

43 Disorders of the thyroid and parathyroid glands

INTRODUCTION

Patients with disorders of the thyroid gland usually present to the surgeon with a mass in the neck. Occasionally patients are referred with hyperthyroidism where medical treatment has failed or radioisotopic treatment is unsuitable. If there is a thyroid mass, malignancy may be suspected or the mass may be causing pressure symptoms or cosmetic deformity. There may be a discrete thyroid lump or the whole gland may be enlarged (goitre). In most cases, the patient is clinically euthyroid (i.e. with normal thyroid hormone activity) and biochemical tests of thyroid function are normal. In contrast, the second group of patients have usually been investigated and found to be hyperthyroid. They are then referred for thyroidectomy after unsatisfactory 'medical' treatment.

Parathyroid disorders usually reach the surgeon because of **hypercalcaemia** caused by excess parathormone secretion. This can only be successfully treated by surgical removal of the cause which is usually parathyroid adenoma or, less commonly, hyperplasia and, very rarely, carcinoma.

DISORDERS OF THE THYROID

Diseases of the thyroid can be divided into four broad pathological categories:

- Developmental abnormalities
- Inflammatory and autoimmune disorders
- Hyperplastic and metabolic disorders
- Neoplasms

The main pathophysiological and clinical features are summarised in Table 43.1, except for thyroid malignancy which is summarised in Table 43.2 later.

MAIN CLINICAL PRESENTATIONS OF THYROID DISEASE IN SURGICAL PRACTICE

Diffuse or generalised enlargement of the thyroid

The term **goitre** is often used to describe any generalised enlargement of the thyroid but it is descriptively and pathologically imprecise. Most large generalised thyroid swellings seen in developed countries are caused by simple, non-toxic **colloid goitre**, i.e. idiopathic diffuse hyperplasia or multinodular hyperplasia. Multinodular goitres usually develop from smooth diffuse goitres over a period of years.

Where the condition is *endemic* (often in isolated, mountainous and underdeveloped regions such as Nepal), iodine deficiency is the usual cause, though this is less common now that iodine is added to the diet. These goitres are often asymmetrical and soft to palpation. They are composed of many large hyperplastic nodules and can reach enormous sizes (see Fig. 43.1a). Although unsightly, endemic goitres cause surprisingly few symptoms and the patient is usually euthyroid.

Table 43.1 Benign diseases of the thyroid

Condition (relative frequency in developed countries)	Pathophysiology	Clinical features
1. Developmental abnormalities		
a. Thyroglossal cyst (*uncommon*)	Cyst formation anywhere along the midline thyroglossal tract. This marks the line of embryological descent of the thyroid from the foramen caecum via the hyoid bone to the normal position in the neck	Smooth, rounded swelling in midline of neck anywhere between the submental area and isthmus of thyroid. Usually found in children and young adults
b. Thyroglossal fistula (*rare*)	Incision into or incomplete removal of a thyroglossal cyst can cause a fistula	Fistulous (or sinus) opening near midline of neck. Intermittently discharges clear fluid or becomes infected and discharges pus
c. Ectopic thyroid (*common*)	Part or all of the thyroid lying anywhere along the thyroglossal tract	Usually symptomless but may present as an unusual swelling near foramen caecum at junction of anterior two-thirds and posterior third of tongue
2. Inflammatory and autoimmune disorders		
a. Hashimoto's thyroiditis (*common*)	Diffuse lymphocytic infiltration of thyroid gland with progressive destruction of thyroid follicles. Over a period of years, leads to progressive atrophy and fibrosis. Various antithyroid antibodies usually present in plasma in high titres. Polygenic inherited disorder which may be associated with other autoimmune disorders e.g. pernicious anaemia. Focal lymphocytic thyroiditis is probably a milder variant of the same condition	Presents in adulthood with mild, diffuse, sometimes tender thyroid enlargement. Often the thyroid is not enlarged. Patient usually euthyroid or hyperthyroid at outset, but later becomes hypothyroid. Affects females much more frequently than males
b. Graves' disease (*fairly common*)	Diffuse thyroid hyperplasia due to the action of a circulating immunoglobulin 'long-acting thyroid stimulator' (LATS). This binds to thyroid acinar cells mimicking the effects of TSH and producing excess thyroid hormone	Diffuse thyroid enlargement, sometimes with a bruit, but main feature is marked hyperthyroidism (thyrotoxicosis) causing weight loss, heat intolerance, tachycardia, hyper-reflexia, tremor and sometimes exophthalmos
c. De Quervain's acute thyroiditis (*uncommon*)	Diffuse inflammation of thyroid gland, probably viral in origin. Neutrophilic and later lymphocytic and histiocytic infiltration of gland occurs	Very tender, diffuse moderate thyroid enlargement, with or without systemic symptoms. Episodes last weeks to months and are often recurrent. Patient usually euthyroid but may be hyperthyroid in acute phase
d. Riedl's thyroiditis (*very rare*)	Dense fibrosis of thyroid gland. Possibly an autoimmune process	Extremely hard ('woody goitre') often asymmetrical thyroid mass suspicious of tumour. Sometimes produces symptoms of compression
3. Hyperplastic and metabolic disorders		
a. Simple non-toxic colloid goitre (*very common*)	Benign, diffuse or multinodular hyperplasia of thyroid follicles. Cause is unknown but possibly minor abnormality of thyroid hormone synthesis	Diffuse or sporadic multinodular thyroid enlargement or single 'adenomatous' nodule or cyst. Patient clinically euthyroid and all thyroid function tests normal. Affects females much more than males
b. Endemic goitre (*very rare in UK*)	Diffuse hyperplasia of thyroid follicles due to dietary iodine deficiency or goitrogenic foods. Endemic in inland, developing countries, especially in mountainous areas	Diffuse, often massive thyroid enlargement which may later become nodular. T4 is low or normal and TSH tends to be elevated

Table 43.1 Continued

Condition (relative frequency in developed countries)	Pathophysiology	Clinical features
c. Drug induced goitre (uncommon)	Diffuse thyroid hyperplasia secondary to interference with thyroid hormone synthesis. Drugs causing this are antithyroid drugs used in therapy (e.g. carbimazole) or others like lithium and aminoglutethimide	Diffuse thyroid enlargement. Patient usually euthyroid. Can be prevented by using replacement dose of T4 concurrently with blocking drugs ('block and replace')
d. Dyshormonogenesis (very uncommon)	Diffuse thyroid hyperplasia caused by a variety of uncommon genetic (recessive) defects affecting thyroid hormone synthesis	Presents at birth or in childhood with thyroid enlargement and severe hypothyroidism (cretinism). In developed countries, these defects are usually diagnosed at birth by neonatal screening tests before any goitre has developed
e. Physiological (common)	Diffuse thyroid hyperplasia often associated with pregnancy and puberty	Mild diffuse thyroid enlargement. Patient euthyroid

Table 43.2 Malignant diseases of the thyroid

MALIGNANT DISEASES OF THE THYROID

Condition (relative frequency in developed countries)	Pathophysiology	Clinical features
Adenocarcinomas		
a. Papillary carcinoma (relatively common — two thirds of all thyroid carcinomas and 90% in children)	Papillary adenocarcinoma forms a complex branching structure with a fibrous stroma (papillary pattern) and psammoma bodies. Variable degree of dysplasia. Commonly metastasises to cervical nodes but distant metastases rare	Slowly growing firm thyroid lump or cervical lymph nodes or both. Occurs in adults and sometimes children, 3F:1M. Excellent prognosis even with local metastases — 90% survival at 10 years
b. Follicular carcinoma (relatively uncommon)	Tumour forms a well-developed follicular pattern reminiscent of normal thyroid. Generally well differentiated but metastasis is usually distant e.g. lungs and bone	Similar presentation to papillary carcinoma but does not involve cervical nodes. Affects slightly older age group than papillary carcinoma, 3F:1M
c. Anaplastic carcinoma (relatively uncommon)	Aggressive tumour rapidly spreading beyond the confines of the gland	Diffuse, hard thyroid enlargement, often with symptoms of tracheal or recurrent laryngeal nerve involvement. Affects elderly patients. Very poor prognosis
d. Medullary carcinoma (very uncommon)	Well differentiated tumour derived from parafollicular calcitonin-secreting cells (C-cells). Tumour contains deposits of amyloid	Stony hard thyroid lump, possibly with secondaries in cervical nodes. Often associated with MEN II. Poor prognosis. Calcitonin in blood is a tumour marker
e. Lymphoma (rare)	Diffuse lymphoid infiltration of thyroid gland	Diffuse thyroid enlargement. Patient euthyroid. Usually occurs in Hashimoto's disease

Anaplastic carcinomas may also cause fairly large thyroid swellings in elderly patients (see Fig. 43.1b). There are usually symptoms of invasion into nearby structures. These include hoarseness if there is recurrent laryngeal nerve involvement and stridor, particularly at night, if there is tracheal displacement or compression. The gland is hard on palpation. The uncommon **lymphomas** of the thyroid also present with diffuse thyroid enlargement.

In **Graves' disease** (primary hyperthyroidism) there is usually a degree of smooth thyroid enlargement (see Fig. 43.1c), often increased by drug treatment. This is almost never the main presenting feature, however. Similarly, in **Hashimoto's** thyroiditis, the thyroid may be moderately enlarged but firmer and finely nodular on palpation.

'Solitary' thyroid nodule

A common presentation of thyroid disease is a **solitary thyroid nodule**, (see Fig. 43.1d) an isolated lump within the thyroid, although 50% turn out to be part of a multi-nodular goitre. These lumps are not usually obvious and are found incidentally by the patient or the doctor. They may first be noticed when the patient swallows. Only about 10% of true solitary nodules are malignant tumours although this rises to about 40% in patients who have undergone previous neck irradiation. Almost all nodules developing in the thyroid in childhood are malignant. Fallout from the nuclear meltdown at Chernobyl produced a huge crop of thyroid cancers in irradiated children. Malignancy must be excluded by investigation, and fine needle aspiration cytology or needle core biopsy is the most effective method for doing so.

An isolated lesion is most commonly a nodule of idiopathic hyperplasia which may be so discrete as to be described as a **thyroid adenoma**. Thyroid cysts are fairly common and fall within the spectrum of the pathological entity '**simple or multinodular colloid goitre**'.

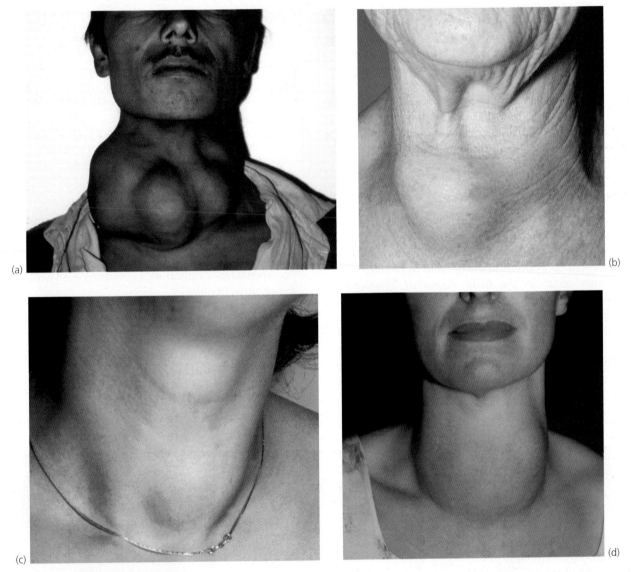

Fig. 43.1 Examples of thyroid swellings

(a) Endemic goitre. This condition, caused by iodine deficiency, is extremely common in isolated mountain regions. The thyroid can reach an enormous size, yet the patient suffers only minimal symptoms and is usually euthyroid. This typical example in a Nepalese man is only of moderate size by local standards! **(b)** Anaplastic carcinoma. Rapidly enlarging hard thyroid mass in an elderly woman; the mass was firmly tethered to strap muscles and deeper structures. **(c)** Solitary thyroid nodule. This asymptomatic nodule had been present for several years. It proved histologically to be a thyroid adenoma. **(d)** Longstanding multinodular goitre in a woman of 40 with a strong family history of thyroid disorders. The thyroid is multinodular on palpation and on ultrasound, there are multiple nodules of various sizes plus some small cysts. Any change in a multinodular goitre may herald malignancy.

As mentioned earlier, an apparent solitary nodule may prove to be a focal accentuation of a generalised thyroid enlargement such as simple multinodular hyperplasia (colloid goitre) or less often, Hashimoto's thyroiditis.

Other features associated with thyroid enlargement

A new area of enlargement in an existing goitre may be caused by haemorrhage into a cyst or nodule, an enlarging hyperplastic nodule or a developing carcinoma. If the thyroid extends behind the sternum (see Fig. 43.4 below) into the anterior mediastinum, the trachea may be compressed or displaced and cause **stridor**. Stridor may only become obvious when the neck is in certain positions, for example, sleeping on one side at night. Hoarseness or stridor may also result from invasion by an anaplastic carcinoma.

Pain and tenderness are uncommon presenting features in thyroid disease, but characterise the rare infective **de Quervain's thyroiditis**. Sometimes in Hashimoto's thyroiditis, the thyroid is painful and tender.

Hyperthyroidism

The clinical manifestations of hyperthyroidism are summarised in Box 43.1. Excessive thyroid hormone production is a feature of Graves' disease, when it is often described as **thyrotoxicosis**. Mild hyperthyroidism may also occur in the early stages of Hashimoto's thyroiditis. A solitary hyperplastic (adenomatous) nodule may produce so much thyroid hormone that it causes hyperthyroidism. This is known as a **toxic or hot nodule**. More often, the patient is euthyroid but blood tests show the thyroid stimulating hormone is low, suppressed by the autonomous production of thyroid hormones by the nodule.

In general, thyroid adenocarcinomas are non-secreting but very occasionally, a well-differentiated carcinoma may cause hyperthyroidism.

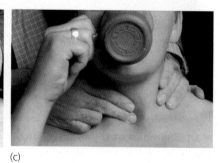

Fig. 43.2 Hyperthyroidism
Exophthalmic eye signs of hyperthyroidism in 43-year-old man with 6-month history of hyperthyroidism. His family had noticed his increasingly staring eyes. He had proptosis and lid lag.

KEY POINTS

Box 43.1 Clinical manifestations of thyrotoxicosis

Metabolic—heat intolerance, increased appetite with weight loss, diarrhoea, menorrhagia

Cardiovascular—palpitations, tachycardia even while asleep, atrial fibrillation

Neuropsychiatric—hyperkinesis, insomnia, emotional instability, tremor, proximal myopathy

Ocular—exophthalmos including proptosis, lid retraction and eventually ophthalmoplegia

Cutaneous—pretibial myxoedema

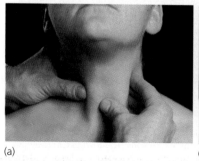
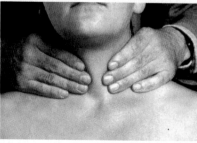

(a)   (b)   (c)

Fig. 43.3 Examination of the thyroid gland
The patient should be sitting upright in a chair with room for the examiner to approach from behind. **(a)** Gentle palpation from the front with slight sideways pressure from the left hand whilst palpating with the right. This is repeated for the right side of the gland. **(b)** General palpation of the gland from behind. Is there enlargement? Is it a single nodule or multinodular? How big is it? **(c)** Palpation of the gland while the patient swallows. Does the gland rise with swallowing? Is there retrosternal extension?

Hypothyroidism

Hypothyroidism is usually the result of either late Hashimoto's thyroiditis or primary thyroid atrophy or else earlier treatment for hyperthyroidism. In either case, the gland is small and fibrous and as such does not present to the surgeon. Hypothyroidism is a late complication in up to 25% of patients after subtotal thyroidectomy for thyrotoxicosis, and is inevitable after total thyroidectomy for carcinoma. Hypothyroidism should be considered in surgical patients presenting with constipation and has also been implicated in abdominal aortic thrombosis in middle-aged women.

SPECIAL POINTS IN EXAMINING A THYROID SWELLING

Examining for a suspected thyroid swelling should begin by seating the patient in a chair (Fig. 43.3) with space to examine the patient from behind and ensuring there is a glass of water for the patient to swallow. First, the front of the neck should be observed while the patient swallows. The characteristic rise and fall of the lump results from the thyroid gland's investment of **pretracheal fascia** which is attached to the larynx above. A normal thyroid is not visible, even on swallowing, and is not normally palpable.

The thyroid area is next palpated from behind with the patient seated. This position is best for examining the size, shape and consistency of the gland. It also allows the lower edge of the swelling to be palpated to identify any retrosternal extension. The lobes of the thyroid lie deep to the sternomastoids and the strap muscles, and these tend to conceal thyroid enlargement and make it difficult to examine the whole gland.

The jugular chain of lymph nodes should be palpated for evidence of lymph node metastases, since this may be the sole presenting feature of papillary carcinoma. In thyrotoxicosis, auscultation of the thyroid may reveal a bruit because of the increased vascularity.

If there is any suspicion of recurrent laryngeal nerve palsy because of hoarseness, tests of vocal cord function should be performed. The patient is asked to cough and to pronounce the sound 'ee', both of which are likely to be abnormal if there is nerve damage. In this case, or if surgery is contemplated, formal assessment of cord function should be performed by indirect laryngoscopy, usually in an ENT department.

General examination should look for signs of hyperthyroidism (tachycardia, atrial fibrillation, fine tremor and hyper-reflexia) and for signs specific to Graves' disease (exophthalmos and ophthalmoplegia).

APPROACH TO INVESTIGATION OF A THYROID MASS

The questions to be answered in investigating a thyroid mass are summarised in Box 43.2 and described in detail

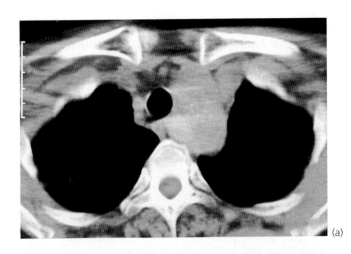

(a)

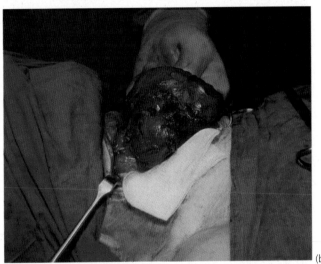

(b)

Fig. 43.4 Retrosternal goitre
This 38-year-old woman had suffered stridor at night for several months. On palpation, the thyroid was not particularly large but the trachea was markedly deviated (Fig. 43.5) and the thyroid did not rise on swallowing, both providing evidence of substantial retrosternal extension. **(a)** CT scan at the level of the clavicles showing enlargement of the left side of the thyroid gland with moderate deviation but no compression of the trachea. **(b)** At operation, this huge retrosternal extension was drawn up out of the anterior mediastinum. As this was a multinodular goitre, a total thyroidectomy was performed. Histopathology confirmed a benign multinodular goitre.

below. Patients who have undergone previous radiotherapy to the neck should be considered at high risk of thyroid carcinoma.

General thyroid status

It should be established whether the patient is **euthyroid**, **hyperthyroid** or **hypothyroid**. Estimations of serum thyroxine (T4) or better, free thyroxine (fT4) as well as thyroid stimulating hormone (TSH) are usually performed in all cases. In pregnancy or puberty, thyroid-binding globulin

Box 43.2 Principles of investigation of a thyroid mass

General thyroid status—thyroid function tests and thyroid autoantibodies

Morphology of the gland, i.e. size, shape and physical consistency, effects upon surrounding structures—ultrasound, plain X-rays of thoracic outlet, CT scanning

Tissue diagnosis—fine needle aspiration cytology or needle biopsy, incision or excision biopsy

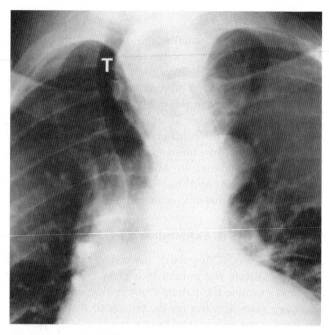

Fig. 43.5 Tracheal displacement by a goitre
This chest X-ray shows gross displacement of the trachea **T** to the right by a large retrosternal goitre. The patient presented with nocturnal stridor when she lay on her left side.

is elevated and knowledge of the free thyroxine level avoids difficulty in interpreting results. Tri-iodothyronine (T3) levels are occasionally measured if the patient is clinically hyperthyroid but the serum thyroxine is normal. TSH level is usually low in hyperthyroidism and elevated in hypothyroidism. Some laboratories prefer to measure just the TSH level initially, and perform more detailed tests if this is abnormal.

Thyroid autoantibodies are assayed if autoimmune disease is a possibility. Although not usually measured clinically, the presence of long-acting thyroid stimulating factor (LATS) is diagnostic of Graves' disease. Hashimoto's thyroiditis is characterised by elevation of other anti-thyroid antibodies such as anti-thyroglobulin or anti-mitochondrial antibodies (anti-thyroid M).

Morphology of the gland

Ultrasound scanning is a useful method of establishing retrosternal extensions or suspected cysts. However, needle aspiration (described below) can easily diagnose a cyst or obtain specimens for cytological examination so the use of ultrasound is declining. Plain X-rays or CT scans of the thoracic outlet are taken if there is suspicion of tracheal displacement or compression (Fig. 43.5).

Tissue diagnosis

Tissue diagnosis using fine needle aspiration cytology (FNA) is usually performed for solitary nodules or recently changed nodules in multinodular goitres. Nowadays, prior ultrasound or radionuclide scans are not generally regarded as helpful. Given a well-trained and interested thyroid cytologist, up to 90% of thyroid nodules can be successfully categorised by this method. An alternative method is to use needle core biopsy under ultrasound guidance. This gives a larger specimen and a higher rate of diagnostic specimens. If a **colloid nodule** is diagnosed, operative excision is not necessary unless the nodule causes compressive symptoms or cosmetic deformity. Lesions which are obviously malignant require

operation. These include **papillary**, **medullary** and early **anaplastic carcinomas**. Most **lymphomas** are inadequately sampled by FNA. **Follicular carcinomas** cannot be distinguished cytologically from **benign follicular adenomas**; both display sheets of follicular cells. Lesions with this appearance must all be removed, although most will be benign.

Incision biopsy at open operation is occasionally used for diagnosing generalised thyroid enlargement where the chances of malignancy are low or lymphoma is suspected.

Functional activity of glandular tissue

Injected radionuclides of iodine are taken up by functioning thyroid tissue and were formerly used widely for thyroid scanning. However, ^{131}I has been found to deliver a high dose of radioactivity to the gland and has been replaced by [99]mTechnetium or ^{123}I which deliver much lower doses. The increasing use of needle cytology and the knowledge that only 10% of cold nodules are malignant have greatly reduced the use of thyroid radionuclide scanning. However, when scanning is employed, the gland is imaged after isotope injection to identify the distribution of isotope activity. This may fall into one of four patterns:

- **Diffuse, homogeneous uptake**—this is found in the normal gland or where there is diffuse hyperactivity, e.g. Graves' disease

- **Generalised but patchy uptake**—this occurs in multinodular goitre where the hyperplastic nodules are less active than the surrounding normal tissue
- **The cold nodule**—an isolated area devoid of isotope uptake indicates non-secreting tissue, i.e. tumour, inactive adenomatous nodule or cyst. This requires tissue diagnosis, usually using fine needle aspiration cytology
- **The hot nodule**—this represents an autonomous focus of excess T4 secretion. The secretory activity of the surrounding normal thyroid tissue is suppressed.

The patient is usually euthyroid but sometimes thyrotoxic ('toxic nodule')

Very occasionally, **thyroid malignancies** secrete thyroid hormone and show up as warm or hot nodules on isotope scanning. Isotope scanning can also identify and localise **ectopic thyroid tissue** (in the tongue or along the course of the thyroglossal duct), **retrosternal extension** of a thyroid swelling and **metastases** of functioning thyroid carcinomas, provided the thyroid has been removed or ablated.

SPECIFIC CLINICAL PROBLEMS OF THE THYROID AND THEIR MANAGEMENT

THYROTOXICOSIS

Thyrotoxicosis most commonly results from Graves' disease. Hashimoto's thyroiditis is a much rarer cause and is self limiting. Occasionally, thyrotoxicosis is caused by a multinodular goitre which has become 'toxic' or an autonomous adenomatous 'hot' nodule.

There are three main treatment options in thyrotoxicosis: **anti-thyroid drugs**, **radioisotope destruction** of functioning thyroid tissue and **subtotal thyroidectomy**.

Carcinoma, a very rare cause of thyrotoxicosis, is occasionally diagnosed unexpectedly when a hot nodule is examined histologically.

ANTITHYROID DRUGS

Most cases of thyrotoxicosis are initially managed with antithyroid drugs which block synthesis of thyroid hormone. **Carbimazole** is the most popular, and restores serum hormone levels to normal over 4–8 weeks. A lower maintenance dose is then prescribed for about 1 year. After this, more than half the patients remain euthyroid without further treatment. The remainder relapse in the succeeding months, necessitating further courses of carbimazole or a different form of therapy. In some patients, stable control cannot be achieved, and hypothyroidism alternates with hyperthyroidism. In these cases, a **block and replace** regimen may succeed, giving a higher dose of carbimazole to block thyroid hormone production altogether, together with a standard replacement dose of thyroxine.

Carbimazole occasionally causes a potentially fatal but reversible neutropenia. The white blood count should therefore be monitored about once every 3 months during treatment. A sore throat or other infection in a patient on carbimazole should alert the patient and the doctor. Rashes, nausea, headache and arthralgia are also common side effects of carbimazole and, if they occur, an alternative antithyroid drug such as **propylthiouracil** may be substituted. Poor control, frequent relapse, side effects and non-compliance lead to eventual surgical referral in up to 40% of patients.

Beta-adrenergic blocking drugs such as **propranolol** rapidly control the distressing and dangerous effects of thyrotoxicosis. These drugs may be used initially in extremely toxic patients until anti-thyroid drugs take effect, or if a patient urgently needs to be stabilised before thyroidectomy.

RADIOACTIVE IODIDE THERAPY

Radioactive iodide (^{131}I or ^{125}I), administered orally in doses 100 times higher than used for diagnostic scanning, (see Fig. 43.6) may be used to treat thyrotoxicosis. This is especially appropriate for middle-aged or elderly patients. Iodide is avidly taken up by the gland, after which emission of radiation destroys the most active thyroid tissue. The treatment is simple but the results are slow to take effect and unpredictable. Late hypothyroidism often occurs, requiring replacement therapy. There is also a small theoretical risk of inducing malignancy, and so the treatment is not advisable in the young. Radioactive iodide therapy is absolutely contraindicated in pregnancy because of the risk of genetic damage to the fetus.

SURGICAL MANAGEMENT

INDICATIONS FOR SURGERY

Surgery for thyrotoxicosis may be indicated as follows:

- When a quick and effective cure is desired which avoids long-term drug therapy and its drawbacks. It is often the best treatment for Graves' disease,

particularly in younger patients, where the disease is not expected to burn itself out for many years
● When anti-thyroid drugs have proved unsatisfactory and radioiodide treatment is unsuitable
● Surgery is usually the most appropriate treatment for

toxic multinodular goitre. Response to drug treatment in this condition is unreliable and surgery also deals with the cosmetic deformity
● Toxic solitary nodules ('hot nodules') are best excised to allow the suppressed normal thyroid to recover

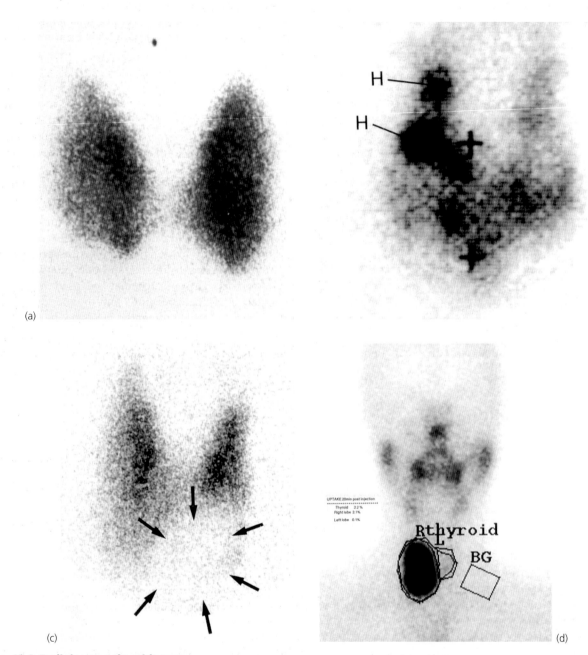

(a)

(b)

(c)

(d)

Fig. 43.6 Radioisotope thyroid scans
(a) This enlarged thyroid shows homogeneous tracer uptake typical of a simple colloid goitre. **(b)** Heterogeneous tracer uptake in a multinodular colloid goitre. The dark areas **H** are 'hot nodules'; to maintain the euthyroid state, the rest of the gland exhibits diminished uptake. The + signs indicate the positions of the thyroid cartilage and the suprasternal notch. **(c)** Solitary 'cold' thyroid nodule. The area of low uptake (outline arrowed) at the lower left pole of the thyroid corresponds with a palpable nodule. In the case of a solid lesion (as confirmed by ultrasound), a cold nodule may indicate malignancy. **(d)** Solitary 'hot' thyroid nodule. The area of high uptake in the lower part of the right lobe corresponds to a palpable mass. This patient was hyperthyroid and the lesion could be described as a 'toxic nodule'. Activity of the rest of the gland is suppressed by pituitary-mediated negative feedback from the high serum thyroxine level. The rectangle marked **BG** measures the background radiation in order to quantify the thyroid uptake.

PREOPERATIVE ASSESSMENT AND MANAGEMENT OF THYROTOXICOSIS

For all thyroid operations, preoperative assessment often includes indirect or direct **laryngoscopy** to demonstrate vocal cord function. This evaluates recurrent laryngeal nerve function should there later be a question of operative damage. Even without demonstrable cord damage, there is often a subtle change in voice quality after thyroidectomy, often due to external laryngeal nerve damage. Patients should be warned of this before operation, especially if they are singers or politicians!

Wherever possible, thyroid function should be brought into the normal range before operation. The thyrotoxic state carries significant anaesthetic risks, especially of cardiac arrhythmias. Furthermore, manipulation of the gland may provoke massive release of thyroid hormone, precipitating a potentially lethal **thyrotoxic crisis** or 'thyroid storm'. Control of thyroid function is usually achieved with antithyroid drugs in the weeks preceding operation. If this fails, or if operation is very urgent, then beta-adrenergic blocking drugs such as propranolol can be used.

Antithyroid drugs cause increased vascularity of the gland which may add to surgical difficulty in toxic enlargement. It is standard practice to administer **Lugol's iodine** solution orally for 10 days before operation while continuing anti-thyroid therapy. This is believed to reduce vascularity and increase the firmness of the gland, making the operation easier.

SUBTOTAL THYROIDECTOMY

Surgery (Fig. 43.7) for hyperthyroidism aims to remove enough thyroid tissue to render the patient euthyroid whilst preserving enough of the gland to prevent hypothyroidism. For Graves' disease or toxic multinodular goitre, about 5–8 g of the gland is left intact. The technique of **subtotal thyroidectomy** leaves the posterior rim of each lobe in situ, thus minimising the risk of parathyroid or recurrent laryngeal damage. A low transverse collar incision along a skin crease gives the best cosmetic result. Meticulous care is required in ligating the **inferior thyroid artery** (after the recurrent laryngeal nerve has been identified) and the **upper pole vessels**. Primary or reactionary haemorrhage is a serious complication causing major blood loss and laryngeal compression. To avoid suffocation from a postoperative bleed, instruments for emergency reopening of the wound should be kept at the patient's bedside after operation. The potential complications of thyroidectomy are summarised in Box 43.3.

THYROID MALIGNANCIES

Thyroid malignancies are uncommon, comprising less than 1% of all malignant tumours. Nearly all originate from thyroid follicular cells and form three distinct pathological entities: **papillary**, **follicular**, and **anaplastic carcinomas**. Each has a characteristic pattern of behaviour and prognosis. With rare exceptions, these tumours do not secrete thyroid hormones.

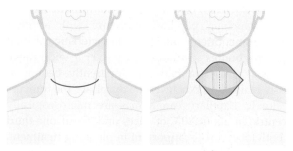

1 'Collar' incision in lines of skin tension 2 cm above suprasternal notch. Platysma divided in same line

2 Flaps mobilised beneath platysma down to suprasternal notch and up to the thyroid cartilage

3 Incision made vertically in midline between strap muscles which are retracted laterally on side of interest

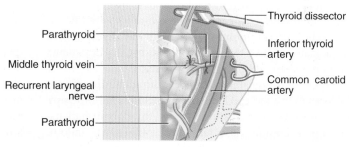

Parathyroid

Middle thyroid vein

Recurrent laryngeal nerve

Parathyroid

Thyroid dissector

Inferior thyroid artery

Common carotid artery

4 Dissection continued deep to strap muscles. Middle thyroid vein ligated and divided

5 Upper pole vessels identified and ligated close to gland

6 Lower pole vessels ligated

7 Lateral lobe displaced anteriorly; inferior thyroid artery located and recurrent laryngeal nerve identified close to inferior thyroid artery. Inferior thyroid artery ligated lateral to nerve. Parathyroids identified

8 *If partial thyroidectomy*, approx 4 g gland left in situ each side and remainder dissected out, arresting bleeding from many small vessels entering gland on tracheal surface. Process repeated with other side
or
If lobectomy or total thyroidectomy, whole lobe(s) excised, carefully preserving recurrent laryngeal nerve and parathyroids

Fig. 43.7 Subtotal thyroidectomy

SUMMARY

Box 43.3 Complications of thyroidectomy

Complications during operation

- *Uncontrollable haemorrhage*—uncommon, usually results from a slipped ligature on the upper pole vessels which then retract
- *Unilateral or bilateral recurrent laryngeal nerve damage*—bilateral nerve damage presents as laryngeal obstruction after tracheal extubation and necessitates immediate tracheostomy
- *Inadvertent damage to other structures*—tracheal or oesophageal perforation or damage to laryngeal muscles or nerves

Early postoperative complications (within the first 12 hours)

- *Major haemorrhage*—presents as rapid swelling of the neck or a large volume of blood loss via the wound drain. This requires emergency surgical exploration of the wound to release the clot and then achieve haemostasis
- *Mediastinal haemorrhage*—presents with hypovolaemic shock
- *Laryngeal oedema*—presents as stridor, rapidly progressing to respiratory obstruction. This requires endotracheal intubation
- *Thyrotoxic crisis*—presents with abrupt onset of extreme agitation and confusion, hyperpyrexia, profuse sweating and rapid tachycardia or other arrhythmia. This requires emergency beta-adrenergic blockade, intravenous hydrocortisone and potassium iodide therapy. The mortality of thyrotoxic crisis is 10% from coma, pulmonary oedema or circulatory collapse. The condition is very rare if the patient has been rendered euthyroid before operation by drug treatment.
- *Tracheomalacia*—removal of a longstanding lesion compressing the trachea may lead to tracheal collapse and stridor

Later postoperative complications

- *Hypoparathyroidism* due to inadvertent parathyroid damage—presents with muscle cramps, paraesthesiae and tetany within 36 hours of operation. Treatment is with calcium and vitamin D analogues
- *Unilateral recurrent laryngeal nerve damage*—presents with hoarseness of voice and defective cough
- *External laryngeal nerve damage*—changes the quality of the voice

Long-term complications

- *Hypothyroidism*—often overlooked because it develops insidiously. Features are loss of energy, weight gain, depression and intellectual deterioration and intolerance of cold weather
- *Recurrent thyrotoxicosis*—insufficient gland removed

About 7% of thyroid carcinomas arise from APUD C-cells which secrete calcitonin. These tumours are known as **medullary carcinomas** of the thyroid. **Lymphomas** occasionally involve the thyroid gland, usually in patients with pre-existing Hashimoto's disease.

Exposure to ionising radiation during childhood predisposes to thyroid carcinoma. This includes radiotherapy (once popular for treating 'status thymolymphaticus' and other benign disorders) and radioactive fallout. Many people exposed at the Hiroshima and Nagasaki bombings and the Bikini atoll nuclear tests developed thyroid tumours and more recently, children exposed to the fallout from Chernobyl. In most cases of thyroid cancer, however, no aetiological factor can be identified.

PAPILLARY CARCINOMA

Papillary carcinomas constitute about two-thirds of thyroid malignancies in adults and nearly all thyroid malignancies in children. Females are affected at least three times as often as males and the peak incidence is between 30–45 years. Histologically, the tumour forms a complex branching papillary structure with a fibrovascular stroma, often containing characteristic calcified '**psammoma bodies**'. Tumours vary over a wide range of epithelial dysplasia between apparently benign to obviously malignant. Whatever the dysplasia, the tumours grow slowly. Papillary carcinomas are microscopically multicentric in about 80% of cases and about one-third affect both lobes; this is important in planning treatment. The tumour occasionally invades locally into trachea or oesophagus. Metastasis is to central cervical and later lateral cervical lymph nodes and only rarely to distant sites such as lung or bone. By the time of presentation, lymph nodes are involved in about 40% of patients (90% in children). Lymph-node enlargement is often the sole presenting feature and the histology of involved lymph nodes is so close to normal thyroid tissue that at one time this condition was known as '**lateral aberrant thyroid**'. The prognosis of papillary carcinoma is the best of all thyroid carcinomas with only about 10% of patients dying of the tumour after 10 years (of remote

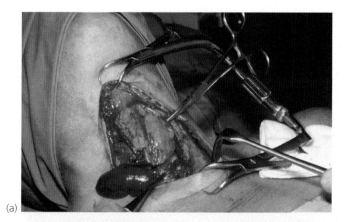

(a)

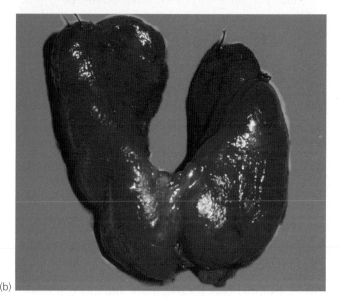

(b)

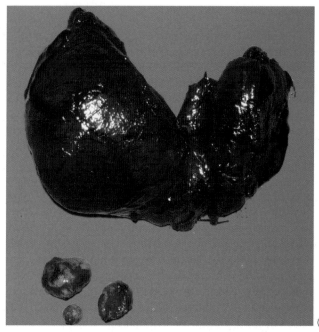

(c)

Fig. 43.8 Thyroid and parathyroid operations
(a) Standard approach to thyroid and parathyroid operations, in this case, neck exploration for hyperparathyroidism. A collar incision has been made and upper and lower flaps are held apart with the specially designed Joll's retractor. **(b)** Subtotal thyroidectomy specimen after operation for hyperthyroidism. **(c)** Total thyroidectomy specimen after operation for right sided medullary carcinoma. Involved lymph nodes were 'cherry picked' and are also shown.

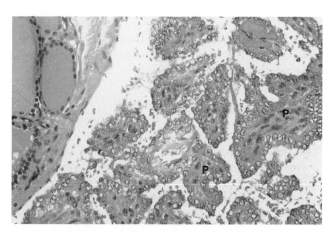

Fig. 43.9 Papillary carcinoma of the thyroid—histopathology
Tumour shows well defined papillae **P** with many cells having large, clear nuclei. Despite its name, the diagnosis is based on these nuclear features, not on the presence of papillae. Normal thyroid tissue is also present.

metastases); it is remarkable that survival is hardly prejudiced by the presence of lymph node metastases. The prognosis is even better for '**minimal papillary carcinoma**', defined as a tumour less than 1 cm in diameter in a young patient with no local invasiveness or metastases.

Symptoms and signs

Clinically, papillary carcinoma presents as a slow-growing solitary thyroid nodule or else an enlarged cervical lymph node close to the gland. The patient is euthyroid. If isotope scanning is performed, it usually shows no uptake in the palpable nodule. Sometimes, other tumour foci in the gland are large enough to also appear as 'cold nodules'. The diagnosis is usually made nowadays by fine needle aspiration cytology of a solitary thyroid nodule. A patient presenting with just an enlarged cervical lymph node may be diagnosed unexpectedly as papillary carcinoma after excision biopsy and histological examination of the node.

Management

The standard management of papillary carcinoma is total thyroidectomy because of the high risk of other foci within the gland. Palpable cervical nodes are removed at the same operation. Technically, the operation is no more difficult than subtotal thyroidectomy but carries a higher risk of postoperative hypoparathyroidism. Total thyroidectomy has the added advantage that recurrent local disease, lymph node or distant metastases can then effectively be treated with radioiodine (^{131}I). This requires a very high TSH level which only occurs if no normal thyroid tissue remains. A further advantage is that thyroglobulin can then be used as a **tumour marker** to detect recurrent disease. After treatment, hormone replacement with oral thyroxine is always necessary at levels necessary to keep TSH close to zero to minimise the risk of stimulating any residual malignant cells. This treatment rarely causes problems. Tumour recurrence in cervical nodes is treated by excision and of itself has little effect on prognosis. External radiotherapy may be employed for local recurrence or chemotherapy with doxorubicin for remote metastases.

Since papillary carcinomas progress so slowly and only about 15% develop contralateral lobe recurrence, some surgeons prefer to retain one thyroid lobe provided the primary tumour is small and there are no palpable or isotope-detectable nodules. Their reasoning is that further tumours can be removed later without reducing life expectancy.

FOLLICULAR CARCINOMA

Follicular carcinoma is another well-differentiated thyroid malignancy. Histologically, the neoplastic cells form a well-developed **follicular pattern** which is impossible to distinguish from benign adenomatous hyperplasia on fine needle aspiration cytology; it may also be difficult to distinguish on histology of the surgical specimen unless there is evident capsular or vascular invasion. Unlike papillary carcinoma, multicentricity is far less common. The peak incidence of follicular carcinoma is between 40 and 50 years of age, older than for papillary carcinoma, but it is still three times more common in women. Generally, follicular carcinoma grows slowly and metastasises at a late stage. In contrast to papillary carcinoma, metastasis tends to occur via the bloodstream to the lungs, bone and other remote sites rather than to local lymph nodes.

Follicular carcinoma is rarely multicentric and management depends on the extent of local invasion (Fig. 43.10). A tumour with only microinvasion of the capsule has a very good prognosis and requires removal of only the thyroid lobe containing the tumour. If, however, there is gross capsular invasion or vascular invasion (or known

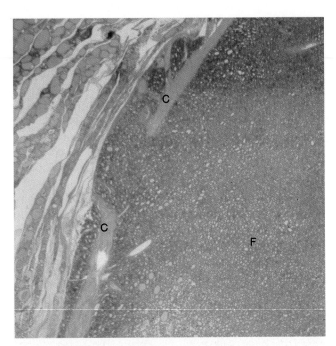

Fig. 43.10 Follicular carcinoma of the thyroid—histopathology
The tumour is made up of numerous small follicles **F** that are cytologically bland. Diagnosis of malignancy requires the demonstration of capsular and/or vascular invasion. In this higher power view, tumour can clearly be seen extending through the capsule **C**.

remote metastases), total thyroidectomy is performed. The purpose of this is not to treat the local tumour but to enhance radioiodine uptake by metastatic lesions should this be required later for diagnosis, and any consequent treatment with high-dose radioiodine.

Prognosis depends on the degree of capsular and vascular invasion by the primary lesion and can be predicted from the histology. If there is no invasion, 10-year survival is close to 100% but this falls to about 30% if there is extensive local invasion.

ANAPLASTIC CARCINOMA

Anaplastic carcinomas are extremely aggressive tumours with an appalling prognosis. Most patients die within 1 year of diagnosis. The tumours are found almost exclusively in the elderly. Most other cancers are less aggressive in this age group but for reasons unknown, thyroid carcinomas are more aggressive.

Anaplastic carcinoma consists of sheets of very poorly differentiated cells which proliferate rapidly. The result is a diffuse, hard thyroid enlargement. The tumour soon invades surrounding structures causing symptoms of tracheal and oesophageal obstruction and recurrent laryngeal nerve damage. There is also early dissemination to regional lymph nodes and haematogenous spread to the lungs, skeleton and brain.

Anaplastic carcinomas respond poorly to both radio-therapy and chemotherapy. The distressing symptoms of tracheal obstruction can be relieved by placing a luminal metal thyroid stent. This avoids the need for surgery but does nothing to slow the tumour growth. Surgical palliation of obstructive symptoms can be undertaken by removing tumour near trachea or by placing an internal stent in the trachea.

MEDULLARY CARCINOMA

This uncommon malignancy arises from parafollicular or C-cells. The tumour often secretes abnormal quantities of **calcitonin**, which can be used as a marker of tumour recurrence after excision. Tumours may also secrete other peptides and amines such as **serotonin** and **ACTH-like peptide**. Medullary carcinoma usually arises sporadically but may be transmitted genetically as part of the **multiple endocrine neoplasia syndrome type II (MEN II)**. This is an autosomal dominant trait with 50% penetrance and is associated with other APUD cell tumours, particularly **phaeochromocytoma** and **parathyroid adenomas**. Thus patients with medullary carcinoma of thyroid should be examined for these conditions before surgery as phaeochromocytoma would take operative precedence.

The tumour is of particular pathological interest because the stroma contains extensive deposits of amyloid. These make the tumour mass stony hard to palpation.

Medullary carcinoma grows relatively slowly, meta-stasising first to regional lymph nodes and later to lungs, bone, liver and elsewhere. The tumour does not take up radioiodine and is resistant to radiotherapy; hence an aggressive surgical approach is required. The standard treatment is total thyroidectomy and clearance of involved anterior cervical and superior mediastinal lymph nodes. Without metastases, operation is often curative but when nodes are involved, 10-year survival falls to about 50%. During follow-up, calcitonin levels are monitored and raised levels indicate tumour recurrence. Surgical re-exploration of the neck may be undertaken to remove involved lymph nodes.

THYROID LYMPHOMA

Lymphomas of the thyroid are rare and usually arise in pre-existing autoimmune (Hashimoto's) thyroiditis. Most are non-Hodgkin's lymphomas. Diagnosis can only be made on histology, either core needle biopsy or open biopsy, as FNA is not usually adequate. Treatment is with radiotherapy and survival depends on whether spread has occurred beyond the thyroid capsule. For lesions confined within the capsule, 5-year survival is 85%, falling to 40% when local spread has occurred.

GOITRES AND THYROID NODULES

As indicated earlier in Table 43.1, several hyperplastic and metabolic disorders cause diffuse or nodular thyroid enlargement.

IDIOPATHIC NON-TOXIC THYROID HYPERPLASIA

Most goitres referred to surgeons in developed countries are caused by simple, idiopathic hyperplasia of thyroid follicles. The condition probably begins with diffuse micronodular enlargement, and the nodules later become heterogeneously enlarged to form a **multinodular colloid goitre**. Within the same spectrum of disease are **solitary hyperplastic nodules** (which may actually be benign thyroid adenomas) and **thyroid cysts**, which are simply huge colloid-filled follicles.

The aetiology of simple thyroid hyperplasia is un-known, but is probably related to disordered sensitivity to TSH. In this sense, the condition may be analogous to fibroadenosis of the breast. The patient is usually clinically euthyroid and thyroid function tests are normal. Sometimes, thyroid hormone secretion escapes from hypothalamic control so the patient becomes hyper-thyroid and occasionally thyrotoxic.

Within the gland, secretory activity is heterogeneous, explaining the patchy distribution of radio-iodine uptake if thyroid scanning is performed. Focal hormone secretion from 'hot' adenomatous nodules may be so great as to completely suppress the rest of the gland. The overall hormone secretion may still be within the euthyroid range; this may be considered the most extreme form of secretory heterogeneity.

Diffuse or multinodular idiopathic goitres develop slowly and cause little trouble until they have been present for many years.

The reasons patients present to surgeons with thyroid enlargement are:

● A goitre has become so large as to be cosmetically unacceptable
● A localised lump has appeared in the thyroid region. This may be a solitary adenomatous nodule, a solitary cyst or, in 10% of cases, thyroid cancer. Alternatively, the apparent solitary lump may be part of an asymmetrical multinodular or multicystic enlargement

- A pre-existing multinodular goitre has undergone rapid asymmetric change. There are several possible causes, i.e. haemorrhage into a cyst or a degenerate area of hyperplasia, or malignant change
- The patient has become hyperthyroid
- The patient has developed stridor from tracheal compression caused by enlargement of a retrosternal extension of the thyroid

SURGICAL MANAGEMENT OF GOITRE

The indications for surgery in idiopathic goitre are:

- Lump suspicious of malignancy
- A compressive retrosternal thyroid
- A solitary toxic nodule
- Toxic multinodular goitre
- Cosmetic deformity

In principle, only enough thyroid tissue is removed to achieve the objective, but in multinodular goitre, recurrence is likely in the long term and a better mode of treatment is total thyroidectomy, with lifetime thyroxine replacement.

Patients presenting for cosmetic reasons, with only moderate thyroid enlargement, have often been treated with thyroxine. The theory is that by suppressing TSH the gland may shrink to an acceptable size. Unfortunately, clinical trials have not shown this approach to be effective. Hyperthyroidism caused by idiopathic thyroid hyperplasia is unresponsive to anti-thyroid drugs and ineffectively treated with radioiodine; hence surgery is required for treatment.

Thyroid cysts are diagnosed as fluid-filled lesions by aspiration. Cytology should be performed to exclude malignancy. Large or recurrent cysts are best treated surgically.

CONGENITAL THYROID DISORDERS

EMBRYOLOGY

The thyroid originates as a diverticulum in the midline between the first two branchial pouches. Its origin is represented in the adult by the **foramen caecum**, visible at the junction of the anterior two-thirds and the posterior third of the tongue. The thyroid diverticulum forms the **thyroglossal duct** which extends caudally through the developing tongue musculature. It passes down in relation to the hyoid bone (in front of, through or behind it) to reach its normal position below the larynx. By this time, it has become a bilobed structure with the lobes connected by a narrow central **isthmus**. The thyroglossal duct later degenerates. The calcitonin-secreting C-cells originate from the **ultimobranchial body** of the fifth pouch.

THYROGLOSSAL CYST AND 'FISTULA'

Part of the thyroglossal duct may persist and become cystic. A thyroglossal cyst presents in children and occasionally adolescents as a smooth, rounded, anterior midline swelling in the neck. Most thyroglossal cysts occur below the hyoid, although rarely they are found in the submental region. A diagnostic feature is that the cyst rises when the patient swallows or protrudes the tongue. Most thyroglossal cysts are asymptomatic but they are prone to inflammation which causes pain and increased swelling. If an inflamed cyst is surgically drained, it may become an intermittently discharging sinus, often incorrectly described as a **thyroglossal fistula** (Fig. 43.11).

Thyroglossal cysts are usually excised along with the thyroglossal tract up to the base of the tongue. This requires removing the middle third of the hyoid bone (**Sistrunk's operation**). A persistent sinus or a recurrent cyst is likely to complicate incomplete excision.

ECTOPIC THYROID GLAND

An ectopic thyroid gland is a rare congenital abnormality which results from interruption of normal descent. It

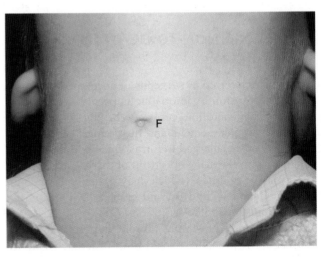

Fig. 43.11 Thyroglossal 'fistula'
This photograph shows the front of the neck in a 14-year-old boy. An attempt had been made to remove a thyroglossal cyst several years previously. The inevitable result of incomplete surgical removal was an intermittently discharging fistula **F** in the midline of the neck.

may present in the same way as a thyroglossal cyst or as a lump in the tongue. As this may be the patient's only thyroid tissue, isotope scanning should be performed to check if there is thyroid tissue in the normal position before proceeding to excision.

DISORDERS OF PARATHYROID GLANDS

HYPERPARATHYROIDISM

SYMPTOMS AND SIGNS

Hyperparathyroidism is the most common clinical disorder of the parathyroid glands. Patients are usually referred to a surgeon after investigation of **recurrent urinary tract calculi** or **hypercalcaemia**.

Hypercalcaemia is often found incidentally on biochemical screening. Many of these 'asymptomatic' patients turn out to have suffered non-specific symptoms of fatigue and malaise for years or have signs of hypertension or renal failure. Symptomatic hypercalcaemia presents with fatigue, polyuria and polydipsia and constipation, and more specifically bone pain (with or without radiological changes), urinary tract stones and abdominal pain (caused by peptic ulcer or pancreatitis)—as an aide mémoire 'bones, stones and abdominal groans'. Mental changes include confusion, depression or even psychosis. **Secondary hyperparathyroidism** with hypercalcaemia also occurs as a response to chronic renal failure. After renal transplantation, hyperparathyroidism may persist and is described as **tertiary hyperparathyroidism**. Note that hyperparathyroidism is only one cause of hypercalcaemia; the other main cause is a variety of malignant diseases which either secrete parathyroid-related protein (PTH-rP) or cause widespread lytic bone metastases.

Raised plasma calcium levels cannot be tolerated for long without causing serious systemic problems or damage to bone. From Figure 43.12, it might seem paradoxical that urinary tract calculi are a common presenting feature of hyperparathyroidism, since parathormone *reduces* urinary calcium excretion. The probable reason for stone formation is the excess phosphate excretion. This is associated with excessive urinary alkalinity, which predisposes to the formation of calcium salts.

CONTROL OF PLASMA CALCIUM (Fig. 43.12)

Plasma calcium level is normally maintained within a very narrow range by the combined effect of parathormone and vitamin D.

Parathormone raises plasma calcium levels in the following ways:

- Increases osteoclastic activity and release of calcium from the bone matrix; this liberates calcium into the circulation

- Enhances renal tubular reabsorption of calcium and diminishes reabsorption of phosphate
- Promotes calcium absorption from the small intestine in the presence of vitamin D

Parathormone also decreases plasma phosphate by increasing renal clearance of phosphate. Vitamin D (as cholecalciferol) is produced by the action of sunlight on cholesterol derivatives in the skin. Cholecalciferol is then converted to 25-hydroxycholecalciferol in the liver, and further hydroxylated by the renal parenchyma to the active compound **1,25-dihydroxycholecalciferol**. This active compound is required for calcium absorption from the intestine. Calcitonin, produced by the C-cells of the thyroid gland, probably plays little part in normal calcium homeostasis.

Calcium homeostasis is thus dependent on normal functioning of parathyroids, liver and kidney, together with an adequate dietary intake of calcium and suitable quantities of vitamin D from diet or exposure to sunlight.

TYPES OF HYPERPARATHYROIDISM

Hyperparathyroidism is classified as follows:

Primary hyperparathyroidism

a. Single parathyroid adenoma

This is the most common cause of primary hyperparathyroidism. One of the four parathyroid glands becomes replaced by a benign neoplasm which secretes parathormone in excessive amounts. Secretion by the other parathyroids is suppressed.

b. Diffuse parathyroid hyperplasia

This is an uncommon cause of primary hyperparathyroidism. The secretory cells of two or more of the glands undergo idiopathic hyperplasia, resulting in excess hormone production.

c. Parathyroid carcinoma

This is extremely rare (1% of primary hyperparathyroid patients) and involves only one of the parathyroid glands. These tumours are often palpable and cause gross elevation of plasma calcium.

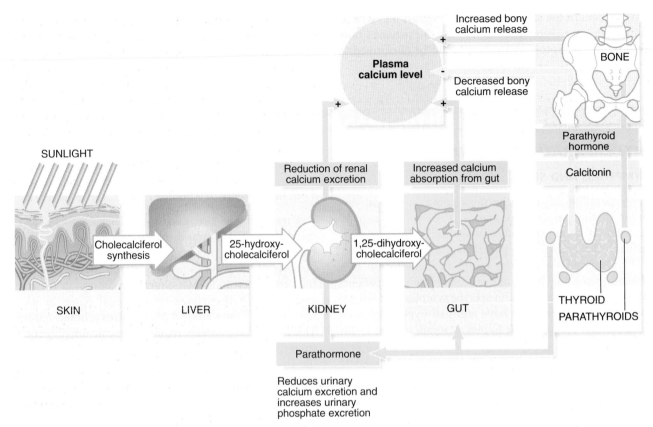

Fig. 43.12 Main control mechanisms for plasma calcium

Secondary hyperparathyroidism

Secondary hyperparathyroidism occurs in response to hypocalcaemia or calcium malabsorption. It is mainly seen in chronic renal failure when there is defective absorption of calcium from the gut. This is probably due to a failure of conversion of 25-hydroxycholecalciferol to 1,25-dihydroxycholecalciferol in the diseased renal parenchyma. These patients are usually undergoing regular renal dialysis. The parathyroid glands undergo **diffuse hyperplasia** in response to the reduced plasma calcium. The output of parathormone increases, thereby mobilising bone calcium and reducing urinary excretion, in an attempt to maintain normal plasma calcium levels. Hyperparathyroidism is usually associated with raised plasma calcium level (and reduced plasma phosphate levels) but in secondary hyperparathyroidism, plasma calcium is normal or even depressed.

Tertiary hyperparathyroidism

Tertiary hyperparathyroidism is a complication of prolonged secondary hyperparathyroidism. If the underlying cause of secondary hyperparathyroidism is corrected by renal transplantation, plasma calcium increases to normal levels yet parathyroid secretion remains abnormally high.

The parathyroid glands remain hyperplastic, having become insensitive to the normal negative feedback from rising plasma calcium levels.

Ectopic parathormone-like protein production

Malignant tumours may cause hypercalcaemia. In 70%, this is due to secretion of parathormone-related protein (PTH-rP) and in the rest to widespread bone destruction. The most common tumours to secrete PTH-rP are squamous cell carcinoma of the lung, renal cell carcinoma and bladder cancer. Tumours causing hypercalcaemia by bone destruction include breast cancer, leukaemias and multiple myeloma.

MANAGEMENT OF HYPERPARATHYROIDISM

Corrected plasma calcium levels are elevated in primary hyperparathyroidism but precise diagnosis was difficult before the advent of immunoassay for parathormone. Modern two-site non-competitive immunoassay recognises different regions of the PTH molecule, producing a robust signal antibody which can be marked by radioactive, luminescent or enzyme labels. Elevated plasma calcium and PTH levels confirm the diagnosis of hyperparathyroidism in virtually all patients, without renal failure or metastatic disease. In primary hyperparathyroidism, distinction between adenoma, diffuse hyperplasia and adenocarcinoma may be best undertaken by surgical exploration of the neck and examination of all four parathyroid glands. Preoperative localisation techniques other than ultrasound are probably appropriate only prior to re-exploratory operations for recurrent hypercalcaemia.

Surgical management

Surgery is the only treatment for primary and tertiary hyperparathyroidism. Secondary hyperparathyroidism is managed by giving oral vitamin D or calcium, although parathyroidectomy may be necessary if there is severe bone resorption. Hypercalcaemia due to ectopic parathormone production is managed medically as it is rarely possible to resect a parathormone-like protein secreting tumour.

There are normally two pairs of parathyroid glands, superior and inferior, lying close to the posterolateral aspect of the lateral lobes of the thyroid. The superior pair usually lie above the inferior thyroid artery at the middle of the gland. The inferior pair are usually located near the lower poles of the thyroid or sometimes within the thymus gland or elsewhere.

Parathyroid surgery is exacting and time-consuming, usually interrupted by histological examination of several frozen section biopsies during the course of the operation. The surgical access is the same as for thyroidectomy. The likely anatomical position of each parathyroid is then meticulously explored in the search for parathyroid tissue. Although the parathyroids have a characteristic yellow-brown colour, they are often difficult to distinguish from thyroid tissue, especially if the tissues have been traumatised.

If one of the parathyroid glands is enlarged and the others are normal, the diagnosis is **parathyroid adenoma**, or rarely, **adenocarcinoma**. In either case, the abnormal gland is completely removed and the other glands left in situ. If no individual gland is disproportionately enlarged, a diagnosis of diffuse hyperplasia can be made. In this case, there is a trend towards total parathyroidectomy rather than incomplete removal, now that plasma calcium can be controlled better medically. The problem is that some parathyroid tissue may remain unidentified, however meticulous the surgery. Surgical practice varies in managing parathyroid hyperplasia. Some surgeons remove all the parathyroid tissue they can find, others remove three and a half glands, while still others remove all the parathyroid tissue and reimplant a small mass of tissue in a forearm muscle pouch. The advantage of this is perceived to be that if hyperparathyroidism persists, then parathyroid tissue is more readily removed from the forearm than from the thyroid area. In fact, it is very difficult to remove.

Complications of parathyroidectomy are similar to those of thyroid surgery (see Box 43.3 earlier). Hypoparathyroidism is more likely, however, and plasma calcium levels must be carefully monitored in the early postoperative period.

HYPOPARATHYROIDISM

The most common cause of hypoparathyroidism is surgical removal or devascularisation of the parathyroid glands during thyroid or parathyroid surgery. It may also be a transient occurrence after excision of a parathyroid adenoma or subtotal parathyroidectomy, lasting until the remaining suppressed parathyroid tissue recovers normal function. Autoimmune hypoparathyroidism may also occur occasionally.

Hypoparathyroidism presents clinically with the effects of hypocalcaemia. A fall in the plasma calcium level increases neuromuscular excitability causing cramps or even **tetany** in severe cases. An early symptom of hypocalcaemia is paraesthesia, especially around the lips. After thyroid or parathyroid operations patients should be asked if they have experienced any tingling around the mouth, and plasma calcium estimations should be performed the morning after operation, then 12-hourly for 48 hours.

Clinical tests for hypocalcaemia include tapping over the parotid gland which provokes transient contraction of the facial muscles (**Chvostek's sign**). A further test involves inflating a sphygmomanometer cuff on the upper arm to above systolic pressure. This induces carpal spasm within about 3 minutes ('*main d'accoucheur*' or obstetrician's hand).

Early postoperative hypocalcaemia is treated with intravenous calcium gluconate. Persistent hypocalcaemia is controlled by oral administration of high doses of calcium and vitamin D.

44 The acute abdomen in children

INTRODUCTION

A large number of surgical conditions in children are treated by general surgeons with a special interest in paediatric surgery, but surgical problems in infants under 1 year, major congenital abnormalities at any age and malignant tumours are usually managed in regional centres by paediatric surgical specialists and urologists. Not only does the range of conditions seen in children differ from that seen in adults but the conditions themselves vary within different age groups. This is particularly true for conditions which present as acute emergencies. Reflecting this, paediatric emergencies may be considered under the headings of the **newborn** (the first few days of life, including premature babies), **infants and young children** (up to about 2 years) and **older children** (up to puberty). During puberty, the conditions merge with those of adulthood. The non-emergency and urogenital disorders tend to be less age specific and are discussed separately later in the chapter.

ABDOMINAL EMERGENCIES IN THE NEWBORN

The more common abdominal emergencies in neonates are summarised in Box 44.1. All are congenital disorders with the exception of necrotising enterocolitis. Successful surgical management requires an understanding of the physiological parameters in small infants; some of these differ substantially from those in adults. For example the basal metabolic rate is particularly high in the newborn, with an oxygen demand of 5–8 ml/kg/min. In older children and adults this falls to 2–4 ml/kg/min.

Temperature regulation in infants is also more critical than in older patients for several reasons: they have a relatively large surface area, poor vasomotor control of skin blood vessels and an inability to generate heat by shivering. A controlled, heated environment is therefore necessary for nursing newborn infants. For those under

KEY POINTS

Box 44.1 Main non-urological abdominal emergencies occurring in the newborn

- Gastrointestinal atresias and stenoses
- Malrotation of the gut
- Anorectal abnormalities
- Meconium ileus and other problems with meconium
- Hirschsprung's disease
- Diaphragmatic hernia
- Deficiencies in the abdominal wall (gastroschisis and exomphalos)
- Necrotising enterocolitis

1 kg, for example, the temperature is set between 34.5–35.5°C and for those over 3 kg, between 31.5–34.5°C. For operations, a specially heated operating theatre is essential, with the infant placed on a heated blanket and all parts of the body except those immediately adjacent to the operating site kept insulated. Intravenous fluids are warmed and anaesthetic gases humidified and warmed.

Fluid requirements are relatively greater in the newborn and in young children than in adults. This is because the kidneys have a lower concentrating power and the obligatory urine output is necessarily higher. Faecal fluid losses are also higher, particularly in children under about 2 years of age, and this has important implications for fluid balance where there is severe diarrhoea in conditions such as gastroenteritis.

The blood volume in young children is approximately 85 ml/kg. Thus, a 20 ml blood loss in a 2.5 kg infant with a blood volume of 212 ml represents 10% of the total blood volume. Even small blood losses are therefore important and need to be accurately measured and replaced during surgery.

Liver function is immature during the newborn period. The common occurrence of physiological jaundice is the result of a high level of unconjugated bilirubin resulting from immaturity of the liver enzyme **glucoronyl transferase**. There is also a reduced ability to detoxify analgesic drugs and these must be used in greatly reduced doses compared with adults. Another reason for reducing drug doses in young infants is the facility with which the drugs cross the blood–brain barrier. Other consequences of liver immaturity include a reduced production of prothrombin (which can be overcome by administration of vitamin K in the perioperative period) and the risk of hypoglycaemia because of relatively low glycogen stores.

In summary, perioperative care of small children demands meticulous attention to fluid and blood balance. Poor temperature control and liver immaturity in the infant can result in problems with metabolism and blood clotting. A specialised knowledge of fluid and electrolyte balance, drug effects and nutritional needs is necessary for safe pre- and postoperative care of these small patients.

INTESTINAL OBSTRUCTION

Intestinal obstruction is the underlying phenomenon in the majority of neonatal abdominal emergencies and occurs approximately once in every 2000 live births. Complete obstruction, particularly of the proximal portion of the intestinal tract, prevents the fetus from swallowing amniotic fluid and this results in **maternal polyhydramnios**. Just as in adults, intestinal obstruction presents with vomiting, constipation and abdominal distension. **Bile-stained vomiting** is a particularly useful sign in this age group as it does not occur in normal full-term infants; it is thus always suspicious of a functional or a mechanical

obstruction beyond the pylorus. The severity of abdominal distension varies from gastric fullness to generalised abdominal distension, depending on the length of bowel affected.

Antenatal ultrasonography is now used as a routine investigation in obstetric departments. In pregnant women with polyhydramnios, 18% of fetuses are found to have congenital abnormalities of the gastrointestinal tract. Surgical abnormalities detectable by antenatal ultrasonography include duodenal atresia, diaphragmatic hernia, meconium peritonitis, and abdominal wall defects such as gastroschisis and exomphalos.

Confirmation of a diagnosis of intestinal obstruction after birth is usually possible with plain abdominal X-rays. The level of occlusion can often be deduced from the position of air and fluid levels. Barium enema examination is particularly useful for identification of distal lesions and for excluding malrotations of the bowel.

If transfer to a specialist centre is necessary, the newborn infant must be placed in a portable incubator which maintains body temperature. Oxygen and suction must be available during the journey, and frequent gastric aspiration via a nasogastric tube reduces the risk of inhalation pneumonitis. Endotracheal intubation is essential for infants with respiratory insufficiency.

GASTROINTESTINAL ATRESIAS AND STENOSES

Atresia is defined as complete obliteration of a segment of the gastrointestinal tract which is thus completely obstructed, whereas a **stenosis** is an indistensible narrowing causing partial obstruction. These problems are most common in the oesophagus and small intestine. Many of these are probably caused by mechanical problems affecting the blood supply in utero of the affected segment.

Oesophageal and duodenal atresias are true embryological abnormalities and often associated with other abnormalities. For example major cardiac, vertebral or renal abnormalities are found in 40% of cases of oesophageal atresia, and 20% of infants with duodenal atresia have Down's syndrome. In contrast, small bowel atresias are largely the result of intra-uterine **mesenteric vascular accidents** and are rarely associated with other congenital abnormalities.

OESOPHAGEAL ABNORMALITIES

Potentially lethal oesophageal abnormalities occur in 1 in 3000 live births and there is an associated **polyhydramnios** in nearly 30%. Oesophageal atresia may occur alone but in 85% of cases it is associated with a fistulous communication between the trachea and the distal oesophageal segment (**tracheo-oesophageal fistula or TOF**), as shown in Fig. 44.1. Fistulae between the trachea and the upper pouch are very rare (1%). A wide variety of oesophageal abnormalities account for the remaining 15% of oesophageal atresia.

The diagnosis is suspected in a newborn infant with excessive amounts of frothy saliva in the mouth. Attempted feeding causes choking or cyanotic attacks and fluid may enter the lungs by aspiration from the blind upper pouch or by regurgitation of gastric acid from the stomach via the fistula. Aspiration pneumonia is a serious complication. Diagnosis of TOF is confirmed by passing a nasogastric tube (10 French gauge) through the mouth. This will be arrested by the distal limit of the blind-ending upper pouch which can be outlined on X-ray by passing a very small quantity of contrast material down the tube. Following the X-ray, the contrast material is aspirated from the pouch to prevent any spill-over into the lungs. If the oesophagus is obstructed and there is gas present in the stomach, this indicates there must be a fistula between the distal oesophagus and the trachea.

Surgical correction is performed soon after diagnosis and after a search for any other congenital abnormalities. The majority are corrected by ligation and division of the fistula and primary oesophageal anastomosis. Oral feeding is started 1 week after surgery in uncomplicated cases.

ANNULAR PANCREAS AND DUODENAL ATRESIA

These two conditions present in an identical manner. **Annular pancreas** is caused by an embryological anomaly in which a portion of the pancreas remains wrapped around the duodenum. The pancreas is normally formed from two separate ventral and dorsal outgrowths of the duodenum and the ventral portion rotates around the bowel to fuse with the dorsal outgrowth. An abnormality in rotation results in annular pancreas. It is important to

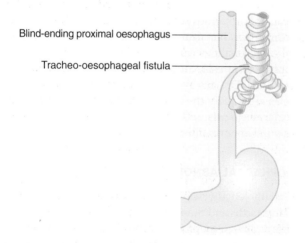

Blind-ending proximal oesophagus ————

Tracheo-oesophageal fistula ————

Fig. 44.1 Tracheo-oesophageal fistula
The most common variant of oesophageal atresia. Air enters the GI tract via the fistula and may be seen on plain X-ray. Gastric secretions may enter the bronchial tree causing 'frothy' breathing.

note that duodenal atresia is associated with Down's syndrome but annular pancreas is not.

The obstruction of **duodenal atresia** is usually below the entry of the common bile duct, resulting in **bile-stained vomiting**. Plain erect abdominal X-ray shows gas in the stomach and proximal duodenum; a gas bubble and fluid level are seen on each side of the upper abdomen ('**double bubble**'—see Fig. 44.2). Urgent surgery is needed to bypass the defect by creating a side-to-side anastomosis between proximal and distal duodenal segments.

JEJUNO-ILEAL ATRESIAS

These atresias are believed to result from damage to the vascular supply of the bowel and are occasionally found in association with intra-uterine occurrence of hernia or volvulus. They occur at any level and are sometimes multiple. Bile-stained vomiting and abdominal distension are often associated with **visible peristalsis** and hypertrophied proximal bowel. The diagnosis is usually evident from the plain abdominal X-ray. Treatment consists of resection (Fig. 44.3) of the affected segment, including the most hypertrophied segment of proximal bowel, and end-to-end anastomosis.

MALROTATION OF THE GUT

During early embryological development, the midgut develops outside the abdominal cavity. By the end of the third month, the midgut has returned to the abdominal cavity having rotated 270° anti-clockwise in the process. **Incomplete rotation** may leave the caecum in front of the duodenum and the two organs are then bound together by peritoneal bands (**Ladd's bands**). These cause duodenal obstruction and bile-stained vomiting. The most serious problem with malrotation is associated with malfixation of the small and large bowel to the posterior abdominal wall. A major portion of the bowel may be suspended by a very narrow mesentery which can twist on its axis and occlude the superior mesenteric vessels, cutting off the blood supply to the whole of the small bowel as well as the proximal half of the large bowel. A sudden onset of duodenal obstruction and peritonitis in a previously well child should suggest a diagnosis of volvulus of this type. Urgent laparotomy is imperative to de-rotate the bowel and any gangrenous bowel must be resected. If less than 50 cm of small bowel can be conserved, a 'short bowel' syndrome is likely, with inadequate absorption of nutrients.

ANORECTAL ABNORMALITIES

The primitive hindgut forms the **cloaca** in the early embryo and a septum then divides it into an **anterior compartment**, from which the urinary tract and part of the genital tract are formed, and a **posterior compartment**

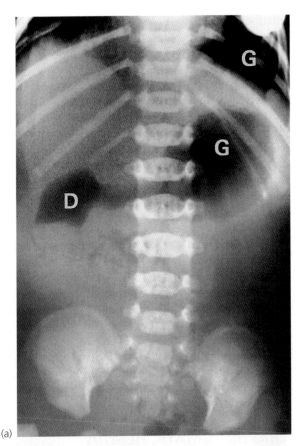

(a)

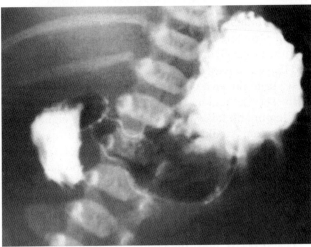

(b)

Fig. 44.2 Duodenal atresia

(a) Supine plain abdominal film in a neonate with duodenal obstruction. This film shows the typical 'double bubble' appearance of gas in the stomach **G** and the first part of the duodenum **D**. Fluid levels would be seen in an erect film. **(b)** A small amount of barium has been passed down the nasogastric tube and confirms that the obstruction in the second part of the duodenum is virtually complete.

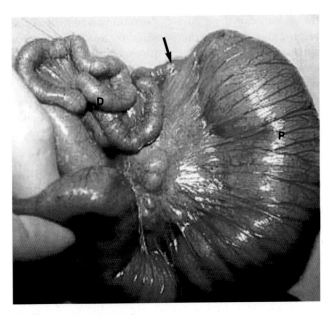

Fig. 44.3 Jejunal atresia

Findings at laparotomy on a neonate presenting with intestinal obstruction. The proximal jejunum **P** is greatly dilated whilst the distal jejunum is collapsed **D**. In between is an atretic segment without a lumen (arrowed). This was resected and the bowel ends joined. The infant thrived soon afterwards.

the levator ani muscle. In **anal agenesis** the virtually blind-ending rectum passes through the puborectalis muscle and ends as a fistula to the perineum—usually to the urethra in the male and to the lower vagina in the female. **Anorectal agenesis** implies that the bowel terminates above the puborectalis. A fistula communicates with the urethra in the male and the upper half of the vagina in the female. Anomalies of the urinary tract are associated with these disorders in 50% of infants with anorectal agenesis and 20% of those with anal agenesis. Several individual congenital abnormalities are often associated with each other: in particular, the **VATER** association of **V**ertebral, **A**norectal, **T**racheo-**O**esophageal and **R**enal abnormalities. Finding one of these abnormalities should lead to a search for others in the group.

In suspected anorectal abnormalities, a combination of careful examination of the perineum, urinalysis for meconium, and lateral X-ray of the pelvis with the infant held upside down allows accurate diagnosis. Water-soluble contrast injected through the perineum into the distal bowel may give more accurate information.

Treatment depends on the level of the distal pouch. In the low lesions (anal agenesis), the main pelvic muscle of continence (puborectalis) is well formed and operations via the perineum are often sufficient. High lesions require a preliminary colostomy and complicated reconstructions later. The currently favoured major reconstruction is performed through a posterior sagittal incision extending from the sacrum to the anal dimple. Any fistula is divided and the rectum mobilised. The essential part of

from which the rectum and upper part of the anal canal are formed. The lower portion of the anal canal is developed from an invagination of ectoderm. There are many types of anorectal anomalies but a simple classification is based on their relationship to the puborectalis portion of

the operation is the accurate apposition and repair of the levator muscles and the muscles of the external anal sphincter. Long-term faecal continence is achieved in most children with low anomalies but in a lesser proportion with high anomalies.

CAUSES OF FAILURE TO PASS MECONIUM

MECONIUM ILEUS

Meconium ileus is an obstruction of the distal ileum by thick, viscid meconium and it occurs in 5–10% of newborn infants with **cystic fibrosis**. These children have an abnormality of mucus-secreting glands which causes secondary changes in the lungs, liver, pancreas and small bowel. Pancreatic enzymes which normally liquefy meconium are deficient and the thick meconium causes severe intestinal obstruction. Clinical examination may reveal thickened loops of hypertrophied bowel and X-rays may show a mottled appearance with a few fluid levels. X-rays are often difficult to interpret. An enema examination with Gastrografin may demonstrate the inspissated meconium in the distal ileum and may also break up the material by a detergent-like action, thereby relieving the obstruction.

Laparotomy is required for unrelieved obstruction and the maximally dilated loop of ileum containing the inspissated meconium is resected. A temporary ileostomy is usually fashioned and closed after 1 month. Pancreatic enzyme supplements are given, as well as antibiotics to prevent pulmonary complications.

OTHER TYPES OF MECONIUM OBSTRUCTION

Occasionally, normal meconium may become inspissated and obstruct either the distal ileum or the large bowel. This complication has been related to early feeding with reconstituted milk feeds and is more frequently encountered in the premature and low birth-weight infant. The obstructing plug of meconium may be evacuated after a rectal examination but occasionally laparotomy and removal of the meconium plug is required; ileostomy is not necessary. Spontaneous ileal perforation is an occasional complication.

HIRSCHSPRUNG'S DISEASE (CONGENITAL AGANGLIONOSIS)

Hirschsprung's disease (Harald Hirschsprung 1830–1916) is a congenital abnormality of part of the bowel which affects all of the intra-mural autonomic nerves. Ganglion cells (neurones) are absent from the inter-myenteric and submucosal plexuses, and the parasympathetic and sympathetic nerves are scattered in a disorderly way throughout the layers of the bowel wall. In 75% of cases the abnormality is restricted to the rectosigmoid area (Fig. 44.4b) but in 8% the whole of the large bowel is involved. Very rarely the condition affects the whole of the intestinal tract. Peristalsis is absent in affected segments and the internal anal sphincter does not relax. The patient therefore has a **functional obstruction of the bowel** that presents either as neonatal intestinal obstruction or as severe constipation in an older child. Ninety-eight percent of normal infants pass meconium within the first 24 hours of life whereas 94% of infants with aganglionosis do not.

Rectal examination may allow an explosive release of air and meconium. Diagnosis is made from the observation on contrast enema of a non-dilated rectum but a dilated proximal colon and is confirmed with mucosal suction biopsies. Histochemical staining of the latter shows absent neurones and an increase in the numbers of cholinesterase-positive (parasympathetic) nerves.

A severe form of enterocolitis may occur in infants where the diagnosis of congenital aganglionosis has been delayed, and death may result from hypovolaemia.

DIAPHRAGMATIC HERNIA

The diaphragm is developed from a complex of embryological structures which include the mesoderm of the septum transversum, the lateral pleuroperitoneal folds and the dorsal mesentery of the embryo. The phrenic nerve arises from the area of origin of the septum transversum in the cervical region. Fusion of the various segments of the diaphragm takes place round about the eighth week of gestation. A failure of closure of the pleuroperitoneal folds results in the most common type of congenital diaphragmatic hernia (Fig. 44.5) which is postero-lateral in position. Bowel occupies part of the thoracic cavity and inhibits development of the lungs. The incidence of this type of hernia is 1 in 3500 live births and 80% are on the left side.

Diagnosis is now frequently made before birth on antenatal ultrasound screening. The infants develop signs of respiratory distress soon after birth and survival depends on the lung volume and its function. Cyanosis, mediastinal shift and an 'empty' (scaphoid) abdomen are the classic signs and the diagnosis is easily confirmed on a chest X-ray. Preoperative nasogastric aspiration and endotracheal intubation are instituted and the hernia is repaired through a subcostal abdominal incision. In many cases a complete diaphragm can be fashioned by suturing diaphragmatic remnants together after lifting the viscera out of the thoracic cavity. Large defects, however, may require a patch of prosthetic material or a flap of abdominal

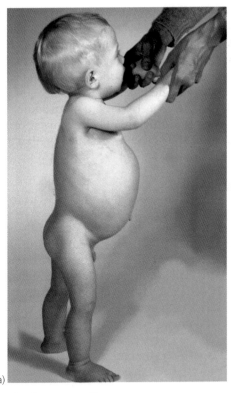

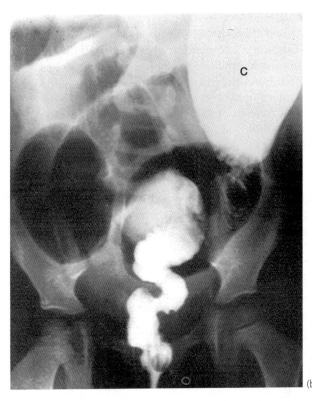

(a)   (b)

Fig. 44.4 Hirschsprung's disease
(a) 3-year-old child demonstrating failure to thrive and a dilated abdomen. **(b)** Barium enema in the same child showing grossly dilated colon C proximal to the recto sigmoid junction. The bowel distal to that point was affected by Hirschsprung's disease.

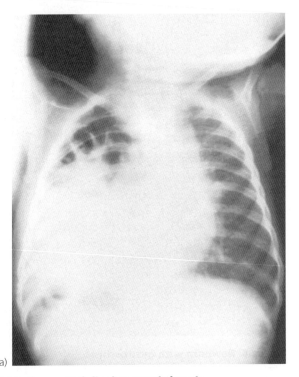

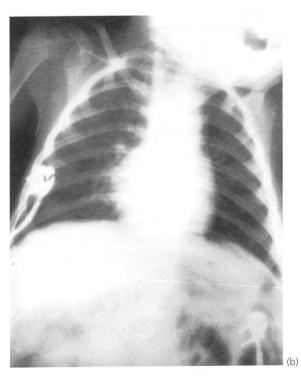

(a)   (b)

Fig. 44.5 Congenital diaphragmatic hernia
(a) Plain chest radiograph of a neonate with respiratory distress. This film shows a large opacity in the right lung field containing obvious loops of bowel caused by a congenital diaphragmatic hernia. This case is unusual as it is on the right side. **(b)** Postoperative chest X-ray of the same infant showing complete lung expansion after repair of the diaphragmatic defect.

wall muscle to achieve satisfactory closure. The overall mortality is still approximately 50% from inadequate lung function. Extra-corporeal membrane oxygenation (ECMO), derived from cardiopulmonary bypass techniques, has recently been introduced to support the infant while the lungs are developing, and initial results have been encouraging. A report of 1000 infants with diaphragmatic hernias treated with ECMO support showed a survival rate of 60%.

OTHER SURGICAL CONDITIONS CAUSING RESPIRATORY PROBLEMS IN THE NEWBORN

VASCULAR RING

This abnormality is caused by the persistence of a posterior aortic arch or by abnormal configurations of the vessels that arise from the aortic arch. Either abnormality results in compression of the trachea and oesophagus. In children with severe symptoms, treatment is essential and consists of division of the smallest moiety of a double aortic arch or by correction of the anatomy of any abnormal vessel. Children with only mild symptoms may improve spontaneously with growth.

CONGENITAL CYSTIC DISEASE OF THE LUNG

The abnormality usually affects one part of the lung—most frequently one or other of the lower lobes. The cysts result from abnormal development of lung parenchyma. Large lesions can cause acute respiratory symptoms from compression of the normal lung. Resection of the affected lobe is curative.

CONGENITAL LOBAR EMPHYSEMA

This condition usually affects an upper lobe of either the right or the left lung. A developmental weakness in a lobar bronchus allows air into the lobe, but bronchial collapse during expiration prevents deflation. Increasing lobar expansion compresses normal lung tissue which leads to deteriorating respiratory function. Surgical excision of the emphysematous lobe is relatively straightforward and curative.

DEFICIENCIES IN THE ABDOMINAL WALL

Major deficiencies in the anterior abdominal wall are an uncommon congenital abnormality and are dramatically obvious at birth (Fig. 44.6). They originate from a midline defect in the abdominal wall so that much of the bowel lies outside the abdominal cavity, with or without a membranous covering. In **gastroschisis**, coils of bare gut are exposed, whereas in **exomphalos**, the gut is invested with a thin layer of peritoneum. **Ectopia vesicae** (extrophy of the urinary bladder) is the rarest of the major abdominal wall defects and is more common in boys. It presents as a defect between the rectus muscles and the pubic bones and a failure of development of the entire front of the bladder, bladder neck and urethra.

GASTROSCHISIS

This abdominal wall defect is characterised by herniation of bowel through a defect to the right of the umbilicus. The defect usually measures about 3 cm in length and there is no peritoneal covering. Exposure to amniotic fluid before birth can result in widespread adhesions and shortened oedematous bowel loops. Gastroschisis may be associated with **small bowel atresias**. Treatment by primary abdominal wall closure is frequently possible but if the abdominal cavity is too small then a temporary covering is fashioned with a Silastic pouch. The bowel is reduced into the abdomen over the next few days and

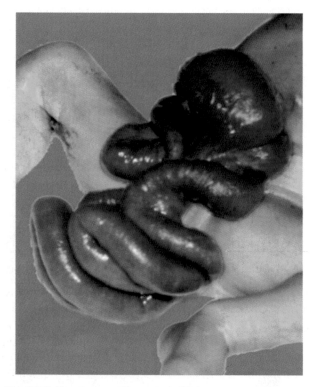

Fig. 44.6 Newborn with gastroschisis
This neonate was born with bowel and stomach protruding as shown. The bowel was covered with a special plastic bag sutured to the wound edges and the bag gradually rolled up day by day until all the bowel had been returned to the abdomen. The abdominal wall was then repaired.

the abdominal wall then repaired. The current mortality rate is approximately 15%. In many cases intravenous nutrition is required for at least 3 weeks before normal bowel activity returns. Gastroschisis is rarely associated with other anomalies.

EXOMPHALOS

Exomphalos major is a defect in the midline of the abdomen and may affect most of the abdominal wall and have a diameter of up to 20 cm. It is often associated with other congenital anomalies such as heart disease, diaphragmatic hernia, abnormalities of the bladder and chromosomal anomalies.

At birth the bowel is covered with a thin sac of amnion and peritoneum which may rupture and allow evisceration of the bowel, infection and septicaemia.

Primary skin cover is the ideal treatment but this may not be possible because the abdominal cavity is too small and causes diaphragmatic splinting and compression of the inferior vena cava. This type of defect may be temporarily closed with a Silastic sac which is rolled up a little each day, returning bowel to the abdominal cavity little by little. A formal repair of the abdomen is then performed. As with gastroschisis, intravenous feeding is usually needed until normal bowel activity returns. The mortality rate for large lesions is approximately 30%.

Exomphalos minor, or herniation of the umbilical cord, does not exceed 4 cm in diameter. The bowel can be reduced with ease and the abdominal wall repaired as a primary procedure.

ECTOPIA VESICAE

Ectopia vesicae is a complex abnormality which presents at birth with exposed bladder mucosa and penile epispadias. The pubic bones may be widely separated with resulting posterior rotation of the hip joints. Closure of the defect, repair of the epispadias and the achievement of urinary continence must be accomplished without producing back-pressure on the kidneys. Urinary diversion may be necessary when continence fails to become established.

NECROTISING ENTEROCOLITIS

This often fatal disorder occurs in newborn babies, who are almost invariably the premature or seriously ill in special care baby units. The pathophysiology is poorly understood but probably involves ischaemia of the large bowel wall which then becomes invaded by gas-producing bacteria. Initially, there is adynamic bowel obstruction, presenting with abdominal distension, vomiting and diarrhoea with blood and mucus. If unrecognised, necrotising enterocolitis soon progresses to large bowel necrosis, perforation and generalised peritonitis.

Plain abdominal X-ray initially shows generalised bowel dilatation with multiple fluid levels. Later, gas shadows may be seen in the bowel wall indicating bowel wall necrosis. Treatment includes vigorous resuscitative measures, broad-spectrum antibiotics and surgical re-section if incipient gangrene is suspected. Mortality remains high.

ABDOMINAL EMERGENCIES IN INFANTS AND YOUNG CHILDREN

In children below the age of about 2 years, there are four main abdominal causes for acute surgical admission; these are listed in Box 44.2.

STRANGULATED INGUINAL HERNIA

PATHOPHYSIOLOGY

Strangulated inguinal hernia is the most common cause of acute surgical admission in boys below the age of 2 years. Strangulation follows incarceration of an indirect inguinal hernia. There is invariably a congenital patent processus vaginalis, although an actual hernia may not have been evident beforehand. Strangulated inguinal hernia may occur at any time from birth onwards and is most common during the first 2 years of life. The high incidence of strangulation in young children is a strong argument in favour of repairing any hernia in this age group soon after it has been discovered. There is a

> **KEY POINTS**
>
> **Box 44.2 Main abdominal emergencies occurring in infants and young children**
> - Strangulated inguinal hernia
> - Hypertrophic pyloric stenosis
> - Intussusception
> - Swallowed foreign body

particularly high incidence of strangulation in premature babies.

CLINICAL FEATURES

Classically, a mother discovers a firm lump in the groin of her crying (usually male) child. He may have vomited once or twice but the diagnosis is usually made before obstruction becomes established. On examination, the child is usually well. There is an obvious, irreducible lump in the groin (Fig. 44.7) which may extend into the scrotum.

MANAGEMENT

In a typical child presenting early, the hernia is not tender or red, and there is no risk that the strangulated bowel has yet become infarcted. Simple sedation and rest in a hospital bed allows most hernias to reduce spontaneously after a few hours. If reduction is successful, the child is kept in hospital and elective hernia repair performed at the earliest scheduled opportunity. If conservative management fails to reduce the hernia within about 6 hours or if there is any clinical evidence of bowel infarction, then operation must be performed as an emergency procedure.

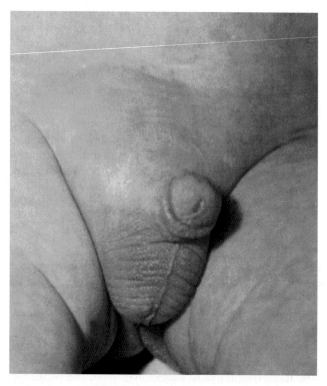

Fig. 44.7 Irreducible inguinal hernia
This 14-month-old boy was known to have a reducible inguinal hernia but after a bout of crying it became irreducible. With sedation and rest, the hernia reduced spontaneously but was repaired on the next available operating list.

HYPERTROPHIC PYLORIC STENOSIS

PATHOPHYSIOLOGY

This common condition of unknown aetiology nearly always presents between 3 and 8 weeks of age. It presents with a sudden onset of complete **pyloric obstruction**. The underlying cause is marked hypertrophy of the circular

muscle in the pyloric region of the stomach. The disorder occurs in about 1 in 400 normal babies and there is a male predominance of 4:1. Firstborn children are most commonly affected. Hereditary factors play a part since it is relatively common for siblings of affected children to develop the condition. It is also common for a parent or other close relative of an affected child to have had infantile pyloric stenosis.

CLINICAL FEATURES

Typically, the infant thrives for the first 3 or 4 weeks and then begins to vomit after every feed. The vomiting characteristically becomes **projectile**, i.e. large amounts of vomitus are hurled from the mouth, rather than running down the baby's front. The vomitus is never bile-stained and this readily distinguishes pyloric stenosis from duodenal stenosis. Apart from the vomiting, the child appears well and is eager for further milk. With sustained vomiting, however, the child becomes progressively dehydrated and electrolyte depleted and loses vigour. Examination often reveals no abdominal abnormality.

DIAGNOSIS

The persistent vomiting leads to hospital admission, where the child's response to feeding is observed. At the same time, the abdomen is palpated. If pyloric stenosis is present, a mass about 2 cm in diameter is usually palpable deeply below the liver during the test feed. If **gastric peristaltic waves** are also visible through the abdominal wall, the diagnosis can be made with confidence (visible peristalsis). If the diagnosis remains in doubt, an ultrasound scan or barium meal examination will reveal typical complete pyloric obstruction.

Treatment is by **Rammstedt's pyloromyotomy** (see Fig. 44.8). Before operation, it is essential that any fluid and electrolyte abnormalities are corrected—the operation should only be performed on a well baby. In addition, the stomach is emptied by nasogastric aspiration and washed out with normal saline. At operation, the muscle of the pylorus is split longitudinally down to but not including the mucosa; the mucosa bulges into the incision when the correct level is reached.

Postoperative recovery is rapid, and graded feeds are reintroduced over 1–2 days, beginning with a standard electrolyte solution.

INTUSSUSCEPTION

PATHOPHYSIOLOGY

Intussusception (Fig. 44.9) is an acquired disorder most common between the ages of 3 months and 2 years. A segment of bowel becomes invaginated into the bowel

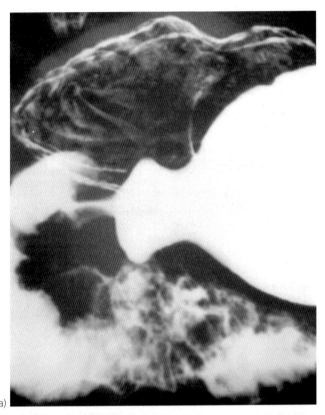

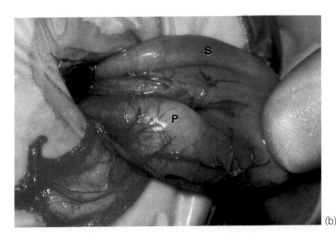

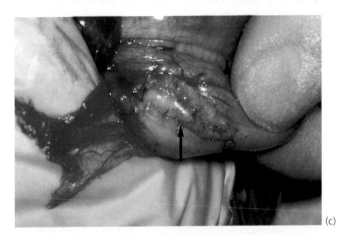

Fig. 44.8 Hypertrophic pyloric stenosis and Rammstedt's operation
(a) Barium meal showing dilated stomach and narrow pyloric channel with apparent shouldering due to pyloric muscle thickening. **(b)** A small transverse abdominal incision has been made and the stomach **S** and pyloric 'tumour' **P** delivered. **(c)** The serosa over the tumour has been incised and the hypertrophic muscle split with forceps. The mucosa is seen bulging through the muscle split (arrowed).

immediately distal to it. The invaginated segment progressively elongates as it is propelled distally by peristalsis. **Ileocaecal intussusception** is the most common variety. It is probably initiated by peristaltic action upon an enlarged Peyer's patch caused by a viral infection. The intussusception commonly extends well into the transverse colon and may even present at the anus.

Intussusception presents with bowel obstruction, but if left untreated for more than about 10 hours, the affected segment undergoes **venous infarction**.

Intussusception sometimes occurs in adults, when the initiating factor is a bowel wall tumour or polyp.

CLINICAL FEATURES

The classic presentation of intussusception is bouts of severe colicky abdominal pain during which the child is doubled-up and screaming. These episodes are separated by periods of about 1 hour when the child appears entirely well. Within the first few hours, the child often

passes a small amount of jelly-like blood described as **redcurrant jelly stool** which is almost pathognomonic of intussusception. Vomiting begins later, consistent with the diagnosis of distal bowel obstruction.

On examination, a sausage-shaped mass is usually palpable, lying across the upper abdomen. The rectum is empty but may contain a little blood.

MANAGEMENT

If intussusception is suspected, barium enema examination should be performed urgently. Diagnosis is confirmed by the typical appearance shown in Figure 44.10. If gentle hydrostatic pressure is applied by elevating the bag containing barium, the intussusception often slowly reduces.

If this fails or infarction is suspected, laparotomy is performed urgently. The intussusception is reduced by gentle manipulation and the appendix is usually removed. If the viability of the segment is in doubt, it must be resected.

597

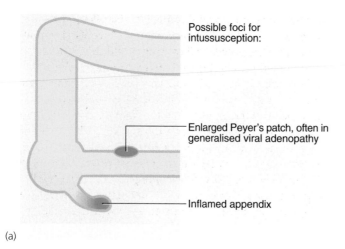

Possible foci for intussusception:

Enlarged Peyer's patch, often in generalised viral adenopathy

Inflamed appendix

(a)

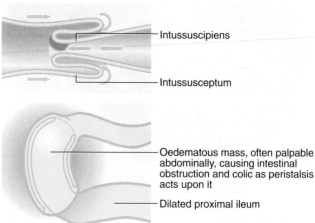

Intussuscipiens

Intussusceptum

Oedematous mass, often palpable abdominally, causing intestinal obstruction and colic as peristalsis acts upon it

Dilated proximal ileum

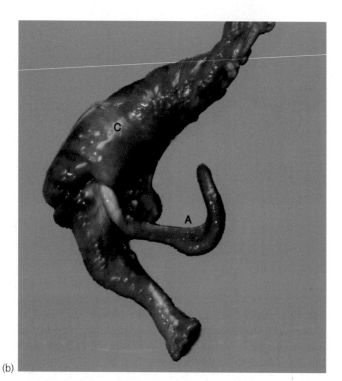

(b)

Fig. 44.9 Intussusception

(a) Mechanism of intussusception **(b)** In this case neither preoperative barium enema nor manual attempts at reduction were successful so the terminal ileum **I** and ascending colon **C** were resected. Note the appendix **A**.

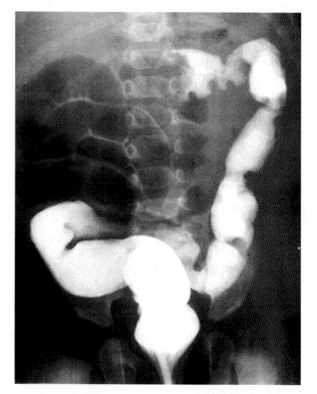

Fig. 44.10 Ileocolic intussusception—barium enema

This 2-year-old child presented as an emergency with spasms of abdominal pain, having passed 'redcurrant jelly' rectally. This barium enema shows the typical appearance of large bowel obstruction by an intussusception of ileum which in this case has progressed to the transverse colon. The barium infusion pressure was increased, resulting in hydraulic reduction of the intussusception which did not recur.

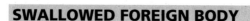

SWALLOWED FOREIGN BODY

Young children examine their environment with their mouths and frequently swallow foreign bodies such as coins, safety pins, buttons or small plastic objects. One of the most dangerous swallowed foreign body is a small button-shaped mercury battery (Fig. 44.11), because it is likely to disintegrate, releasing toxic mercury salts.

The narrowest part of the gastrointestinal tract is the cricopharyngeus sling at the upper end of the oesophagus. Foreign bodies (other than mercury batteries) that pass beyond this level are likely to pass all the way through the tract without incident. Only rarely does an object

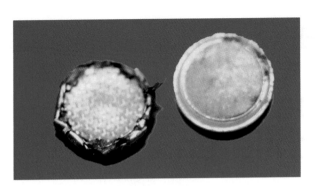

Fig. 44.11 Ingested mercury battery
Young children often put small hearing aid-type batteries into their mouths. They are at risk from inhalation and bronchial obstruction, and also from mercury poisoning if the battery disintegrates. This battery was removed endoscopically from the stomach of a toddler and had already disintegrated.

become arrested, usually in the terminal ileum or sometimes at the pylorus. Occasionally a sharp foreign body penetrates the bowel wall causing peritonitis.

Provided the child is well, management involves plain radiography which will show any metal-containing object and confirm that it is not in the bronchial tree. X-rays only need to be repeated if the foreign body has not passed spontaneously after 5 days. If the child develops abdominal pain, vomiting or bleeding, the object must be retrieved. If it is proximal to the pylorus, this may be by flexible endoscopy, but if more distal, laparotomy is required. Swallowed **mercury batteries** are extremely dangerous and must be removed as soon as possible.

ABDOMINAL EMERGENCIES IN OLDER CHILDREN

THE ACUTE ABDOMEN

DIFFERENTIAL DIAGNOSIS

From childhood to adolescence, acute abdominal pain is a common cause of surgical admission. Usually, **appendicitis** is suspected and this condition is described in detail in Chapter 12. The major differential diagnosis is **constipation**, closely followed by **mesenteric adenitis** (Box 44.3). The child with constipation is afebrile and systemically well. Mesenteric adenitis causes a higher fever than appendicitis and the signs and symptoms settle quickly, usually within 24 hours. There is often a recent history of viral upper respiratory tract infection and enlarged cervical lymph nodes may be palpable.

Less commonly, acute abdominal pain in this age group is caused by a **lower urinary tract infection**, or occasionally a right lower lobe **pneumonia**. Both these diagnoses should be considered and the urine tested. **Testicular torsion** (Ch. 27) sometimes presents solely with abdominal pain; the genitalia must always, therefore, be examined in boys with abdominal pain, although it should be noted that testicular torsion is uncommon before adolescence.

KEY POINTS

Box 44.3 Differential diagnosis of acute abdominal pain in pre-adolescent children

- **Acute appendicitis**
- **Constipation**
- **Mesenteric adenitis**
- **Lower urinary tract infection**
- **Right lower lobe pneumonia**

PRINCIPLES OF MANAGEMENT

If acute appendicitis is diagnosed when the child is first seen, operation should be performed without delay. More commonly, the diagnosis of appendicitis is uncertain. In these children, urinary tract infection should be excluded by urine microscopy. The child should be kept under close review and re-examined at intervals of several hours. Soon, a worsening or improving trend will become apparent. This approach may be used both in family practice and after surgical admission. It reduces the psychological trauma and the rate of unnecessary operations to a minimum and also ensures that appendicitis is not missed until peritonitis has become all too obvious.

45 Non-acute abdominal problems in children

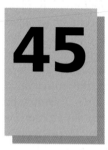

INTRODUCTION

The most common non-acute reasons for surgical referral in children are hernias and associated problems, abnormalities of testicular descent and foreskin problems, mainly phimosis. Less often, surgeons are asked to manage chronic or recurrent abdominal pain, chronic constipation, rectal bleeding, an abdominal mass or rectal prolapse. Many of these children present first to a paediatrician. Finally, there is a range of urological problems that occur in infancy and childhood, most of them unique to young patients. These are discussed later in this chapter.

Unlike most of the acute conditions described earlier, non-acute conditions may present across the whole age spectrum of childhood.

PROBLEMS WITH GROIN AND MALE GENITALIA

HERNIAS AND ASSOCIATED PROBLEMS

Persistence of the peritoneal sac that is associated with testicular descent causes three very common problems in boys: inguinal hernia, patent processus vaginalis (PPV) and hydrocoele. These conditions all present as inguinal or scrotal swellings, usually in babies and preschool children. They are illustrated in Figure 45.1.

INGUINAL HERNIA

Inguinal hernias in children arise because the processus vaginalis fails to close after testicular descent. They are therefore true congenital abnormalities. Anatomically, they are identical to indirect inguinal hernias in adults (see Ch. 27). Inguinal hernias are very common in premature infants and may become obstructed or strangulated.

In childhood, an inguinal hernia usually presents as a lump at the external inguinal ring. The lump appears when the child cries but reduces spontaneously between times, so that when the child is seen by the surgeon, no abnormality may be detectable. Most surgeons would accept a mother's clear history of hernia even if no abnormality is found, and arrange surgical repair. Where the defect is larger, the lump is always present and simply expands during bouts of crying. Childhood inguinal hernias are prone to strangulation when they present with pain and obstructive symptoms, Thus, inguinal hernias in children should be electively repaired without long delay.

In adult inguinal hernias, a repair or inlay patch (**herniorrhaphy**) is necessary because an anatomical abdominal wall defect is important in the pathogenesis. In babies and children, there is rarely a permanent abdominal wall defect and usually the peritoneal sac only needs to be removed (**inguinal herniotomy**) (Fig. 45.1).

PATENT PROCESSUS VAGINALIS

The term patent processus vaginalis should be reserved to describe a hydrocoele which communicates with the peritoneal cavity via a remnant too narrow to admit bowel. Children with these **communicating hydrocoeles** present with a history of scrotal swelling which increases during the day (as peritoneal fluid accumulates) and subsides during the night when the child lies flat (Fig. 45.2). The condition is usually seen in toddlers up to the age of about 3 years.

Treatment is surgical excision of the peritoneal remnant as in herniotomy.

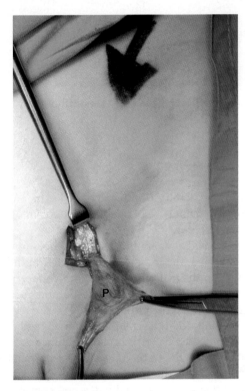

Fig. 45.1 Inguinal hernia
At operation, the peritoneal sac **P** is being held up before it is excised. No other procedure is necessary in this 4-year-old child. Unusually, the patient was female.

INFANTILE HYDROCOELE

Non-communicating hydrocoeles surrounding the testis are mostly seen in neonates and young babies. The hydrocoele (Fig. 45.3) results from incomplete reabsorption of fluid from within the tunica vaginalis after closure of the processus. The fluid will usually resorb slowly if untreated. Alternatively, it can be removed by needle aspiration, after which it does not usually recur.

UMBILICAL HERNIA

Many newborn babies have umbilical hernias, particularly if premature. Most will spontaneously shrink and disappear over the first 2 years of life. Those that remain substantial after that age should be repaired as there is little chance of further spontaneous improvement (see Fig. 45.4). A small subumbilical incision allows emptying and ligation of the peritoneal sac and placement of a few non-absorbable repair sutures. The umbilicus is usually sutured to the repair to restore its normal recessed cosmetic appearance.

TESTICULAR MALDESCENT

In up to 4% of normal full-term newborn males, one or both testes has failed to reach the scrotum. This percentage is greatly increased with prematurity. By the age of 1 year, full descent will have occurred in most boys, leaving about 0.3% with maldescended testes.

Maldescent is associated with up to 30 times the normal risk of later testicular malignancy (although the risk is still small); surgical correction probably does not reduce this risk. In addition, maldescended testes tend to be **subfertile** and have an increased risk of traumatic injury or torsion. There is histological evidence that mal-

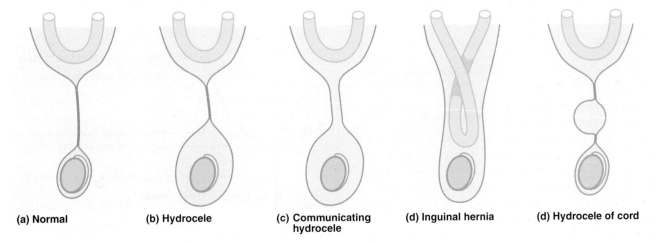

| (a) Normal | (b) Hydrocele | (c) Communicating hydrocele | (d) Inguinal hernia | (d) Hydrocele of cord |

Fig. 45.2 Abnormalities associated with the processus vaginalis

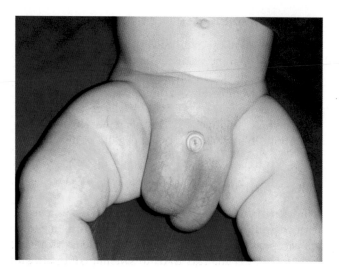

Fig. 45.3 Hydrocoeles
This 11-month-old boy had an enlarged scrotum confirmed by transillumination to be the result of hydrocoeles.

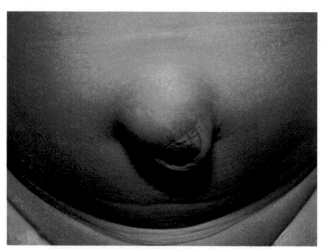

Fig. 45.4 Umbilical hernia in a 14-month-old boy
This was repaired surgically.

descent may be a result of structural abnormalities of the testis rather than vice versa.

To minimise the risk of complications, boys are examined regularly from birth through school age to identify problems of maldescent and allow timely surgical correction (**orchidopexy**). It is now known that previously descended testes can later ascend and doctors should be alert to this possibility. Although orchidopexy has little influence on the predisposition to malignancy, a testicular tumour is more likely to be discovered early if the testis is in the scrotum. The influence of orchidopexy on fertility is probably marginal except for any benefit gained from the cooler environment of the scrotum.

The maldescended testis may be arrested at any point on its path of descent from the posterior abdominal wall to the scrotum. Nearly all lie in the groin area, outside the external inguinal ring in the **superficial inguinal pouch**. In addition, the testis may be deflected from its normal

path into the scrotum and come to lie in an ectopic position. The main sites of incomplete descent or ectopia are shown in Figure 45.5.

In most boys in whom the testis does not appear to be fully descended, the testis can be palpated in the scrotal neck and gently manipulated into its correct position. This is described as a **retractile testis** and requires no treatment provided the testis become less retractile as the boy grows. Indeed, if the child is examined by the parents after a warm bath, the testis is usually fully descended.

In other boys, the testis can only be manipulated into the upper part of the scrotum. Although a small proportion of these will eventually descend completely (the 'high retractile' testis), the majority are truly incompletely descended and require surgical correction.

The optimum age for orchidopexy is debated, but the procedure is probably best performed between the ages of 2 and 3 years. The usual technique of orchidopexy

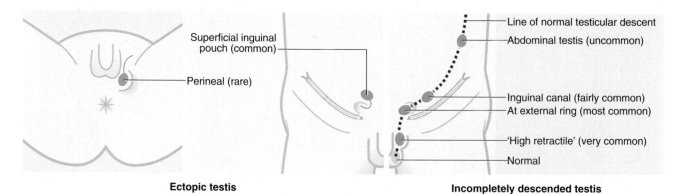

Superficial inguinal pouch (common)

Perineal (rare)

Line of normal testicular descent
Abdominal testis (uncommon)
Inguinal canal (fairly common)
At external ring (most common)
'High retractile' (very common)
Normal

Ectopic testis

Incompletely descended testis

Fig. 45.5 Testicular maldescent

involves mobilising the spermatic cord and placing the testis in a subcutaneous scrotal pouch outside the dartos muscle.

FORESKIN PROBLEMS

The foreskin is normally adherent to the glans until about the age of 2 years. For this reason, parents should be advised not to attempt to retract the foreskin before this age as this may excite a fibrotic response. Some young boys develop stenosis of the preputial orifice (**phimosis**), probably the result of a combination of recurrent low-grade balanoposthitis, chronic ammoniacal inflammation and ill-judged attempts at retraction by the parents.

Phimosis presents with chronic foreskin irritation or 'spraying' on micturition, often accompanied by 'ballooning' of the foreskin. There is often a recent history suggestive of acute balanoposthitis.

Most boys with phimosis do not require circumcision. In cases followed up for several years, nearly all revert to normal retractile foreskins without operation. In cases where the orifice is very tight or meatal stenosis is suspected operation is often required. A lesser operation than circumcision is **preputioplasty** which involves dividing the tight band longitudinally and suturing it transversely. Attempts to simply dilate the phimosis under anaesthesia are usually unsuccessful as this causes further scarring and rapid relapse.

Paraphimosis (see Ch. 27) sometimes occurs in children, especially if there is a degree of phimosis. This causes the foreskin to become trapped in the coronal sulcus after it has been retracted. This leads to swelling and pain and requires urgent reduction.

ABDOMINAL PROBLEMS

CHRONIC AND RECURRENT ABDOMINAL PAIN

Chronic or recurrent abdominal pain is a common problem in children of school age but in most, no cause is discovered and the problem gradually resolves; these children are often managed by paediatricians. The main organic causes are summarised in Box 45.1, but psychological factors are fairly common and should not be overlooked (**periodic syndrome**).

CHRONIC CONSTIPATION

Chronic constipation is among the most common abdominal problems in children; it may present as **faecal soiling**, i.e. faecal overflow incontinence. In most children, the aetiology is unknown, but the condition usually responds to simple measures like a high-fibre diet, regular attempts at defaecation and, if necessary, a small daily dose of a laxative (lactulose or senna derivative). The problem should not be neglected as it may otherwise lead to lifelong problems. A tiny proportion of children with severe constipation have **ultra-short segment Hirschsprung's disease**, described earlier (p. 592).

RECTAL BLEEDING

Rectal bleeding is a common problem in childhood, but is rarely caused by tumour or haemorrhoids; the usual causes are shown in Box 45.2.

KEY POINTS

Box 45.2 Main causes of rectal bleeding in childhood

Conditions marked with a bullet point are discussed in this section of the book

Painful
● Anal fissure
  Intussusception (discussed earlier, see p. 596)
● Meckel's diverticulum
  Gastroenteritis—*Campylobacter* more common than *Shigella* or *Salmonella*
  Henoch–Schönlein purpura—rash on lower limbs
  Inflammatory bowel disease—Crohn's disease or ulcerative colitis
  Trauma—consider sexual abuse

Painless
● Polyps—usually solitary hamartomas, sometimes familial adenomatous polyposis
  Arteriovenous malformations

KEY POINTS

Box 45.1 Organic causes of chronic or recurrent abdominal pain in children
● Chronic constipation—common
● Hydronephrosis—uncommon
● Recurrent appendicitis—rare
● Crohn's disease—rare
● Gallstones—rare, sometimes associated with haemolytic anaemia
● Peptic ulceration—rare

ANAL FISSURE

Anal fissure occurs at any age during infancy and childhood and is probably initiated by straining to pass a large hard stool. The condition is readily diagnosed when digital rectal examination is found to be impossible because of extreme tenderness; the posterior end of the fissure may sometimes be seen by parting the buttocks. Treatment involves gentle anal dilatation under general anaesthesia, followed by measures to prevent constipation.

MECKEL'S DIVERTICULUM

Meckel's diverticulum is present in less than 2% of the population. It represents the embryological remnant of the **vitello-intestinal duct** which joined the fetal midgut and yolk sac. The diverticulum is situated on the antimesenteric border of the distal ileum about 60 cm from the ileo-caecal junction. Meckel's diverticula are usually asymptomatic but may cause rectal bleeding or become inflamed and perforate.

Meckel's diverticula often contain a variety of gut-related tissues. These include **ectopic acid-secreting gastric mucosa**, which may cause peptic ulceration. In children below 2 years, this is an important cause of rectal bleeding which may require transfusion. In older children, the ectopic gastric mucosa more often causes chronic occult bleeding, leading to iron deficiency anaemia. Much less commonly, peptic ulceration in a Meckel's diverticulum results in **perforation**.

If a Meckel's diverticulum is suspected as the cause of rectal bleeding, an attempt is made to confirm the diagnosis by radionuclide Meckel's scanning. An isotope is chosen which is concentrated in gastric mucosa. A negative scan does not, however, exclude the diagnosis and laparotomy may have to be performed to examine the bowel directly.

If the neck is narrow, a Meckel's diverticulum may become inflamed in a manner identical to appendicitis and cause similar symptoms and signs (see Fig. 19.4, p. 270). The diagnosis is only made at operation. As with appendicitis, the complications of gangrenous inflammation are perforation and peritonitis. Unlike the complications of peptic ulceration and bleeding, Meckel's diverticulitis is uncommon in children under 10 years of age and occurs in older children, adolescents and young adults.

POLYPS

Hamartomatous polyps are a common cause of rectal bleeding in children. They are nearly always single and usually occur in the rectum or sigmoid colon. They may occur elsewhere in the colon and occasionally in the small intestine. Polyps in children are almost never malignant. **Familial adenomatous polyposis** may present in childhood with rectal bleeding. As described in Chapter 20, polyps of this type inevitably turn malignant from about the age of 16 onwards. There may be a family history.

Rectal bleeding is investigated as for adults with digital examination followed by proctoscopy and sigmoidoscopy. If a polyp is seen, it is removed by diathermy snare. If no polyp is visible, colonoscopy is performed and any identified polyps removed by snare.

RECTAL PROLAPSE

Transient rectal prolapse is a common and alarming childhood problem, usually occurring during the first 2 years of life. The most common cause is excessive straining during defecation but it may be a presenting feature of cystic fibrosis. The majority of prolapses can be gently manipulated back into position without causing pain and will not recur if the stool is kept soft. If the problem is persistent or recurrent, proctoscopy and sigmoidoscopy are indicated. A rectal polyp is occasionally responsible, and can be removed by diathermy snare. If simple stool-softening measures fail to prevent recurrence, submucosal injections of phenol in oil are used to induce fibrosis. In the rare event of this failing, a perianal subcutaneous suture may be inserted.

ABDOMINAL MASS

An abdominal mass is an uncommon reason for surgical referral in children. It may be caused by a malignant embryonal tumour, most often a **nephroblastoma** (Wilms' tumour). Other causes of a mass include **hydronephrosis** and **post-traumatic pancreatic pseudocyst**.

NEPHROBLASTOMA

Nephroblastoma presents in early childhood, usually before the age of 3 years. The tumour arises in the kidney from embryonal renal tissue, hence the term nephroblastoma. The tumours are locally invasive and metastasise to the regional nodes, liver, lungs and bone. Often, a large abdominal mass is noticed by the mother as the child is bathed (see Fig. 45.6). The mass is sometimes so large as to obscure its site of origin. Less common presenting features include haematuria, anorexia, weight loss, pyrexia and hypertension.

When surgery was the only treatment available, the cure rate was only about 10%. The modern combination of surgical resection, radiotherapy and chemotherapy

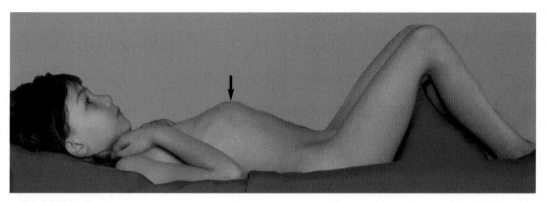

Fig. 45.6 Nephroblastoma
This 9-year-old girl presented with a large unilateral mass (arrowed), which was later confirmed to be arising from the left kidney (Wilms' tumour or nephroblastoma).

gives an excellent chance of complete cure even when distant metastases are present.

NEUROBLASTOMA

Another embryonal tumour occurring in early childhood is the neuroblastoma. This is a highly malignant tumour arising from embryonal sympathetic nervous tissue in the adrenal gland or sympathetic chain. A less aggressive variant is the **ganglioblastoma**. This tumour sometimes presents as an abdominal mass but the usual presentation is failure to thrive. The standard treatment is a combination of surgical resection, chemotherapy and radiotherapy, but the prognosis is poor.

UROLOGICAL DISORDERS IN CHILDREN

All of the important urological disorders in children have a congenital origin, although not all congenital disorders of the urinary system present in childhood. The congenital urinary tract disorders and their clinical presentations are illustrated in Table 45.1 and the important remediable disorders are described below.

VESICOURETERIC REFLUX

As described in detail in Chapter 33 and elsewhere, anatomical and functional abnormalities of the urinary tract strongly predispose to urinary tract infections. This is particularly true in children, where the commonest abnormality is **vesicoureteric reflux**. For this reason, a single bacteriologically proven urinary tract infection in a boy, and two or more in a girl, are indications for radiological or radionuclide investigation. Indeed, between 30 and 50% of children so investigated are found to have vesicoureteric reflux.

PATHOPHYSIOLOGY

In the normal individual, the distal ureter takes an oblique course through the muscular bladder wall so that detrusor contraction during voiding acts as a sphincter, preventing urine from refluxing from the bladder into the ureters (the **anti-reflux mechanism**). Vesicoureteric reflux most commonly results from a minor congenital (often familial) abnormality of ureteric insertion, but may also be caused by other morphological abnormalities such as ectopic or duplex ureters, congenital megaureter (a peristaltic abnormality), bladder outlet obstruction, neuropathic bladder or previous surgical procedures to the lower end of the ureter.

Reflux of sterile urine into the pelvicalyceal system during early childhood probably causes impairment of normal renal development and function. This is exacerbated by rises in back-pressure and is greatly enhanced by bacterial infection, possibly even a single episode. Vesicoureteric reflux of grade I and II (see Box 45.3) appears to cause little damage but grades III and IV are associated with radiological 'clubbing' and distortion of calyces and patchy loss of renal cortical substance; this is known as **reflux nephropathy**. Untreated reflux nephropathy may cause progressive irreversible renal damage and, if bilateral, may eventually result in renal failure.

CLINICAL PRESENTATION AND INVESTIGATION

Children of any age may present with isolated or recurrent upper urinary tract infections. Girls are more

Table 45.1 Congenital urinary tract disorders and their presentation (conditions presenting at birth or in childhood are marked with an asterisk)

Nature of abnormality	Presentation
a. Kidney	
Bilateral agenesis (Potter's syndrome)	Oligohydramnios in pregnancy, stillborn infant with characteristic appearance of face and ears
Unilateral agenesis, aplasia or hypoplasia	Usually an incidental finding at any age. Often some abnormality on the other side
Multicystic kidney: usually unilateral dysplasia of kidney with multiple cysts	Usually presents in the neonate as abdominal mass. Fatal if bilateral
Infantile polycystic disease: bilateral inherited disorder in which multiple small cysts replace renal parenchyma. Liver and pancreatic cysts often present also	Usually presents as gross abdominal distension in the neonate due to huge non-functioning kidneys. Invariably fatal.
Medullary sponge kidney: cystic dilatation of collecting ducts of one or more medullary pyramids in one or both kidneys	May be found incidentally or during investigations for urinary infection. Cysts tend to become calcified and have characteristic X-ray appearance
Adult polycystic kidney: autosomal dominant disorder with multiple cysts throughout the parenchyma	Usually presents after age 30 with chronic renal failure, hypertension, haematuria or recurrent urinary tract infections
Solitary cysts: usually develop at one pole	Often incidental finding. May present with loin swelling or pain
Horseshoe kidney: fusion of lower poles of kidneys preventing normal developmental ascent	Often found incidentally but may cause hydronephrosis due to pelviureteric obstruction
Ectopic kidneys and abnormalities of rotation due to failure of developmental ascent	Found incidentally or during investigation of complications such as pelviureteric obstruction
b. Pelvicalyceal system and ureters	
Pelvic hydronephrosis: dilatation of pelvicalyceal system due to congenital stenosis at pelviureteric junction	Usually presents in childhood or adolescence with loin pain or mass
Megaureter: abnormality of peristalsis of lower ureter resulting in gross proximal dilatation	Presents in young children as recurrent urinary tract infections
Ureterocoele: cystic dilatation of intravesical part of ureter due to stenosis of ureteric orifice	Incidental finding or may cause infection or symptoms of obstruction
Vesicoureteric reflux: unilateral or bilateral abnormality of ureteric insertion into bladder	Presents in children as recurrent pyelonephritis which can cause severe damage to developing kidney
Duplex systems: partial or complete duplication of a ureter	Often incidental finding or cause of recurrent infection
Ectopic ureter: ureter does not open into the bladder but into some other part of the genital tract e.g. vagina	In females presents as dribbling incontinence and in males as recurrent urinary tract infections
c. Bladder and urethra	
Agenesis of bladder: associated with other major abnormalities of genitourinary system	Present at birth and often fatal; very rare
Bladder hypoplasia: associated with some cases of hypospadias in boys or ectopic ureters in girls	Bladder distends once ureters or hypospadias is corrected
Urachal abnormalities i.e. cyst, sinus, patent urachus: due to persistence of urachal remnants	Patent urachus usually presents in childhood with urine dribbling from umbilicus. Cysts and sinuses may present in adulthood. Adenocarcinoma sometimes develops in the urachal remnant
Bladder diverticulum: forms by herniation of mucosa through defect in muscular wall. In adults, usually due to bladder outlet obstruction; in children, due to congenital urethral valves	Usually presents as recurrent urinary tract infection
Bladder exstrophy: incomplete closure of lower abdominal wall in midline	Gross abnormality of genitourinary system obvious at birth
Urethral valves: usually occur in posterior urethra causing varying degrees of obstruction. More distal valves cause less obstruction	Severe cases present in the neonate with gross obstructive effects, renal failure and infection. Milder cases present later with recurrent infection

Table 45.1 Continued

Nature of abnormality	Presentation
Epispadias: urethral meatus located in abnormal position somewhere on dorsum of penis. Often associated with major abnormality of penis	Obvious at birth
Hypospadias: urethra opens in abnormal position on ventral aspect of penis due to defective urethral fold. The prepuce is 'hooded' and incomplete ventrally. Distal urethra hypoplastic and shortened. The abnormally placed external urethral opening may be on the corona of the glans or further back, even as far as the penoscrotal junction. In this position, the possibility of intersex should be considered.	Major cases obvious at birth. Minor cases have downward deviation of urinary stream. Sometimes a degree of *chordee* (downward bend of the penis)

prone to infection than boys because of short urethra and its proximity to the anus. Infants or young children with urinary tract infections may not exhibit symptoms and signs specific to the urinary tract and the diagnosis is often made on investigation of vomiting, fever or failure to thrive. Older children more typically suffer incontinence, frequency or dysuria or abdominal pain and tenderness.

Clinical examination seeks evidence of abnormal external genitalia, spina bifida and impaired perineal innervation (perineal sensation and anal sphincter tone).

To demonstrate reflux, two methods can be used: micturating cystography or radionuclide cystography. **Micturating cystography** (Fig. 45.7) has been the standard investigation and involves injecting contrast medium into the bladder via a urinary catheter. The catheter is then removed and X-rays are taken while the child voids urine. The radiological grades of reflux severity are shown in Box 45.3 and provide a useful guide to the likelihood of future renal damage. More recently, static and dynamic **isotope studies** have been introduced, particularly for investigating children suspected of reflux and for long-term follow-up of children known to have reflux. Isotope studies also provide additional information. DMSA, bound to renal tubules, demonstrates cortical scarring, while DTPA estimates glomerular filtration rate in each kidney

(differential function) and reveals sites of urinary tract obstruction. Other isotopes are also employed (see Ch. 2).

MANAGEMENT OF VESICOURETERIC REFLUX

If there are no other anatomical abnormalities and the ureter is not dilated (i.e. grades I and II), then there is an 85% chance of spontaneous resolution of vesicoureteric reflux as the child grows. In the meantime, the urinary tract must be kept free of infection. This is done by encouraging regular voiding and a high fluid intake,

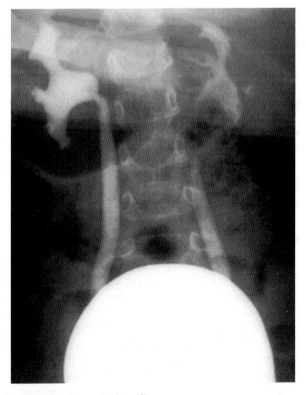

Fig. 45.7 Vesicoureteric reflux
Micturating cysto-urethrogram (MCU) in a child with recurrent urinary tract infections. On voiding, the right ureter and pelvicalyceal system filled with contrast. This is defined as grade IV reflux.

KEY POINTS

Box 45.3 Grades of vesicoureteric reflux on micturating cystography

Grade I—reflux into lower ureter only on micturition

Grade II—reflux into renal pelvis on micturition but no ureteric dilatation

Grade III—constant reflux into renal pelvis but no ureteric dilatation

Grade IV—constant reflux into renal pelvis with ureteric dilatation

avoiding constipation and maintaining perineal hygiene. At the same time, the child is maintained on continuous **anti-bacterial chemotherapy** (such as cotrimoxazole) until the danger of reflux is past. The child is followed up regularly, charting the progress of growth and development, blood pressure and serum creatinine. Radiography or radionuclide investigation of the urinary tract is repeated annually.

Surgical correction is required for more severe reflux with dilated ureters (i.e. grades III and IV) and for other obvious anatomical abnormalities. Surgery is also indicated for children who fail to progress on conservative management. The operations for simple reflux aim to **reimplant the ureter** in the bladder wall so that a length of it lies deep to the bladder mucosa; this is flattened by intraluminal pressure during voiding, thus restoring an anti-reflux mechanism.

After operation, if there is no renal scarring, the child can be discharged from follow-up. If there is unilateral scarring, the blood pressure should be monitored long-term because of the risk of hypertension. If both kidneys are damaged, renal function must be monitored as well because of the risk of deterioration.

PELVIURETERIC JUNCTION OBSTRUCTION

PATHOPHYSIOLOGY

Obstruction at the pelviureteric junction (PUJ) may appear at any age from birth through to the end of the fourth decade. It presents with dilatation of the renal pelvis and calyces (**hydronephrosis**). The cause of obstruction may not be physical narrowing but instead a functional abnormality of the 'sphincter' mechanism. This normally prevents reflux of ureteric urine into the kidney when the ureters contract.

Obstruction at the PUJ increases the pressure in the collecting system and causes deterioration in renal function. Stasis predisposes to infection.

CLINICAL PRESENTATION AND DIAGNOSIS

Many patients with PUJ obstruction go undetected. Many others are discovered by chance on urography during investigation of an unrelated condition. Even in symptomatic patients, the condition may be intermittent. Some patients complain of aching pain in the renal area; others suffer bouts of severe abdominal or loin pain, sometimes with haematuria. The precipitating factor is often not identifiable, but symptoms are sometimes exacerbated by drinking large volumes of fluid or by changes in posture.

In many patients, the diagnosis can be made on a standard IVU. The typical changes on the affected side are a **prolonged nephrogram** and a **negative pyelogram** (i.e. contrast persists in the renal cortex without opacifying the pelvis), **delayed drainage of contrast** from an often dilated renal pelvis, or a combination of these features. The only reliable sign, however, is **spontaneous extravasation** of contrast into parenchymal lymphatics. This is seen as 'contrast streaking' in the renal cortex.

A dilated renal pelvis on a standard urogram may just represent harmless stasis without obstruction, and diagnostic features of PUJ obstruction may become apparent only if a diuretic is given at the same time. A **radionuclide diuretic renogram** is a better way of distinguishing between simple stasis and stasis with obstruction: a characteristic isotope excretion curve is seen in about 80% of PUJ obstructions. The remainder are difficult to diagnose, requiring percutaneous intubation of the renal pelvis and sophisticated pressure and flow measurements (**the Whitaker test**).

MANAGEMENT

If PUJ obstruction is proved in symptomatic patients, particularly if renal function is impaired, operative treatment is required. The aim is to enlarge the pelviureteric junction; this is known as **pyeloplasty**. Results are generally favourable but recovery of renal function may be incomplete.

HYPOSPADIAS AND EPISPADIAS

Hypospadias is a common congenital abnormality of the penis and urethra. It occurs in about 1 in 400 male births. The distal urethra fails to develop normally, so that the urethral meatus lies somewhere along the ventral surface of the penis from the glans to the perineum (see Fig. 45.8). The remnant of urethral tissue distal to the meatus is fibrotic, causing the penis to bend downwards on erection. This is known as **chordee**. The more proximal the urethral meatus, the worse the chordee. In addition, the ventral part of the foreskin is absent giving rise to a hooded appearance.

Repair is a highly specialised procedure and utilises the hood of the foreskin; thus circumcision should **never** be carried out without specialist advice.

Epispadias is much less common and may be associated with other major genitourinary abnormalities. In epispadias, the urethral meatus is on the dorsal aspect of the penis.

URETHRAL VALVES

Urethral valves are congenital mucosal folds which may occur in the posterior male urethra. They impede or

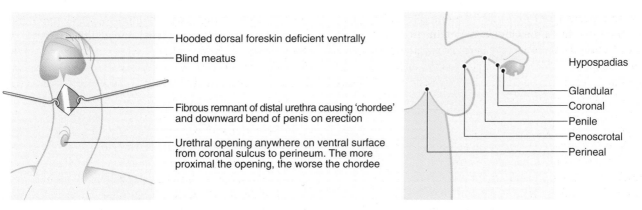

Hooded dorsal foreskin deficient ventrally

Blind meatus

Fibrous remnant of distal urethra causing 'chordee' and downward bend of penis on erection

Urethral opening anywhere on ventral surface from coronal sulcus to perineum. The more proximal the opening, the worse the chordee

Hypospadias

Glandular
Coronal
Penile
Penoscrotal
Perineal

Fig. 45.8 Hypospadias

completely obstruct urinary flow. Complete obstruction becomes apparent soon after birth but partial obstruction may easily be overlooked. In either case, the back-pressure effects on the urinary tract soon lead to renal failure. Treatment is by endoscopic division of the valves as soon as possible.

Management problems of surgical in-patients

Medical problems in surgical patients

INTRODUCTION

'Medical' disorders appear in surgical practice in four main ways:

- A pre-existing medical condition may cause a surgical admission because of progression, exacerbation or complications: for example, foot problems in patients with diabetes
- A surgical condition may be complicated by an unrelated medical disorder. For example, a patient with rheumatoid arthritis on steroid therapy is vulnerable to impaired healing and recurrent infection
- A pre-existing medical condition may be exacerbated by operation. In chronic bronchitis (chronic obstructive pulmonary disease), for example, general anaesthesia and postoperative sputum retention may precipitate a life-threatening pneumonia.
- An occult condition can become manifest under the stress of anaesthesia and operation. For example, postoperative myocardial infarction can be caused by occult ischaemic heart disease

CARDIAC AND CEREBROVASCULAR

Many surgical patients are elderly and thus have an increased risk of cardiovascular disease. Together with respiratory disorders, cardiovascular disorders account for most postoperative medical complications. Atherosclerosis is the most common cause of cardiovascular disease complicating surgery.

In this context, there are six main categories of cardiovascular disorder (although more than one may occur in the same patient):

1. Ischaemic heart disease
2. Cardiac failure
3. Arrhythmias
4. Hypertension
5. Cerebrovascular disease
6. Valvular heart disease

Emergency surgery in patients with cardiac disease is about four times more likely to result in death compared with the same operation done electively. Thus, pre-operative assessment is particularly important in emergency patients so that any cardiac condition can be stabilised, electrolyte imbalance corrected and appropriate anaesthesia, surgical technique, monitoring and aftercare employed to minimise risk.

1. ISCHAEMIC HEART DISEASE

The most common clinical manifestations of ischaemic heart disease are:

- Angina and previous myocardial infarction
- Cardiac failure
- Arrhythmias such as atrial fibrillation

Asymptomatic myocardial ischaemia may progress to infarction under the various stresses of anaesthesia and operation. These stresses include laryngoscopy and endotracheal intubation, pain, hypoxia, rapid blood loss, anaemia, hypotension, hypocarbia and fluid overload. For major operations, general anaesthesia and spinal anaesthesia carry similar risks; for minor procedures, local anaesthesia is far safer.

Clinical problems

a. Unstable coronary syndromes
Stable angina poses little increased risk during operation but unstable or severe angina or a myocardial infarction within the previous 30 days is a major risk factor and indicates the need for intensive management and delaying the operation, if practicable. Nitrates, which dilate

the coronary arteries and reduce preload and left ventricular work, protect the heart during general anaesthesia and should not be stopped in the perioperative period. A transdermal patch is a useful alternative to tablets. Beta-adrenergic blockers, which reduce cardiac work and oxygen demand, should be continued unless non-ischaemic cardiac failure develops.

b. Myocardial infarction

Myocardial infarction associated with surgery usually occurs during the first few days after operation, not during the operation. Typical chest pain is not always a feature—postoperative infarction may present 'silently' with acute hypotension, cardiac failure, arrhythmias or cardiac arrest, particularly in diabetics. Diagnosis can usually be made by typical electrocardiograph (ECG) changes, especially if a preoperative ECG is available. Creatine kinase (CK) and lactate dehydrogenase (LDH) are released from surgically damaged skeletal muscle, but measurement of the cardiospecific isoenzyme CK-MB is helpful in making a diagnosis of myocardial infarction, particularly when its value is expressed as a percentage of total creatine kinase.

Preoperative assessment of ischaemic heart disease

The cardiac history should include questions about previous myocardial infarction, angina and particularly exercise tolerance—for example, on stairs.

An ECG should be performed before operation on all patients over 60 years of age and on any patient with cardiac symptoms or signs. Preoperative ECGs may show arrhythmias, ischaemic changes or evidence of previous infarction. They are also worth their weight in gold during the 3 a.m. assessment of a postoperative patient with chest pain!

In patients undergoing major surgery, particularly vascular surgery, a preoperative exercise test with ECG may give useful information about the patient's ability to exercise and about exercise-induced ischaemic changes. However, ECG changes and symptoms of angina come relatively late in the evolution of myocardial ischaemia. If there is concern from the history or the resting or exercise ECG that there may be a major risk of cardio-vascular disease, then angiography with appropriate revascularisation (if possible) is the best course of action.

2. CARDIAC FAILURE

Cardiac failure needs to be stabilised before operation, but even if it is, it is important to be aware that there is still a significantly higher mortality rate after major surgery of up to 5%. Causes, symptoms and signs of cardiac failure are shown in Box 46.1.

KEY POINTS

Box 46.1 Cardiac failure

Causes
- Ischaemic heart disease*
- Hypertension*
- Valvular disease
- Arrhythmias
- Thyrotoxicosis
- Severe anaemia

Symptoms
- Dyspnoea
- Lethargy
- Loss of appetite

Signs
- Dependent oedema
- Raised jugular venous pressure
- Tachycardia
- Peripheral cyanosis

*Common

Clinical problems

a. Treated cardiac failure

Treatment may be inadequate and, if so, must be corrected before operation. Plasma urea, electrolytes and creatinine should be measured before operation because patients taking diuretics and angiotensin-converting enzyme (ACE) inhibitors may have abnormalities of fluid and electrolytes, such as chronic dehydration or hypokalaemia.

Over-treatment with diuretics may cause:

- Thirst
- Postural hypotension
- Low serum sodium concentration
- Raised serum urea and creatinine
- Low serum potassium (usually due to potassium-losing diuretics prescribed without potassium supplements)

b. Cardiac failure discovered before operation

Operation should be postponed until cardiac failure is treated and stabilised. Hasty preoperative diuretic therapy is dangerous because it may provoke dehydration and electrolyte abnormalities. Vasodilatation caused by general anaesthesia lowers the blood pressure and may precipitate acute myocardial infarction or a cerebrovascular accident.

c. Cardiac failure developing during or after operation

This problem most often results from poor tolerance of intravenous fluids or unaccustomed supine posture. Prompt and vigorous diuretic therapy with intravenous frusemide is required to prevent worsening cardiac failure, hypoxia, renal failure or other potentially lethal complications. Postoperative cardiac failure is best managed in an intensive care unit, using a central venous pressure (CVP) line to guide fluid replacement. In severe cases, a pulmonary flotation catheter (Swann– Ganz catheter) should be used to monitor left atrial pressure. Perioperative cardiac failure may also be precipitated by myocardial infarction, severe angina or arrhythmias such as atrial fibrillation.

Preoperative assessment of cardiac failure

Chest X-ray will demonstrate cardiomegaly and may show signs of pulmonary oedema. These include upper lobe diversion, hilar congestion, septal Kerley B lines and pleural effusions. ECG may show an arrhythmia, myocardial ischaemia, ventricular hypertrophy, left bundle branch block or loss of R waves. If there is any doubt about the fitness of a patient for operation, a cardiological opinion should be sought.

3. CARDIAC ARRHYTHMIAS

Clinical problems

a. Atrial fibrillation
This is usually secondary to ischaemic heart disease but may be caused by mitral valve disease or thyrotoxicosis. Atrial fibrillation with a controlled ventricular rate (i.e. a pulse rate of less than 90 beats per minute at rest) causes minimal extra risk. Uncontrolled fibrillation may cause perioperative cardiac failure. Even controlled atrial fibrillation increases the risk of **arterial embolism** from any thrombus present in the left atrium. Adequate control of ventricular rate should be achieved before operation with digoxin, occasionally supplemented with verapamil, amiodarone or beta-adrenergic blockade. Digoxin can be given intravenously if rapid control is necessary. The question of anticoagulation should be considered, particularly if the patient has experienced any arterial embolic events. In such cases, stabilising the patient on long-term warfarin prior to operation and maintaining it over the perioperative period and afterwards may be the best option. The use of perioperative heparin is favoured by some, but the anticoagulation is more brittle, with greater risk of over-anticoagulation.

The therapeutic range of digoxin is narrow. Toxicity occurs if the dose is excessive or if renal excretion is impaired. The elderly and those with hypokalaemia are particularly prone to toxicity. Symptoms include anorexia, nausea and vomiting, which may be wrongly attributed to the operation. The chief concern, however, is the risk of potentially fatal ventricular arrhythmia. Assessment of patients on digoxin should include tests of renal function (plasma urea, electrolytes and creatinine) and, if toxicity is suspected, plasma digoxin levels taken 6 hours after the last dose.

b. Tachycardia
Postoperative sinus tachycardia is usually associated with hypotension, sepsis, cardiac failure, fluid overload, anxiety or, occasionally, thyrotoxicosis. Tachycardia may be the first sign of any of these problems. Primary cardiac abnormalities or phaeochromocytoma must be considered if the cause of tachycardia during operation is not apparent.

c. Bradycardia
Bradycardia may be caused by complete heart block and can be diagnosed on electrocardiography. This requires urgent **transvenous pacing** except in patients in whom it results from an acute myocardial infarction without haemodynamic compromise. If the onset of sinus bradycardia or another atrial arrhythmia (particularly atrial fibrillation) is associated with right bundle branch block, this suggests a diagnosis of pulmonary embolism.

Excessive digoxin or beta blockade may cause bradycardia. If the apex rate is below 60 beats per minute, that day's dose should be omitted and the regular dose reviewed.

A temporary or permanent **cardiac pacemaker** is not a particular problem for general anaesthesia. However, a surgical diathermy machine used too close to the control box may cause inhibition of a permanent system. In this

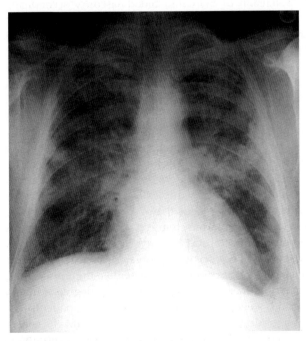

Fig. 46.1 Heart failure
This plain PA chest X-ray in a patient with heart failure shows cardiomegaly, upper lobe diversion and hilar congestion. Kerley B septal lines were present in the original film but are not visible in this reproduced image.

case, a bipolar diathermy machine may be safely used instead.

d. Other arrhythmias

Bifascicular block, in which conduction is impaired down two of the three main fascicles (right bundle plus anterior or posterior divisions of the left bundle), may progress to complete heart block (and low cardiac output) under anaesthesia. For these patients, a prophylactic temporary transvenous pacemaker should be considered before operation.

e. Arrhythmias developing during general anaesthesia

Arrhythmias developing under general anaesthesia may be precipitated by hypoxia, hypercapnia and hypo- or hyperkalaemia. Inadequately treated cardiac failure also predisposes to atrial arrhythmias. Preoperative investigations include ECG, full blood count, plasma electrolytes and digoxin level if appropriate.

4. HYPERTENSION

About one in four patients coming to surgery is either hypertensive or receiving antihypertensive therapy. Most have **essential hypertension**, but other causes include oral contraceptives, renal parenchymal disease, renal artery stenosis and phaeochromocytoma.

Clinical problems

a. Mild-to-moderate essential hypertension

Patients with a systolic pressure of less than 180 mmHg and a diastolic less than 110 mmHg are at minimal risk of cardiac complications unless there is some other cardiovascular disease. Sometimes, anxiety about the operation contributes to the hypertension and the blood pressure falls with preoperative bed rest. A labile blood pressure may, however, indicate widespread atherosclerosis.

b. Treated hypertension

Diuretic therapy may cause fluid and electrolyte abnormalities. These should be corrected before operation. Most common antihypertensive drugs are cardioprotective and should not usually be stopped prior to general anaesthesia. These drugs include beta-adrenergic blockers, calcium antagonists, ACE inhibitors, vasodilators and methyldopa. Postural hypotension may occur after operation, especially if there is dehydration.

Despite the patient being 'nil by mouth' in the immediate preoperative period, the normal dose of oral antihypertensive drugs should usually be given with a small amount of water. Sudden withdrawal of hypotensive drugs may cause rebound hypertension. Withdrawal of beta

blockers may trigger autonomic hyperactivity and lability of blood pressure.

c. Severe or poorly controlled hypertension

These patients are at high risk of perioperative cardiac failure or stroke, particularly if there are swings of blood pressure. Unrecognised phaeochromocytoma may also cause uncontrollable cardiovascular abnormalities during anaesthesia and has a high mortality rate. Severely hypertensive or poorly controlled hypertensive patients should not undergo general anaesthesia and surgery until adequately treated.

Preoperative assessment of hypertensive patients

Chest X-ray may identify cardiomegaly or cardiac failure. An ECG may reveal signs of ventricular hypertrophy and ischaemia. Serum urea and electrolytes should be measured in all patients on diuretics and in any patient with suspected chronic renal failure. Most hypertensive patients can be stabilised on an outpatient basis but occasionally, a severely hypertensive patient may need to be admitted to hospital a few days before operation for stabilisation.

5. CEREBROVASCULAR DISEASE

Cerebral atherosclerosis may render the blood flow to the brain precarious. These patients have a high risk of stroke during the perioperative period from hypoxia, hypotension or increased blood viscosity secondary to dehydration. Cerebrovascular disease should be suspected if there is a history of stroke or transient ischaemic attacks (TIAs). Patients with ischaemic heart disease or peripheral vascular disease should also be assumed to have cerebrovascular disease and, at the least, the carotid arteries should be auscultated for bruits. Ideally, a duplex Doppler examination of the carotids should be performed in high-risk patients.

The main surgical problems relate to patients who have had a previous stroke or who give a history of transient ischaemic attacks. In these, the carotid arteries should be assessed by duplex Doppler scanning. Patients with a stenosis greater than 70% should be considered for carotid endarterectomy if conditions permit. An asymptomatic carotid bruit discovered on preoperative examination is a separate problem. About 12% of people over 60 will have a bruit but neither the presence of a bruit nor its quality correlates with the degree of internal carotid stenosis. Indeed, about 30% of patients with high-grade (70–90%) stenosis have no bruit. In general, management is conservative, particularly if the stenosis is less than 60%. However, a large trial comparing prophylactic surgery against conservative management in patients with > 60% stenosis showed surgery reduced risk of ipsilateral stroke from 11% in the medically treated group to 5%, even after taking surgical deaths into account.

If possible, operation should be avoided for at least 2 months after a stroke. Other than that, there are very few specific measures which will reduce cerebrovascular complications, although there are good reasons for prescribing low-dose aspirin (75–150 mg daily) to inhibit platelet aggregation. However, patients on aspirin tend to bleed excessively when undergoing major surgery. The anaesthetist should be warned of any signs or symptoms suggestive of carotid artery disease so that special care can be taken to avoid hypotension during surgery.

6. VALVULAR HEART DISEASE

The common valvular abnormalities are listed here in decreasing order of frequency: mitral regurgitation, aortic stenosis, aortic regurgitation and mitral stenosis. Any of these may dangerously alter cardiovascular dynamics, but stenotic lesions are more serious than regurgitant ones.

Under perioperative stress, valvular disease may precipitate acute myocardial ischaemia, hypotension, cardiac failure, arrhythmias or thromboembolism. Valvular heart disease also predisposes to infective endocarditis. Thus certain operations need to be covered by antibiotic prophylaxis.

Aortic stenosis

Aortic stenosis is potentially the most serious valvular disorder in a surgical patient because it limits the cardiac output. The patient may already be functioning close to the limit, with little reserve. Aortic stenosis usually occurs in elderly patients and must be distinguished from the innocent flow murmur of **aortic sclerosis**, which is more common. Innocent aortic murmurs are systolic (and never diastolic), soft, short and localised.

Clinical signs of aortic stenosis are:

● Slow rising upstroke of carotid pulse
● A systolic murmur radiating into the neck
● Hyperdynamic apex beat indicating left ventricular hypertrophy. (*Note*: the apex beat is only displaced laterally if aortic stenosis coexists with aortic regurgitation or is complicated by cardiac failure)
● Left ventricular hypertrophy on ECG

If aortic stenosis is suspected, an echocardiogram with Doppler assessment of the gradient across the valve is an important part of preoperative assessment.

Clinical problems of valvular heart disease

a. History of rheumatic heart disease without significant symptoms or signs
The patient may or may not have a cardiac murmur, but when a murmur is present, this has often been assessed previously and any functional deficit documented. If not,

specialist preoperative cardiological assessment is essential. In most patients, there is no special risk for general anaesthesia or surgery but antibiotic prophylaxis must be considered. Rheumatic heart disease is becoming a rarity in developed countries but is still common in many developing countries.

b. Murmur found at preoperative examination without evidence of rheumatic heart disease
This may be an innocent flow murmur, as in aortic sclerosis of the elderly, or may indicate a hyperdynamic circulation associated with anxiety or pregnancy. If there is doubt about the innocence of the murmur, a specialist opinion should be obtained. Operation may have to be deferred.

c. Symptomatic valvular disease
These conditions are potentially dangerous and require full preoperative assessment and treatment. Major valvular heart disease may be discovered in recent immigrants from under-developed countries where **rheumatic heart disease** is prevalent. Patients with valvular heart disease undergoing general anaesthesia require monitoring of cardiac function during operation and probably intensive care afterwards.

d. Prosthetic valves
Replacement valves carry the greatest risk of infective endocarditis. For these patients, antibiotic prophylaxis is required for most invasive procedures.

Patients with mechanical valves are usually maintained on permanent oral warfarin anticoagulation and it is important to maintain this to prevent valve thrombosis, which is a potentially fatal condition. Patients with bioprosthetic valves (pig valves) do not usually require anticoagulation.

Anticoagulation is often reduced before operation; for many operations it is safe to continue warfarin therapy in the lower range of prothrombin ratios (1.5–2.0). Agreement with a haematologist or the patient's anticoagulant clinic is advisable. If much bleeding is anticipated, some surgeons prefer to stop warfarin 2 days before operation and substitute intravenous heparin. For patients with mitral valve prostheses where the risk of thrombosis is high, full heparinisation is carefully maintained throughout the operative period. For other patients, heparin can be stopped 12 hours before operation and restarted once the danger of bleeding is over. The advantage of heparin over warfarin is that its effects can be quickly reversed by stopping the infusion or with **protamine** if bleeding is excessive.

INFECTIVE ENDOCARDITIS AND INDICATIONS FOR ANTIBIOTIC PROPHYLAXIS
When blood is forced under pressure through a narrow

orifice, laminar flow is disrupted, and eddy currents predispose to local thrombus formation and deposition of circulating bacteria. The vegetations of infective endocarditis are thus formed on the low-pressure side of the jet of blood passing through a damaged valve or a ventricular septal defect. The left side of the heart is more susceptible than the right because of the higher pressures and greater potential for turbulence.

Streptococcus viridans is the most common causative organism. Other bacteria such as coliforms, or fungi such as *Candida*, may also be responsible. Many types of operation and some invasive investigations cause a transient bacteraemia. Although the incidence of infective endocarditis following such procedures is small, the consequences may be catastrophic. The efficacy of prophylactic antibiotics is not absolutely proven, but it is all that is available. The relative risks associated with various cardiac and valvular lesions are summarised in Box 46.2. The procedures most likely to cause bacteraemia are shown in Box 46.3.

The choice of prophylactic antibiotics and the dose regimen depend on the anticipated organisms and the operative procedure. Local protocols may be available. Alternatively, a hospital microbiologist may be consulted or a regimen from a national publication such as the *British National Formulary* used.

RESPIRATORY DISEASES

Respiratory complications occur in up to 15% of surgical patients and are the leading cause of postoperative mortality in the elderly. The main postoperative complications are atelectasis, aspiration pneumonitis and pneumonia. The risk of a respiratory complication is associated with the duration of the anaesthetic. It is greatly increased by pre-existing respiratory disease like chronic airflow limitation, asthma or bronchiectasis. Other important factors include smoking, cardiac failure, obesity, old age and general debility.

CLINICAL PROBLEMS

a. Chronic obstructive pulmonary disease (also known as chronic obstructive airway disease and chronic bronchitis)
Chronic bronchitis and emphysema are common. They strongly predispose to postoperative chest complications, particularly bronchopneumonia, lobar collapse and pneumothorax. There is often a degree of reversible bronchoconstriction, and this can be assessed before operation by measuring peak expiratory flow before and after treatment with a bronchodilator.

Other chronic lung diseases include bronchiectasis, pneumoconiosis, pulmonary fibrosis, sarcoidosis and pulmonary tuberculosis.

KEY POINTS

Box 46.2 Cardiovascular lesions at risk of infective endocarditis and indications for perioperative antibiotic prophylaxis

High-risk conditions requiring prophylaxis
- Prosthetic valve or other intracardiac surgery
- Rheumatic valve disease
- Congenital heart disease and aortic coarctation, whether or not corrected (Note: atrial septal defect is not a high risk)
- Degenerative valve disease
- Previous infective endocarditis

Low-risk conditions—need for prophylaxis depends on likelihood of the operative procedure inducing a bacteraemia
- Mitral valve prolapse
- Haemodialysis shunts
- Transvenous pacemakers
- Ventriculo-atrial and ventriculo-peritoneal shunts for hydrocephalus

Minimal-risk conditions not requiring antibiotic prophylaxis
- Coronary bypass grafts
- Closed patent ductus arteriosus
- Closed atrial septal defect
- Established prosthetic arterial grafts

KEY POINTS

Box 46.3 Procedures frequently associated with bacteraemia and requiring antibiotic cover in patients at risk of bacterial endocarditis

Surgical operations
- Dental extractions and other procedures involving the gums
- Tonsillectomy
- Oesophageal dilatation
- All gastrointestinal and biliary tract surgery
- Most urological procedures including endoscopy, catheter insertion and removal, transrectal prostatic biopsy
- Hysterectomy, dilatation and curettage, termination of pregnancy
- Surgery of infected wounds and tissues
- Cardiac surgery

Other procedures
- Sigmoidoscopy, colonoscopy, barium enema and liver biopsy—prophylaxis is only required for patients at high risk, e.g. prosthetic valves

The complication rate in chronic lung diseases can be greatly improved by careful preoperative assessment (including lung function tests) and treatment designed to bring the patient into optimum physical condition.

b. Cigarette smoking

Smokers have a five times greater risk of postoperative respiratory problems. This is partly due to pre-existing respiratory disease attributable to smoking. Smoking should be stopped at least 4 weeks and ideally 8 weeks before operation if any benefit is to be achieved. This gives time for recovery of respiratory functions such as bronchial ciliary activity. Stopping smoking just before surgery may actually be detrimental because of an increase in bronchial mucus production.

c. Current respiratory infections

Acute viral or bacterial upper respiratory tract infections are common in preoperative patients. The main question is whether the operation should be deferred. Patients with significant upper respiratory infections have reduced resistance to surgical trauma and infection. This alone may be grounds for cancelling an elective operation.

In children there is a particularly high risk of acute airways obstruction because of swelling of the bronchial mucosa in the narrow airways, and also because of increased secretions. This may result in lobar collapse or bronchopneumonia. There is also an element of bronchospasm in childhood infections which, when added to the already narrowed airways, leads to a difficult and dangerous anaesthetic. A 'wet' cough with a wheeze and a fever is an indication for postponing the operation until normal function is recovered. Similar factors apply in adults but to a lesser extent.

Chronic conditions associated with infection, such as bronchiectasis and cystic fibrosis, are more difficult problems. Elective operations should be carried out during periods of remission, with intensive physiotherapy and prophylactic antibiotics perioperatively.

d. Asthma

Asthma is common in children and adolescents but may occur later in life, particularly as a component of chronic airflow limitation. The main elements of asthma are bronchoconstriction, bronchial wall oedema, excessive mucus production and airway plugging. All these factors predispose to atelectasis, infection and hypoxia.

Asthmatic problems can be exacerbated by the following factors associated with general anaesthesia and surgery:

- Endotracheal intubation—causing increased airways sensitvity
- Increased airways secretions due to instrumentation or the autonomic side effects of anaesthetic drugs such as muscle relaxants

- Dehydration (increases mucus viscosity)
- Limitation of movement and posture because of pain (inhibits clearance of secretions)
- The direct effects of other drugs, e.g. bronchoconstriction with beta blockers or non-steroidal anti-inflammatory drugs (NSAIDs), or respiratory depression with morphine

In asthmatic patients, the usual medication should be continued in the perioperative period if practicable. Alternatively, inhaled preparations may be given via a nebuliser for the first 24 hours. The operation should be postponed during acute exacerbations.

e. Previous chest problems

A previous spontaneous pneumothorax may recur during anaesthesia or in the postoperative period. If respiratory function deteriorates postoperatively, the diagnosis of pneumothorax must be considered.

Previous chest surgery or radiotherapy increases the risk of postoperative infection. Physiotherapy before and after operation minimises the risk and should be arranged routinely for these patients.

f. Previous pulmonary embolus or deep venous thrombosis

These patients have a greatly increased risk of recurrent thromboembolism. Prophylactic measures are mandatory for all but the most minor procedures.

PREOPERATIVE INVESTIGATION OF RESPIRATORY DISEASE

A chest X-ray should be performed on any patient with symptoms or signs of chest disease or dysfunction or a cardiac problem. There is no need to take 'routine' chest X-rays on all preoperative patients. Studies have shown that undirected screening of asymptomatic patients has an extremely low yield of abnormalities likely to influence surgical outcome.

Appropriate lung function tests should be performed in patients with chronic lung disease. Peak flow measurements are useful to determine the extent of airflow limitation. The reversible element of bronchospasm can be assessed using peak flow measurements before and after bronchodilators. Blood gas measurements are indicated if hypoxaemia or carbon dioxide retention is likely.

PERIOPERATIVE MANAGEMENT OF RESPIRATORY DISEASE AND HIGH-RISK PATIENTS

The following measures will maximise respiratory function and reduce the risk of postoperative complications:

- **Preoperative physiotherapy**—helps to prevent postoperative chest complications. Physiotherapy

should include teaching the patient breathing exercises and correct posture
- **Drug therapy**—may need to be adjusted to achieve the optimum respiratory function. Theophyllines may be added to the therapy of asthma patients, for example, and nebulised salbutamol may improve the reversible component of chronic bronchitis. Prophylactic antibiotics are not commonly used for patients with chronic airflow limitation, but their prophylactic use in abdominal surgery may have the additional benefit of reducing infective chest complications. Preoperative bronchodilators given by inhaler or nebuliser may help to prevent an exacerbation of asthma perioperatively. Adequate hydration reduces the risk of retained secretions which might cause airways obstruction
- **Encouragement of smokers to quit**—should be started at time of booking for elective surgery. Smoking should be stopped at least 4 weeks before operation to achieve the optimum beneficial effect
- **Alternative methods of anaesthesia—local, regional or spinal**—should be considered for patients with chronic respiratory disorders but they are not necessarily the best solution. Physiotherapy and other supportive measures should be the same as for general anaesthesia. With the use of newer anaesthetic drugs and techniques, these patients may be better off with endotracheal intubation and ventilation using short-acting muscle relaxants. These techniques allow good bronchial toilet at the end of operation. In some patients, the respiratory function is better after the operation than before! Certain operations, such as transurethral resection of the prostate, are made more difficult under spinal anaesthesia if a patient with chest trouble coughs persistently during the procedure. General anaesthesia avoids this
- **Early postoperative physiotherapy**—aims to enhance deep breathing, coughing and general mobility, reducing the incidence of respiratory complications
- **Perioperative administration of intravenous steroids**—for patients on long-term steroid therapy for airways obstrution

GASTROINTESTINAL DISORDERS

The main gastrointestinal conditions giving rise to complications in surgical patients are dental problems, peptic ulcer disease and inflammatory bowel disease. Previous abdominal surgery may also complicate in-patient treatment.

DENTAL PROBLEMS

Teeth and artificial fixed crowns and bridges are vulnerable to damage during intubation. This causes not only cosmetic and medicolegal problems, but also exposes the patient to the risk of aspirating foreign bodies into the bronchi. Similarly, infected material from carious (decayed) teeth or inflamed gums may be aspirated. This causes a particularly grave aspiration pneumonia. Dentures should routinely be removed before operation for the same reason. In unconscious accident victims, the possibility of aspiration, swallowing or pharyngeal obstruction by a dental prosthesis should always be considered.

PEPTIC ULCER DISEASE

Peptic ulcer disease can be a surgical problem in its own right, but surgical patients admitted for other reasons may also have an active peptic ulcer. Whether the ulcer is causing symptoms or not, it may be exacerbated by the stresses of surgical admission. These stresses include serious illness and trauma, operations, and drugs such as aspirin, NSAIDs and corticosteroids. The result may be a sudden catastrophic **haemorrhage** (presenting as haematemesis or melaena), or occasionally **perforation**. Bleeding may also result from acute stress ulceration in the seriously ill patient. Stress ulceration is distinct from chronic peptic ulcer disease; impaired splanchnic perfusion is probably an important factor, but acid-pepsin does play a part in its pathogenesis (see Ch. 14).

Patients with known peptic ulcer disease or strongly suggestive symptoms should receive perioperative prophylaxis with **sucralfate** (a mucosal protective agent). H_2-receptor antagonists and proton pump inhibitors are also used. NSAIDs and irritant oral drugs should be avoided.

Previous gastrectomy is associated with a number of long-term side effects. These include anaemia (due to deficiency of iron, vitamin B_{12} and occasionally folate) and, rarely, osteomalacia. A full blood count should be included in the preoperative assessment of these patients.

INFLAMMATORY BOWEL DISEASE

Patients with chronic inflammatory bowel disease may be anaemic or malnourished if the disease is active. Patients may also be **steroid-dependent** because of adrenal suppression from long-term steroid therapy. Occasionally immunosuppressive drugs such as azathioprine are being taken and may increase the predisposition to infection.

PREVIOUS ABDOMINAL SURGERY

Previous abdominal surgery results in scarring and sometimes multiple adhesions in the peritoneal cavity. Further operations on the same area are more difficult and take longer. In addition, there is greater risk of damage to structures which are adherent to the operation site. These include gut, ureters and major vessels.

HEPATIC DISORDERS

Pre-existing liver disease may have important consequences in the surgical patient and generally increases the risk of postoperative morbidity and mortality. A history of jaundice must be evaluated as it may be a clue to serious risks for both patient and medical staff.

CLINICAL PROBLEMS

a. History of jaundice

A past history of jaundice raises the possibility that the patient may be a carrier of hepatitis B or C which can readily be transmitted to surgical, nursing or laboratory staff. The main danger is from needle-stick injuries. Vaccination against hepatitis B is now mandatory for health workers at occupational risk of infection. Hepatitis carriers among patients should be identified if practicable and special precautions adopted.

Most previously jaundiced patients will have suffered acute infective hepatitis (hepatitis A) which poses no risk to staff because the infective agent does not cause a chronic carrier state. In contrast, lifetime chronic hepatitis develops in 5–10% of those infected with hepatitis B virus (HBV) and in 80% of those infected with HCV.

These diseases should be suspected if the illness associated with the previous jaundice was prolonged or serious. Jaundice contracted in developing countries should be regarded with suspicion because hepatitis B and C are often endemic. Hepatitis C is becoming more common and, because of its chronicity, causes a high rate of cirrhosis in the long term; some patients progress to hepatocellular cancer. Hepatitis B and C are also common among male homosexuals and intravenous drug abusers who share syringes. The history should include questions to determine whether the patient falls into a high-risk group, and clinical examination of patients should include searching for intravenous injection sites characteristic of drug abuse. In high-risk patients, screening for hepatitis B surface antigen (HBsAg) and hepatitis C antibody should ideally be performed before any other blood test (see Ch. 1, pp. 20–21).

b. History of jaundice following anaesthesia

The anaesthetic agent halothane is believed to cause an idiosyncratic hepatotoxicity in about 1 in 30 000 patients. It is prudent to record exposure to halothane when jaundice occurs days or weeks after an operation. Suspicion of previous halothane-induced jaundice should be reported to the anaesthetist. Halothane is much less commonly used nowadays, but further exposure to the drug in a sensitised patient may produce a more serious and more rapidly developing response.

c. Presence of obstructive jaundice

Surgery in this situation is usually performed to relieve an obstruction in patients where endoscopic stenting of the bile ducts has failed or is unavailable. This surgery carries a number of special risks and management problems which are described in Chapter 11. These include ascending cholangitis, clotting disorders, deep vein thrombosis and acute renal failure.

d. The patient with known hepatitis

Patients with any form of hepatitis, whether viral or alcoholic, tolerate general anaesthesia and surgery badly and there is a distinct mortality risk. Surgery should be avoided unless absolutely essential. If alcoholism is suspected, a CAGE questionnaire should be completed. Positive answers to two or more of the four questions suggest a drinking problem. The questions are given in Box 46.4.

An elevated serum gamma glutaryl transferase level is a fairly good indicator of excessive alcohol intake. Mean corpuscular volume (MCV) may also be raised, and should alert the doctor to the possibility of concealed alcoholism.

e. The patient with known cirrhosis

Patients with cirrhosis have a high risk of perioperative morbidity and mortality. The main factors are:

- Anaemia
- Portal hypertension
- Defective synthesis of clotting factors and thrombocytopenia
- Malnutrition
- Electrolyte disturbances (particularly hyponatraemia)
- Defective energy metabolism (gluconeogenesis and glycogenolysis)
- Abnormal drug metabolism and distribution (due to hypoalbuminaemia)
- Ascites

The main postoperative complications of cirrhosis are excessive bleeding, defective wound healing, hepato-

---

KEY POINTS

Box 46.4 CAGE questionnaire

- Have you ever felt you ought to **C**ut down on your drinking?
- Have people **A**nnoyed you by criticising your drinking?
- Have you ever felt bad or **G**uilty about your drinking?
- Have you ever had a drink first thing in the morning to steady your nerves or get rid of a hangover (**E**ye-opener)?

cellular decompensation leading to encephalopathy, and susceptibility to infection.

Excessive bleeding results from several factors:

- Defective synthesis of clotting factors (all but factor VIII are synthesised in the liver)
- Thrombocytopenia (due to hypersplenism and depressed platelet production)
- Abnormal polymerisation of fibrin
- Portal hypertension (greatly expanded intra-abdominal venous network under high pressure). This, together with numerous vascular adhesions, makes dissection tedious, difficult and bloody

Portal hypertension may initially be discovered because of ascites, an acute upper gastrointestinal haemorrhage or splenomegaly. (Note that only about half of such episodes of haematemesis/melaena in patients with portal hypertension are due to oesophageal varices. The rest are largely caused by gastric erosions.) If a patient with known oesophageal varices requires an operation, preoperative endoscopic assessment and sclerotherapy or banding may be appropriate.

Preoperative assessment and management

Preoperative blood tests for patients with liver disease are listed in Box 46.5.

If prothrombin time is prolonged, intravenous vitamin K injections are given for several days before operation. If this fails to correct the abnormal clotting (as in severe hepatic impairment), **fresh-frozen plasma** is given during the operation. If the patient is thrombocytopenic, platelet transfusion may also be required.

RENAL DISORDERS

Renal impairment is commonly encountered in general surgical patients. It is characterised by impaired homeostasis of fluid and electrolytes and reduced excretion of nitrogenous compounds. The risk of perioperative complications increases with the degree of renal failure. Patients can be divided into two groups: mild chronic renal failure (CRF) and severe chronic renal failure. Acute renal failure is usually a postoperative complication, often with several contributory causes including hypovolaemia, and is described in the next chapter. Patients with pre-existing renal disease are particularly vulnerable to acute renal failure ('acute-on-chronic renal failure').

CLINICAL PROBLEMS

a. Mild chronic renal failure
This is common in the elderly and may be caused by hypertension. The main management problems in surgical patients are:

> **KEY POINTS**
>
> **Box 46.5 Preoperative blood tests for patients with liver disease**
>
> **Initial tests**
> - Serological testing for hepatitis B and C
>
> **Further tests**
> - Full blood count
> - Clotting screen and platelet count
> - Plasma urea and electrolytes
> - Bilirubin
> - Transaminases
> - Calcium
> - Phosphate
> - Gamma glutaryl transferase
> - Albumin

- **Impaired excretion of drugs**—such drugs must therefore be given in smaller doses or less frequently, as documented in publications such as the *British National Formulary*. In practice, digoxin and gentamicin pose the main problem. Gentamicin dosage is worked out from a nomogram according to blood levels measured immediately pre-dose ('trough' level) and then 15 minutes after intravenous or 1 hour after intramuscular administration ('peak' level)
- **Fluid and electrolyte homeostasis**—only becomes a problem in mild CRF if fluid balance is not carefully monitored in the perioperative period. Monitoring should include regular checks of serum urea, electrolytes and creatinine, especially if the patient is receiving diuretic therapy
- Reduction in renal reserve—even mild renal failure implies a drastic reduction in renal reserve. For example, major reconstructive surgery to the abdominal aorta in a patient with mild renal failure may interfere with renal function because of aortic cross-clamping near the renal arteries. This is exacerbated by transient hypotension caused by blood loss. The lack of renal reserve in these patients may then progress to acute renal failure. Thus, renal function must be properly assessed before these operations by measuring serum urea and creatinine. If these are abnormal, renal arteriography may be needed to exclude renal artery stenosis. In addition, special precautions must be taken during anaesthesia and surgery to avoid precipitating acute renal failure

b. Severe chronic renal failure
These patients are usually under the care of specialist physicians who should be involved in perioperative management. Patients may be receiving regular haemo-

dialysis or ambulatory peritoneal dialysis; in such patients, surgery is usually for renal transplantation.

The main perioperative problems of severe CRF are:

- **Fluid overload**—this is caused by impaired glomerular filtration and may require correction with large doses of diuretics and fluid restriction and haemofiltration if necessary. Fluid requirements in the perioperative period may be difficult to assess. They are best controlled by monitoring central venous pressure in an intensive care unit
- **Regulation of serum osmolality**—this is disordered in patients with severe CRF who are particularly vulnerable to hypo- and hypernatraemia. Care must be taken that the sodium content of intravenous fluids is appropriate for the individual
- **Hyperkalaemia**—this is a particular risk of advanced CRF. Patients with lesser degrees of CRF are vulnerable to increase in potassium load (due to transfusion, tissue damage or hypoxia) or changes in glomerular filtration rate (caused by cardiac failure or hypotension). Hyperkalaemia may cause cardiac standstill and susceptibility is best assessed by monitoring the ECG. To minimise this risk, the preoperative plasma potassium level should be stabilised below 5.0 mmol/L
- **Metabolic acidosis**—this tends to develop in CRF but it is usually compensated by respiratory alkalosis. This compensation is disrupted by general anaesthesia and also by additional metabolic acidosis due to tissue ischaemia or hypoxia
- **Chronic normochromic normocytic anaemia**—this results from decreased erythropoietin production by the kidney. Cardiovascular function is usually well adapted to this anaemia and preoperative transfusion

is unnecessary. Transfusion adds the further risk of precipitating fluid and electrolyte problems, and may complicate tissue typing for future kidney transplantation

PREOPERATIVE ASSESSMENT

Hydration should be assessed by looking for clinical evidence of dehydration or fluid overload (particularly jugular venous pressure). Plasma urea, electrolytes, creatinine and bicarbonate should be checked for abnormalities. Full blood count is checked for anaemia.

DIABETES MELLITUS

Patients with diabetes are at special risk from general anaesthesia and surgery for the following reasons:

- Diabetic complications are associated with a higher perioperative risk. These are summarised in Box 46.6
- Stress (including surgery, trauma and infections) causes increased production of catabolic hormones which oppose the action of insulin (see Ch. 2). This makes diabetic control more difficult

---

KEY POINTS

Box 46.6 Specific perioperative problems in patients with diabetes

Predisposition to ischaemic heart disease
- Greater risk of postoperative myocardial infarction which has higher mortality in diabetics
- Infarction may be painless or 'silent', (possibly due to autonomic neuropathy)

Increased danger of cardiac arrest
- Due to autonomic neuropathy

Predisposition to diabetic nephropathy
- Tendency to chronic renal failure

Predisposition to peripheral vascular disease
- Greater risk of perioperative strokes and lower limb ischaemia

Predisposition to heel pressure sores
- Especially if there is peripheral neuropathy

Increased incidence of postoperative infection
- In the wound, chest or urinary tract

Obesity
- Particularly common in non insulin-dependent diabetes
- Associated with increased operative morbidity

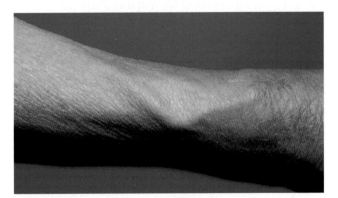

Fig. 46.2 Cimino-Brescia arteriovenous fistula
This recently constructed fistula performed for chronic renal failure in a diabetic woman of 56, involved dividing the cephalic vein and suturing the proximal end to the side of the radial artery. It was performed under local anaesthesia through the incision visible on the wrist. Already the wrist veins are dilating and will soon be usable for renal dialysis.

- General anaesthesia, surgery, deprivation of oral intake and postoperative vomiting disrupt the delicate balance between dietary intake, exercise (energy utilisation) and diabetic therapy
- Diabetic ketoacidosis may cause an elevated leucocyte count and amylase level, which may confuse the diagnosis of an acute abdomen. Indeed, ketoacidosis may sometimes present with abdominal pain
- Diabetic patients are at greater risk of hospital-acquired infection, which may be elusive as a cause of deterioration

CLINICAL PROBLEMS

For the purposes of perioperative management, patients with diabetes fall into three groups: **insulin-dependent**, those taking **oral hypoglycaemic** medication and those who are **diet-controlled**. Preoperative assessment should include evaluation of current diabetic control by serial blood glucose and **glycosylated haemoglobin** measurements. Potential cardiovascular and renal complications should be assessed by performing an ECG (with Valsalva manoeuvre) and estimating plasma urea and electrolytes.

Perioperative management should maintain blood glucose level between 4 and 10 mmol/L, but it is particularly important to avoid hypoglycaemia. Surgery should be deferred if the blood glucose cannot be stabilised below 13 mmol/L. Above this level, there is an unacceptable risk of ketoacidosis or a hyperosmolar non-ketotic state.

a. Insulin-dependent diabetics

Insulin-dependent diabetics, as the name indicates, depend for their metabolism on administered insulin. If the blood glucose level is low, insulin is not withheld but glucose infusion is increased. The general principles of perioperative management are:

- Establish good diabetic control before operation
- Give insulin as a continuous intravenous infusion during the operative period
- Give an infusion of dextrose (glucose) throughout the operative period to balance the insulin given and to make up for lack of dietary intake
- Add potassium to the dextrose infusion
- Monitor blood glucose and electrolytes frequently throughout the operative and early postoperative period

A typical management protocol is given in Box 46.7 and a recommended insulin infusion regimen in Box 46.8. The key to successful management of diabetes is adjusting the dose of insulin against frequent measurement of blood glucose. Finger-prick tests on the ward are adequate provided they are performed correctly by properly trained staff. The insulin dose is adjusted hourly according to the blood glucose results.

KEY POINTS

Box 46.7 Perioperative management of insulin-dependent diabetes

Before operation

1. Arrange outpatient stabilisation of diabetes with diabetes physician and specialist nurse in advance, if available
2. Admit patient to hospital 2–3 days before operation if outpatient preparation unavailable or unsatisfactory
3. Establish good preoperative control—a twice-daily mixture of short- and intermediate-acting insulin is usually adequate. If not, extra doses of short-acting insulin can be added
4. Monitor blood glucose throughout the day, e.g. before and after meals and at bedtime
5. Arrange for the operation to take place as early as possible in the day

Operation day

1. Starve from midnight and omit first dose of insulin
2. Check blood glucose and electrolytes before operating list commences—postpone if glucose level greater than 13 mmol/L or electrolyte abnormalities are found
3. Commence intravenous dextrose and insulin infusions
4. Check blood glucose and electrolytes at conclusion of operation (or at 1–2-hour intervals in a long operation)
5. Adjust concentration of infusions and rate of administration as required

After operation

1. Check glucose 2–4-hourly and electrolytes 6–12-hourly and adjust infusion as indicated
2. Continue infusion until full oral diet is established, then reintroduce subcutaneous insulin, using the preoperative regimen

---

KEY POINTS

Box 46.8 Perioperative management of diabetics using insulin infusion

1. Intravenous 5% or 10% glucose infusion at 125 ml per hour
2. Constant pump-controlled intravenous soluble insulin infusion. This is adjusted according to 2–4-hourly blood glucose estimations
3. If there is a need to limit fluids, use 20% dextrose solution and infuse at 50 ml per hour

b. Diabetics controlled on oral hypoglycaemic drugs

Many of these patients are receiving short-acting sulphonylureas such as glipizide. Patients on long-acting drugs such as chlorpropamide or metformin (or both) should be changed several days before operation to a short-acting sulphonylurea. If this fails to provide adequate control, an insulin regimen can be used as above.

On the morning of the operation, the patient is starved in the usual manner and the short-acting sulphonylurea omitted. This drug is reintroduced when oral intake is resumed. Blood glucose should be monitored regularly as for insulin-dependent patients because it may still reach unacceptable levels, despite the lack of carbohydrate intake. If glucose rises above 13 mmol/L, it can be controlled by small subcutaneous doses of short-acting insulin, e.g. 6 units of soluble insulin. If a major operation is planned or if postoperative 'nil by mouth' is likely to be prolonged, it is best to use insulin and glucose infusions as for insulin-dependent diabetics.

c. Diabetics controlled by diet alone

These patients require no special perioperative measures if preoperative control is adequate; they do not become hypoglycaemic and blood glucose rarely drifts above acceptable levels. Finger-prick blood glucose measurement may be used if there is any doubt.

d. Diabetics poorly controlled on emergency admission

Any diabetic patient may present with uncontrolled diabetes, particularly if admitted as an emergency. This may be due to infection or vomiting. The diabetes must first be brought under control with infusions of insulin, glucose and potassium. Rehydration will also be required before operation can proceed.

e. Abdominal pain and vomiting in a diabetic child

This may be due to diabetic ketoacidosis rather than an 'acute abdomen'. If so, symptoms will resolve when diabetic control is re-established by rehydration and insulin therapy. As a general rule, the vomiting precedes the abdominal pain in diabetic ketoacidosis, whereas the opposite occurs in an acute abdomen. (*Note*: emergency laparotomy in uncontrolled diabetes is extremely dangerous and must be avoided at all costs.) Conversely, an acute abdomen may precipitate diabetic ketoacidosis. If the abdominal symptoms fail to respond to diabetic therapy, a diagnosis of acute abdomen must be reconsidered.

THYROID DISEASE

THYROTOXICOSIS

Surgery in untreated thyrotoxicosis carries a risk of thyrotoxic crisis, which has a high mortality. In surgery for

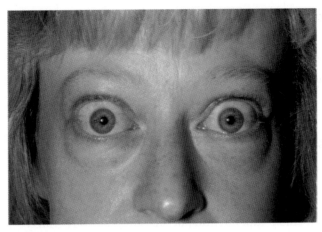

Fig. 46.3 Thyrotoxic eye signs
This woman of 36 presented with a typical history of primary thyrotoxicosis (Graves' disease), with weight loss, irritability and menstrual irregularity. In addition her eyesight had become blurred. She had fairly florid exophthalmos with protruding eyeballs (proptosis) and lid lag. She was barely able to close her eyelids and would soon be at risk of corneal drying.

thyrotoxicosis, the patient should be rendered euthyroid before operation by using antithyroid drugs or beta blockers. Non-selective beta blockers rapidly control the cardiovascular effects of thyrotoxicosis and can be used for urgent preoperative preparation. A thyrotoxic crisis may also occur if an undiagnosed thyrotoxic patient has an operation for another reason. Any patient with symptoms or signs of thyrotoxicosis should have a serum thyroxine measurement included in the preoperative assessment.

HYPOTHYROIDISM

Untreated hypothyroid patients are at moderate risk when undergoing surgery. They are more sensitive to CNS depressants and have a decreased cardiovascular reserve. They are also susceptible to electrolyte disorders. Severe infection, especially accompanied by trauma, a cold environment or depressant drugs, may precipitate myxoedema coma which, though very rare, is often fatal.

Hypothyroidism is common, particularly in women, and increases with age. Many patients are maintained on replacement therapy and are at no special risk. Patients previously treated for thyrotoxicosis may become insidiously hypothyroid. Features of hypothyroidism include weight gain, bradycardia, psychomotor depression, thinning eyebrows, coarse hair and skin, chronic constipation and hoarse voice. The most useful clinical sign is tendon reflexes which are slow to relax.

If there is clinical suspicion of hypothyroidism, operation should be postponed and thyroid function checked by measuring free thyroxine (T4) and thyroid stimulating hormone (TSH) levels. If hypothyroidism is diagnosed, oral replacement therapy is commenced. If surgery must be performed urgently, it is usually best to proceed with the operation and begin oral treatment later.

DISORDERS OF ADRENAL FUNCTION

ADRENAL INSUFFICIENCY

The most common cause of adrenal insufficiency is hypothalamo-pituitary-adrenal suppression by long-term corticosteroid therapy. It is occasionally caused by primary adrenal failure (**Addison's disease**) or pituitary ablation (due to tumour or surgery). Very rarely, it results from previous adrenalectomy. This may have been carried out for palliation of breast cancer, treatment for a hypersecretion syndrome or primary surgery for bilateral adrenal tumours.

In primary or secondary adrenal failure, the patient is usually already on oral steroid replacement therapy. In any case, the adrenals are unable to respond to the stress of trauma, surgery or infection, which would normally lead to increased secretion of glucocorticoids. The lack of adrenal response in these patients may cause acute postoperative cardiovascular collapse with hypotension and shock (**Addisonian crisis**).

Perioperative 'steroid cover'

Patients with potential adrenal insufficiency must be given steroid cover during the perioperative period. This is usually in the form of intravenous hydrocortisone, e.g. 100–200 mg prior to the operation, and 100 mg daily until recovery. It is better to give prophylactic hydrocortisone in doubtful cases than risk acute hypo-adrenalism. For any steroid-dependent patient, a doctor should write clearly in the notes *'Treat any unexplained collapse with hydrocortisone.'*

CUSHING'S SYNDROME

Cushing's syndrome results from excess secretion of cortisol. This may be in response to excess adreno-corticotropic hormone (ACTH) secretion by a pituitary tumour. Occasionally, it is due to ectopic ACTH secretion (usually by a malignant tumour) and rarely due to a primary tumour of the adrenal. Clinically the patient may be plethoric, moon-faced, hypertensive, hirsute and obese with abdominal striae. There may be a characteristic 'buffalo hump'. The most common cause of Cushingoid features is long-term steroid therapy for conditions such as rheumatoid arthritis or asthma. The main surgical problems in Cushingoid patients are hypertension, poor wound healing, infection and peptic ulceration. If the condition is due to steroid therapy, there is an additional risk of secondary adrenal insufficiency.

PHAEOCHROMOCYTOMA

Phaeochromocytoma is rare, and is usually diagnosed during investigation of paroxysmal hypertension. Sometimes, a phaeochromocytoma is discovered after wild swings of blood pressure are encountered during an operation. Phaeochromocytomas are usually located in the adrenal medulla but can occur retroperitoneally in embryological remnants of the organ of Zuckerkandl. Diagnosis is made by finding high levels of catecholamine metabolites such as **vanillylmandelic acid** (VMA) in the urine. Nowadays, the tumour is usually localised by radionuclide scans and by computed tomography or magnetic resonance imaging.

In the surgical management of phaeochromocytoma, there are two main problems: to control dangerous rises in blood pressure during operation and to prevent hypotension afterwards. The former are caused by handling the tumour which increases catecholamine release, while the latter is the effect of vasoconstriction leading to chronic hypovolaemia. Hypovolaemia results from the high levels of circulating catecholamines before operation, which rapidly fall once the tumour is removed. Management involves gradual preoperative control of hypertension with **alpha-adrenergic blocking drugs** (e.g. phenoxybenzamine). As alpha blockade is increased, vasoconstriction is reduced and chronic hypovolaemia corrected, which minimises postoperative hypotension. During operation, short-acting alpha- and beta-adrenergic drugs are used and a range of other drugs is kept ready to control swings in blood pressure. These patients are best managed in specialist centres.

DIABETES INSIPIDUS

Diabetes insipidus is uncommon. Its causes can be divided into **cranial** (with reduced production of antidiuretic hormone (ADH), also known as vasopressin, and **nephrogenic**, in which the renal tubules are unresponsive to ADH. Renal diabetes insipidus may be caused by hypercalcaemia, hypokalaemia or drugs such as lithium. Cranial diabetes insipidus is often idiopathic but may be due to trauma (either surgical or following head injury) which disrupts the secretory pathway from the hypothalamus via the pituitary stalk to the posterior pituitary (neurohypophysis). Most patients receive replacement therapy in the form of **vasopressin or desmopressin** by nasal insufflation. Patients with diabetes insipidus are prone to abnormalities of plasma electrolytes, particularly sodium, which should be checked before operation.

MUSCULOSKELETAL AND NEUROLOGICAL DISORDERS

Musculoskeletal and neurological disorders influence the outcome of surgery in two main ways. Firstly, any condition which hinders mobility predisposes to chest infection, deep venous thrombosis and pulmonary embolism, aspiration pneumonitis and pressure sores. The last is even more likely if there is also sensory impairment due to stroke or diabetic peripheral neuropathy. Secondly, specific aspects of these disorders must be considered in relation to general anaesthesia, positioning of the patient on the operating table and the use of drugs.

RHEUMATOID ARTHRITIS

Rheumatoid arthritis poses special problems related to chronic anaemia, drug therapy and spinal complications (Some of these problems are shared by other collagen disorders.):

● **Normochromic normocytic anaemia**—common in chronic inflammatory disorders, including rheumatoid arthritis. The anaemia is refractory to iron therapy and there is no benefit from preoperative transfusion unless haemoglobin concentration is extremely low

● **Gastrointestinal disorders**—most rheumatoid patients are taking aspirin or other NSAIDs, all of which predispose to peptic ulceration, ulceration and perforation of small and large bowel and small bowel strictures. Long-term steroid therapy may contribute to peptic ulceration. Chronic low-grade bleeding from the upper gastrointestinal tract may exacerbate the existing anaemia in these patients. Operative stress may also precipitate acute gastrointestinal haemorrhage

● **Long-term steroid therapy**—may result in adrenal insufficiency under stress. Gold and penicillamine cause renal parenchymal damage and bone marrow depression; NSAIDs may exacerbate chronic renal failure

● **Odontoid subluxation**—if rheumatoid arthritis involves the atlanto-axial joint, the transverse ligament may be destroyed, allowing the odontoid process to sublux. During general anaesthesia, the protective reflexes are lost. If the neck is hyperextended during intubation, there is a serious risk of injury to the spinal cord by the unrestrained odontoid

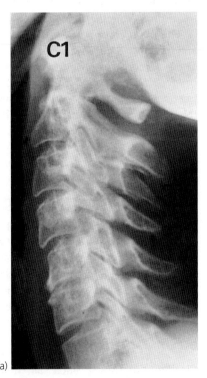
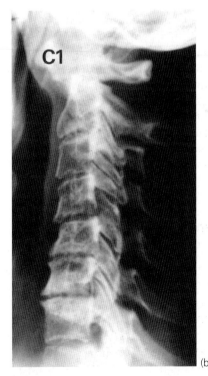

(a)   (b)

Fig. 46.4 Subluxation of the atlanto-axial joint in rheumatoid arthritis
This 62-year-old woman with long-standing severe rheumatoid arthritis required a major abdominal operation. Cervical radiographs were taken before operation to anticipate problems during anaesthesia. **(a)** Cervical spine in extension. **(b)** The same patient in flexion. Anterior subluxation is most obvious if the anterior border of the body of the atlas **C1** is compared with that of the axis in the two pictures. This mobility is caused by destruction of the transverse axial ligament of the odontoid by pannus (excessive granulation tissue) from the synovial joint. Under general anaesthesia, muscle relaxation may allow exaggeration of the subluxation, causing damage to the cervical cord

Preoperative assessment of the rheumatoid patient

Full blood count is essential to check for non-specific anaemia or iron deficiency anaemia. Serum urea, electrolytes and creatinine are measured if there is any suspicion of chronic or drug-induced disturbance of renal function. Preoperative assessment must include examination of neck movements and cervical spine X-rays.

EPILEPSY

Epilepsy is common and many routine surgical patients will therefore be taking anticonvulsive therapy. Fortunately, there is no particular risk from general anaesthesia or surgery. Indeed, the central depressive effect of general anaesthetic drugs is a powerful anticonvulsant!

HAEMATOLOGICAL DISORDERS

ANAEMIAS

Severe anaemias are associated with increased perioperative morbidity and mortality. General anaesthesia poses the greatest single problem. Moderate anaemia, in which the haemoglobin concentration is more than 10 g/dl, appears to impose no excess risk. For elective surgery, the haemoglobin concentration should ideally be above this level before operation but long-standing chronic anaemias probably pose little increased risk.

Management of anaemic patients depends on the cause of the anaemia. For patients on renal dialysis, there is no point in trying to raise the haemoglobin level by transfusion as it rapidly falls again, but these patients can be treated with **erythropoietin**.

The cause of the anaemia may be the reason for the operation. Whether or not to transfuse before operation depends on the level of anaemia, whether the anaemia is acute and the expected blood loss during the operation. Transmission of human immunodeficiency virus (HIV) by transfusion is a very small risk in developed countries with sophisticated screening of donors but remains a serious risk in countries without such precautions. It is good policy to reappraise former indications for transfusion and transfuse donor blood only when strictly necessary. It is usually possible to avoid transfusion in young, fit patients but elderly or very ill patients with less cardiorespiratory reserve are more likely to need transfusion. Transfusions should be given at least 24 hours before operation to allow fluid balance to stabilise and to ensure optimal red cell function. For deficiency anaemias, treatment as appropriate with iron, vitamin B_{12} or folate may be all that is necessary before operation.

HAEMOGLOBINOPATHIES

Patients with sickle cell disease and beta thalassaemia

have a high operative mortality and morbidity. They require intensive perioperative management with particular avoidance of hypoxia, infection, acidosis, dehydration and hypothermia. Patients with sickle cell trait are at much lower risk, and develop complications only if they become severely hypoxic. Sickle cell trait and disease occur amongst black people, who should always be asked specifically about sickle cell disease. A sickle cell test must be performed before operation on any black patient so that the anaesthetist can be prepared.

POLYCYTHAEMIA

Polycythaemia may be caused by a primary myelo-proliferative disorder such as polycythaemia rubra vera (PRV) or be secondary to chronic cardiac or pulmonary disease. Heavy cigarette smoking itself may cause polycythaemia. There is an increased red cell mass in both primary and secondary polycythaemia, which causes a high haematocrit and increased blood viscosity. In PRV, the platelet count may be abnormally high, which, paradoxically, is associated with defective haemostasis as well as the risk of thrombosis.

Some patients found to have a raised haematocrit do not have an increased red cell mass but rather a reduced plasma volume. This is sometimes known as **stress polycythaemia**. The increased blood viscosity may lead to thromboembolic problems.

The main complications of polycythaemia rubra vera are **haemorrhage**, and **arterial or venous thrombosis**. The risk increases once the haematocrit rises above 50%. In general, operation should be postponed to allow treatment by venesection or myelosuppression. If possible, the cardiovascular system should be allowed to stabilise for about 1 month after treatment. In an emergency, the haematocrit may be reduced by preoperative venesection, restoring the volume by colloid infusion.

LEUKAEMIA, LEUCOPENIA AND THROMBOCYTOPENIA

Patients with these haematological disorders may need surgery for unrelated conditions. Prophylactic antibiotics may be required in neutropenia and haematologists give specific advice in patients at risk because of chemotherapy. In thrombocytopenia, haemorrhage can be minimised by transfusing platelet concentrates.

BLEEDING DISORDERS

Bleeding diatheses such as thrombocytopenia, von Willebrand's disease (abnormal platelet function and factor VIII deficiency) and haemophilia are occasionally encountered in general surgical practice. Most surgical bleeding problems, however, are caused by poorly controlled anticoagulant therapy, liver disease, aspirin therapy and sometimes vitamin K malabsorption. The last occurs in obstructive jaundice and malabsorption syndromes.

A history of abnormal bleeding or factors which may predispose to abnormal bleeding are the most important pointers to a likely bleeding problem at operation. They should be sought from every surgical patient as follows:

- Excessive bleeding from simple cuts, previous surgery, dental extractions or childbirth
- Current use of anticoagulant drugs or aspirin
- A family history of bleeding disorders
- Intercurrent haematological or liver disease, cystic fibrosis or other malabsorption syndromes
- Recent jaundice
- Previous intestinal resection or bypass surgery

Any clotting abnormality may lead to excessive bleeding at operation or recurrent bleeding in the early postoperative period. This may simply require additional care during surgical haemostasis but may well lead to runaway haemorrhage when clotting factors become exhausted. If this occurs, bleeding may be very difficult to control so preoperative diagnosis and treatment is vital.

If a bleeding disorder is suspected, a **platelet count** and a **clotting screen** must be performed. A clotting screen includes prothrombin time or ratio and activated partial thromboplastin time. If an abnormality is revealed, further special investigations such as assay of individual clotting factors may be necessary. Operation should be deferred until the problem is overcome.

Clotting abnormalities (where platelet function is unaffected) are often responsible for recurrent bleeding after initial haemostasis has been achieved. In contrast, an abnormality in platelet numbers or function tends to cause excessive bleeding at operation and postoperative oozing. Other complications of clotting disorders include retroperitoneal or muscle haematomas and bleeding into joint cavities (haemarthroses). In contrast, platelet abnormalities tend to cause spontaneous bruising.

CLINICAL PROBLEMS OF BLEEDING DISORDERS

a. Inherited clotting disorders
Haemophilia occurs in males. The disorder is an X-linked deficiency of factor VIII, or less commonly, factor IX. The appropriate antihaemophilic factor is administered before operation and for up to 2 weeks after operation until the danger of secondary haemorrhage is over. Von Willebrand's disease is an autosomal dominant condition with abnormalities of both factor VIII and platelet function. It is managed perioperatively with fresh-frozen plasma or cryoprecipitate.

b. Anticoagulant therapy
Long-term anticoagulant therapy with warfarin is commonly used in venous thromboembolism, for patients with mechanical heart valve prostheses and in elderly patients with atrial fibrillation. Patients on anticoagulants have a small extra risk of perioperative haemorrhage, particularly if control is poor. For most patients, some form of anticoagulation needs to be continued, particularly if a mechanical heart valve is in situ. Many doctors prefer to continue oral warfarin, reducing the prothrombin ratio somewhat during the perioperative period. An alternative approach is to discontinue warfarin about 4 days before operation and convert to intravenous heparin infusion. This can be closely adjusted or even reversed.

If anticoagulation has been prescribed for treatment of venous thromboembolism, some doctors prefer to discontinue warfarin 2 or 3 days before operation. The perioperative period is then covered with prophylactic subcutaneous low-dose heparin (see Ch. 47).

c. Liver disease
Bleeding disorders in cirrhosis are described earlier in this chapter and disorders in the jaundiced patient are described in detail in Chapter 11.

d. Aspirin therapy
Aspirin has an irreversible inhibitory effect on platelet aggregation which persists clinically for at least 10 days. The effect is reversed only when the affected platelets have been replaced. Most NSAIDs act on platelets in the same way. A similar but short-lived effect is also produced by high doses of intravenous penicillin. Aspirin ingestion, even in low doses, tends to result in oozing during and after operation, although this is rarely serious. Bleeding following dental extraction is a common manifestation of aspirin ingestion and can usually be controlled by sutures and pressure. For major arterial surgery, aspirin should be stopped at least 2 weeks before elective operations.

e. Malabsorption of fat-soluble vitamins
Vitamin K absorption may be impaired in pancreatic dysfunction, after resection of the proximal ileum or in malabsorption syndromes. The problem is readily overcome by preoperative injections of vitamin K.

PSYCHIATRIC DISORDERS

MENTAL ILLNESS AND LEARNING DISABILITY

Behavioural problems associated with mental illness and learning disability can be minimised by a sympathetic and consistent approach from medical and nursing staff. Any procedure or investigation must be carefully explained to the patient in terms which can be understood. Patients should not be moved from bed to bed around the ward as this produces disorientation.

The patient's usual oral medication should be continued whenever possible. A parenteral substitute may be required if oral intake is restricted and behaviour is known to be unstable. Side effects and drug interactions are common with psychoactive drugs and these should be anticipated by checking with a formulary. Monoamine oxidase inhibitors (used as antidepressants) interact with sympathomimetic amines and opiate analgesics to cause severe hypertension. They should be discontinued at least 2 weeks before operation. Tricyclic antidepressants and phenothiazines also have a wide range of interactions. Serum urea, electrolytes and thyroid function should be checked in patients taking **lithium**, which may cause renal parenchymal damage and disturbed thyroid function.

ALCOHOLISM AND DRUG ADDICTION

Alcoholics are prone to cirrhosis, malnutrition and peripheral neuropathies. Drug addicts are at risk of hepatitis, acquired immunodeficiency syndrome (AIDS) and other infections.

Alcohol potentiates general anaesthetic agents, and the inebriated patient needs smaller doses. In contrast, chronic alcohol abuse induces liver enzymes which break down anaesthetic agents and also increase tolerance to central nervous sysyem depressants. Higher doses of anaesthetic agents will therefore be required. Similarly, larger doses of intravenous sedatives are required for procedures such as gastrointestinal endoscopy.

Opiate addiction leads to similar dosage problems. Doctors must be aware of feigned illness as a means of obtaining restricted drugs.

Problems of drug withdrawal

Withdrawal symptoms may develop unexpectedly during the postoperative period if drug or alcohol addiction has been concealed.

Alcohol withdrawal is characterised initially by irritability and tremors. Convulsions may develop after 24–48 hours. Full-scale delirium tremens may appear as long as 10 days after alcohol withdrawal. It is characterised by mental confusion and visual hallucinations accompanied by fever, tachycardia, pallor, vomiting and sweats. Such signs also occur in other postoperative complications and alcohol withdrawal is an easily overlooked cause.

Alcoholic cirrhosis may cause **episodic hypoglycaemia**, the symptoms of which may be confused with those of delirium tremens. Hypoglycaemia should be excluded by measuring blood glucose.

Mild alcohol withdrawal states may be managed with regular oral doses of chlormethiazole or benzodiazepines. Parenteral B vitamins are usually given daily. If symptoms become pronounced, chlormethiazole can be administered by continuous intravenous infusion. A bolus dose is used initially, and the subsequent rate of administration is adjusted according to response. Oral drugs can usually be substituted after 48–72 hours. If the patient has a history of convulsions, phenytoin should also be given.

Opiate withdrawal symptoms are broadly similar to those of alcohol. Treatment is usually with a substitute drug such as methadone.

DEMENTIA

Patients with dementia become even more confused when subjected to the strange and ever-changing environment of the surgical ward. They poorly tolerate the stress of general anaesthesia and operation. The potential benefit of any elective procedure must be carefully weighed against the possible adverse effects. Unfortunately, these patients often fail to become rehabilitated in their own homes after operation.

Sudden deterioration in mental state or increasing confusion may be provoked by infection, dehydration, electrolyte disturbances, hypoxia or overdose of drugs such as digoxin, hypnotics and sedatives. All these causes should be considered in any patient who undergoes mental deterioration in the perioperative period.

OBESITY

Gross obesity carries 2–3 times the normal risk of perioperative death or morbidity, as outlined in Box 46.9. Whenever possible, weight should be reduced before operation, particularly if the operation is not urgent. Referral to a dietitian may be helpful although self-help groups often provide stronger motivation. Preoperative investigations for obese patients include blood glucose measurement and ECG, even if the patient is asymptomatic.

CHRONIC DRUG THERAPY

Many drugs prescribed for 'medical' conditions may complicate the management of the surgical patient. The most important of these commonly encountered in practice are summarised in Box 46.10.

KEY POINTS

Box 46.9 Surgical complications of obesity

Cardiopulmonary complications such as cardiac failure and chest infections
- Predisposing factors are atherosclerosis, increased demands on the cardiovascular system, decreased chest wall compliance, inefficient respiratory muscles and shallow breathing

Wound complications such as infection, dehiscence
- Poor-quality abdominal wall musculature with fat infiltration. Large 'dead space' in which fat predisposes to haematoma formation

Deep venous thrombosis and pulmonary embolism
- Due to poor peripheral venous return and general inertia

Complications with general anaesthesia
- Physiological problems, e.g. intravenous cannulae are difficult to insert and intubation is more difficult. Clinical signs of dehydration and hypovolaemia are more difficult to elicit
- Metabolic problems, e.g. altered distribution of drugs

Predisposition to various medical disorders
- Hypertension, ischaemic heart disease, diabetes, gallstones, gout

Operative difficulties
- Operations take longer to perform because of difficult access and vital structures obscured by fat

KEY POINTS

Box 46.10 Potentially dangerous drugs in the surgical patient

Glucocorticoids
- Predispose to peptic ulceration, delayed wound healing and infection
- May lead to acute adrenal insufficiency causing cardiovascular collapse

Antihypertensive and anti-anginal drugs
- Not hazardous unless abruptly stopped; this may cause rebound hypertension or angina

Antidepressants
- Monoamine oxidase inhibitors (MAOIs) interact with tyramine-containing foods (such as cheese and yeast extracts), as well as sympathomimetic amines and narcotic analgesics; this interaction may cause a hypertensive crisis and potentiate narcotic effects

Oral contraceptives
- Increased risk of deep venous thrombosis and pulmonary embolism

Anticoagulants
- Predispose to haemorrhage

Diuretics
- May cause electrolyte abnormalities and dehydration

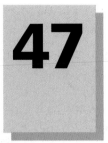

47 Complications of surgery and trauma and their prevention

INTRODUCTION

Any operation, major trauma or other surgical admission may be attended by one or more complications. These not only cause additional pain and suffering to the patient but may put the patient's life at risk. Furthermore, complications place extra demands upon medical and nursing time and often prolong surgical admissions, thus imposing additional costs on already overstretched budgets. For example, an anastomotic leak or a wound dehiscence can double the cost of an elective colonic resection.

While some complications are to an extent inherent in the condition being treated (e.g. deep venous thrombosis following multiple lower limb fractures) or arise from some comorbid condition such as myocardial ischaemia, others arise from inefficiency or errors of judgement (e.g. misdiagnosis), poor management practices (e.g. allowing pressure sores to develop) or even frank negligence (e.g. operation on the wrong side); many of these can be attributed to lack of appropriate training or an absence of local management guidelines (or a failure to follow them). Poor communication between hospital staff is a common cause of avoidable complications, e.g. failing to record penicillin allergy in the case record, or neglecting to inform the operating theatre about changes to an operating list.

A large proportion of complications can be prevented or minimised by appropriate prophylactic measures, careful attention to detail and by early recognition and treatment of problems as they develop. Early diagnosis and treatment of potentially serious complications (e.g.

bowel anastomotic leak) is essential, as delay often leads to catastrophic 'snowballing' multi-organ dysfunction. Once three or more body systems become involved, mortality is extremely high, e.g. acute respiratory distress syndrome (ARDS) and renal failure, complicating an operation for obstructive jaundice with liver impairment.

In respect of operative surgery, complications can be divided into the **general** complications of any operation and the **specific** complications of individual operations. Both groups of complications can be subdivided into **immediate** (during operation or within the next 24 hours),

---

SUMMARY

Box 47.1 Principal categories of surgical complications

1. Complications predisposed to by intercurrent 'medical' disorders, whether symptomatic or occult, e.g. ischaemic heart disease, chronic respiratory disease or diabetes mellitus (discussed in Ch. 46)
2. Complications of anaesthesia
3. General complications of operations, e.g. haemorrhage or wound infection
4. Complications of any surgical condition, e.g. pulmonary embolism, pneumonia or urinary tract infection
5. Complications of specific disorders and operations (complications of operations involving bowel are discussed here; the rest are discussed in Chs 11–45, as relevant)

early postoperative (during the first postoperative week or so), **late postoperative** (up to 30 days after operation) and **long-term**.

The complications of surgery can be divided into five broad categories as shown in Box 47.1. This chapter covers categories 2, 3, 4 and the complications of abdominal surgery from category 5; 'medical' complications are discussed in Chapter 46. The complications associated with specific operations are discussed in Chapters 11–45, as appropriate.

COMPLICATIONS OF ANAESTHESIA

GENERAL PRINCIPLES OF ANAESTHESIA

Complications of anaesthesia are essentially the responsibility of the anaesthetist, although the surgical team usually bears responsibility for recognising potential problems in advance. The exception is local anaesthesia, which is usually administered by the surgeon. Much of the preoperative assessment for an anaesthetic, whether spinal, epidural or general, falls to the junior members of the surgical or anaesthetic team, who by anticipating complications, can prevent many of them. The main complications of anaesthesia are summarised in Box 47.2.

KEY POINTS

Box 47.2 Complications of anaesthesia

Local anaesthesia
- Injection site—pain, haematoma, delayed recovery of sensation (direct nerve trauma), infection
- Vasoconstrictors—ischaemic necrosis (if used in digits or penis)
- Systemic effects of local anaesthetic agent
  — idiosyncratic or allergic reactions (very rare)
  — toxicity due to either excess dosage (see Ch. 6) or inadvertent intravenous injection. The same effect is produced by premature release of a Bier's block cuff. Toxic effects include: dizziness, tinnitus, nausea and vomiting, fits, central nervous system (CNS) depression, bradycardia and asystole

Spinal, epidural and caudal anaesthesia
- Failure of anaesthetic—anatomical difficulties or technical failure
- Headache—loss of cerebrospinal fluid because of dural puncture
- Epidural or intrathecal bleeding (especially if the patient is on anticoagulants)
- Unintentionally wide field of anaesthesia
  — in epidural anaesthesia, injection of local anaesthetic into the wrong tissue plane may give a spinal anaesthetic
  — in spinal anaesthesia, if the anaesthetic agent flows too far proximally, respiratory paralysis may occur
- Permanent nerve or spinal cord damage—injection of incorrect drug
- Paraspinal infection—introduced by the needle
- Systemic complications—severe hypotension or postural hypotension

General anaesthesia
- Direct trauma to mouth or pharynx, e.g. teeth, artificial crowns and bridges
- Inherited disorders
  — malignant hyperpyrexia (MH)—any inhalational anaesthetic or suxamethonium may trigger MH
  — pseudocholinesterase deficiency (prolonged apnoea after succinylcholine)
- Idiosyncratic or allergic reactions to anaesthetic agents
  — minor effects, e.g. postoperative nausea and vomiting
  — major effects, e.g. cardiovascular collapse, respiratory depression, halothane jaundice
- Slow recovery from anaesthetic
  — poor cardiac, hepatic and renal function
  — drug interactions
  — inappropriate choice of drugs or dosage in relation to age or the requirements of day-case surgery
  — inadequate reversal
- 'Awareness' during anaesthetic—effective paralysis but ineffective anaesthesia (very expensive medicolegally!)
- Disorders of fluid balance—inadequate or excessive replacement of fluids

KEY POINTS

Box 47.2 Continued

General anaesthesia

- Hypothermia
  - long operations with extensive fluid loss
  - large-volume transfusion of cold blood
  (*Note*: neonates and small infants are especially vulnerable to hypothermia)
- Inadvertent trauma
  - initiation of pressure sores
  - pressure injury to nerves (especially ulnar and lateral popliteal)
  - diathermy pad burns
  - corneal abrasions

GENERAL COMPLICATIONS OF OPERATIONS

The main complications of any operation are haemorrhage, infection, delayed wound healing, surgical damage to related structures and inadvertent trauma to the patient in theatre.

HAEMORRHAGE

PERIOPERATIVE HAEMORRHAGE

Haemorrhage occurring during an operation (primary haemorrhage) should be controlled by the surgeon before the operation is completed; the methods are described in Chapter 6.

EARLY POSTOPERATIVE HAEMORRHAGE

Haemorrhage during the immediate postoperative period usually indicates inadequate operative haemostasis or a technical mishap such as a slipped ligature or unrecognised trauma to a blood vessel.

If an operation involves major blood loss which requires large-volume transfusion of stored blood, post-operative haemorrhage may be perpetuated by **consumption coagulopathy**, in which platelets and coagulation factors have been 'consumed' in a vain attempt at haemostasis. Occasionally bleeding results from the pre-operative use of aspirin or, aspirin-like drugs, uncontrolled anticoagulant drugs or, less commonly, a pre-existing but unrecognised bleeding diathesis. Any patient with a history of excess bleeding should have a platelet count and a coagulation screen before operation.

Operations at particular risk of early postoperative haemorrhage include the following:

- Major operations involving highly vascular tissues such as the liver or spleen
- Major arterial surgery (in which the patient is usually heparinised)
- Operations which leave a large raw surface such as abdomino-perineal resection of the rectum

This type of postoperative haemorrhage has been traditionally described as reactionary haemorrhage in the belief that it was a 'reaction' to the recovery of normal blood pressure and cardiac output. This concept is misleading and should now be discarded, especially since it may hinder the decision to re-explore a wound as a matter of urgency.

Management of early postoperative haemorrhage

It should be remembered that early postoperative haemorrhage is really a form of primary haemorrhage and, if it is substantial, the patient must be surgically re-explored and the source of haemorrhage treated as at the original operation. It is wise to perform a clotting screen (including platelet count) and order an appropriate amount of bank blood as a preliminary measure. Good intravenous access should be ensured and a central venous pressure catheter inserted for monitoring. If heparin has been used at the original operation, protamine can be given to reverse any residual activity. If the clotting screen is abnormal, specific clotting factors such as fresh-frozen plasma or platelet concentrates should be given. Many of these patients will stop bleeding with supportive measures and blood transfusion, but re-exploration must be considered at every stage.

LATER POSTOPERATIVE HAEMORRHAGE

Haemorrhage occurring several days after operation is usually related to infection which erodes vessels at the operation site; this is known as **secondary haemorrhage**. Treatment involves managing the infection, but exploratory operation is often required to ligate bleeding vessels.

INFECTION RELATED TO THE OPERATION SITE

MINOR WOUND INFECTIONS

The most common operative infection is a superficial wound infection occurring within the first postoperative week. This relatively trivial infection presents as localised pain, redness and a slight discharge. The organisms are usually *Staphylococci* derived from the skin. The infection usually settles without treatment. The exception is the patient in whom a prosthesis such as an arterial graft or artificial joint has been inserted. For these patients, antibiotics must be given to prevent the devastating consequences of infection around the prosthesis.

WOUND CELLULITIS AND ABSCESS

More severe wound infections occur most commonly after bowel-related surgery, when faecal organisms are usually incriminated. The majority present in the first postoperative week but they may occur as late as the third postoperative week, sometimes after the patient has left hospital. These infections commonly present first with a pyrexia; examination of the wound reveals either a spreading **cellulitis** or localised **abscess formation**.

Cellulitis is treated with appropriate antibiotics after taking a wound swab for culture and sensitivity, whereas a wound abscess is treated by surgical drainage. This may simply involve suture removal and probing of the

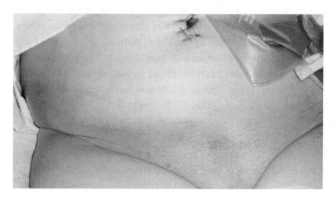

Fig. 47.1 Abdominal cellulitis
This woman of 73 presented with faecal peritonitis due to a diverticular perforation of the sigmoid colon. She was resuscitated and underwent a laparotomy and sigmoid loop colostomy (note bag). She remained toxic with a high fever and tachycardia and developed spreading cellulitis in the left groin and flank. This proved to be due to continuing leakage from the perforation. Nowadays, a Hartmann's operation is likely to be performed so there is no longer a perforation able to leak faecal matter within the peritoneal cavity.

wound, but deeper abscesses are likely to require re-exploration under general anaesthesia. In either case, the wound is left open to heal by secondary intention (see Fig. 47.2).

Intra-abdominal infection is discussed under complications of abdominal and bowel surgery later in this chapter.

GAS GANGRENE

Gas gangrene is an uncommon, acute, life-threatening wound infection, in which the anaerobic organisms multiply in necrotic tissue, particularly muscle (see Ch. 1).

LATE INFECTIVE COMPLICATIONS

A late infective complication of surgery is a chronically discharging **wound sinus** which emanates from a deep chronic abscess. It usually relates to foreign material such as a non-absorbable suture or mesh or sometimes necrotic fascia or tendon. These sinuses commonly follow wound infections where healing is delayed and incomplete. Wound sinuses occasionally appear after apparent normal healing, particularly after insertion of a prosthesis.

Sinuses rarely heal spontaneously unless the foreign material is discharged, and the usual treatment is therefore re-exploration of the wound and removal of the offending substance. In groin sinuses following aorto-femoral bypass grafts, removal of the graft would impair the arterial supply of the lower limb unless the infected graft can be replaced or bypassed.

IMPAIRED HEALING

FACTORS RETARDING WOUND HEALING

The vast majority of wounds heal without complication. It is a popular misconception that wounds heal slowly in the elderly; this is not so unless there are specific adverse factors or complications. Wound healing in general is retarded if blood supply is poor (as in arterial insufficiency of the lower limb) or if the wound is under excess suture tension. Other factors which may retard wound healing are long-term corticosteroid therapy, immunosuppressive therapy, previous radiotherapy, severe rheumatoid disease, malnutrition and vitamin deficiency, especially of vitamin C.

WOUND DEHISCENCE ('BURST ABDOMEN')

Wound dehiscence, i.e. total wound breakdown, is an uncommon problem. It affects about 1% of abdominal wounds and usually occurs about 1 week after operation, preceded by profuse discharge of sero-sanguinous fluid

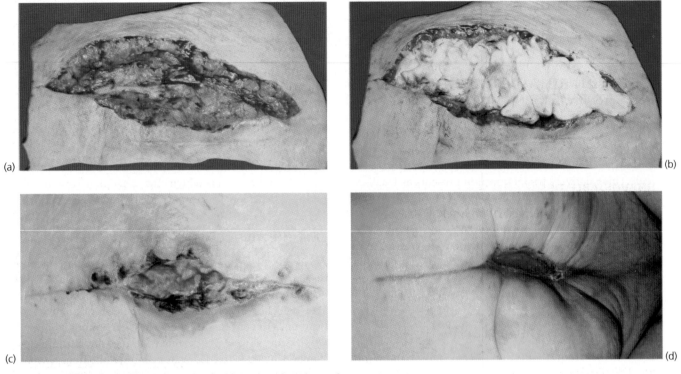

(a)

(b)

(c)

(d)

Fig. 47.2 Deep wound infection healed by secondary intention

This 80-year-old diabetic woman underwent laparotomy and the wound became infected with *Staphylococcus aureus*. This resulted in a wound abscess and necrosis of the wound edge. **(a)** The wound after all necrotic tissue has been excised. **(b)** It was then packed with gauze and allowed to heal by secondary intention. **(c)** and **(d)** The wound at 3 weeks and 8 weeks. It was completely healed after 2 further weeks. Note the degree of wound contraction, which plays a major part in overcoming the tissue defect.

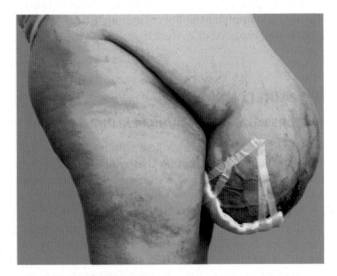

Fig. 47.3 Incisional hernia

This 55-year-old woman presented with a massive incisional hernia through an old umbilical hernia repair scar. Her only complaint was of skin breakdown at its lowermost extent. Repair presented a huge challenge but was achieved using mesh.

from the wound. The sudden bursting open of the abdomen revealing coils of bowel is alarming to nurses and junior doctors but is remarkably pain-free for the patient. Infection and other factors already described may play a part but the usual cause is inadequate abdominal wall repair. This may be compounded by mechanical disruption caused by coughing or abdominal distension.

The wound should initially be covered with sterile swabs soaked in saline and the patient returned to the operating theatre within a few hours for repair. This usually involves placement of tension sutures which incorporate large 'bites' of the whole thickness of the abdominal wall (see Fig. 47.4).

INCISIONAL HERNIA

Incisional hernia is a late complication of abdominal surgery. These hernias usually become apparent within the first postoperative year but sometimes develop as long as 15 years later; the overall incidence is about 10–15% of abdominal wounds. The hernia is caused by breakdown of the repair to the abdominal wall muscle and fascia. Predisposing factors are abdominal obesity, distension and poor muscle quality, poor choice of incision, inadequate closure technique, postoperative wound infection and multiple operations through the same incision.

An incisional hernia usually presents as a bulge in the abdominal wall near a previous wound. The condition is usually asymptomatic but occasionally a narrow-necked hernia presents with pain or strangulation. Once an incisional hernia has appeared, it tends to enlarge progressively and may become a nuisance cosmetically or for dressing (see Fig. 47.3). Repair is indicated for strangulation, pain or inconvenience.

SURGICAL INJURY

UNAVOIDABLE TISSUE DAMAGE

Anatomical structures, particularly nerves, blood vessels and lymphatics, may be unavoidably damaged during operation. This is particularly true in cancer surgery, illustrated by facial nerve damage during total parotidectomy. This may have to be accepted as part of the operative risk and discussed with the patient beforehand. Sometimes the integrity or location of vulnerable structures can be established before operation, thus allowing better planning of the operation. For example, intravenous urography (IVU) may be carried out to identify the course of the ureters in patients with colonic cancer, or indirect laryngoscopy may be done to assess vocal cord integrity prior to thyroid surgery.

INADVERTENT TISSUE DAMAGE

Structures may be inadvertently damaged during operation. Examples include recurrent laryngeal nerve damage during thyroidectomy and trauma to the common bile duct during laparoscopic cholecystectomy. The main factors are inexperience, anatomical anomalies, attempts at arresting precipitate haemorrhage and the obscuring of tissue planes by inflammation or malignancy. Signs of damage to structures at risk during specific operations should be sought in the postoperative period; for example, hoarseness after thyroidectomy or jaundice after cholecystectomy.

INADVERTENT OPERATING THEATRE TRAUMA

Apart from surgical trauma, patients are at risk of injury when being transported in the operating theatre and when under anaesthesia. Special training should be given to all who handle patients in operating theatres to minimise these risks.

The most common complications caused by trauma in the operating theatre are:

- Injuries resulting from falls from trolleys or operating table during positioning
- Injury to diseased bones and joints from manipulation or positioning. These include dislocation of a

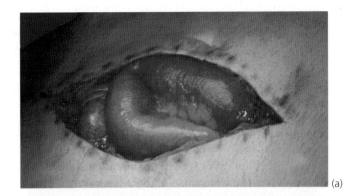
(a)

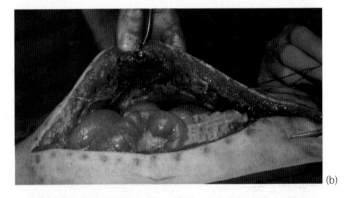
(b)

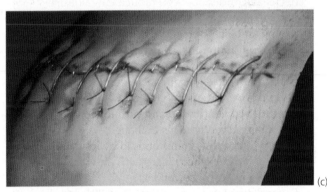
(c)

Fig. 47.4 Burst abdomen and repair with tension sutures
(a) Complete wound dehiscence 6 days after laparotomy for peritonitis. Note the exposed bowel spilling out of the wound.
(b) Operative photograph showing insertion of 'tension sutures' through the whole thickness of the abdominal wall. **(c)** The completed wound repair.

rheumatoid atlanto-axial joint and dislocation of a prosthetic hip joint
- Ulnar and lateral popliteal nerve palsies
- Electrical burns from wet or poorly contacting diathermy pads or misuse of the diathermy probe
- Excess pressure on the calf causing deep venous thrombosis
- Excess heel pressure causing pressure sores
- Cardiac pacemaker disruption by diathermy equipment

COMPLICATIONS OF ANY SURGICAL CONDITION

RESPIRATORY COMPLICATIONS

Up to 15% of patients suffer from respiratory complications associated with general anaesthesia and major operations. The most common of these are **atelectasis**, **pneumonia**, **aspiration pneumonitis** and **aspiration pneumonia**. Pre-existing lung disease greatly increases the risk of complications. Severely ill patients, including those with acute pancreatitis, and burns or trauma victims, are susceptible to the development of **acute respiratory distress syndrome**.

EFFECTS OF ANAESTHESIA AND SURGERY ON RESPIRATORY FUNCTION

Anaesthesia and surgery predispose to postoperative complications by altering lung function and compromising normal defence mechanisms as follows:

- **Lung tidal volume**—may be reduced by as much as 50%, depending on the incision site. Thoracic, upper abdominal and lower abdominal incisions (in decreasing order of effect) reduce lung volume
- **Lung expansion**—reduced by the **supine posture** during and after operation, pain, abdominal distension, abdominal constriction by bandages and the effects of sedative drugs
- **Ventilation rate**—usually increases and there is loss of normal periodic hyperinflation
- **Diminished ventilation and pulmonary perfusion**—result in reduced gaseous exchange
- **Airway defences**—compromised by loss of the cough reflex and diminished ciliary activity, which both lead to accumulation of secretions
- **Several problems are associated with laparoscopic abdominal surgery**: the pneumoperitoneum and head-down position lead to diaphragmatic splinting, a reduction in functional residual capacity and changes in intrathoracic blood volume. These lead to atelectasis, pulmonary shunting and hypoxaemia. Raised airways pressure may lead to pulmonary barotrauma

ATELECTASIS

Pathophysiology and clinical features

Atelectasis or alveolar collapse occurs when airways become obstructed and air is absorbed from the air spaces distal to the obstruction. Bronchial secretions are the main cause of this obstruction. Predisposing factors include shallow ventilation, loss of periodic hyperinflation, inhibition of coughing and pooling of mucus. All of these are particular problems after thoracic and upper abdominal

surgery. The resulting **ventilation/perfusion mismatch** produces a degree of right-to-left shunting of blood, and tends to cause a fall in PaO_2. If the obstructed airways are small, there is only minor segmental collapse, in which case localising signs are minimal and X-ray appearance is unremarkable. Despite this, the overall extent of collapse may be large and cause significant hypoxaemia.

Obstruction of a major airway causes collapse and consolidation of a whole lobe, resulting in the typical clinical signs of dullness to percussion and reduced breath sounds or **bronchial breathing**. Chest X-ray will show the lobe to be contracted and, opacified with mediastinal shift and compensatory expansion of other lobes.

Most cases of atelectasis are relatively mild and pass undiagnosed, although the patient may be slow to recover from operation. The patient may have a poor colour resulting from mild hypoxaemia, mild tachypnoea, tachycardia and low-grade pyrexia, which all resolve spontaneously within a few days. Sputum culture (if any is produced) is usually negative but infection may complicate severe cases.

Prevention and treatment of atelectasis

Atelectasis is best prevented by preoperative and postoperative physiotherapy for patients undergoing major surgery. This includes deep breathing exercises, regular adjustments of posture and vigorous coughing. During physiotherapy, wounds should be supported by the patient's hand. Effective analgesia facilitates physiotherapy and mobility, e.g. infiltration of the wound with local anaesthetic or epidural analgesia. Nebulised bronchodilators such as salbutamol may assist the patient to cough up secretions. Severe cases of diffuse atelectasis may require endotracheal intubation and positive-pressure ventilation. Lobar or whole lung collapse requires intensive physiotherapy and sometimes **flexible bronchoscopy** to aspirate occluding mucus plugs.

PNEUMONIAS

Bronchopneumonia is the usual form of chest infection seen in surgical patients. It occurs secondarily to chronic lung disease or following atelectasis or aspiration of gastric contents. *Haemophilus* and *Streptococcus pyogenes* are the common infecting organisms but coliforms may be responsible in elderly, debilitated or seriously ill patients. *Pseudomonas* bronchopneumonia occurs in patients on ventilators or with bronchiectasis.

Infection is manifest by pyrexia, tachypnoea, tachycardia and a raised leucocyte count. The mucopurulent sputum is thick, copious and green. Antibiotics, usually amoxycillin or co-trimoxazole, are given on a 'best-guess' basis until sputum culture and sensitivities are available. Physiotherapy and encouragement to cough are equally important for recovery.

ASPIRATION PNEUMONITIS

Aspiration pneumonitis (Mendelson's syndrome) is a sterile, chemical inflammation of the lungs resulting from inhalation of acidic gastric contents. There is often a clear history of vomiting or regurgitation, followed by a rapid onset of breathlessness and wheezing. This may later become complicated by infection, i.e. broncho-pneumonia, with its typical symptoms and signs. Chest X-ray shows characteristic 'fluffy' opacities, particularly in the lower lobes, which are most affected for anatomical and postural reasons.

Aspiration occurs when protective laryngeal reflexes are suppressed or when there is intestinal obstruction and regurgitation. Laryngeal suppression may be due to impairment of consciousness (e.g. during recovery from general anaesthesia or in alcoholic intoxication) or loss of consciousness after head injury.

Emergency anaesthesia in the non-starved patient poses special risks. Whenever possible, anaesthesia should be postponed for 4–6 hours after the last food or drink. In accident victims, it is important to note the time of last eating with respect to the time of the accident, and to remember that stress and anxiety may greatly delay gastric emptying. In pregnancy, gastric emptying is also much slower.

A patient with **intestinal obstruction** is at particular risk of inhalation of gastric contents. If possible, the stomach should be emptied by nasogastric tube. If general anaesthesia must be performed on the non-starved or otherwise at-risk patient, a **crash induction** technique is employed: the supine patient is tilted head-up and an endotracheal tube is inserted to protect the airway. At the same time, an assistant applies **cricoid pressure** to flatten the pharynx against the cervical spine, preventing reflux. Oral antacids may be given beforehand to neutralise gastric acidity. Metoclopramide, given by injection, may also be used to hasten gastric emptying.

The mortality from aspiration pneumonitis approaches 50% and urgent treatment must be started should it occur. This involves thorough bronchial suction via an endo-tracheal tube (or bronchoscope if necessary), followed by positive-pressure ventilation and prophylactic antibiotics. Intravenous steroids are usually given to try to limit the inflammatory process, but their efficacy is unproven.

ASPIRATION PNEUMONIA

Aspiration pneumonia may complicate aspiration pneu-monitis, but more often it develops insidiously, following chronic aspiration of infected food and oropharyngeal secretions. In the surgical context, debilitated, confused or elderly patients are the usual victims, but aspiration pneumonia is also seen in alcoholics, drug addicts and stroke patients. Achalasia of the oesophageal cardia and large hiatus hernias can lead to chronic aspiration, par-ticularly occurring at night. The clinical features are of infection and lobar consolidation (usually of the lower lobe) progressing to **lung abscess** formation. The organ-isms are usually mixed oral anaerobes sensitive to penicillin, but prognosis depends more on the patient's general condition and is usually poor.

ACUTE RESPIRATORY DISTRESS SYNDROME

This syndrome of acute respiratory failure, formerly known as adult respiratory distress syndrome, is characterised by rapid, shallow breathing, severe hypox-aemia, stiff lungs and diffuse pulmonary opacification on X-ray. It can develop in response to a variety of systemic and direct insults to the pulmonary alveoli and microvasculature.

Acute respiratory failure has long been known to occur in many disparate conditions and has been given many different names such as shock lung, wet lung, post-traumatic respiratory insufficiency, Da Nang lung (Vietnam war) and white lung (after the typical X-ray appearance). In 1976, it was finally realised that the underlying pathological phenomena were similar, and were directly related to the well-recognised respiratory distress syndrome of newborn babies. The main con-ditions with which acute respiratory distress syndrome (ARDS) is associated are summarised in Box 47.3.

Pathophysiology of ARDS

The causative insults to the lung all have the effect of increasing the permeability of pulmonary capillaries leading to leakage of protein-rich fluid into the alveolar interstitium. This causes interstitial oedema which in turn **reduces lung compliance** and causes 'stiff lungs' and reduced alveolar ventilation.

The alveolar lining cells (**type I pneumocytes**) are also damaged in some way. The damage, combined with increased interstitial hydrostatic pressure, causes leakage of fluid into the alveolar spaces until they are filled. The result is disruption of the lung ventilation to perfusion ratio (V/Q ratio), causing effective **right-to-left shunting** of blood. The intra-alveolar fluid later condenses to form a **hyaline membrane** which lines the alveoli. This is similar histologically to the neonatal form of the disease.

The full clinical syndrome often takes 24–48 hours to develop after the initial insult. If the patient eventually recovers, the interstitial damage may result in diffuse **interstitial fibrosis**. It is important to note that cardiac

KEY POINTS

Box 47.3 Conditions associated with acute respiratory distress syndrome (ARDS)

Common causes in surgical patients are emphasised in *italic* type

Direct insults to the lung
- Lung contusion
- Near-drowning
- Aspiration of gastric acid
- Inhalation of smoke and corrosive chemicals, e.g. chlorine, phosgene, nitrogen dioxide or ammonia
- Radiation pneumonitis

Systemic insults to the lung
- *Multiple trauma with shock*
- *Septic shock, e.g. after a colonic anastomotic leak*
- *Severe acute pancreatitis*
- Major head injuries ('neurogenic pulmonary oedema')
- Fat, air and amniotic fluid embolism
- Major blood transfusion reaction or massive blood transfusion
- Disseminated intravascular coagulation
- Cardiopulmonary bypass
- Eclampsia
- Severe allergic reactions
- Drug overdose or sensitivity, e.g. heroin, barbiturates, paraquat, bleomycin

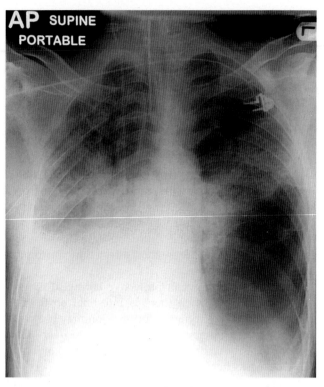

Fig. 47.5 Acute respiratory distress syndrome (ARDS)
Chest X-ray from a 62-year-old man admitted to intensive care with severe head injuries and multiple fractures. There is diffuse bilateral pulmonary shadowing typical of 'shock lung'. Note inadvertent placement of the endotracheal tube (identified by its radiopaque line) into the right main bronchus.

failure plays no part in the development of ARDS, although cardiac failure may later complicate the condition.

Clinical features of ARDS

The main clinical finding is rapid shallow respiration with only scattered crepitations heard on auscultation. There is usually no cough, chest pain or haemoptysis. Blood gas analysis reveals low PaO_2 but the $PaCO_2$ remains normal, except in the most severe cases. Chest X-ray may be normal in the early stages, progressing rapidly through increased interstitial markings to complete 'white-out' or partial (see Fig. 47.5). ARDS may be difficult to distinguish from cardiac failure except that cardiac diameter is normal in ARDS, and cardiac failure usually responds to diuretic therapy.

Treatment of ARDS

The overall objective is to maintain respiratory function and cardiovascular stability while the underlying cause (e.g. sepsis) is brought under control. This should be carried out under intensive care conditions. The sooner the treatment is begun, the greater the chance of recovery.

Most patients require mechanical **ventilation** with **positive end-expiratory pressure** (PEEP) to achieve adequate oxygenation and to try to reverse alveolar oedema and collapse. Fluid balance is complex in these patients and usually requires monitoring of both **right and left atrial pressures**; a central venous line is used to measure right atrial pressure, but left atrial pressure is measured indirectly as **pulmonary artery wedge pressure** via a **Swann–Ganz catheter**. Cardiac output can also be measured using the Swann–Ganz catheter. One of the treatment aims is to produce a negative fluid balance and thus help minimise lung water. Loop diuretic infusions or continuous veno-venous haemofiltration can be used to achieve this. Any associated renal failure can also be treated by this form of haemofiltration. In these patients, diuretics alone do not control pulmonary oedema but instead aggravate the hypovolaemia and shock associated with the underlying cause.

Renal failure is a common complication, sometimes prevented by early use of drugs such as dopamine. The mortality rate for complicated cases of ARDS approaches 90%.

THROMBOEMBOLISM

Pathophysiology

Venous thromboembolism is a major cause of complications and death after surgery or trauma. Venous blood is normally prevented from clotting within the veins by a complex series of mechanisms which include local inhibition of the clotting cascade, prompt lysis of small clots that do form, and continuous flow of blood. In 1856, Virchow proposed in his 'triad' that venous thrombosis could be caused by abnormalities in the vein wall (trauma, inflammation), alterations in blood flow (stasis) and changes in the blood (hypercoagulability), and this explanation largely holds good today. The subtle balance within the veins can be disturbed by several local and systemic factors, many incompletely understood. Imbalance results in thrombus formation within the venous sinuses of the calf muscles and sometimes primarily in the pelvic veins. More often, distal thrombi form first, then propagate proximally to involve the femoral and pelvic veins. If thrombi in the larger vessels become detached, they circulate proximally to impact in the pulmonary arteries as **pulmonary emboli**.

The main predisposing factors to venous thromboembolism are summarised in Box 47.4, but thromboembolism can also occur in healthy individuals with no apparent predisposing factors. It should be remembered that patients may have been ill and dehydrated at home for some time before hospital admission and venous thrombosis may have been initiated before admission.

The risk of thromboembolism increases incrementally as the number and severity of local and systemic risk factors increase; this is neatly illustrated in Table 47.1. The impact of many of the predisposing factors can be minimised by early mobilisation and prevention of local venous stasis. A number of specific preventive measures for high-risk groups are described later.

DEEP VEIN THROMBOSIS

Deep vein thrombosis (DVT) in the lower limbs is often silent, with the classic clinical features found in only half of cases. These include swelling of the leg, tenderness of the calf muscles, increased warmth of the leg, and calf pain on passive dorsiflexion of the foot (**Homans' sign**). The presence of these features indicates that venous occlusion has extended at least as far as the popliteal veins.

Occlusion of the ilio-femoral veins tends to produce diffuse and sometimes massive swelling of the whole lower limb (see Fig. 47.6a). In addition, there is tenderness over the femoral vein in the groin. In severe cases, the leg becomes painful and white, and boggy with oedema; this is known as **phlegmasia alba dolens**

Box 47.4 Predisposing factors for deep vein thrombosis and pulmonary embolism

- **Previous venous thromboembolism**
- **Trauma and surgery (complex systemic effects)**
- **Increasing age**
- **Direct trauma to the pelvis and lower limbs, especially fractures**
- **Pre-existing lower limb venous disorders causing stasis**
- **Venous stasis during general or regional anaesthesia (loss of calf muscle pump and postural pressure on the calves)**
- **Malignant disease**
- **Immobility, e.g. bed-bound patients after operation or stroke**
- **Cardiac failure**
- **High-oestrogen oral contraceptive pill, oestrogen treatment**
- **Pregnancy**
- **Pelvic masses causing venous obstruction**
- **Groin masses obstructing femoral vein, e.g. femoral aneurysm, malignant lymph nodes**
- **Obesity**
- **Dehydration**
- **Blood disorders, e.g. polycythaemia, thrombocythaemia and pro-thrombotic disorders**

Table 47.1 Varying risk of deep vein thrombosis

Age	Grade of surgery	Other risk factors	Risk of DVT (%)
20	Minor		1
40	Minor		3
60	Minor		10
60	Major		20
60	Major	Previous DVT	50
80	Major		40
80	Major	Previous DVT + infection or malignancy	96

(painful white leg). In extreme cases, the limb becomes more painful and blue, with incipient venous infarction (**phlegmasia caerulea dolens**).

Asymptomatic DVTs have the same potential for causing both pulmonary embolism and long-term chronic venous insufficiency as symptomatic venous thromboses. To complicate the problem, as many as half of the patients who develop swelling and pain in the calf after operation do not have deep vein thrombosis.

Diagnostic tests for DVT

Venography (phlebography) has long been the standard diagnostic technique when deep venous thrombosis is suspected; it is however, gradually being superseded by colour duplex imaging. Venography involves cannulating a small vein in the foot and injecting contrast material. Before the procedure, tourniquets are applied at the ankle and below the knee to direct superficial venous blood into the deep system. A typical venogram showing obstructed deep venous architecture is shown in Figure 47.7. Where local expertise is available duplex Doppler ultrasonography (preferably with colour) is the preferred diagnostic method. This technique allows scanning of all the major lower limb deep veins for flow and contained thrombus; the test is probably safer then venography. Both techniques are highly operator-dependent as regards making an accurate diagnosis. Another technique, mainly used for research purposes, is detection of thrombi using **radionuclide-labelled fibrinogen** given before operation. **Thermography** may have a value for screening all patients after operation to select those for further investigation.

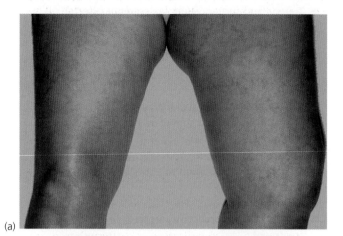

(a)

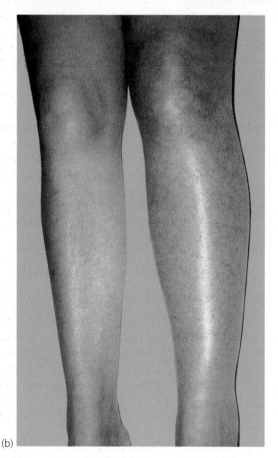

(b)

Fig. 47.6 Clinical obvious deep vein thrombosis
This woman of 45 suffered swelling and bursting pain in the whole of her left leg after radical surgery for ovarian cancer. The left thigh **(a)** and leg **(b)** are both visibly swollen and blueish. On palpation, the limb felt warm. A massive ilio-femoral venous thrombosis was diagnosed on venography and the patient was anticoagulated. Luckily she did not suffer a pulmonary embolism and the limb returned to normal diameter over six months. She will be at lifetime risk of post-thrombotic deep venous insufficiency.

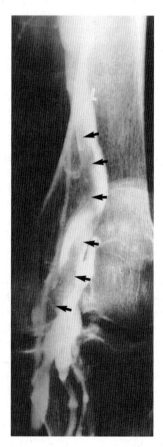

Fig. 47.7 Venogram (phlebogram) of deep vein thrombosis
Venogram showing the popliteal veins in a patient who complained of calf pain 5 days after a laparotomy for obstructive jaundice. There is extensive thrombus in the deep veins (arrowed) which is only loosely attached to the vein wall and therefore in danger of embolisation to the lung.

PULMONARY EMBOLISM

The classic picture of pulmonary embolism ('PE') is sudden dyspnoea and cardiovascular collapse, followed by pleuritic chest pain, development of a pleural rub and haemoptysis. The electrocardiogram (ECG) may show evidence of right heart strain (S wave in lead I, Q wave and inverted T wave in leads III–S1, Q3, T3). This clinical presentation, however, is uncommon and occurs only when 50% or more of the pulmonary arterial system is occluded. More extensive occlusion usually results in sudden death.

Smaller pulmonary emboli are more common and are often 'silent', presenting as non-specific episodes of general deterioration, confusion, breathlessness or chest pain. The patient often has a tachycardia and low-grade fever, and there are no diagnostic changes on ECG. The condition may be attributed to chest infection, atelectasis or cardiac failure unless a diagnosis of pulmonary embolism is considered. More specific diagnostic symptoms may occur with small pulmonary emboli, including localised **pleuritic chest pain** and small **haemoptyses** in the form of blood-streaked sputum. A small pulmonary embolus may herald a massive or fatal embolus, and must therefore always be treated seriously.

Venous thromboembolism is most common from about the fourth to the seventh postoperative day but may present at any time during the postoperative month, often after the patient has left hospital.

Diagnostic tests for pulmonary embolism

Chest X-ray rarely shows specific changes. A useful method of confirming the diagnosis is radioisotope **ventilation/perfusion scanning** (V/Q scanning), as shown in Figure 47.8. This involves two separate imaging procedures designed to demonstrate **ventilation/perfusion mismatch**. Firstly, the patient inhales radioactive gas and a gamma camera is used to detect the distribution of radioactivity within the air spaces of the lungs. This **ventilation scan** is followed by the **perfusion scan** in which an intravenous injection of radionuclide-labelled albumen microspheres is given. These lodge evenly throughout the pulmonary bed except where the pulmonary arteries are occluded by thrombus. This is again detected by gamma camera. In pulmonary embolism, distribution of isotope in the ventilation scan is normal, but areas of pulmonary under-perfusion (embolism) show as defects in the perfusion scan. In areas of infection or atelectasis (which are under-ventilated), the ventilation scan is deficient but the perfusion scan is normal.

Pulmonary angiography provides a more precise anatomical demonstration of the occluded vessels, as well as access to the pulmonary circulation for clot aspiration or thrombolysis. It should be performed if embolism is strongly suspected but cannot be proved by other means. Dynamic spiral computed tomography (CT) scanning using intravenous contrast is a minimally invasive means of detecting pulmonary embolism and has become the preferred diagnostic method in many centres (Fig. 47.8c).

MANAGEMENT OF VENOUS THROMBOEMBOLISM

For most patients, removing or lysing lower limb thrombus or pulmonary embolus is impractical. The main objective, therefore, in managing deep vein thrombosis and pulmonary embolism is to halt the coagulation process with the aim of preventing established thrombi from propagating and new thrombi from forming. Removal of thrombus is left to the normal body processes of lysis.

In the lower limbs, venous thrombi eventually become organised and firmly attached to the vessel wall, posing no further risk of embolisation. The thrombus is later invaded by granulation tissue and the veins eventually become recanalised, thus restoring venous flow. In the process, the valves are often destroyed, leading in the long term to **chronic venous insufficiency** (see Ch. 34). After pulmonary embolism, if the patient survives the initial embolic episode, the emboli are efficiently removed by local thrombolysis, leaving little functional deficit.

Initially, anticoagulation is achieved with **intravenous heparin**, commencing with a bolus dose of 10 000 units. This is followed by a continuous infusion of 24 000–48 000 units over each 24-hour period, with the dose adjusted to maintain the **partial thromboplastin time** 2–3 times normal. Heparin anticoagulation takes effect immediately and is continued for about 5 days, by which time acute symptoms have usually subsided. Often, nowadays, full anticoagulation is affected using subcutaneous doses of low molecular weight heparin alone. This has the advantage that it does not require monitoring by blood tests and hence can be employed on an ambulatory basis. In the mean time, oral **warfarin therapy** (which takes several days to become fully effective) is begun. Warfarin therapy is continued for 3–6 months, the period of highest risk of recurrent thromboembolism. Patients who suffer repeated thromboembolic episodes may have to be maintained on warfarin for life. In addition, a **filter** (e.g. a Greenfield filter) may be placed in the inferior vena cava via a percutaneous route.

In the rare case of massive but non-fatal pulmonary embolism, surgical **embolectomy** may be appropriate. This is performed under cardiopulmonary bypass and is therefore no small undertaking. Systemic thrombolytic therapy with **streptokinase** has been employed in this situation, but the high rate of serious bleeding in surgical patients precludes its use. The newer technique of manipulating a pulmonary artery catheter into the embolus and instilling high doses of **local thrombolytic drugs** or

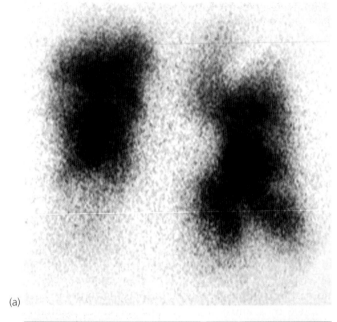

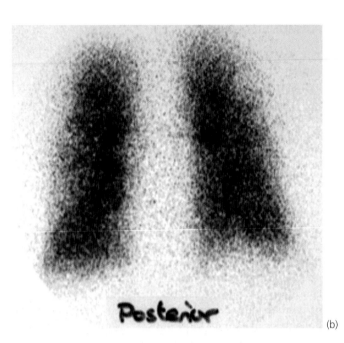

Posterior

(a)

(b)

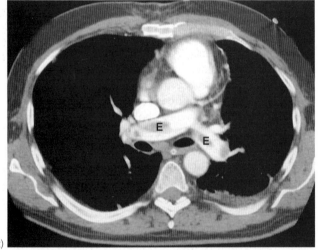

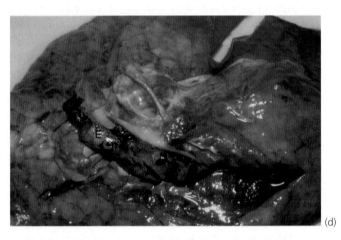

(c)

(d)

Fig. 47.8 Ventilation/perfusion scan in pulmonary embolism
(a) Perfusion scan showing multiple filling defects typical of pulmonary embolism. **(b)** Ventilation scan from the same patient, which is normal. Impaired perfusion with normal ventilation is typical of pulmonary embolism. **(c)** Thoracic CT scan with intravenous contrast showing large emboli **E** in the pulmonary arteries. This is becoming the investigation of choice for suspected PE. **(d)** Post-mortem specimen of lung from a patient who died of massive pulmonary embolism. Embolic material has been removed **E**, but some remains in the pulmonary arteries.

performing clot suction is more promising. Note that thrombolytic therapy takes several hours to act.

PREVENTION OF VENOUS THROMBOEMBOLISM

The importance of general measures in preventing venous thrombosis cannot be over-emphasised. These include **early postoperative mobilisation, adequate hydration** and **avoiding pressure on the calves**. In addition, patients on oestrogen-containing oral contraceptives should ideally stop taking them at least 6 weeks before major operations or be given heparin prophylaxis for intermediate and minor operations.

For patients at higher risk, as shown in Box 47.4 earlier, specific prophylactic measures should be taken to reduce the risk of deep venous thrombosis (and consequent pulmonary embolism). Prophylactic measures include the following:

● **Low-dose subcutaneous heparin**—this may be given as standard **unfractionated heparin** or as **low molecular weight heparin**. Both types are as effective for preventing deep venous thrombosis and pulmonary embolism but the chief advantage of low molecular weight heparin is that it is given only once a day instead of two or three times. Low-dose heparin is the most effective method of reducing venous thromboembolism in at-risk patients. It has been shown to reduce the rate of postoperative DVT by 70% in general surgical, urological, gynaecological, orthopaedic and trauma patients. Similar reductions are achieved in the rate of pulmonary embolism. The intravascular antithrombotic effect is not due to anticoagulation, but results from stimulation of platelet factor **antithrombin III**; there should be no detectable in vitro anticoagulant effect or any clinically significant effect on haemostasis during or after operation, although patients bleed about 10% more when on low-dose heparin

- **Calf compression devices**—several pneumatic and electrical devices are available for intraoperative calf compression to simulate normal muscle pump activity. These have the advantage of being non-invasive and easily applied to all patients, even those at low risk, but their efficacy is less than low-dose heparin
- **Graduated compression 'anti-embolism' stockings**— the use of these stockings is simple and widely practised. Provided they are correctly fitted, graduated compression stockings offer a suitable level of prophylaxis for patients at low or moderate risk. The stockings must be worn during operation as well as during the early postoperative period
- **Intravenous dextran**—dextrans are high molecular weight polysaccharides, which were once used as plasma substitutes. Intravenous Dextran 70 has been shown to provide prophylaxis against deep venous thrombosis almost as effectively as low-dose heparin; 500 ml of a standard solution is given daily from the time of operation until the third postoperative day. The main disadvantages are the need for an intravenous line, the large volume of fluid and the occasional hypersensitivity reaction. All of these have limited its more general use
- **Warfarin anticoagulation**—this is one of the best methods of prophylaxis for elective operations, and is widely used for major elective surgery in the Netherlands. It is considered impractical by many surgeons, not least because of the supposed risk of incidental and operative haemorrhage. In addition, the logistics of establishing preoperative anticoagulation and continuing dose monitoring afterwards require a great deal of resources

FLUID AND ELECTROLYTE DISTURBANCES

Fluid and electrolyte disturbances such as **dehydration** or **fluid overload**, **hyponatraemia**, **hypokalaemia** and **hyperkalaemia** frequently develop in the postoperative period. Fluid and electrolyte abnormalities are particu-

larly common after major surgery of the bowel, especially if there have been massive fluid losses through vomiting, diarrhoea or sequestration in obstructed or adynamic bowel, or surgical complications. These problems are discussed in Chapter 50.

TRANSFUSION COMPLICATIONS

The management of blood transfusion and its complications is described in detail in Chapter 3.

URINARY RETENTION

Acute retention of urine is common in the immediate postoperative period. The usual problem is that the patient has been unable to pass urine following operation. The anuria is often drawn to the doctor's attention by a nurse several hours after operation but before the patient becomes distressed. Acute retention needs to be distinguished from true oliguria resulting from poor renal perfusion or acute renal failure; if this cannot be resolved clinically, ultrasonography will show whether the bladder is full of urine.

Pathophysiology

Postoperative retention is much more common in men, particularly when there is a degree of prostatic hypertrophy. Patients with symptoms of bladder outflow obstruction ('prostatism') are at high risk of developing acute retention, although young male patients can also be affected.

Acute postoperative urinary retention seems to result from a combination of the following factors:

- Pre-existing bladder outlet obstruction
- Difficulty in passing urine in the supine position
- Embarrassment at passing urine without sufficient privacy
- Accumulation of a large volume of urine during the operation and recovery from anaesthesia, causing overfilling of the bladder
- Transient disturbance of the neurological control of voiding by general or spinal anaesthesia
- Pain from an abdominal or inguinal wound inhibiting normal contraction of the abdominal musculature and relaxation of the bladder neck
- Problems after certain operations which predispose to acute retention, e.g. abdomino-perineal resection of rectum or bilateral inguinal hernia repair
- Constipation—gross faecal loading is common in the elderly in hospital and is probably the most frequent cause of acute retention (and faecal incontinence)

Management of postoperative urinary retention

Conservative measures

Most cases of postoperative acute retention can be managed conservatively, bearing in mind the precipitating factors mentioned above. If the problem is dealt with early, the patient is less likely to require catheterisation and this should be avoided if possible. However, if there is a history of symptoms of bladder outlet obstruction or previous prostatectomy, catheterisation is more likely to be needed. The first step is to ensure there is adequate **postoperative analgesia** and this may be all that is needed to enable the patient to pass urine. The next step is to help the patient out of bed in order to use a commode at the bedside or use a urine bottle standing at the bedside.

The patient will often need continuous support to stand if still 'groggy' from the anaesthetic or analgesia. For young male patients, a male assistant should be at hand if possible, as the presence of a young female can have a marked inhibitory effect!

If these measures fail, the patient should be wheeled into a bathroom for privacy and left alone for a while, if he (or she) is fit enough. The familiar sound of a tap left running often encourages micturition. If the patient still does not pass urine, it may be appropriate to encourage a bowel movement by means of a lubricant glycerine suppository. Defaecation is usually accompanied by bladder neck relaxation and micturition, so this may help. In women, where the risk of bladder neck obstruction or urethral stricture is small, a single injection of **carbachol** is worth trying and may initiate micturition.

Catheterisation

If conservative measures fail, catheterisation will usually be necessary. In females, bladder drainage and immediate removal of the catheter is often all that is required. In males, the catheter is usually left in situ until the following morning or until the patient is well. In patients with prostatic obstruction, a suprapubic catheter is a better option as it avoids urethral trauma and can easily be temporarily clamped to check if normal micturition has returned. Recurrent problems of retention are usually caused by bladder outlet obstruction and are managed as described in Chapter 29.

URINARY TRACT INFECTIONS

Urinary tract infections are extremely common in the postoperative period, especially in women. The most obvious predisposing factor is catheterisation, although urinary tract infections commonly occur without urethral instrumentation. The cause is probably a combination of reduced urinary output, reducing 'flushing' of the bladder, incomplete bladder emptying in the supine posture, bacteraemia induced by operation or infection, and finally inadequate perineal hygiene.

Typical symptoms of dysuria and frequency may be less apparent or absent altogether. The diagnosis of urinary tract infection is often made on investigation of an unexplained pyrexia or septicaemia. Treatment is by ensuring adequate fluid input and prescription of appropriate antibiotics such as trimethoprim.

ANTIBIOTIC-ASSOCIATED COLITIS

Pathophysiology and clinical features

Colonic inflammation and other diarrhoeal disorders may be side effects of almost any antibiotic treatment. The conditions are probably due to selective overgrowth of intestinal organisms which then produce toxins which cause damage. The clinical picture may range from a mild attack of diarrhoea to profuse, life-threatening, haemorrhagic colitis. **Pseudomembranous colitis** can take a particularly virulent form (see below). Antibiotic-associated colitis may develop suddenly or gradually and occasionally becomes chronic or relapsing.

Surgical patients are most likely to be affected in the postoperative period. *Clostridium difficile* is responsible for many of these cases and in severe form, the full picture of pseudomembranous colitis may develop. **Staphylococcal enterocolitis** is less common.

If a surgical patient on antibiotics develops diarrhoea which is worse or more prolonged than might be expected after an operation, antibiotic-associated colitis should be suspected. Stool specimens should be examined by microscopy and culture and by measuring levels of *Clostridium difficile* toxin. Sigmoidoscopic inspection and biopsy of the rectum should also be performed. Treatment is based on the results of these tests. If *Clostridium difficile* infection is diagnosed, it is treated with oral metronidazole or, in resistant cases, with oral (non-absorbed) vancomycin.

ACUTE RENAL FAILURE

Acute renal failure is defined clinically as the abrupt onset of oliguria or anuria, associated with a steep rise in blood urea concentration. This is caused by failure to excrete nitrogenous waste products. The usual cause is **acute tubular necrosis**, but acute renal failure is sometimes caused by nephrotoxins. These include the **aminoglycoside antibiotics** gentamicin and tobramycin, myoglobin (released in the crush syndrome) and the 'hepatorenal syndrome' associated with obstructive jaundice (see Ch. 11). Acute renal failure is also a particular complication of surgery of the abdominal aorta, in which the renal arteries may be occluded by inadvertent damage or occult embolism.

Pathophysiology

The renal tubules are acutely sensitive to a variety of metabolic insults, particularly hypoxia and certain toxins. Hypoxia readily occurs if renal perfusion falls significantly. The usual surgical cause is an episode of severe or prolonged **hypotension**. This may be the result of hypovolaemic shock (haemorrhage or dehydration), cardiovascular collapse (postoperative cardiac failure or myocardial infarction) or septic shock. In the last, endotoxic and cytokine-initiated renal cell damage is probably an important factor. Pre-existing **chronic renal disease** increases a patient's susceptibility to acute renal failure.

Provided the insult to the renal tubules is not overwhelming, the damage to the tubular cells is confined to disruption of cellular metabolism rather than tissue necrosis. This is potentially reversible, provided the patient can be maintained in good general condition while tubular recovery takes place. The usual sequence is that poor urine output continues for a period (**oliguric phase**), followed by **spontaneous diuresis** of large volumes of unconcentrated urine consisting of unmodified glomerular filtrate (**diuretic phase**). Urinary concentrating power then slowly improves as the tubules recover normal metabolic function. In contrast, if tubular damage is more extensive, the patient remains anuric or severely oliguric.

Prevention of acute renal failure

Acute renal failure is largely preventable by careful attention to preoperative assessment, fluid balance, and prevention and prompt management of hypotension and sepsis, as well as dose monitoring of potentially nephrotoxic drugs. In high-risk patients (with pre-existing renal disease or obstructive jaundice and those undergoing cardiopulmonary bypass or aortic surgery), **intravenous renal dose dopamine** given during operation helps protect renal function.

Diagnosis of oliguria

When urinary retention has been excluded and true **oliguria** or **anuria** is diagnosed, the problem is to differentiate between acute tubular necrosis and reduced renal perfusion. As a first step, a **urinary catheter** should be inserted to monitor the hourly rate of urine production, which should ideally be at least 30 ml/hour. *Note*: if a catheter is already in situ and stops draining, it may have become blocked.

Low urine output is most often caused by **reduced renal perfusion**, resulting from relative hypovolaemia or low cardiac output. This leads to diminished glomerular filtration and enhanced tubular reabsorption. The usual reason is inadequate replacement of a perioperative fluid deficit. To test this, an intravenous fluid challenge of 250 ml can be infused over a few minutes. If this restores urinary output, under-hydration is confirmed and the fluid balance must be corrected to prevent acute tubular necrosis. Potentially more serious causes of reduced renal perfusion include cardiac failure and acute myocardial infarction; these need to be considered in postoperative patients with a low urinary output. Only if poor renal perfusion can be excluded should acute renal failure be diagnosed.

Management of acute renal failure

When acute renal failure is mild, simple conservation measures such as fluid restriction may sustain the patient until tubular function recovers. When complete (oliguric) renal failure occurs, serum urea, creatinine and potassium concentrations rise inexorably and the patient usually requires **haemofiltration** or **renal dialysis**. Fortunately, many of these patients recover renal function gradually over a few weeks or months and do not require permanent renal support.

PRESSURE SORES

Pathophysiology

Elderly, debilitated and other bed-bound patients are extremely susceptible to pressure sores ('bed sores'), particularly over bony prominences such as the sacrum and heels (see Figs. 47.9 and 47.10). Pressure sores occur because the frequent spontaneous adjustment of position that normally occurs is lost through obtunded sensation and immobility. Diminished protective pain response plays an important part. Tissue necrosis and subsequent failure to heal result from a combination of factors including recurrent pressure ischaemia, poor tissue perfusion (from cardiac or peripheral vascular disease) and malnutrition. Note that patients who have undergone substantial weight loss and patients with relatively ischaemic lower limbs are at particular risk.

Prevention and management of pressure sores

Once established, pressure sores are difficult to eradicate and prevention must be given high priority in patients at risk. Relatively hard surfaces such as accident and emergency department trolleys and operating tables may initiate pressure sores in susceptible patients in less than 1 hour. Likewise, pressure sores can develop in a remarkably short time in a hospital bed, particularly if the patient is incontinent of urine or faeces. Prevention of pressure sores on the ward is mainly a nursing

647

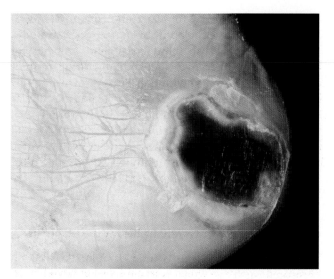

Fig. 47.9 Typical heel pressure sore
This elderly man presented with a ruptured abdominal aortic aneurysm and had a stormy post-operative course. At some stage, this heel was allowed to remain too long in one position, resulting in deep necrosis. He had no evidence of occlusive peripheral arterial disease.

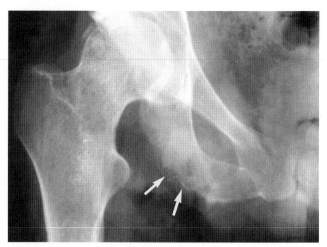

Fig. 47.10 Osteomyelitis of the ischial tuberosity secondary to pressure ulceration
X-ray of the pelvis in an elderly immobile woman showing osteomyelitis of the ischial tuberosity (arrowed) underlying a deep long-standing sacral pressure ulcer.

responsibility; indeed, the incidence of pressure sores is a good indicator of the quality of nursing care.

Prevention of pressure sores involves the following procedures:

● **Special bed surfaces to spread the load**—these include (in ascending order of cost and complexity) pressure-relieving foam mattresses, electric ripple mattresses, water beds, suspended net beds and sophisticated low pressure continuous airflow beds
● **Relieving pressure on the heels**—use of ankle rests while on the operating table, use of heel pads, orthopaedic foam gutters and 'bean-bags' on return to the ward
● **Regular change of posture**—for most patients, this involves encouragement to get out of bed, at least into a bedside chair, and to mobilise beyond this as much as possible. A bed-bound patient requires regular turning so that the same skin area is not subjected to constant pressure
● **Regular checking of pressure areas and local massage**
● **Management of incontinence**

Treatment of established pressure sores is unsatisfactory unless the causative factors can be eliminated. This is often impossible in the permanently disabled patient. Avoiding pressure is the mainstay of treatment, supplemented by local cleansing and dressings designed to remove necrotic tissue and control secondary infection. For a deep sacral sore, major plastic surgery involving a rotational buttock flap is occasionally justified.

COMPLICATIONS OF OPERATIONS INVOLVING BOWEL

These include delayed return of bowel function, mechanical bowel obstruction, anastomotic failure, intra-abdominal abscesses, peritonitis, bowel fistula and acute bowel ischaemia.

DELAYED RETURN OF BOWEL FUNCTION

TEMPORARY INTERRUPTION OF PERISTALSIS

Any abdominal operation may temporarily disrupt peristalsis. This is particularly true where the operation is for peritonitis, an abscess or intestinal obstruction, or if the operation involves extensive handling of the bowel. Operations involving the retroperitoneal area, such as aortic surgery, may also disrupt peristalsis. The mechanism is probably via a disturbance of parasympathetic activity. The problem is usually minor and mostly affects the small intestine. Patients may complain of nausea, anorexia and vomiting. This becomes obvious after oral fluids are reintroduced early in the postoperative period. This condition is often loosely described as **ileus** and is the reason for gradual reintroduction of fluids, followed by solids after abdominal operations. However, if ileus is prolonged another cause such as an intraperitoneal collection should be sought.

ADYNAMIC OBSTRUCTION

Occasionally, a much more prolonged and extensive form of adynamic bowel obstruction occurs. This presents with vomiting and protracted intolerance to oral intake. **Adynamic obstruction** must be distinguished from true mechanical obstruction, which may require reoperation (see Ch. 12).

Acute gastric dilatation

Occasionally, adynamic obstruction involves the stomach, causing acute gastric dilatation and accumulation of large volumes of gastric and duodenal reflux secretions. The warning feature is when the patient suddenly vomits a large volume of fluid which may, even on the first occasion, result in fatal bronchial aspiration. Preventing acute gastric dilatation is the main reason nasogastric tubes are used after upper gastrointestinal surgery or relief of mechanical bowel obstruction. If acute gastric dilatation is suspected in any patient in whom recovery is unexpectedly slow, the abdomen should be examined daily for a **succussion splash**, and a nasogastric tube passed if the result is positive.

'Pseudo-obstruction'

Adynamic obstruction involving the large bowel is conventionally described as pseudo-obstruction. It may follow any abdominal operation, especially if the retroperitoneal area has been disturbed, as in nephrectomy or aortic surgery. Pseudo-obstruction is also a recognised complication of *non-abdominal operations* such as fractured neck of femur, especially in frail patients. Pseudo-obstruction may even occur without operation as a complication of severe hypokalaemia, trauma involving the lower spine and retroperitoneal area, or anti-Parkinsonian and other drugs. The diagnosis can rapidly be made on an 'instant' unprepared barium enema by excluding mechanical causes of obstruction. Treatment involves supportive measures until function returns.

MECHANICAL BOWEL OBSTRUCTION

EARLY POSTOPERATIVE MECHANICAL OBSTRUCTION

Postoperative mechanical obstruction of the bowel is uncommon. It may be caused by a loop of bowel becoming twisted or trapped in a peritoneal defect, unwittingly created at open operation or laparoscopy.

Fibrinous adhesions may also cause obstruction and these usually develop about 1 week after operation. In both cases, the obstruction may be transient and settle with conservative measures (nasogastric aspiration and intravenous fluids), or may progress to full-blown intestinal obstruction requiring laparotomy. If tenderness and systemic signs of toxicity appear, reoperation becomes urgent to exclude strangulation. Obstruction occurring after gastrectomy or gastroenterostomy may be due to oedema of the mucosa surrounding the anastomosis; this usually settles eventually with conservative measures although reoperation may be required.

LATE POSTOPERATIVE MECHANICAL OBSTRUCTION

Fibrinous adhesions may organise and persist as broad **fibrous adhesions** between adjacent loops of bowel or as isolated fibrous bands traversing the peritoneal cavity. These fibrous adhesions are a common cause of an isolated episode of small bowel obstruction or even infarction. Adhesions may also cause recurrent bouts of bowel obstruction months or years after abdominal operations. Most episodes will resolve spontaneously with conservative treatment, i.e. nasogastric aspiration and intravenous fluids, but failure of resolution or signs of strangulation (tenderness, toxaemia) will necessitate laparotomy. Adhesive obstruction has become less common since talc powder on surgical gloves was discontinued in the 1970s and possibly since the declining use of starch on surgical gloves more recently. However, patients with recurrent intestinal obstruction due to adhesions present a serious surgical challenge. Each laparotomy becomes more difficult and hazardous for the patient. Therapeutic agents to prevent adhesions forming, often in the form of films, are currently under trial but conclusive evidence of their benefit is awaited.

ANASTOMOTIC FAILURE

Anastomotic leakage or breakdown is a major cause of postoperative morbidity after bowel surgery. Inadequate diagnosis and surgical intervention may lead to snowballing complications including sepsis, multi-organ dysfunction and failure, and fistulae.

Small anastomotic leaks are relatively common and lead to small **localised abscesses** which are walled off by surrounding gut and omentum. Small leaks are clinically manifest by delayed recovery of bowel function due to local peristaltic dysfunction. Usually, the problem eventually settles with continued intravenous fluids and delayed reintroduction of oral intake. Reoperation, however, should be considered regularly if recovery is slow.

Major anastomotic breakdown results in generalised peritonitis, large abdominal abscesses, progressive sepsis and fistula formation. Most of these are described here; systemic sepsis is described in Chapter 2.

INTRA-ABDOMINAL ABSCESSES

ABSCESS ASSOCIATED WITH BOWEL ANASTOMOSIS

An anastomotic leak from any part of the bowel may be walled off by small bowel and omentum as a vigorous intraperitoneal response (see Fig. 47.11). This results in formation of an abscess near the anastomosis. The patient will either be non-specifically unwell with delayed recovery, a swinging pyrexia and signs of local peritonitis, or more seriously ill with early signs of septicaemia. A detailed description of the clinical features is given in Chapter 12. For systemic inflammatory response syndrome, see p. 25.

Early reoperation is usually necessary to drain the abscess and prevent continued contamination of the peritoneal cavity. Where the anastomosis has broken down, both ends of the bowel should be brought out to form temporary stomas, since reanastomosis will almost certainly fail. The bowel can often be rejoined once the local infection and metabolic disruption have resolved.

OTHER INTRA-ABDOMINAL ABSCESSES

Intra-abdominal abscesses may also develop at sites remote from an anastomosis—for example, in the pelvis (**pelvic abscess**) or beneath the diaphragm (**subphrenic abscess**). These abscesses occur most commonly as a complication of treated peritonitis, particularly faecal peritonitis. They may also develop because of contamination of the operative site by faeces or other infected material, or by 'tracking' of an anastomotic abscess within the abdomen. Abscesses of this type usually produce a less severe illness than do those in direct communication with the bowel.

If an abscess is suspected, ultrasound or CT scanning may help to identify its location and guide needle aspiration or placement of a percutaneous drain, if appropriate. Surgical exploration may, however, be necessary.

PERITONITIS

Peritonitis in the postoperative period usually results from a major anastomotic breakdown causing wide-

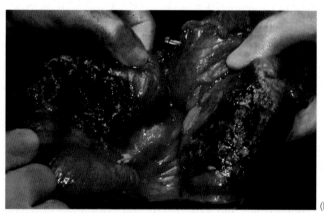

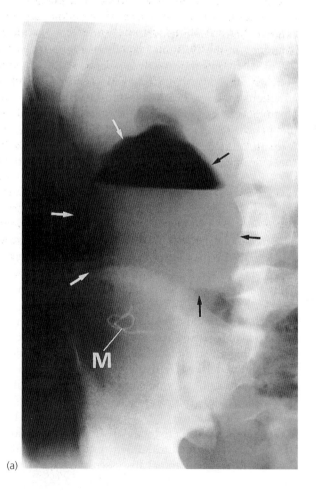

(b)

(a)

Fig. 47.11 Intra-abdominal abscess
Intraperitoneal abscess following appendicectomy. **(a)** Erect abdominal X-ray from a 16-year-old boy 1 week after removal of a perforated gangrenous appendix. He remained ill with anorexia and intermittent vomiting, general malaise and a swinging pyrexia. A large mass was palpable in the right side of the abdomen. The X-ray shows a huge abscess cavity (outline arrowed) with a gas bubble above a fluid (pus) level. Note the radiopaque marker **M** in a gauze swab packed into the open abdominal wound. **(b)** At operation, the abscess was surrounded by adherent small bowel, shown here.

spread peritoneal contamination. Sometimes the cause of peritonitis is perforation of **obstructed or ischaemic bowel** or perforation of an incidental **peptic ulcer**. The clinical picture may develop rapidly over a few hours or, if infection spreads from an intraperitoneal abscess, more insidiously over a few days. The patient is systemically ill with severe, generalised abdominal pain; the abdomen is tender and rigid to palpation (see Ch. 12 for more details). *Note*: elderly patients with peritonitis may have surprisingly little tenderness. Generalised peritonitis progresses to septicaemia and multiple organ failure unless promptly treated.

The patient is resuscitated and commenced on intravenous antibiotics and then returned to theatre for laparotomy. The abdomen is explored, the underlying cause is treated and peritoneal toilet is carried out. Early and vigorous treatment will usually save the patient's life.

BOWEL FISTULA

Fistula formation as a complication of surgery usually results from an anastomotic leak or infarction of a segment of bowel. A local abscess first develops then discharges to the surface via the wound or along the track of an abdominal drain. Anastomotic breakdown is more likely when there is obstruction of bowel distally, and the fistulous tract provides a means of drainage for the obstructed bowel contents. With time, the drainage tract slowly becomes lined with epithelium from the bowel and the skin surface and the fistula becomes permanent. Occasionally a fistula develops in a patient after an operation for bowel cancer. In this case the fistula may be lined with malignant cells. Proximal small bowel fistulae result in the loss of large volumes of intestinal secretions containing digestive enzymes. This rapidly leads to dehydration and major electrolyte disturbances and usually causes gross intra-abdominal inflammation and skin destruction. The more proximal the origin of the fistula, the greater the volume and the more destructive its consequences.

The general state of the patient with a fistula depends on the extent of intra-abdominal infection. If this is minimal and there is no distal obstruction, the fistula usually closes spontaneously within weeks or months, provided the patient can be sustained in the interim. Proximal small bowel fistulae require **total bowel rest** (i.e. nil by mouth and a nasogastric tube) with full **parenteral fluid replacement and nutrition**. Somatostatin analogues may be given to reduce the volume of secretion into the small bowel substantially. Distal small bowel or large bowel fistulae may be managed with **enteral feeding** using low-residue elemental or semi-elemental fluid diets. These are often given via a fine-bore nasogastric tube.

When a fistula is associated with intra-abdominal infection, the patient is desperately ill, septicaemic and hypercatabolic. These patients need intensive care management and reoperation. Laparotomy is required to bring the disrupted bowel ends to the surface as stomas and to drain the gross foci of infection; further laparotomies, even daily, may still be required before the intra-abdominal infection is brought under control. Mortality from these complicated fistulae is high.

ACUTE BOWEL ISCHAEMIA

Acute bowel ischaemia is an uncommon postoperative complication, usually occurring after abdominal aortic surgery. Infarction of the sigmoid colon follows inferior mesenteric artery ligation (usually a necessary part of the operation) if the collateral blood supply is compromised by obliterative atherosclerosis of the remaining mesenteric arteries. Fortunately, this problem is rare. The patient has usually progressed satisfactorily at first and then deteriorates unexpectedly several days after operation, often passing fresh blood per rectum. If untreated at this stage, the patient collapses with peritonitis due to colonic necrosis and perforation. Clinical signs are non-specific, but plain abdominal X-ray may show 'thumb printing' of the affected bowel or the characteristic appearance of gas in the bowel wall. If acute bowel ischaemia is suspected, laparotomy must be performed urgently as perforation will soon occur and is nearly always fatal. Even with timely surgery, the prognosis is bleak.

48 Preoperative assessment and preparation

INTRODUCTION

When a patient is admitted to hospital for surgical investigation or treatment, a detailed history and examination (**clerking**) is usually undertaken by a junior hospital doctor. This is often performed at a separate **pre-clerking visit** prior to admission to hospital. Clerking is mainly concerned with anticipating complications and taking preventive action rather than with diagnosing the primary disorder. If an anaesthetic other than a simple local is required, the anaesthetist will additionally make his or her own assessment.

PRINCIPLES OF ASSESSMENT

In preparing a patient for operation, the doctor needs to answer a series of questions, summarised in Box 48.1. Answers from the history and examination may reveal the need for tests or some other action.

The majority of surgical cases are straightforward but preventable disasters occur unless a thorough and systematic approach is used.

KEY POINTS

Box 48.1 Preoperative assessment and planning

1. **Diagnosis**
   - What is the (provisional) diagnosis and how confident is the diagnosis?
   - What are the important facets of the history?
   - What are the findings on examination?
   - What are the results of investigations already performed?
   - If appropriate, have tissue diagnoses been obtained before admission to hospital?
   - Are any further investigations needed to confirm the primary diagnosis?

2. **Operation**
   - What operation or procedure is planned?
   - Have any circumstances changed relating to the planned operation?
   - Has the patient got better or worse?
   - Has any new diagnostic information appeared? (e.g. pulmonary metastases on a chest X-ray)
   - Is the planned operation still appropriate?
   - Are there any special risks attending this particular operation, intraoperative or postoperative? (e.g. risk of DVT after pelvic surgery)
   - Are there any 'routine' procedures that need to be performed in relation to the operation? (e.g. ordering blood if heavy blood loss is anticipated)

Box 48.1 (Continued)

2. Operation
- Are there operation-specific actions that need to be performed? (e.g. examining vocal cord movement before thyroid surgery, arranging peroperative cholangiogram for open cholecystectomy)

3. Anaesthesia
- What type of anaesthesia is to be employed?
- Can any anaesthetic complications be anticipated? (e.g. risk of postoperative chest infection after thoracotomy or upper abdominal surgery, risk of a patient with bowel obstruction inhaling vomitus during anaesthetic induction)

4. Fitness for operation
- Is the patient fit for the planned anaesthetic and operation?
- Are there any intercurrent diseases which are currently inadequately treated, or which might pose special problems? (e.g. insulin-dependent diabetes, rheumatoid arthritis with cervical spine involvement)
- Are any preoperative investigations or treatments needed for intercurrent disease? (e.g. lung function tests and physiotherapy for chronic bronchitis, cervical spine radiology for rheumatoid arthritis)
- Does the surgical condition itself pose special problems? (e.g. fluid or electrolyte disturbances as a result of vomiting)
- Is the patient taking any drugs which might cause problems with anaesthesia or operation? (e.g. MAOIs or steroids)

5. High risk
- Is this patient particularly predisposed to anaesthetic or surgical complications (Table 48.1)?

6. After the operation
- Can any special problems be anticipated for this patient during the postoperative period and after discharge from hospital? (e.g. elderly patients living alone)
- Are there any problems specific to this anaesthetic or operation with respect to recovery and rehabilitation? (e.g. prostheses after mastectomy, stoma care, limb fitting and rehabilitation following amputation)
- Is any planning required for operation-specific problems?

PATIENTS AT HIGH RISK OF COMPLICATIONS

The history and examination will identify patients with medical comorbidity who are at risk of specific problems in the perioperative period. Special investigations may be needed to identify and characterise potential problems and to provide baseline information against which later changes can be measured. The common problems of high-risk groups of patients are summarised in Table 48.1.

Table 48.1 High risk groups for perioperative complications

Group	Particular risks	Management
Premature or tiny babies, neonates and infants	Fluid and electrolyte loss Heat loss in operating theatre	Careful measurement and replacement Warming blanket, temperature monitoring
Patients over 60	Cardiovascular disease	Chest X-ray and ECG preoperatively and monitoring during operation
Very elderly patients	Confusion Hyponatraemia Immobility	Multifactorial—see Chapter 46 Preoperative electrolyte estimations and correction Good nursing and rehabilitation
Smokers	Postoperative chest infection and atelectasis Increased risk of myocardial infarction	Stop smoking before operation — ideally at least four weeks beforehand. Preoperative chest X-ray. Preoperative and postoperative physiotherapy Preoperative ECG; avoid hypoxia during and after operation; postoperative oxygen therapy
Obese patients	Increased risk of DVT Reduced mobility	DVT prophylaxis (see Chapter 47) Early mobilisation with assistance
Patients with intercurrent medical disease	Depends on medical condition	Early referral to anaesthetist (Problems discussed in Chapter 46)

653

ESSENTIALS OF PREOPERATIVE ASSESSMENT

Although procedures vary in different hospitals, certain basic steps must be taken to ensure the maximum safety of a patient before operation (see Box 48.2). These steps depend on the nature of the operation and the condition of the patient. The **need for an operation** must be reviewed on admission to hospital, since circumstances can change substantially between booking and the time of operation. **Overt and occult illnesses** must also be considered in every patient.

EXPLANATIONS TO THE PATIENT AND INFORMED CONSENT

The surgeon must carefully explain the diagnosis and the proposed operation to the patient beforehand. Patients often absorb very little of what has been said, however, and fail to understand the full ramifications. This is because they are often anxious and disorientated when admitted, and most have little understanding of how their bodies work. Ideally, the patient would have been given information leaflets or if appropriate, put in contact with self-help groups. This provides a basis for obtaining informed consent. The doctor must adopt a sympathetic and unhurried approach, and must often explain things more than once. By this means, the surgeon or junior doctor can ensure that the patient is giving genuinely informed consent. This requires an explanation of any potential complications which have more than a 1–5% risk of arising as a result of the procedure, or of any less common procedure-specific risks.

If the immediate postoperative period is likely to be unpleasant or unfamiliar, such as admission to an intensive care unit, it is prudent to forewarn the patient and arrange a visit to the unit beforehand. Patients with learning difficulties and the elderly have particular difficulty in adapting to changing circumstances and care should be taken to familiarise them with facilities and staff.

At the time of obtaining consent, the **operation site should be marked** on the patient's skin with an indelible pen. This is particularly important if the operation could be performed on either side of the body, for example an inguinal hernia or limb amputation. This marking procedure also gives the patient an opportunity to agree which operation is to be done and on which side!

LIAISON WITH ANAESTHETIST

The anaesthetist (anaesthesiologist) should be informed in advance of the proposed operation and the condition of the patient; anaesthetists see patients preoperatively to anticipate problems, discuss their plans and prescribe premedication if appropriate. The anaesthetist is ultimately responsible for ensuring that the patient is fit for the operation and that anaesthetic procedures have been explained.

OPERATING THEATRE ARRANGEMENTS

The house surgeon (intern) is usually responsible for informing the operating department about the operation and the need for any special arrangements. A formal **operating list** should be prepared, giving full details of the name, age, sex, ward, and proposed operation for each patient. The side of the body to be operated on should be clearly (and correctly!) indicated. In addition, any special requirements for instruments, intra-operative radiography or patient positioning must be noted on the list. In some hospitals, the amount of bank blood ordered for a patient is also recorded on the list.

PLANNING THE RECOVERY PERIOD

Plans for rehabilitation and convalescence should be discussed with the patient and relatives in advance. The

---

SUMMARY

Box 48.2 Essential steps in preoperative assessment and preparation

- History taking
- Physical examination
- Collating pre-admission information about diagnosis
- Arranging any further diagnostic investigations
- Making special preparations for the particular operation
- Investigating any intercurrent or occult illness suggested by medical clerking, enlisting appropriate specialist help
- Discussing the operation and the recovery period with the patient and obtaining signed consent
- Marking the operation site
- Making arrangements for the operation with the operating theatre staff
- Arranging and informing the anaesthetist
- Prescribing medication, prophylactic antibiotics and treatment to prevent thromboembolism, as appropriate
- Planning rehabilitation and convalescence

patient should be advised about the likely rate of recovery and the level of activity possible on discharge. In this way, social, business and domestic arrangements can be made in good time. If necessary, domestic or home nursing help can be arranged. Uncertainty about these matters often causes anxiety and hampers recovery.

PREPARATION FOR MAJOR OPERATION—CASE HISTORY

This case history illustrates the way a patient might be prepared for a major operation and the considerations which guide the preoperative management.

HISTORY

James Brown, a 70-year-old retired farmer, admitted electively for an anterior resection of the rectum for carcinoma at the rectosigmoid junction.

Present complaint

Seen urgently in outpatient clinic 3 weeks ago with a 5-week history of loose stools three to five times a day, without blood or mucus. GP reported three stool specimens were positive for occult blood. Lost about 4 kg in weight over the last 3 months, but has been trying to lose weight anyway.

Results of outpatient investigations:

- Flexible sigmoidoscopic examination—obvious fungating tumour of upper rectum. Scope could not be passed beyond it. Biopsies confirmed adenocarcinoma
- Barium enema—'apple-core' lesion at recto-sigmoid junction; no other lesions in the rest of the colon
- Chest X-ray—normal
- Ultrasound examination of liver—no metastases
- Full blood count-haemoglobin 11.6 g/L, otherwise normal
- Urea and electrolytes, liver function tests—normal

Systems enquiry

Generally well, but systems enquiry reveals recent onset of shortness of breath after walking 200 yards on flat ground and occasional fast palpitations. No other cardio-respiratory symptoms. Poor stream on micturition. Nil else on systemic enquiry.

Past medical history

Appendicectomy aged 14; no anaesthetic complications. Serious farming injury to left elbow aged 20. Jaundiced during the Second World War in Asia, nil since. Hypertensive for 10 years and on drug treatment for 5. Diabetes discovered 3 years ago on routine urine testing, controlled by diet alone.

Family history

Mother was obese; died age 55 from complications of diabetes (gangrene). Older brother had major stroke at 64 but partially recovered. No family history of bowel cancer.

Social history

Widowed for 2 years, wife died of breast cancer. Has one son and one daughter, both married with young children, but living far away. Lives in own house with an upstairs lavatory, on a smallholding with a few stock animals. Lives independently, and uses his car for shopping. Smoked 20 cigarettes a day since age 15; drinks alcohol occasionally, average 4 units a day.

Drug history

Takes propranolol 40 mg o.d. (a beta blocker) and chlorothiazide (a diuretic) with potassium supplement each morning for hypertension. Takes aspirin 75 mg o.d. 'for his heart'. Told in the past not to have penicillin, but cannot recall why; does not remember when he last had penicillin. Not allergic to iodine.

EXAMINATION

General. Fit-looking man of 70, not obviously anxious. Tanned; no anaemia, cyanosis, jaundice, lymphadenopathy or clubbing; no thyroid enlargement. Fingers tobacco stained. Not febrile.

Cardiovascular and respiratory system. Pulse 68 beats per minute and regular. BP 150/110 mmHg. Soft systolic murmur at the left sternal edge. No ankle swelling and JVP not elevated. Extensive bilateral varicose veins.

Chest examination unremarkable apart from a few crepitations which do not clear with coughing.

Abdomen. Moderately obese. Appendicectomy scar. Soft to palpation. No organomegaly. Possible mass in left iliac fossa—not indentable. No groin hernias. External genitalia normal. Rectal examination—moderately enlarged smooth prostate and normal-coloured stool.

Central nervous system and locomotor system. Fixed flexion deformity of left elbow at 90°, otherwise normal.

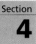

SUMMARY

A 70-year old man with proven rectosigmoid carcinoma without obvious dissemination, admitted for anterior resection of the recto-sigmoid.

A problem list was constructed from this information, which led to further investigations and a management plan. The reasoning is shown in Table 48.2.

Table 48.2 Example of preoperative assessment of a patient admitted for a major operation (case history given above)

Problem	Surgical significance	Plan of action for each problem
1. 'Mild' diabetes mellitus	Is it under good control?	All urine samples to be tested for glucose
		Random blood glucose estimation
		May need sliding scale insulin perioperatively
2. Obesity	Multiple potential problems	Early referral to anaesthetist
	May make access difficult at operation	Ensure adequate theatre time available plus at least two assistants
	Predisposes to wound infection	Consider delayed primary closure of wound if contaminated
	Increased risk of deep vein thrombosis or pulmonary embolism	Prophylaxis, e.g. low dose heparin plus graduated compression stockings
3. Hypertension	How well is hypertension controlled on present medication?	Monitor blood pressure 4-hourly on admission and then decide about drug therapy
	Is elevated BP on admission just due to anxiety?	Check pulse rate and BP several times
	Are there other complications of hypertension such as ventricular hypertrophy or dilatation?	Perform (and check) ECG and chest X-ray
4. Recent shortness of breath on exertion and palpitations	Are these merely symptoms of anxiety about the diagnosis or do they represent significant cardiac or respiratory disease?	Consult internal physician re palpitations ECG and chest X-ray Possibly needs lung function tests
5. Poor urinary stream and large prostate	Possible carcinoma of prostate	Prostate should be palpated and possibly biopsied. Measured plasma PSA
	Possible difficulty with catheterisation that will be required at operation	Anticipate
	Risk of postoperative urinary retention when catheter removed	Anticipate
6. Jaundice in the past	History suggestive of Hepatitis A	Serological tests for hepatitis antigen?
7. Smoker	Possible occult lung cancer	Chest X-ray
	Increased risk of postoperative chest infections	Preoperative physiotherapy and breathing exercises
	Increased risk of myocardial infarction	Postoperative oxygen therapy
8. Left elbow injury	May cause inconvenience during operation	Inform theatre staff about need for careful positioning on the operating table
9. Diuretic therapy	Are electrolytes and renal function normal?	Plasma urea, electrolytes and creatinine estimations
10. Aspirin therapy	Could gastric irritation partly account for the mild anaemia?	Use non gastric irritant analgesics
	May cause excess bleeding at operation	Anticipate—stop 10–14 days before surgery if possible
11. Possible penicillin allergy	A penicillin is often used for prophylaxis or treatment of postoperative infections	Record possible penicillin allergy; alternative drugs may have to be used
12. Cardiac murmur	Is this clinically significant?	Consult anaesthetist or cardiologist
	Is antibiotic prophylaxis necessary?	

Table 48.2 Continued

Problem	Surgical significance	Plan of action for each problem
13. Lives alone, looks after animals	Who will look after his animals while he is in hospital? Who will look after him when he returns home?	Discuss domestic arrangements and convalescence plans
14. Low haemoglobin	Not low enough to need preoperative transfusion but there is less reserve for the operation Potentially extensive operation—may have large blood loss	Cross match at least two units of blood to cover operation Cross match extra blood, i.e. at least 4 units in all
15. May need temporary or even permanent colostomy	Will he be able to cope? What does he understand about stomas?	Needs counselling and possible preoperative 'trial' of colostomy appliance (see Chapter 20)
16. Bowel will be opened during operation	Potential for faecal contamination of abdominal cavity and wound	Needs preoperative bowel preparation and perioperative prophylactic antibiotics
17. Lesion at pelvic brim	Does it involve the ureter?	Consider ultrasound of kidneys in case of hydronephrosis
18. Varicose veins	Increases risk of DVT (already high because of major pelvic operation and age 70)	Give prophylaxis—low dose heparin, antiembolism stockings Early mobilisation

49 Common postoperative problems — diagnosis and management

INTRODUCTION

Despite the best endeavours at diagnosis, preoperative assessment, surgical technique and perioperative management, unexpected symptoms and signs arise in the postoperative period which may herald a postoperative complication. Complications can be minimised by regular and close postoperative patient observation. For example, daily auscultation of the chest may reveal a chest infection before symptoms appear.

Managing the common problems of fever, pain and collapse requires accurate diagnosis and early treatment if the complication is not to get out of hand. Making the diagnosis is often difficult as the doctor called to see a postoperative patient with problems may not know the patient's history. In addition, the patient may be anxious, in pain or not fully recovered from an anaesthetic. It is vital to conduct a thorough and systematic clinical assessment and if necessary, investigation—whatever the hour—of these potentially serious but often remediable complications.

The following problems commonly develop in the postoperative period, often 'after hours', and are the immediate responsibility of junior surgical doctors.

POSTOPERATIVE PAIN

Pain can be expected from most surgical wounds but, in most cases, this gradually subsides over the first few days after operation and can be controlled by planned analgesia. Some types of wound are more painful than others, for example vertical abdominal incisions and skin graft donor sites. Postoperative analgesia is far better managed nowadays, with the recognition that it is better to prevent pain than to react to established pain.

METHODS OF PERIOPERATIVE PAIN RELIEF

Postoperative pain can be reduced by preoperative counselling, peroperative measures and postoperative analgesia. Counselling involves letting the patient know in advance what to expect after the operation in terms of wounds, intravenous lines, catheters and so on. The patient should also be told the likely extent of pain, the plans for pain relief and the degree of mobility he or she might expect after operation. During operation, a great deal can be achieved by using **pre-emptive analgesia**. This involves a variety of methods to ensure that pain does not become established after operation. It includes long-acting analgesic drugs given intravenously, local anaesthetic infiltration into the wound edges at the end of the operation with long-acting **bupivacaine**, regional nerve blocks (e.g. intercostal nerves for upper abdominal surgery), epidural analgesia using morphine and local anaesthetic agents during and after abdominal and pelvic surgery, and non-steroidal analgesic agents given before the patient awakes by means of suppository or intramuscular injection. With non-steroidal agents, care must be taken not to give them to patients with known allergy to aspirin or other NSAIDs, a history of severe asthma or angioedema, bleeding disorders, renal impairment, hypovolaemia or pregnancy. Mild asthma is not a contraindication. It is also unwise to use these drugs in operations that carry a high risk of haemorrhage, e.g. major arterial surgery. Commonly used oral and parenteral analgesic drugs are listed in Box 49.1. Postoperative analgesia is discussed in the next two sections.

MINOR AND INTERMEDIATE SURGERY

Patients vary greatly in their tolerance of pain and their need for analgesics. For minor and intermediate surgery, pre-emptive techniques described above usually mean that simple analgesic tablets are sufficient. However, the

Box 49.1 Postoperative analgesics and their indications (approximate ascending order of analgesic strength)

Mild-to-moderate pain:
- Paracetamol
- Compounds of paracetamol and codeine, e.g. co-codamol
- Aspirin

Moderate pain:
- Paracetamol plus dextropropoxyphene (co-proxamol)
- Codeine or dihydrocodeine

Moderate-to-severe pain:
- Non-steroidal anti-inflammatory drugs as tablets or suppositories, e.g. ibuprofen, indomethacin
- Non-steroidal anti-inflammatory drugs by intramuscular injection, e.g. diclofenac
- Morphine slow-release tablets
- Pethidine (usually intramuscular)
- Morphine, diamorphine or papaveretum (patient-controlled, pump-controlled intravenous or rarely intramuscular)

amount of analgesia must be tailored to the individual need. Anxiety, exhaustion and sleep deprivation may greatly reduce pain tolerance; these should be considered in any patient who fails to respond to a reasonable amount of analgesia.

MAJOR SURGERY AND TRAUMA

Many hospitals now provide an **acute pain service**, usually run by a specialist nurse and one or more anaesthetists. This team can plan an analgesic strategy for individual patients and ensure it is carried out with at least twice-daily ward visits. The team also serves an important educational function, making sure clinicians and nurses are pain-relief aware as well as helping to deal with individual problems as they arise.

For major abdominal and many perineal operations **epidural analgesia** using drugs such as bupivacaine and morphine can be invaluable. A single dose can be given to provide anaesthesia for the operation, e.g. transurethral prostatectomy, and can provide several hours of complete postoperative analgesia. For more extensive surgery, e.g. abdominal aortic aneurysm grafting, an epidural cannula can be left in situ to allow 'topping-up' for prolonged postoperative analgesia. These patients need to be carefully observed for signs of toxicity or severe hypotension and respiratory depression, usually in a high-dependency

unit. Note that moderate hypotension is an indication of a satisfactory block caused by sympathetic blockade.

For major surgery and trauma where epidural analgesia is inappropriate, the dose of analgesic needs to be sufficient to eliminate the pain without dangerous side effects, and the drug needs to be given frequently enough to maintain continuous pain relief. The old practice of writing up intermittent intramuscular opiates 'at 4-hourly intervals, as required' has been recognised as inadequate and ineffective for relieving pain associated with major surgery. Given the enormous variation in analgesic requirements, standard regimens of this type are too inflexible and usually inadequate. Much more effective pain control can be achieved by using a **continuous low-dose infusion of opiates**, with the dose varied according to need with a programmable infusion pump. An even better alternative is to allow patients to give themselves small intravenous increments of opiates as soon as they are needed using a **patient-controlled analgesia** (PCA) device. This allows presetting of the incremental dose (often 1 mg of morphine), with lockout to prevent it being given too frequently, as well as control of the total dose given. Continuous effective pain relief is thus easily achieved and, paradoxically, the total dose of drug used is often less than with intermittent injections. Furthermore, this technique causes minimal sedation and respiratory depression while maintaining excellent continuous analgesia, although it can cause opiate-induced nausea.

EXCESSIVE POSTOPERATIVE PAIN

If the pain is not controlled by what appears to be an adequate dose and frequency of analgesia, complications should be suspected.

- The dose should be reviewed in relation to the expected severity of pain and the weight of the patient.
- **Local postoperative complications** should be considered. Wound pain may be caused by pressure from a **haematoma**. In limb trauma, bleeding into a fascial compartment must be diagnosed before ischaemia ensues ('**compartment syndrome**'). Wound pain increasing after the first 48 hours may be caused by **infection**. The wound will be unusually tender even before redness and induration develop. There is usually a pyrexia. Other complications to consider with lower limb pain include deep vein thrombosis and acute ischaemia. Lastly, major comorbid conditions may be the cause of pain, for example myocardial ischaemia, or a fractured neck of femur may follow a fall from a bed.

Major complications in the area of the operation may need to be considered. After an abdominal operation, excessive pain may be caused by intra-abdominal complications. These include haemorrhage, anastomotic leakage, biliary leakage, abscess formation, gaseous distension due to ileus or air swallowing, urinary retention and bowel ischaemia. Constipation may also cause late postoperative pain. These complications are all described in Chapter 47.

As a general rule, serious complications cause deterioration in the patient's general condition, whereas the patient remains well with less serious complications such as urinary retention or constipation.

PYREXIA

Fever is a common postoperative observation which is not always caused by infection. Nonetheless, a search should always be made for a focus of infection. The common ones are **superficial** or **deep wound infection, chest infection** (pneumonia), **urinary tract infection** and infection of an **intravenous cannula site**. If there is a central venous line, infection of this should always be suspected in a patient with unexplained pyrexia. Unfortunately, this can only be properly diagnosed by removing the line and culturing the tip for organisms. Blood cultures are often positive but do not reveal the source of infection. Patients usually recover spontaneously once the cannula is removed.

Unrelated infections such as viral **upper respiratory tract infections** are easily overlooked. **Malaria** should be considered in a recent immigrant or traveller from an endemic area.

Common non-infective causes of pyrexia include **transfusion reactions, wound haematomas, deep venous thrombosis** and **pulmonary embolism**. Pyrexia is sometimes the only sign of an idiosyncratic or allergic **drug reaction**. Other rare causes of pyrexia include thyrotoxic crisis, phaeochromocytoma and malignant hyperpyrexia following general anaesthesia.

TACHYCARDIA

Tachycardia may simply indicate **pain** or **anxiety** but it is also a feature of **infection, circulatory disturbances** and **thyrotoxicosis**. Mild tachycardia may be a sign of incipient **hypovolaemic shock** as a result of haemorrhage or dehydration. It may also herald **cardiac failure** which, if missed, may progress to a life-threatening complication. Tachycardia may be a sign of recent onset **atrial fibrillation or flutter**; this is confirmed by electrocardiography, and may indicate the patient has suffered a myocardial infarction. In postoperative bowel surgery patients, this change is often a sign of **anastomotic leakage**, presumably mediated by cytokines released as a result of the leakage.

COUGH, SHORTNESS OF BREATH AND TACHYPNOEA

These symptoms are often associated with an overt respiratory problem such as **acute bronchopneumonia, aspiration of gastric contents, lobar collapse, pneumothorax** or an exacerbation of a pre-existing chronic lung disorder. Clinical examination and chest X-ray will rapidly diagnose most of them.

Shortness of breath and rapid shallow breathing are a feature of alveolar collapse (**atelectasis**) which may not be detected by clinical examination or chest X-ray. Atelectasis usually responds to chest physiotherapy. **Abdominal distension** may also cause rapid shallow breathing by inhibiting diaphragmatic movement. Shortness of breath and tachypnoea may be early features of **cardiac failure** or **fluid overload** but there are usually other clues such as tachycardia and basal crepitations.

A sudden onset of shortness of breath and tachypnoea may indicate **pulmonary embolism**, and this must be recognised, investigated and treated vigorously. **Acute respiratory distress syndrome** may occur in chest trauma, acute pancreatitis or systemic sepsis and should be anticipated in these patients. Finally, respiratory symptoms may be due to **hyperventilation** induced by pain, anxiety or hysterical reaction to stress.

COLLAPSE OR RAPID DETERIORATION

The junior doctor on call is commonly asked to deal with a patient who has 'collapsed' or 'gone off' in a non-specific way. To make matters more difficult, the patient is often under the care of another surgical team and is not well known to the emergency doctor. An urgent diagnosis must be made. The more serious general possibilities are summarised in Box 49.2.

In practice, the problem is tackled in the following order, which usually leads to a logical diagnosis:

- Brief history of the collapse and postoperative course to date
- Rapid clinical appraisal, i.e. general appearance and changes in temperature, pulse, blood pressure and respiratory rate. Urinary output and fluid balance review
- Review of:
  — Reason for admission and preoperative state
  — Other pre-existing comorbid conditions
  — The nature and extent of operation, including any particular operative problems
  — Extent of perioperative blood and other fluid losses (including sequestration in the gut)
  — Adequacy of fluid replacement
  — Drug therapy—what drugs have been prescribed? Have important drugs been given or omitted?

Box 49.2 Important causes of postoperative collapse or rapid deterioration

Cardiovascular
- Myocardial infarction
- Other cause of rapid deterioration of cardiac function, e.g. sudden arrhythmia or fluid overload
- Pulmonary embolism
- Stroke (may be without obvious limb paralysis)

Respiratory
- Failure to reverse anaesthesia adequately (early)
- Drug induced respiratory depression
- Hypoxia due to a respiratory disorder or respiratory depressant drugs

'Surgical' and infective
- Hypovolaemic shock from acute blood loss or sudden decompensation in unrecognised hypovolaemia
- Bowel strangulation or obstruction
- Systemic sepsis (often caused by anastomotic leakage)
- Severe local infection, e.g. chest or operation site

Metabolic
- Electrolyte disturbances, e.g. hyponatraemia
- Hypoglycaemia or hyperglycaemia associated with diabetes
- Adrenal insufficiency, e.g. adrenal suppression by steroids

Drug effects
- Drug reactions, e.g. anaphylaxis

- Detailed physical examination
- Special tests as suggested by clinical findings, e.g. ECG, chest X-ray, serum electrolyte estimation, full blood count

NAUSEA AND VOMITING

IMMEDIATE POSTOPERATIVE PERIOD

- Vigorous handling of the patient in moving around the operating department and in the recovery room may stimulate vestibular input causing motion sickness
- Oropharyngeal stimulation—NG tube, early postoperative aspiration of secretions
- Hypoxia
- Hypotension
- Pain
- Anxiety, higher CNS function with regard to the operative event

DRUGS

Nausea and vomiting are common postoperative problems. The usual causes are side effects from drugs used for premedication, general anaesthesia and postoperative analgesia. The major culprits are **opiates**. Anti-emetics such as prochlorperazine or metoclopramide are usually given with opiates and are prescribed 'as required' for the early postoperative period. Nausea and sometimes vomiting later in the postoperative period may also be caused by drugs. The worst offenders are the antibacterial agents erythromycin and metronidazole, and **digoxin** overdosage (which should be anticipated in the elderly and in chronic renal failure).

BOWEL OBSTRUCTION (see Chapter 47)

Serious or sustained vomiting 48 hours or more after operation is usually caused by failure of normal peristalsis of stomach, small bowel or large bowel. This may be caused either by **mechanical obstruction** or by **adynamic bowel**. Acute gastric dilatation, an adynamic problem, may follow any abdominal operation and any patient who vomits should be examined for a 'succussion splash'. If present, immediate nasogastric intubation is necessary; 2 or more litres of fluid may need to be aspirated which might otherwise be vomited and inhaled. Aspiration of gastric contents can cause mild aspiration pneumonia, severe aspiration pneumonia (Mendelson's syndrome); if massive aspiration occurs, it can effectively drown the patient causing sudden death. Other adynamic bowel problems may be a response to local factors (e.g. bowel handling, a bowel-wall haematoma or a collection of pus in contact with bowel) or to systemic abnormalities, particularly **hypokalaemia**. Adynamic large bowel (pseudo-obstruction) sometimes occurs in a debilitated patient with a severe non-abdominal illness, such as fractured neck of femur. Finally, **faecal impaction** is a common problem in the elderly or immobile patient. It may cause vomiting from what amounts to physical obstruction plus adynamic bowel.

Mechanical obstruction, usually of small bowel, may follow any abdominal operation. Early obstruction due to fibrinous adhesions occurs within 4 days of operation and may respond to conservative treatment but often requires a further operation.

SYSTEMIC DISORDERS

Electrolyte disturbances, uraemia, hypercalcaemia and other systemic disorders may cause vomiting because of their central effects. Centrally mediated vomiting also occurs in **raised intracranial pressure**. This must be considered following head injuries, neurosurgical operations or in patients with cerebral metastases.

HAEMATEMESIS

Elderly postoperative patients sometimes produce a small quantity of **'coffee ground' vomit** which is positive for blood on 'stick' testing. This rightly causes concern to nurses but rarely indicates a major haematemesis. It probably results from trivial bleeding from mild, stress-related gastritis or reflux oesophagitis. No special treatment is usually required but the patient should be closely observed for signs of internal bleeding, and mucosal protective agents such as sucralfate given.

Occasionally, a major upper gastrointestinal haemorrhage occurs in the postoperative patient. If there has been forceful vomiting, a Mallory–Weiss oesophageal tear may be the cause. Major bleeding may also arise from exacerbation of a peptic ulcer or even oesophageal varices. Seriously ill patients and the victims of burns and head injuries are susceptible to **acute stress ulceration**, which may cause catastrophic gastrointestinal haemorrhage (see Ch. 14).

DISORDERS OF BOWEL FUNCTION

The main bowel function disorders which develop in the postoperative period are constipation, diarrhoea, adynamic bowel problems and intestinal obstruction.

CONSTIPATION

Constipation is common and becomes apparent several days after operation. It usually represents a failure to re-establish normal bowel function. The causes include restriction of oral fluids and fibre, difficulty or reluctance in using a bed pan, slow recovery of normal peristalsis and general lack of mobility. Anal pain is a powerful disincentive to defecation following surgery for anal conditions. Constipation causes great distress, especially in the elderly. It should be anticipated and prevented if possible by prescribing **bulk-forming agents** (e.g. methylcellulose or ispaghula husk preparations), **osmotic laxatives** (e.g. lactulose) or **lubricant laxatives** (e.g. liquid paraffin). Irritant laxatives and bowel stimulants can be used if there is still no progress.

For colonic surgery, large-bowel cleansing procedures (enemas, osmotic laxatives and restriction of solid foods) are usually carried out beforehand to prevent solid faecal matter disrupting the anastomosis. Bowel cleansing also reduces the risk of faecal contamination during operation. Impacted faeces may result in **overflow incontinence** which must not be confused with diarrhoea from other causes. Thus any patient with abnormal bowel function must undergo rectal examination.

DIARRHOEA

Transient diarrhoea frequently follows abdominal operations, and should be regarded as normal following bowel resections or operations to relieve intestinal obstruction.

Diarrhoea may also complicate **antibiotic therapy**. Several days after the onset of treatment, loose, frequent stools are passed, probably as a result of bacterial or fungal overgrowth. Less commonly, **antibiotic-associated diarrhoea** may develop, and even become life-threatening. These are characterised by severe and persistent diarrhoea, sometimes containing blood (see Ch. 47).

After surgery of the abdominal aorta, blood-stained diarrhoea may sometimes occur several days post-operatively. This may indicate **large-bowel ischaemia** due to surgical interference with its blood supply. This is a dangerous complication and requires urgent surgical exploration.

POOR URINE OUTPUT

RETENTION OF URINE

Abnormally low urinary output or complete failure to pass urine is a frequent postoperative problem. The most common cause is urinary retention, which usually occurs in males. It is readily diagnosed if there is a palpable suprapubic mass which is dull to percussion. Retention can readily be confirmed by ultrasound examination or more invasively by passing a urinary catheter.

BLOCKED CATHETER

If the patient is already catheterised, the catheter may have become blocked. The catheter can be checked for patency using a bladder syringe and flushed or replaced as necessary.

DIMINISHED URINE PRODUCTION

Poor urine output commonly results from poor renal perfusion due to **hypotension** during the operation or **hypovolaemia** caused by inadequate fluid replacement. If untreated, this may progress to acute renal failure.

If hypovolaemia is suspected, then an intravenous **fluid challenge** of 250 ml of dextrose or dextrose-saline should be given over 15 minutes or so, while monitoring urine output. If the patient is hypotensive, the cause (cardiac failure or hypovolaemia, for example) must be identified and treated as soon as possible. If oliguria persists or worsens, then a urinary catheter should be

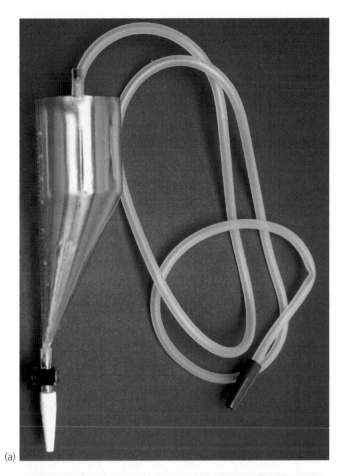

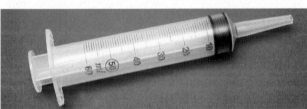

Fig. 49.1 Urine burette and bladder syringe
(a) A urine burette is attached to a urinary catheter when urine output must be measured accurately and when volumes may be small. **(b)** Bladder syringe used to flush urinary catheters suspected of blockage with debris. The nozzle is specially shaped to fit the end of a Foley catheter. Note that full sterile precautions must be employed to reduce the risk of urinary infection.

inserted to ensure that the bladder is emptying and to measure hourly urine output. If urine output is still poor, a central venous line should be placed for monitoring of CVP. If CVP is satisfactory, many patients will respond to a small intravenous dose of a loop diuretic, e.g. 40 mg of frusemide. If these simple measures fail to improve urine output, then acute renal failure must be suspected.

Lastly, bilateral ureteric obstruction should be considered. This is extremely rare as a cause of postoperative low urine output. It can be diagnosed by renal ultrasound which will usually reveal bilateral hydronephrosis.

CHANGES IN MENTAL STATE

Marked mental changes may occur in the early postoperative period and are most common in the elderly. These changes are often loosely called 'confusion'. Common phenomena include clouding of consciousness, perceptual disturbances, incoherent speech and agitation or destructive behaviour, such as pulling out cannulas or catheters. Other features are loss of orientation, apathy and stupor, and stereotyped movements such as plucking at the bedclothes.

ELDERLY PATIENTS

The elderly are vulnerable to dementia or cerebrovascular insufficiency. There may thus be little tolerance of systemic insults which tip the balance against cerebral equilibrium.

Factors which predispose to postoperative mental changes in the elderly include:

- Disorientation brought about by rapid changes of environment (from ward to operating theatre and on to ITU, for example)
- Dehydration
- Hyponatraemia
- Hypoxia (from pneumonia or cardiac failure, for example)
- Infection (especially of the urinary tract)
- Drugs (particularly opiates and hypnotics)
- Uraemia
- Hypoglycaemia

In addition, pain, anxiety and sleep deprivation may precipitate confusion.

OTHER CAUSES OF MENTAL CHANGE

Marked alterations in behaviour in younger patients may indicate alcohol withdrawal or craving for drugs such as cocaine or heroin. The history has usually been concealed at the time of admission. Patients with a recent history of head injury may behave abnormally if hypoxic or if intra-cerebral bleeding develops.

JAUNDICE

GENERAL CAUSES

Jaundice may develop several days postoperatively in a patient with no history of biliary disease. In these patients, the cause is usually a prehepatic or hepatic disorder. Causes of **prehepatic jaundice** include large blood transfusions, absorption of large haematomas or exacerbation

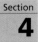
of a haemolytic disorder such as thalassaemia or sickle-cell trait (exacerbated by postoperative hypoxia, dehydration or hypothermia).

Hepatic causes are less common. They include cholestasis (caused by infection near the liver or drug idiosyncrasy), hepatitis and liver cell toxicity from drug idiosyncrasy and visceral ischaemia caused by shock.

CAUSES RELATED TO BILIARY OR LIVER SURGERY

Patients subjected to biliary tract or liver surgery may become jaundiced after operation. The most likely cause is **obstruction** of the extrahepatic bile ducts due to retained stone, unrecognised surgical trauma or inadvertent duct ligation. Other causes include **infection** such as ascending cholangitis, and systemic absorption of an intra-abdominal collection of bile (biliary peritonitis).

50 Fluid, electrolyte, acid-base and nutritional management

INTRODUCTION

Most problems of fluid, electrolyte, acid–base management are relatively straightforward and can be worked out with reasoning and common sense. Problems are minimised if high-risk patients are assessed properly before operation and their cardiovascular status and fluid balance is closely monitored before and after operation. Plasma urea, electrolytes and haematocrit should be checked at least once a day in patients undergoing major surgery or receiving intravenous fluids, and at least once after preoperative bowel preparation before operation.

Recognising pre-existing malnutrition and preventing postoperative malnutrition are important aspects of inpatient management. Simple scoring systems help with the former and awareness of the problem allows action to be taken to prevent the latter in the form of enteral or parenteral nutrition.

Severely ill patients with abdominal infection and fistulae are likely to suffer major problems of fluid balance and nutrition. These are increasingly managed with the help of experienced anaesthetists in intensive care or high-dependency units, where monitoring and therapy can be rigorously managed. Patients with extensive burns are at particular risk of hypovolaemia and require early and vigorous fluid replacement before transfer to a specialist burns unit.

NORMAL FLUID AND ELECTROLYTE HOMEOSTASIS

An average adult normally loses between 2.5 and 3 litres of fluid in 24 hours. About 1 litre is lost insensibly from skin and lungs, 100 ml are lost in the faeces and the remaining 1300–1800 ml are passed as urine (about 60 ml/hour). Fluid mainly enters the body by oral intake of both fluids and food but about 200 ml of water is produced as a by-product of metabolism. About 100–150 mmol of sodium ions and 50–100 mmol of potassium ions are lost each day in the urine and this is balanced by normal dietary intake (see Table 50.1).

When a patient is deprived of all oral intake—as occurs in the perioperative period or in coma—isotonic electrolyte solutions of different types are given intravenously as a replacement.

WATER AND SODIUM

In an uncomplicated patient, the daily water and sodium requirements can be given as 2.5–3 litres of a standard

Table 50.1 Summary — normal daily fluid and electrolyte input and output

NORMAL DAILY INTAKE	NORMAL DAILY OUTPUT
Water	
Diet 2300 ml	Urine 1400 ml (minimum obligatory volume = 4000 ml)
Metabolism 200 ml	Skin loss 500 ml (obligatory diffusion and vaporisation). *Note: sweating in pyrexia or a high ambient temperature can cause several litres extra loss each day*
	Lung loss 500 ml (obligatory)
	Faecal loss 100 ml
Sodium	
Diet 150 mmol/day (range 50–300 mmol)	Stool 5 mmol/day
	Skin transpiration 5 mmol/day (in the absence of sweating)
	Urine 140 mmol/day (can fall down to 15 mmol/day if required)
Potassium	
Diet 100 mmol/day (range 50–200 mmol)	Stool 10 mmol/day (obligatory)
	Skin < 5 mmol/day
	Urine 85 mmol/day (rarely falls below 60 mmol/day)

dextrose–saline solution containing 4% dextrose and 0.18% sodium chloride (Note: this has only one-fifth the salt content of 'normal', i.e. physiological saline). This fluid regimen is often, however, prescribed automatically without considering the special requirements of individual patients. For this reason, its general use should be discouraged except when an intravenous infusion is required for only a day or two and there are no special fluid or electrolyte problems.

For most patients, the daily water and sodium requirements are best met by using appropriate quantities of **normal saline** solution (0.9% sodium chloride) and **5% dextrose** (glucose) solution. Normal saline contains 154 mmol of sodium ions per litre. 750–1000 ml will thus satisfy the daily sodium requirement of uncomplicated patients. The additional water requirement is made up with 2–2.5 litres of 5% glucose (Box 50.1). The small amount of glucose present contributes little to nutrition but renders the solution isotonic. This prescription is altered for patients with electrolyte abnormalities by varying the volume of normal saline given.

POTASSIUM

Basic potassium requirements are met by infusing 60–80 mmol of potassium chloride in divided doses over each 24-hour period. Premixed intravenous fluids are generally available with 20 mmol of potassium chloride per 500 ml container. If premixed containers are not available, potassium chloride can be added to intra-

SUMMARY

Box 50.1 Sample daily intravenous fluid regimens as a substitute for oral intake in uncomplicated cases

Prescription (1) for 24 hours (each bag to be given over 4 hours):

500 ml 0.9% sodium chloride + 20 mmol KCl

500 ml 5% dextrose

500 ml 5% dextrose + 20 mmol KCl

500 ml 5% dextrose

500 ml 5% dextrose + 20 mmol KCl

500 ml 5% dextrose

Prescription (2) for 24 hours (each bag to be given over 4 hours):

500 ml dextrose–saline (i.e. 4% dextrose + 1.8% NaCl) + 20 mmol KCl

500 ml dextrose–saline

500 ml dextrose–saline + 20 mmol KCl

500 ml dextrose–saline

500 ml dextrose–saline + 20 mmol KCl

500 ml dextrose–saline

venous solutions but care must be taken to ensure thorough mixing. Concentrations of potassium chloride greater than 40 mmol in 500 ml should be avoided for general use, and bolus injections of KCl must *never* be given because rapid increases in plasma potassium cause cardiac arrest.

Note that added potassium is not usually required in the immediate postoperative period because potassium is released from damaged cells and raises the plasma potassium concentration.

LIMITS OF COMPENSATORY MECHANISMS

The kidneys are normally able to maintain fluid and electrolyte homeostasis in spite of large variations of fluid intake from hour to hour and day to day. The same also applies to fluid and electrolytes given intravenously. Note that the kidneys' compensating capacity is reduced by renal parenchymal disease and by chronic renal insufficiency.

The total blood volume in an adult male is about 6 litres of which about 55–60% is water (about 3.5 litres). Falls in blood volume which are not too rapid or extensive can be compensated by fluid movement from the extracellular compartment. This compartment has a volume of more than 10 litres. A deficit of more than 3 litres in whole body fluid volume cannot be sustained and intravascular volume inevitably becomes depleted. This is reflected in compensatory cardiovascular changes. Vasoconstriction causes cold peripheries and this is an important warning sign of hypovolaemia and more reliable than early tachycardia, particularly in children. Initially, there is a mild **tachycardia** but when the overall fluid deficit reaches about 3 litres, the pulse rate becomes very rapid and hypotension develops. Note that patients on beta-adrenergic blocking drugs or with cardiac conduction defects may not be able to increase the heart rate and will therefore decompensate earlier. With 4 or more litres of fluid deficit, the limit of cardiovascular compensation is reached and the patient develops **hypovolaemic shock** (see Ch. 2). Note that fit young men are able to sustain normal vital signs for longer than other patients but when they do decompensate, they do so abruptly.

In neonates, children, the elderly and the chronically ill, cardiovascular compensation capacity is greatly reduced. A relatively small fluid and electrolyte imbalance may cause life-threatening complications.

PROBLEMS OF FLUID AND ELECTROLYTE DEPLETION

Surgical patients may suffer large losses of fluid and electrolytes as a result of disease, trauma, burns, surgical operations or surgical complications. These causes are summarised in Box 50.2. In addition, many surgical patients are deliberately deprived of oral intake during the perioperative period.

LOSS OF WHOLE BLOOD OR PLASMA

Rapid and copious blood loss in traumatic injury or operative surgery initially affects the intravascular compartment. Rapid loss of only 1 litre may cause hypotension or even hypovolaemic shock. When haemorrhage is less rapid, there is time for the extracellular compartment to replace the loss. Thus greater volumes can be lost before the cardiovascular system becomes compromised. The lost blood volume, though compensated for by extracellular fluid shift, is still a loss to the system and must be restored either physiologically or by transfusion. If blood loss has ceased, the need for transfusion is based on the volume lost and on the previous haemoglobin concentration. Furthermore, the possibility of further blood loss must be anticipated by ensuring good venous access and obtaining bank blood. Acute blood loss of 500–1000 ml is usually treated by transfusing plasma substitutes such as **gelatin solutions**. These remain longer in the circulation than crystalloids but there is debate about whether these are better than crystalloids for treating acute surgical blood loss. Larger volume losses ideally require whole blood but unfortunately whole blood for transfusion is becoming an increasingly rare commodity and packed cells plus plasma volume equivalent should be given. Slow chronic blood loss does not lead to fluid balance problems but may cause symptoms and signs of anaemia.

Plasma loss from **severe burns** should be anticipated by using a standard formula based on the area burnt to guide plasma replacement (see burns, Ch. 8). Infusion requirements can be seriously underestimated unless an accepted formula or a suitable alternative system is used.

> ### KEY POINTS
>
> **Box 50.2 Sources of excess fluid loss in surgical patients**
>
> **Blood loss**—traumatic or surgical
> **Plasma loss**—burns
> **Gastrointestinal fluid loss**—vomiting, nasogastric aspiration, sequestration in obstructed or adynamic bowel, loss through a fistula or an ileostomy, diarrhoea
> **Inflammatory exudate into the peritoneal cavity**—generalised peritonitis or acute pancreatitis
> **Sepsis syndrome (septicaemia)**—massive peripheral vasodilatation and third space losses due to increased capillary permeability causing relative hypovolaemia
> **Abnormal insensible loss**—fever, excess sweating or hyperventilation

GASTROINTESTINAL FLUID LOSS

Between 5 and 9 litres of electrolyte-rich fluid is normally secreted into the upper gastrointestinal tract each day as saliva, gastric juice, bile, pancreatic fluid and succus entericus (see Table 50.2). Most of the fluid is reabsorbed lower in the intestine.

Large volumes of water and electrolytes may be lost from the body by vomiting, nasogastric aspiration, diarrhoea, sequestration in obstructed or adynamic bowel or drainage via a fistula or an ileostomy. If there is widespread **inflammation of the bowel** as in gastroenteritis or ulcerative colitis, inflammatory exudate may greatly increase the fluid lost as diarrhoea. Cholera can cause the loss of up to 10 litres of electrolyte-rich fluid in one day.

Abnormal fluid losses must be measured or estimated as accurately as possible. This enables intravenous replacement to be anticipated and the consequences of fluid and electrolyte depletion prevented. From Table 50.2, it can be seen that vomitus and nasogastric aspirate usually contain about 120 mmol of sodium ions per litre and up

Table 50.2 Daily gastrointestinal secretions and electrolyte composition

SECRETION	VOLUME (L)	Na$^+$ (mmol/L)	K$^+$ (mmol/L)	Cl$^-$ (mmol/L)	HCO3$^-$ (mmol/L)
Saliva	1–1.5	20–80	10–20	20–40	20–160
Gastric juice	1–2.5	20–100	5–10	120–160	nil
Bile	up to 1	150–250	5–10	40–60	20–60
Pancreatic juice	1–2	120	5–10	10–60	80–120
Succus entericus	2–3	140	5 (increases up to 40 in inflammatory diarrhoea)	variable	variable

to 10 mmol potassium ions per litre. Inflammatory diarrhoea contains a slightly lower concentration of sodium ions, but more than 40 mmol of potassium ions per litre. As a general rule, gastrointestinal fluid losses should be replaced by an equivalent volume of normal saline, with potassium chloride added as necessary. In intestinal obstruction or adynamic ileus, fluid sequestrated in the bowel is replaced in a similar manner, although volume requirements cannot be measured accurately and have to be estimated, aided by observation of urine output and blood pressure and, if necessary, central venous pressure. Fistulae and overactive ileostomies cause chronic loss of fluid which is high in chloride and bicarbonate.

INTRA-ABDOMINAL LOSS OF INFLAMMATORY FLUID

Severe intra-abdominal inflammation, as in peritonitis or acute pancreatitis, may cause several litres of fluid, rich in plasma proteins and electrolytes, to be lost into the peritoneal cavity. There is also an important element of 'third-space loss' in systemic inflammatory response syndrome (SIRS) likely to occur in these conditions, i.e. fluid leached into the extra-cellular or interstitial space. This is best replaced during resuscitation, as well as can be estimated, by a combination of plasma substitutes and physiological saline.

SYSTEMIC SEPSIS (SIRS AND MULTIPLE ORGAN DYSFUNCTION SYNDROME)

Systemic sepsis is associated with widespread endothelial damage and a large increase in capillary permeability mediated by a range of cytokines and other circulating substances. The result is extensive loss of protein and electrolyte-rich fluid from the circulation into the extracellular space, which, combined with a loss of peripheral resistance, results in cardiovascular collapse and shock. This fluid deficiency should be replaced with a combination of plasma substitutes and physiological saline in the same way as for fluid loss into the peritoneal cavity.

The required fluid volume is difficult to estimate and replacement is usually given so as to maintain cardio-vascular stability (pulse rate and blood pressure) and urinary output (at least 0.5 ml/kg body weight/hour), whilst avoiding fluid overload and cardiac failure. In the severely ill patient, in whom the volume requirements are particularly difficult to judge, a central venous pressure line (and perhaps a Swann–Ganz catheter in cardiac failure) make treatment safer and more precise. These patients are best managed in high-dependency or intensive care units.

ABNORMAL INSENSIBLE FLUID LOSS

Abnormal insensible fluid loss can greatly increase overall fluid loss, particularly in the seriously ill patient. Insensible losses must be included in the fluid balance equation, especially if losses are sustained for more than a short period. Pyrexia increases insensible loss by approximately 20% for each degree Celsius rise in body temperature, mainly in the form of exhaled water vapour. A pyrexia of 38.5° C for 3 days would therefore cause an extra litre of fluid loss. **Sweating** causes loss of sodium-rich fluid which can be easily overlooked in patients with fever and when the ambient ward temperature rises in summer. The elderly are particularly vulnerable when denied oral fluids before operation.

PREVENTING ACUTE RENAL FAILURE

Maintaining fluid balance in surgical patients depends on anticipating problems before they cause harm and put the patient at risk of acute renal failure. This is a serious complication with a high mortality in surgical patients. Prevention involves observing changes in pulse rate, blood pressure and hourly urine output in patients at risk, measuring fluid losses to guide replacement and seeking clinical signs of fluid imbalance (both dehydration and overload). Regular estimations of plasma urea and electrolytes should be made.

In patients with cardiac failure or shock, monitoring and treatment is best carried out in an intensive care or high-dependency unit, using invasive monitoring to help determine the required volume of fluid replacement.

PHYSIOLOGICAL CHANGES IN FLUIDS AND ELECTROLYTES IN RESPONSE TO SURGERY AND TRAUMA

The stresses of trauma or surgery cause a rise in the level of circulating **catecholamines**. Stress also stimulates the hypothalamo–pituitary–adrenal axis, which increases secretion of **cortisol** and **aldosterone**. These hormones promote renal conservation of sodium and water and a reduction in both urine volume and urine sodium concentration.

Several factors contribute to a fall in renal perfusion. These include haemorrhage, loss of oedema fluid into a site of trauma or operation, third-space losses and cardiovascular responses to anaesthesia. Abdominal aortic surgery may greatly alter the dynamics of renal artery flow, while raised intra-abdominal pressure (e.g. in gross bowel distension) disturbs renal blood flow by collapsing renal veins. A fall in renal perfusion activates the **renin–angiotensin–aldosterone** mechanism to sustain the blood pressure. This also promotes reabsorption of sodium and water from the renal tubules and, by way of exchange, more potassium and hydrogen ions are lost in the urine. Postoperative urine output thus falls by several hundred millilitres per day, and the urine is low in sodium (less than 40 mmol/L), high in potassium (greater than 100 mmol/L) and acidic.

Water conservation is further enhanced by stress-mediated **ADH secretion** from the posterior pituitary (neurohypophysis). Normally, ADH release is mediated only by a rise in plasma osmolality, i.e. an elevated plasma sodium concentration.

At the site of trauma or operation, a volume of fluid is effectively though temporarily removed from the circulation in the form of inflammatory oedema (isotonic third-space losses). The displaced volume is compensated for by fluid retained as a result of the hormonal changes described above. More potassium is released by damaged tissues than the excess lost by exchange via the kidney. Thus, the postoperative plasma potassium level tends to rise in the first day or two. This is particularly true if stored blood has been transfused as this releases potassium from elderly red cells. For these reasons, potassium supplements are not usually needed for the first few days after operation provided the preoperative plasma potassium level is normal and potassium-losing diuretics are not being prescribed.

COMMON FLUID AND ELECTROLYTE PROBLEMS

INTERMEDIATE ELECTIVE AND STRAIGHTFORWARD EMERGENCY OPERATIONS

Most operations fall into this category. The majority of patients are in fluid and electrolyte equilibrium before operation although some have problems caused by diuretic therapy (for cardiac failure, hypertension or chronic renal failure). For these patients, plasma urea and electrolytes should be checked before operation. Loop and thiazide diuretics may cause **hypokalaemia** whilst potassium-sparing diuretics such as spironolactone may cause **hyperkalaemia**. If serious abnormalities are found, operation must be postponed until the problem is corrected. Hypokalaemia can usually be treated by oral potassium supplements or by adding a potassium-sparing diuretic. Hyperkalaemia is usually corrected by substituting a loop or thiazide diuretic.

Mild renal dysfunction (plasma urea up to about 15 mmol/L and creatinine up to about 170 mmol/L) is not usually a contraindication to surgery. These patients tend to be mildly dehydrated, however, and oral fluid intake should be strongly encouraged.

Management

For elective surgery, the patient is often kept 'nil by mouth' for 6–12 hours before operation and will take very little oral fluid for up to 6 hours after operation. A fluid deficit of 1000–1500 ml is therefore common. There is a trend, however, towards encouraging clear fluids by mouth up to 3 hours before operation. Mild fluid deficits can usually be accommodated and are quickly made up once the patient is drinking normally. Intravenous fluids are therefore not required for most uncomplicated minor operations in adults. For patients with **mild renal failure**, an infusion should be set up at the outset of the 'nil by mouth' period to prevent the dire consequences of acute-on-chronic renal failure. Most anaesthetists place an intravenous cannula for any operation involving general or regional anaesthesia to ensure venous access; this can be removed as soon as the patient is drinking satisfactorily. Occasionally, and despite the use of anti-emetics, patients vomit after operation and intravenous fluids should be employed if vomiting is prolonged.

Children and especially infants and neonates are much more vulnerable to fluid deprivation because of their small total body fluid volume and disproportionate insensible losses. Even relatively minor operations can cause dehydration and intravenous fluids may be necessary, with the rate and volume calculated according to body weight and measured blood loss.

As a rule, the sooner the body can assume control over its own fluid and electrolyte homeostasis the better. Intravenous fluids should be discontinued as soon as normal oral intake has been resumed and urine output is satisfactory.

MAJOR OPERATIONS

Major operations, especially those involving bowel, pose particular problems of fluid management whether the operation is elective or an emergency. The principal reasons are:

- Patients are often elderly and are likely to have a diminished cardiovascular reserve and may have pre-existing fluid and electrolyte abnormalities
- Preoperative vomiting, restricted fluid intake (and bowel preparation with osmotically active preparations such as magnesium sulphate or mannitol) may result in dehydration and electrolyte abnormalities

- Blood loss during and after operation may be large
- Operations may take several hours with consequent insensible losses from the open wound
- Third-space losses of 500–1000 ml can occur after major surgery or trauma as a result of the systemic hormonal responses to trauma
- The recovery period when oral intake is nil or restricted may be long—several days following uncomplicated bowel surgery (e.g. hemicolectomy or gastrectomy) and longer after peritonitis (e.g. perforated diverticulitis or an anastomotic leak)

Careful preoperative and postoperative assessment of patients having major surgery is essential so that problems can be recognised early. This should include clinical examination for evidence of **dehydration** (dry mouth and loss of normal skin turgor) or **overhydration** (elevated jugular venous pressure or cardiac failure). Plasma urea and electrolytes, creatinine and full blood count should be measured. An elevated urea concentration with little elevation of creatinine is characteristic of dehydration. An abnormally high haemoglobin concentration (providing polycythaemia is not present) also indicates dehydration, especially if it was normal beforehand.

Management

If the patient is dehydrated, has significant electrolyte abnormalities or has been vomiting, an intravenous infusion is set up to resuscitate and stabilise the patient before operation. Dehydration should normally be corrected with normal saline. Blood loss from trauma or gastrointestinal bleeding is replaced with whole blood (or packed cells plus plasma substitute) although plasma substitutes can be used in an emergency as a holding measure.

Fluid management during the operation is the responsibility of the anaesthetist. An isotonic electrolyte infusion such as Hartmann's solution is usually set up at the outset, often followed by a plasma substitute such as a gelatin solution. If operative blood loss exceeds about 1000 ml or 20% of blood volume, blood is usually given to make up the loss. If the blood loss is less than 1000 ml, the risks of transfusion usually outweigh the benefit. The exception is patients who were anaemic before operation (haemoglobin concentration less than about 10 g/dl). Children and infants are less tolerant of blood loss and transfusion would normally be begun at about 10% loss of blood volume.

A fluid regimen is planned for the 24 hours following operation taking into account the sources of fluid loss described earlier. For example, a further 500 ml blood loss may be expected from the drain after total hip replacement. In general, only 3 litres of intravenous fluids are required in the first 24 hours. It is safer to err on the side of underhydration rather than overhydration, especially if there is a risk of exacerbating cardiac failure with fluid overload. For major surgery, a urinary catheter allows accurate monitoring of urine output and avoids the common complication of postoperative acute urinary retention.

Intravenous fluids are continued after operation until bowel function has returned and free oral fluids resumed. The basic regimens shown in Box 50.1 earlier is usually satisfactory. In the meantime, plasma urea and electrolytes should be checked daily. Potassium supplements may not be needed until the third postoperative day, depending on the blood results.

ABNORMALITIES OF PLASMA SODIUM CONCENTRATION

Plasma sodium abnormalities are usually discovered incidentally on 'routine' measurement of electrolytes.

Hyponatraemia

A measured low plasma sodium may be real or spurious. Spurious results commonly arise when blood is taken from an arm receiving an intravenous infusion; less commonly, false laboratory results can occur if there is **lipaemia** resulting from parenteral nutrition. If in doubt, the test should be repeated with appropriate precautions.

In hyponatraemia (except in severe hyperglycaemia or infusion of mannitol), the plasma becomes **hypotonic**. This causes cellular overhydration which in severe cases results in cerebral oedema. Mild hyponatraemia is symptomless but when the plasma sodium falls below about 120 mmol/L, patients often become confused. Convulsions and coma occur when sodium concentrations fall below about 110 mmol/L. If hyponatraemia is confirmed biochemically, the next step is to clinically assess the **state of hydration** (i.e. the extra-cellular fluid volume) and this will guide therapy.

There are three possibilities:

- **Water deficit with a larger sodium deficit** (clinical signs—dry mouth, poor skin turgor, poor urine output, high urine osmolality): sodium insufficiency is usually due to diuretic therapy, vomiting, diarrhoea or other excessive losses of body fluids with inadequate replacement. Treatment involves rehydration with appropriate sodium-containing intravenous fluids
- **Sodium excess with a larger water excess** (clinical signs—weight gain, ankle swelling, raised jugular venous pressure): this usually results from organ dysfunction. Cardiac failure is the most common cause, followed by renal, liver and respiratory failure. Overhydration is compounded by excessive intravenous fluid administration. Management is based primarily on treating the organ failure, e.g. diuretics for cardiac failure

● **Water excess**: this is uncommon and is usually due to **inappropriate antidiuretic hormone (ADH) secretion**. This is rare on a surgical ward except for TUR syndrome in which excess fluid is absorbed during transurethral resection of the prostate. It can also occur following head injury or neurosurgery, or may occur in pneumonia, empyema, lung abscess or oat-cell carcinoma of the lung. Excess ADH increases water reabsorption by the renal tubules independently of sodium. The result is water overload and dilutional hyponatraemia. Inappropriate ADH secretion is the likely diagnosis if the urine osmolality is found to be high and the plasma osmolality low. Hyponatraemia caused by inappropriate ADH secretion is managed by restricting fluid intake.

Hypernatraemia

This is an uncommon problem and in the surgical patient is usually iatrogenic. The usual cause is either excess administration of sodium via intravenous fluids, or inadequate water replacement. Hypernatraemia is more likely to occur after operation because increased aldosterone secretion causes sodium to be conserved by the kidney. Very rarely, hypernatraemia is caused by **Conn's syndrome** (primary hyperaldosteronism).

Treatment involves encouraging the patient to drink more water, or infusing fluids with a low sodium content.

ABNORMALITIES OF PLASMA POTASSIUM CONCENTRATION

Plasma potassium abnormalities, like abnormalities of sodium, are often discovered incidentally. A cause can usually be found and treatment is straightforward. Acid–base abnormalities (see below) can have a profound effect on plasma potassium concentration but the latter is likely to correct spontaneously as the acid–base problem is treated.

Hypokalaemia

In the preoperative patient, hypokalaemia usually results from poor dietary intake, diuretic therapy, chronic diarrhoea, losses from a malfunctioning ileostomy or rarely, excess mucus secretion from a rectal villous adenoma. Rarely, hypokalaemia may be caused by **primary hyperaldosteronism** (Conn's syndrome).

Postoperatively, hypokalaemia is usually caused by inadequate potassium supplementation in intravenous infusions. The lack of intake is compounded by increased urinary losses from stress-induced **secondary hyperaldosteronism**.

Hypokalaemia causes skeletal muscle weakness and reduces gastrointestinal motility, with paralytic ileus in extreme cases. When severe, there is also a risk of sudden cardiac arrhythmias or even cardiac arrest. Hypokalaemia can usually be corrected with oral potassium supplements (effervescent or slow-release tablets). For patients on intravenous fluids, potassium supplements are added as appropriate. The infusion rate should not generally exceed 15–20 mmol per hour, but larger quantities may be required following operations involving cardiopulmonary bypass.

Hyperkalaemia

This is less common in surgical patients than hypokalaemia. In the preoperative patient, it is most commonly caused by chronic renal failure or high doses of ACE inhibiting drugs or potassium-sparing diuretics. Occasionally, non-steroidal anti-inflammatory drugs cause hyperkalaemia. Post operative hyperkalaemia is usually iatrogenic, caused by excessive intravenous potassium administration, although it may be associated with acute renal failure or large transfusions of old stored blood.

Hyperkalaemia is asymptomatic in the early stages but there is a high risk of sudden death from asystole when the plasma potassium concentration reaches about 7.0 mmol/L. Potassium concentration at this level is a medical emergency especially if there are typical ECG changes (i.e. peaked T-waves) and it should be treated initially by intravenous infusion of insulin and glucose. This causes a shift of potassium from the extracellular to the intracellular fluid compartment. Lesser degrees of hyperkalaemia may be treated with **cation exchange resins** (e.g. calcium resonium) given orally or rectally. Severe renal failure may require haemofiltration treatment.

ACID–BASE DISTURBANCES

Major acid–base abnormalities are rare in uncomplicated surgical patients and usually arise in seriously ill patients being managed in an intensive care unit.

METABOLIC ACIDOSIS

Metabolic acidosis usually follows an episode of severe tissue hypoxia resulting from hypovolaemic shock, myocardial infarction or systemic sepsis. The most common cause is inadequate tissue oxygenation leading to accumulation of lactic acid. In surgical patients in the intensive care unit, the onset of metabolic acidosis is often an indicator of serious intra-abdominal problems such as an anastomotic leak. Metabolic acidosis is also seen in acute renal failure and uncontrolled diabetic ketoacidosis. Clinically, the patient has rapid, deep respirations (a respiratory compensatory mechanism). Arterial blood gas estimations show the characteristic picture of raised hydrogen ion concentration and low standard bicarbonate with a low arterial PCO_2. Plasma potassium concentration is elevated because of a shift from the intra-cellular compartment to the extra-cellular compartment.

Treatment is directed at the underlying cause. Bicarbonate infusion was formerly considered appropriate in severe cases but this does not address the underlying cause.

RESPIRATORY ACIDOSIS

This results from carbon dioxide retention in respiratory failure. The usual causes are underlying chronic respiratory disease made worse by postoperative chest complications or prolonged respiratory depression due to sedative, hypnotic or narcotic drugs. Plasma hydrogen ion concentrations and PCO_2 are elevated but standard bicarbonate is normal. Treatment is directed at the underlying cause and to providing assisted ventilation.

METABOLIC ALKALOSIS

Metabolic alkalosis is usually caused by severe and repeated vomiting or prolonged nasogastric aspiration for intestinal obstruction. The latter classically occurs in pyloric stenosis with gross loss of gastric acid. The patient becomes severely dehydrated and depleted of sodium and chloride ions; the condition is thus known as **hypochloraemic alkalosis** or **chloride-sensitive alkalosis**. The kidney attempts to compensate by conserving hydrogen ions but this occurs at the expense of potassium ions lost into the urine. Patients become hypokalaemic not only from excess urinary loss but also because potassium shifts into the cells in response to the alkalosis. Treatment of hypochloraemic alkalosis involves rehydration with normal saline infusion with potassium supplements; large volumes up to 10 litres are often required. Renal excretion of bicarbonate ions eventually corrects the alkalosis.

RESPIRATORY ALKALOSIS

This occurs when carbon dioxide is lost via excessive pulmonary ventilation. The usual cause in surgical practice is prolonged mechanical ventilation during general anaesthesia or in the intensive care unit without adequate monitoring.

NUTRITIONAL MANAGEMENT IN THE SURGICAL PATIENT

ESSENTIAL PRINCIPLES

Most surgical patients have no special nutritional requirements and easily withstand the short period of starvation associated with their illness and operation. A few patients need nutritional support which can range in complexity upwards from easily prepared oral diets (e.g. liquidised normal food), through specialised types of enteral nutrition (available in a variety of proprietary formulations) to **total parenteral nutrition** (TPN) for patients unable to absorb nutrients from the gastro-intestinal tract.

RECOGNITION OF THE PATIENT AT RISK

Malnutrition is common in surgical patients and is often unrecognised. The problem is complicated by the fact that many major surgical operations are required urgently and that correction of recognised malnutrition is difficult, particularly if the patient is unable or unwilling to eat because of anorexia or nausea or the intestinal tract cannot be used for mechanical reasons such as obstruction. Thus there is a fine balance between the need to get on with the operation and the need to optimise the patient's nutritional state. Even if it is impracticable to improve nutrition before operation, the problem should be recognised. Attention can then be given to the problem in the postoperative period so as not to extend the period of starvation and malnutrition, and thereby contribute to improved healing and resistance to infection and other complications.

A variety of simple scoring systems have been developed to assess a patient's nutritional state and these are becoming regularly employed in enlightened units. These systems look at how far an individual varies from the normal in several aspects, for example: body weight, body mass index, appetite, ability to eat, intestinal function, medical condition/treatment. Weight loss alone of 4.5 kg in the 6 months before surgery is associated with a 20-fold increase in mortality. There may be a **nutritional support team** that can be called upon for assistance. A typical team consists of four members with overlapping responsibility—clinician, dietician, nurse and pharmacist.

Protein-energy malnutrition can be recognised by assessing dietary intake, general cellular or muscular dysfunction (e.g. grip strength) or body composition (weight loss, plasma albumin concentration, lymphocyte count, skin fold thickness or muscle circumference). Low plasma albumin concentrations (less than 35 g/L) are associated with a 5-fold increase in complications, and critically ill patients, with a 10-fold increase in death.

When both plasma albumin and total lymphocyte count are low, there is a 20-fold increase in deaths.

ENTERAL FEEDING AND DIETARY SUPPLEMENTS

Enteral feeding is much cheaper than parenteral nutrition and is intrinsically safer. Enteral feeding can also provide nutrition directly to the bowel mucosa if appropriate formulations containing glutamine are employed. If normal food can be given in some suitable form, this is preferable to a proprietary enteral diet; parenteral nutrition should be reserved for conditions where it is specifically indicated. For example, new enteral diets have been designed to help treat individual diseases and support specific organ systems. Certain patients (who are not receiving full enteral or parenteral feeding) may benefit from vitamin supplements; these include folic acid and thiamine supplements for alcoholics and vitamin K injections for patients receiving prolonged antibiotic therapy where disturbance of normal gut flora may impair intestinal absorption of vitamin K.

Box 50.3 summarises the range of nutritional regimens and their main surgical indications.

COMPLETE FLUID DIETS

Complete fluid diets were developed after research into the special requirements of manned space travel. These are mostly based on **hydrolysed casein** with certain additives and have proved valuable for nutritional support of patients unable to take nutrition by mouth but with an otherwise intact gut. Apart from their general nutritive role, enteral feeding appears to protect the integrity and function of the intestinal mucosa by direct nutrition of enterocytes. This helps to prevent systemic inflammatory response syndrome caused by microbial invasion across the intestinal wall (**translocation**) in seriously ill patients.

Elemental feeding is required much less commonly and is indicated in patients with seriously impaired intestinal absorptive function, e.g. after massive small bowel resection.

If the patient is able to eat, fluid diets can be given orally, either as the sole means of nutrition or as dietary supplements, usually with advice from a dietician. Even if the patient is unable to swallow (for example, because of bulbar palsy, unconsciousness or facial fractures), complete enteral nutrition can be delivered by means of a fine-bore nasogastric tube. These tubes cause minimal nuisance to the patient and can be left in place for long periods. A fluid diet is planned and formulated for the individual and is delivered at a controlled rate using a pump, often overnight. Fine-bore tubes can also be placed percutaneously into the stomach or jejunum,

SUMMARY

Box 50.3 Special methods of nutrition and their indications

1. **Selective diets for specific indications**, e.g. diabetic, low-protein (renal and liver failure), low-fat (gallstones), high-fibre (constipation, diverticular disease) or weight reducing (obesity)

2. **Liquidised normal diet**—for patients with partial oesophageal obstruction (e.g. stricture, tumour or oesophageal intubation for cancer) or teeth wired together for fractured mandible or gross obesity

3. **High-protein, high-calorie dietary supplements**—for chronically malnourished patients capable of a normal diet or debilitated convalescent patients

4. **Complete fluid diet**, e.g. lactose-free isotonic diets containing a full range of nutritional requirements often including fibre. These can be administered orally via a fine-bone nasogastric tube or via a fine-bore gastrostomy or jejunostomy tube—for nutritional support of patients unable to eat or drink such as the unconscious, ventilated and seriously ill patient in intensive care or patients unwilling to take adequate nutrition following major surgery or trauma

5. **Elemental feeds**, i.e. mixture of amino acids, glucose and triglycerides requiring no digestion and minimal absorptive capacity (usually given by fine-bore tube)—for patients with minimal remaining bowel after massive resection or in the early stages of an exclusion diet for Crohn's disease

6. **Total parenteral nutrition (TPN)**, i.e. comprehensive intravenous nutrition—for patients with prolonged ileus or a very proximal fistula

either at operation or with endoscopic help. Fine-bore gastrostomies are often employed in patients after stroke. The usual technique nowadays is a percutaneous endoscopic gastrostomy (PEG) in which a combination of gastroscopy and percutaneous placement is used. For jejunostomy placement, devices are available which allow the tube to be tunnelled submucosally for a distance before entering the lumen to minimise the risk of leakage. These tubes can be placed under direct vision after, for example, total gastrectomy, or laparoscopically. Nutrition is delivered in all of these as for fine-bore NG tubes.

TOTAL PARENTERAL NUTRITION (TPN)

TPN formulations principally contain a mixture of glucose, amino acids, lipids, minerals and vitamins. The osmolality is usually high so that administration via a dedicated central venous line is required, although formulations for peripheral administration are available. The usual aim is to provide sufficient nitrogen and energy to offset the catabolic demands of surgery and/or trauma and their complications. In calculating requirements, nitrogen intake is matched to estimated nitrogen losses and this is complemented by providing non-nitrogenous sources of energy in the form of glucose and lipids which have a **protein-sparing** effect and minimise the consumption of protein as energy.

The nitrogen requirements can be calculated by measuring urinary nitrogen loss as urea or else a standard formula can be employed. For example, basic daily adult requirements are 100 g protein (in the form of amino acids) and 350 g glucose and 50 g lipid to provide energy. Standard supplements of vitamins and minerals are usually incorporated in the mix.

Excessive nutrition can be a problem. Hyperglycaemia can be corrected with modest doses of insulin but in the longer term, disturbances of liver function may reflect intrahepatic cholestasis caused by fatty infiltration (tests show elevated plasma alkaline phosphatase and gamma glutaryl transferase).

Parenteral nutrition is reserved for patients in whom the gastrointestinal tract is not functional or is inaccessible and who are malnourished or who are likely to become malnourished. These may include:

- Postoperatively (enteral feeding for more than 5 days may be contraindicated)
- Short bowel syndrome
- Gastrointestinal fistulae
- Prolonged paralytic ileus
- Acute pancreatitis
- Multiple injuries involving viscera
- Major sepsis
- Severe burns
- Inflammatory bowel disease

Patients receiving parenteral nutrition require close monitoring. This should include:

- Fluid balance and weight—daily
- Temperature—twice daily
- Line entry site—daily
- Every 8 hours—blood glucose (finger-prick sticks)
- Daily—plasma urea, electrolytes and creatinine
- Alternate days—liver function tests
- Weekly—plasma zinc, magnesium and phosphate

Parenteral nutrition is costly in materials and in staff time and is prone to complications; it should be continued for as short a time as possible.

Complications of parenteral nutrition

These include:

Catheter problems
- Problems associated with placement of the central venous catheter e.g. trauma to great arteries or veins, pneumothorax
- Infection of the central venous catheter—a common cause of fever and tachycardia which is likely to progress to systemic inflammatory response syndrome
- Blockage or leakage of catheter
- Central venous thrombosis

Metabolic problems
- Hypophosphataemia ($PO_4 < 0.5$ mmol/L)
- Hypernatraemia (Na > 150 mmol/L)
- Hyponatraemia (Na < 130 mmol/L)
- Hyperglycaemia
- Overnutrition (see earlier)
- Long-term—fatty degeneration of the liver

Index

Page numbers in **bold** indicate main discussions; those in *italics* refer to Figures, Tables or Boxes.

675

R

U

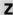